Pathophysiologic
Foundations of Critical Care

Pathophysiologic Foundations of Critical Care

Editors

Michael R. Pinsky, MD, CM, FCCP, FCCM

Professor of Anesthesiology and Critical Care Medicine
Director of Research
Department of Anesthesiology and Critical Care Medicine
Presbyterian-University Hospital
University of Pittsburgh
Pittsburgh, Pennsylvania

Jean-François A. Dhainaut, MD, PhD

Professor of Critical Care Medicine and Clinical Pharmacology
Director of Department of Intensive Care Medicine
Cochin Port-Royal University-Hospital
Paris V University
Paris, France

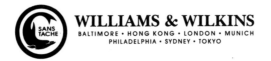

WILLIAMS & WILKINS
BALTIMORE · HONG KONG · LONDON · MUNICH
PHILADELPHIA · SYDNEY · TOKYO

Editor: Timothy H. Grayson
Project Manager: Marjorie Kidd Keating
Copy Editor: Klementyna L. Bryte, S. Gillian Casey, and E. Ann Donaldson
Designer: Norman W. Och
Illustration Planner: Ray Lowman

Copyright © 1993
Williams & Wilkins
428 East Preston Street
Baltimore, Maryland 21202, USA

Accurate indications, adverse reactions, and dosage schedules for drugs are provided in this book, but it is possible that they may change. The reader is urged to review the package information data of the manufacturers of the medications mentioned.

Printed in the United States of America

Chapter reprints are available from the Publisher.

Library of Congress Cataloging-in-Publication Data

Pathophysiologic foundations of critical care / editors, Michael R. Pinsky, Jean-François A. Dhainaut.
   p.   cm.
   Includes bibliographical references and index.
   ISBN 0-683-06888-1
   1. Critical care medicine. 2. Physiology, Pathological.
I. Pinsky, Michael R. II. Dhainaut, J.-F. (Jean-François)
   [DNLM: 1. Acute Disease. 2. Critical Care—methods. WB 105
P297]
RC86.7.P368 1993
616'.028–dc20
DNLM/DLC
for Library of Congress   92-15867
                                        CIP

92 93 94 95 96
1 2 3 4 5 6 7 8 9 10

To Janis, Daniel, Stephanie, and Jill
Annie, Stephanie, Thomas, and Mathieu

Preface

Critical care medicine has come of age as a defined field of medicine. Increasing numbers of intensive care unit beds, departments of critical care medicine within hospitals, and training programs in critical care medicine have been established. Certification processes underwritten by all the specialty boards in medicine have been conferring Certificates of Special Qualifications in Critical Care Medicine for the last few years. National and international organizations representing critical care health providers have existed for over 20 years, and the national meetings are a forum for the presentation of new information. Furthermore, periodicals and textbooks in critical care medicine exist and are widely read. Yet, with all these trappings of academia, the teaching and practice of critical care medicine is largely based on empiric experience. Only a small percentage of all critical care practices are supported by objective scientific evidence. These are the "False Columns of the Temple" of Critical Care Medicine.

Is there a scientific basis for the practice of critical care medicine? Yes. The underlying principles that direct care are based on an understanding of the pathophysiologic basis of disease and its interaction with treatment. Thus, although we may not have sound clinical data to support the use of a treatment in a certain circumstance, we do have a vast fund of knowledge acquired over many years and validated by several laboratories throughout the world defining and continuing to define the pathophysiologic basis of disease. Within this framework and without good clinical data to support the use of one therapy over another, the physician may select from several reasonable options in the management of the critically ill. Furthermore, unless these basic pathophysiologic concepts are challenged, such an approach in the management of the critically ill will be valid into the future, even as new therapies and approaches are introduced into the clinical area.

The conceptual basis for the practice of critical care monitoring is rooted in an understanding of the pathophysiologic processes that are in play. What specific inotropic agent, antibiotic, diuretic, vasodilator, mode of ventilation, or volume expander used in a given clinical situation is relative less important than is the understanding that specific modulations of the endogenous physiology and of the exogenous disease process are required. In essence, it is the *whys* and not the *hows* of therapy that change slowly and need to be taught and practiced. These lessons are learned to a variable degree by all physicians during their training. These lessons are taught every day in academic centers. Yet even the best of training programs can have deficits in specific areas of training regarding the principles that underscore clinical applications. Furthermore, physicians often need to be reminded that specific therapies are usually less important than the underlying principles that define their application. Thus, a textbook that addresses these issues systemwide could function as an adjunct to this training. We decided to address these issues directly by this novel approach to the presentation of critical care medicine. We did not wish to catalog disease processes and therapies, but to describe the pathophysiological processes that underlie these disease states and the principles of management that reflect an understanding of these processes.

The management of the critically ill requires an understanding of: 1) the pathophysiologic processes at work, 2) the abilities and limitations of monitoring and other diagnostic techniques to follow and interpret both these processes and their responses to therapies, 3) potential process-specific therapies, and 4) unwanted intra- or interorgan side effects of therapies or changes in responsiveness to therapy related to disease progression. Perhaps no field of medicine has evolved faster in the last 15 years than has critical care medicine. What was once considered reasonable management may now be considered inadequate. The issues involved with this change are protean to the very basis of medical science. Therapies, monitoring capabilities and even the diseases have changed. Thus, it seems reasonable to redefine management based on our present understanding of pathophysiology, monitoring, and therapeutic options.

In order to prevent the antiquation of such a volume before it is published, we have attempted to define management based on physiologic rationale that allows the reader to modify his or her approach to patient care as new information becomes available. The introductory chapters of each section briefly define pathophysiology, as currently known, then list therapeutic options in a pathophysiologic manner. Each author of each section was selected as an expert in both the theory and practice of each specific topic. The authors attempted to relate new and future trends within the context of the introductory pathophysiology chapters. To do this, they defined the role of hemodynamic monitoring and other diagnostic techniques, and their strengths and limitations within this context. Then they suggested reasonable scenarios for management. No one treatment schedule will care for all patients. Therefore, a more generalized systematic approach to management based on continual monitoring tends to be the one recommended most. Finally, specific therapeutic goals, monitoring, treatments, and logical end-points are listed in the clinical application sections of each chapter.

Pathophysiologic Foundations of Critical Care, therefore, is not exhaustive in its description of clinical treatments of disease, but it is very nearly complete in its description of mechanisms of disease, limitations of diagnostic and monitoring systems, and the principles underscoring the treatment goals. We hope the reader feels, as we do, that this approach, the pathophysiologic approach to the management of the critically ill, reflects a balanced method of handling new information from the literature and integrating it into a reasonable treatment plan with an appropriate level of expectation for success.

Michael R. Pinsky, M.D.
Pittsburgh

Jean-François Dhainaut, M.D., Ph.D.
Paris

Acknowledgments

The editors would like to thank Lisa Cohn for her review of the final manuscripts; Wendy Bouton and Carole Maillet for their secretarial support; Tim Grayson, Editor, and Margie Keating, Project Manager, at Williams & Wilkins for their support and encouragement; and the faculties of the Division of Critical Care Medicine of the University of Pittsburgh and the Department of Intensive Care Medicine of Paris V University for giving them the stimulation and the time to complete this work.

Contributors

Derek C. Angus, M.B., Ch.B., M.P.H., M.R.C.P.(U.K.)
Investigator
Critical Care Medicine Division
Department of Anesthesiology/CCM
University of Pittsburgh Medical Center
Pittsburgh, Pennsylvania

Michel Aubier, M.D.
Professor of Medicine
Bichat University Hospital
Paris, France

Michel Azizi, M.D.
Assistant in Cardiology
Division of Hypertension
Broussais University Hospital
Paris, France

Jacques Belghiti, M.D.
Professor of Surgery
Beaujon University Hospital
Clichy, France

Jean-Pierre Belot, M.D.
Senior Cardiologist
Department of Anesthesiology and
    Critical Care Medicine
Surgical Intensive Care Unit
Lariboisière University Hospital
Paris, France

Sadek Beloucif, M.D.
Assistant Professor
Department of Anesthesiology and
    Critical Care Medicine
Lariboisière University Hospital
Paris, France

Franklin A. Bontempo, M.D.
Associate Professor of Medicine
Director of Clinical Coagulation
Medicine Blood Bank
Pittsburgh, Pennsylvania

Pascale Borensztein, M.D.
Assistant Professor
Department of Clinical Physiology and
    Nuclear Medicine
Pierre et Marie Curie University
Broussais University Hospital
Paris, France

Jean-Pierre Bourdarias, M.D., F.A.C.C.
Professor of Cardiology
Director, Department of Cardiology
Ambroise Paré University-Hospital
Boulogne, France

Fabrice Brunet, M.D.
Assistant Professor
Medical Intensive Care Unit
Cochin Port-Royal University Hospital
Paris, France

Hilmar Burchardi, M.D.
Department of Anesthesiology
Rettungs-u. Intensivmedizin
Gottingen, Germany

James E. Calvin, M.D.
Associate Professor of Medicine
Director of Coronary Care Unit
Rush-Presbyterian-St. Luke's Medical
    Center
Chicago, Illinois

Jean Chastre, M.D.
Professor of Critical Care Medicine
Medical Intensive Care Unit
Bichat University-Hospital
Paris, France

Marie Emilie Chauveau, M.D.
Assistant in Department of
    Endocrinology and Metabolism
Cochin University Hospital
Paris, France

Lakshmipathi Chelluri, M.D., F.C.C.M., F.C.C.P.
Associate Professor of Anesthesiology/ CCM
Director, General Intensive Care Unit
University of Pittsburgh Medical Center
Pittsburgh, Pennsylvania

Deborah J. Cook, M.D., F.R.C.P.C., M.Sc.
Assistant Professor of Medicine
Clinical Epidemiology and Biostatistics
McMaster University
Hamilton, Ontario
Canada

Pierre Corvol, M.D.
Professeur au Collège de France
Collège de France
Paris, France

Frank Cosentino, D.O.
Staff Physician
Department of Hypertension/Nephrology
Cleveland Clinic Foundation
Cleveland, Ohio

Jean-François A. Dhainaut, M.D., Ph.D.
Professor and Chairman
Medical Intensive Care Unit
Cochin Port-Royal University Hospital
Paris V University
Paris, France

William M. Davies, M.D.
Practice of Cardiology
Santa Fe Cardiology Associates
Santa Fe, New Mexico

Martin Day, M.D.
Assistant in Internal Medicine
Hypertension Department
Hôpital Broussais
Paris, France

Marie-Christine Dombret, M.D.
Assistant Professor
Service de Pneumologie
Hôpital Bichat
Paris, France

Jean-Marc Duclos, M.D.
Médecin de l'Hôpital Saint Joseph
Department of Urology
Hôpital Saint-Joseph
Paris, France

Aldo Fabris, M.D.
Chief of Nephrology and Dialysis Service
City Hospital
Bassano del Grappa, Italy

Jean-Yves Fagon, M.D.
Chief, Medical Intensive Care Unit
Broussais University Hospital
Paris, France

Bruce F. Farber, M.D.
Department of Medicine
North Shore University Hospital
Cornell University Medical College
Manhasset, New York

Mariano Feriani, M.D.
Associate Professor
Department of Nephrology
Ospedale San Bortolo
Vicenza, Italy

Jean Paul Gardin, M.D.
Department of Clinical Physiology and Nuclear Medicine
Pierre et Marie Curie University
Broussais University Hospital
Paris, France

Luciano Gattinoni, M.D.
Professor in Anesthesia and Intensive Care
Instituto di Anestesia e Rianimazione
Università di Milano
Monza, Italy

Deborah A. Hayek, M.D.
Assistant Director of Clinical Research
Department of Critical Care Medicine
St. John's Mercy Medical Center
St. Louis, Missouri

Pascal Houillier, M.D.
Assistant Professor
Department of Clinical Physiology and Nuclear Medicine
Pierre et Marie Curie University
Broussais University Hospital
Paris, France

François Jardin, M.D.
Professor of Critical Care Medicine
Director, Medical Intensive Care Unit
Ambroise Paré University-Hospital
Boulogne, France

Horst Kierdorf, M.D.
Medizinische Klinik II
Aachen University of Technology
Aachen, Germany

David J. Kramer, M.D.
Assistant Professor of Anesthesiology,
  Critical Care Medicine, and Surgery
Co-Director, Liver Transplant ICU
  Service
Presbyterian University Hospital
Pittsburgh, Pennsylvania

Martin LeWinter, M.D.
Professor of Medicine
Director, Cardiology Unit
University of Vermont
Burlington, Vermont

Peter Linden, M.D., D.M.D.
Assistant Professor of Anesthesiology
  and Medicine
Department of Anesthesiology
Division of Critical Care Medicine
University of Pittsburgh Medical Center
Pittsburgh, Pennsylvania

Jean-Pierre Luton, M.D.
Professor and Chairman
Dean of the Cochin Port-Royal Faculty of
  Medicine
Department of Endocrinology and
  Metabolism
Hôpital Cochin
Paris, France

Sheldon Magder, M.D.
Associate Professor
Chief, Division of Critical Care
Department of Medicine
Royal Victoria Hospital
Montreal, Quebec
Canada

Marc D. Malkoff, M.D.
Assistant Professor of Neurology and
  Anesthesiology
Head, Section of Neurological Intensive
  Care
St. Louis University School of Medicine
St. Louis, Missouri

Helmut Mann, M.D.
Medizinische Klinik II
Aachen University of Technology
Aachen, Germany

John J. Marini, M.D.
Professor of Medicine
University of Minnesota
Director of Pulmonary and Critical Care
  Medicine
St. Paul Ramsey Medical Center
St. Paul, Minnesota

Luis H. Martinez, M.D.
Research Fellow, Department of Critical
  Care Medicine
St. John's Mercy Medical Center
St. Louis, Missouri

George M. Matuschak, M.D., F.C.C.M.
Associate Professor of Medicine
Division of Pulmonology and Pulmonary
  Occupational Medicine
Department of Internal Medicine
St. Louis University School of Medicine
Co-Director, Medical Intensive Care Unit
St. Louis University Hospital
St. Louis, Missouri

Alan H. Morris, M.D.
Professor of Medicine
University of Utah
Director of Research, Pulmonary Division
LDS Hospital
Salt Lake City, Utah

Loren D. Nelson, M.D.
Associate Professor of Surgery and
  Anesthesiology
Director of Surgical Critical Care
Vanderbilt University
Nashville, Tennessee

Alain Nitenberg, M.D.
Professor and Chairman
Explorations Fonctionnelles
Hôpital Louis Mourier
Colombes, France

Gerard Nitenberg, M.D.
Chief, Medical Intensive Care Unit
Gustave Roussy Institute
Villejuif, France

Michel Paillard, M.D.
Professor and Chairman
Department of Clinical Physiology and
  Nuclear Medicine
Pierre et Marie Curie University
Broussais University Hospital
Paris, France

Y. Panis, M.D.
Resident Head
Department of Digestive Surgery
Hôpital Beaujonra
Clichy, France

Didier M. Payen, M.D., Ph.D.
Professor and Chairman
Department of Anesthesiology and
  Critical Care Medicine
Lariboisière University Hospital
Paris, France

Andrew B. Peitzman, M.D.
Associate Professor of Surgery
University of Pittsburgh School of
  Medicine
Director, Trauma/Emergency Services
Presbyterian University Hospital
Pittsburgh, Pennsylvania

Maria Valentina Pellanda, M.D.
Assistant Professor
Nephrology and Dialysis Service
City Hospital
Bassano del Grappa, Italy

Claude Perret, M.D., F.C.C.M., F.C.C.P.
Professor of Pathophysiology
Director of Medical Intensive Care
  Department
University Hospital
Lausanne, Switzerland

**Michael R. Pinsky, M.D., C.M.,
F.C.C.P., F.C.C.M.**
Professor of Anesthesiology and Critical
  Care Medicine
Director of Research
Department of Anesthesiology and
  Critical Care Medicine
University of Pittsburgh
Pittsburgh, Pennsylvania

Pierre-François Plouin, M.D.
Professor of Internal Medicine
Division of Hypertension
Broussais University Hospital
Paris, France

Thomas A. Raffin, M.D.
Associate Professor and Chief
Division of Pulmonary and Critical Care
  Medicine
Stanford University Medical Center
Stanford, California

**Graham Ramsey, M.B. Ch.B., M.D.,
F.R.C.S.**
University Department of Surgery
Western Infirmary
Glasgow, Scotland

Mary B. Ramundo, M.D.
Department of Medicine
North Shore University Hospital
Cornell University Medical College
Manhasset, New York

Max Rattes, M.D.
Resident, Cardiology
University of Ottawa Heart Institute
Ottawa, Ontario
Canada

Emmanuel Rene, M.D.
Professor of Medicine
Bichat-Claude Bernard University
  Hospital
Paris, France

Robert Rodriguez-Roisin, M.D.
Chief of Service
Hospital Clinic
Professor of Medicine
Universitat de Barcelona
Barcelona, Spain

Claudio Ronco, M.D.
Associate of Clinical Nephrology
Department of Nephrology
St. Bortolo Hospital
Vicenza, Italy

Edmund J. Rutherford, M.D.
Assistant Professor of Surgery
Vanderbilt University
Nashville, Tennessee

Robert Schlichtig, M.D.
Associate Professor of Anesthesiology
  and Critical Care Medicine, Internal
  Medicine and Surgery
University of Pittsburgh
Co-Director of Surgical ICU
Veterans Administration Medical Center
Pittsburgh, Pennsylvania

Paul T. Schumacker, Ph.D.
Section of Pulmonary and Critical Care
  Medicine
The University of Chicago
Chicago, Illinois

Jean-Louis Selam, M.D.
Professor of Medicine
Division of Diabetology
Hôtel Dieu de Paris
Paris, France

Hans G. Sieberth, M.D.
Medizinische Klinik II
Aachen University of Technology
Aachen, Germany

Gérard Slama, M.D.
Professor and Chairman
Division of Diabetology
Hôtel Dieu de Paris
Paris, France

Pierre Squara, M.D.
Assistant Professor
Medical Intensive Care Unit
Victor Dupouy Hospital
Argenteuil, France

Keith L. Stein, M.D.
Associate Professor of Anesthesiology
Critical Care Medicine & Surgery
Director, Cardiothoracic Surgical ICU
University of Pittsburgh Medical Center
Pittsburgh, Pennsylvania

David P. Strum, M.D., F.R.C.P.(C.)
Assistant Professor of Anesthesiology
   and Critical Care Medicine
University of Pittsburgh
Pittsburgh, Pennsylvania

**Peter M. Suter, M.D., F.C.C.P.,
   F.C.C.M.**
Professor and Chief of the Division of
   Surgical Intensive Care
University Hospital of Geneva
Geneva, Switzerland

Pierre Thomopoulos, M.D.
Professor of Medicine
Department of Endocrinology and
   Metabolism
Hôpital Cochin
Paris, France

**H. K. F. van Saene, M.D., Ph.D.,
   M.R.C. Path.**
University Department of Microbiology
Royal Liverpool Hospital
Liverpool, England

Christopher Veremakis, M.D.
Clinical Assistant Professor of Medicine
St. Louis University School of Medicine
Chairman, Department of Critical Care
   Medicine
St. John's Mercy Medical Center
St. Louis, Missouri

Simon Weber, M.D.
Professor of Cardiology
Cochin Port-Royal University Hospital
René Descartes University
Paris, France

Serge Witchitz, M.D.
Clinique de Réanimation
Maladies Infectieuses
Hôpital Bichat-Claude Bernard
Paris, France

Michel Wolff, M.D.
Assistant Professor
Division of Critical Care and Infectious
   Disease
Bichat-Claude Bernard University
   Hospital
Paris, France

Contents

Preface . . . . *vii*
Acknowledgments . . . . *ix*
Contributors . . . . *xi*

Section 1

Integrated Therapeutic Approach in Critical Care Medicine   1

PART A
MONITORING **3**

1. Principles of Hemodynamic Monitoring 3
   Loren D. Nelson, Edmund J. Rutherford
   PART B
NUTRITION **23**

2. Substrate Metabolism and Resting Energy Expenditure 23
   Robert Schlichtig

3. Enteral and Parenteral Nutrition 42
   Gerard Nitenberg
   PART C
INFECTION AND THE IMMUNOCOMPROMISED HOST **82**

4. The Role of Selective Decontamination of the Digestive Tract 82
   Graham Ramsey, H. K. F. van Saene

5. Bacteremia and Sepsis: Clinical Perspectives 96
   Derek C. Angus, David J. Kramer
   PART D
SHOCK AND MULTIPLE SYSTEMS ORGAN FAILURE **112**

6. Physiologic Regulation of Systemic Blood Flow 112
   Paul T. Schumacker

7. O$_2$ Uptake, Critical O$_2$ Delivery, and Tissue Wellness 119
   Robert Schlichtig

8. Shock Physiology 140
   Sheldon Magder

9. Hypovolemic Shock 161
   Andrew B. Peitzman

10. Sepsis Syndrome: Pathogenesis, Pathophysiology, and Management 170
    George M. Matuschak, Luis H. Martinez

PART E
ETHICAL ISSUES IN CRITICAL CARE MEDICINE **188**

11. Brain Death, Donor Management, and Withdrawal of Life Support 188
    Lakshmipathi Chelluri

12. Paradigms in Management 193
    Alan H. Morris

Section 2

Organ System Approach to the Management of the Critically Ill 207

PART A
CARDIAC FUNCTION AND IMPAIRMENT **209**

13. Determinants of Left Ventricular Performance 209
    Alain Nitenberg

14. Acute Left Ventricular Failure 230
    Didier M. Payen, Sadek Beloucif

15. Acute Myocardial Ischemia 245
    Claude Perret

16. Acute Left-Sided Valvular Regurgitation 262
    Jean-Pierre Belot

17. Determinants of Right Ventricular Performance 280
    Michael R. Pinsky

18. Acute Right Ventricular Failure 284
    Pierre Squara, Jean-François A. Dhainaut, Fabrice Brunet

19. Acute Pulmonary Hypertension 312
    Max Rattes, James E. Calvin

20. Cardiac Tamponade 337
    William M. Davies, Martin LeWinter

21. Pharmacologic Cardiovascular Support 348
    Simon Weber

22. Postoperative Care of the Cardiac Surgical Patient 363
    Keith L. Stein

23. Infective Endocarditis 372
    Michel Wolff, Serge Witchitz

PART B
PULMONARY FUNCTION AND INSUFFICIENCY **389**

24. Ventilation-Perfusion Relationships 389
    Robert Rodriguez-Roisin

25. Acute Hypoxemic Respiratory Failure 414
    Deborah J. Cook, Thomas A. Raffin

26. Acute Exacerbation of Chronic Airflow Obstruction 427
    Michel Aubier, Marie-Christine Dombret

27. Weaning from Respiratory Support in Hypoxemic Pulmonary
    Parenchymal Failure 447
    Peter M. Suter

28. Ventilatory Management of Severe Airflow Obstruction 453
    John J. Marini

29. Heart-Lung Interactions 472
    Michael R. Pinsky

30. Acute Asthma 491
    François Jardin, Jean-Pierre Bourdarias

31. Cardiopulmonary Resuscitation 502
    Sheldon Magder

32. Community-Acquired Acute Pneumonia and Respiratory Failure 525
    Jean Chastre, Jean-Yves Fagon

33. Hospital-Acquired Pneumonia 545
    Jean-Yves Fagon, Jean Chastre

PART C

RENAL DISEASE 571
Associate Editor, Claudio Ronco

34. Etiology and Pathophysiology of Acute Renal Failure 571
    Maria Valentina Pellanda, Aldo Fabris, Claudio Ronco

35. Clinical Manifestations of Acute Renal Failure and Their Patho-
    physiologic Bases 586
    Frank Cosentino

36. Electrolyte Derangements in Acute Renal Failure 601
    Aldo Fabris

37. Acid-Base Derangements in Acute Renal Failure 610
    Luciano Gattinoni, Mariano Feriani

38. Management of Acute Renal Failure in the Critically Ill Patient 630
    Claudio Ronco, Hilmar Burchardi

39. Acute Complications in Patients with Chronic Renal Failure 677
    Hans G. Sieberth, Helmut Mann, Horst Kierdorf

PART D

GASTROINTESTINAL DISEASE 696

40. Esophageal Problems 696
    Jacques Belghiti, Y. Panis

41. Stress Ulcer Prophylaxis 699
    Deborah J. Cook, Thomas A. Raffin

42. Acute Abdominal Processes 716
    Jacques Belghiti, Y. Panis

43. Severe Diarrhea 729
    Emmanuel Rene

PART E

NEUROLOGICAL DISEASE AND TRAUMA **738**

44. Pathophysiologic Mechanisms of Brain Injury 738
    Deborah A. Hayek, Christopher Veremakis

45. Cerebral Resuscitation 753
    Deborah A. Hayek, Christopher Veremakis

46. Neuromuscular Disease 778
    Marc D. Malkoff

47. Trauma Critical Care 789
    David P. Strum

PART F

HEMATOLOGICAL DISEASE **805**

48. Coagulation Abnormalities: Bleeding and Thrombosis 805
    Franklin A. Bontempo

49. General Hematology and Transfusion 815
    Franklin A. Bontempo

50. Management of the Immunocompromised Host 823
    Peter Linden

51. HIV Infection and Acquired Immunodeficiency Syndrome 851
    Mary B. Ramundo, Bruce F. Farber

PART G

ENDOCRINOLOGICAL DISEASE **863**
Associate Editors, Pierre Thomopoulos and Jean-Pierre Luton

52. Diabetes 863
    Gérard Slama, Jean-Louis Selam

53. Thyroid Dysfunction 891
    Pierre Thomopoulos

54. Acute Adrenal Insufficiency 902
    Marie Emilie Chauveau

55. Pathology of Posterior Pituitary 910
    Marie Emilie Chauveau

56. The Pathophysiological Basis of Current Pheochromocytoma Management ... 917
    *Pierre-François Plouin, Michel Azizi, Martin Day, Jean-Marc Duclos,
    Pierre Corvol*

57. Abnormalities in Calcium Metabolism 925
    Michel Paillard, Jean Paul Gardin, Pascale Borensztein, Pascal Houillier

    Index 945

INTEGRATED THERAPEUTIC APPROACH IN CRITICAL CARE MEDICINE

1

Principles of Hemodynamic Monitoring

Loren D. Nelson
Edmund J. Rutherford

HISTORY OF MONITORING

Hemodynamic monitoring has evolved over the three decades of critical care practice in this country. The history of monitoring parallels the history of our understanding of the shock state and of shock resuscitation. In the 1960s, shock was believed to be very closely linked to hypotension, and monitoring techniques of the 1960s were aimed at the assessment of pressure. Arterial catheters (9) came into widespread use, and percutaneous placement of central venous catheters to estimate central venous pressure (16) also became common. When it was recognized that correction of hypotension was not necessarily associated with appropriate resuscitation from shock, monitoring needs evolved and the "golden age of vasopressors" came to an end.

In the 1970s, the physiologic understanding of shock was related to "perfusion" and therefore to blood flow. After the introduction of the flow-directed pulmonary artery catheter in 1970, widespread use was accepted, and monitoring in the intensive care unit (ICU) turned toward the thermodilution measurement of cardiac output (12, 47, 49). The 1970s were the "golden age of inotropes."

As the definition of shock evolved further in the 1980s to that of an imbalance between the supply and demand of oxygen, monitoring needs again changed. In the 1980s, a continuous assessment of the relative balance between oxygen supply and demand (27) became available through continuous monitoring of mixed venous oxygen saturation (Svo_2).

Although monitoring needs will no doubt continue to evolve, in the early 1990s clinicians are faced with technical limitations requiring us to look at "whole body" hemodynamics rather than those of individual tissues. The direction of monitoring research in the 1990s appears to be moving toward better understanding of tissue oxygenation by less invasive and more continuous, real-time monitoring.

GOALS OF MONITORING

Fundamental goals of hemodynamic monitoring have actually changed very little over the past several years (29). The first goal of monitoring is to assure the adequacy of perfusion in patients who appear to be relatively stable (Table 1.1). Optimal monitoring of this large number of patients in critical care units allows the intensivist to be quite cost-effective in the selection of intermittent tests and therapy.

The second goal is the early detection of the *in*adequacy of perfusion that may occur as a patient becomes hemodynami-

3

Table 1.1
Goals of Hemodynamic Monitoring

Assurance of adequacy of perfusion
Early detection of the inadequacy of perfusion
Titration of therapy to specific hemodynamic
  endpoints
Quantification of the magnitude of illness
Differentiation between various organ system
  dysfunctions

cally unstable (52). The early detection role is particularly important in differentiating between those "monitor only" patients and those who will require active intervention. It has long been assumed (often with little supporting data) that early intervention will prevent the progression of organ system dysfunction to system failure.

The third goal of hemodynamic monitoring is to titrate therapy to specific hemodynamic endpoints in unstable patients (32). Although this represents the most challenging group of critically ill patients, it is a small group, which tends to receive the highest level of monitoring.

The fourth goal of monitoring, which has eluded us for several years, is to quantify the magnitude of illness. Whereas it is relatively easy to measure individual hemodynamic variables, it is, in fact, difficult to assess the magnitude of illness of an individual patient. Accurate estimation of the magnitude of illness may allow, in the future, a more precise prediction of outcome than is currently available.

Finally, hemodynamic monitoring is useful to differentiate between various organ system dysfunctions. Classically, hemodynamic monitoring combined with oxygen transport assessment has been used to differentiate the relative magnitude of pulmonary and cardiovascular dysfunction that contributes to hypoxemia (32). The differentiation is of critical importance since therapy directed to correct pulmonary dysfunction may have adverse effects on hemodynamic function.

Hemodynamic monitoring for individual patients should be physiologically based and goal-oriented. Monitoring of all possible parameters in all patients is expensive, dangerous, and undesirable. Selecting the appropriate level of monitoring for the appropriate degree of illness should result in optimal monitoring.

HOW TO MONITOR PRESSURE
Technology

Bedside hemodynamic monitoring is generally based around a relatively complex electronic amplifier circuit, which is connected to analog and digital display systems and usually a "hard copy" recording device (20). Although many aspects of the selection of this "black box" fall into the realms of ease of use, ease of teaching, flexibility, available functions, and asthetics, the most important characteristic of a pressure monitoring system is its frequency response. The monitor must be sensitive enough to detect the smallest clinically significant pressure change that may be created by the patient. In addition, it must be capable of measurements far beyond the fundamental frequencies that are generated. A general estimate has been made that the frequency response of a monitoring system should be capable of detecting up to the 10th harmonic of the fundamental frequencies generated (4). For example, if a patient has a heart rate of 120 beats/min (i.e., 2 Hz) the detection of all significant pressure changes would require a frequency response of the system of 20 Hz. Since pressure displays are complex with multiple elements contributing to the waveform, it is generally accepted that a frequency response of 30 Hz is required for clinical purposes. Fortunately, today nearly all electronic monitoring systems are capable of obtaining this frequency response.

The electromechanical pressure transducer serves as the interface between the sterile patient components of the system and the nonsterile electronic components of the system. Transducers have evolved greatly in the last few years to solid-state devices, which tend to minimize the cost and fragility associated with the older diaphragm/strain gauge devices used prior to the mid-1980s. The newer devices are less expensive, disposable, and better suited for the harsh environment of the intensive care unit. The purpose of the transducer is to convert a mechanical pressure wave to an electronic signal that may be amplified and displayed by the monitor. In the older diaphragm-type systems, this required a significant volume of fluid between the intravascular catheter and the transducer to move toward the transducer during periods of rising pressure and away from the transducer during falling pressure. The to-and-fro movement of fluid in the monitor tubing contributed to the development of artifacts described in the following sections. The more modern solid-state devices eliminate much of the to-and-fro movement and, therefore, tend to decrease the amount of artifact seen when compared with the older systems.

Design of the catheters used for invasive hemodynamic monitoring is dependent upon the type of pressure measurement required. Generally, short, nonthrombogenic, nontapered catheters, which can be placed by either an over-the-needle approach or by using a Seldinger guidewire, are used for arterial catheterization (43, 55). The thrombotic/embolic complications of arterial catheters are related to the relative sizes of the catheter and vessel. Generally, larger diameter, longer catheters have a higher complication rate in small vessels such as the radial artery (7). Underlying vascular disease, shock, hypovolemia, and the use of vasopressors increase the risk of thrombotic complications. The avoidance of end arteries (such as the brachial) and assurance of adequate collateral flow will help to minimize the chances of significant distal ischemia if thrombosis occurs in the catheterized artery.

Arterial catheters are generally connected to a length of low compliance tubing that transmits the pressure signal to the electromechanical transducer. Within this system is installed a flush device that provides a low constant flow (generally 1–3 ml/hr) of a heparinized saline solution to maintain patency of the catheter. The flush device also allows a rapid infusion of fluid (30 ml/min) to clear any blood or air in the tubing. The intravascular portion of the catheter has little effect on the accuracy of pressure monitoring. The extravascular portion of the catheter and any overly compliant elements (injection ports, air bubbles, etc.) or high resistance elements (stopcocks, connectors, etc.) within the system may affect the dynamic response characteristics (13, 14).

Pitfalls of Pressure Monitoring

A number of artifacts are commonly seen during pressure monitoring. One of the most commonly described artifacts is "catheter whip." Catheter whip artifact is generally seen in situations where the catheter is moving. Therefore, true catheter whip artifact is extremely uncommon in the measurement of either central venous pressure or arterial pressure using standard techniques. Catheter whip may become a significant problem when the catheter traverses the chambers of the heart. During systole, the catheter may be accelerated in a manner that produces pressure changes at the tip of the catheter independent from pressure changes surrounding the catheter. Similarly, during diastole as the catheter decelerates and then accelerates in a retrograde fashion, the pressure at the tip of the catheter may be lower than that surrounding the catheter. These artifacts produce a very "busy" pressure signal, which may confuse the observer. Stabilization of the tip of the catheter to minimize the acceleration and deceleration seen throughout the cardiac cycle may be accomplished by putting a small volume of gas into the pulmonary artery catheter balloon. The balloon should not be inflated to the point where the catheter will move into the occluded position, but a small volume of gas may minimize the to-and-fro movement caused by the cardiac cycle.

The two most common causes of pressure monitoring artifacts are related to the dynamic response characteristics of the monitoring system (13, 19). *Over*damping occurs when the response characteristics of the system impede the magnitude of pressure change that is sensed at the transducer. This artifact causes a convergence of the systolic and diastolic pressures toward the mean pressure. *Under*damping is a situation that causes an accentuation of the systolic and diastolic pressure changes so that the observed pressures diverge away from the mean, causing an overestimation of systolic pressure and an underestimation of diastolic pressure. In both cases, the mean pressure remains relatively accurate.

Overdamping may be caused by any element in the monitoring system that causes increased resistance or increased compliance of the system. The use of high compliance tubing, tubing with rubber injection ports, or multiple stopcocks may lead to overdamping (Table 1.2). The most common cause of overdamping, however, is the presence of air bubbles within the fluid pathway of the monitoring system. Since gas is compressible and the liquid is not compressible, the movement of the pressure wave toward the transducer is attenuated by the presence of gas in the system (Fig. 1.1). This produces a typical overdamped pressure wave, which is usually observed to be broad, slurred, and often loses the dicrotic notch. Systolic and diastolic pressures converge toward the

Table 1.2
Causes of Dynamic Response Artifacts

Overdamping
Air bubbles
Compliant tubing
Stopcocks
Injection ports
Underdamping
Tubing length
Tubing diameter

mean pressure and may lead to therapeutic mismanagement if not detected.

Although air bubbles may be inadvertently introduced into the monitoring system during flushing of the system or withdrawal of blood from the system, the most common source of air bubbles is gas coming out of solution at the flush device. Since the flush devices are dependent upon fluid being compressed to high levels (often 300 mm Hg), gas present in the flush so-

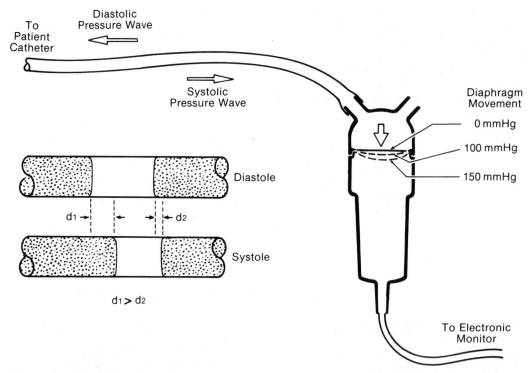

Figure 1.1. Overdamping is frequently caused by compression of gas bubbles in the transducer dome or tubing. As overdamping increases, the systolic and diastolic pressures converge toward the mean pressure. (From Nelson LD. In: Snyder JV, Pinsky MR, eds. Oxygen transport in the critically ill. Chicago: Year Book, 1987:212.)

lution bag becomes dissolved in the solution. When the pressure is released at the flush device (to approximate mean arterial pressure), the increased volume of dissolved gas comes out of solution and may be deposited in the transducer dome, connectors, or the tubing itself. Large bubbles in the monitoring system are usually obvious and easily corrected; however, multiple very small bubbles will have a very large compressible surface area and may lead to equally large artifacts. The typical tracing seen in an overdamped signal is demonstrated in Figure 1.2.

The cause of underdamping is more complex. In general, underdamping is thought to be the result of "harmonic amplification" caused by an improperly configured monitoring system (Table 1.2). In addition to the normal high amplitude, low frequency pressure signals identified at the tip of the intravascular catheter, multiple low amplitude, high frequency signals are also present. Since the pressure monitoring system follows the usual laws of physics, the length and diameter of the monitoring tubing determine the natural resonant frequency of the system. When the frequencies generated by the patient approach the natural frequency of the monitoring system, the low amplitude signals become superimposed on the normal high amplitude pressure signals that are

being monitored. This induces an additive effect on the systolic pressure and causes the observed pressures to diverge away from the mean, thus overestimating true systolic pressure and underestimating true diastolic pressure.

This phenomenon is similar to that which occurs with a musical instrument such as the flute. When the flutist plays the instrument, multiple low amplitude signals are generated at the mouthpiece. Harmonics of these signals are selected by changing the functional length (natural frequency) of the instrument using the keys. Therefore, high amplitude tones may be created at frequencies inversely proportional to the functional length of the flute. In the pressure monitoring system, these signals distort the actual high amplitude signal that is being measured. The overestimation of systolic pressure may lead to inappropriate overtreatment of systolic hypertension, and the low observed diastolic pressure may cause concern about low coronary perfusion pressures.

The typical underdamped signal shows a rapid upstroke toward systolic pressure. The systolic peak is narrow with a rapid fall and usually a late and prominent dicrotic notch. The systolic pressure is overestimated and the diastolic pressure is underestimated (Fig. 1.3).

Interpretation of Pressure Data

Arterial Blood Pressure

The determinants of systolic, diastolic, and mean pressures differ. It is important to recognize that the dynamic response characteristics of the monitoring system have little effect on mean pressure but may have significant effects on both systolic and diastolic pressures. Therefore, most calculations of derived hemodynamic indices use the mean arterial pressure.

The systolic blood pressure is determined primarily by myocardial contractility, great vessel compliance, and the diastolic pressure (Table 1.3). A common clinical problem in the ICU is the assessment of patients with isolated or predominantly systolic hypertension. Since great vessel compliance is relatively fixed, the

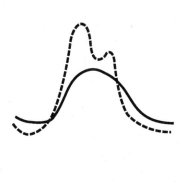

OVER-DAMPED

Figure 1.2. The overdamped waveform *(solid line)*, when compared with an ideal waveform *(dashed line)*, is noted to be slow in upstroke and downstroke, broad, slurred, and has lost the dicrotic notch. Systolic and diastolic pressures converge toward the mean pressure.

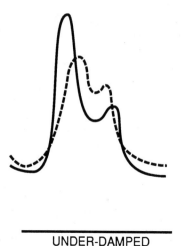

UNDER-DAMPED

Figure 1.3. The underdamped waveform *(solid line)*, when compared with an ideal waveform *(dashed line)*, has a rapid upstroke to a narrow systolic peak. The downstroke of the wave is rapid and often has a late and prominent dicrotic notch. Systolic and diastolic pressures diverge from the mean pressure.

major determinant of systolic pressure is the stroke volume of the ventricle.

Perhaps the best way to assure that true systolic hypertension is present is to confirm the systolic pressure by the restoration of flow method. A blood pressure cuff is placed on the arm proximal to the arterial line. The cuff is inflated until the arterial pressure wave form is attenuated to the mean circulatory pressure (slightly above venous pressure) of the extremity. The cuff is then gradually deflated until a systolic upstroke is noted. At this point, it is assumed that flow is reestablished to the extremity and the reading on the manometer can be interpreted as the true systolic pressure in that extremity. Once systolic hypertension is confirmed, manipulations of systolic pressure must begin with a careful evaluation of diastolic pressure.

The primary determinants of diastolic blood pressure are systemic vascular resistance, peripheral run-off into the distal circulation, and heart rate (Table 1.3). Maintenance of adequate diastolic pressure is especially important when one considers that coronary perfusion (in the presence of atherosclerotic disease) is

Table 1.3
Determinants of Blood Pressure

Systolic
    Myocardial contractility
    Great vessel compliance
    Diastolic pressure
Diastolic
    Systemic vascular resistance
    Peripheral run-off
    Heart rate

determined almost completely by the difference between diastolic blood pressure and the intracavitary pressure of the ventricle. Significant diastolic *hypo*tension should not be allowed in patients at risk for coronary artery disease since this may compromise myocardial perfusion and precipitate subendocardial ischemia. Overly aggressive control of systolic hypertension with vasodilators may result in impairment of coronary blood flow because of falls in diastolic blood pressure. The perfusion of other organ systems is primarily dependent upon mean arterial pressure and the relative resistances of each of the vascular beds.

When treating systolic hypertension, diastolic pressure is first optimized. Following optimization of diastolic pressure, the systolic peak must be controlled by modulating ventricular contractility since the compliance of the great vessels cannot be altered significantly. This implies that isolated systolic hypertension is best treated with calcium channel blockers or β-adrenergic blockers.

It is important to note that a great deal of information can be obtained by careful observation of the analog waveform. Changes in waveform upstroke, pulse pressure, and downstroke can be used to follow changes in a patient's cardiovascular status. The slope of the upstroke of the waveform is proportional to contractility of the ventricle. The peak pressure is determined by the relationship between the volume ejected and the compliance of the great vessels. The downstroke of the waveform is proportional to both the compliance of the great vessels and the systemic vascular resistance, which controls peripheral run-off. However, given conditions at a specific point in time, a waveform can be nonspecific and cannot in and of itself be used to imply cardiovascular function. Changes in the waveform of an individual patient can indicate a change in hemodynamic status and can be useful in detecting dynamic response artifacts of the monitoring system as described previously.

The area described by the systolic pressure curve is proportional to the volume of blood ejected from the ventricle during systole (51). Multiple means have been used to estimate average cardiac output by summing the values of the individual stroke volumes estimated from the arterial waveform (8) Although this monitoring technique is fraught with a number of artifacts related to changes in total aortic impedance, the values may be useful when impedance is stable (54).

Central Venous Pressure

Central venous pressure (CVP) is often measured in conjunction with other hemodynamic information so that systemic vascular resistance and its index may be calculated (35). CVP by itself gives little significant information as to overall hemodynamic performance of the patient. The CVP is an estimate of right atrial pressure and therefore, in the absence of significant tricuspid valve disease, of the right ventricular end-diastolic pressure. The CVP, therefore, gives the clinician information about the relative relationship between effective circulating volume and right ventricular function. It is important to note that CVP does not measure intravascular volume or right ventricular function as an independent parameter. Only the relative relationship between these two factors can be assessed by CVP.

A number of investigations have looked for correlations between right and left ventricular function in critically ill patients. Unfortunately, the relationship often changes quickly and very little correlation can be found between CVP and pulmonary artery occlusion pressure ("wedge" pressure) in any group of critically ill patients (5, 41). Since there is no reliable correlation between CVP and pulmonary artery occlusion pressure in critically ill

patients, CVP cannot be used as an estimate of left ventricular function (3, 6, 10, 37, 39).

Although central venous pressure was commonly measured as an isolated parameter in the 1960s and early 1970s, it gives no significant information about any of the determinants of stroke volume and, therefore, of cardiac output. CVP has no known correlation with preload, afterload, or contractility and cannot serve as an isolated hemodynamic monitor.

Pulmonary Artery Occlusion Pressure

Occlusion of a proximal branch of the pulmonary artery allows the temporary establishment of a no-flow state. When the flow is interrupted in the distribution of the pulmonary artery, the vessel itself becomes a conduit for the measurement of pressure in the left atrium. Since there is no flow during the measurement of the occluded pressure, resistance of the pulmonary vasculature has no significant impact on the pressure measurement (4). In the absence of mitral valve disease, the left atrial pressure correlates with the left ventricular (LV) end-diastolic pressure. Therefore, a properly transduced pulmonary artery occlusion pressure in the absence of significant mitral valve disease is an index of LV end-diastolic pressure and, therefore, of the relative relationship between the effective circulating volume of the patient and left ventricular function. As with CVP, the pulmonary artery occlusion pressure does not give information regarding volume status of the patient independent of its relationship with left ventricular function but is only an index of the relative balance between these two factors.

Additionally, the measurement of CVP and pulmonary artery occlusion pressure gives only an estimate of the absolute value of the end-diastolic pressure of the respective ventricles. Since the true transmural pressure across the ventricle is dependent upon intrapleural pressure or mediastinal pressure, CVP and pulmonary artery occlusion pressure do not estimate transmural pressures. During positive-pressure mechanical ventilation, pleural pressure rises from its normal negative value. This will result in an increase in the absolute value of pulmonary artery occlusion pressure that is measured but will not increase (and may decrease) the transmural pressure.

Proper positioning of the pulmonary artery catheter tip is crucial for the estimate of pulmonary artery occlusion pressure (and cardiac output). Ideally, the catheter tip should be as proximal in the pulmonary vasculature as possible and yet still yield an appropriate occluded waveform with inflation of the balloon and distal migration of the catheter. The catheter should lie across the pulmonic valve so that irritation of the ventricle and the right ventricular (RV) outflow tract are minimized. The adequacy of the position of the catheter is probably best assessed by the volume of gas required in the balloon to achieve an occluded pressure waveform. The volume of gas introduced in the balloon should be near the maximum capacity of the balloon (1.5 ml) when the waveform change is noted. When the pulmonary artery occlusion pressure waveform changes and balloon volume is substantially less than 1.25 to 1.5 ml, the catheter position is too distal (35). A distal catheter predisposes to many problems associated with pulmonary artery catheterization (Fig. 1.4A). In particular, a distal catheter may result in rupture of the pulmonary artery if the balloon is inflated to normal volumes. Furthermore, a distal position of the pulmonary artery catheter makes the pressure measurement more dependent on a small area of the pulmonary vasculature and, therefore, more susceptible to local pathology in the distribution of that vasculature. If the catheter remains in a distal position for too long, it may predispose the patient to occlusion of the vessel, thrombosis, and even lung infarction (Fig. 1.4B). Finally, a very distally placed pulmonary artery catheter may lead to artifacts in the measurement of cardiac output by the thermodilution method and artifacts in the measurement of mixed venous oxygen saturation at the tip of the catheter. Generally, the transverse segment of the pulmonary artery catheter after it has entered one of the main pulmonary arteries should be confirmed on chest radiography to be very close to the midline of the patient. An excessively long transverse segment (greater than the width of the vertebral body) generally means the catheter is too distal.

One of the most difficult problems to differentiate when trying to place a pulmonary artery catheter in the proper position is the presence of a LV wave (V-wave) transmitted retrograde from the left ventricle (4). In the presence of mitral insufficiency or significant mitral valve prolapse, a large V-wave may be superimposed on the occluded pulmonary artery pressure tracing. This V-wave may be interpreted as a right ventricular-generated pulmonary systolic pressure wave even though the catheter is in the fully occluded position. This can predispose to artifacts in the estimate of pulmonary artery occlusion pressure and may predispose to pulmonary artery rupture caused by a distal catheter tip.

A V-wave should be suspected whenever the pulmonary artery occlusion pressure waveform cannot be easily identified on a catheter that is felt to be properly positioned. In this situation, the catheter is best pulled back into the right ventricle and refloated with the balloon inflated into a branch of the pulmonary artery. If a pulmonary artery occlusion pressure tracing is not observed at an appropriate distance from the pulmonic valve, a V-wave should be suspected.

The V-wave can be confirmed by superimposing the electrocardiogram (ECG) on the pulmonary artery tracing. In a normal pulmonary artery tracing, the upstroke toward pulmonary artery systolic pressure begins near the end of the QRS of the ECG. Since in the normal situation, the left ventricle contracts after the right ventricle, a delay of approximately 200–300 msec is often seen between the QRS and the left ventricular-generated V-wave (Figs. 1.5 and 1.6). When a V-wave is identified, the pulmonary artery occlusion pressure should be read just prior to the upstroke of the V-wave. A V-wave may appear intermittently over time due to

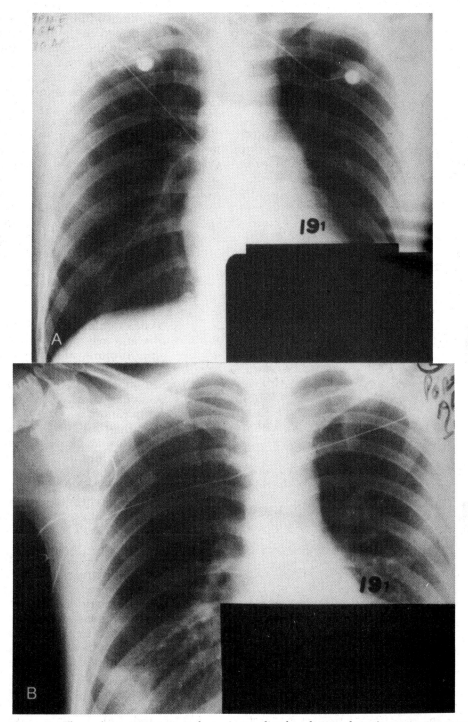

Figure 1.4.   **A,** The pulmonary artery catheter is too distal and may place the patient at increased risk of pulmonary artery rupture if the balloon is inflated. **B,** This radiograph taken 24 hours later shows evidence of a pulmonary infarction.

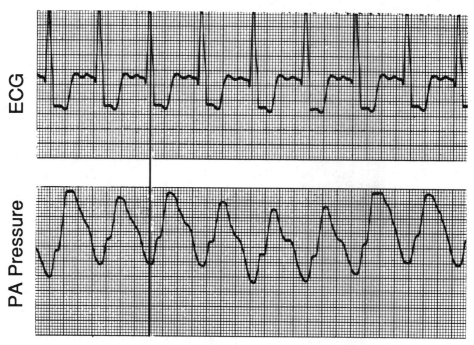

Figure 1.5. A V-wave can be identified by timing the pulmonary artery tracing with the ECG. As indicated in this figure, normally the upstroke of the pulmonary artery *(PA)* trace starts near the end of the QRS.

changes in cardiac size caused by changes in circulating volume, ventricular compliance, or ventilatory support.

HOW TO MONITOR FLOW

Indicator Dilution Technology

Cardiac output has been estimated by variations of indicator dilution since the early 1960s. The first method that received widespread popularity was the indocyanine green dye dilution method employing the Stewart-Hamilton equation and an injection of a known volume of dye at a known concentration into the central circulation. The dye concentration density changes were then measured in a peripheral artery and integrated over time. Precise measurement of the original concentration and volume injected and measurement of arterial concentration changes allowed the calculation of volume over time or flow. Because this technique required ex vivo densitometry to calculate the dye concentration, it was cumbersome

and prone to many complications and calculation errors.

Thermodilution measurement of cardiac output, introduced clinically in the early 1970s (11), has virtually replaced all other invasive measurements of cardiac output. The thermodilution measurement is similar to dye dilution in that a known volume of solution at a known temperature is introduced in the central circulation. A thermistor in the pulmonary artery measures the temperature change in the blood flowing by the catheter, and this value is integrated over time to yield flow. The measurement is relatively accurate (within about 10%) and is easily performed to yield a reproducible number (22, 40). The temperature change integrated over time is inversely proportional to the blood flow into which the initial injection was made. Therefore, a very high cardiac output will result in a very small temperature change in the pulmonary arterial blood, and a low cardiac output will allow a very large temperature change (Fig. 1.7).

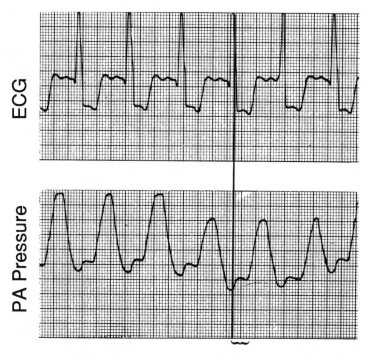

Figure 1.6. A V-wave is delayed 200–300 msec after the QRS. In this tracing the pulmonary artery (*PA*) catheter balloon is inflated and the positive-pressure wave is noted to move to a later position following the QRS. Without the "timing signal" provided by the ECG, the occluded waveform would be indistinguishable from the pulmonary artery waveform in Figure 1.5.

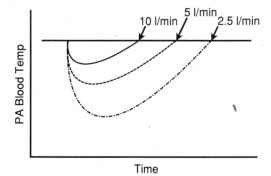

Figure 1.7. During measurement of a thermodilution cardiac output, temperature in the pulmonary artery (PA) is measured over time. Assuming identical injectate temperatures and volumes, a large measured temperature change indicates a low cardiac output and a small temperature change indicates a high cardiac output.

Pitfalls of Cardiac Output Measurement

Proper position of the pulmonary artery catheter is important for the accurate measurement of cardiac output by thermodilution. Once the catheter has been properly positioned, the computer must be given the injectate volume and temperature range as well as the characteristics of the catheter that determine the computation constant. These catheter characteristics are available in the package insert for all commonly available pulmonary artery catheters. The temperature of the injectate and the volume of injectate must be precisely determined. A slightly high injectate volume will produce a greater temperature change in the pulmonary circulation, which will be interpreted by the computer as a lower cardiac output. Similarly, a low injectate volume will produce a smaller temperature change, which will be interpreted as a higher cardiac output (22).

The injectate temperature must be appropriate to give an adequate signal-to-noise ratio at the thermistor (48, 53). If too small a volume is injected at too high a temperature, the resultant temperature change in the pulmonary arterial blood will be small and will yield a small absolute signal relative to the random noise in background temperature with spontaneous and mechanical ventilation. Most of the computers available today will alert the operator when an inadequate thermal curve or temperature change is detected.

It is clear from a number of studies that room temperature injectate yields values equal to those of ice temperature injectate (31, 44, 45). The theoretic advantage of room temperature injectate is that there will be less injectate temperature change from the time that the solution is drawn until it is injected, thereby giving more reproducible cardiac output values. The practical reason for using room temperature injectate is that it is much simpler and does not require the cumbersome iced injectate. The practical disadvantage of room temperature injectate is that it may produce too small a temperature change, especially in patients with high cardiac output, hypothermia, or who are in very warm rooms (31).

Several systems are currently available that measure the temperature of the injectate at the time it enters the proximal port of the pulmonary artery catheter. These systems minimize injectate temperature errors and may improve the reproducibility of the measurement. The nearly closed systems also may minimize the chance of bacterial contamination of the injectate solution (34).

The volume of injectate also determines the magnitude of temperature change measured in the pulmonary artery. A larger volume (10 ml) of injectate will produce a greater temperature change and therefore a greater signal-to-noise ratio than a smaller volume (5 ml). However, a smaller volume may be required in patients who cannot tolerate large amounts of intravenous fluids. Also, it may be technically easier to inject with a smaller syringe. A smaller syringe allows more precise measurement of the injectate volume, but an error in measurement of injectate volume causes a greater percentage of error in cardiac output.

The timing of injection in relation to the patient's ventilatory cycle on mechanical ventilation has been an area of considerable debate. It appears that, when the mechanical ventilatory rate is relatively high, the mean value of random injections throughout the ventilatory cycle will yield a cardiac value that is closest to the actual cardiac output of the patient (17, 46). On the other hand, timing of the injection during a particular point in the ventilatory cycle may yield more consistent (i.e., reproducible) values (1, 56). At low ventilatory rates, it would seem to be most appropriate to inject the thermal indicator at a fixed point in the ventilatory cycle, and at high ventilatory rates, to inject at random (17, 36). Most studies would indicate that multiple injections will give more consistent values than single injections. This may be more dependent upon operator technique and the conditions of the injection than on the fact that multiple injections were made (33).

Interpretation of Flow Data

Errors made in the interpretation of flow data fall into two common areas. First, the clinician may be lulled into a sense of complacency thinking that a onetime "snapshot" of cardiac output represents a steady-state picture of the patient. In fact, flow can vary widely over a short period of time, and isolated measurements of cardiac output should not be thought of as monitoring in the continuous sense.

The other common errors made in the interpretation of flow data are the failure to normalize the data to patient size and the failure to interpret the data in light of the patient's clinical condition. Once an accurate measurement of cardiac output is made, a host of derived cardiopulmonary parameters becomes available to the clinician. It is important to recognize that there are no normal values for either cardiac

Table 1.4
Hemodynamic Variables Commonly Used in Critical Care Patients

Term	Abbreviation	Calculation[a]	Normal Range
Mean arterial pressure	MAP	$MAP = DBP + \left(\dfrac{SBP - DBP}{3}\right)$	80–100 torr
Mean pulmonary artery pressure	MPAP	$MPAP = DPAP + \left(\dfrac{SPAP - DPAP}{3}\right)$	9–16 torr
Cardiac output	CO	(Measured)	(Varies with size)
Cardiac index	CI	$CI = CO/BSA$	2.8–4.2 liters/min/m²
Stroke volume	SV	$SV = CO/HR$	(Varies with size)
Stroke index	SI	$SI = CI/HR$	30–65 ml/beat/m²
Pulmonary artery occlusion pressure	PAOP	(Measured)	6–12 torr
Systemic vascular resistance index	SVRI	$SVRI = \dfrac{MAP - CVP}{CI} \times 80$	1600–2400 dyne·sec·cm⁻⁵/m²
Pulmonary vascular resistance index	PVRI	$PVRI = \dfrac{MPAP - PAOP}{CI} \times 80$	250–430 dyne·sec·cm⁻⁵/m²
Left ventricular stroke work index	LVSWI	$LVSWI = SI \times (MAP - PAOP) \times 13.6$	44–64 g·m/m²
Right ventricular stroke work index	RVSWI	$RVSWI = SI \times (MPAP - CVP) \times 13.6$	7–12 g·m/m²

[a]DBP, diastolic blood pressure (torr); SBP, systolic blood pressure (torr); DPAP, diastolic pulmonary artery pressure (torr); SPAP, systolic pulmonary artery pressure (torr); HR, heart rate (beats/min); BSA, body surface area (m²); CVP, central venous pressure (torr).

output or stroke volume. A normal range often quoted, many times in error, represents normal values for "normal"-sized patients. Cardiac index does have a normal range, as does the stroke index (Table 1.4). Since the stroke index is a primary determinant of total flow (cardiac output) and is the single parameter most often manipulated clinically, it represents an important index. The ability to calculate stroke index may be one of the most important factors leading to the current popularity of the flow-directed pulmonary artery catheter.

The volume of blood ejected by the left ventricle during each contraction is determined by three physiologic constructs: preload, afterload, and contractility. The pulmonary artery catheter gives some insight into each of these parameters and allows the derivation of indices reflective of the relative states for each ventricle.

Preload is related to the resting fiber length of the myocardial muscle (38). In a given geometric shape, this fiber length is proportional to the left ventricular end-diastolic volume. When ventricular compliance is static (often not the case in critically ill patients), there is a relationship between left ventricular end-diastolic volume and left ventricular end-diastolic pressure. In the absence of significant mitral valve disease, the left ventricular end-diastolic pressure is equal to the mean left atrial pressure. Finally, when the pulmonary artery catheter is properly positioned, the pulmonary artery occlusion pressure will be equal to the absolute value of the mean left atrial pressure. Thus, in this very circuitous situation when all of the assumptions are valid, the pulmonary artery occlusion pressure gives the clinician an index of relative changes in left ventricular preload. It must be clearly stated that the pulmonary artery occlusion pressure does not represent absolute preload and must be viewed in the context of factors that affect left ventricular compliance and transmural pressure (35).

The effect of ventricular compliance on preload estimates is an especially important concern in the ICU. Two common factors that decrease ventricular compliance are myocardial ischemia and increases in the inotropic state from endogenous or exogenous sympathomimetic stimuli. When ventricular compliance is reduced, higher filling pressures are needed to achieve the same ventricular end-diastolic volume (preload). This must be carefully considered when adding inotropes to patients with marginal or low filling pressures.

Ventricular afterload is defined as the impedance to blood flow from the ventricle (21, 35, 38). For the left heart, this includes ventricular compliance, aortic compliance, aortic valve resistance, systemic vascular resistance, and the mass and viscosity of blood. Since systemic vascular resistance is the impedance factor that may vary the most in a clinical situation and since it is the factor that we have the most control over with pharmacologic agents, systemic vascular resistance has been popularized as an indicator of left ventricular afterload. Resistance is typically calculated as a pressure gradient divided by mean flow (i.e., $(MAP - CVP)/CO$) where MAP is mean arterial pressure and CO is cardiac output. Since there are no normal values for cardiac output, there can be no normal values for systemic vascular resistance. Therefore, the systemic vascular resistance is indexed to body surface area (i.e., $SVRI = (MAP - CVP)/CI$) where SVRI is the systemic vascular resistance index and CI is the cardiac index. Since the pressure change is being divided by the cardiac index rather than cardiac output, systemic vascular resistance is, in effect, multiplied by body surface area rather than divided by body surface area (Table 1.4). The same indices can be applied to right-sided afterload by calculating the pulmonary vascular resistance index ($PVRI = (MPAP - PAOP)/CI$) where MPAP is the mean pulmonary arterial pressure and PAOP is the pulmonary artery occlusion pressure.

Contractility is one of the most difficult constructs to assess at the patient's bedside. Contractility, in general, is assessed by wall motion velocity of the ventricle or as the derivative of the intrachamber pressure change over time. Since neither of these is easily available in a reproducible fashion at the bedside, several assumptions must be made when assessing ventricular contractility (35).

Starling has related the amount of work performed by a muscle to the resting fiber length of that muscle. When assessing cardiac muscle, one generally plots the incremental work performed by the ventricle against either the end-diastolic volume or, more commonly, the filling pressure as estimated on the left side by the pulmonary artery occlusion pressure. The work performed by the ventricle is usually assessed by the stroke work index. The three fundamental factors that determine stroke volume and, therefore, ventricular performance are preload, afterload, and contractility. If two of these factors are kept constant, the third becomes the determinant of ventricular function. Therefore, in situations where both preload and systemic vascular resistance are fixed, changes in left ventricular stroke work index ($LVSWI = SV \times (MAP - PAOP)/BSA$), where SV is stroke volume and BSA is body surface area, at a given filling pressure will reflect changes in contractility. When all of the previous assumptions are valid, LVSWI can be used to assess the contractile function of the left ventricle, and the right ventricular stroke work index ($RVSWI = SV \times (MPAP - CVP)/BSA$) can be used for the right ventricle (Table 1.4).

HOW TO MONITOR OXYGEN TRANSPORT

Oxygen Transport Terminology

Oxygen transport has been defined in many ways (Table 1.5). Current thinking relates oxygen transport to the overall balance between the supply and demand of oxygen (24). The supply of oxygen from the left ventricle is generally equal to the oxygen delivery, which should be indexed to body surface area ($Do_2I = Cao_2 \times CI \times 10$) (Table 1.5) where Do_2I is the oxygen delivery index and Cao_2 is the arterial oxygen content. The demand for oxygen is much more difficult to assess. Generally, the Fick equation is used to calculate oxygen consumption indexed to body surface area

Table 1.5
Oxygen Transport Variables Commonly Used in Critically Ill Patients

Term	Abbreviation	Definition/Calculations[a]	Normal Range
Transport		Balance between supply and demand	
Delivery	Do_2	O_2 volume ejected from left ventricle $Do_2I = CI \times Cao_2 \times 10$	500–650 ml/min/m^2
Consumption	Vo_2	O_2 volume used by tissue $Vo_2I = CI \times C(a\text{-}v)o_2 \times 10$	110–150 ml/min/m^2
Uptake		O_2 volume taken up by lungs	110–150 ml/min/m^2
Demand		O_2 volume need by tissues	110–150 ml/min/m^2
Utilization	OUC	Fraction of delivered O_2 consumed $OUC = Vo_2/Do_2$	0.22–0.30

[a]CI, cardiac index (liters/min/m^2); Cao_2, arterial oxygen content (ml/dl); $C(a\text{-}v)o_2$, arterial-venous oxygen content difference (ml/dl).

$(Vo_2I = C(a\text{-}v)o_2 \times CI \times 10)$ where Vo_2I is the oxygen consumption index and $C(a\text{-}v)o_2$ is the arterial-venous oxygen content difference. Vo_2I yields information regarding the amount of oxygen that is actually *used* by the patient. In most situations, oxygen consumption is equal to oxygen demand.

Oxygen consumption may differ slightly from oxygen uptake, which is the volume of oxygen extracted from inspired gas, often measured using metabolic carts during nutritional assessment.

Oxygen demand describes how much oxygen is *needed* by the tissues to function aerobically (18). When the demand for oxygen exceeds the actual use of oxygen (consumption), anaerobic metabolism will occur and lactate acidosis may result. Oxygen demand cannot be measured directly in the clinical situation but indirect indicators of anaerobic metabolism (lactic acid) demonstrate that the need for oxygen (demand) has exceeded the use of oxygen (consumption) (18).

The oxygen utilization coefficient or extraction ratio describes the fraction of delivered oxygen that is consumed $(OUC = Vo_2/Do_2)$. The oxygen utilization coefficient, therefore, is an indication of the relative balance between oxygen supply and demand and, therefore, of oxygen transport. The variables in the Fick equation are used to calculate the oxygen utilization coefficient. When arterial saturation is maintained at a high level, the oxygen utilization coefficient is inversely related to mixed venous oxygen saturation (Svo_2) (28).

Clinical Determinants of Svo_2

Mixed venous oxygen saturation measurements are fundamental to understanding oxygen transport balance in critically ill patients. The Svo_2 is determined by the elements of the Fick equation and, therefore, by the balance between oxygen supply and demand. When the Fick equation is solved for Svo_2, it can be seen that there are four primary determinants: cardiac output, hemoglobin, Sao_2, and Vo_2 (28).

1) $Vo_2 = C(a\text{-}v)o_2 \times CO \times 10$ [Fick equation]
2) $Vo_2/(CO \times 10) = C(a\text{-}v)O_2$ [divide by $CO \times 10$]
3) $Vo_2/(CO \times 10) - Cao_2 = -Cvo_2$ [subtract Cao_2]
4) $Cvo_2 = Cao_2 - Vo_2/(CO \times 10)$ [multiply by -1]
5) $Cvo_2/Cao_2 = 1 - Vo_2/(Cao_2 \times CO \times 10)$ [divide by Cao_2]
6) $Svo_2 = 1 - Vo_2/(Cao_2 \times CO \times 10)$ [assume Sao_2 approaches 1]
7) $Svo_2 = 1 - Vo_2/Do_2$ [substitute definition of Do_2]
8) $Svo_2 = 1 - OUC$ [substitute definition of OUC]

Uncompensated increases in oxygen consumption or uncompensated decreases in cardiac output, hemoglobin concentration, or Sao_2 will reduce Svo_2. Similarly, oxygen delivery increases in excess of oxygen consumption changes will result in an increase in Svo_2.

Technology of Continuous Svo_2 Monitoring

Mixed venous oxygen saturation can be monitored continuously using fiberoptic technology incorporated into a flow-directed thermodilution pulmonary artery catheter. Two fiberoptic bundles are used to transmit and receive narrow wavebands of light selected for reflectance characteristics of total hemoglobin and oxyhemoglobin. The relative fraction of total hemoglobin that is oxyhemoglobin is the oxyhemoglobin saturation. When red blood cells are flowing past the tip of the fiberoptic pulmonary artery catheter, light is reflected back to the catheter, and Svo_2 may be calculated (2, 23, 42, 50).

Several systems are available that allow this type of monitoring. Controversy continues regarding the use of a two- versus three-wavelength system. Although only two wavelengths of light are necessary to calculate the oxyhemoglobin saturation, changes in total hemoglobin concentration and reflectance characteristics of the fiberoptics may vary (15). For this reason, a third wavelength of light (white light) may be added to correct the overall reflectance for changes in hemoglobin concentration and fibrin deposition over the tip of the catheter. Studies have suggested that the three-wavelength technology is superior to the two-wavelength technology, at least in some situations (15).

Pitfalls of Continuous Svo_2 Monitoring

The most common problem associated with mixed venous oxygen saturation monitoring is an error induced by malpositioning of the tip of the pulmonary artery catheter. If the catheter drifts into a distal branch of the pulmonary artery or close to a bifurcation of the vessel or a vessel wall, an abnormal reflectance of light will occur that can alter the Svo_2 value (26). Therefore, the tip of the catheter should be positioned as proximal as possible, as described earlier in this chapter.

The continuous Svo_2 monitoring system is generally precalibrated prior to insertion into the patient. This in vitro calibration is valid over a very wide range of venous oxygen saturations. However, if the instrument is disconnected from the catheter at the optical module, recalibration may become necessary. It is recommended that the calibration be checked by an in vivo method, at least every 24 hours and prior

to any major therapeutic changes made on the basis of Svo_2 changes (27). The in vivo calibration is performed by slowly drawing a blood sample through the distal port of the pulmonary artery catheter and sending it for laboratory cooximetry. If the values indicated on the instrument are within 4% of the laboratory value, the system does not require recalibration (26, 28).

The final issue that must be addressed regarding technical problems with continuous Svo_2 monitoring is that of functional versus fractional saturation measurements (30). The functional oxyhemoglobin saturation is defined as the fractional oxyhemoglobin saturation divided by 1 minus the dyshemoglobins (functional So_2 = fractional $So_2/(1 - COHb - MetHb)$. Therefore, the functional oxyhemoglobin saturation is always greater than the fractional saturation by an amount proportional to the amount of dyshemoglobin present. The Svo_2 devices used today measure functional saturation but are often calibrated to fractional saturation. This must be taken into account when calculating derived oxygen transport parameters.

Interpretation of Oxygen Transport Data

Each of the elements of oxygen transport can be independently assessed when the proper definitions are used (Table 1.5). The delivery of oxygen is assessed by measuring the Sao_2, Pao_2, hemoglobin concentration, and cardiac index. The consumption of oxygen is assessed by calculating the $C(a-v)o_2$ and multiplying this by the cardiac index. The overall oxygen transport balance is assessed by calculating the oxygen utilization coefficient. As indicated earlier in this section, the Svo_2 can also be used to assess relative oxygen transport balance as long as arterial saturation is maintained at a high level (25).

When the oxygen transport balance is disrupted (i.e., oxygen utilization coefficient > 0.35 or Svo_2 < 0.65), further information is needed to better understand which of the four determinants of oxygen transport balance (Sao_2, hemoglobin, cardiac index, oxygen consumption) should be addressed. When oxygen consumption is fixed, the $C(a-v)o_2$ is inversely proportional to the cardiac index. When oxygen consumption increases without a concomitant increasing cardiac index, the C(a-v)o$_2$ increases (> 5.5 ml O$_2$/dl) (25).

While oxygen demand cannot be directly assessed, an inference can be made that oxygen demand has exceeded oxygen consumption when markers of anaerobic metabolism are present. The lactic acid concentration may serve as a clinically useful marker to demonstrate that the demand for oxygen has exceeded the amount of oxygen used and some tissues have converted to anaerobic metabolism (18).

Three important balances help to describe the clinical adequacy of oxygen transport (Fig. 1.8). The Svo$_2$ or oxygen utilization coefficient describes the adequacy of oxygen delivery relative to oxygen consumption. The C(a-v)o$_2$ describes adequacy of cardiac index relative to oxygen consumption. The arterial lactate concentration describes the adequacy of oxygen consumption relative to oxygen demand. When oxygen consumption increases to meet the demand for oxygen at the cellular level, markers of anaerobic metabolism will not be present.

A useful goal of clinical critical care is to treat the patient in such a way that oxygen consumption can rise to meet the body's oxygen demand. Since oxygen demand can never be known precisely, many practitioners would consider increasing the delivery of oxygen until consumption no

longer rises. At this point, it is assumed that consumption equals demand.

Since total body oxygen consumption is the product of cardiac output and extraction (C(a-v)o$_2$), consumption can increase only by increases in output or C(a-v)o$_2$. Increases in cardiac output or C(a-v)o$_2$ are therefore "protective" in that they allow (at least temporarily) oxygen consumption to increase to meet oxygen demand and prevent lactic acidosis secondary to anaerobic metabolism. A reasonable therapeutic goal in critically ill patients would be to maximize oxygen consumption while decreasing (or at least not increasing) oxygen demand.

Priorities in Treatment

With the nearly overwhelming number of measured and calculated oxygen transport and hemodynamic variables available, the question often arises "What is most important?". The answer is not simple and varies greatly from patient to patient. However, a common question in nearly all critically ill patients regards not the *value* but rather the *adequacy* of cardiac output. A second common question when cardiac output is inadequate is "What is likely to be the most effective treatment?".

The adequacy of cardiac output is defined by the adequacy of oxygen transport. The final pathway of oxygen transport is the cellular consumption of oxygen to meet metabolic needs. Therefore, whenever

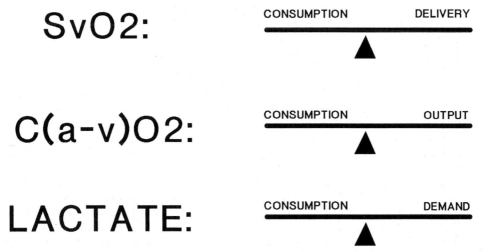

Figure 1.8. Assessment of oxygen consumption: The three balances relating oxygen consumption to delivery, cardiac output, and demand.

oxygen demand exceeds consumption and a progressive lactic acidosis is present, oxygen delivery is (by definition) inadequate. The cause of the inadequacy can be assessed by measuring the Svo_2 or calculating the oxygen utilization coefficient. This will help to determine if the lactic acidosis is caused by an ongoing oxygen consumption-delivery imbalance, reperfusion and delayed washout, or decreased lactate metabolism. Next, calculation of the $C(a-v)o_2$ will help to determine if the imbalance is due to inadequate cardiac output for the current oxygen consumption or if it is more likely related to other factors such as low hemoglobin, low Sao_2, or a combination of problems.

Various pathologic states change oxygen consumption significantly. Typically, hypodynamic shock states (cardiogenic, hypovolemic, and obstructive shock) cause a marked decrease in oxygen consumption. This is felt by many investigators to be caused by intense peripheral reflex vasoconstriction as the body attempts to maintain central arterial blood pressure.

The vasoconstriction reduces nutrient blood flow initially from nonessential and later from essential vascular beds. Reduced availability of oxygen in these beds caused by low blood flow results in an initial increase in oxygen extraction ($C(a-v)o_2$) in an attempt to maintain oxygen consumption. Increased extraction in the face of a fixed arterial oxygen content results in a decreased venous oxygen content and therefore Svo_2. When Svo_2 falls, a critical driving pressure for oxygen to diffuse to the mitochondria is reached (at about 26 mm Hg). Without oxygen, the mitochondria switch to anaerobic pathways in a final attempt to maintain cell viability. Lactic acid is released, which (for a short time) improves the availability of oxygen by shifting the oxyhemoglobin dissociation curve to the right raising the P_{50} and therefore the partial pressure of oxygen at a given saturation (content) (where P_{50} is the partial pressure of O_2 at which 50% of the hemoglobin is bound with oxygen).

In this example the low cardiac output from the hypodynamic shock state is inadequate to maintain the oxygen delivery-consumption balance and has resulted in a low Svo_2. The oxygen transport crisis is caused by the low cardiac output as indicated by the high $C(a-v)o_2$. Oxygen consumption is low and inadequate for cellular demand, resulting in a lactic acidosis.

Oxygen transport calculations indicate when cardiac output is inadequate and *when* treatment is needed. However, these variables are sensitive but not specific, and hemodynamic variables must be calculated to determine *how* to treat the patient most effectively.

The hemodynamic manifestations of hypodynamic forms of shock include a low cardiac index, tachycardia, a low stroke index and a high systemic vascular resistance index. The hypovolemic form of hypodynamic shock manifests low ventricular filling pressures, suggesting that the most appropriate therapy would be to augment preload by volume expansion.

Cardiogenic and obstructive forms of hypodynamic shock are manifest by high ventricular filling pressures. Cardiogenic shock is produced by very poor ventricular contractility and always produces a low left ventricular stroke work index. The therapy implied by this hemodynamic profile would be to reduce afterload and enhance contractility.

Obstructive shock is somewhat more complex, depending on the initiating event. Absolute filling pressures are high on both the right side (CVP) and the left (pulmonary artery occlusion pressure) in obstructive shock due to pericardial tamponade or tension pneumothorax. However, the transmural pressures are usually normal or low. When obstructive shock is caused by massive pulmonary emboli, right-sided pressures (CVP and mean pulmonary artery pressure) are usually high and left-sided filling pressure (pulmonary artery occlusion pressure) is usually normal or low. Treatment is aimed at correcting the primary problem.

Hyperdynamic forms of shock are far more complex and beyond the scope of this chapter to discuss in detail. Most forms of hyperdynamic shock are associated with intense vasoderegulation in the peripheral vasculature. This is manifested by vasodilation and low systemic vascular resistance index (at least in normovolemic subjects). The low systemic resistance unloads the ventricle, allowing a high stroke index and, in the presence of tachycardia, a very high cardiac index. Filling pressures are usually normal or low.

Oxygen consumption is quite variable in subjects with hyperdynamic shock. Fever and stress in these patients may increase oxygen demand. Because of inhomogeneity of peripheral blood flow, some vascular beds may be overperfused and some underperfused. Underperfused beds may release lactic acid because consumption cannot increase to meet increased oxygen demands. At the same time, oxygen extraction ($C(a-v)o_2$) in overperfused tissue may be low, resulting in a high Cvo_2 and therefore high Svo_2.

This leads to the apparent paradox of progressive lactic acidosis in a patient with high oxygen delivery, low extraction and utilization, and normal consumption. These complex patients have a high mortality. Therapy is aimed at restoring perfusion to all tissues and reversing the process leading to vasoderegulation.

CONCLUSION

While monitoring goals in critical care have changed over the last three decades, our current understanding of the importance of oxygen transport balance mandates an accurate assessment of hemodynamics. Hemodynamic monitoring using invasive techniques is the mainstay of today's practice of critical care. When accurate information is obtained, most clinicians will act in a similar manner to achieve reasonable physiologic endpoints. If accurate hemodynamic monitoring is not available, we are left in a state where clinical judgment and personal opinion dictate random management of complex clinical problems.

Acknowledgment. The authors wish to express their greatest appreciation to Christy McRae for the careful preparation of this manuscript.

References

1. Armengol J, Man GCW, Balsys AJ, Wells AL. Effects of the respiratory cycle on cardiac output measurements: reproducibility of data enhanced by timing the thermodilution injections in dogs. Crit Care Med 1981;9:852–854.
2. Baele PL, McMichan JC, Marsh HM, et al. Continuous monitoring of mixed venous oxygen saturation in critically ill patients. Anesth Analg 1982;61:513–517.
3. Brisman R, Parks LC, Benson DW. Pitfalls in the clinical use of central venous pressure. Arch Surg 1967;95:902–907.
4. Civetta JM. Pulmonary artery catheter insertion. In: Sprung CL, ed. The pulmonary artery catheter: methodology and clinical applications. Baltimore: University Park Press, 1983.
5. Civetta JM, Gabel JC, Laver MB. Disparate ventricular function in surgical patients. Surg Forum 1971;22:136–139.
6. DeLaurentis DA, Hayes M, Matsumoto T, Wolferth CC. Does central venous pressure accurately reflect hemodynamic and fluid volume patterns in the critical surgical patient? Am J Surg 1973;126:415–418.
7. Downs JB, Rackstein AD, Klein EF, Hawkins IF. Hazards of radial-artery catheterization. Anesthesiology 1973;38:283–286.
8. English JB, Hodges MR, Sentker C, et al. Comparison of aortic pulse-wave contour analysis and thermodilution methods of measuring cardiac output during anesthesia in the dog. Anesthesiology 1980;52:56–61.
9. Ersoz CJ, Hedden M, Lain L. Prolonged femoral arterial catheterization for intensive care. Anesth Analg 1970;49:160–164.
10. Forrester JS, Diamond G, McHugh TJ, Swan HJC. Filling pressures in the right and left sides of the heart in acute myocardial infarction: a reappraisal of central venous pressure monitoring. N Engl J Med 1971;285:190–192.
11. Forrester JS, Ganz W, Diamond G, McHugh T, et al. Thermodilution cardiac output determination with a single flow-directed catheter. Am Heart J 1972;83:306–311.
12. Ganz W, Swan HJC. Measurement of blood flow by thermodilution. Am J Cardiol 1972;29:241–246.
13. Gardner RM. Direct blood pressure measurement—dynamic response requirements. Anesthesiology 1981;54:227–236.
14. Gardner RM, Hollingsworth KW. Optimizing the electrocardiogram and pressure monitoring. Crit Care Med 1986;14:651–658.
15. Gettinger A, DeTraglia MC, Glass D. In vivo comparison of two mixed venous saturation catheters. Anesthesiology 1987;66:373–375.
16. Hartong JM, Dixon RS. Monitoring resuscitation of the injured patient. JAMA 1977;237:242–244.
17. Jansen JRC, Versprille A. Improvement of cardiac output estimation by the thermodilution method during mechanical ventilation. Intensive Care Med 1986;12:71–79.
18. Kandel G, Aberman A. Mixed venous oxygen saturation: its role in the assessment of the critically ill patient. Arch Intern Med 1983;143:1400–1402.
19. Kleinman B. Understanding natural frequency and damping and how they relate to the measurement of blood pressure. J Clin Monit 1989;5:137–147.
20. Lantiegne K, Civetta JM. A system for maintaining invasive pressure monitoring. Heart Lung 1978;7:610–621.

21. Lappas DG, Fahmy NR. The heart. In: Burke JF, ed. Surgical physiology. Philadelphia: WB Saunders, 1983.
22. Levett JM, Replogle RL. Thermodilution cardiac output: a critical analysis and review of the literature. J Surg Res 1979;27:392–404.
23. McMichan JC. Continuous monitoring of mixed venous oxygen saturation: theory applied to practice. In: Schweiss JF, ed. Continuous measurement of blood oxygen saturation in the high risk patient. San Diego: Beach International, 1983.
24. Nelson LD. Application of venous saturation monitoring. In: Civetta JM, Taylor RW, Kirby RR, eds. Critical care. Philadelphia: JB Lippincott, 1988.
25. Nelson LD. Bedside application of Svo_2 measurements. O_2 transport. (in press).
26. Nelson LD. Continuous venous oximetry: Part I: Physiology and technical considerations. Curr Rev Resp Ther 1986;8:99–103.
27. Nelson LD. Continuous venous oximetry in surgical patients. Ann Surg 1986;203:329–333.
28. Nelson LD. Mixed venous oximetry. In: Snyder JV, Pinsky MR, eds. Oxygen transport in the critically ill. Chicago: Year Book, 1987.
29. Nelson LD. Monitoring and measurement in shock. In: Barrett J, Nyhus LM, eds. Treatment of shock: principles and practice. 2nd ed. Philadelphia: Lea & Febiger, 1986.
30. Nelson LD. Real-time monitoring of gas exchange. In: Vincent JL, ed. Update in intensive care and emergency medicine. Vol 10. Update 1990. Heidelberg: Springer-Verlag, 1990.
31. Nelson LD, Anderson HB. Patient selection for iced versus room temperature injectate for thermodilution cardiac output determinations. Crit Care Med 1985:13:182–184.
32. Nelson LD, Civetta JM, Judson-Civetta J. Titrating positive end-expiratory pressure therapy in patients with early, moderate arterial hypoxemia. Crit Care Med 1987;15:14–19.
33. Nelson LD, Houtchens BA. Automatic vs manual injections for thermodilution cardiac output determinations. Crit Care Med 1982;10:190–192.
34. Nelson LD, Martinez OV, Anderson HB. Incidence of microbial colonization in open versus closed delivery systems for thermodilution injectate. Crit Care Med 1986;14:291–293.
35. Nelson LD, Snyder JV. Technical problems in data acquisition. In: Snyder JV, Pinsky MR, eds. Oxygen transport in the critically ill. Chicago: Year Book, 1987.
36. Okamoto K, Komatsu T, Kumar V, Sanchala V, et al. Effects of intermittent positive-pressure ventilation on cardiac output measurements by thermodilution. Crit Care Med 1986;14:977–980.
37. Rice CL, Hobelman CF, John DA, Smith DE, et al. Central venous pressure or pulmonary capillary wedge pressure as the determinant of fluid replacement in aortic surgery. Surgery 1978;84:437–440.
38. Ross J. Role of vasodilator therapy. In: Karliner JS, Gregoratos G, eds. Coronary care. New York: Churchill Livingstone, 1981.
39. Rubin LR, Bongiovi J. Central venous pressure: an unreliable guide to fluid therapy in burns. Arch Surg 1970;100:269–274.
40. Runciman WB, Ilsley AH, Roberts JG. An evaluation of thermodilution cardiac output measurement using the Swan-Ganz catheter. Anaesth Intensive Care 1981;9:208–220.
41. Samii K, Conseiller C, Viars P. Central venous pressure and pulmonary wedge pressure. Arch Surg 1976;111:1122–1125.
42. Schweiss JF. Continuous measurement of blood oxygen saturation in the high risk patient. San Diego: Beach International, 1983.
43. Seldinger SI. Catheter replacement of the needle in percutaneous arteriography: a new technique. Acta Radiol 1953;39:368–376.
44. Shellock FG, Riedinger MS. Reproducibility and accuracy of using room-temperature vs. ice-temperature injectate for thermodilution cardiac output determination. Heart Lung 1983;12:175–176.
45. Shellock FG, Riedinger MS, Bateman TM, Gray RJ. Thermodilution cardiac output determination in hypothermic postcardiac surgery patients: room vs ice temperature injectate. Crit Care Med 1983;11:668–670.
46. Snyder JV, Powner DJ. Effects of mechanical ventilation on the measurement of cardiac output by thermodilution. Crit Care Med 1982;10:677–682.
47. Sorensen MB, Bille-Brahe NE, Engell HC. Cardiac output measurement by thermal dilution: Reproducibility and comparison with the dye-dilution technique. Ann Surg 1976;183:67–72.
48. Stoller JK, Herbst TJ, Hurford W, Rie MA. Spuriously high cardiac output from injecting thermal indicator through an ensheathed port. Crit Care Med 1986;14:1064–1065.
49. Swan HJC, Ganz W, Forrester JS, et al. Catheterization of the heart in man with use of a flow-directed balloon-tipped catheter. N Engl J Med 1970;283:447–451.
50. Waller JL, Kaplan JA, Bauman DI, et al. The left shifted oxyhemoglobin curve in sepsis: a preventable defect. Ann Surg 1974;180:213–220.
51. Warner HR, Swan HJC, Connelly DC, et al. Quantitation of beat-to-beat changes in stroke volume from the aortic pulse contour in man. Am J Physiol 1953;5:495–507.
52. Watson CB. The PA catheter as an early warning system. Anaesth Rev 1983;10:34–35.
53. Weisel RD, Berger RL, Hechtman HB. Measurement of cardiac output by thermodilution. N Engl J Med 1975;292:682–684.
54. Wesseling KH, deWit B, Weber JAP, Smith NT. A simple device for the continuous measurement of cardiac output. Adv Cardiovasc Phys 1983;5:16–52.
55. Wilkins RG. Radial artery cannulation and ischemic damage: a review. Anesth Forum 1985;40:896–899.
56. Woods M, Scott RN, Harken AH. Practical considerations for the use of a pulmonary artery thermistor catheter. Surgery 1976;79:469–475.

2

Substrate Metabolism and Resting Energy Expenditure

Robert Schlichtig

Unlike most patients, those who are critically ill depend largely on intensive care unit (ICU) practitioners for exogenous nutrients needed to support vital metabolism. Failure to ensure adequate oxygen (O_2) transport (see Chapter 7, "O_2 Uptake, Critical O_2 Delivery, and Tissue Wellness") is rapidly catastrophic, so the intensivist is most immediately occupied with the monitoring and maintenance of adequate O_2 transport parameters. Less pressing, but potentially equally important, is provision of fuel and protein. Tissues of most patients contain sufficient energy and protein reserves to permit survival for many weeks in the absence of nutritional therapy. Failure to provide fuel and protein, however, will permit the progressive erosion of proteinaceous host defense to become an increasingly important independent risk factor for death. Nutritional therapy is therefore a necessary, if insufficient, therapeutic modality in many instances. The purpose of this chapter is to review current understanding of fuel and protein metabolism in normal and stressed states, so as to facilitate appropriate implementation of nutritional therapy.

DEFINITION OF TERMS

The vocabulary used by nutritionists is sometimes confusing to those unfamiliar with nutritional literature, so it may be useful to review briefly a few key phrases.

Protein turnover describes the continuous synthesis and catabolism that characterizes all body proteins; some (such as serum proteins) turn over relatively rapidly, and others (such as skeletal muscle) turn over more slowly (78). This process costs somewhere between 10 and 40% of resting metabolic expenditure but permits plasticity of structure and function, so that disused protein can be disposed of and new protein synthesized as needed (78) (Fig. 2.1). *Biologic value* is a rating of protein sources based on the ability of tissues to utilize them for new protein synthesis. Because humans can synthesize a relatively limited number of amino acids, exogenous protein that is relatively deficient in one or more essential amino acids is of low biologic value. The natural protein of highest biologic value, not surprisingly, is contained within human breast milk. Commercially available crystalline amino acid formulas and most enteral formulas are carefully designed high biologic value preparations that are composed of approximately half essential amino acids and half nonessential amino acids.

Nitrogen is frequently used interchangeably with "protein" or "amino acid," because urea nitrogen is easy to measure in the urine and provides a rough estimate of protein catabolism. One gram of urinary nitrogen is equivalent to the catabolism of 6.25 g of high biologic value protein. *Balance* (nitrogen balance, caloric balance) is

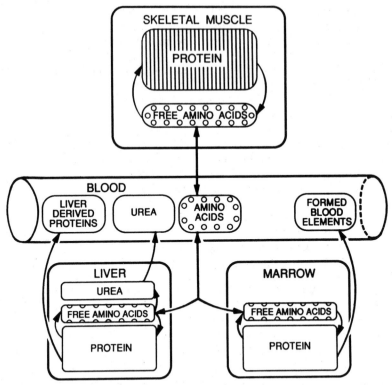

Figure 2.1. Protein turnover. Normally, all body protein is continuously catabolized and resynthesized at varying rates depending on the tissue type and prevailing metabolic conditions. During stress, muscle catabolism outweighs synthesis as muscle-derived amino acid is translocated to liver and marrow for synthesis of proteins needed acutely for survival. Although considerable urea is also formed, whole body protein synthetic rate is actually somewhat higher than normal.

simply the quantity of substance that enters a tissue minus the quantity that exits. Like O_2 consumption, another balance (see Chapter 53), balance measurements often provide woefully little information regarding the responsible mechanisms.

Lean body mass refers to tissues other than the adipose reserve. *Catabolism* properly refers to degradation of any endogenous substance but this term is more commonly used by nutritionists to describe catabolism of lean body mass, a phenomenon generally viewed as the most deleterious by-product of emaciation. *Stress* is loosely defined as a condition characterized by a higher than normal protein catabolic rate, an abnormal hormonal milieu, and alterations in blood content of fuel substrate, but is not easily quantified. Most commonly, this term refers to abnormalities observed in septic, burned, or multi-

ply traumatized conditions. However, it is important to recognize that many ICU patients are not stressed, but simply being weaned from mechanical ventilation or otherwise recovering from illness. It should also be noted that alterations of substrate utilization of severely burned patients tend to be considerably more profound than those seen in patients who are simply septic.

In this chapter, little distinction is drawn between intravenous and enteral nutrients, because administration of protein, carbohydrate, and lipid by either route generally produces a very similar balance. However, for reasons that remain mystifying, intravenous administration of the same substances tends to produce hepatic parenchymal abnormalities that are rarely seen during enteral alimentation (78). Though not stated elsewhere in this chapter, it is important to recognize that virtually all nutritionists favor feeding by the enteral route whenever possible.

STARVATION

Acute starvation represents a metabolic emergency equally as serious as dysoxia (abnormal oxygen metabolism), because endogenous tissues must quickly release sufficient quantities and appropriate species of fuel to support vital metabolism. Acute intervention by the intensivist is rarely needed, because the hormonal-tissue interactions that sustain fuel supply are rarely sufficiently perturbed to produce a cellular fuel deficit. However, an understanding of these interactions helps to explain some of the metabolic disturbances seen in many patients and assists in developing appropriate nutritional regimens.

Approximately 180 g of glucose is needed daily to support oxidative phosphorylation in brain and formed blood elements (9). During acute starvation, this requirement imposes several strategic difficulties. Liver and muscle glycogen can support this requirement, but only briefly, for about 12–18 hr. Thereafter, adequate gluconeogenic substrata cannot be scavenged from adipose reserves, because only the glycerol moiety of triglyceride, representing a calorically small proportion of triglyceride fuel, can be used for glucose synthesis. Thus only glucogenic amino acids (i.e., those that can be catabolized by the Embden-Myerhof pathway) can provide the needed substrate for gluconeogenesis. At odds with this urgent need to catabolize tissue protein is the need to sustain protein mass, of which there is no reserve. As noted, protein that is disused is not resynthesized during the process of protein turnover. During starvation, endogenous proteins may still be needed, but are sacrificed to serve the need for energy demand.

During "normal" starvation (i.e., starvation in the absence of stress), protein catabolism is gradually minimized, and adipose reserves maximally support the organism's need for fuel. Thus, humans who starve in the absence of other illness tend to become malnourished in a balanced manner, resulting in a condition termed "marasmus," or "protein-calorie malnutrition." During many critical illnesses, however, protein is catabolized to a much greater degree, resulting in "kwashiorkor." Though seemingly the result of deranged metabolism, kwashiorkor may actually represent the end product of metabolic adaptations to needs other than simply provision of cellular fuel.

Normal Starvation

Following complete intestinal absorption of a meal, as well as cellular storage of the excess caloric equivalents, a healthy individual becomes briefly hypoglycemic. Under normal conditions, this appears to represent the initial trigger of the ensuing hormonal and metabolic response to starvation. Low blood glucose is sensed by the adrenals, which are thereby stimulated to synthesize epinephrine. Epinephrine, in turn, simultaneously promotes lipolysis in adipose tissue and glycogenolysis in the liver, thereby permitting stored glucose and free fatty acids to enter the circulation. These metabolic properties of epinephrine are frequently encountered by intensivists who make use of its inotropic properties, and who subsequently observe hyperglycemia in these patients. Hypoglycemia is also sensed in the pancreas, where islet cells release increased quantities of glucagon and decreased quantities of insulin, further stimulating glycogenolysis. As noted, glycogen stores can support the individual's glucose needs for approximately 12–18 hr.

When glycogen stores have been depleted, insulin secretion diminishes further, while glucagon secretion increases. A hallmark of this phase is ketonuria, which represents accelerated lipolysis (owing to decreased blood insulin that normally entraps triglyceride within adipocytes) and formation of ketone bodies of the liver (28). To prevent life-threatening ketoacidosis, blood insulin must be maintained sufficiently elevated. It is this restriction, combined with the low glycerol content of triglyceride, that renders lipids insufficient to serve the glucose needs. Therefore it is

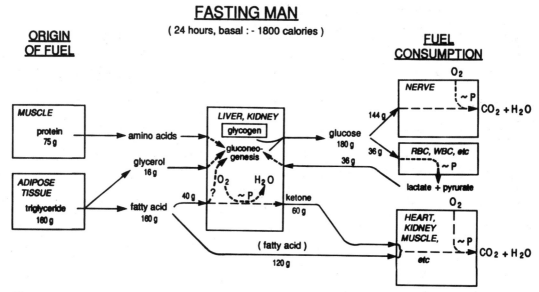

FASTING MAN

(24 hours, basal : - 1800 calories)

Figure 2.2. Acute starvation in an otherwise healthy individual. Seventy-five grams of muscle-derived protein is catabolized, providing gluconeogenic substrate for nervous tissue and formed elements. (From Cahill GF. Starvation in man. N Engl J Med 1970;282:668–675.)

important that amino acids are also permitted to escape from native protein during this period. This phenomenon may relate partially to decreased blood insulin, as insulin appears to function as an important anticatabolic hormone (7, 10, 30, 59). Alternatively, amino acid efflux may simply represent the expected imbalance of protein synthesis and catabolism, in the absence of protein intake. During early starvation, protein turnover is characterized by synthesis of approximately 3 g of protein/kg/day, but protein catabolism is 4.5 g/kg/day (51). As a consequence of these various adaptations, a 75-kg man catabolizes approximately 160 g of fat and 75 g of protein/day during the early phase of fasting (Fig. 2.2) (9).

If net protein catabolism were to continue at the initial fasting rate, body protein deficiency would become life-threatening within several weeks. Instead, urinary nitrogen efflux decreases to two thirds of the initial value, i.e., from 12 g/day to 8 g/day, during the first week. During the ensuing several weeks, urinary nitrogen loss gradually declines to 25% of the initial value, or 3 g/day (Fig. 2.3). This

adaptation appears to result from increased consumption of ketone bodies by nervous tissue, and decreasing need for gluconeogenic substrate (9). Concurrent with these hormonal adaptations is a slowing of protein turnover, which may also account for decreased nitrogen loss. Therefore, the gradual decline of protein catabolism may represent not only a decreasing glucose requirement of brain, but a slowing of the normal rate of protein breakdown as well.

Starvation during Stressed States

In contrast to the relatively gradual erosion of body protein during normal starvation, stressed states are associated with a more rapid rate of protein catabolism. Thus, starving patients who are severely traumatized, burned, or septic catabolize body protein at approximately two to three times the normal starving rate (50). Since each gram of net nitrogen loss represents catabolism of 30 g of lean tissue (27), a patient with a net urinary nitrogen loss of 20 g/day catabolizes half a kilogram of lean body tissue! This figure seems unbelievably high but is supported by body cell

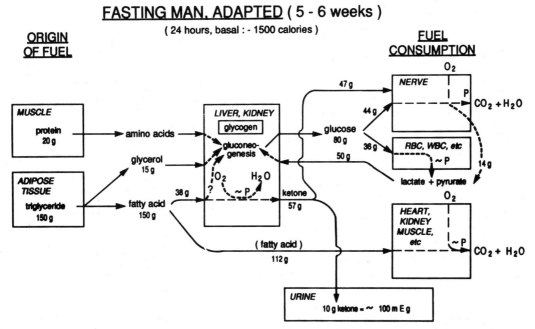

Figure 2.3. Starvation in an otherwise healthy individual, after a period of adaptation. Less muscle protein is catabolized, and nervous tissue utilizes an increased proportion of ketone to support its metabolism. (From Cahill GF. Starvation in man. N Engl J Med 1970;282:668–675.)

mass measurements in postoperative surgical patients who lost 3.2 kg of lean body mass in 5 days (81), or 9.1% of total body nitrogen 2 weeks after surgery, despite normal nutritional intake during the second week (16, 101). However, it is important to note that the catabolic rate, even of stressed patients, decreases progressively as they become malnourished (23, 48, 58).

Unlike "normal" starvation, "stressed starvation" is not initiated by hypoglycemia, but rather is associated with hyperglycemia, as well as with increased blood insulin (11, 21). Blood insulin is normal or low during shock, increasing to supranormal values only after resuscitation (11), thereby permitting increased glucose substrate for anaerobic energy metabolism. The trigger of increased catabolic rate during stress could be simply related to increased blood concentrations of cortisol, glucagon, and epinephrine, which counteract the protein-preserving action of insulin. However, infusion of these hormones in normal volunteers to simulate stress conditions increased protein catab-

olism to only a fraction of that seen in stressed patients (2, 51). Another hypothesis is that increased protein catabolism results from a fuel deficit in skeletal muscle, because it appears that skeletal muscle of stressed patients consumes inadequate blood-borne substrate to satisfy skeletal muscle energy demand (5, 24, 65). Since muscle can consume only the branched-chain amino acids (BCAA) of its protein store, it appears that increased patient nitrogen loss represents skeletal muscle "autocannibalism" of BCAA needed to support muscle oxidative phosphorylation. Nevertheless, the relative proportions of amino acids released from skeletal muscle are quite similar during normal and stressed starvation (14). These data suggest either that a muscular fuel deficit characterizes both conditions, or that muscle autocannibalism of BCAA is simply a by-product of a more generalized need for amino acid substrate. Preliminary evidence suggested that skeletal muscle proteolysis represents an adaptive response to injury, because cytokines such as interleukin-1 simultaneously stimulate production of acute phase reactants as well as skeletal muscle proteolysis (3, 15, 70). Although the potential role of cytokine mediators now appears less clear (51), it is quite apparent that the stressed starving individual must synthesize a large number of proteinaceous substances (mucus, granulocytes, clotting factors, etc.) and requires a mechanism for liberating amino acid substrate from endogenous tissue (Fig. 2.1). Indeed, the total body synthetic rate during stressed states is actually somewhat higher than normal, so that the increased net nitrogen loss actually results from a rate of catabolism that exceeds synthesis (51). Another hypothesis under investigation is that increased cellular need for glutamine, a preferred fuel of many cells (72, 95–97), during stress (72, 85, 94) may stimulate skeletal muscle proteolysis, because muscle proteolysis appears quite sensitive to intracellular glutamine concentration (73).

SUBSTRATE UTILIZATION

The goal of nutritional supplementation is to reverse the protein catabolism that would otherwise occur with starvation. In so doing, however, it is considered important to provide fuel, protein, and other needed substrates in balanced proportions to ensure efficient cellular utilization commensurate with the patient's ability to utilize various nutrients. When critically ill patients are fed excessive quantities of nutrients that they cannot immediately oxidize, they are burdened by the need to dispose of the unused substrate by metabolic pathways that may already be overwhelmed. For example, the human liver contains the only known enzymatic machinery for converting glucose to lipid (54, 67, 102) and is therefore required to transport the manufactured very low density lipoproteins to adipose tissue. Owing in part to the concern that some patients may be intolerant to various nutrients, considerable research has focused on patterns of substrate utilization in various disease states. Few definitive statements can yet be made; however, a brief review of this literature will alert the reader to areas of concern.

Normal Utilization of Exogenous Substrate

Carbohydrate

During a carbohydrate meal, glucose homeostasis is initially attained by reducing the rate of hepatic gluconeogenesis. This is achieved by a slight increase of pancreatic insulin production, sufficient to inhibit hepatic glucose production, but insufficient to increase uptake of glucose by muscle (99). When diminished hepatic production alone becomes insufficient to maintain normal blood glucose concentration, blood insulin rises twofold, allowing muscle and liver to clear glucose from the circulation (99). Glucose is then oxidized preferentially, sparing dietary and endogenous lipid (12, 62, 63). Preferential glucose oxidation appears cost-effective, as it precludes the need for conversion of glucose to lipid, an energy-consuming process.

Exogenously administered dextrose normally suppresses protein catabolism considerably. One hundred fifty to 200 g of dextrose (equivalent to infusion of 3–4 liters of 5% dextrose) is normally sufficient to reduce urinary nitrogen loss by one half (98). This quantity of dextrose appears sufficient to arrest hepatic gluconeogenesis, but insufficient to prevent "oxidative deamination" of amino acids by other tissues (49). Oxidative deamination of amino acids refers to direct catabolism of the carbon skeleton, without prior conversion to glucose (Fig. 2.4). Infusion of dextrose equivalent to a patient's metabolic rate (approximately 600 g of dextrose, or 860 ml of 70% dextrose) further reduces urinary nitrogen loss, apparently by decreasing oxidative deamination of amino acids (80), to about one quarter of the starving value. However, even this quantity of dextrose is insufficient to eradicate protein catabolism entirely (64, 98).

Lipid

Like glucose metabolism, lipid metabolism is normally closely regulated in a cost-efficient manner. During oral/intestinal feeding, lipid particles enter the circulation as chylomicrons that are synthesized by

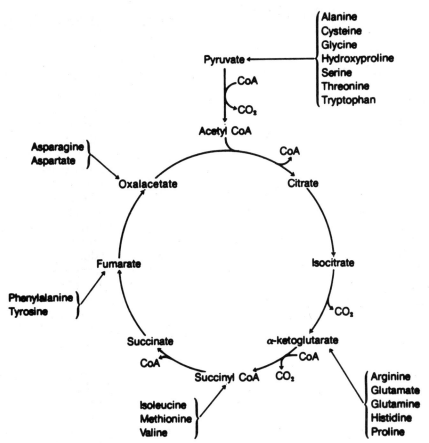

Figure 2.4. Catabolism of amino acids. Carbon skeletons of glucogenic amino acids may be converted to pyruvate, and then may undergo conversion to glucose via the Embden-Meyerhof pathway. Alternatively, all amino acid carbon may be oxidized directly, a phenomenon referred to as "oxidative deamination." (From Devlin T. Textbook of biochemistry with clinical correlations. New York: John Wiley & Sons, 1982.)

enterocytes and secreted into lymph. Lipid particles of intravenous emulsions are in many respects quite similar to chylomicrons and are metabolized in a similar manner. Lipid particles are cleared primarily by skeletal muscle (47%), intestine (25%), and heart (25%) during intravenous administration (74). Liver normally does not clear lipid particles, possibly owing to absence of lipoprotein lipase in hepatic endothelium. However, at high concentrations the hepatic reticuloendothelial system may clear lipid particles (35).

Clearance of blood triglyceride is dependent on liproprotein lipase, an enzyme contained within capillary endothelium, and hormone-sensitive lipase, which resides within adipocytes (Fig. 2.5). Triglyc-eride cannot enter adipocytes directly, requiring lipoprotein lipase for its digestion into three free fatty acid moieties and one glycerol. Predictably, lipoprotein is stimulated by insulin. The hormone-sensitive lipase residing within adipose cells governs net fatty acid efflux. During ingestion of a meal, this enzyme is inhibited by insulin, to prevent inappropriate release of fatty acids. Insulin also permits adipocyte uptake of small quantities of glucose, which produces glycerol-3-phosphate, required to rejoin with three free fatty acid moieties to form a single adipose triglyceride. Conversely, during starvation (see above), hormone-sensitive lipase is stimulated by catecholamines and glucagon and releases fatty acids to other tissues.

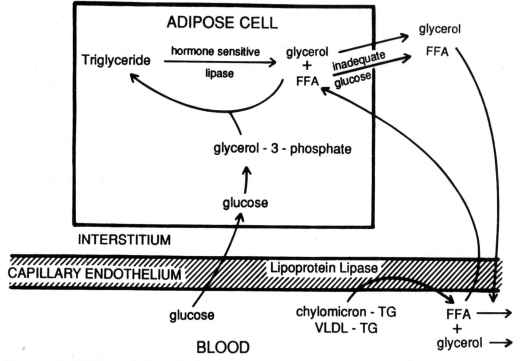

Figure 2.5. Lipid metabolism. Triglyceride is catabolized and resynthesized continuously. Net synthesis or release depends on concentrations of glucose, insulin, catecholamines, and glucagon. (From Schlichtig R, Ayres SM. Nutritional support of the critically ill. Chicago: Year Book, 1988.)

Limited data suggest that the anticatabolic properties of lipid are minor. Data from one investigation suggest that lipid emulsion alone reduces protein catabolism only to the extent that it contains glycerol (a gluconeogenic precursor) (6). Many subsequent investigators have substituted varying proportions of lipid for dextrose caloric equivalents in complete nutritional regimens and have observed nearly identical nitrogen balance. However, because these regimens included substantial protein, which alone can retard net protein catabolism considerably (see below), it may be incorrect to conclude that lipid infusion impacts nitrogen balance to the same degree as does dextrose infusion (78).

Amino Acids/Protein

Ingested protein is reduced to amino acids by intestinal mucosa and released to the portal circulation. The liver catabolizes a portion of these, permitting movement of the remaining amino acids to peripheral tissues in proportion to their need. As the liver has little capacity to catabolize BCAA, these are almost entirely released in hepatic venous efflux and are primarily taken up by skeletal muscle (61).

As noted earlier, body protein continues to turn over during acute starvation, with synthesis of approximately 3.0 g/kg/day and catabolism of approximately 4.5 g/kg/day, suggesting considerable reutilization of catabolized lean body mass. The goal of protein therapy is to increase body protein synthesis, so as to offset the protein catabolic rate. Normally, intake of approximately 1.0 g of high biologic value protein/kg/day, together with noncaloric protein substrate, is adequate for this goal, even when administered with a low-calorie diet (31, 78, 90). After a period of adaptation, humans can maintain protein mass by ingesting as little as 0.4 g/kg/day (86), owing to a rapid reduction of body protein turnover (90). This value of protein intake is generally recommended for patients with chronic renal insufficiency.

Exogenous Substrate Utilization during Stress

During stressed states (sepsis, burns, trauma), exogenous administration of carbohydrate, lipid, and protein is considerably less likely to prevent erosion of lean body mass. For this reason, it is very important to begin nutritional supplementation early in those patients who appear likely to remain severely ill for prolonged periods. Indeed, it is generally possible to arrest lean body catabolism only partially in patients characterized by a generalized inflammatory response (23, 48, 51, 58). Only during the anabolic recovery phase are administered nutrients efficiently utilized to replenish scavenged protein stores.

Carbohydrate

While three liters of 5% dextrose reduces net nitrogen efflux by approximately 50% in normal individuals, this quantity is of relatively little nutritional value, even in uncomplicated postoperative surgical patients, reducing urinary nitrogen loss in that population to approximately 8–9 g/day (4, 29, 32). In septic and/or multiply traumatized individuals, low dose dextrose infusion has no appreciable influence on protein catabolism. Dextrose infusion alone at higher (isocaloric) quantities succeeds only in suppressing hepatic gluconeogenesis (25, 34, 49, 80), while oxidative deamination of amino acids is relatively unaffected (25, 80). Consequently, isocaloric dextrose infusion alone reduces nitrogen loss by only one third to one half (40, 41, 80). More importantly, infusion of dextrose at a rate higher than the patient's metabolic expenditure does not appear to improve nitrogen retention significantly (41).

It is important to recognize that the influence of dextrose with respect to protein catabolic rate appears to be less striking when it is administered with adequate quantities of amino acids. Thus, while isocaloric dextrose may reduce nitrogen loss by one third to one half in the absence of amino acid, provision of only half the quantity of dextrose would diminish the effect on nitrogen retention by only a few grams when amino acids are also provided (40). This consideration is important when calculating caloric requirements of ICU patients, who are often intolerant of dextrose infusion.

The fact that isocaloric dextrose suppresses hepatic gluconeogenesis in stressed patients suggests that it merely satisfies the body's need for glucose, so that amino acid substrate is no longer needed for gluconeogenesis. Inconsistent with this hypothesis, however, is the observation that only about half of dextrose infused at most rates is actually oxidized by stressed patients (25, 80). Thus it appears that dextrose does not simply "substitute" for amino acid or lipid as a cellular fuel. These data are in agreement with the finding that dextrose incompletely suppresses endogenous lipid oxidation in stressed patients (63). In other words, lipid is still used as a fuel substrate when isocaloric dextrose is provided. In this regard, it is interesting to note that isocaloric dextrose infusion is also associated with increased metabolic rate and increased production of catecholamines, which would seem to be needed to liberate free fatty acid fuel from adipose tissue in the face of dextrose-enhanced insulin secretion (25).

Some data suggest that dextrose helps to conserve body mass indirectly, by stimulating secretion of insulin, a potent anticatabolic hormone. Infusion of insulin sufficient to increase blood insulin to eight times the basal value (the "insulin clamp" technique) can nearly abolish amino acid efflux from the limbs of critically ill patients (7). Considerable clinical data further indicate that administration of insulin sufficient to maintain blood sugar less than 150 g/dl reduces urinary nitrogen loss by one third to one half of the value of that in patients who did not receive supplemental insulin (38, 100). However, this method appears to benefit protein metabolism of only the most highly catabolic patients.

If only 50% of administered dextrose is oxidized, the remainder must be converted to glycogen and/or lipid. Thus the knowledge that only hepatocytes can synthesize lipid from glucose (see above) may be of concern in patients with hepatic failure and/or those with marginal perfusion states. Though incompletely investigated, it is conceivable that provision of excessive nutrients could produce an energy drain on the liver (44). Fatty liver is an abnormality commonly associated with infusion of large quantities of dextrose and can often be partially reversed when lipid calories are substituted for a portion of dextrose calories in a total parenteral nutritional regimen (8, 56). In this regard, it is interesting to note that a respiratory quotient in excess of 1.0 has been reported when profoundly septic patients received isocaloric dextrose, strongly suggesting substantial conversion of glucose to lipid (33). For these reasons, it may be inadvisable to provide isocaloric dextrose and insulin: although nitrogen loss may be thereby minimized, the effects on hepatic parenchyma are uncertain. Many intensivists routinely provide one half of total parenteral nutrition calories as lipid and one half as dextrose to patients with suspected inability to oxidize dextrose. Though not yet completely studied, it appears that administration of human growth hormone may prove a superior alternative to insulin (69, 93).

When beginning infusion of carbohydrate-containing formulas, it is important to recognize the impact on cellular electrolyte balance. Following the second World War, many released prisoners died suddenly during refeeding, possibly because they received insufficient phosphorus and potassium to fill expanding intracellular stores (46). Similarly, malnourished Jamaican children were characterized by abnormal cellular sodium-potassium ATPase activity, and some developed severe tachycardia and tachypnea during refeeding unless digoxin was administered (46). Sometimes, critically ill patients also develop severe blood deficiencies of intracellular ions—potassium, magnesium, and phosphorus—when nutritional supplementation is begun. These electrolytes should be monitored closely in all patients at the initiation of feeding.

Lipid

The role of lipid infusion in critically ill patients is uncertain. As noted, lipid infusion may spare some of the undesirable effects of dextrose, but appears to have little influence on nitrogen loss. Of lipid administered intravenously to stressed patients, only a small fraction appears to be oxidized immediately, and the remainder is presumably stored in adipose reserves (63). Nevertheless, isocaloric lipid-dextrose formulas generally appear to reduce erosion of lean body mass as effectively as do isocaloric dextrose formulas when combined with appropriate quantities of amino acids, and are commonly used by many intensivists. Indeed, exclusive provision of a nonprotein caloric substrate such as dextrose is unsupportable, as patients will then develop essential fatty acid deficiency, characterized by acral rash and blood lipid abnormalities. This abnormality does not occur in starving patients, but is observed during caloric repletion with dextrose, possibly because adequate endogenous release of essential fatty acids from the adipose reserve is inhibited by increased insulin concentrations (78).

Potentially undesirable effects of intravenous lipid emulsion include hypoxemia and diminished immune function. Hypoxemia of significant clinical consequence is quite unusual, and is rarely noted by ICU practitioners, but diminished immune function produced by long-chain triglyceride emulsions is of increasing concern (43, 77). Unfortunately, few attractive alternatives are currently available. For example, intravenous medium-chain triglyceride (MCT) formulas are controversial, as they appear to promote increased thermogenesis. MCT cannot be stored, and then becomes an obligate fuel, suggesting that only limited quantities can be administered (53). In addition, MCT infusion in animal models replicates serum abnormalities associated with Reye's syndrome and has been associated with central nervous system toxicity (57). Thus, long-chain triglyceride emulsions currently seem to provide the best therapeutic option in most patients. While no firm recommendations can be made, it appears advisable to monitor serum triglyceride concentration when adjusting the infusion rate of long-chain triglyceride emulsion, and to infuse it slowly so as to minimize immune deficits (43, 77).

Amino Acids/Protein

By far the most important determinant of nitrogen retention in critically ill patients is the quantity of amino acids infused. Indeed, it appears foolish to subject a patient to the risks of central venous nutrition or of enteral nutrition, unless optimum quantities of amino acids are included in the regimen. For example, many enteral formulations provide only 1.0 g of protein/kg/day when infused to provide 2000 caloric equivalents.

Many practitioners view amino acids simply as fuel that will be ineffective unless nonprotein fuel, equivalent to the patient's metabolic rate, is also infused. This belief is not supported by available evidence, as amino acids alone can promote near-complete protein retention in many patient populations, including those postoperative from major surgery (16, 78). Highly stressed patients tend to retain a considerably smaller proportion of administered amino acids than do routine postoperative patients (40). Nevertheless, the amino acid infusion rate remains the single most important determinant of nitrogen balance for these individuals (42). The optimum quantity of amino acids for highly catabolic patients is approximately 1.5 to 2.0 g/kg/day (78). Branched-chain amino acid-enriched formulas can be tried; however, the improvement of nitrogen retention is generally unremarkable and can usually be replicated by providing slightly increased quantities of conventional high biologic value formulas (78).

The major adverse consequences of amino acid/protein administration are azotemia and hepatic encephalopathy. The former can be at least partially avoided when nitrogen is provided in the form of essential amino acids (78). In so doing, however, it is very important never to exceed 0.7 g/kg/day, because essential amino acids are, gram for gram, twice as effective as high biologic value amino acid/protein mixtures (88), and because numer-

ous clinicians have reported hyperammonemic encephalopathy when larger quantities have been infused. The latter observation may relate in part to the fact that these mixtures are deficient in arginine, which is needed for urea synthesis (78). Similarly, patients with compromised hepatic function need not be deprived of necessary protein. Hepatic encephalopathy can be avoided when amino acid mixtures enriched with BCAA and depleted of aromatic amino acids are used (78). These hepatic formulations are based on the belief that aromatic amino acids serve as precursors of encephalogenic false neurotransmitters, and the belief that aromatic and branched-chain amino acids compete for passage across the blood-brain barrier (78). However, because these mixtures are expensive, they should generally be reserved for patients with a well-documented predisposition to encephalopathy. In other words, clinicians are frequently surprised to find that adequate quantities of simple high biologic value amino acid formulas do not precipitate encephalopathic states in patients with liver impairment.

In spite of the major influence of amino acid and relatively minor influence of dextrose and/or lipid infusion on patient protein retention, few (if any) nutritionists infuse only amino acids. Many ICU patients possess limited adipose reserve and, if deprived of nonprotein fuel, must eventually develop a life-threatening fuel deficiency. In addition, it is generally suspected that the nonprotein component of a nutritional regimen exerts beneficial effects on functions other than protein retention. For example, patients postoperative from major surgery displayed excellent protein retention when given only amino acids, but developed more complications than similar patients who also received nonprotein caloric substrate (16).

RESTING ENERGY EXPENDITURE, CALORIC REQUIREMENTS, AND THE RESPIRATORY QUOTIENT

As noted, it appears important to provide patients with as many generic caloric equivalents as are needed to maintain energy balance, if only to prevent an eventual body energy deficiency. While this reasoning is incompletely supported by hard evidence, it is contradicted by little evidence and is firmly embraced by the majority of nutritionists, including those who care for critically ill patients. Nevertheless, this tendency should be weighed against the concern that excess caloric equivalents will overburden metabolic disposal pathways of severely ill patients. Consequently, the energy expenditure and respiratory quotient of ICU patients are of considerable interest.

Resting Energy Expenditure

Resting energy expenditure, as the name indicates, is simply the quantity of energy expended in the resting state. This value can be estimated in a number of different ways and is used as a frame of reference when determining caloric needs. Direct measurement of resting energy expenditure, as the quantity of heat produced, is no longer employed in modern times but illustrates the principle that heat production (calorigenesis) is "coin of the realm" of nutritionists. Those interested in O_2 transport physiology are more concerned with $\dot{V}o_2$; however, these parameters are closely related (if not completely inter-

changeable (82)), as they are coupled in the process of oxidative phosphorylation (Fig. 2.6).

When amino acid catabolism is assumed to represent 12% of caloric expenditure, calorigenesis can be estimated by the De Weir formula, using measured $\dot{V}o_2$ and $\dot{V}co_2$ (22). However, methodologic problems frequently preclude accurate measurement of $\dot{V}o_2$ and $\dot{V}co_2$ in the ICU setting, and this method is considered by many to be too impractical for routine clinical use (78). The Harris-Benedict formula estimates caloric expenditure of healthy individuals, using age, sex, and weight, but may inaccurately reflect rate in critically ill patients.

Because of difficulties inherent in estimation of metabolic expenditure in ICU patients, many investigators have attempted to develop empiric formulas. Early investigators concluded that resting metabolism in the critically ill is considerably higher than normal, and stress factors were applied to Harris-Benedict values to provide representative estimates of resting metabolic expenditure (50). In contrast, a number of recent observations suggest that metabolic rate in mechanically ventilated critically ill patients (with the important exception of burned patients (18)) is little different from the normal rate (78). Most likely, these differences represent different

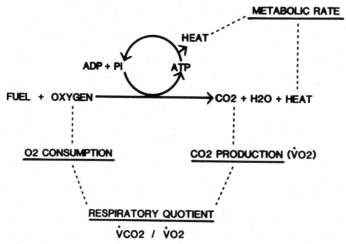

Figure 2.6. Relation between oxygen consumption, metabolic rate, generation of ATP, and generation of heat. (From Schlichtig R, Ayres SM. Nutritional support of the critically ill. Chicago: Year Book, 1988.)

contributions to resting metabolism that arise from differences in work of breathing, thermogenesis of fever, nonrespiratory skeletal muscle O_2 demand, ambient temperature of the ICU, and possibly even O_2 supply-limited states (see Chapter 51). However, because of striking variability among patients within the same disease category, stress factors should be viewed with some caution. For example, a profoundly septic patient who is truly O_2-supply-dependent is characterized by both a metabolic rate that is less than 1.6 times the Harris-Benedict predicted value and a marked inability to oxidize glucose.

Several considerations may help to place this controversy in perspective. First, only comatose or deeply sedated ICU patients rest completely, so that metabolic cart-derived parameters obtained at rest are unlikely to represent actual 24-hr metabolic expenditure (91, 92). Even accurate measurements derived from metabolic carts would need to be modified according to an estimation of the patient's nonresting activity to provide an accurate assessment of a patient's 24-hr metabolic expenditure. Second, the relation between caloric balance and protein retention (see above) is such that over- or underestimation of caloric expenditure by 500–1000 cal is unlikely to impact net nitrogen balance by more than a few grams daily when adequate protein is provided (40, 41). Thus, overestimation of caloric needs produces a marginal improvement of protein retention, but may overburden fuel disposal pathways; a slight underestimation is unlikely to produce any harm. Conversely, well-adapted patients generally do not suffer from considerable overfeeding, which is often quite appropriate during the anabolic recovery phase. Third, current evidence suggests that metabolism in critically ill patients is rarely limited by inadequate provision of exogenous nutrients: clinical estimates of the cellular redox state of patients in shock have generally implied increased NADH/NAD ratio, suggesting that fuel is adequate, and O_2 deficient (see Chapter 51). With this reasoning in mind, some busy ICU practitioners simply provide approximately 2000 nonprotein calories to all their critically ill patients, adjusting this value upwards or downwards, depending on state of resuscitation and nitrogen balance measurements.

The Respiratory Quotient

Respiratory quotient is of interest, because different quantities of carbon dioxide are produced by the combustion of different foodstuffs, which may tax respiratory muscle reserve to different degrees. During the process of oxidation, glucose produces 1.0 mol of carbon dioxide per mole of O_2 consumed, and lipid produces 0.7. If one individual oxidized only glucose to support metabolism, and another oxidized only lipid to support the same quantity of metabolism, there would be a 25% difference in the quantity of carbon dioxide produced. (Students of O_2 transport physiology please note: this figure seems to differ from 1 divided by 0.7, or 43%, because different quantities of O_2 consumption and carbon dioxide production would be associated with manufacture of the same quantity of ATP (82)). Accordingly, minute ventilation would need to increase by an equivalent amount to maintain blood carbon dioxide homeostasis and could conceivably precipitate respiratory distress in an individual with marginal respiratory muscle reserve. This difference is of no concern in humans with normal respiratory muscle reserve, because a 300% increase in metabolic rate (and therefore carbon dioxide production) is routinely achieved during minimal activities of daily living, and a 900% increase is seen during heavy exercise.

Of somewhat greater concern is the fact that hepatocytic conversion of glucose to lipid, a consequence of overfeeding, is associated with a respiratory quotient between 2.8 and 8.7, depending on the species of free fatty acid synthesized (82). This phenomenon is a consequence of the need to excise two of every six dextrose carbons during conversion to lipid. The highest values of respiratory quotient reported in critically ill patients fed isocaloric dextrose were observed in those who were profoundly septic, and averaged 1.23 (33). However, even this value represents an

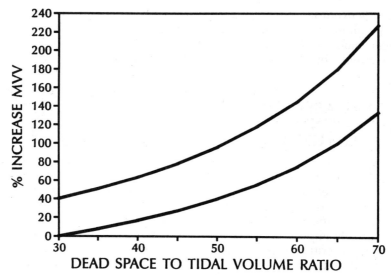

Figure 2.7. Approximate increase of minute ventilation *(MVV)* as dead space to tidal volume ratio *(VD/VT)* increases. *Curve A,* CO_2 production is constant at a fixed value. *Curve B,* CO_2 production is also constant, but is 40% higher than *curve A.* This representation assumes that end-tidal P_{CO_2} is 40 torr, and neglects the increased CO_2 that would result from the increased work of breathing.

increase in carbon dioxide production of only 50% above the normal fasting value (assuming constant O_2 consumption). Given the normal physiologic range of carbon dioxide production (300–900% above the resting value), it appears unlikely that even these values of respiratory quotient would alone provoke respiratory failure. Thus a value of respiratory quotient greater than 1.0 would seem to indicate a stress of *hepatic* disposal pathways more so than *respiratory* disposal pathways.

Theoretical considerations suggest that the burden imposed upon the respiratory musculature by increased carbon dioxide production is somewhat greater for those patients with a higher dead space to tidal volume ratio (VD/VT). Normally, VD/VT is approximately 30%, and end-tidal P_{CO_2}, 40 torr, resulting in a mean expired carbon dioxide concentration in expired air of roughly 3.7%. However, for a patient with VD/VT of 50% and end-tidal P_{CO_2}, 40 torr, mean expired carbon dioxide concentration is approximately 2.65%, so that 40% more tidal volume must be exchanged to support the same value of carbon dioxide production. Accordingly, the percent increase of minute ventilation rises more

rapidly as VD/VT increases (Fig. 2.7). It is also important to recognize that VD/VT increases as tidal volume decreases during the progression of respiratory failure.

These theoretical considerations support the clinical observation that excessive carbohydrate feeding occasionally provokes respiratory failure in patients (17). However, this generally occurs only when patients with very limited respiratory reserve are grossly overfed, because the increase of carbon dioxide production produced by overfeeding is generally only a fraction of that precipitated by normal activities of daily living (see above). Nevertheless, it has now become customary for many practitioners to substitute lipid for dextrose caloric equivalents when weaning patients from mechanical ventilation. Whether ventilator weaning is significantly facilitated by this process is uncertain; however, it is no more expensive and certainly less risky than many other modalities routinely employed. On the other hand, it may be extremely important to reduce carbon dioxide production by any means possible when caring for patients with extremely high VD/VT who cannot be ventilated. In these circumstances, it is usually advisable to employ chemical muscular paralysis, allow $Paco_2$ to rise to supraphysiologic values, and reduce the carbohydrate content of the nutritional formula.

NUTRITIONAL ASSESSMENT AND THE RESPONSE TO NUTRITIONAL THERAPY

As noted, nutritional therapy should be provided as early as possible to all ICU patients who are expected to remain unable to eat for extended periods. This reasoning is based on the observation that anabolism is virtually impossible to achieve during the stress of critical illness. Nutritional assessment at the onset of sepsis, burns, or trauma is somewhat irrelevant, as it is known that these individuals will become rapidly malnourished. Nevertheless, many clinicians place considerable emphasis on nutritional assessment parameters, both to measure the nutritional state on admission to the ICU, and to follow the response to nutritional therapy.

Available evidence strongly indicates that most nutritional assessment parameters are unreliable and should be viewed with scepticism in the ICU setting. Serum proteins are commonly measured on the assumption that serum concentration reflects the mass and/or function of the organ that produced them. However, serum albumin, for example, is generally normal or slightly elevated in patients with anorexia nervosa, who have lost considerable proportions of lean body mass (39, 45, 89). Conversely, multiply traumatized, burned, or septic patients manifest low serum albumin, long before equivalent proportions of lean body mass have been catabolized (71, 75, 87). These contradictions of conventional wisdom are probably related to differences in the balance of synthesis and catabolism. During anorexia nervosa, albumin catabolism decreases resulting in normal serum albumin concentration (39, 45), while stressed states are associated with increased albumin catabolism (71, 75, 87). In fact, no correlation between serum albumin concentration and albumin synthetic rate could be demonstrated in injured and septic patients (19, 20). Similar

problems are encountered with the use of serum transferrin (83) and thyroxin-binding prealbumin (83) as nutritional assessment parameters. Unreliability of serum proteins as nutritional markers in acutely ill patients may result from a reprioritization of protein synthesis with decreased production of relatively nonessential proteins and increased production of proteinaceous substances needed for survival. For example, the decrease of serum albumin concentration that occurs with acute illness is also associated with increased concentration of acute phase reactants (79).

Other parameters routinely used to assess nutritional status are generally either impractical or unreliable in the ICU setting. Mid-arm muscle circumference and triceps skin fold measurements are cumbersome, may be influenced by skin edema, and are unlikely to respond perceptibly within short periods of time (37). Cutaneous reactivity may be diminished in severely malnourished patients (47), but is nonspecific in acutely ill patients who uniformly become anergic independently of nutritional status (52, 55). Total lymphocyte count is also occasionally employed; however, this parameter has not been validated as a nutritional assessment parameter (26). Sophisticated measures of body composition, such as in vivo neutron activation analysis and radionuclide estimations, directly measure body nitrogen content and lean body mass, respectively, but are clearly impractical in the ICU setting.

A time-honored, simple, and practical approach to bedside nutritional assessment is illustrated by the children's fable, "Hansel and Gretel" (recall the myopic witch who daily assessed Hansel's nutritional status by attempting to squeeze his finger). In an analogous fashion, ICU practitioners frequently discover that simply drawing back the patient's bedclothes reveals more information than do many purported nutritional assessment parameters. In support of this approach, investigators recently reported that "subjective global assessment," a nutritional scoring system based on history and physical examination, predicted development of complications better than commonly employed nutritional parameters (1). In performing physical examinations, however, it is important to recall that patients who have suffered prolonged catabolic illness tend to retain body fat to a greater degree than muscle (see above); ample quantities of adipose tissue may mislead the cursory examiner to believe that body protein has also been preserved.

The most appropriate goal of nutritional assessment in the ICU setting is to determine the direction of change. Nitrogen balance measurements provide the most practical approach and should be determined weekly, with some appreciation of their imprecision. Nitrogen intake measurements suffer from the problem that many ICU patients receive considerable protein in the form of blood products, which are not easily assimilated within nutritional calculations. Nitrogen output measurements are plagued with more serious problems. Urinary nitrogen, assessed as urea nitrogen, accounts for only approximately 85% of all urinary nitrogen loss. In addition, many patients lose considerable quantities of protein from other sources, including bronchial secretions, wound exudate, and fistulae, that cannot practically be measured. During intravenous feeding, stool protein loss is generally minimal, so that the customary 4 g of fecal protein loss may be an overestimate. During enteral feeding, on the other hand, fecal losses may be several times higher than 4 g/day for patients who develop diarrhea (13, 60).

More disturbing is the problem that some sources of nitrogen loss cannot be accounted for in normal individuals, even when hair and fingernail clippings and all other proteinaceous substances are carefully collected and analyzed. In several investigations, normal volunteers fed large quantities of protein (similar to quantities routinely administered to ICU patients) manifested 1.5–3 g of positive nitrogen balance for extended periods, although lean body mass did not appear to be increasing (36, 66, 84). These data suggest that nitrogen balance measurements may routinely overestimate true nitrogen retention, even at their most accurate. One should also consider the problem that retained (or lost) nitrogen reflected by a nitrogen balance measurement may partly reflect blood urea nitrogen if the blood urea nitrogen value changes substantially during the collection period. Because urea is evenly distributed throughout all body water, blood urea measurements are insensitive indicators of this form of nitrogen retention over a 24-hr period.

In spite of these limitations, nitrogen balance measurements are frequently and appropriately obtained to assess the response to nutritional intervention, for lack of a better substitute. While positive values may not necessarily reflect protein retention, markedly negative values can generally be taken as evidence of catabolism. Thus the starting formula containing 1.5 g of amino acid/kg/day, 1000–1500 carbohydrate caloric equivalents, and 500–1000 lipid caloric equivalents (total 2000 nonprotein calories), may then be modified based on nitrogen balance measurements as well as on a clinical assessment of the patient's ability to utilize additional substrates.

References

1. Baker JP, Detsky AS, Wesson DE. Nutrition assessment: a comparison of clinical judgement and objective measurements. N Engl J Med 1982; 306:969–971.
2. Bessey PQ, Watters JM, Aoki TT, et al. Combined hormonal infusion simulates the metabolic response to injury. Ann Surg 1984;200:264–281.
3. Beutler B, Cerami A. Cachetin: more than a tumor necrosis factor. N Engl J Med 1987;316:379–385.
4. Blackburn GL, Flatt JP, Clowes GHA, et al. Protein sparing therapy during periods of starvation with sepsis or trauma. Ann Surg 1973;177:588–593.
5. Border JR, Chenier R, McMenany RH, et al. Multiple systems organ failure: muscle fuel deficit with visceral protein malnutrition. Surg Clin North Am 1976;56:1147–1167.
6. Brennan MF, Fitzpatrick GF, Cohen KH, et al. Glycerol: major contributor to the short term protein sparing effect of fat emulsions in normal man. Ann Surg 1975;182:386–394.
7. Brooks DC, Bessey PQ, Black PR, et al. Insulin stimulates branched chain amino acid uptake and diminishes nitrogen flux from skeletal muscle of injured patients. J Surg Res 1986;40:395–405.
8. Buzby GP, Mullen JL, Stein TP, et al. Manipulation of TPN caloric substrate and fatty infiltration of the liver. J Surg Res 1981;31:46–54.
9. Cahill GF. Starvation in man. N Engl J Med 1970;282:668–675.
10. Cahill GF. Physiology of insulin in man. Diabetes 1971;20:785–799.

11. Carey LC, Lowery BD, Cloutier CT. Blood sugar and insulin response of humans in shock. Ann Surg 1970;172:342–347.
12. Chen WJ. Effects of hypertonic glucose on the rates of plasma clearance and CO_2 production of intravenously administered intralipid emulsion in dogs. JPEN 1983;7:6–10.
13. Cheng AHR, Gomez A, Berghan JG, et al. Comparative nitrogen balance study between young and aged adults using three levels of protein intake from a combination wheat-soy mixture. Am J Clin Nutr 1978;31:12–22.
14. Clowes GHA, Randall HT, Cha CJ. Amino acid and energy metabolism in septic and traumatized patients. JPEN 1980;4:195–205.
15. Clowes GHA, George BC, Villee CA, et al. Muscle proteolysis induced by a circulating peptide in patients with sepsis or trauma. N Engl J Med 1983;308:545–552.
16. Collins JP, Oxby CB, Hill GL. Intravenous amino-acids and intravenous hyperalimentation as protein-sparing therapy after major surgery. A controlled clinical trial. Lancet 1978;1:788–791.
17. Covelli HD, Black JW, Olsen MS, et al. Respiratory failure precipitated by high carbohydrate loads. Ann Intern Med 1981;95:569–581.
18. Cunningham JJ. Factors contributing to increased energy expenditure in thermal injury: a review of studies employing indirect calorimetry. JPEN 1990;14:649–656.
19. Dahn MS, Jacobs LA, Mitchell RA, et al. Significance of hypoalbuminemia following injury and infection. Surg Forum 1984;35:92–94.
20. Dahn MS, Jacobs LA, Smith S. The significance of hypoalbuminemia following injury and infection. Am Surg 1985;51:340–343.
21. Datey KK, Nanda NC. Hyperglycemia after acute myocardial infarction. N Engl J Med 1967;276:262–265.
22. De Weir JB. New methods for calculating metabolic rate with special reference to protein metabolism. J Physiol, Lond 1949;109:1–9.
23. Dinarello CA. Interleukin-1 and the pathogenesis of the acute-phase response. N Engl J Med 1984;311:1413–1418.
24. Duff JG, Viidik T, Marchuk JB, et al. Femoral arteriovenous amino acid differences in septic patients. Surgery 1979;85:344–348.
25. Elwyn DH, Kinney JM, Malayappa J, et al. Influence of increasing carbohydrate intake on glucose kinetics in injured patients. Ann Surg 1979;190:117–127.
26. Fischer JE, Ghory MJ. Protein deficiency and immunity in the hospitalized patient. In: Wright RA, Heymsfield S, eds. Nutrition assessment. London: Blackwell Scientific Publications, 1984.
27. Folin O. Laboratory manual of biological chemistry, 5th ed. New York: Appleton-Century-Crofts, 1934.
28. Foster DW, McGarry JD. The metabolic derangements and treatment of diabetic ketoacidosis. N Engl J Med 1983;309:158–168.
29. Freeman JB, Stegink LD, Wittine MF, et al. The current status of protein sparing. Surg Gynecol Obstet 1977;144:843–849.
30. Fulks RM, Li JB, Goldberg AL. Effects of insulin, glucose and amino acids on protein turnover in rat diaphragm. J Biol Chem 1975;350:290–298.
31. Garlick PJ, Clugston GA, Waterlow JC. Influence of low-energy diets on whole body protein turnover in obese subjects. Am J Physiol 1980;238:E235–E244.
32. Gazzaniga AB, Day AT, Bartlett RH, et al. Endogenous caloric sources and nitrogen balance. Arch Surg 1976;111:1357–1361.
33. Giovannini I, Bolderini G, Castagneto M, et al. Respiratory quotient and patterns of substrate utilization in human sepsis and trauma. JPEN 1983;7:226–230.
34. Gump FE, Long C, Killian PI, et al. Studies of glucose intolerance in septic injured patients. J Trauma 1974;14:378–388.
35. Hallberg D. Elimination of exogenous lipids from the blood stream. Acta Physiol Scand 1965;(suppl 254):5–23.
36. Hegsted DM. Assessment of nitrogen requirements. Am J Clin Nutr 1978;31:1669–1677.
37. Heymsfield SB, McManus CB II, Setiz SB, eds. Nutritional assessment. London: Blackwell Scientific Publications, 1984:27–82.
38. Hinton P, Allison SP, Littlejohn S, et al. Insulin and glucose to reduce catabolic response to injury in burned patients. Lancet 1971;1:767–769.
39. Hoffenberg R, Black E, Brock JF. Albumin and gamma-globulin tracer studies in protein depletion states. J Clin Invest 1966;45:143–152.
40. Iapichino G, Solca M, Radrizzani D, et al. Net protein utilization during total parenteral nutrition of injured critically ill patients: an original approach. JPEN 1981;5:317–321.
41. Iapichino G, Gattiononi L, Solca M, et al. Protein sparing and protein replacement in acutely injured patients during TPN with and without amino acid supply. Intensive Care Med 1982;8:25–31.
42. Iapichino G, Radrizzani D, Solca M, et al. The main determinants of nitrogen balance during total parenteral nutrition in critically ill injured patients. Intensive Care Med 1984;10:251–254.
43. Jensen GL, Mascioli EA, Seidner DL, et al. Parenteral infusion of long- and medium-chain triglycerides and reticuloendothelial system function in man. JPEN 1990;14:467–471.
44. Katayama T, Tanaka M, Tanaka K, et al. Alterations in hepatic mitochondrial function during total parenteral nutrition in immature rats. JPEN 1990;14:640–645.
45. Kirsch R, Frith L, Black E, et al. Regulation of albumin synthesis and catabolism by alteration of dietary protein. Nature 1966;217:578–579.
46. Knochel JP. The pathophysiology and clinical characteristics of severe hypophosphatemia. Arch Intern Med 1977;137:203–220.
47. Law DK, Dudrick SJ, Abdou NI. Immunocompetence of patients with protein calorie malnutrition: the effects of nutritional repletion. Ann Intern Med 1973;139:257–266.
48. Levenson SM, Watkin DM. Protein requirements in injury and certain acute and chronic diseases. Fed Proc 1959;18:1155.
49. Long CL, Kinney JM, Geiger JW. Nonsuppressibility of gluconeogenesis by glucose in septic patients. Metabolism 1976;25:193–210.

50. Long CL, Schaffel N, Geiger JW, et al. Metabolic response to injury and illness: estimation of energy and protein needs from indirect calorimetry and nitrogen balance. JPEN 1979;3:452–456.

51. Long CL, Lowry SF. Hormonal regulation of protein metabolism. JPEN 1990;14:555–562.

52. MacLean LD, Meakins JL, Taguchi K, et al. Host resistance in sepsis and trauma. Ann Surg 1975; 182:207–216.

53. Mascioli EA, Randall S, Porter KA. Thermogenesis from intravenous medium-chain triglycerides. JPEN 1991;15:27–31.

54. Masoro EJ. Fat metabolism in normal and abnormal states. Am J Clin Nutr 1977;30:1311–1320.

55. McLoughlin GA, Wu AV, Saporoschetz I, et al. Correlation between anergy and a circulating immunosuppressive factor following major surgical trauma. Ann Surg 1979;190:297–304.

56. Meguid MM, Schimmel E, Johnson WC, et al. Reduced metabolic complications in total parenteral nutrition: pilot study using fat to replace one-third of glucose calories. JPEN 1982;6:304–307.

57. Miles JM, Cattalini M, Sharbrough FW. Metabolic and neurological effects of an intravenous medium-chain triglyceride emulsion. JPEN 1991; 15:37–41.

58. Miller JDB, Bistrian RR, Blackburn GL, et al. Failure of postoperative infection to increase nitrogen excretion in patients maintained on peripheral amino acids. Am J Clin Nutr 1977;30:1523–1527.

59. Morgan HE, Rannels KE, Wolpert EB, et al. In: Fritz IB, ed. Insulin action. New York: Academic Press, 1972.

60. Mueller KJ, Crosby LO, Oberlander JL, Mullen JL. Estimation of fecal nitrogen in patients with liver disease. JPEN 1983;7:266–269.

61. Munro HN. Differences in metabolic handling of orally versus parenterally administered nutrients. In: Green M, Greene HL, eds. The role of the gastrointestinal tract in nutrient delivery. New York: Academic Press, 1984.

62. Nordenstrom J, Carpentier YA, Askanazi J, et al. Metabolic utilization of intravenous fat emulsion during total parenteral nutrition. Ann Surg 1982;196:221–231.

63. Nordenstrom J, Carpentier YA, Askanazi J, et al. Free fatty acid mobilization and oxidation during total parenteral nutrition in trauma and infection. Ann Surg 1983;198:725–735.

64. O'Connell RC, Morgan AF, Aoki TT, et al. Nitrogen conservation in starvation: graded responses to intravenous glucose. J Clin Endocrinol Metab 1974;39:555–563.

65. O'Donnell TF, Clowes GHA, Blackburn GL, et al. Proteolysis associated with a deficit of peripheral energy fuel substrates in septic man. Surgery 1976;80:192–200.

66. Oddoye EA, Margen S. Nitrogen balance studies in humans: long-term effect of high nitrogen intake on nitrogen accretion. J Nutr 1979;109:363–367.

67. Patel MS, Owne OE, Goldman LI, et al. Fatty acid synthesis by human adipose tissue. Metabolism 1975;24:161–173.

68. Patrick J. Death during recovery from severe malnutrition and its possible relationship to sodium pump activity in the leukocyte. Br Med J 1977;1:1051–1054.

69. Ponting GA, Ward HC, Halliday D, Sim AJW. Protein and energy metabolism with biosynthetic human growth hormone in patients on full intravenous nutritional support. JPEN 1990;14:437–441.

70. Powanda MC, Beisel WR. Hypothesis: leukocyte endogenous mediator/endogenous pyrogen/lymphocyte-activating factor modulates the development of nonspecific and specific immunity and affects nutritional status. Am J Clin Nutr 1982;35:762–767.

71. Powanda M, Moyer ED. Plasma proteins and wound healing. Surg Gynecol Obstet 1981; 152:749–755.

72. Proceedings of an international glutamine symposium—Glutamine metabolism in health and disease: basic science and clinical aspects. JPEN 1990;14(suppl):39S–146S.

73. Rennie MJ, Babij P, Taylor PM, et al. Characteristics of a glutamine carrier in skeletal muscle have important consequences for nitrogen loss in injury, infection, and chronic disease. Lancet 1986;2:1008–1011.

74. Rossner S. Studies on an intravenous fat tolerance test: methodological experimental and clinical experiments with Intralipid. Acta Med Scand 1974;196(suppl):564.

75. Rothschild MS, Oratz M, Schreiber SS. Albumin synthesis: Part 1. N Engl J Med 1972;286:748–757.

76. Roza AM, Tuitt D, Shizgal HM. Transferrin: a poor measure of nutritional status. JPEN 1984;8:493–496.

77. Salo M. Inhibition of immunoglobulin synthesis in vitro by intravenous lipid emulsion. JPEN 1990;14:459–462.

78. Schlichtig R, Ayres SM. Nutritional support of the critically ill. Chicago: Year Book, 1988.

79. Sganga G, Siegel JH, Brown G, et al. Reprioritization of hepatic plasma protein release in trauma and sepsis. Arch Surg 1985;120:187–199.

80. Shaw JHF, Klein S, Wolfe RR. Assessment of alanine, urea, and glucose interrelationships in normal subjects and in patients with sepsis with stable isotopic tracers. Surgery 1985;97:557–568.

81. Shizgal HM, Milne CA, Spanier AH. The effect of nitrogen-sparing intravenously administered fluids on postoperative body composition. Surgery 1979;85:496–503.

82. Silberman H, Silberman AW. Parenteral nutrition, biochemistry, and respiratory gas exchange. JPEN 1986;10:151–154.

83. Socolow EL, Woeber KA, Purdy RH, et al. Preparation of I-131 labeled human serum prealbumin and its metabolism in normal and sick patients. J Clin Invest 1965;44:1600–1609.

84. Soroff HS, Pearson E, Artz CP. An estimation of the nitrogen requirements for equilibrium in burned patients. Surg Gynecol Obstet 1961;159–172.

85. Souba WW, Smith RJ, Wilmore DW. Glutamine

metabolism by the intestinal tract. JPEN 1985; 9:608–617.

86. Steffee WP, Goldsmith RS, Pencharz PB, et al. Dietary protein intake and dynamic aspects of whole body nitrogen metabolism in adult humans. Metabolism 1976;25:281–297.

87. Sterling K, Lipsky SR, Freeman LJ. Disappearance curve of intravenously administered I-131 tagged albumin in the postoperative injury reaction. Metabolism 1955;4:343–349.

88. Tempel G, Jelen S, Jekat F. Investigation of protein metabolism with respect to amino acid administration. JPEN 1985;9:725–731.

89. Waterlow JC. Observations on the mechanism of adaptation to low protein intakes. Lancet 1968; 2:1091–1097.

90. Waterlow JC. Nutrition and protein turnover in man. Br Med Bull 1981;37:5–10.

91. Weissman C, Kemper BA, Elwyn DH, et al. The energy expenditure of the mechanically ventilated critically ill patient. Chest 1986;89:254–259.

92. Weissman C, Kemper M. The oxygen uptake-oxygen delivery relationship during ICU interventions. Chest 1991;99:430–435.

93. Wilmore DW, Moylan JA, Bristow BF, et al. Anabolic effects of human growth hormone and high caloric feedings following thermal injury. Surg Gynecol Obstet 1974;138:875–884.

94. Wilmore DW, Smith RJ, O'Dwyer ST, et al. The gut: a central organ after surgical stress. Surgery 1988;104:917–923.

95. Windmueller HG, Spaeth AE. Uptake and metabolism of plasma glutamine by the small intestine. J Biol Chem 1974;249:5070–5079.

96. Windmueller HG, Spaeth AE. Identification of ketone bodies and glutamine as the major respiratory fuels in vivo for postabsorptive rat small intestine. J Biol Chem 1978;253:69–76.

97. Windmueller HG, Spaeth AE. Respiratory fuels and nitrogen metabolism in vivo in small intestine of fed rats. J Biol Chem 1980;255:107–112.

98. Wolfe BM, Culebras JM, Sim AJW, et al. Substrate interaction in intravenous feeding: comparative effects of carbohydrate and fat on amino acid utilization in fasting man. Ann Surg 1977; 186:518–540.

99. Wolfe RR. Glucose metabolism in burn injury: a review. J Burn Care Rehabil 1985;6:408.

100. Woolfson AMJ, Heatley RV, Allison SP. Insulin to inhibit protein catabolism after injury. N Engl J Med 1979;300:14–17.

101. Young GA, Hill GL. A controlled study of protein-sparing therapy after excision of the rectum: effects of intravenous amino acids and hyperalimentation on body composition and plasma amino acids. Ann Surg 1980;192:183–191.

102. Zakim D. Integration of energy metabolism by the liver: the role of the gastrointestinal tract. In: Morris G, Green HL, eds. Nutrient delivery. Orlando, FL: Academic Press, 1984.

3

Enteral and Parenteral Nutrition

Gerard Nitenberg

Modern monitoring and support of vital organ systems have led to the survival of patients with major organ failures. Resuscitation is the first priority in the management of these critically ill patients, followed by treatment of the specific injured structures. A major factor that may improve outcome is the preservation of nutritional status, although the role of nutrition (enteral or parenteral) as a life-support modality remains controversial in many instances. This is probably due to the remarkable heterogeneity of disease states grouped under the term "critical illness." Any clinician dealing with nutritional support must have an understanding of the metabolic response to injury and sepsis, with particular emphasis on alterations in regional and whole body substrate metabolism, to intervene effectively with specialized nutritional support during a prolonged course of treatment, recuperation, hypermetabolism, and immobilization. The aim of this chapter is to provide practical guidelines for nutritional management of critically ill patients and to present recent developments with particular relevance to future treatment modalities.

RATIONALE OF NUTRITIONAL SUPPORT

During the initial period of trauma, injury, or sepsis, which lasts from 1 to 4 days, the priority is the management of the patient's hemodynamic and respiratory requirements, with an overall and regional increase in oxygen consumption ($\dot{V}o_2$). Above all, it is necessary to seek and treat rapidly the basic cause. Such treatment will consist of antibiotics for infectious conditions, the reduction of multiple fractures, abscess drainage, etc. This period is often assimilated to the "ebb phase" described by Cuthbertson (64) and is characterized by an activation of the neurohormonal system, together with cytokine production (148, 182); there is rapid metabolism of glucose and the triglycerides of the fatty tissues. As long as the situation remains unstable, it is probably unnecessary, and possibly detrimental, to initiate complex nutritional support (161, 253). The nutrient supply can consist simply of glucose in sufficient quantities (200–300 g/day) to meet the requirements of glucose-dependent tissues, i.e., the brain, but also the renal medullary and blood cells; electrolytes are also necessary, particularly phosphorus (68). However, it is best not to delay the start of nutritional support for too long, as has been shown in burn patients (156); at all events, it should be started before the onset of severe metabolic disorders and/or complications, especially infections, which can engender irreversible multiple organ failure.

When the initial insult does not rapidly lead to death and reanimation has ensured the vital functions, the patient enters a period of relative stability, in general a satellite of lung injury, characterized by hypermetabolism with increased energy consumption, muscle hypercatabolism qualified as "autocannibalism," and an increase in endogenous lipolysis (48, 132, 215, 245) (Table 3.1). Within a few days or weeks, a state of postinjury wasting sets in unless countered by nutritional and metabolic support. Nitrogen excretion can reach more than 20 g/day, i.e., the equivalent of 600 g of muscle. The duration of this phase varies between a few days and several weeks, according to the gravity of

Table 3.1
Metabolic Alterations Commonly Observed in Simple Starvation and at Different Levels of Stress

Metabolic Abnormalities	Starvation	Stress State		
		Injury and Trauma (T)	T and S	Sepsis (S)
Basal metabolism	↓ [a]	↑		⇑
Blood glucose	↓	↑		⇑
Lactate	=	↑		⇑
Insulin	↓		= or ↑	
Glucagon	↑		⇑	
Insulin resistance	↑	↑		⇑
Glucose recycling (Cori cycle)	=	↑		⇑
Nitrogen losses	↓	↑		⇑
Aminoacidemia	↓		↑	
Protein turnover	↓		↑	
Protein synthesis	↓	= or ↑		↑
Protein catabolism	=	↑		⇑
Gluconeogenesis	↑		⇑	
Endogenous lipolysis	↑		⇑	
Ketosis	⇑		↑	

[a] ↓, significantly decreased; =, unchanged or normal; ↑, significantly increased; ⇑, major augmentation; ⇓, major diminution.

the initial insult, its persistence, or the onset of secondary complications. A better understanding of metabolic and neurohormonal alterations and the role of cell mediators (107, 148, 182) should form the basis for the rational management of this hypermetabolic phase, to which we shall return later. Nutritional (metabolic) support is aimed at preventing malnutrition and its consequences, particularly on the immune system (56), and correcting immediate deficiencies that can be cofactors in the morbidity and mortality associated with critical illness and multiple organ failure. Nutritional support contributes to gaining the time necessary for restoring adequate microcirculation and treating the underlying cause. One should not expect miraculous effects, nor an action in terms of morbidity or mortality in these patients in whom the exact cause of death is often difficult to establish and in whom a favorable outcome clearly results from the combined effects of the therapeutic measures applied. The future lies in the prospective evaluation of multiple metabolic and nutritional approaches specific to these acute conditions; several protocols are currently under investigation.

NUTRITIONAL ASSESSMENT

Assessment of the critically ill patient requires an estimation of the nutritional status before injury and the nutritional requirements during recovery. The traditional markers of nutritional status of patients with simple starvation are of limited usefulness in the critical care setting (164); the most commonly referenced are body weight and history of weight loss, anthropometric measurements of tissue masses, urinary nitrogen excretion (reflecting net protein losses), creatinine and 3-methylhistidine excretion (reflecting, respectively, lean tissue and muscle protein loss), serum protein levels (indicators of visceral protein synthesis), and delayed cutaneous hypersensitivity (Table 3.2). However, all these parameters can be obscured during sepsis or following injury. Fluid retention inevitably occurs during resuscitation, expanding the extravascular (interstitial) water compartment; these changes lead to wide

Table 3.2
Anthropometric, Biochemical, and Immunological Measurements Commonly Used in Assessment of Nutritional Status

Body Compartment	Measurement[a]	Type
Somatic protein and fat stores	Height, weight Weight/height indexes	Anthropometric
Fat stores	Triceps Subscapular } skin fold thickness	Anthropometric
Lean body mass		
Skeletal muscle mass	Midarm muscle {circumference area	Anthropometric
	Creatinine/height index	Laboratory
Visceral protein stores	Albumin, transferrin	Laboratory
	transthyretin,[a] RBP[b]	
	CRP, α_1 acid glycoprotein[c]	
Immune functions	Cell mediated = DHT[d]	Skin testing
	Humoral = Total lymphocyte count	Laboratory

[a] Prealbumin.
[b] Retinol-binding protein.
[c] Acute phase proteins.
[d] Delayed hypersensitivity testing.

inaccuracies in the interpretation of body weight and anthropometry (62). Redistribution of plasma volume with altered capillary permeability can similarly lower the levels of circulating serum proteins, mainly albumin and transferrin. Visceral proteins with shorter half-lives, such as transthyretin (prealbumin) ($t_{1/2} = 3$ days) and retinol-binding protein ($t_{1/2} = 12$ hr), have a smaller volume of distribution and may therefore reflect alterations in nutritional status faster than albumin (214) and may also be less susceptible to modifications of fluid status. Other serum markers of potential interest for monitoring the adequacy of nutritional intake in acute illness include fibronectin (203) and somatomedin-C (77). Delayed hypersensitivity is affected by many factors such as anesthesia, surgery, corticosteroids, chemotherapeutic agents, inflammation, and sepsis without implying previous or current nutritional depletion (60, 236); moreover, skin tests are almost always unresponsive for at least 10–15 days following trauma or sepsis (168).

Several authors have combined multiple measurements into nutritional indexes for use in intensive care units (ICUs) (31) or to estimate the risk of complications after surgery (90, 168, 240). These indexes are of limited interest because of both the interdependence of their components and the uncertain validity because of the variability of norms for each country (e.g., triceps skin fold) or each laboratory (e.g., serum albumin). Although a variety of scoring systems have been developed to classify the severity of injury and to predict morbidity and mortality, few authors have attempted to correlate scores with nutritional requirements; in addition, the results of the few existing studies are divergent and no definitive conclusions can be drawn (119).

Because of the problems with anthropometric and laboratory measurements for the assessment of nutritional status, Baker et al. have developed a "subjective global assessment" scoring system. This method predicts development of (infectious) complications more accurately than the measurement of albumin, transferrin, delayed cutaneous hypersensitivity, anthropometry, and the creatinine-height index (19). Moreover, interobserver agreement between members of the nutritional team was very high. However, although the method appears useful for initial assessment, it is not easily transferable to other groups of clinicians and is insensitive for following nutritional progression during treatment.

Therefore, from a clinical point of view,

the logical approach to nutritional assessment of the critically ill must rely on the recent dietary history, physical examination, and nature and course of the illness. In general, any injured or septic patient in the hypermetabolic phase who cannot eat at least two thirds of his or her nutritional needs, already has had more than 5 days of diminished nutritional intake, or is likely to spend a prolonged period (>5–7 days) before returning to "normal" dietary intake will require some type of nutritional support. This should be tailored to meet the total caloric and nitrogen requirements for the individual patient. As we have seen above, we have no "gold standard" to measure the efficacy of nutritional support in the critical care setting. In the future, bedside determination of body composition may provide an accurate and precise measure of both nutritional status and the response to nutritional therapy. Measures of total-body potassium (reflecting the cellular mass) with a whole-body counter or by the isotope dilution technique, as well as total-body nitrogen (reflecting the body cell mass) by means of neutron activation analysis, are at present tedious, expensive, and reserved for research protocols. Recently a relationship has been demonstrated between whole-body bioelectric impedance and the lean body mass (32), permitting the indirect determination of body fat, extracellular mass, and body cell mass (115). However, although the measurement is simple and noninvasive, its accuracy remains to be demonstrated, especially in critical care patients with unpredictable and rapid changes in metabolic status and fluid compartments (61).

THERAPEUTIC APPROACHES

Traditionally, metabolic and nutritional support in the hypermetabolic phase of injury and sepsis is aimed at correcting, at least partially, the metabolic alterations (Table 3.1) that have been detailed in the previous chapter.

Optimal Energy Supply

Resting energy expenditure (REE), similar to the basal metabolism, can be estimated or measured. The standard formulas, such as those proposed by Harris and Benedict (106), were established for healthy volunteers and cannot simply be extrapolated to the intensive care setting in which the metabolic state fluctuates according to the temperature, treatment (229), ventilation, etc. (239). Differences of the order of 25–50% between the calculated REE and energy expenditure (EE) measured by means of indirect calorimetry have been reported (237, 242). The correction of such differences, such as that proposed by Long et al. (146) by the introduction of an activity factor and a stress factor and, more recently, the elegant approach proposed by Rime et al. (191) for intensive care patients, can help to avoid excessively inappropriate caloric support. In the study by Rime, the originality was to establish a new estimation of EE as a function of paraclinical parameters, the pathological setting, and the treatment. This approach was validated prospectively in comparison with measured EE:

$$EE \text{ (kcal/day)} = 33 \times T + 387^{(1)} + 457^{(2)} - 294^{(3)} - 3591$$

where T is height in cm—(1) if active, (2) in case of nitrogen support, (3) in case of mechanical ventilation and nitrogen support.

The measurement of EE by means of indirect calorimetry is possible, even in patients under mechanical ventilation, as long as strict conditions of measurement are respected (21, 43). The use of technical devices permits a satisfactory estimation on the basis of $\dot{V}o_2$ alone, but the most expensive and efficient equipment uses $\dot{V}o_2$, carbon dioxide production ($\dot{V}co_2$), and urinary urea excretion, giving a precision of the order of 5% (153, 178). Surprising results have been obtained. While EE can reach twice the normal value in patients with deep and extensive burns, it is generally no more than 1.5–1.7 higher in those with septicemia or peritonitis; in patients having stabilized following multiple trauma or major surgery, the value exceeds the normal by only about 12–15% (21, 201) (Fig. 3.1). The various clinical and therapeutic factors influencing EE are given in Table 3.3. If an indirect calorimeter is not available, some authors have advocated the use of a Swan-Ganz catheter to give a reasonable estimation of $\dot{V}o_2$; however, in

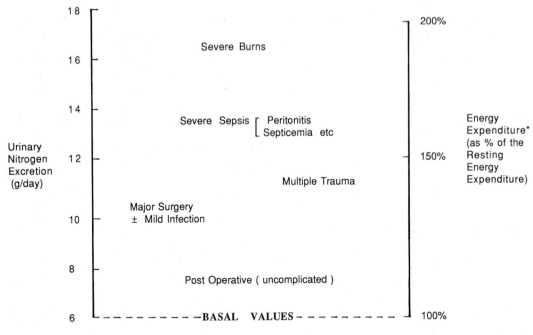

Figure 3.1. Effects of injury, sepsis, and nutritional depletion on energy expenditure and protein catabolism. Protein catabolism is estimated from urinary nitrogen losses. *, energy expenditure is measured by indirect calorimetry or estimated from basal energy expenditure (Harris-Benedict formulas) with adjustments based on fever and stress factors.

Table 3.3
Modifications of Energy Expenditure (EE) and Oxygen Consumption ($\dot{V}O_2$) Related to Metabolic Stress and Treatment

$\uparrow$ EE $\dot{V}O_2$	$\downarrow$ EE $\dot{V}O_2$
Fever	Hypothermia
Artificial nutrition (TPN > EN?)[a]	(Partial) fasting
Encephalopathy	Profound coma
	Stable quadriplegia
Hyperkinetic states ($\Uparrow$ catecholamines)[b]	Barbiturates, sedatives
	Anesthesia
	Muscle relaxants
Severe burns[c]	Mechanical ventilation
>Sepsis (early phase)	Sepsis (late phase)
>Multiple trauma	
>Major surgery	

[a] Thermogenesis induced by artificial nutrition is significantly higher by the parenteral than by the enteral route.
[b] $\Uparrow$, major augmentation.
[c] > indicates the approximate level of energy expenditure, from the highest (burns) to the lowest (uncomplicated major surgery), in different clinical settings.

our experience, calculation of $\dot{V}O_2$ by this method does not correlate well with indirect calorimetry, especially in unstable patients, where differences (usually underestimation of $\dot{V}O_2$ by the Swan-Ganz method) can reach 20–30%.

In practice, an energy supply of 30–40 g/kg/day, i.e., 1800–2400 kcal/day for a patient weighing 60 kg, is sufficient in 90% of cases and corresponds to 1.3–1.5 the estimated EE. In the context of critical care, and especially when multiple organ failure occurs, the most important thing is not to act to the patient's disadvantage. As there appears to be no correlation between total calorie supply and mortality (49), it is preferable to avoid excess that has known detrimental effects, including hyperosmolarity, hepatocyte steatosis, adrenergic stimulation (dependent on concomitant amino acid supply (120)), a risk of lactic acidosis, absence of inhibition of gluconeogenesis and nitrogen catabolism, abnormal in-

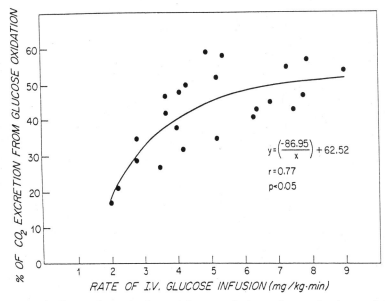

$$y = \left(\frac{-86.95}{x}\right) + 62.52$$

$$r = 0.77$$

$$p < 0.05$$

Figure 3.2. Using the hyperglycemic glucose clamp technique, the maximal rate of glucose uptake approximates 6–7 mg/kg/min (in the absence of exogenous insulin), which corresponds to the plateau reached by the percentage of CO_2 from the direct oxidation of infused glucose. At infusion rates less than 2 mg/kg/min, the curve is expected to plateau at about 18%. (From Burke JF, Wolfe RR, Mullany CJ, Matthews DE, Bier DM. Glucose requirements following burn injury. Ann Surg 1979;190:274–285.)

crease in $\dot{V}o_2$ and $\dot{V}co_2$, problems with weaning from artificial ventilation, and intestinal meteorism in the case of enteral nutrition (54).

Energy Supply: Glucose or Lipids?

The relatively poor tolerance of carbohydrates in the early frank hyperglycemic phase of aggression is related to the increased hepatic production via protein gluconeogenesis (147), the increased glucose turnover (mainly due to the activation of Cori's cycle (250)), and a partial (and controversial) fall in peripheral oxygenation despite the fact that cellular uptake is preserved (147). These factors, together with the well-known risks of excessive glucose perfusion (see above), mean that it must be used only with care, particularly in case of severe sepsis (228). A minimum supply of about 150 g/day is, however, necessary to furnish glucose-dependent tissues, particularly since peripheral amino acid utili-

zation is altered when the glucose supply is inadequate (145). As the maximum rate of glucose oxidation is of the order of 4–6 mg/kg/min (29, 41, 249) (Fig. 3.2), i.e., 350–500 g/day for a patient weighing 60 kg, the recommended supply is about 3–5 g/kg/day (200–300 g/day for 60 kg). To increase the nonprotein energy supply, there are two alternatives: exogenous insulin supply or mixed (glucose-lipid) caloric supply.

The addition of insulin when the endogenous blood insulin is elevated does not appear to be justified, with the exception of checking osmotic polyuria in cases of severe hyperosmolarity (29, 93). Insulin resistance induced by aggression is complex (93): it can be related to a lack of intracellular glucose metabolism, to competition with the peripheral utilization of lipids released by the action of glucagon and catecholamines (Randle's cycle) or to an increase in insulin turnover (67). In practice, insulin increases peripheral uptake of glucose up to 9 mg/kg/min but does not improve its utilization (oxidation) (29, 245) by the cells, or the protein balance.

Postinsult lipid metabolism appears to be characterized by a large increase in endogenous lipolysis and long-chain triglycerides (LCTs) and medium-chain triglycerides (MCTs) turnover, although it has not been established whether or not lipid oxidation is increased in absolute terms (144, 171). The essential element is the absence of any correlation between the circulating free fatty acid (FFA) concentration and lipid turnover, i.e., the loss of lipolysis regulation, during severe insult. Another important observation made in burn patients, as well as in those with multiple trauma and severe sepsis, is the inhibition of normal fasting hyperketonemia, no doubt related to the reesterification of FFA by the liver—a metabolic situation probably favored by postinsult hyperglycemia and hyperinsulinemia (27), which hinder the complete oxidation of lipids into ketone bodies, although the metabolic capacities for hepatic ketogenesis appear to be spared (25). Lipid emulsions appear therefore to be the most logical alternative for parenteral nutrition (PN), avoiding the risk of glucose overload when the calorie input exceeds 1200 kcal/day. Such emulsions provide a high degree of energy support in a small volume (9 kcal/g) and reduce the osmolarity of nutritional mixtures. In fact, there is no "preferential energy substrate": Nordenstrom et al. (171), Roulet et al. (201), and Baker et al. (19) have clearly shown that the traumatized and/or infected patient's metabolism is oriented according to the energy supply (149, 211). Glucose oxidation is favored when the glucose supply is elevated, whereas glucose/lipid support leads to reductions in thermogenesis, catecholamine secretion, and $\dot{V}CO_2$ (171), with a drop in the nonprotein respiratory quotient (RQ), reflecting the existence of a certain degree of lipid oxidation (121). The nitrogen-sparing effects of glucose and a mixed energy supply appear to be identical and may even favor the glucose-lipid system, as suggested by Baker et al. (19) and Long et al. (149). Finally, the available lipid emulsions, given the fact that they contain polyunsaturated fatty acids (PUFAs), can

help to avoid or correct rapidly essential fatty acid deficiencies that occur at an early stage (5). However, although the accumulation of oleic acid (nonessential) observed in these situations is avoided, the deficiencies in linoleic acid and arachidonic acid (ω-6-PUFA) are sometimes only partially corrected (5, 48).

Some teams hesitate to use lipid emulsions because of their potential toxicity in the severely ill patient, although this point is controversial. Excessive (>3 mg/kg/day or 80% of energy input) and prolonged lipid supply can cause kupfferian hepatic steatosis, but the risk disappears if 25% of the lipid energy equivalent is replaced by glucose (99); indeed, a balanced supply appears to reduce the risk of fatty infiltration both in hepatocytes (reduction in sugars) and Kupffer cells (moderate lipid supply). Above all, there is a great deal of controversy surrounding the possible immunosuppressive effect of lipids in the acutely ill and/or septic patient. The uptake of lipid particles by the reticuloendothelial system could induce an alteration

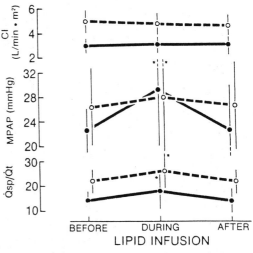

Figure 3.3. Effect of lipid infusion on cardiac index *(CI)*, mean pulmonary artery pressure *(MPAP)*, and intrapulmonary shunt *(Qsp/Qt)* in septic (– – –) and nonseptic (——) patients. *$p<0.05$. Lipids (20% Intralipid) are infused over a 10-hr period. (From Venus B, Prager R, Patel CB, Sandoval E, Sloan P, Smith RA. Cardiopulmonary effects of intralipid infusion in critically ill patients. Crit Care Med 1988;587–590.)

of polymorphonuclear leukocyte, lymphocyte (209), and macrophage (118) functions leading to an increased susceptibility to bacteremia and abnormal results from in vitro immunologic tests (48). Alterations of alveolar macrophages could partially explain the abnormal pulmonary vascular tone and transitory desaturations observed during discontinuous perfusion of lipid emulsions (217, 238) (Fig. 3.3). However, in clinical practice, chemotactic responses and phagocytosis are not diminished in intensive care patients with severe infections, as long as the perfusion rate is not excessive (<83 ml/hr for 20% emulsions) (80,

81, 174) (Fig. 3.4); it is even better to give a continuous 24-hr perfusion, for example, with a glucose-lipid-protein mixture (122).

In practice, it seems reasonable within the context of acute stress to limit the lipid supply to 20–35% of the nonprotein calorie input, or even less in patients who are very seriously ill (burns, septicemia) or when there is reduction in the activity of peripheral lipoprotein lipases. An initial supply of 1 g/kg/day of LCT seems to be best; this can be increased to 2 g/kg/day as long as plasma lipid clearance is regularly monitored (triglyceridemia, serum lactescence) and the perfusion is given contin-

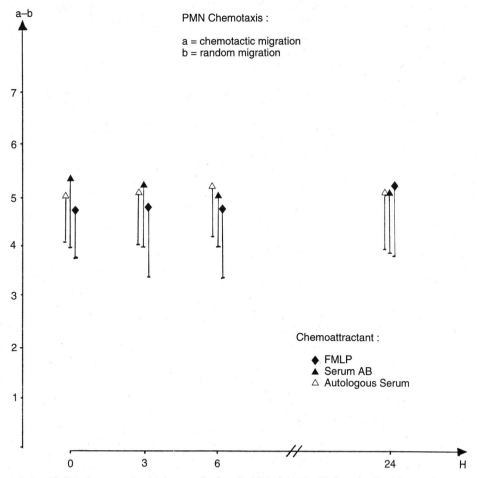

Figure 3.4. PMN chemotaxis during and after lipid infusion. *H*, hours. Random migration and chemotaxis of PMN are measured under agarose with three different chemoattractants; no significant change in chemotaxis (as well as in phagocytosis, data not shown) is observed during and after Intralipid infusion when compared to the basal state. (From Escudier B, Escudier E, Mina E, et al. Effects of intralipid and heparin on neutrophil (PMN) functions during total parenteral nutrition (TPN) [Abstract]. Clin Nutr 1986;5(suppl):41a.)

uously over a 24-hr period. We shall see later the approaches in nutritional pharmacology that have recently led to the use of mixed LCT-MCT emulsions and LCT emulsions with a modified PUFA content.

Is a High Nitrogen Supply Justified?

Postinsult protein metabolism is characterized by net peripheral catabolism, with a lesser increase in synthesis then in breakdown (28, 78, 129). The muscle is the main site of production for amino acids initially destined for gluconeogenesis (more than half is represented by alanine and glutamine) (213). However, interorgan exchanges reveal the significant role of the kidney, lung (181), and intestine. In contrast, hepatic amino-acid uptake is increased, with a stimulation of protein synthesis, essentially that of inflammatory proteins (complement C_3, α_1-acid glycoprotein, haptoglobin, C-reactive protein, etc.) (224), rather than so-called anabolic proteins (albumin, transthyretin or prealbumin, transferrin, retinol-binding protein, etc.) (60).

The therapeutic approach to this metabolic profile is delicate. To a certain extent, muscle proteolysis to the benefit of the hepatic factory is a favorable mechanism, but it is unacceptable because the degree of catabolism is correlated with morbidity and mortality in these patients, especially when multiple organ failure occurs, with the onset of infectious and respiratory complications (49). The main goal of nitrogen supply is therefore to limit muscle catabolism, while at the same time maintaining an adequate nutrient supply to the liver, particularly essential amino acids, so that the synthesis of certain proteins, especially those involved in immune defenses (78, 86, 129), can be maintained. In this context, equilibrium or positivity of nitrogen balance (Table 3.4) is not an end in itself and can even be detrimental if it leads to an accumulation of urea (100). Correctly adapted supplies can, however, reduce the myofibrillar breakdown (142) and, above all, stimulate protein synthesis, generally without upsetting the balance in hypermetabolic patients (212). A simple and relatively reliable way of evaluating nutritional efficacy in this population of patients in whom all the usual markers are inappropriate (180) is the Prognostic Inflammatory and Nutritional Index (PINI) proposed by Ingenbleek and Carpenter, which takes into account both the nutritional and inflammatory components of the response to the aggression and to its metabolic basis (116):

$$PINI = \frac{CRP \times AAG}{Alb \times PA}$$

where CRP = C-reactive protein; AAG = α-$_1$-acid glycoprotein; Alb = albumin; and PA = prealbumin (transthyretin).

Table 3.4
Nitrogen Balance

N intake	Oral feeding = Evaluation 1 g of N = 6.25 g protein[a] $\left.\begin{array}{l}\text{Enteral}\\\text{Parenteral}\end{array}\right\}$ Nutrition = measurement
N output Usually 2–3 g/day	Nonurinary N losses $\left\{\begin{array}{l}\text{Perspiration and sweat: 0.2–1.5 g/day or 0.1–0.5 g/m}^2\\\text{Fecal N}\\\quad\text{Normal transit: 0–2 g/day ($\rightarrow$ 0 in bowel rest)}\\\quad\text{Diarrhea, fistula, enteropathy: $\rightarrow$ 15 g/day}\\\quad\text{(measurement)}\end{array}\right.$ Urinary N losses (g/day) $\quad$ Measurement: Chemiluminescence or Kjeldahl method $\quad$ Estimation from UU: UU (mmol/day) $\times 0.028 + 1$–2 g $\quad$ Proposed formula in hypercatabolic situations $\quad\quad$ (>350 mmol UU/day): UU (mmol/day) $\times 0.035$

[a]N, nitrogen; UU, urinary urea.

The value of this index oscillates between less than one in the healthy subject and more than 30 according to the severity of the condition and the response to therapy.

In practice, the optimal nitrogen supply cannot be determined at present, since the response of each patient depends on the type of insult, hepatic and renal function, and the severity of stress. A nitrogen supply of 200 mg/kg/day, i.e., 1.2 g of protein/kg/day, appears to be a minimum. Above this value, opinions diverge. For certain authors, an increase in nitrogen supply to 40 mg/kg/day does not improve the nitrogen balance (14, 78, 100) nor largely decrease net protein breakdown, and leads to a significant increase in EE (100). Other authors consider that the nitrogen balance is a priority and an input of the order of 0.35–0.40 g/kg/day (2–2.4 g of protein/kg/day) could be necessary in case of major hypercatabolism (47, 121). The calorie/nitrogen ratio (cal/N = nonprotein calories/g N) corresponding to high protein supplies is no longer 150, as in conventional nutrition, but 120 or even 100. In a recent randomized study of bone marrow transplant recipients with severe hypercatabolism, we found that for the same calorie input (REE x 1.7), only a cal/N ratio of 100 clearly rendered positive the cumulative nitrogen balance over the period of aplasia, but at the price of a significant increase in protein turnover, with no increase in blood urea concentrations (3).

Is There a Preferred Nitrogen Substrate?

At the beginning of the 1980s, the peculiar metabolism of branched-chain amino acids (BCAAs) raised high hopes. The BCAAs (leucine, isoleucine, and valine) are mainly metabolized by skeletal muscle (218), not by the liver like the other essential amino acids. Their metabolic fate is triple:

Stimulation of protein synthesis, either directly or after transanimation;

Transfer of the animated radical, with the formation of alanine for hepatic gluconeogenesis, and glutamine destined for the kidney and intestine;

Complete muscular oxidation or transformation into ketoanalogs, which are then metabolized by the liver.

The fact that leucine and its ketoanalog, α-ketoisocaproate, have been implicated in the regulation of muscular protein synthesis and degradation (44, 108) has led to clinical trials of amino acid solutions enriched in BCAA (35, 36, 50). Although a recent meta-analysis has suggested that BCAA could improve the comatose state of patients with hepatic encephalopathy (166), the results are somewhat contradictory and disappointing in patients with severe insult, be it infectious or not (218): the nitrogen balance is improved, but only partially and transiently (50). Protein synthesis was found to be increased in one study with a solution containing 45% of BCAA and enriched in leucine (35), but most available studies suffer from important methodological biases (166). Finally, it is difficult to separate the direct effects of BCAA from those obtained either by increased insulin secretion or by modifications of energy metabolism. In practice, the overriding impression is that there are no firm arguments sufficient to recommend the use of BCAA in hypermetabolic states, including in cases of multiple organ failure, instead of the various balanced amino acid solutions currently available (63, 151).

Finally, the choice of an injectable solution of amino acids can be based on the general characteristics of the products currently available (Fig. 3.5). A major consideration is the number of amino acids contained in the solution: certain products contain fewer than 18 amino acids. The nitrogen content varies greatly from one solution to another (from 6 to 30 g of nitrogen/liter) and is often the factor that determines the choice. The osmolality of the solution (from 400 to 1500 mOsm/kg) should be taken into consideration since it determines the route of administration. The quantities of the eight essential amino acids per gram of nitrogen (E/T) is another element of choice and divides the solutions into two categories: those (the majority) with a ratio greater than 3 and those with a ratio closer to 2. Certain solutions of amino acids also contain glucose and electrolytes (Fig. 3.5).

These relatively simple criteria of choice are not always sufficient to discriminate between the products. In certain cases, the

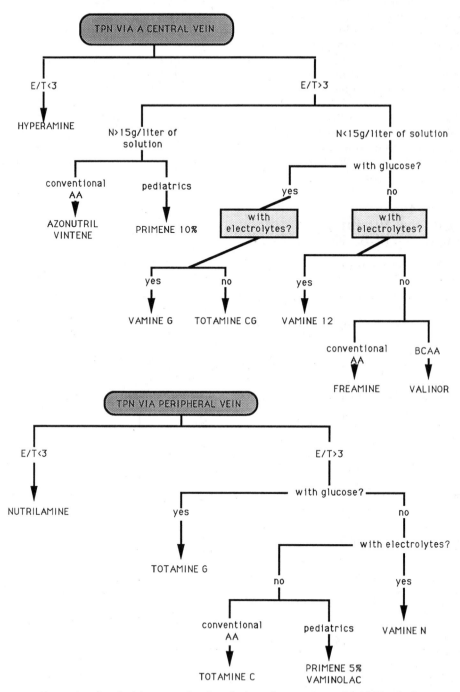

Figure 3.5. Example of a decision tree for the choice of an amino acid *(AA)* solution as used in France. *E/T* represents the quantities of the eight essential amino acids per gram of nitrogen *(N)*. *TPN*, total parenteral nutrition; *BCAA*, branched-chain amino acids. (Modified from Corriol O. Les solutés injectables d'acides aminés pour nutrition parentérale; critères de choix pharmaceutiques. Nutr Clin Metabol 1987;1:17–30.)

amino acidogram, i.e., the quantity of each amino acid per gram of nitrogen, must be considered for each solution. Notable differences sometimes appear in the quantities of branched-chain, aromatic, sulphurated, diacidic, and dibasic amino acids and others such as glycine and alanine (63).

The compositions of these solutions are complex. The choice can be made only after a critical comparative study, particularly when long-term PN is involved and the metabolic profile of the patient is changing.

Electrolytes, Vitamins, and Trace Elements Must Be Kept in Mind

While the requirements of the healthy subject are relatively well known (88) (Table 3.5), the situation in severe aggression, infection, and multiple organ failure is somewhat empiric (158). One or two recent notions merit attention.

In the case of severe infection, there are early deficiencies in intracellular phosphorus (68), magnesium (84), and potassium, even though plasma levels of these remain normal. Phosphorus requirements are par-

ticularly high in patients with respiratory distress and when the glucose input is large (16, 139).

Deficiencies in zinc, which is sequestered by the tissues and excreted in excess in the urine, can occur despite normal blood zinc levels and can lead to the persistence, and even the onset, of sepsis due to immune deficiency (56). Zinc losses are correlated with the severity of stress and intestinal disturbances (diarrhea), and requirements are increased when exogenous amino acids are administered (185).

Vitamin B_1 (thiamine) requirements are considerably increased by insult and by PN, particularly in malnourished patients. Indeed, there have been well-documented cases of acute beriberi and Wernicke's encephalopathy in ICUs (94). Vitamin C requirements are multiplied by at least 100 in order to ensure cicatrization. Finally, an association of adult respiratory distress syndrome (ARDS) and vitamin E deficiency has recently been reported; a lack of vitamin E would seem to favor lipoperoxidation, to be correlated with the level of circulating lipids and to be aggravated during the development of ARDS via poorly understood mechanisms (190).

Table 3.5
Suggested Doses for Enteral and Parenteral Administration of Electrolytes, Vitamins, and Trace Elements in Stable Hypermetabolic Adult Patients

Sodium		>60[a]	Vitamin A		(IU)	2000–5000
Potassium		>80[a]	Vitamin D		(IU)	200–400
Calcium	(mmol)	20–30	Vitamin E			8–15
Phosphorus		15–40	Vitamin K		(mg)	0.15–1
Magnesium		12–16				
Sulfur (methionine)		300–400	Vitamin B_1 (thiamine)			3–50
Iron		1–2	Vitamin B_2 (riboflavin)			3–10[b]
Zinc		2.5–5	Vitamin B_3 (PP or niacin)		(mg)	40–100
Copper	(mg)	0.2–0.5	Vitamin B_5 (pantothenic acid)			15–40
Manganese		1–3	Vitamin B_6 (pyridoxine)			4–100[c]
Fluoride		1–2	Vitamin C (ascorbic acid)			50–200
Molybdenum		0.1–0.2				
Chromium		1–10	Vitamin B_8 (biotin)			60–300
Cobalt		1–3	Vitamin B_{12}		(μg)	5–60
Iodine	(μg)	>20	Folic acid			400
Selenium		50–150				

[a] Average recommended doses for stable patients during total parenteral nutrition.
[b] Needs dependent on glucose load.
[c] Needs dependent on nitrogen intake.

Table 3.6
Basis for Nutritional Support at the Onset of Hypermetabolic Syndrome

Caloric requirements
  30–40 kcal/kg/day (indirect calorimetry)
  Glucose ≤5 g/kg/day
  0.5 g/kg/day ≤lipids (LCT) ≤2 g/kg/day, continuous infusion on 24 hr recommended[a]
Amino acids or proteins
  1.5–2 g/kg/day
  Adaptation based on level of catabolism {BUN / Nitrogen balance
  Conventional crystalline amino acid solutions
  BCAA enriched solutions?
Vitamins
  Standard balanced formulas
    + vitamin K (10 mg/day)
    + vitamin B_1 and vitamin B_6 (100 mg/day)
    + vitamins A, C, E?
Trace elements (provided there is normal renal function)
  Complete standard solutions
    + Zn (15–20 mg/day)
    + Se (120 μg/day)
Electrolytes
  Based on daily evaluation (Na^+, K^+, Ca^{2+})
    + P^{2-} (>16 mmol/day)
    + Mg^{2-} (>200 mg/day)

[a]LCT, long-chain triglycerides; BCAA, branched-chain amino acids; BUN, blood urea nitrogen.

Table 3.6 summarizes the nutritional and metabolic recommendations that can serve as a basis for nutritional support early in the onset of hypermetabolic syndrome. They must be adjusted to each individual case according to the type of insult, the metabolic surveillance that is feasible (calorimetry, nitrogen balance), and the possible onset of side effects.

CAN THIS THERAPEUTIC SCHEMA BE IMPROVED IN THE NEAR FUTURE?

It is clear that present nutritional support can only limit the process of stressed starvation that accompanies injury and sepsis and has no impact on the syndrome itself. However, over the last few years, new methods of nutrition and/or new substrates have been undergoing trials with the aim of correcting specific metabolic immunological disturbances, which are partially dependent on capillary hyperpermeability and cell activation induced by mediators. The impact of this "nutritional pharmacology" is being evaluated, not only in terms of biological and immunological parameters, but also in terms of morbidity/mortality in critically ill patients at risk or having developed multiple organ failure (8, 52, 215).

PARENTERAL OR ENTERAL NUTRITION?

Paradoxically, although most of our current knowledge has been acquired with PN, it is clear that PN is not an ideal substitute for the physiological use of the digestive tract (9, 89, 150, 204). Except in cases of occlusion, enteral nutrition (EN) is almost always feasible (170, 216) (Fig. 3.6), even following major intestinal surgery, by means of the jejunostomy "a minima" technique (205, 232) (Fig. 3.7). EN is the sole guarantor of intestinal motility and villous protein content and is necessary for the maintenance of bile secretion, as well as that of secretory IgA, which plays a major role as a barrier against the intestinal translocation of bacteria (9). Finally, EN itself reduces the hypermetabolic response to insult by about 20% by maintaining the enteroinsulinic axis and reducing neuroendocrine stimulation (11, 204).

In addition, the use of antacids and/or

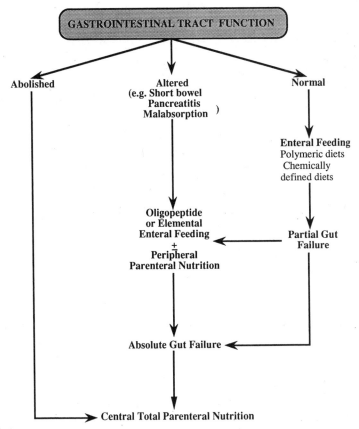

Figure 3.6. Example of a decision tree for selecting the type of nutritional support. It must be kept in mind that at least a part of the nutrition can be delivered by the enteral route in about 75% of the cases.

H_2 blocking agents to prevent acute stress ulceration may lead to bacterial overgrowth by Gram-negative rods, increasing the risk of both severe aspiration pneumonia and diarrhea (163). Moreover, the absence of intragastric nutrients in combination with stress increases the risk of ulceration. EN has been reported to be as effective as antacids in the prophylaxis of stress ulcers in ICU patients (79, 220). The mechanisms potentially involved in this effect include dilutional alkalinization of luminal acidity, trophic effects of nutrients, and stimulation of prostaglandin secretion.

In practice, EN alone or associated with PN is clearly efficacious when started at an early stage. After the 2nd or 3rd day, when the hypercatabolic phase is well established, the two types of nutrition appear to give similar results (54). The only serious complication of EN in the patient with an acute condition and/or infection is the onset of diarrhea.

Approximately half of all patients in ICUs develop diarrhea (128). Each of the factors that correlates with the occurrence of diarrhea, i.e., broad-spectrum antibiotics, H_2 blocking agents, and EN either directly or indirectly affects the intestinal ecology (102). Intestinal atrophy could also lead to refeeding diarrhea after starvation (98). Finally, hypoalbuminemia-induced diarrhea could be due to a decrease in oncotic pressure giving rise to intestinal edema and either secretory or malabsorptive diarrhea (37). However, whether or not hypoalbuminemia alone produces intestinal edema is uncertain, and even more controversial is the hypothesis that intestinal edema may cause diarrhea (38, 194).

Diarrhea in the critically ill patient is

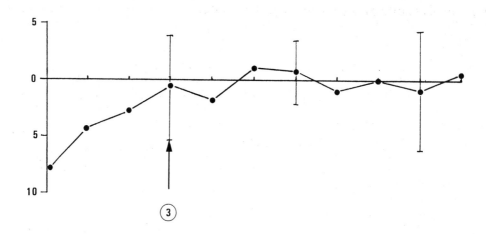

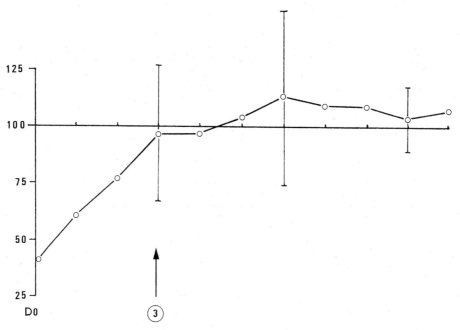

Figure 3.7. Results of immediate postoperative enteral nutrition (jejunostomy "a minima"), using polymeric or oligopeptide isotonic diets, in 80 patients undergoing esogastric surgery. An effective caloric intake of 36 kcal/kg/day corresponding to mean caloric requirements was achieved and nitrogen equilibrium was reached on average by day 3. Central TPN was never used, and withdrawal from peripheral venous access was usually possible by day 2. (From Nitenberg G, Tandonnet F, Henry-Amar M, et al. Immediate postoperative enteral nutrition (EN) in esogastric surgery: a three years experience [Abstract]. Clin Nutr 1986;5(suppl):41a.)

one of the most difficult problems involved in the decision on feeding (197). In the majority of cases, diarrhea can easily be controlled by reducing the flow rate and the osmolarity of the mixture and by providing sufficient intraluminal sodium (above 80 mmol/liter) (216). Several complementary approaches are of interest, including fecal bulking agents (202), pectin, narcotics, substitution of MCT oil for LCT, etc.; manipulation of the serum albumin concentration is rarely effective (103). But diarrhea may also indicate gut failure, with underlying ischemia and bacterial overgrowth (197), and EN is contraindicated in this setting. The patient should be closely monitored not only for signs of diet intolerance but also for worsening of the underlying disease and/or entry into multiple organ failure. Intolerance to EN is associated with increased mortality in critically ill patients (197). EN may thus be considered a "stress test": the development of symptoms of gut failure usually indicates a poor prognosis, and EN should be formally withheld. Research is under way into the provision of "specific" intestinal fuels for these types of patients with intestinal barrier failure (see below).

Factors such as severe hypercatabolism, renal or hepatic failure, pulmonary insufficiency, and malnutrition alter nutrient metabolism, thereby theoretically necessitating a more specific formulation (197). Most critical care patients, however, can be fed with polymeric or oligopeptide isotonic diets and seldom require elemental or "specialized" diets (199) (Fig. 3.8).

There have been numerous recent modifications of EN support with some notable successes. A simple increase in protein content (15–23% of total energy supply) significantly improves survival in patients with deep and extensive burns, whereas a deleterious effect occurs with an excessive calorie input (40–60 kcal/kg/day) (6). The enrichment of nutrient mixtures with arginine (204) and vitamin C (8), the reduction in ω-6-PUFA (linoleic and arachidonic acids), and the enrichment with ω-3-PUFA (linolenic acid), all considered to be immunomodulatory, have given interesting results in animal models (176) and are currently undergoing clinical trials (7). Starting EN at an early stage appears to be an essential prognostic factor, particularly in burn patients (59, 156): Moore et al. have

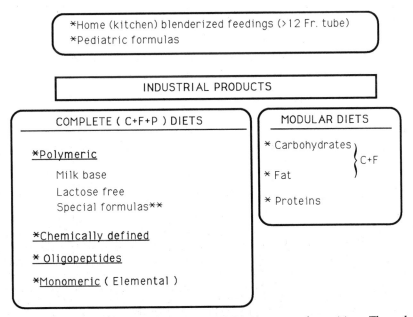

Figure 3.8. Classification of feeding formulas available for enteral nutrition. The selection of a diet is based on the individual patient's absorptive capacity, caliber and location of the feeding tube (gastric or postpyloric), substrate tolerance, and any specialized requirements.

shown that EN significantly diminishes the incidence of infection relative to that in patients treated with equivalent PN (9 versus 37%) when it is started within 12 h of injury (162). On the basis of these findings, a nutritional mixture has been developed with the aim of restoring the immune status in septic and intensive care patients (33). The protein source (Na and Ca caseinate) provides 23% of total energy supply, with a calorie:nitrogen ratio of 100, and the mixture is enriched with arginine and nucleotides at supposedly immunomodulatory doses. The lipid supply is modified by the incorporation of structured MCT and by a balanced content of ω-3- and ω-6-PUFA (see below). A prospective multicenter trial is under way to evaluate if this product can reduce the length of hospital and intensive care stay, and at the same time improve the nutritional and immune status and reduce financial costs (secondary evaluation criteria) (33). The principal investigator recently provided very promising preliminary results at a European Society of Parenteral and Enteral Nutrition meeting (Athens, 1990).

The prevention of endogenous septicemia due to intestinal bacterial translocation has been the object of several studies, mainly concerning the value—albeit highly controversial—of selective gut decontamination. Certain nutritional manipulations in EN could reduce this phenomenon, which is now considered a major factor in the onset and persistence of multiple organ failure (74, 222, 246); in contrast, PN would appear to be ineffective (10). Enrichment with glutamine, the preferred fuel for the enterocyte, which utilizes a large proportion of what is released during muscle proteolysis (221, 246), has reduced the incidence of endotoxinemia in a model of necrotizing enterocolitis (8), and well-designed human studies are beginning (223). Similarly, the enteral (or parenteral) administration of short-chain fatty acids, the preferred fuel of the colonocyte, e.g., β-hydroxybutyrate, appears to reduce the atrophy of the colonic mucosa and could thereby avoid another potential source of endogenous infection (112, 136, 137).

Adjustment of the Energy Supply

Severe alterations of intracellular energy metabolism appear late in the course of postaggressive metabolic alterations, so that the energy supply has long been adequate and sufficiently well used (72, 143). In the later stages, phosphorylating oxidation can become uncoupled, with a drastic fall in phosphate-rich cellular components, e.g., ATP, phosphocreatinine, associated with a large drop in intracellular potassium and magnesium (145). The breakdown of the ATP-ADP-AMP system could be effectively countered at this late phase by continuous hemofiltration, which permits sufficient nutritional support but avoids hypervolemia, associated with the administration of a mixture of ATP-magnesium (113).

When lactic acidosis, which usually accompanies liver failure, appears imminent dichloroacetate has been proposed for its direct and indirect activating effects on pyruvate dehydrogenase, the enzyme responsible for the orientation of pyruvate toward the Krebs cycle (226). The results obtained were not homogenous because this compound has no effect when the lactic acidosis reflects only the presence of mitochondrial asphyxia, preventing the normal functioning of the oxidative cycle.

Alexander et al. (6) and Yamazaki et al. (252) have pointed out the increased risk of infection associated with excessive energy supply. In experimental studies on rodents, the mortality rate and incidence of infectious complications were found to be inversely proportional to the energy supply; the best results were obtained when it remained below the REE, even though the animals that survived longest lost weight! Even more surprisingly, the optimal protein input was only one third of the theoretical optimum, and the lipid calorie supply could be increased without detriment up to 50% of the total energy input; indeed, the best survival rate was obtained in the group of animals in which the nitrogen balance was least favorable (175)! These experimental data are in relative agreement with observations in patients with severe, deep suppurative infections, made by Baker et al. (19) and Greig et al. (100), and may indicate that the type of nutrition should be adapted to the initial aggression (sepsis versus trauma), even if the most detrimental risk, i.e., multiple organ failure, is the same.

Adjusting the Lipid Supply

Lipid emulsions for PN consist of LCT with 16- to 20-carbon fatty acids. Their penetration into mitochondria for β-oxidation is dependent on carnitine, which can be deficient in acutely ill patients (179). MCT, in which the fatty acids have 6–12 carbon atoms, have therefore been proposed because of potential advantages in intensive care patients at risk for multiple organ failure, i.e., rapid clearance from the plasma, limited storage, and more rapid oxidation than LCT, which is relatively independent of carnitine (18, 124). In fact, their oxidation is not always complete, as was initially thought, and MCT can undergo a degree of elongation and accumulation. The risks related to their potential direct neurotoxicity and the accumulation of dicarboxylic acids by microsomal ω-oxidation is, however, theoretical in adults in intensive care. Only one mixed emulsion, containing 50% MCT and 50% LCT, is at present available in France, and there are few studies evaluating this type of emulsion. Recently, Ball and White found that balanced PN with LCT/MCT in intensive care patients under mechanical ventilation showed excellent clinical and biological tolerance relative to a conventional lipid emulsion and induced a 60% higher blood insulin level, a higher concentration of FFA and a certain degree of ketonemia (20). Together with other preliminary studies, the metabolic profile obtained appears to be favorable in such patients, although further substantial clinical confirmation is required.

Some of the most promising recent work suggests that LCTs (both in EN and PN), in addition to their role as an energy source, substrates for essential fatty acids and transporters of fat-soluble vitamins, are powerful immunomodulators (130). Constitutive PUFAs are progressively inte-grated into the membrane of immuno-competent cells (polymorphonuclear neutrophils, lymphocytes, macrophages, and monocytes), the composition of which eventually reflects alimentary fatty acids. These alterations of membrane phospholipids affect cell functions and membrane fluidity (130), a phenomenon that may be fundamental in the response to antigens and local cell-to-cell interactions, e.g., between hepatocytes and Kupffer cells (55, 244). Conventional lipid emulsions are relatively rich in ω-6-PUFAs (linoleic and arachidonic acids); it is the degradation products of arachidonic acid (eicosanoids—PGE_2 and leukotrienes) that are mainly responsible, particularly in macrophages, for the immunosuppressive properties and for the generation of free oxygen radicals (48, 130) (Fig. 3.9). On the contrary, such emulsions are poor in ω-3-PUFAs (linolenic acid), which inhibit the degradation of arachidonic acid via the cyclooxygenase pathway and, thus, the synthesis of PGE_2; they lead, via the eicosapentanoids, to the synthesis of PGI_3 and thromboxane A_3 (127). ω-3-PUFAs therefore give rise to a decrease in platelet activation and thrombogenesis and inhibit the inflammatory reaction related to the activation of target cells by cytokines (interleukin-1, interleukin-6, and tumor necrosis factor-α) (26, 183).

In practice, reducing the ω-6-/ω-3-PUFA ratio in the lipid supply is the most promising approach in clinical pharmacology in the setting of intensive care. This can be achieved by balancing soya lecithins (rich in ω-6-PUFA) and fish lecithins (rich in ω-3-PUFA) (52, 130). Studies are under way in burn patients, intensive care patients (multiple organ failure + ARDS), and organ transplant recipients (177).

Adjusting the Protein Supply

The importance of glutamine in post-aggression conditions has recently been underlined (109, 187, 221, 222). In this setting, glutamine becomes an essential amino acid and the preferred fuel for rapidly dividing cells, such as lymphocytes, macrophages, and enterocytes (70). Glu-

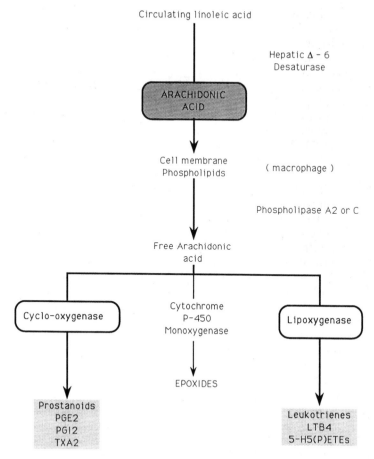

Figure 3.9. Metabolism of free arachidonic acid, released from membrane macrophage phospholipids by the action of phospholipases A₂ and C. Free arachidonic acid is rapidly metabolized through three pathways. Prostanoids (prostacyclin or PGI₂, prostaglandins *(PG)*, and thromboxane *(TXA₂)*) are synthetized by cyclo-oxygenase; leukotrienes *(LT)* and different hydroxyeicosatetraenoic *(HETE)* acids are formed by lipoxygenase. Both these pathways yield superoxides. (Modified from Kinsella JE, Lokesh B. Dietary lipids, eicosanoids, and the immune system. Crit Care Med 1989;18:94–113.)

tamine requirements increase considerably after multiple trauma, severe infection, and major surgery (109, 221). In addition, glutamine is essential for tissue repair and wound healing. In the absence of food intake, these increased requirements are met by muscle proteolysis, and the glutamine stores (25 g) are reduced by half within a few days of the insult. This process is considered a beneficial adaptation in the early stages, but in the hypermetabolic phase, proteolysis releases increasing quantities of alanine destined to the liver and cuts down glutamine supplies. It is therefore during this period that endoge-

nous glutamine supplies become essential, particularly to meet intestinal requirements (40, 221), since blood glutamine levels are at a minimum. We have already seen the importance of the glutamine contained in EN in limiting bacterial translocation, but its metabolic role in the control of proteolysis is also fundamental. The most suitable enteral mixtures at this stage will therefore be those richest in glutamine. Nontoxic and efficacious artificially enriched preparations should eventually become available. The supply of glutamine by PN is hindered by the instability of this amino acid during industrial sterilization of solutions of crystalline amino acids. The use of dipeptides, particularly alanine-glutamine and glycyl-glutamine, has enabled this problem to be circumvented (4). Dipeptides are perfectly soluble, totally hydrolyzed within minutes, and are nontoxic; however, the preparation of amino acid solutions rich in dipeptides is costly. Stehle et al. (227) and, more recently, Hammarqvist et al. (105), have shown the clinical efficacy of such a solution in intestinal surgery patients in terms of nitrogen balance, and the sparing effect on the muscle glutamine pool. However, the value of such an approach in truly hypercatabolic situations remains to be demonstrated.

Ornithine α-ketoglutarate (OKG) is a very old product but its anabolic (i.e., stimulation of insulin and growth hormone (GH) secretion) and anticatabolic properties (i.e., stimulation of glutamine and arginine synthesis) (66) are theoretically adapted to the hypermetabolic states (Fig. 3.10). OKG is easy to administer enterally or parenterally, in short or 24-hr perfusions. Particularly favorable results

have been obtained when OKG was added to EN in severely burned patients, in terms of both metabolic parameters and morbidity (65); in addition, there was a large (but not significant) increase in survival relative to a control group of burn patients. As is the case for glutamine, some authors have found that OKG is effective in noncomplicated postoperative patients (104, 140), with the maintenance of muscle ribosome and polyribosome levels apparently reflecting a sparing effect on the capacity for muscle protein synthesis (243).

OTHER POTENTIAL HORMONAL AND IMMUNOLOGICAL MANIPULATIONS

Arginine is a semiessential amino acid in the adult, but is essential in the child, and becomes indispensable during severe hypermetabolic and septic states (131, 167). Arginine is required for collagen synthesis, and its supplementation in animal

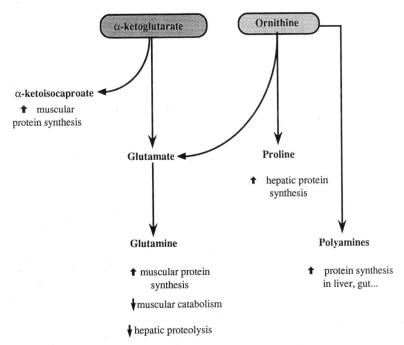

Figure 3.10. Metabolites of ornithine α-ketoglutarate potentially implicated in its action on protein metabolism. (Modified from Cynober L. Ornithine α-ketoglutarate in nutritional support. *Nutrition* 1991; 7 (in press).)

studies has been found to accelerate wound healing and to stimulate thymus growth, lymphocyte proliferation, and the response of mononuclear cells to mitogens (8). We have already seen the probable efficacy of arginine in experimental infections in animals. T cell stimulation has also been observed in intensive care patients receiving arginine-rich EN (53).

A supply of nucleotides (purines and pyrimidines) is essential in EN for maintaining normal immune function (138). Their absence leads to a selective loss of helper T cells and reduced interleukin-2 production; uracil appears to be the most important nucleotide in these respects. In clinical nutrition, adequate supplies of RNA or nucleotides seem to be at least as important as those of ω-3-PUFA to restore immune status, as suggested by animal models (173) and studies in critical care patients (33).

Numerous pharmacological and hormonal substrates appear to be effective in modulating the hypermetabolic response to aggression (210, 247). GH (now produced by genetic manipulation) has been extensively studied in recent years. In association with conventional (184) and even hypocaloric PN (247), GH improves protein synthesis, nitrogen balance, and lipid oxidation during the postoperative period in patients undergoing major gastrointestinal surgery (in the absence of complications). A very recent controlled study of intensive care patients with severe insult has given similar results and showed a lack of toxicity (255). A multicenter study is also under way in the United States to evaluate the impact of this approach on the duration of hospital stay and on the survival of patients with multiple organ failure.

Other growth factors, such as epidermal growth factor are being evaluated. In vitro, epidermal growth factor accelerates enterocyte proliferation, stimulates intestinal protein synthesis, and increases luminal enzyme activity (8). Its mode of action is different from and no doubt complementary to that of glutamine, but its utility in the clinical situation has not so far been studied.

Finally, great hope has been placed in the use of cyclooxygenase inhibitors, and chiefly ibuprofen (192), as adjuvant treatment or, preferably, as preventative treatment of ARDS and multiple organ failure. This type of nonsteroidal antiinflammatory drug has shown beneficial effects in animal models of septic shock, as well as in ARDS, as an immunomodulator. At the metabolic level, its early administration following the onset of sepsis can inhibit the increased splanchnic output but does not prevent the emergence of hyperglycemia or the accumulation of glycerol and lactate in the plasma (23). The effect and precise mode of action of nonsteroidal antiinflammatory drugs, particularly on cytokine secretion, remain poorly understood. At the clinical level, there is no convincing evidence that nonsteroidal antiinflammatory drugs influence the course of hypermetabolic states, particularly in patients with ARDS or multiple organ failure (192).

Figure 3.11 summarizes the potential role of all these proposed metabolic adjustments and novel substrates in modifying the cycle of adaptation to stress and/or sepsis (101).

NUTRITIONAL SUPPORT DURING ORGAN FAILURE IN SPECIFIC PATIENT GROUPS

Nutritional support of the critically ill patient is frequently complicated by the presence of coexisting organ dysfunction. Respiratory compromise, renal failure, acute liver failure, and circulatory disorders are the main situations encountered in injury and sepsis. Each of these entities superimposes characteristic disturbances upon the hypermetabolic status. Nutrition must thus be tailored to limit the harmful effects of organ failure, while still providing an adequate supply of nutrients to promote recovery (206).

Respiratory Failure

Ventilatory insufficiency in most critically ill patients is due to either direct chest trauma with pulmonary contusion or to increased capillary permeability, associated with ARDS, pneumonia, sepsis, or the fat embolism syndrome. Adequate nu-

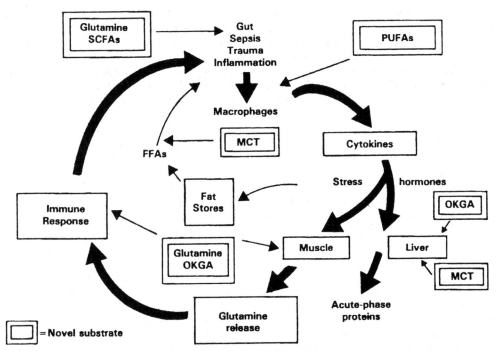

Figure 3.11. The role of novel substrates in modifying the cycle of adaptation at stress or infection. *PUFAs*, polyunsaturated fatty acids; *OKGA*, ornithine α-ketoglutarate; *MCT*, medium-chain triglycerides; *SCFAs*, short-chain fatty acids. (From Grimble G, Payne-James JJ, Rees R, Silk DBA. Enteral nutrition: novel substrates. Intensive Ther Clin Monitoring 1989;10:51–57.)

tritional support is important to maximize the potential for recovery of respiratory muscle function and resumption of normal clearance of bronchiolar secretions. Unfortunately, data are lacking in the literature on the precise nutrition required for patients with acute respiratory failure. Some recommendations, however, can be formulated concerning the quantitative and qualitative aspects of nutritional support for these patients.

About one-quarter of patients admitted for acute respiratory failure are malnourished (body weight of less than 80% of ideal). Body weight and diphragmatic muscle mass are reduced in parallel (13). Muscle atrophy due to malnutrition, prolonged mechanical ventilation, or neuromuscular disease may predispose the patient to the development of respiratory fatigue. The increased work of breathing is believed to be the primary reason for hypermetabolism in these patients. The normal work of breathing accounts for about 5% of resting energy expenditure,

but in acute respiratory failure it may increase up to 25% (85). Although most of this increase is abolished by mechanical ventilation, assist-control or control ventilation permits $\dot{V}_{O_2}$ to be reduced more than intermittent ventilation modes (intermittent mandatory ventilation and assist/controlled ventilation) (186).

Malnourished patients on mechanical ventilation have a higher mortality rate than well-nourished patients in similar circumstances, possibly due to inadequate nutritional support. Bassili and Deitel (22) reported that 93% of patients receiving adequate nutritional support (2000 to 3000 kcal/day) were weaned from the ventilator, whereas it was the case for only 53% of the patients on an inadequate diet (400 kcal/24 hr); this difference was most significant for postoperative patients (91 versus 36%).

The RQ ($\dot{V}_{CO_2}/\dot{V}_{O_2}$) reflects the individual substrate that is being metabolized. For example, pure carbohydrate metabolism is associated with an RQ ratio of 1.0, whereas pure fat metabolism is associated with an RQ of 0.70. Protein metabolism gives an RQ ratio of 0.82. When glucose intake exceeds oxidation, the RQ ratio rises above 1.0 because lipogenesis releases CO_2 and has an RQ ratio of approximately 8.0, and this increases demands upon the ventilatory system (193, 248). Elevated CO_2 production, which is usually well tolerated by patients with normal respiratory function, could be harmful for patients with marginal respiratory reserves, leading to an elevation of $Paco_2$ (69, 110). As noted above, care should be taken not to overfeed these patients, and indirect calorimetry may be necessary to document daily energy requirements and ensure that the RQ is <1.0 during nutritional support.

Weaning from a ventilator may be more difficult during the administration of a glucose-based total parenteral nutrition (TPN) solution if the patient is being overfed (15, 22). Usually, this can be easily avoided with an intake of around 1500 kcal/day of a mixed fuel load with no more than 60% (900 kcal) provided by carbohydrates and at least 30–40% by a fat emulsion as the nonprotein energy (15). Theoretically, this regimen reduces ventilatory demands and may facilitate ventilatory weaning in marginal patients. Enteral feeding preparations that are relatively low in carbohydrates and high in fats are commercially available, but fat malabsorption and ensuing diarrhea, which leads to decreased fat utilization, occur frequently in these patients.

As noted above, lipids should be administered at a slow rate to patients with acute respiratory failure. Rapid administration can induce pulmonary vasoconstriction, presumably because of an alteration in lung prostaglandin metabolism, promoting a proinflammatory response (225). Prostaglandins have effects on both vascular and bronchial tone, and the changes fat emulsions induce in eicosanoid production are thus of major clinical importance (217). Recently, Venus et al. (238) reported that 100 g of fat emulsion infused over 10 hr in ventilated patients increased mean pulmonary arterial pressure (MPAP) and decreased oxygenation (Fig. 3.3). Unpublished data from Venus

and Kinney's groups suggest that a 24-hr infusion modality does not increase MPAP, but decreases $\dot{V}o_2$ relative to a rapid (8-hr) infusion. Increases in vasodilating and antiinflammatory prostaglandin I_2 and E_2 synthesis could be the most plausible explanation. This may result in changes in ventilation/perfusion ratio and may explain the decrease in diffusion capacity often described with intravenous fat emulsions (217).

Amino acids alter ventilatory drive (241); this effect may be related to the BCAA content (230), although this hypothesis has been questioned (75). Both standard amino acids and BCAA increase minute volume, the mean inspiratory flow rate, $\dot{V}o_2$, and the ventilatory response to CO_2 inhalation, and decrease $Paco_2$. Many patients with borderline respiratory function will not tolerate excessive levels of amino acids since their minute ventilation cannot increase in response to an increase in ventilatory drive, and this effect may lead to respiratory muscle fatigue and precipitate respiratory arrest. Particular caution should be exercised when combining high glucose content with a high protein content.

Acute Renal Failure

Acute renal failure is a common complication in severely ill and highly catabolic patients; its etiology is complex and frequently multifactorial, including administration of nephrotoxic agents (e.g., anticancer chemotherapy, aminoglycosides), circulatory shock, and Gram-negative septicemia. The presence of a nephropathy considerably changes whole-body carbohydrate, fat, and protein metabolism. It is not clear whether nutritional support influences survival in patients with acute renal failure, because of the heterogeneity of the populations so far studied. However, individualized nutrient formulations are required, according to the state of renal failure (157, 189). The high catabolic rate associated with injury and/or sepsis can precipitate rapid increases in potassium, phosphorus, and blood urea nitrogen (BUN) levels.

In oliguric renal failure one nutritional

goal is to control the rapid accumulation of metabolic by-products and delay or avoid the need for hemodialysis or hemofiltration (45). Acute renal failure could be associated with increased measured energy expenditure up to 20–50% above normal (154, 208). The use of low nitrogen content diets containing high-quality protein and adequate-to-excess calories was pioneered in the early 1960s for the treatment of chronic uremia (96) and later applied to patients with acute renal failure (2, 235). In a double-blind randomized study, Abel et al. (2) compared infusions of dextrose with dextrose plus essential amino acids and showed clear metabolic benefits, e.g., decreases in phosphate, magnesium, potassium, and serum urea nitrogen levels. This was associated with better wound healing, decreased frequency of dialysis, and improved survival. However, it is unclear whether amino acids per se could have achieved the same results. Since these studies were performed, many randomized prospective trials have compared the effects of glucose with essential amino acids and glucose with essential and nonessential amino acids. No conclusive improvements in terms of recovery of renal function, the severity of the catabolic response, or patient survival were demonstrated using any specific formula (82, 159, 165). A likely explanation is that the advantages of essential amino acid solutions, which provide only about 40 g/day of amino acids, are offset, in stressed patients, by their inability to meet gluconeogenic and synthetic demands. Nevertheless, positive energy and nitrogen balances can be achieved, and this correlates with overall survival in the critically ill patient (21).

Finally, increasing the calorie-to-nitrogen ratio to above 250/liter can slow the rate of BUN and metabolic by-products accumulation, although this has little effect on creatinine accumulation. In this situation, potassium, phosphorus, and/or magnesium can be driven back into the cell, and, despite severe renal failure, these electrolytes must usually be supplemented during feeding. Serum BUN can often be maintained at or below an acceptable concentration of 28–36 mmol/liter with this regimen, particularly if the clinical condition of the patient stabilizes (45). The main purpose of aggressive nutritional care in this patient population is to avoid volume overload. Nutritional solutions are frequently limited and are dependent on other fluid losses and the need for antibiotics and other drugs. In oliguric acute renal failure, a solution that contains 350 g of dextrose and 21 g of amino acids in a total volume of 750–1000 ml with the appropriate electrolytes, vitamins, and trace elements is well tolerated until dialysis is started or renal output increases (45). As renal function improves, the amount of administered amino acids is no longer restricted as serum BUN and creatinine levels decrease.

When some form of instrumentation for fluid removal becomes necessary, the clinician faces the choice between hemodialysis and hemofiltration (206). Our experience is that continuous arteriovenous or venovenous hemofiltration, in association with "free" nutritional support, is the best method of maintaining intravascular volume without precipitating hypotension. Amino acid administration is no longer restricted with either method since hemodialysis and hemofiltration reduce the toxic metabolic by-products and remove, respectively, up to 2.4 g of protein/hr (134) and approximately 4 g/day at an ultrafiltration rate of 160 ml/hr (71). Moreover, when glucose-free hemodialysis is instituted, amino acids, glucose, and water-soluble vitamins are lost. A total of 25–30 g of dextrose can be lost in the dialysate per session, and higher concentrations of glucose are needed in the nutrient formula. This may explain why some authors have found that 50 kcal/kg/day is required to maintain positive nitrogen balance in patients undergoing hemodialysis (30).

Because protein is also lost in the dialysate, as a reasonable guide, protein intake may be brought as close to 1.5 g/kg/day as possible while maintaining the serum urea nitrogen below 30 mmol/liter. Patients who become anabolic may develop life-threatening deficiencies; it is therefore often better not to withhold potassium, magnesium, phosphorus, and/or zinc (185).

Because renal failure does not allow accurate estimation of nitrogen breakdown by a 24-hr urine analysis, a calculation of the rate of urea appearance can be used to quantitate catabolism and adjust the protein dosage. The urea appearance rate is calculated as follows: change in body urea pool = (change in BUN) × (0.6 IBW) × 10/1000 (g/day), where IBW is the ideal body weight in kilograms (45).

Other special considerations are pertinent in patients with renal failure. By the use of the glucose clamp technique, it has been shown that uremic patients have higher insulin levels for a given blood glucose content than nonuremic patients (73). The presence of this insulin resistance provides a potential explanation for hyperglycemia in renal failure as well as increased serum triglyceride levels. Hence, insulin resistance in trauma is likely to be intensified by uremia, accentuating the need for careful monitoring of glucose and triglyceride levels. Histidine administration is recommended in renal failure because a specific histidine deficiency syndrome has been described in these patients related to absent de novo synthesis and increased plasma clearance of this amino acid (83, 231). Nitrogen balance improves in renal failure patients when they are given histidine supplementation. Vitamin C may need to be curtailed in oliguric patients.

Special feeding formulas for patients with renal failure contain essential amino acids and histidine as the protein source. Since the purpose is to decrease urea production by recycling nitrogen into the synthesis of nonessential amino acids, they are mainly indicated to avoid dialysis (96). Otherwise, their superiority over standard feedings is unproved, and even their theoretical ability to decrease urea accumulation in vivo has been questioned (159).

The mortality associated with acute renal failure in critically ill patients may still be as high as 60% (49, 234). Efforts continue to be made to improve all facets of treatment, including new forms of nutritional support. Hypertonic solutions of amino acids and glucose, but not lipids, have been infused directly during hemodialysis (251) and peritoneal dialysis. Both of these techniques may prove to be useful as options in feeding patients with renal failure.

Several modifications of the composition of amino acid formulas have been suggested specifically for uremia and include enrichment in valine (11), histidine, tyrosine, serine, and ornithine, but the value of these nutritional manipulations remains to be demonstrated. In theory, the provision of ketoacid analogs of amino acid could also be of use because their amination should result in a reduction of the urea pool while at the same time enhancing the supply of amino acids needed for protein synthesis. However, the clinical consequences of this approach are controversial (95).

Hepatic Failure

The considerable confusion in this area seems to continue. One must be careful to distinguish adequately between acute liver failure (frequently associated with so called "septic encephalopathy") of injury and sepsis, and hepatic (or portasystemic) encephalopathy. This confusion is encouraged by the similarities existing between the symptoms of septic encephalopathy (irritability, disorientation, confusion, somnolence, stupor, and even frank coma) and those of hepatic encephalopathy.

The etiology of *hepatic encephalopathy* is still uncertain (92). It has been hypothesized that excess ammonia and related compounds exert a toxic effect on the brain. Alternatively, an amino acid imbalance has been said to cause central nervous system depression. Investigations concerning cirrhotics have revealed an elevation in the plasma concentrations of the aromatic amino acids phenylalanine, tyrosine, and tryptophan, whereas BCAA levels are decreased (34). The failing liver is presumably no longer able to catabolize surfeit aromatic amino acids while, at the same time, there is an imbalance of insulin and glucagon, resulting in an activation of BCAA uptake by muscle (34, 92). The elevation of aromatic amino acid concentrations and the absence of BCAA competing for the same transport system (system L) ultimately results in an excess of brain levels of tryptophan, phenylalanine, and tyrosine. Both the production of false neurotransmitters and the conversion of tryptophan to serotonin, a central nervous system depressant, may result (87).

On the basis of these data, an enriched BCAA solution associated with hypertonic glucose was used by Fisher and Baldessarini (87) to treat hepatic encephalopathy. Many randomized prospective studies of BCAA-supplemented formulas (arginine is usually added because it may help to reduce hyperammonemia) have now been carried out and have recently been examined with respect to the amelioration of encephalopathy and survival (166). Despite the different treatments used and the different types of cirrhosis studied, patients receiving BCAA came to more rapidly wake up than controls or those receiving neomycin lactulose treatment; in particular, the results for hepatic encephalopathy remain consistently favorable to BCAA, independently of such factors as the length of follow-up and the amount of calories from lipid emulsions. However, differences in study design and other methodologic considerations greatly obscure the interpretation in terms of survival (166). It remains to be determined if a subset of encephalopathics could benefit from these formulas or from other combinations of treatments.

In the injured patient, hepatic decompensation may be precipitated by sepsis, hypotension, surgery, anesthesia, and direct injury, especially if chronic disease is already present (34). The liver is essential for appropriate metabolic responses to trauma. In the presence of hepatic insufficiency, energy expenditure, gluconeogenesis, lipogenesis, production of ketone bodies, synthesis of acute-phase proteins, and the removal of various drugs and toxins (126) are all potentially disturbed. The regulatory role of the liver in the maintenance of micronutrient and amino acid concentrations may also be affected.

Since critically ill patients with hepatic failure are frequently both severely malnourished and highly catabolic, nutritional supplementation should generally be initiated as early as possible. Liver disease is associated with many features observed in marasmus and kwashiorkor. Refeeding should be undertaken with caution since these critically ill patients are water, sodium, and protein intolerant and may accumulate ascites and develop encephalopathy.

In cases of acute hepatocellular damage, plasma high density lipoprotein levels decrease and plasma cholesterol and triglyceride levels increase. In cases of prolonged cholestasis, plasma unesterified cholesterol and phospholipid levels are elevated, due to the presence of a lipoprotein termed lipoprotein "X." Liberal administration of intravenous lipids, e.g., soybean oil or safflower oil emulsions, is not theoretically recommended for patients with multiple organ failure and/or severe hepatic dysfunction because LCTs are metabolized by the liver. However, despite concern that intravenous lipid emulsions might be poorly tolerated, neither the literature that we have reviewed nor our clinical experience indicates general intolerance in this patient population at common rates of infusion (1–1.5 g/kg ideal body weight/day). Serum turbidity and plasma FFA levels should be monitored routinely, and clinicians should maintain awareness of a theoretical potential exacerbation of encephalopathy. Medium- and short-chain triglycerides may be better utilized by these patients, but emulsions of these triglycerides still require a minimal amount of added linoleic acid. Studies evaluating efficacy and innocuity of mixed (MCT-LCT) and structured lipid emulsions are presently under way (18, 124).

Of equal theoretical concern is overfeeding with intravenous carbohydrates, which may increase hepatic metabolic demands. Glucose intolerance may be secondary to a deficient regulation of insulin receptors in the liver, and elevated levels of FFAs, GH, and glucagon. On the other hand, glucose should be monitored closely in the septic patient with advancing liver failure, particularly in the cirrhotic patient in whom severe hypoglycemia may occur.

Finally, even though altered lipid and carbohydrate metabolism is altered in hepatic failure, caloric infusion at a rate closely approximating the estimated metabolic rate and composed of 150–200 g of dextrose and 125–250 ml of a 20% fat emulsion/day is not associated with significant complications. The clearance of this amount of lipid is possible even in the presence of severe cirrhosis (200). Cyclic nutrition, which involves the administration of hypertonic glucose solutions for only 12–18 hr each day, promotes lipolysis and minimizes fatty infiltration of the liver (125) and is hence theoretically of additional benefit to patients with hepatic insufficiency. The increased energy demands in severe injury, however, usually reduce the effectiveness of this latter approach.

Rationale for the use of BCAA formulas in metabolic stress states has been discussed above. The effects of this type of metabolic support on protein metabolism in the patient with injury and hepatic failure are controversial. The overall conclusions are clouded by the heterogenous nature of the patient groups and the variability of their responses to injury and sepsis (35, 50, 218). It is noteworthy, however, that improved survival with BCAAs has not been reported (160, 218). The failure to detect a benefit with BCAA in these patients may have several explanations, including the insufficient amounts of leucine and the inadequacy of nitrogen balance as a nutritional index to measure the usefulness of amino acid infusions (36). In summary, although the physiologic implications are intriguing, these formulations are expensive, and prospective studies have failed to demonstrate unequivocal improvements in terms of morbidity and mortality relative to balanced amino acid solutions. The trauma/septic patient with liver failure requires essential amino acids, which are best delivered in a balanced amino acid solution.

Patients who are encephalopathic may be fed intravenously or by the enteral route, provided that they have not recently bled. Although commercial enteral mixtures are now available specifically for patients with liver dysfunction (199), their use in trauma is problematic. Not only is their efficacy uncertain, but their low content of the essential amino acids phenylalanine and tryptophan makes them unsuitable for supporting protein synthesis in the stressed patient. Extrapolating from studies on alcoholic hepatitis, it would seem that patients showing an abrupt deterioration in liver function but without premorbid cirrhotic disease have similar amino acid requirements to normal subjects and clearly benefit from standard amino acid solutions (117).

Circulatory Failure

We shall restrict our analysis to the nutritional problems posed by patients in medical and surgical ICUs and who develop hemodynamic failure. Nutritional support in patients suffering primarily from exacerbations of congestive heart failure or coronary disorders has recently been reviewed (1, 188). It is generally accepted that the heart ultimately fails in critically ill patients. However, it is not clear whether the heart is affected primarily in injury or sepsis and fails relatively early due to metabolic phenomena, exerting a negative inotropic effect, or whether heart failure is a late event, resulting from durable hemodynamic failure, and leading to inadequate coronary perfusion. The most troublesome complication for nutritional support in the injured patient with heart disease is sodium and fluid overload. This is best addressed by restricting sodium input and by using concentrated (hypertonic) parenteral formulas to minimize volume delivery of nonprotein calories and amino acids. Enteral formulas containing 2 kcal/ml may be of interest. Close monitoring of magnesium, calcium, potassium, and phosphorus is critical in these patients who are frequently on inotropic agents and diuretic therapy and can manifest life-threatening rhythm disturbances with abnormal concentrations of electrolytes (97). Renal dysfunction in the trauma patient with heart failure can require the nitrogen density to be reduced.

The effect of nutritional supplementation in these stressed patients with hemodynamic failure is poorly documented (206). In low cardiac output states, all efforts must be directed toward avoiding unnecessary increases in $\dot{V}_{O_2}$ (17). Casper et al. (46) described the cardiopulmonary effects of EN. Bolus administration and increased infusion rates of an enteral formula increased the metabolic rate, $\dot{V}_{O_2}$, $\dot{V}_{CO_2}$, minute volume, and respiratory quotient. Myocardial $\dot{V}O_2$ was also increased. The authors recommended continuous nasogastric feeding, which was relatively free of side-effects. In unstable patients, especially in those with a compromised myocardium, high-output congestive heart failure may occur following an increase in metabolic demand due to a poorly adapted nutritional intervention.

No single fuel is ideal for the myocardium in all conditions. Glucose is not normally a myocardial fuel substrate. In experimental ischemia, glucose is undesirable, as anaerobic glycolysis leads to tissue acidosis. However, it can be a useful fuel in vivo in hypoxic states and during myocardial ischemia (97). A glucose-insulin-potassium solution, tried with various degrees of success in patients with acute myocardial infarction (195, 196) and during septic shock (39), produces a markedly better myocardial utilization of glucose than glucose alone (195) and reduces FFA combustion and plasma FFA levels, which are toxic for the damaged myocardium (196).

Because intravenous fat emulsions are associated with increased FFA levels in the plasma, there has been some concern regarding potential adverse cardiac effects (1). During ischemia, elevation of plasma FFAs induces depression of contractility, increased $\dot{V}O_2$, and an increased frequency of serious rhythm disturbances. Although controversy persists, fat emulsions can be used as accessory caloric sources in patients with severe cardiac dysfunction, at up to 30–40% of the nonnitrogen caloric contribution. During ischemia, the glucose-insulin-potassium regimen, which increases membrane stability, may be preferred. Because of the high incidence of fat malabsorption in patients with malnutrition and cardiac failure, MCTs should be used as the source of enteral and parenteral fat calories. However, no truly conclusive data are available.

Although carnitine administration may improve FFA utilization and myocardial performance (219); its routine clinical use must await results of further studies on safety and efficacy (179). Similarly, although selenium deficiency may cause car-diomyopathy (123), there is no evidence that routine supplementation improves or "protects" myocardial function.

NUTRITIONAL SUPPORT IN SPECIFIC PATIENT GROUPS

It is beyond the scope of this chapter to discuss in detail the theory, techniques, and cost-effectiveness of nutritional support for a multitude of situations, such as burns, pancreatitis, enterocutaneous fistulas, neurological disorders, bone marrow transplantation, AIDS, etc. We refer the reader interested in these subjects to the abundant and recent literature available (24, 42, 58, 91, 141, 197, 198, 207). We will concentrate on two special problems that are frequently encountered by the intensivists.

THE CASE FOR PERIOPERATIVE NUTRITIONAL SUPPORT

From the provocative paper by Koretz (135) to a recent issue of the American Journal of Clinical Nutrition (240), contradictory data concerning the value and efficacy of perioperative nutritional support are abundant in the international literature. The main questions are the following:

Is there a "gold standard" to accurately assess malnutrition in the surgical patient?
Can perioperative nutritional support maintain or improve nutritional status in the days immediately before and after surgery?
If such a direct benefit exists, does it lead to a reduction in postoperative morbidity and/or mortality, without an excessive iatrogenic risk?

We have already reviewed the current limitations and lack of precision in nutritional assessment. Several nutritional indexes have been developed in recent years worldwide, including the well known "PNI" of Buzby et al. (169, 240). However, for a number of methodological reasons, none of them can be used universally (169), and they can engender major discrepancies in the classification of patients with regard to the risk of postoperative complications (90, 169, 240). Finally, nutritional indexes, overall in the setting of digestive tract cancer patients, cannot separate the nutritional and immunological consequences of the tumor burden from those of the malnutrition itself (168). Clearly, nutritional assessment needs to move beyond static measurements and statistical manipulations to the evaluation of cell and organ functions in relation to nutritional status (119).

Although improved nutritional status is a legitimate objective in itself, in most cases it will not justify the potential morbidity and expense of perioperative enteral or parenteral feeding unless there are convincing data showing a reduction in postoperative complications or death.

In the preoperative period, nutritional support (enteral or parenteral) should be considered in two settings. First, given the high morbidity and mortality associated with preoperative malnutrition, malnutrition cannot be allowed to develop or progress during preoperative starvation of patients who cannot undergo immediate surgery or for whom bowel rest is indicated. This is the case for benign esophageal stenosis, radiation enteritis, acute inflammatory bowel diseases, acute pancreatitis, gastrointestinal and pancreatic fistulas, etc. There is no firm agreement as to how long a patient can starve before significant nutritional deficits develop. On the basis of the current literature and our own experience, it seems reasonable to provide nutritional support in these circumstances (if possible at home via the enteral route) when preoperative starvation is likely to exceed 4 or 5 days in an unstressed patient, or 3 or 4 days in a stressed patient.

Second, numerous clinical studies have attempted to define the efficacy of nutritional support (usually parenteral) in patients who can undergo operation immediately but who have severe preexisting nutritional deficits. The issue is to determine whether preoperative nutritional support is warranted even if it necessitates delaying the operation. These studies have been cautiously reviewed in two recent sophisticated meta-analyses (76, 133) (Fig. 3.12). Despite multiple methodological biases and the wide heterogeneity of the data, both of these reviews found a potential benefit of preoperative support *in severely malnourished patients* undergoing major surgery (particularly for gastrointestinal cancer), but the data were not conclusive. They also seemed to rule out any benefit in well-nourished patients. Existing published studies do not provide conclusive data concerning patients with mild to moderate malnutrition.

A recent Veterans Administration cooperative trial addressed the issue of efficacy in this patient population (240). Definitive results have been recently published (233) and show that the incidence of major noninfectious complications (such as anastomotic leak) was reduced only in moderately to severely malnourished patients who received 7–15 days of preoperative TPN prior to major abdominal or noncardiac thoracic procedures. In contrast, there was a substantially higher infection rate (pneumonia, wound infections, etc.) in patients who received preoperative TPN, independently of catheter-related sepsis. Finally, only in the small subset of severely malnourished patients (the worst 5–6% of the population studied), the substantial improvement in noninfectious complications outweighed the minimal increase in infections and yielded a substantially lower overall complication rate (26% for TPN patients versus 47% for control patients). This confirms that surgery should be delayed for perioperative nutritional support only in this limited subgroup of patients.

Postoperative Nutritional Support

Data are limited with regard to the circumstances when nutritional support should be provided in the postoperative period (152). The objective of such support is to minimize nutritional deterioration during the period of mandatory postoperative ileus and/or in those normal and moderately malnourished patients exposed to a high risk of complications. The period before clinically significant malnutrition develops will clearly depend on the preoperative nutritional status.

Although definitive studies are lacking (152), the guidelines published by the American Society of Parenteral and Enteral Nutrition provide a reasonable approach to postoperative nutritional support (12).

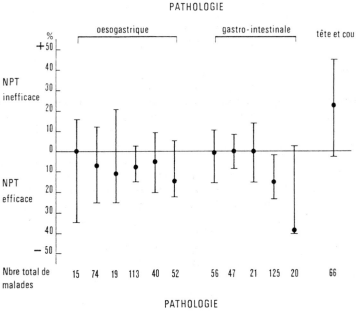

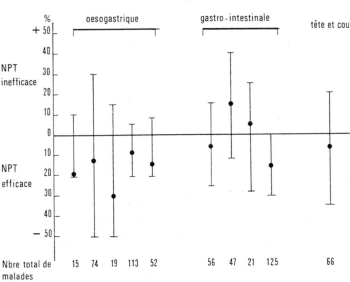

Figure 3.12. Comparison of the rates of fatal outcomes *(top)* and complications *(bottom)* in the main randomized controlled studies of perioperative nutritional support in major surgery. Absolute differences between the rate for the control group and the rate for the group receiving total parental nutrition (NPT) are indicated by ●, with 95% confidence intervals for these differences. Note that two studies did not report the number of complications. (From Nitenberg G, Misset B, Escudier B, et al. L'assistance nutritionnelle péri-opératoire en chirurgie digestive. Approche rationnelle, méthodologique et économique. In: Belghiti J, ed. Chirurgie digestive et réanimation. Paris: Masson, 1989:57–82.)

These guidelines recommend nutritional support (via the enteral route when feasible) following major surgery if adequate oral intake is not anticipated within 7–10 days. If the patient is severely catabolic or if severe preoperative malnutrition is present, the guidelines recommend support when 7 days of postoperative starvation is anticipated.

In these settings, protein-sparing therapy for preservation of endogenous protein stores appears reasonable (207). The potential advantage of this practice is that volume infused can be minimized and central venous access may not be required. Amino acids alone seem to be the most effective of the single-modality therapies for postoperative patients, producing nitrogen equilibrium in many studies of postoperative patients (207). However, limited data suggest that amino acids alone do not significantly enhance the nutritional status of patients who are more highly catabolic. Glucose alone reduces nitrogen losses but is progressively less effective with increasing degrees of stress.

TPN or, preferably, immediate postoperative EN via a jejunostomy catheter (205, 232) is thus recommended after major operations and, obviously, when complications occur (Fig. 3.7). The caloric requirements, the proportion of fuel administered as glucose or lipid, as well as the protein needs, clearly depend on the nutritional status and on the degree of stress; this point has been extensively reviewed. For EN, some recent data appear to give a substantial metabolic advantage to oligopeptide diets in comparison with whole-protein diets (254).

MULTIPLE ORGAN FAILURE

Multiple organ failure is characterized by an association of respiratory, hepatic, renal, cardiac, intestinal, and neurological failures combined with a hyperkinetic, hypermetabolic, and hypercatabolic state (49, 52). Classically, these failures occur in a cascade following the initial insult, be it infectious, traumatic, or inflammatory—in the broad sense of the term—and the usual sequence is ARDS, liver failure, and acute kidney failure. The association of at least two organ system failures, regardless of the chronology, is classified as multiple organ failure; this syndrome is therefore considered more as the consequence of progress in the treatment of shock and single organ failure with the resulting decrease in the rate of early death, than as a pathological entity in its own right. The main interest of the multiple organ failure concept is that it provides a relatively homogenous approach to the consequences of acute stress, with inflammatory cell activation (macrophages, lymphocytes, and polymorphonuclear neutrophils) at both the local and systemic level, in response to stimuli engendered by infection, the neuroendocrine system, and mediators such as tumor necrosis factor, as well as the induction of generalized abnormalities in endothelial cell function and microcirculation (55, 155).

Metabolic and nutritional support in multiple organ failure must be approached within a dynamic context, which can change at any time. Shock or acute insult gives way to a stabilization with a hypermetabolic and hyperkinetic state, followed by a phase of recuperation or, on the contrary, a degradation leading to irreversible multiple organ failure (49). Within this continuum, it is important to note that most data concerning nutrition and metabolism in this setting concern only stabilized hypermetabolic states; there have been few experimental or clinical studies on the acute phase, due to a lack of investigative methods. If one simplifies the situation and envisages the three periods one by one, it must be borne in mind that a given patient will not necessarily follow the course anticipated, and one must be ready to adapt rapidly to any changes in clinical status that may occur.

The metabolic and nutritional approach of the early phase and of the hypermetabolic phase following aggression have been discussed above. The hypermetabolic-hypercatabolic state constitutes a watershed for the patient. Either the clinical course is favorable and leaves the patient in a state of destruction (at the muscular level, inter alia), which can be quite impressive and require lengthy convalescence and "simple" nutritional support (outside the scope of this chapter), with a progressive return to anabolic processes, or multiple organ failure develops, usually in association with a fibrotic process and ARDS. The transition to multiple organ failure is generally irreversible and is usually preceded by the onset of hepatic and renal failure (49). At the metabolic level, there is a sudden or progressive reduction in energy consumption, together with the onset of a hyperkinetic state, hepatic lipid synthesis, a reduction in triglyceride clearance due to the inhibition of muscular and fatty tissue lipoprotein lipase (172), hyperglycemia with insulin resistance (which precedes terminal hypoglycemia) and hyperlactacidemia of mixed origin (143). In the terminal phase, hepatic and muscular synthesis are virtually nil, overall catabolism augments and exogenous amino acids only serve to increase ureagenesis, with a more rapid increase in blood nitrogen levels and the onset of functional then organic renal failure. At this stage, therapeutic (including nutritional) intervention is useless and death is inevitable.

CONCLUSION

There is at present no specific nutritional or metabolic support for critically ill patients. All our efforts must be concentrated on the immediate treatment of the triggering factor and precise and well-adapted symptomatic treatments.

The main preoccupation in the initial phase of stress is the maintenance of hemodynamic status, together with local and systemic oxygen supplies; metabolic (nutritional) support is required as soon as the patient's condition has stabilized in order to prevent severe postinsult malnutrition. It is clear that, in the present state of the art, such "metabolic support," in conjunction with other supportive care, can only help to gain time. Some principles have emerged from conventional nutrition, based on improved—though still incomplete—knowledge of postinsult hypermetabolism. These include the restriction of energy supplies (both carbohydrates and lipids); careful increase in nitrogen supply; and prevention of cellular deficiencies in electrolytes (phosphorus,

magnesium), trace elements (zinc, selenium), and vitamins (E, K). There remain disagreements and unknowns in conventional nutrition, e.g., the amount and nature of the nitrogen supply, or the risk/benefit ratio of lipids in severe sepsis. There is an enormous lack of information with regard to well-conducted prospective clinical trials in which the only therapeutic variable is the nutritional support and in which the judgment criteria include not only the improvement of nutritional parameters, but also morbidity and mortality. The selection and stratification of the patients in the rare acceptable studies suffer from the absence in usual severity indices (SAPS, APACHE, and OSF) of metabolic parameters that might have real weight in these settings (51, 57). This could partly explain the disagreement on the results obtained (114, 256).

Metabolic support of the critical care patient in general is at a watershed; only the future can tell if the change from traditional therapeutic support to specific nutrition of an organ or a function will find practical applications. Nutritional pharmacology, aimed at immunomodulation and/or antiinflammatory effects, together with the consideration of the gastrointestinal tract as a key organ in stress, are the major axes of such an approach. For example, this should enable the various components of multiple organ failure to be viewed as the "exploded" cellular response to insult and to reperfusion phenomena, and to envisage the integrated and possibly unified management of multiple organ failure.

References

1. Abel RM. Nutritional support and the cardiac patient. In: Rombeau JL, Caldwell MD, eds. Parenteral feeding (Clinical nutrition; v. 2). Philadelphia: WB Saunders, 1986:575–585.
2. Abel RM, Beck CH, Abbott WM, et al. Improved survival from acute renal failure after treatment with intravenous essential L amino acids and glucose. N Engl J Med 1973;233:696–699.
3. Abitbol JL, Nitenberg G, Fuerxer F, et al. Effects of varying intake of total parenteral nutrition in bone marrow transplant recipients. A randomized prospective trial [Abstract]. Clin Nutr 1989;8(supp):70a.
4. Albers S, Wernerman J, Stehle P. Availability of amino acids supplied intravenously in healthy

man as synthetic dipeptides: kinetic evaluation of L-alanyl-L-glutamine and glycyl-L-tyrosine. Clin Sci 1988;75:463–468.

5. Alden PB, Svingen BA, Johnson SB, et al. Partial correction by exogenous lipid of abnormal patterns of polyunsaturated fatty acids in plasma phospholipids of stressed and septic surgical patients. Surgery 1986;100:671–678.

6. Alexander JW, Gonce SJ, Miskell PW, et al. A new model for studying nutrition in peritonitis: the adverse effect of over-feeding. Ann Surg 1989;209:334–340.

7. Alexander JW, Gottschlich MM. Nutritional immunomodulation in burn patients. Crit Care Med 1990;18:149–153.

8. Alexander JW, Peck MD. Future prospects for adjunctive therapy: pharmacologic and nutritional approaches to immune system modulation. Crit Care Med 1990;18:159–164.

9. Alverdy JC, Burke D. Influence of nutrient administration on the structure and function of the small intestine. Probl Gen Surg 1991;8:111–117.

10. Alverdy JC, Ayos E, Moss G. Total parenteral nutrition promotes bacterial translocation from the gut. Surgery 1988;104:185–190.

11. Alvestrand A, Ahlberg M, Bergstrom J, et al. The effect of nutritional regimens on branched chain amino acid antagonism in uremia. In: Metabolism and clinical implications of branched chain amino and keto acids. Walser M, Williamson JR, eds. New York: Elsevier/North-Holland, 1981:605–613.

12. American Society of Parenteral and Enteral Nutrition Board of Directors. Guidelines for use of total parenteral nutrition in the hospitalized patient. JPEN 1986;10:441–445.

13. Arora D, Rochester DF. Effect of body weight and muscularity on human diaphragm muscle mass, thickness and area. J Appl Physiol 1982;52:64–70.

14. Askanazi J, Carpentier YA, Elwyn DH, et al. Influence of total parenteral nutrition on fuel utilization in injury and sepsis. Ann Surg 1980;191:40–45.

15. Askanazi J, Nordenstrom J, Rosenbaum SH, Elwyn DH, Hyman AI, Carpentier YA. Nutrition for the patient with respiratory failure: glucose vs fat. Anesthesiology 1981;54:373–377.

16. Aubier M, Murciano D, Lecocqguic Y, et al. Effects of hypophosphatemia on diaphragmatic contractility in patients with acute respiratory failure. N Engl J Med 1985;313:420–424.

17. Aubier M, Vires N, Syllie G, et al. Respiratory muscle contribution to lactic acidosis in low cardiac output. Am Rev Respir Dis 1982;126:648–652.

18. Bach AC, Frey A, Lutz O. Clinical and experimental effects of medium-chain-triglyceride-based fat emulsions—a review. Clin Nutr 1989;8:223–235.

19. Baker JP, Detsky AS, Stewart S, Whitvel IJ, Marliss EB, Jeejeebhoy KN. Randomized trial of total parenteral nutrition in critically ill patients: metabolic effects of varying glucose-lipid ratios as the energy source. Gastroenterology 1984;87:53–59.

20. Ball MJ, White K. Metabolic effects of intravenous medium and long chain triacylglycerols in critically ill patients. Clin Sci 1989;76:165–170.

21. Barlett RH, Dechert RE, Mault JR, Ferguson SK, Kaiser AM, Erlandson EE. Measurement of metabolism in multiple organ failure. Surgery 1987;92:771–779.

22. Bassili HR, Deitel M. Effect of nutritional support on weaning patients off mechanical ventilators. JPEN 1981;5:161–163.

23. Beck RR, Abel FL. Effect of ibuprofen on the course of canine endotoxin shock. Circ Shock 1987;23:59–70.

24. Bessey PQ, Wilmore DW. The burned patient. In: Kinney JM, Jeejeebhoy KN, Hill GL, et al, eds. Nutrition and metabolism in patient care. Philadelphia: WB Saunders, 1988:672–700.

25. Beylot M, Guiraud M, Grau G, Bouletreau P. Regulation of ketone body flux in septic patients. Am J Physiol 1989;15:E665–E674.

26. Billiar TP, Bankey PE, Svingen BA, et al. Fatty acid intake and Kupffer cell function: fish oil alters eicosanoid and monokine production to endotoxin stimulation. Surgery 1988;104:343–349.

27. Birkhahn RH, Long CL, Fitkin DL, et al. A comparison of skeletal trauma and surgery on the ketosis of starvation in man. J Trauma 1981;21:513–519.

28. Birkhahn RH, Long CL, Fitkin D, et al. Effects of major skeletal trauma or whole body protein turnover in man measured by $L^{1,14}C$-leucine. Surgery 1980;88:294–300.

29. Black PR, Brooks DC, Bessey PQ. Mechanisms of insulin resistance following injury. Ann Surg 1982;196:420–435.

30. Blumberg A, Keller G. Oxygen consumption during hemodialysis. Nephron 1979;23:276–279.

31. Boles JM, Garre MA, Youinon PY, et al. Nutritional status in intensive care patients: evaluation in 84 unselected patients. Crit Care Med 1983;11:87–90.

32. Boulier A, Fricker J, Thomasset AL, Apfelbaum M. Fat-free mass estimation by the two electrode impedance method. Am J Clin Nutr 1990;52:581–585.

33. Bower RH. A unique enteral formula as adjunctive therapy for septic and critically ill patients. Multicenter study: design and rationale. Nutrition 1990;6:92–95.

34. Bower RH, Fischer JE. Hepatic indications for parenteral nutrition. In: Rombeau JL, Caldwell MD, eds. Parenteral feeding (Clinical nutrition; v. 2). Philadelphia: WB Saunders, 1986:602–614.

35. Bower RH, Muggia-Sullam M, Vallgren S, Fisher J. Branched chain amino acid-enriched solutions in the septic patient: a randomized prospective trial. Ann Surg 1986;203:13–21.

36. Brennan MF, Cerra F, Dalyu JM, et al. Report of a research workshop: branched chain amino acids in stress and injury. JPEN 1986;10:446–452.

37. Brinson RR, Pitts WM. Enteral nutrition in the critically ill patient: role of hypoalbuminemia. Crit Care Med 1989;17:367–370.

38. Brinson RR, Kolts BE. Diarrhea associated with severe hypoalbuminemia: a comparison of a peptide-based chemically defined diet and standard

enteral alimentation. Crit Care Med 1988;16:130–136.

39. Bronsveld W, Bos GC, Thijs LG. Use of glucose-insulin-potassium (GIK) in human septic shock. Crit Care Med 1985;13:566–570.

40. Burke DJ, Alverdy JC, Aoys E, Moss GS. Glutamine-supplemented total parenteral nutrition improves gut immune function. Arch Surg 1989;124:1396–1399.

41. Burke JF, Wolfe RR, Mullany CJ, Matthews DE, Bier DM. Glucose requirements following burn injury. Ann Surg 1979;190:274–285.

42. Burns HGJ, ed. Nutritional support. Baillière's clinical gastroenterology. 1988;2:715–954.

43. Bursztein S. Methods of measurement and interpretation of indirect calorimetry. In: Bursztein S, Elwyn DH, Askanazi J, Kinney JM, eds. Energy metabolism, indirect calorimetry and nutrition. Baltimore: Williams & Wilkins, 1989:173–209.

44. Buse MG, Reid SS. Leucine: a possible regulator of protein turnover in muscle. J Clin Invest 1975;56:1250–1261.

45. Bynoe RP, Kudsk KA, Fabian TC, Brown RO. Nutrition support in trauma patients. Nutr Clin Pract 1988;137–144.

46. Casper K, Matthews D, Heymsfield S. Overfeeding: cardiovascular and metabolic response during continuous formula infusion in adult humans. Am J Clin Nutr 1990;52:602–609.

47. Cerra F, Blackburn G, Hirsch J, et al. The effect of stress level, amino acid formula, and nitrogen dose on nitrogen retention in traumatic and septic stress. Ann Surg 1987;205:282–287.

48. Cerra FB, Alden PB, Negro F, et al. Clinical sepsis, endogenous and exogenous lipid modulation. JPEN 1988;12:S63–S69.

49. Cerra FB. Hypermetabolism organ failure syndrome: a metabolic response to injury. In: Charbonneau P, ed. Le syndrome de défaillance multiviscérale. Paris: Expansion Scientifique, 1991:47–55.

50. Cerra FB, Mazuski J, Teasley K, et al. Nitrogen retention in critically ill patients is proportional to the branched chain amino acid load. Crit Care Med 1983;11:775–778.

51. Cerra FB, Negro F, Adams A. Apache II score does not predict MOF or mortality in postoperative surgery patients. Arch Surg 1990;125:519–522.

52. Cerra FB, Holman RT, Bankey PE, Mazusky JE. Nutritional pharmacology: its role in the hypermetabolism-organ failure syndrome. Crit Care Med 1990;18:S154–S158.

53. Cerra FB, McPherson JP, Konstantinides FN, Konstantinides NN, Teasley KM. Enteral nutrition does not prevent multiple organ failure syndrome (MOFS) after sepsis. Surgery 1988;104:727–733.

54. Cerra FB, Shronts EP, Raup S, Konstantinides N. Enteral nutrition in hypermetabolic surgical patients. Crit Care Med 1989;17:619–622.

55. Cerra FB, West M, Keller G, Mazuski J, Simmons RL. Hypermetabolism/organ failure: the role of the activated macrophage as a metabolic regulator. Prog Clin Biol Res 1988;264:27–42.

56. Chandra RK. Nutrition, immunity and infection: present knowledge and future directions. Lancet 1983;1:688–691.

57. Chang RW, Lee B, Jacobs S. Identifying ICU patients who would not benefit from total parenteral nutrition. JPEN 1989;13:535–538.

58. Chen MK, Souba WW, Copeland EM. Nutritional support of the surgical oncology patient. Hematol Oncol Clin North Am 1991;5:125–145.

59. Chiarelli A, Enzi G, Casadei A, Baggio B, Valerio A, Mazzoleni F. Very early nutrition supplementation in burned patients. Am J Clin Nutr 1990;52:1035–1039.

60. Christou NV, Tellado Rodriguez J, Chartrand L, et al. Estimating mortality risk in preoperative patients using immunologic, nutritional, and acute phase response variables. Ann Surg 1989;69–77.

61. Cochran W, Fiorotto M, Ping Sheng H, et al. Reliability of fat-free mass estimates derived from total body electrical conductivity measurements as influenced by changes in extracellular fluid volume. Am J Clin Nutr 1989;49:29–32.

62. Constans T, Bacq Y, Bertrand P, et al. The American anthropometric norms are not suitable to assess the nutritional status of a French population. Am J Clin Nutr 1990;93:163–167.

63. Corriol O. Les solutés injectables d'acides aminés pour nutrition parentérale; critères de choix pharmaceutiques. Nutr Clin Metabol 1987;1:17–30.

64. Cuthbertson DP. Post traumatic metabolism: a multidisciplinary challenge. Surg Clin North Am 1978;58:1045–1054.

65. Cynober L. Amino acid metabolism in thermal burns. JPEN 1989;13:196–205.

66. Cynober L. Ornithine α-ketoglutarate in nutritional support. Nutrition 1991;7 (in press).

67. Dahn MS, Lange P, Mitchell RA, Lobdell K, Wilson RF. Insulin production following injury and sepsis. J Trauma 1987;27:1031–1037.

68. Daily WH, Tonnesen AS, Allen SJ. Hypophosphatemia. Incidence, etiology and prevention in the trauma patient. Crit Care Med 1990;18:1210–1214.

69. Dark D, Pingleton SK, Kerby GR. Hypercapnia during weaning a complication of nutritional support. Chest 1985;88:141–143.

70. Darmaun D. Métabolisme de la glutamine in vivo chez l'homme: implications pour la nutrition artificielle. Nutr Clin Metabol 1990;4:203–214.

71. Davenport A, Roberts N. Amino acid losses during continuous high flux hemofiltration in the critically ill patient. Crit Care Med 1989;17:1010–1014.

72. Davies AO, Samuelson WM. Assessing redox status in human plasma: experiences in critically ill patients. Crit Care Med 1986;14:942–946.

73. Defronzo RA, Felip P. Amino acid metabolism in uremia. Insights gained from normal and diabetic man. Symposium on nutrition in renal disease. Am J Clin Nutr 1980;33:1978–1986.

74. Deitch EA. The role of intestinal barrier failure and bacterial translocation in the development of systemic infection and multiple organ failure. Arch Surg 1990;125:403–404.

75. Delafosse B, Bouffard Y, Bertrand O, Viale JP, Annat G, Motin J. Effects of protein intake on

pulmonary gas exchange and ventilatory drive in postoperative patients. Anesthesiology 1989;70:26–29.

76. Detsky AS, Baker JP, O'Rourke K, et al. Perioperative parenteral nutrition: a meta-analysis. Ann Intern Med 1987;107:195–203.

77. Donahue SP, Phillips L. Response of IGF-1 to nutritional support in malnourished hospital patients; a possible indicator of short term changes in nutritional status. Am J Clin Nutr 1989;50:962–969.

78. Elwyn DH. Protein metabolism and requirements in the critically ill patient. Crit Care Clin 1987;3:57–69.

79. Ephgrave KS, Kleiman-Wexler RL, Adair CG. Enteral nutrients prevent stress ulceration and increase intragastric volume. Crit Care Med 1990;18:621–624.

80. Escudier B, Escudier E, Mina E, et al. Effects of intralipid and heparin on neutrophil (PMN) functions during total parenteral nutrition (TPN) [Abstract]. Clin Nutr 1986;5(suppl):41a.

81. Escudier E, Escudier B, Henry-Amar M, et al. Effects of infused intralipids on neutrophil chemotaxis during total parenteral nutrition. JPEN 1986;10:596–598.

82. Feinstein EI, Blumenkrantz MJ, Healy M, et al. Clinical and metabolic responses to parenteral nutrition in acute renal failure. Medicine 1981;60:124–137.

83. Feinstein EI, Kopple JD, Siberman H, et al. Total parenteral nutrition with high or low nitrogen intakes in patients with acute renal failure. Kidney Int 1983;26:S319–S323.

84. Fiaccadori E, DelCanale S, Coffrini E, et al. Muscle and serum magnesium in pulmonary intensive care unit patients. Crit Care Med 1988;16:751–753.

85. Fields S, Kelly SM, Macklem PT. The oxygen cost of breathing with cardiorespiratory disease. Am Rev Respir Dis 1982;126:9–13.

86. Fischer JE. A teleological view of sepsis. Clin Nutr 1991;10:1–9.

87. Fisher JE, Baldessarini JR. False neurotransmitters and hepatic failure. Lancet ii;1971:75–80.

88. Fleming R. Trace element metabolism in adult patients requiring total parenteral nutrition. Am J Clin Nutr 1989;49:573–579.

89. Fong Y, Marano MA, Barber A, et al. Total parenteral nutrition and bowel rest modify the metabolic response to endotoxin in humans. Ann Surg 1989;210:449–457.

90. Fourtanier G, Prevost F, Lacaine F, et al. Etat nutritionnel des malades atteints d'un cancer digestif. Valeur pronostique pré-opératoire. Gastroenterol Clin Biol 1987;11:748–752.

91. François G, ed. Nutrition artificielle de l'adulte en réanimation. Paris: Masson, 1986.

92. Fraser CL, Arieff AI. Hepatic encephalopathy. N Engl J Med 1985;313:865–873.

93. Frayn KN. L'insulino-résistance en nutrition artificielle. Nutr Clin Metab 1988;2:76–82.

94. Fried R, Levy M, Andrew B, et al. Wernicke's encephalopathy in the intensive care patient. Crit Care Med 1990;18:779–780.

95. Giordano C. Amino acids and ketoacids, advan-

tages and pitfalls. Am J Clin Nutr 1980;33:1649–1653.

96. Giordano C. The use of exogenous and endogenous urea for protein synthesis in normal and uremic subjects. J Lab Clin Med 1963;62: 231–246.

97. Gottdiener JS, Gross HA, Henry WI, et al. Cardiac abnormalities in cachetic patients before and during nutritional repletion. Am Heart J 1978;58:425–433.

98. Gottschlich MM, Warden GD, Michel MA, et al. Diarrhea in tube fed patients. Incidence, etiology, nutritional impact and prevention. JPEN 1988;12:338–345.

99. Grant JP, Cox CE, Kleinman LM, et al. Serum hepatic enzyme and bilirubin elevations during parenteral nutrition. Surg Gynecol Obstet 1977;145:573–580.

100. Greig PD, Elwyn DN, Askanazi J, Kinney JM. Parenteral nutrition in septic patients: effect of increasing nitrogen intake. Am J Clin Nutr 1987;46:1040–1047.

101. Grimble G, Payne-James JJ, Rees R, Silk DBA. Enteral nutrition: novel substrates. Intensive Ther Clin Monitoring 1989;10:51–57.

102. Grube BJ, Heimbach DM, Marvin JA. Clostridium difficile diarrhea in critically ill burned patients. Arch Surg 1987;122:655–661.

103. Guthrie R, Hines C. Use of intravenous albumin in the critically ill patient. Am J Gastroenterol 1991;86:255–263.

104. Hammarqvist F, Wernerman J, Von der Decken A, et al. Alpha ketoglutarate preserves protein synthesis and free glutamine in skeletal muscle after surgery. Surgery 1991:28–36.

105. Hammarqvist F, Wernerman J, Von der Decken A, Vinnars E. Alanyl-glutamine counteracts the depletion of free glutamine and the postoperative decline in protein synthesis in skeletal muscle. Ann Surg 1990;212:637–644.

106. Harris JA, Benedict FG. A biometric study of basal metabolism in man. Carnegie Institute of Washington publication. Washington, DC, 1919: No. 279.

107. Hasselgren PO, Hall-Angeras M, Angeras U. Cytokines et régulation de la protéolyse musculaire au cours des états septiques. Nutr Clin Metab 1990;4:99–104.

108. Hasselgren PO, James JH, Warner BW, Hummel RP, Fischer JE. Protein synthesis and degradation in skeletal muscle from septic rats: response to leucine and α-ketoisocaproic acid. Arch Surg 1988;203:360–365.

109. Herskowitz K, Souba WW. Intestinal glutamine metabolism during critical illness: a surgical perspective. Nutrition 1990;6:199–206.

110. Hervé P, Simonneau G, Girard P, et al. Hypercapnic acidosis induced by nutrition in mechanically ventilated patients; glucose versus fat. Crit Care Med 1985;13:537–540.

111. Heymsfield SB, Hill JO, Evert M, Casper K, DiGirolamo M. Energy expenditure during continuous intragastric infusion of fuel. Am J Clin Nutr 1987;45:526–533.

112. Hiraide A, Katayama M, Sugimoto H, et al. Effect of 3-hydroxybutyrate on posttraumatic metabolism in man. Surgery 1991:176–181.

113. Hirasawa H, Sugai T, Ohtake Y, Inaba H, Aoe T, Shiga H. Metabolic abnormalities and nutritional management in postoperative multiple organ failure. Nippon Geka Gakkai Zasshi 1988;89:1351–1354.

114. Hopefl AW, Taaffe CL, Herrmann VM. Failure of APACHE II alone as a predictor of mortality in patients receiving total parenteral nutrition. Crit Care Med 1989;17:414–417.

115. Horwill CA, Geeseman R, Boileau RA, et al. Total body electrical conductivity (TOBEC): relationship to estimates of muscle mass, fat-free, and lean body mass. Am J Clin Nutr 1989;49:593–598.

116. Ingenbleek Y, Carpentier YA. A prognostic inflammatory and nutritional index scoring critically ill patients. Int J Vitam Nutr Res 1985;55:91–101.

117. Jaksic T, Blackburn GL. Nutritional support. In: Clowes GHA, ed. Trauma, sepsis and shock. The physiological basis of therapy. New York and Basel: Marcel Dekker, 1988:493–526.

118. Jastrend C, Berghelm X, Lahnborg G. Human granulocyte and reticuloendothelial cell function during intralipid infusion JPEN 1987;2663–2670.

119. Jeejeebhoy KN, Detsky AS, Baker JP. Assessment of nutritional status. JPEN 1990;14:193–199.

120. Jeevanandam M, Grote-Holman E, Chikenji T, Askanazi J, Elwyn DH, Kinney JM. Effects of glucose on fuel utilization and glycerol turnover in normal and injured man. Crit Care Med 1990;18:125–135.

121. Jeevanandam M, Young DH, Schiller WR. Influence of parenteral nutrition on rates of net substrate oxidation in severe trauma patients. Crit Care Med 1990;18:467–473.

122. Jensen GL, Mascioli EA, Seidner DL, et al. Parenteral infusion of long and medium chain triglycerides and reticulo-endothelial system function in man. JPEN 1990;14:467–471.

123. Johnson RA, Baker SS, Fallon JT, et al. An occidental case of cardiomyopathy and selenium deficiency. N Engl J Med 1981;304:1210–1212.

124. Johnson RC, Young SK, Cotter R, Lin L, Rowe WB. Medium-chain-triglyceride lipid emulsion: metabolism and tissue distribution. Am J Clin Nutr 1990;52:502–508.

125. Just B, Messing B, Darmaun D, Rongier M, Camillo E. Comparison of substrate utilization by indirect calorimetry during cyclic and continuous total parenteral nutrition. Am J Clin Nutr 1990;51:107–111.

126. Ke J, Tam YK, Koo WWK, Gray MR, Coutts RT. Effects of parenteral nutrition on hepatic elimination of lidocaine. A study using the isolated perfused rat liver. J Pharmacol Exp Ther 1990;255:351–356.

127. Kelley DS, Branch LB, Love JE, Taylor PC, Rivera YM, Iacono JM. Dietary α-linolenic acid and immunocompetence in humans. Am J Clin Nutr 1991;53:40–46.

128. Kelly TWJ, Patrick MR, Hillman KM, et al. Study of diarrhea in critically ill patients. Crit Care Med 1983;11:7–9.

129. Kinney JM. Clinical biochemistry. Implications for nutritional support. JPEN 1990;14:148–156.

130. Kinsella JE, Lokesh B. Dietary lipids, eicosanoids, and the immune system. Crit Care Med 1989;18:94–113.

131. Kirk SJ, Barbul A. Role of arginine in trauma, sepsis and immunity JPEN 1990;14:226S–229S.

132. Kirvela O, Singer P, Askanazi J, Kvetan V. Metabolism in the intensive care unit. Baillière's Clinical Anaesthesiology 1989;3:423–446.

133. Klein S, Simes J, Blackburn GL. Total parenteral nutrition and cancer clinical trials. Cancer 1986;58:1378–1386.

134. Kopple JD, Swendseid ME, Shinaberger JH, et al. The free and bound amino acids removed by hemodialysis. Trans Am Soc Artif Intern Organs 1979;19:309–313.

135. Koretz RL. What supports nutritional support? Dig Dis Sci 1984;29:577–588.

136. Koruda MJ, Rolandelli RH, Settle RG, et al. The effect of pectin-supplemented elemental diet on intestinal adaptation to massive small bowel resection. JPEN 1986;10:343–350.

137. Koruda MJ, Rolandelli RH, Bliss DZ, Hastings J, Rombeau JL, Settle RG. Parenteral nutrition supplemented with short-chain fatty acids: effect on the small-bowel mucosa in normal rats. Am J Clin Nutr 1990;51:685–689.

138. Kulkarni AD, Fanslow WC, Rudolph FB, et al. Effect of dietary nucleotides on response to bacterial infections. JPEN 1986;10:169–171.

139. Laaban JP, Grateau G, Psychoyos I, et al. Hypophosphatemia induced by mechanical ventilation in patients with chronic obstructive pulmonary disease. Crit Care Med 1989;17:1115–1120.

140. Leander U, Furst P, Vesterberg K, Vinnars E. Nitrogen sparing effect of Ornicetil in the immediate postoperative state. Clinical biochemistry and nitrogen balance. Clin Nutr 1985;4:43–51.

141. Lenssen P, Cheney C. Enteral feeding of the immunocompromised patient. In: Rombeau JL, Caldwell MD, eds. Enteral and tube feeding (Clinical nutrition; v. 1). Philadelphia: WB Saunders, 1990:361–385.

142. Leverve X, Guignier M, Carpentier F, Serre JC, Caravel JP. Effect of parenteral nutrition on muscle amino-acid output and 3-methylhistidine excretion in septic patients. Metabolism 1984;33:471–477.

143. Leverve X, Guignier M. Role du lactate dans le métabolisme intermédiaire. Intérêt en réanimation. Rean Soins Intens Med Urg 1990;6:491–500.

144. Levinson MR, Groeger JS, Jeevanandam M, Brennan MF. Free fatty acid turnover and lipolysis in septic mechanically ventilated cancer-bearing humans. Metabolism 1988;37:618–625.

145. Liaw KY, Askanazi J, Michelson CB, Kantrowitz LR, Furst P, Kinney JM. Effect of injury and sepsis on high-energy phosphates in muscle and red cells. J Trauma 1980;20:755–759.

146. Long CL, Schaffel N, Geiger JW, et al. Metabolic response to injury and illness: estimation of

energy and protein needs from indirect calorimetry and nitrogen balance. JPEN 1979;452–456.

147. Long CL, Spencer JL, Kinney JM, et al. Carbohydrate metabolism in man: effect of elective operations and major injury. J Appl Physiol 1971;31:110–116.

148. Long CL, Lowry SF. Hormonal regulation of protein metabolism. JPEN 1990;14:555–562.

149. Long CL, Nelson KM, Akin JM, Merick HW, Blakemore WS. A physiologic basis for the provision of fuel mixtures in normal and stressed patients. J Trauma 1990;9:1077–1086.

150. Lowry SF. The route of feeding influences injury responses. J Trauma 1990;30:10–15.

151. Lundhom K, Bennegard K, Wickstorm I, et al. Is it possible to evaluate the efficacy of aminoacid solution after major surgical procedures or accidental injuries? Evaluation in a randomized prospective study. JPEN 1986;10:29–33.

152. Lundholm K, Sandstrom R, Drott C, et al. The effect of post-operative intravenous feeding (TPN) on outcome following major surgery evaluated in a randomized study [Abstract]. Clin Nutr 1991;10(suppl 2):1a.

153. Makk LJK, Mcclave SA, Creech PW, et al. Clinical application of the metabolic cart to the delivery of total parenteral nutrition. Crit Care Med 1990;18:1320–1327.

154. Mault JR, Dechert RE, Barlett RH, et al. Oxygen consumption during hemodialysis for acute renal failure. Trans Am Soc Artif Intern Organs 1982;28:510–513.

155. Mazuski JE, Platt JL, West MA, et al. Direct effects of endotoxin on hepatocytes. Arch Surg 1988;123:340–344.

156. McDonald S, Sharp C, Deitch E. Immediate enteral feeding in burn patients is safe and effective. Ann Surg 1991;213:177–183.

157. Mirtallo JM, Kudsk KA, Ebbert ML. Nutritional support of patients with renal disease. Clin Pharm 1984;3:253–263.

158. Mirtallo JM. Assessing the nutritional needs of the critically ill patient. Ann Pharmacol 1990;24:20–23.

159. Mirtallo JM, Schneider PJ, Marko K, et al. A comparison of essential and general amino acids infusions in the nutritional support of patients with compromised renal function. JPEN 1982;6:109–114.

160. Mizock BA. Branch-chained amino acids in sepsis and hepatic failure. Arch Intern Med 1985;145:1284–1288.

161. Moore EE. Total parenteral nutrition versus total enteral nutrition or resuscitation versus nutrition? Crit Care Med 1991;19:7.

162. Moore FA, Moore EE, Jones TN, et al. TEN versus TPN following major abdominal trauma: reduced septic morbidity. J Trauma 1989;29:916–923.

163. More DG. Randomized prospective trial of cimetidine and ranitidine for control of intragastric pH in the critically ill. Surgery 1985;97:215–223.

164. Murray MJ, Marsh M, Wochos D, et al. Nutritional assessment of intensive care unit patients. Mayo Clin Proc 1988;63:1106–1115.

165. Naylor CD, Detsky AS, O'Rourke K, Fonberg E. Does treatment with essential amino acids and hypertonic glucose improve survival in acute renal failure? A meta-analysis. Ren Fail 1987–88;10:141–152.

166. Naylor CD. Parenteral nutrition with branched-chain amino acids in hepatic encephalopathy. A meta-analysis. Gastroenterology 1989;97:1033–1042.

167. Newsholme EA, Newsholme P, Curi R. The role of the citric acid cycle in cells of the immune system and its importance in sepsis, trauma and burns. Biochem Soc Symp 1987;54:145–161.

168. Nitenberg G, Henry-Amar M, Escudier B, et al. Nutritional and immunological assessment in oesogastric cancer is predictive of tumoral extension not of postoperative complications [Abstract]. Clin Nutr 1984;4(suppl):34a.

169. Nitenberg G, Misset B, Escudier B, et al. L'assistance nutritionnelle périopératoire en chirurgie digestive. Approche rationnelle, méthodologique et économique. In: Belghiti J, ed. Chirurgie digestive et réanimation. Paris: Masson, 1989:57–82.

170. Nitenberg G, Tandonnet F, Henry-Amar M, et al. Immediate post-operative enteral nutrition (EN) in esogastric surgery: a three years experience [Abstract]. Clin Nutr 1986;5(suppl):41a.

171. Nordenstrom J, Carpentier YA, Askanasi J, et al. Metabolic utilization of intravenous fat emulsion during total parenteral nutrition. Ann Surg 1982; 196:211–231.

172. Nordenstrom J, Carpentier YA, Askenazi J, et al. Free fatty acid mobilization and oxidation during total parenteral nutrition in trauma and sepsis. Ann Surg 1983;198:725–735.

173. Numez MC, Ayudarte MV, Morales D, Suarez MD, Gil A. Effect of dietary nucleotides on intestinal repair in rats with experimental chronic diarrhea. JPEN 1990;14:598–604.

174. Ota DM, Jessup JM, Badcock GF, et al. Immune function during intravenous administration of a soy bean emulsion. JPEN 1985;9:23–27.

175. Peck MD, Alexander JW, Gonce SJ, et al. Low protein diets improve survival from peritonitis in guinea pigs. Ann Surg 1989;209:448–454.

176. Peck MD, Ogle CK, Alexander JW, et al. The effects of dietary fatty acids on response to *Pseudomonas* infection in burned mice. J Trauma 1990;30:445–452.

177. Perez RV, Munda R, Alexander JW. Dietary immunoregulation of transfusion-induced immunosuppression. Transplantation 1988;45:614–617.

178. Phang PT, Rich T, Ronco J. A validation and comparison study of two metabolic monitors. JPEN 1990;14:259–261.

179. Pichard C, Roulet M, Schutz Y, et al. Clinical relevance of L-carnitine-supplemented total parenteral nutrition in postoperative trauma. Metabolic effects of continuous or acute carnitine administration with special reference to fat oxidation and nitrogen utilization. Am J Clin Nutr 1989;49:283–289.

180. Pittiruti M, Siegel JH, Sganga G, Coleman B, Wiles CE, Placko R. Determinants of urea nitrogen production in sepsis. Muscle catabolism,

total parenteral nutrition, and hepatic clearance of amino acids. Arch Surg 1989;124:362–372.

181. Plumley DA, Souba WW, Hautamaki RD, Martin TD, Flynn TC, Rout WR, Copeland EM. Accelerated lung amino acid release in hyperdynamic septic surgical patients. Arch Surg 1990;125:57–61.
182. Pomposelli JJ, Flores EA, Bistrian BR, et al. Role of biochemical mediators in clinical nutrition and surgical metabolism. JPEN 1988;12:212–218.
183. Pomposelli JJ, Flores EA, Hirschberg Y, Teo TC, Blackburn GL, Zeisel SH, Bistrian BR. Short term TPN containing N-3 fatty acids ameliorate lactic acidosis induced by endotoxin in guinea pigs. Am J Clin Nutr 1990;52:548–552.
184. Ponting GA, Ward HC, Halliday D, Sim AJW. Protein and energy metabolism with biosynthetic human growth hormone in patients on full intravenous nutritional support JPEN 1990; 14:437–441.
185. Pradad AS. Clinical, endocrinological and biochemical effects of zinc deficiency. Clin Endocrinol Metab 1985;14:567–589.
186. Prakash O, Meij SH. Oxygen consumption and blood gas exchange during controlled and intermittent mandatory ventilation after cardiac surgery. Crit Care Med 1985;13:556–559.
187. Proceedings of an international, glutamine symposium. Glutamine metabolism in health and disease: basic science and clinical aspects. JPEN 1990;14(suppl):40S–146S.
188. Quinn T, Askanasi J. Nutrition and cardiac disease. Crit Care Clin 1987;3:167–184.
189. Rainford DJ. Nutritional management of acute renal failure. Acta Chir Scand 1981; 507(suppl):327–329.
190. Richard C, Lemonnier F, Thibault M, Couturier M, Auzepy P. Vitamin E deficiency and lipoperoxidation during adult respiratory distress syndrome. Crit Care Med 1990;18:4–9.
191. Rime A, Mangalaboy J, Boniface M, et al. Estimation et mesure des dépenses énergétiques (EE): validation d'une formule prédictive [Abstract]. Rean Soins Intens Med Urg 1990;6: 527a.
192. Rockwell WB, Ehrlich HP. Ibuprofen in acute care therapy. Ann Surg 1990;211:78–83.
193. Rodriguez J, Askanasi J, Weissman C, et al. Ventilatory and metabolic effects of glucose infusions. Chest 1985;88:512–518.
194. Roediger WEW. Metabolic basis of starvation diarrhea. Implications for treatment. Lancet 1986;1:1082–1084.
195. Rogers WJ, Russel RO, McDaniel HG, et al. Acute effects of glucose-insulin-potassium infusion on myocardial substrates, coronary blood flow and oxygen consumption in man. Am J Cardiol 1977;40:421–428.
196. Rogers WJ, Stanley AW, Breinig JG. Reduction of hospital mortality rate of acute myocardial infarction with glucose-insulin-potassium infusion. Am Heart J 1976;92:441–454.
197. Rolandelli R, DePaula J, Guenter P, Rombeau JL. Critical illness and sepsis. In: Rombeau JL, Caldwell MD, eds. Enteral and tube feeding (Clinical nutrition; v. 1). Philadelphia: WB Saunders, 1990:288–305.
198. Rombeau JL, Caldwell MD, eds. Parenteral feeding (Clinical nutrition; v. 2). Philadelphia: WB Saunders, 1986.
199. Rombeau JL, Caldwell MD, eds. Enteral and tube feeding (Clinical nutrition; v. 1). Philadelphia: WB Saunders, 1990.
200. Rossner S, Johanssen C, Walldins G, Ally A. Intralipid clearance and lipoprotein pattern in men with advanced alcoholic liver cirrhosis. Am J Clin Nutr 1979;32:2022–2026.
201. Roulet M, Detsky AS, Marliss EB, et al. A controlled trial of the effect of parenteral nutrition support on patients with respiratory failure and sepsis. Clin Nutr 1983;2:97–105.
202. Royall D, Wolever TMS, Jeejeebhoy KN. Clinical significance of colonic fermentation. Am J Gastroenterol 1990;85:1307–1312.
203. Saba TM, Kiener JL, Holman JM. Fibronectin and the critically ill patient: current status. Int Care Med 1986;12:350–358.
204. Saito H, Trocki O, Alexander JW, et al. The effects of route of nutrient administration on the nutritional state, catabolic hormone secretion, and gut mucosal integrity after burn injury. JPEN 1986;11:1–7.
205. Sarr MG, Mayo S. Needle catheter jejunostomy: an unappreciated and misunderstood advance in the care of patients after major abdominal operations. Mayo Clin Proc 1988;63:565–572.
206. Schlichtig R, Ayres SM. Nutritional considerations for specific disease states. In: Schlichtig R, Ayres SM, eds. Nutritional support of the critically ill. Chicago: Year Book, 1988:185–209.
207. Schlichtig R, Ayres SM, eds. Nutritional support of the critically ill. Chicago: Year Book, 1988.
208. Schneeweiss B, Graninger W, Stockenhuber F, Druml W, Ferenci P, Echinger S, Grimm G, Laggner AN, Lenz K. Energy metabolism in acute and chronic renal failure. Am J Clin Nutr 1990;52:596–601.
209. Sedman PC, Ramsden CW, Brennan TG, et al. Pharmacological concentrations of lipid emulsions inhibit interleukin-2 dependent lymphocyte responses in vitro. JPEN 1990;14: 12–17.
210. Shaw JHF, Wolfe RR. Metabolic intervention in surgical patients. Ann Surg 1988;207:274–282.
211. Shaw JHF, Wolfe RR. Response to glucose and lipid infusions in sepsis: a kinetic analysis. Metabolism 1985;34:442–449.
212. Shaw JHF. Influence of stress, depletion, and/or malignant disease on the responsiveness of surgical patients to total parenteral nutrition. Am J Clin Nutr 1988;48:144–147.
213. Shaw JHF, Wildbore M, Wolfe RR. Whole body protein kinetics in severely septic patients. Ann Surg 1987;205:288–294.
214. Shetty PS, Watrasiedwicz KE, Jung RT, et al. Rapid turnover transport proteins: an index of subclinical protein energy malnutrition. Lancet 1979;2:230–232.
215. Siegel JH, Vary TC, Rivkind A, Bilik R, Coleman B, Tall BE, Morris JG. Abnormal metabolic control in the septic multiple organ failure syndrome: pharmacotherapy for altered fuel control

mechanisms. Prog Clin Biol Res 1989;308:535–543.

216. Silk DBA. Towards the optimization of enteral nutrition. Clin Nutr 1987;6:61–74.

217. Skeie B, Askanazi J, Rothkopf M, et al. Intravenous fat emulsions and lung function, Crit Care Med 1988;16:183–194.

218. Skeie B, Kvetan V, Gil KM, Rothkopf MM, Newsholme EA, Askanazi J. Branched-chain amino acids: their metabolism and clinical utility. Crit Care Med 1990;18:549–571.

219. Silverman NA, Schmitt G, Vishwanath M, et al. Effect of carnitine on myocardial function and metabolism following global ischemia. Ann Thorac Surg 1985;40:20–24.

220. Solem DD, Strate RG, Fischer JE. Antacid therapy and nutritional supplementation in the prevention of Curling's ulcer. Surg Gynecol Obstet 1979;190:189–191.

221. Souba W, Austgen T. Interorgan glutamine flow following surgery and infection. JPEN 1990;14,4:90–93.

222. Souba WW, Herskowitz K, Klimberg S, Salloum RM, Plumley DA, Flynn TC, Copeland EM. The effects of sepsis and endotoxemia on gut glutamine metabolism. Ann Surg 1990;543–555.

223. Spaeth G, Specian RD, Berg RD, Deithc EA. Bulk prevents bacterial translocation induced by the oral administration of total parenteral nutrition solution. JPEN 1990;14:442–447.

224. Spanga G, Siegel JH, Brown G, et al. Repriorization of hepatic plasma protein release in trauma and sepsis. Arch Surg 1985;120:187–199.

225. Spannhake E, Hyman AL, Kadowitz PL. Dependence of the airway and pulmonary vascular effects of arachidonic acid upon route and rate of administration. J Pharmacol Exp Ther 1980;212:584–590.

226. Stacpool PW. The pharmacology of dichloroacetate. Metabolism 1989;38:1124–1144.

227. Stehle P, Zander J, Mertes N, et al. Effect of parenteral glutamine peptide supplements on muscle glutamine loss and nitrogen balance after major surgery. Lancet 1989;1:231–233.

228. Stoner HB, Little RA, Frayn KN, Elebute AE, Tresadern J, Gross E. The effect of sepsis on the oxidation of carbohydrate and fat. Br J Surg 1983;70:32–35.

229. Swinamer D, Phang P, Jones R, et al. Effect of routine administration of analgesia on energy expenditure in critically ill patients. Chest 1988;13:4–10.

230. Takala J, Askanazi J, Weissman C, et al. Changes in respiratory control induced by amino acid infusions. Crit Care Med 1988;16:465–469.

231. Takala J. Nutrition in acute renal failure. Crit Care Clin 1987;3:155–166.

232. Tandonnet F, Nitenberg G, Henry-Amar M, et al. Immediate postoperative enteral (EN) versus parenteral nutrition (PN) in eoso-gastric surgery for cancer: a controlled prospective study [Abstract]. Clin Nutr 1985;4(suppl):103a.

233. The Veterans Affairs Total Parenteral Nutrition Cooperative Group. Perioperative total parenteral nutrition in surgical patients. N Engl J Med 1991;325:525–532.

234. Tilney NL, Lazarus JM. Acute renal failure in surgical patients, causes, clinical patterns, and care. Surg Clin North Am 1983;63:357–377.

235. Toback FG. Amino acid enhancement of renal regeneration after acute tubular necrosis. Kidney Int 1997;12:193–198.

236. Twomey P, Ziegler D, Rombeau J. Utility of skin testing in nutritional assessment: a critical review. JPEN 1982;6:50–58.

237. Van Lanshot JJB, Feenstra BWA, Vermeij CG, et al. Accuracy of intermittent metabolic gas exchange recordings extrapolated for diurnal variation. Crit Care Med 1988;16:737–742.

238. Venus B, Prager R, Patel CB, Sandoval E, Sloan P, Smith RA. Cardiopulmonary effects of intralipid infusion in critically ill patients. Crit Care Med 1988;16:587-590.

239. Vermeij CG, Feenstra BWA, van Lanschot JJB, Bruining HA. Day-to-day variability of energy expenditure in critically ill surgical patients. Crit Care Med 1989;17:623–626.

240. Veterans Administration cooperative trial of perioperative total parenteral nutrition in malnourished surgical patients. Background, rationale, and study protocol. Am J Clin Nutr 1988;47:351–391.

241. Weissman C, Askanasi J, Rosenbaum SH, et al. Amino acids and respiration. Ann Int Med 1983;98:41–43.

242. Weissman C, Kamper M, Askanazi J, Hyman AI, Kinney JM. Resting metabolic rate of the critically ill patient: measurement versus predicted. Anesthesiology 1986;64:673–679.

243. Wernerman J, Hammarqvist F, Alexandra Von der Decken, Vinnars E. Ornithine-alpha-ketoglutarate improves skeletal muscle protein synthesis as assessed by ribosome analysis and nitrogen use after surgery. Ann Surg 1987;206:674–678.

244. West MA, Billiar TR, Mazuski HE, et al. Endotoxin modulation of hepatocyte secretion and cellular protein synthesis is mediated by Kupffer cells. Arch Surg 1988;123:1400–1405.

245. Wilmore DW, Goodwin CW, Aulick LH, et al. Effect of injury and infection in visceral metabolism and circulation. Ann Surg 1980;192:491–504.

246. Wilmore DW, Smith RJ, O'Dwyer ST, Jacobs DO, Ziegler TR, Wang XD. The gut: a central organ after surgical stress. Surgery 1988;104:917–923.

247. Wilmore DW. Catabolic illness. Strategies for enhancing recovery. N Engl J Med 1991;325:695–702.

248. Wolfe RR, O'Donnell TF, Stone MD, et al. Investigation of factors determining the optimal glucose infusion rate in total parenteral nutrition. Metabolism 1980;29:892–900.

249. Wolfe RR. Carbohydrate metabolism in the critically ill patient. Crit Care Med 1987;3:11–24.

250. Wolfe RR, Herndon DN, Jahoor F, Mizashi H, Wolfe M. Effect of severe burn injury on substrate cycling by glucose and fatty acids. N Engl J Med 1987;317:403–408.

251. Wolfson M, Jones MR, Kopple JD. Amino acid losses during hemodialysis with infusion of

amino acids and glucose. Kidney Int 1982;21:500–506.

252. Yamazaki K, Maiz A, Moldawer LL, et al. Complications associated with the overfeeding of infected animals. J Surg Res 1986;40:152–158.

253. Zaloga GP, Knowles R, Black KW, Prielipp R. Total parenteral nutrition increases mortality after hemorrhage. Crit Care Med 1991;19:54–59.

254. Ziegler F, Olivier JM, Masini JP, Coudray-Lucas C, Levy E, Giboudeau J. Efficiency of enteral nitrogen support in surgical patients: small peptides vs. non-degraded proteins. Gut 1990; 31:1277–1283.

255. Ziegler TR, Young LS, Ferraribaliviera E, Demling RH, Wilmore DW. Use of human growth hormone combined with nutritional support in a critical care unit. JPEN 1990;14:574–581.

256. Zimmerman JE. Severity measurement and efficacy of nutritional support: neither success nor failure. Crit Care Med 1989;17:479–480.

4

The Role of Selective Decontamination of the Digestive Tract

Graham Ramsay
H. K. F. van Saene

The incidence of nosocomial infection in a general ward situation averages 5–10%; the infection rate in intensive care units (ICUs), however, can be as high as 36%. The incidence of unit-acquired infection increases with the length of stay and, in some units, rates exceeding 80% have been reported in long-stay patients (56). This high occurrence of infection appears to be associated with increased mortality (26) and, until recently, it was thought that infection contributed directly to multiple organ failure (MOF) in many instances (22); both of these associations are now open to debate. It has become clear that, often, critically ill patients die *with* but not *of* infection, and nonbacterial sepsis is now recognized as a trigger of MOF, a fact proven by the successful use of selective decontamination of the digestive tract (SDD) as an infection prevention regime.

A great number of factors contribute to the high acquired infection rate in ICU: severe underlying disease; extremes of age; widespread use of broad-spectrum antimicrobial agents; invasive procedures for therapy or monitoring; and an elevated gastric pH (pH > 4) often present even in the absence of therapy with antacids or H_2 receptor antagonists.

Until recently, most ICUs employed traditional infection control measures (based on antiseptic and aseptic techniques) such as the use of gowns and gloves, careful handling and regular changing of intravascular access lines, the use of sterile breathing circuits and ventilators, and even full isolation of high risk patients. All of these traditional infection control measures are really only effective in reducing the incidence of *exogenous* infection. Most acquired infections within ICU, however, are now thought to be *endogenous*, with abnormal colonization of the patient's gastrointestinal tract by Gram-negative aerobic bacilli (GNB) preceding colonization and infection of the major organ systems (2, 13, 15). This *abnormal carrier state* (qualitative and quantitative change in the carriage of GNB within the gastrointestinal tract) is almost invariably found in critically ill patients after 2 or 3 days in ICU. This abnormal carrier state and high incidence of acquired infection largely reflects the state of the patient's host defenses as the infections, in many cases, are caused by opportunistic organisms of low inherent pathogenicity.

SDD is defined, and its role in ICU practice described, in the subsequent sections of this chapter. SDD is generally thought of as a prophylactic regimen, aimed at infection prevention, but should more correctly be thought of as a regime aimed at the prevention of the abnormal carrier state that characterizes critically ill patients.

DEFINITION AND CLINICAL CLASSIFICATION OF COLONIZATION AND INFECTION IN ICU

It has already been stated that, currently, most acquired infections in ICU are thought to be endogenous, preceded by abnormal colonization of the gastrointestinal tract with the infecting organism (usually a GNB). The terms endogenous and exogenous, when used to describe infections, tend to be used inaccurately, and for the purposes of clarity within this chapter, warrant definition.

Colonization

Colonization describes a purely microbiological phenomenon, since, by definition, no clinical features are evident. It can be defined as the isolation of an identical microorganism in at least two consecutive samples (spanning 1 week), from the same site, without clinical signs of infection. The microbial counts in samples are low (typically $\leq 10^4$ colony-forming units/ml or g of specimen), accompanied, in some cases, by a few leukocytes.

A patient who is colonized is exhibiting a state of *carriage*. Any carrier colonized with pathogenic strains represents a cross-infection risk to other patients within the unit.

Infection

Infection is best described as a microbiologically proven clinical diagnosis. As distinct from colonization, the number of microorganisms in a sample is higher (typically $>10^5$ colony-forming units/ml or g of specimen) in association with a greater number of leukocytes (25 or more per low power field). In the case of urinary tract infection and bacteremia there is little difficulty in defining the presence of infection—$\geq 10^5$

colony-forming units/ml of urine and the presence of any microorganism in an aseptically taken blood culture. The only difficulty in diagnosing bacteremia arises when an organism is isolated from a blood culture that may represent contamination from skin, e.g., a coagulase-negative *Staphylococcus*, in which case two further cultures are generally required for confirmation.

Difficulty arises with the diagnosis of bronchopulmonary infection. Critically ill patients are often subjected to invasive monitoring and therapeutic devices, including endotracheal intubation. The presence of these foreign bodies can be associated with inflammatory reactions to the device itself resulting in samples containing leukocytes with sterile cultures. Furthermore, conditions such as adult respiratory distress syndrome can, in the absence of infection, mimic the clinical signs of pneumonia: purulent sputum, infiltrates on chest x-ray, and deterioration in gas exchange. Similarly, antibiotic administration prior to admission to ICU can make the microbiological findings difficult to interpret in a patient with suspected infection. It is always conceivable that the antibiotics, either topical or systemic, might remove organisms from the site of sampling giving a false-negative result. Topical antisepsis, as with SDD regimes, may render the oropharynx and upper trachea sterile in a patient who is harboring pathogenic organisms in the lower airways. It is important to remember these difficulties in diagnosis of infection (particularly nosocomial pneumonia) when interpreting trials of SDD or other antisepsis regimens in the ICU.

Basing diagnosis of bronchopulmonary infection solely on clinical criteria will circumvent the possibility that poor sampling techniques or local antisepsis might be responsible for negative microbiological results. This will, however, have the effect of overdiagnosing respiratory tract infection by including some patients with adult respiratory distress syndrome or pulmonary contusion. The use of techniques such as the protected specimen brush may be useful in this situation, as it allows sampling from the lower airways without the risk of contamination from microbes in the oropharynx or upper trachea. (See Chapter 33, "Hospital-Acquired Pneumonia.")

Endogenous and Exogenous Infections

Infections in intensive care patients may be classified into three groups.

Primary Endogenous Infections

These infections are caused by both community and hospital microorganisms that are already carried on admission to the ICU (e.g., *Haemophilus influenzae* pneumonia following intubation in a trauma patient, or a postsurgical intraabdominal infection caused by *Proteus mirabilis*).

Secondary Endogenous Infections

Such infections are caused by microorganisms acquired after admission to the ICU, and the microorganisms invariably belong to the hospital group of bacteria (e.g., an *Acinetobacter* pneumonia caused by a strain originating in another long-stay patient and transferred, via the hands of staff to the second patient). The transferred organism first colonizes the gastrointestinal tract of the patient prior to producing colonization and infection of adjacent organ systems— the respiratory tract in the case of the above example. It is known that colonizing organisms carried in the upper gastrointestinal tract (oropharynx and stomach) tend to cause bronchopulmonary infections and wound infections of the upper torso while organisms carried in the lower gastrointestinal tract (colon and rectum) tend to cause urinary tract infections and wound infections of the lower torso. This has been particularly clearly exhibited in burn patients (65).

Exogenous Infection

In such an infection, the microorganism is introduced into the patient from the environment, either animate or inanimate. In this case, bacteria are transferred directly, with no intermediate stage of gastrointestinal carriage, to a site where col-onization and infection occur (e.g., a *Pseudomonas* pneumonia following the use of a contaminated bronchoscope).

Sepsis

Sepsis is a clinical state typically characterized by cardiovascular instability, pyrexia, oliguria, mental obtundation, tissue edema, and leukocytosis, all usually in the absence of any positive blood cultures (nonbacterial sepsis). Sepsis is commonly *associated* with infection but is less often *caused* by infection; in this situation infection is merely an epiphenomenon, reflecting impaired host defenses and commonly caused by low-virulence organisms. Nonbacterial sepsis is now a well recognized clinical entity and, in the absence of any infection, can follow trauma, burns, major surgery, and severe or prolonged hemorrhage. Although many mediator systems are involved, sepsis is best described as a state of macrophage activation resulting in malignant intravascular inflammation that leads to impairment of organ function through: central cardiovascular effects; regional perfusion imbalance; endothelial damage; and impaired microcirculatory flow.

COLONIZATION AND INFECTION RATES IN A TRADITIONALLY MANAGED ICU

As already discussed, the incidence of acquired infection in ICUs is extremely high, with some units reporting infection rates exceeding 80% in patients ventilated beyond 5 days. However, the incidence of infection in different types of ICUs can vary widely (5, 8). The use of SDD as an infection prevention regimen may be appropriate in a general ICU with an infection rate above 30% but would clearly be inappropriate in a coronary care or cardiac ICU, where infection rates would typically be below 2%. Therefore, before considering the introduction of SDD into a particular ICU, it is first necessary to carry out a prospective assessment of the unit's infection rate and the attendant morbidity and mortality. The introduction of SDD would then be indicated only if the unit's infection rate was sufficiently high, or if subgroups of patients, among whom the infection rate was high, could be identified, in which case SDD should be considered for selective application to that particular patient group.

The abnormal carrier state exhibited by a typical ICU patient has already been alluded to. A large number of trials have now observed that colonization of the gastrointestinal tract with GNBs rapidly occurs following admission to ICU—usually within 48–72 hr (reviewed in Ref. 38). In day-to-day life the gastrointestinal tract is constantly exposed to large quantities of potentially pathogenic GNBs. Except in situations of extremely high bacterial concentrations, a variety of factors, together constituting *colonization defense* (68), act to prevent invasion of the mucosal surfaces of the digestive tract. In health, motility, an anatomically intact mucosal surface, low gastric pH, and the presence of indigenous, predominantly anaerobic flora are the most important factors in preventing abnormal colonization. The ICU patient should be considered to be an immunosuppressed host, with multiple factors contributing to impairment of normal defense.

Colonization Defense in ICU

Colonization defense factors and reasons for their impairment in an ICU patient have been described in some detail elsewhere (68). However, several factors involved in the production of abnormal colonization are worthy of individual mention.

Nature of Underlying Disease

A patient's host defense can be adversely affected by a number of underlying diseases such as diabetes (35), renal and liver failure (64), and malnutrition (9, 11). In addition, patients suffering from physical trauma show impaired host defense whether the trauma is skeletal, thermal, or a consequence of major surgery (20, 31, 33, 63).

Antimicrobial Therapy

In a national survey of infection in hospitals (30) it was reported that 60% of patients in ICUs at any given time were receiving broad-spectrum systemic antibiotics. It has long been known that the widespread use of broad-spectrum antibiotics can predispose to colonization by GNBs as a result of alterations in normal indigenous flora. Such an effect was reported in 1968 (47) in association with large dose penicillin therapy. The same authors were able to prevent abnormal colonization by inducing a state of resistance in the normal flora of the gastrointestinal tract (46). More recently, increasing importance has been attached to the role of native anaerobic flora in the preservation of colonization resistance of the gastrointestinal tract (62). It is probably fair to say that the existence of colonization resistance is now generally accepted, but the role played by the indigenous anaerobic flora is still open to debate.

Extremes of Age

Host defense factors are known to be impaired in neonates and the elderly. With the exception of trauma patients, the average age of patients in ICU is high. There is some evidence to suggest that colonization resistance is decreased in elderly patients, with abnormal GNB colonization being found in a proportion of this group, even in health, especially if they are institutionalized (61).

Invasive Instrumentation

Medical intervention, such as endotracheal intubation, bladder catheterization, and the insertion of intravascular lines, predispose to infection by breaching physical barriers. The presence of an endotracheal tube or nasogastric tube can lead to abrasion of mucosal membranes, thus increasing the risk of bacterial adherence and colonization. Nasogastric tubes can also increase the risk of gastroesophageal reflux and microaspiration into the respiratory tract. This is particularly likely to occur in the supine position.

Abnormal Gut Motility

Lack of oral food intake, the inability of an intubated patient to swallow or chew, and decreased or absent peristalsis all tend to predispose to abnormal colonization.

Gastric Colonization: Relationship to pH

Atherton and White, in 1978, showed that gastric colonization was a preceding and predisposing factor for tracheal colonization and subsequent pneumonia (2) and, in critically ill patients, a gastric pH > 4 has been shown to be a major risk factor for gastric colonization (19). One obvious reason why critically ill patients in ICU may have a gastric pH > 4 is the use of H_2 receptor antagonists or antacids, administered as prophylaxis against stress ulceration and hemorrhage. Interest in the role of gastric pH with regard to colonization and subsequent risk of nosocomial pneumonia has been heightened by the introduction of the mucosal protective agent, sucralfate, as an alternative to H_2 receptor antagonists. In a controlled trial, Tryba demonstrated a significantly higher incidence of nosocomial pneumonia in patients treated with antacids than in those treated with sucralfate (58), though this reached statistical significance only after excluding patients with primary thoracic trauma and those with signs of pneumonia on admission. In the antacid group, 90% of patients had a pH > 4, while in the sucralfate group, 53% of patients had a pH > 4. In another study (12) Driks et al. showed a nosocomial pneumonia rate twice as high in an antacid/H_2 receptor antagonist group compared with a sucralfate group, but this difference was not statistically significant on primary analysis.

It is worth stressing that critically ill patients frequently have a gastric pH > 4 even in the absence of therapy with antacids or H_2 receptor antagonists; this was the case in sucralfate-treated patients in 52% in Driks' study and 53% in Tryba's study. In a recent controlled study (12), SDD and H_2 receptor antagonist therapy was compared with sucralfate therapy in a cardiac ICU. Patients in the SDD group had significantly lower colonization of the oropharynx and stomach by GNBs and significantly fewer infections due to GNB. In the sucralfate group, Gram-negative bacillary infection was preceded by colonization with the causative organism in 86% of cases. Only 23% of sucralfate patients had an average mean daily gastric pH < 4. Sucralfate patients with elevated gastric pH (mean daily ≥4) were twice as likely to have positive surveillance cultures as were those with a low pH. There was, however, no direct correlation between gastric pH and the risk of pneumonia.

In summary, it would appear that where gastric mucosal protection is deemed necessary, the use of sucralfate will result in a reduction in nosocomial pneumonia, although further controlled trials are necessary. Sucralfate can contribute to prevention of nosocomial pneumonia only for patients in whom gastric pH is <4. This is often not the case, and gastric pH > 4 is frequently seen as a function of the patient's illness. SDD would appear to be superior to sucralfate as a technique for prevention of nosocomial pneumonia, though again, further comparative studies would be useful. Despite potential, logistical problems (relating to binding of antibiotics by sucralfate) sucralfate and SDD have been used together successfully (14). (See Chapter 41, "Stress Ulcer Prophylaxis.")

RATIONALE FOR THE USE OF SDD

The pathogenesis of infection in ICU is complicated and multifactorial. Recent thinking on the pathogenesis of these infections is reflected in the classification of ICU infection given earlier in this chapter and such a classification is crucial to understanding the role played by SDD.

SDD is primarily an anticarriage regimen that is used not in isolation, but rather as part of an overall package for infection prevention. The overall package is as follows:

SDD, itself, describes the topical application of nonabsorbable antimicrobials given to patients throughout their ICU stay in order to abolish the oropharyngeal and gastrointestinal carriage of potentially pathogenic microorganisms (including GNBs, *Staphylococcus aureus*, and yeasts);

Short-term parenteral antimicrobial therapy is given during the first few days of admission to treat patients who are admitted with established infection, as early empirical therapy in cases where infection is incubating at the time of admission and as prophylaxis in patients who are not infected on admission;

Finally, careful screening of surveillance cultures by a clinically involved microbiologist is essential to ensure the efficacy of the decontamination procedure and also to screen for possible development of resistance. Cultures are typically taken from the oropharynx, tracheal aspirate, gastric aspirate, urine, and rectum on admission and thereafter twice or three times weekly.

In the context of ICU practice it is important not to consider SDD in isolation. Experience has shown that the decontamination effect takes 2–3 days to achieve, even in the upper gastrointestinal tract. During endotracheal intubation, organisms may be carried into the airway resulting in an early pneumonia. The short-term parenteral antibiotic provides prophylaxis for this and other invasive instrumentation.

Referring to the classification of ICU infection given earlier, an overall concept for the prevention of infection can be considered as follows. *Exogenous infection* is relatively rare in ICU practice. It refers to the direct transmission of microorganisms to the site of infection from the environment. Prevention of exogenous infections depends upon traditional infection control maneuvers including the careful application of good aseptic and antiseptic technique. *Primary endogenous infections* generally occur early after admission to ICU and may be caused by either community or hospital microorganisms carried in the gastrointestinal tract on admission to ICU. Treatment of these infections relies upon the short-term parenteral agent given as part of an overall SDD package. *Secondary endogenous infection* is caused by microorganisms acquired following admission to ICU; the infection is preceded by a phase of carriage within the gastrointestinal tract. It is this large group of infections that SDD

aims to prevent through its action as an anticarriage regimen.

From the above, it can be seen to be illogical to use SDD in isolation. There is a paucity of reports regarding the relative importance of SDD and the short-term parenteral agent, but this was the subject of a publication by Stoutenbeek et al. (51) that strongly supported the view that SDD and short-term parenteral therapy should be combined. Thus, SDD alone can only contribute to the control of ICU infection.

The isolated use of SDD, however, may be indicated in some situations: through suppression of GNBs, SDD has been shown to significantly reduce fecal endotoxin levels (69) and may therefore have a role to play in the prevention of gut-origin sepsis and MOF; SDD has been successfully used to control outbreaks of multiresistant GNBs, as is discussed later in this chapter; SDD alone has also been successfully applied preoperatively to certain high risk surgical groups, notably patients undergoing esophageal resection (55).

In summary, SDD is an anticarriage regimen that has a potential role to play in the prevention of infection, limitation of gut-origin sepsis and MOF, and control of outbreaks of resistance. However, for the control of ICU infection, SDD must be combined with short-term parenteral antibiotic therapy and careful attention to traditional infection control maneuvers.

CHOICE OF ANTIMICROBIAL AGENTS FOR SDD

To be suitable for use in an SDD regimen, antimicrobial agents should ideally meet the following criteria. The antimicrobial spectrum should cover all *Enterobacteriaceae* (including *Serratia* species, *Pseudomonas*, and *Acinetobacter*). The spectrum should not include anaerobes in order to establish a *selective flora elimination*. The antimicrobials should ideally have low minimum bactericidal concentrations for the GNBs listed above, because there are no leukocytes in the lumen of the intestinal canal to assist microbial killing. The agents should be nonabsorbable (or absorbed to only a minimal extent) in order both to achieve high intraluminal levels and to avoid having fluctuating levels of plasma and tissue antimicrobial concentration. The agents show minimal inactivation by food and fecal compounds and no degradation by fecal enzymes. The interactions among feces, bacteria, and antimicrobial agents are of potentially great importance in deciding the success of a given SDD regimen (67). The original trial of SDD, in an ICU setting, from Groningen, utilized a mixture of polymyxin E, tobramycin, and amphotericin B (PTA) (Table 4.1).

Prior to the introduction of SDD into ICU practice, a large background of literature existed dealing with the moderately successful use of SDD in neutropenic patients (4, 40, 48). Many different regimens for both selective and complete decontamination have been used in neutropenic patients and, on occasion, their use was associated with the development of microbial resistance, particularly in regimens that included gentamicin. Retrospectively, it has been claimed that resistance and other failures using these regimens can be explained on the basis of flaws in the chosen regimen (66). One potentially important point is that gentamicin appears to be moderately inactivated by feces while this is not the case with tobramycin (67).

The PTA regimen (described in Table

Table 4.1
Prophylactic Regimen Based on a Combination of Topical and Systemic Antimicrobials

Topical antimicrobials (PTA regimen), administered throughout the ICU stay
  Oropharyngeal cavity: A small volume of a 2% mixture of polymyxin E, tobramycin, and amphotericin B in a paste with carboxymethylcellulose (Orabase) is applied to the buccal mucosa with a gloved finger 4 times daily.
  Gastrointestinal canal: 9 ml of a suspension of polymyxin E (100 mg), tobramycin (80 mg), and amphotericin B (500 mg) is administered via the gastric tube 4 times daily.
Systemic antimicrobial, administered for the first 4 days of the ICU stay
  Cefotaxime 50–100 mg/kg body weight/day given intravenously

4.1) can therefore be thought of as a logical extension of previous decontamination regimens. The spectrum of polymyxin E excludes *Proteus*, *Morganella*, and *Serratia* species, but these gaps in the spectrum are covered by the addition of tobramycin. *Pseudomonas* species are difficult to eradicate from the gut following oral polymyxin E as monotherapy, because it is substantially inactivated by feces; tobramycin, however, is only minimally inactivated. The combination of polymyxin E and tobramycin is synergistic against *Proteus* and *Pseudomonas* species; moreover, tobramycin is also active against *S. aureus*. Emergence of resistance to polymyxin E is rare, while tobramycin can be inactivated by some bacterial enzymes; polymyxin E is thought to protect tobramycin from being destroyed by such enzymes (49).

TRIALS OF SDD IN ICU PRACTICE

Groningen was the first center to publish results of SDD applied to ICU patients (50), and the authors also first described the PTA regimen. To date, a total of 21 trials of SDD in ICU practice have been published (1, 3, 6, 10, 14, 16, 17, 21, 23–25, 28, 34, 39, 42, 50, 53–55, 59, 60); additional observational reports have also been published but these did not include a control group. These trials do not easily lend themselves to meta-analysis because of substantial differences in study design—notably ICU type, patient groups studied, criteria for diagnosis of infection, and, perhaps most importantly, variations from the original PTA regimen. Changes to the regimen include the following: tobramycin was replaced by gentamicin in the trials published by Unertle, Cockerill, Flaherty, and colleagues (10, 14, 60); tobramycin was replaced by neomycin and nalidixic acid in the study by Brun-Buisson et al. (6) and by norfloxacin in the studies by Aerdts, Ulrich, and colleagues (1, 59). Systemic cefotaxime was used in the majority of studies as short-term prophylaxis. Cefotaxime was substituted by trimethoprim in one study (59). Cefotaxime was excluded in several studies (10, 14, 42, 55) and was not indicated in two studies where

SDD was used for outbreak control (6, 54), and in two studies where oropharyngeal decontamination alone was assessed (34, 39).

Impact of SDD on Gastrointestinal Carriage of GNBs

SDD is primarily a regimen aimed at eradicating or preventing abnormal carriage of GNBs within the gastrointestinal tract. Of the 21 trials listed above, 20 showed a significant reduction in GNB carriage with SDD. The exception was the trial by Brun-Buisson et al. (6), which utilized neomycin and nalidixic acid; in this study, carriage of enterobacteria was replaced by carriage of pseudomonads. In the studies mentioned above that utilized gentamicin and norfloxicin, carriage of pseudomonas also occurred, but overall there was a significant reduction in GNB carriage.

All trials utilizing polymyxin E and tobramycin reported a highly effective eradication of enterobacterial and pseudomonal carriage. This may be due to the synergism between polymyxin E and tobramycin and also the lesser degree of inactivation by salivary and fecal compounds as compared with other combinations. In addition, the high tobramycin concentrations achieved, by utilizing a 2% paste for oropharyngeal decontamination, is usually successful in eradicating *S. aureus*.

The *selective* nature of the decontamination effect was also highlighted by the results of surveillance cultures looking at isolation rates of normal flora (25).

Effect of SDD on Acquired Infection

SDD had a statistically significant beneficial effect on acquired infection rates in 20 of the 21 studies listed, the exception again being the study by Brun-Buisson et al. (6). The greatest impact was on Gram-negative respiratory tract infections, though infection rates in other organ systems were also reduced. Schardey et al.'s study (42) showed a significant reduction in infection in the SDD group, but the addition of sucralfate to SDD appeared to confer an

additional advantage, with a respiratory infection rate of 7% compared to one of 14% in patients receiving SDD with H_2 receptor antagonists. Many of the studies report some infections in decontaminated patients, by enterococci and coagulase-staphylococci, as a result of a gap in the antimicrobial cover of the agents used. Where these infections did occur, they were amenable to therapy with standard antimicrobial agents such as ampicillin and vancomycin.

Mortality Rates in SDD Studies

Not all of the studies listed above evaluated mortality. From the results of those that did, the fact that many ICU patients die *with* but not necessarily *of* infection has been highlighted. In most of the studies the endpoint was elimination of carriage or prevention of acquired infection and the majority of the trial designs were quite inappropriate to evaluate the effect of SDD on mortality. Nevertheless, of the trials that did evaluate mortality, four reported a significant reduction in overall mortality (21, 42, 53, 59) and two others reported a significant reduction in infection-related mortality (23, 60). Ledingham et al.'s study (25) reported a highly significant reduction in mortality in trauma patients and post-hoc stratification revealed an apparent mortality benefit in patients with mid-range acute physiology and chronic health evaluation (APACHE) scores and in long-stay patients. The study by Godard et al. (16) also showed a reduction in mortality in patients with midrange APACHE scores and in those whose stay exceeded 7 days, again on post-hoc stratification. In a more recent study by Blair et al. (3), patients were prospectively analyzed according to APACHE score ranges and, in patients with midrange APACHE scores, mortality was lower in the SDD group, although this just failed to achieve statistical significance.

In summary, mortality may not be the most appropriate endpoint by which to judge a regimen that aims to prevent abnormal gastrointestinal carriage of GNBs. Subgroups of ICU patients, in whom infection contributes significantly to outcome, need to be identified and trials designed to examine the effect on mortality in these groups. Such studies will, of necessity, be large and multicenter in nature in order to provide sufficient analytical power to answer the mortality question. However, it appears reasonable to assume from existing studies that trauma patients and long-stay patients do benefit from SDD. The apparent effect on patients with midrange APACHE scores is interesting. It may reflect the fact that patients with low APACHE scores tend to be short stay and those with the higher scores tend to die of MOF, and prevention of infection in this latter group may not significantly alter outcome.

SDD and Microbial Resistance

There is an understandable concern often expressed (41) that SDD, representing the widespread prophylactic use of antibiotics in ICU, must of necessity carry a high risk of contributing to the development of microbial resistance. Such a statement ignores the fact that in a traditionally managed ICU very large quantities of parenteral therapeutic antibiotics are administered to treat suspected or proven infections. SDD should not be compared with a situation in which no antibiotics are used. In fact, the introduction of SDD produces a reduction in the usage of therapeutic parenteral antimicrobials (23, 25, 42) and therefore will reduce the selection pressure for resistance, since fluctuating antibiotic levels within the gastrointestinal tract, after parenteral administration, is one of the recognized factors in the emergence of resistance.

All units have isolated GNB that are resistant to one or another of the agents used, but these tend not to persist, often disappearing without a change in the antibiotic regimen. In Groningen, the pattern of microbial resistance over a 30-month period during which an SDD regimen was used has been the subject of a separate publication (52) that reported no increase in resistance to any of the agents used.

An increase in resistant enterobacteria or pseudomonas was reported in two studies (24, 32). However, in these two studies, analysis of resistance has been based on the inclusion of *copy* isolates (identical isolates, with the same identification and sensitivity pattern, from the same site of the same patient were included in the analysis of resistance). It is probably more accurate to use *patient controlled* data for the reporting of resistance, i.e., a single patient colonized with a single organism at a single site should be counted once, rather than counting the number of isolations, which may represent multiple sampling. In another study, an apparent increase in the isolation of resistant bacteria was shown to be false when copy isolates were excluded (17).

SDD AS A METHOD OF OUTBREAK CONTROL

Since the 1970s, *Klebsiella* species showing plasmid-mediated resistance to multiple antibiotics have caused many hospital epidemics, especially in ICU (7). Intestinal colonization has been shown to be an important reservoir for these organisms and transfer from patient to patient is primarily via the hands of health care personnel.

Two centers have reported the successful control of outbreaks of multiresistant *Klebsiella* species by means of SDD (6, 54). In Taylor and Oppenheim's study (54) the outbreak was caused by a *Klebsiella aerogenes* resistant to ceftazidime, cefuroxime, cefotaxime, ampicillin, and piperacillin. The outbreak occurred in a busy general ICU over a 3-month period. Traditional infection control methods failed to eradicate the outbreak. As an additional outbreak control measure, all patients were then treated with an SDD regimen; PTA in a gel form was applied to the oropharynx, nose, and rectum and a suspension of the same agents was also given via a nasogastric tube. Introduction of the SDD regimen resulted in rapid disappearance of the *Klebsiella*, with no evidence of superinfection or appearance of other resistant isolates. In the French study by Brun-Buisson et al. (6) only half of the patients were treated with SDD, but this still resulted in control of the outbreak. It would appear that the abolition of carriage of multiresistant *Klebsiella* strains is associated with a significant reduction in its transmission, followed by the control of outbreaks. Clearly, there is no role for a parenteral agent in this situation, unless systemic antibiotics are otherwise clinically indicated.

THE APPLICATION OF SDD TO HIGH RISK SURGICAL GROUPS

The SDD regimen described in this chapter was adapted and developed for use in the ICU. SDD is now being increasingly adopted for use in groups of high-risk surgical patients, including application to some individual patients outside ICU. In a general ICU setting many patients are infected at the time of admission. SDD is essentially a prophylactic regimen aimed against colonization, making its application to high-risk surgical groups prior to surgery or ICU admission entirely appropriate.

Esophageal Surgery

Tetteroo et al. (55) have reported on the successful use of SDD, utilizing the PTA regimen, to reduce Gram-negative colonization and infections after esophageal resection. Patients undergoing esophageal resection have a particularly high frequency of lower respiratory tract infections with GNB. In their trial, Tetteroo et al. observed that 32 of 58 control patients acquired 51 infections while only 12 of 56 SDD treated patients acquired 18 infections, a significant difference. In addition, the requirement for postoperative therapeutic antibiotics was significantly lower in the SDD group and no endogenous infections caused by GNBs were seen in the SDD patients.

Transplantation

Transplant patients are at increased risk of infection because of the immunosuppressive treatment given to prevent rejection of the transplant. All patients consequently have T cell suppression. Among the most severely compromised of transplant patients are those receiving allogenic bone marrow transplantation who require strong immunosuppression in order to mitigate or prevent graft versus host disease. SDD has been reported to have been successful in infection prevention in bone marrow transplant patients (18, 43).

Liver transplant patients are also extremely prone to infection. In addition to immunosuppression, these patients also have a 2–3-week period before the Kupffer cells repopulate the sinusoids. During this period, spillover of gastrointestinal tract organisms is likely. The successful use of SDD as a prophylactic regimen has been reported in patients undergoing liver transplantation (70), and additional trials in this field are currently ongoing.

Burn Patients

Patients suffering from severe burns are often treated within ICU, where they suffer from the same nosocomial infections as other patients. In addition, burn patients are also extremely prone to infection of the burn wound, particularly with endogenous GNBs (65). Organisms derived from the upper gastrointestinal tract tend to contaminate burn wounds of the upper limbs and trunk, while organisms derived from the lower gastrointestinal tract and rectum tend to contaminate the lower limbs and lower half of the trunk. Again, SDD has been shown to be of benefit to burn patients (27).

Head and Neck Cancer

Head and neck cancer patients undergoing radiotherapy are prone to develop a reactive inflammatory-like process of the oropharyngeal mucous membrane, a problem known as irradiation mucositis. Mucositis causes serious complaints such as pain and difficulties with swallowing, eating, and speech. This can lead to serious systemic toxicity and weight loss (45).

It is now known that colonization of the oropharyngeal tissues with GNBs significantly contributes to the process of mucositis. It has also been shown that SDD can lead to a highly significant reduction of mucositis, when compared to a control group (44).

Cardiothoracic Surgery

In general, infection rates in cardiac surgery ICU are rather low. However, SDD has been successfully used for longer stay cardiac ICU patients (those in whom postoperative organ failure occurs) leading to a significant reduction in infection (14, 57).

EFFECT OF SDD ON MOF

SDD was introduced to the ICU setting because of the very high incidence of unit-acquired infections, and there can be little doubt that SDD does have significant impact on the incidence of acquired Gram-negative infections, with 20 of the 21 trials currently published showing a statistically significant reduction. Despite unsuitable trial design, some studies on SDD show an impact on mortality. However, it has become clear that, despite the use of SDD, many patients still die of MOF in the absence of infection. Therefore, it has to be assumed that the previously observed link between infection, MOF, and late deaths in ICU was not a causative one. Patients may die of MOF secondary to "nonbacterial sepsis." There is now increasing evidence to suggest that such patients are suffering from absorption of mediators, such as endotoxin, from the gastrointestinal tract (29). If gut-origin endotoxin is a major mediator (37), then SDD may have a role in reducing the gut load of endotoxin by reducing GNB colonization. However, as presently administered, the reduction of lower bowel GNB by SDD is both slow and incomplete (particularly in postoperative surgical patients) suggesting that further synergistic therapy may be required if gut-mediated MOF is to be prevented (36, 37).

CONCLUSIONS

There seems little doubt from the published evidence that SDD can successfully reduce the incidence of acquired infection in ICU. However, it is increasingly obvious that, in critically ill patients, infection contributes significantly to mortality in only a proportion of some types of patient. In many others, both abnormal gastrointestinal carriage of the GNBs and resulting infection (often with low virulence organisms) can be regarded as almost an epiphenomenon reflecting the state of the patient's host defenses and occurring as a function of the degree of illness.

SDD successfully prevents the abnormal gastrointestinal carriage of GNBs and prevents secondary endogenous infections, but in some patient groups the impact on mortality is limited, as would be expected from the above. It takes 2–3 days for the decontamination effect to be achieved, even in the oropharynx, and therefore short-stay patients, in particular those admitted for overnight observation postoperatively, are unlikely to benefit from the regimen. There is, therefore, a strong argument for the selective administration of SDD; there would appear to be clear evidence of a significant benefit for trauma patients and patients undergoing esophageal resection as well as a strong suggestion that other long-stay groups in a general ICU would also benefit. Further trials are required, properly designed to address the question of mortality and cost-benefit analysis.

Finally, as outlined earlier in this chapter, SDD should be thought of within the context of a total infection control package, including good aseptic and antiseptic technique, adequate staff-patient ratios, and a clinically oriented and involved microbiology service.

References

1. Aerdts SJA, van Dalen R, Clasener HAL, Vollaard DJ. The effect of a novel regimen of selective decontamination on the incidence of unit-acquired lower respiratory tract infections in mechanically ventilated patients. In: van Saene HKF, Stoutenbeek CP, Lawin P, Ledingham IMcA, eds. Infection control by selective decontamination. Berlin: Springer-Verlag, 1989:123.
2. Atherton ST, White DJ. Stomach as a source of bacteria colonising respiratory tract during artificial ventilation. Lancet 1978;ii:968–969.
3. Blair P, Rowlands BJ, Lowry K, Webb H, Armstrong P, Smillie J. Selective decontamination of the digestive tract: a stratified randomised prospective study in a mixed ICU. Surgery 1991; 110:303–310.
4. Bodey GP. Antibiotic prophylaxis in cancer patients: regimens of oral non-absorbable antibiotics for prevention of infection during induction or remission. Rev Infect Dis 1981;3:S259–268.
5. Brown RB, Hosmer D, Chen HC, et al. A comparison of infections in different ICU within the same hospital. Crit Care Med 1985;13:472–476.
6. Brun-Buisson G, Legrand P, Rauss A, et al. Intestinal decontamination for control of nosoco-

mial multi-resistant Gram-negative bacilli. Ann Intern Med 1989;110:873–881.

7. Casewell MW, Phillips I. Aspects of the plasmid-mediated antibiotic resistance and epidemiology of *Klebsiella* species. Am J Med 1981;70:459–462.

8. Chandrasetar PM, Kruse JA, Matthews MF. Nosocomial infection among patients in different types of intensive care units at a city hospital. Crit Care Med 1986;14:508–510.

9. Christou NV, McLean APH, Meakins JL. Host defense in blunt trauma: inter relationships of kinetics of anergy and depressed neutrophil function, nutritional status and sepsis. J Trauma 1980;20:833–841.

10. Cockerill FR, Muller SM, Anhalt JP, Thompson RL. Reduction of nosocomial infections by selective digestive tract decontamination in the ICU. International Congress on Antibiotic Antimicrobial Chemotherapy. 1989;Abstract 785.

11. Dionigi R, Zonta A, Diminioni L, Gnes F, Ballabio A. The effects of total parenteral nutrition on immuno-depression due to malnutrition. Ann Surg 1977;185:467–474.

12. Driks MR, Craven DE, Celli BR, et al. Nosocomial pneumonia in intubated patients given sucralfate as compared with antacids or histamine type 2 blockers: the role of gastric colonisation. N Engl J Med 1987;817:1376–1382.

13. du Moulin GC, Patterson DG, Hedley-Whyte J, Lisbon A. Aspiration of gastric bacteria in antacid treated patients: a frequent cause of post-operative colonization in the airway. Lancet 1982;i:242–245.

14. Flaherty J, Nathan C, Kabins SA, Weinstein RA. Pilot trial of selective decontamination for prevention of bacterial infection in an ICU. J Infect Dis 1990;162:1393–1397.

15. Flynn DM, Weinstein RA, Nathan C, Gaston MA, Kabins SA. Patients endogenous flora as the source of nosocomial *Enterobacter* in cardiac surgery. J Infect Dis 1987;156:363–368.

16. Godard J, Guillaume C, Reverdy ME, Bachmann P, Bui-Xuan B, Nageotte A, Motin J. Intestinal decontamination in a polyvalent ICU: a double blind study. Intensive Care Med 1990;16:307–311.

17. Hartenauer U, Thulig B, Diemer W, Lawin P, Fegeler W, Kehrel R, Ritzerfeld W. Effect on selective flora suppression on colonisation, infection, and mortality in critically ill patients: a one year prospective consecutive study. Crit Care Med 1991;19:463–473.

18. Heimbhal A, Gahrton G, Groth CG, et al. Selective decontamination of the alimentary tract microbial flora in patients treated with bone marrow transplantation: a microbiological study. Scand J Infect Dis 1984;16:51–60.

19. Hillman KM, Riorda T, O'Farrell SM, Tabaqchal S. Colonisation of the gastric contents in critically ill patients. Crit Care Med 1982;10:444–447.

20. Howard RJ, Simmons RL. Acquired immunologic deficiencies after trauma and surgical procedures. Surg Gynecol Obstet 1974;139:771–782.

21. Hunefeld G. Klinische studie zur selektiven darmdekolonisation bei 204 langzeitbeatmeten abdominal- und unfallchirurgischen intensivpatienten. Anaesthesiol Reanim 1989;3:131–153.

22. Kaplan ES, Hoyt N. Infection surveillance and control in the severely traumatized patient. Am J Med 1981;70:638–640.

23. Kerver AJH, Rommes JH, Mevissen-Verhage EAE, Hultsaert PF, Voa A, Verhoerf J, Wittebol P. Prevention of colonisation and infection in critically ill patients: a prospective randomised study. Crit Care Med 1988;16:1087–1093.

24. Konrad F, Schwalbe B, Heeg K, Wagner H, Wiedeck H, Kilian J, Ahnefeld FW. Kolonisations, pneumoniefrequenz und resistenzentwicklung bei langzeitbeatmeten intensivpatienten unter selektiver dekontamination des verdauungstraktes. Anaesthesist 1989;38:99–109.

25. Ledingham IMcA, Alcock SR, Eastaway AT, McDonald JC, MacKay IC, Ramsay G. Triple regimen of selective decontamination of the digestive tract, systemic cefotaxime, and microbiological surveillance for prevention of acquired infection in intensive care. Lancet 1988;i:785–790.

26. Machiedo GW, Lo Verme PJ, McGovern PJ, Blackwood JM. Patterns of mortality in a surgical ICU. Surg Gynecol Obstet 1981;152:757–759.

27. Manson WL, Westerveld AW, Klasen HJ, Sauer EW. Selective intestinal decontamination of the digestive tract for infection prophylaxis in the severely burned patient. Scand J Plast Reconstr Surg Hand Surg 1987;21:269–272.

28. McClelland P, Murray AE, Williams PS, van Saene HKF, Gilbertson AA, Mostafa SM, Bone JM. Reducing sepsis in severe combined acute renal and respiratory failure by selective decontamination of the digestive tract. Crit Care Med 1990;18:935–939.

29. Meakins JL, Marshall JC. The gastrointestinal tract: the motor of multiple organ failure. Arch Surg 1989;121:197–201.

30. Meers PD, Ayliffe GAJ, Emmerson AM, et al. Report on the national survey of infection in hospitals. J Hosp Infect 1980;2:1–51.

31. Münster AM. Post traumatic immunosuppression is due to activation of suppressor T-cells. Lancet 1976;i:1329–1330.

32. Nau R, Ruchel R, Mergerian H, Wegener U, Winkelmann T, Priange HW. Emergence of antibiotic-resistant bacteria during selective decontamination of the digestive tract. J Antimicrob Chemother 1990;25:881–883.

33. Ninnemann JL, Condie JT, Davies SE, Crocket RA. Isolation of immunosuppressive serum components following thermal injury. J Trauma 1982;22:837–844.

34. Pugin J, Auckenthaler R, Lew PD, Suter PM. Oropharyngeal decontamination decreases incidence of ventilator associated pneumonia. JAMA 1991;265:2704–2710.

35. Raefield EJ, Ault MJ, Keusch GT, Brothers MJ, Nechemias C, Smith H. Infection and diabetes: the case for glucose control. Am J Med 1982;72:439–450.

36. Ramsay G. Endotoxaemia in multiple organ failure: a secondary role for SDD? In: van Saene HKF, Stoutenbeek CP, Lawin P, Ledingham IMcA, eds. Infection control by selective decontamination. Berlin: Springer-Verlag, 1989;135–142.

37. Ramsay G, Ledingham IMcA. Management of multiple organ failure: control of the microbial environment. In: Bihari DJ, Cerra FD, eds. Multiple organ failure. Fullerton, California: Society of Critical Care Medicine, 1989:327–336.

38. Reidy JJ, Ramsay G. Clinical trials of selective decontamination of the digestive tract: Review. Crit Care Med 1990;18:1449–1456.

39. Rodriguez-Roldan JM, Altuna-Cuesta A, Lopez A, Carrillo A, Garcia J, Leon J, Martinez-Pellus AJ. Prevention of nosocomial lung infection in ventilated patients: use of an antimicrobial pharyngeal non-absorbable paste. Crit Care Med 1990;18:1239–1242.

40. Rozenberg-Arska M, Dekker AW, Verhoef J. Colistin and trimethoprim-sulfamethoxazole for the prevention of infection in patients with acute lymphocytic leukaemia. Infection 1983;11:167–169.

41. Sanderson PJ. Selective decontamination of the digestive tract. Br Med J 1989;299:1413–1414.

42. Schardey M, Meyer G, Kern M, Marre R, Hohlbach G, Schildberg FW. Nosocomial respiratory tract infections: preventive measures in surgical intensive care patients (English abstract translation). Intensivmed Notfallmed 1989;26:242–249.

43. Schmeiser TH, Kurrle E, Arnold R, Kriger D, Heit W, Heinpol H. Antimicrobial prophylaxis in neutropenic patients after bone marrow transplantation. Infection 1988;16:19–24.

44. Spijkervet FKL. Irradiation mucositis and oral flora [Thesis]. Groningen, Netherlands: Rijksuniversiteit, 1989:95–104.

45. Spijkervet FKL, van Saene HKF, Planders KK, Vermey A, Mahta VM. Scoring irradiation mucositis in head and neck cancer patients. J Oral Pathol Med 1989;18:167–171.

46. Sprunt K, Leidy GA, Redman W. Prevention of bacterial overgrowth. J Infect Dis 1971;123:1–10.

47. Sprunt K, Redman W. Evidence suggesting importance of role of interbacterial inhibition in maintaining balance of normal flora. Ann Intern Med 1968;68:579–580.

48. Storring RA, Jameson B, McElwain TJ, Wilshaw E, Spears ASD, Gaya H. Oral absorbed antibiotics prevent infection in acute lymphoblastic leukaemia. Lancet 1977;ii:837–840.

49. Stoutenbeek CP, van Saene HKF. Infection prevention in intensive care by selective decontamination of the digestive tract. J Crit Care 1990;5:137–156.

50. Stoutenbeek CP, van Saene HKF, Miranda DR, Zandstra DF. The effect of selective decontamination of the digestive tract on colonisation and infection rate in multiple trauma patients. Intensive Care Med 1984;10:185–192.

51. Stoutenbeek CP, van Saene HKF, Miranda DR, Zandstra DF, Langrehr D. The effect of oropharyngeal decontamination using topical non-absorbable antibiotics on the incidence of nosocomial respiratory tract infections in multiple trauma patients. J Trauma 1987;27:357–364.

52. Stoutenbeek CP, van Saene HKF, Zandstra DF. The effect of oral non-absorbable antibiotics on the emergence of resistant bacteria in patients in an ICU. J Antimicrob Chemother 1987;19:513–520.

53. Sydow M, Burchardi H, Crozier TA, Ruchel R, Busse C, Seyde WC. Einfluss der selektiven dekontamination auf nosokomiale infektionen, erregerspektum und antibiotikaresistenz bei langzeitbeatmeten intensivpatienten. Anasth Intensivther Notfallmed 1990;25:416–423.

54. Taylor ME, Oppenheim BA. Selective decontamination of the gastrointestinal tract as an infection control measure. J Hosp Infect 1991;17:271–278.

55. Tetteroo GWM, Wagenvoort JAT, Castelein A, Tilanus HW, Ince C, Bruining HA. Selective decontamination to reduce Gram negative colonisation and infections after oesophageal resection. Lancet 1990;335:704–707.

56. Thorp JM, Richards WC, Telfer ABM. A survey of infection in an intensive care unit. Anaesthesia 1979;68:457–467.

57. Thulig B, Harteneur U, Diemer W, et al. Effektive Infektionskontrolle durch selektive Darm-dekontamination (SDD) bei thoraxchirurgischen Intensivpatienten [Abstract]. Der Anaesthetist 1989; 38:S352.

58. Tryba M. Risk of acute stress bleeding and nosocomial pneumonia in ventilated ICU patients. Am J Med 1987;83(suppl 3b):117–124.

59. Ulrich C, Harinck-de-Weerd JE, Bakker NC, Jacz K, Doornbos L, de Ridder VA. Selective decontamination of the digestive tract with norfloxacin in the prevention of ICU-acquired infection: a prospective randomised study. Intensive Care Med 1989;15:424–431.

60. Unertl K, Rückdeschel G, Selbmann HK, Jensen J, Forst H, Lenhart FP, Peter K. Prevention of colonisation and respiratory infections in long-term ventilated patients by local antimicrobial prophylaxis. Intensive Care Med 1987;13:106–113.

61. Valenti WM, Trundell RG, Bentley DW. Factors predisposing to oropharyngeal colonisation with Gram negative bacilli in the aged. N Engl J Med 1978;298:1108–1111.

62. van der Waaij D. Berghuis-Devries JM, Lekkerkerk-van der Wees JEC. Colonization resistance of the digestive tract in conventional and antibiotic treated mice. J Hyg 1971;69:405–411.

63. van Dijk WC, Verbrugh HA, van Rijswijk REN, Vos A, Verhoef J. Neutrophil function, serum opsonic activity, and delayed hypersensitivity in surgical patients. Surgery 1982;92:21–29.

64. van Epps DE, Strickland RD, Williams RC. Inhibitors of leukocyte chemotaxis in alcoholic liver disease. Am J Med 1975;59:200–207.

65. van Saene HKF, Nicolay GPA. The prevention of wound infection in burn patients. Scand J Plast Reconstr Surg Hand Surg 1979;13:63–67.

66. van Saene HKF, Stoutenbeek CP. Selective decontamination. J Antimicrob Chemother 1987; 20:462–465.

67. van Saene HKF, Stoutenbeek CP, Lerk CF. Influence of faeces on the activity of antimicrobial agents used for decontamination of the alimentary canal. Scand J Infect Dis 1985;17:295–300.

68. van Saene HKF, Stoutenbeek CP, Zandstra DF, Gilbertson AA, Murray A, Hart CA. Nosocomial infections in severely traumatized patients: mag-

nitude of problem, pathogenesis, prevention and therapy. Acta Anaesthesiol Belg 1987;38:347–353.

69. van Saene JJM, Stoutenbeek CP, van Saene HKF. Significant reduction of faecal endotoxin pool by oral polymyxin E and tobramycin in human volunteers. In: van Saene HKF, Stoutenbeek CP, Lawin P, Ledingham IMcA, eds. Infection control in ICU by SDD. Heidelberg: Springer Verlag, 1989:128–134.

70. Wiesner RH, Hermans PE, Rakela J, Washington JA, Perkins JD, DiCecco S, Crom R. Selective bowel decontamination to decrease Gram-negative aerobic bacterial and candidal colonisation and prevent infection after orthotopic liver transplantation. Transplantation 1988;45:570–574.

5

Bacteremia and Sepsis: Clinical Perspectives

Derek C. Angus
David J. Kramer

Sepsis is the systemic response to tissue inflammation. As this systemic response evolves, characteristic changes occur in multiple system organ function and hemodynamics. If unchecked, these changes progress to refractory hypotension, multiple systems organ failure, or death (5, 36, 69). Despite considerable advances in our understanding of the mechanisms and processes involved, we continue to be faced by a disease with a mortality that fails to decrease despite technological advances and an incidence that continues to rise due to these same advances (69). Traditionally, management of the septic patient has consisted of antimicrobial therapy and organ system support (vasopressors, intravenous fluids, respiratory support, and hemodialysis). However, new treatment modalities, such as blockade and inhibition of sepsis mediators, are on the horizon and may come to revolutionize our management of these patients in the next decade (69).

To assess the efficacy and significance of such therapies we must first agree on more accurate definitions of sepsis and related conditions (9). Specifically, we should differentiate between bacteremia, septicemia, sepsis, septic syndrome, and septic shock.

DEFINITIONS

Bacteremia is the presence of viable bacteria in the blood and is not an infection per se, but rather the laboratory diagnosis of a positive blood culture.

Septicemia is a term used to suggest blood-borne infection. However, it is not clear whether microorganisms must be isolated from the blood, or whether the suspicion alone of systemic disease of infective origin constitutes the diagnosis. Furthermore, there are no uniformly accepted criteria for defining "infection" in this category. Thus, though commonly used, the term is probably of limited value (9).

Sepsis is defined by *Webster's Medical Dictionary* as "a toxic condition resulting from the spread of bacteria or their products from a focus of infection" (91). Like septicemia, there has been liberal interpretation of its meaning in the past. In an attempt to define sepsis more objectively, Bone has suggested the clinical criteria summarized in Table 5.1 (10).

Sepsis syndrome has been proposed as a distinct clinical entity that precedes septic shock (Table 5.1) (11). Its importance in diagnosis is based on the premise that aggressive intervention before the development of frank shock may result in improved survival rate (11, 21). It is also proving to be a useful diagnosis from the perspective of establishing criteria by which to compare different treatment modalities between studies.

Septic shock can be regarded as the development of hypotension (systolic blood pressure < 90 mm Hg, or a 40 mm Hg decrease from baseline systolic blood pressure) in the presence of the septic syndrome (9). There is debate as to whether the responsiveness of the hypotension should be measured in the definition of septic shock. In a recent editorial, Bone

Table 5.1
A Uniform System for Defining the Spectrum of Disorders Associated with Sepsis [a]

Disorder	Requirements for Clinical Diagnosis
Bacteremia	Positive blood cultures
Sepsis	Clinical evidence suggestive of infection plus signs of a systemic response to the infection (all of the following): Tachypnea (respiration >20 breaths/min (if patient is mechanically ventilated, >10 liters/min)) Tachycardia (heart rate >90 beats/min) Hyperthermia or hypothermia (core or rectal temperature >38.4°C (101°F) or <35.6°C (96.1°F))
The sepsis syndrome (may be considered incipient septic shock in patients who later become hypotensive)	Clinical diagnosis of sepsis outlined above, plus evidence of altered organ perfusion (one or more of the following): Pao_2/Fio_2 no higher than 280 (in the absence of other pulmonary or cardiovascular disease) Lactate level above the upper limit of normal Oliguria (documented urine output <0.5 ml/kg body weight for at least 1 hr in patients with catheters in place) Acute alteration in mental status Positive blood cultures are not required [b]
Early septic shock	Clinical diagnosis of sepsis syndrome outlined above, plus hypotension (systolic blood pressure below 90 mm Hg or a 40 mm Hg decrease from baseline systolic blood pressure) that lasts for less than 1 hr and is responsive to conventional therapy (intravenous fluid administration or pharmacologic intervention)
Refractory septic shock	Clinical diagnosis of the sepsis syndrome outlined above, plus hypotension (systolic blood pressure below 90 mm Hg or a 40 mm Hg decrease below baseline systolic blood pressure (that lasts for more than 1 hr despite adequate volume resuscitation and that requires vasopressors or higher doses of dopamine (>6 μg/kg/hr))

[a] Adapted from Bone RC. The pathogenesis of sepsis. Ann Intern Med 1991;115:457–469.
[b] The sepsis syndrome may result from infection with Gram-positive or Gram-negative bacteria, pathogenic viruses, fungi, or rickettsia; however, an identical physiologic response may result from such noninfectious processes as severe trauma or pancreatitis. Blood cultures may or may not be positive.

suggested that septic shock should be defined only if the hypotension responded to intravenous fluids and/or pressors within 1 hr (9). Hypotension beyond this time period would be indicative not of septic shock but of supervening *refractory shock* and would be associated with a higher mortality. It is Bone's premise that variability in mortality rates in studies assessing septic shock may in part be due to failure to distinguish between these entities. At the present time, such distinction has not been widely adopted in clinical and animal studies nor has its usefulness been proven.

For the purposes of this chapter, we will use the terms *sepsis* and *septic state* as global expressions for sepsis, septic syndrome, or septic shock.

EPIDEMIOLOGY

The incidence of sepsis and septic shock has been rising throughout this century (99). The Centers for Diseases Control reported a 139% increase in septicemia rates between 1979 and 1987 (20). The reasons include increased use of broad-spectrum antibiotics; increased instrumentation and use of invasive procedures (intravenous and bladder catheters, endotracheal intubation, pleural and peritoneal catheters); use of immunosuppressive therapy, steroids, chemotherapy, and radiotherapy; and an increased survival of patients at risk for such infections (11, 51, 67, 71). In the United States, it is estimated that over 400,000 cases of sepsis occur annually, while septic shock occurs in about 200,000 with a mortality of 30–70% (71). Much clinical and laboratory research is focused upon elucidating the mechanisms of and formulating treatment strategies for sepsis and septic shock.

ETIOLOGICAL AND PATHOPHYSIOLOGICAL ASPECTS

The most common etiology for sepsis is infection (Table 5.2). The most common organisms responsible are Gram-negative bacteria though Gram-positive bacteria, *Rickettsiae*, fungi, viruses, and protozoa can also produce the sepsis syndrome. Bacteremia is present in less than half of all cases, but a localized site of infection or tissue injury can usually be identified and pathogenic organisms can often be recovered. The mechanisms by which localized infection (e.g., pneumonia, pyelonephritis, etc.) progresses to a generalized septic state are complex, but certain steps have become clearer in recent years. An initial focus of microorganisms multiplies, producing toxins and further microorga-

Table 5.2
Common Etiological Agents in Sepsis

Infective	Noninfective
Gram-negative bacteria	Major trauma
Escherichia coli	Extensive burns
Enterobacteriaceae	Pancreatitis
Pseudomonadaceae	End-stage liver disease
meningococci	Allograft rejection
Gram-positive bacteria	
Rickettsiae	
Viruses	
Fungi	

nisms. This process stimulates the host immune system resulting in cellular activation and the release of various mediators of inflammation. The principal cell line involved is the reticuloendothelial system (tissue macrophages) while the most important noncellular mediators are the cytokines (36, 45). Once stimulated, this response, if unchecked, may progress beyond local control processes and result in a characteristic systemic response, leading to local and remote tissue dysfunction. Thus, the septic state is the manifestation of the effects of both the invading pathogen and the host response.

In the latter stages of septic shock, when end-organ dysfunction has developed, defining a specific microbe as the etiologic agent may be problematic. The possible explanations for this apparent dissociation between bacterial infection and sepsis are listed below.

Nonviable cell wall fragments of the offending microbe perpetuate the septic state, e.g., endotoxin (25).

Ongoing local inflammation with cellular ischemia and necrosis liberates additional proinflammatory substances which result in the systemic expression of the septic state (82).

The combination of reasons one and two above may overwhelm the basic immunoregulatory control mechanisms, allowing phlogistic mediators to continue to circulate.

Tissues initially not involved in the infectious processes may become dysfunctional (specifically the gut). Leak of gut-derived substances into the peritoneal cavity and portal circulation may result in subclinical bacteremia or endotoxemia, overwhelming the clearance mechanism of the liver thus further contributing to inappropriate circulating levels of phlogistic mediators (3).

In addition, though the development of the septic state would seem to imply underlying infection, the initial insult may not be of an infective nature (95). Indeed, the hemodynamic derangements and clinical signs (fever, leukocytosis, and even end-organ dysfunction) of sepsis may be seen with multiple trauma, extensive burns, severe pancreatitis, end-stage liver disease, and acute graft rejection. Such catastrophic insults are not clearly related to infection in the early stages. However, there is extensive tissue destruction and this may activate a cascade of immunologic and phlogistic mediators similar to primary infection. Therefore, a final common pathway to the septic syndrome, shock, and death ensues from both infectious and noninfectious causes.

An alternative explanation, known as the "gut hypothesis," states that an insult such as severe trauma or extensive burns results in gut dysfunction enabling increased translocation of bacteria and cell wall products, such as endotoxin, across the bowel wall (19, 93). These products gain subsequent entry to the systemic circulation either via lymphatic drainage or, perhaps more importantly, due to impaired hepatic clearance mechanisms (a result of the primary shock coupled with Kupffer cell overload) (29, 72, 93). This influx of bacteria and cell wall products into the systemic circulation triggers the typical cascade of mediators seen with primary infection. Thus, a primary insult that results in gut dysfunction may be the common pathway for both initiating and maintaining the septic state (29).

Both overwhelming systemic infection and the "gut hypothesis" place the burden for modulating the systemic response to infection or inflammation squarely upon the liver clearance and detoxifying mechanisms. If these mechanisms are impaired, the liver will be unable to effectively clear proinflammatory mediators (72). However, liver function as assessed by standard liver function tests is often not deranged despite significant impairment in hepatic host defense (59). Indeed, while cholestasis may develop later in the course of multiple systems organ failure, liver function tests are usually normal early on in the course of the septic state unless severe hepatic ischemia or direct hepatic injury occurs (59).

Patients with severe liver impairment have, by definition, hepatocellular dysfunction. This impairment can be identified crudely by standard liver function tests including measures of synthetic function such as prothrombin time and serum albumin. However, these patients also have abnormalities in fixed tissue macrophage (Kupffer cell) function (82). Tissue macrophage function, which is of prime impor-

tance in clearing bacteremia and endotoxin, is poorly assayed by current laboratory tests. Patients with end-stage liver disease often have derangements in systemic hemodynamics, thermoregulation, and end-organ function that are similar, if not identical, to the sepsis syndrome (8, 13, 22, 27, 28, 31, 48, 49, 55, 59, 63, 65, 75, 98). In addition, the presence of portal hypertension results in passive gut congestion (edema) that facilitates translocation of bacteria (spontaneous bacterial peritonitis) and endotoxin. Portosystemic collateral blood flow facilitates the systemic presentation of these inflammatory factors, which may explain the classic hyperdynamic clinical state seen in patients with end-stage liver failure (59).

To understand sepsis, it is important to consider a common clinical sequence of events: a severe physiological insult that is initially treated effectively by resuscitation is followed by progressive organ dysfunction in multiple organ systems and eventually death (19). This inexorable progression may be mediated in part by the amplifying effect of endotoxin on intestinal permeability and the failure of the liver to clear endotoxin and bacteria from the portal circulation, which results in further hepatic insult (13, 27, 28, 59, 75). The development of jaundice with hyperbilirubinemia is an ominous sign in the progression of multiple systems organ failure and is associated with a particularly high mortality (8, 48, 55). The interaction between circulating endotoxin and hepatocellular function has been demonstrated in the setting of liver transplantation. Allograft function is clearly related to the level of circulating endotoxin in the recipient at the time of implantation (98). The pivotal role of the liver in multiple systems organ failure is also suggested by the resolution of multiple systems organ failure including the adult respiratory distress syndrome (ARDS) after liver transplantation (31, 59).

CLINICAL FEATURES

The clinical features of sepsis comprise those resulting from the primary insult, those pertaining to systemic activation, and those resulting from end-organ dysfunction. The most common insult resulting in sepsis is primary infection. Virtually any organ or system may be the source, but certain sites such as the lower respiratory tract, the urinary tract, wounds, and catheter-related sources are the most common. For further reading, the reader is referred to the excellent review by Norwood and Civetta, where the clinical features and diagnostic criteria of primary infections are succinctly summarized (65). The systemic response to infection produces the classical features of fever (or hypothermia), apprehension, tachypnea, and malaise. Although fever is more common, hypothermia confers a worse prognosis (52, 99).

End-Organ Dysfunction

Systemic hypotension and regional microcirculatory deficits in oxygen delivery, particularly when associated with endotoxemia, result in end-organ dysfunction. Respiratory failure and renal failure are recognized at an early stage in part because objective markers of their function are routinely assessed. Disorders of cerebral and peripheral neurologic function and derangements in the coagulation process are later recognized. Progression of the septic process results in multiple systems organ failure (Table 5.3).

Cardiovascular Function

The most common cardiovascular presentation is a generalized hyperdynamic response with tachycardia, wide pulse pressure, warm extremities, and an increased cardiac output as confirmed by pulmonary arterial catheterization. Hypotension and shock develop, despite a high cardiac output, due to profound peripheral vasodilation. Since fluid resuscitation is universally given to these patients, it is not clear if the hyperdynamic state would develop without fluid resuscitation.

Though the usual picture is that of high cardiac output with hypotension, 10% of patients may present with myocardial dysfunction evidenced by normal or low cardiac output (84). Furthermore, even in those with an elevated cardiac output, there is usually impaired ventricular function with ventricular dilatation and a reduction in

Table 5.3
End-Organ Dysfunction

System	Manifestation
Cardiovascular	Microcirculatory defects Hyperdynamic cardiac output Myocardial impairment Hypotension Shock
Pulmonary	Tachypnea Respiratory alkalosis Hypoxia Ventilation-perfusion mismatching Adult respiratory distress syndrome Late pulmonary fibrosis
Renal	Oliguria Isosthenuria Acute tubular necrosis Uremia
Neurological	Altered consciousness Peripheral neuropathy Coma
Gastrointestinal	Gastric paresis Ileus Stress ulceration Mucosal dysfunction Bacterial translocation
Hepatic	Cholestasis Decreased protein synthesis Impaired Kupffer cell function
Hematological	Leukocytosis (or leukopenia) Multifactorial anemia Multifactorial thrombocytopenia Disseminated intravascular coagulopathy
Metabolic	Hyperglycemia Hyperlactemia Metabolic acidosis

the ventricular ejection fraction (84). Parrillo and colleagues have demonstrated that myocytes in vitro have depressed function when patent in serum from patients with sepsis (70). They have also demonstrated in patients with sepsis that the depression of left ventricular (LV) ejection fraction and LV dilatation are reversible (68). Interestingly, these changes appear to correlate with outcome. Survivors of sepsis are more likely to have had a reduced LV ejection fraction and LV dilatation during the acute phase of the illness suggesting this dilatation may indeed be a normal compensatory mechanism. This reversibility had initially been thought to be secondary to myocardial ischemia but recent work by Cunnion et al. and Dhainaut et al. counters this hypothesis by demonstrating normal or higher coronary flow in septic shock and no difference in lactate extraction between those in septic shock with and without myocardial depression (23, 30). Instead, it has been hypothesized that this phenomenon is induced by myocardial depressant substances though the exact nature of these substances remains elusive (18, 40, 53).

Stroke volume may change little in sepsis, and tachycardia is the primary mechanism for elevated cardiac output. This produces an elevated oxygen delivery providing adequate fluid resuscitation has been achieved. Oxygen consumption, however, may be variable and perhaps dependent upon delivery (16, 17, 24, 43, 61). This has been called a pathologic oxygen supply relationship (73, 89). The mechanisms by which this occurs are discussed elsewhere in this book (see Chapter 10, "Sepsis Syndrome: Pathogenesis, Pathophysiology, and Management"). The clinical manifestation of impaired peripheral oxygen extraction is of a narrow arteriovenous oxygen content difference, high mixed venous oxygen saturation, and paradoxical progressive hyperlactemia.

Pulmonary Function

One of the earliest signs of sepsis is tachypnea with a resultant respiratory alkalosis. Contributing factors include fever, apprehension, and nonhydrostatic pulmonary edema. High protein fluid accumulates in the pulmonary interstitium and alveoli resulting in a marked elevation of the alveolar-arterial oxygen gradient and decrease in lung compliance. The early edematous phase is followed by a cellular reparative phase, which may progress to pulmonary fibrosis. Pulmonary dysfunction may persist and worsen if the septic process fails to resolve. Subsequent pulmonary nosocomial infection may significantly contribute to morbidity and mortality (62).

Renal Function

In part because renal function can be evaluated in an objective fashion, derangements are commonly appreciated in sepsis. Early on, a hypotensive episode may be associated with decreased renal blood flow and sodium avidity. However, hypoperfusion with or without concomitant infection and endotoxemia results in an ischemic insult and resultant tubular dysfunction. This may be seen initially as isothenuria with a loss of concentrating ability followed by a significant decrease in the glomerular filtration rate and creatinine clearance (60). Serum creatinine and urea nitrogen levels may be normal initially and measurements of creatinine clearance, calculation of the fractional excretion of Na^+, and measurement of urine specific gravity or osmolarity may be more sensitive (14). The development of renal failure is associated with a marked increase in morbidity and mortality despite dialytic therapy.

Neurologic Function

Alterations in the level of consciousness are common in patients with the sepsis syndrome and may range from mild confusion to stupor and coma. While coexistent hypotension may compromise cerebral perfusion, particularly in the setting of diffuse atherosclerosis, cerebral ischemia is an uncommon etiology of central nervous system (CNS) dysfunction. Cerebral blood flow and cerebral oxygen consumption are depressed (12), however, other factors, such as hepatic and renal dysfunction, alterations in the circulating amino acid pattern with an excess of aromatic amino acids, and altered balance of neutrotransmitters are a more likely (though poorly characterized) explanation of CNS dysfunction (41).

Peripheral nerve function is often compromised, as detected by nerve conduction studies (101). This may be missed during the intensive care management of these patients due to concomitant depressed central function and sedation; it may, however, dominate the recovery phase (97). The exact mechanism underlying critical illness polyneuropathy remains unclear though theories include hypoxic damage due to hyperglycemia, hypoalbuminemia and loss of microcirculatory autoregulation (97).

Gastrointestinal Function

Abnormal gastrointestinal function is common. Delayed gastric emptying, gastric paresis, and stress ulceration may be precipitated by shock and last throughout the septic phase. Small bowel function is usually initially preserved though several histologic studies demonstrate marked compromise of structural integrity with mucosal and submucosal bacteria invasion and subsequent translocation of bacteria (93). Diarrhea is common and may relate to infection (e.g., with *Clostridium difficile*), ischemia, catheters, hyperosmolar loads, and electrolyte abnormalities (32, 85).

Hepatic Function

Hepatocellular function in the absence of prior liver disease or severe shock resulting in hepatic ischemia or infarction does not appear to deteriorate until later in the course. Cholestasis, manifested by hyperbilirubinemia in the absence of obstruction of the biliary system, is an ominous finding and is associated with a very high mortality (8, 55). Unfortunately, standard liver function tests do not assay Kupffer cell function, and tests of colloidal extraction are not routinely employed (7). Hepatic blood flow may be decreased when cardiac output is low or when mesenteric blood flow is limited due to endogenous or exogenous vasoconstrictors. Passive congestion may result when hepatic venous pressures are markedly elevated in volume overload, ventricular failure, tamponade, and perhaps when intrathoracic pressure is significantly elevated with the application of positive end-expiratory pressure (PEEP) (47). Synthetic function is usually initially preserved, but standard markers such as prothrombin time and serum albumin become inaccurate as disseminated intravascular coagulation, malnutrition, and persistent stress develop.

Hematologic Function

Hematologic abnormalities and coagulation deficits are common. Typically, leukocytosis is present, though profound leukopenia occurs and may be more ominous. Lymphopenia may result from endogenous corticosteroid and catecholamine release. A leftward shift to more immature forms such as bands, myelocytes, and metamyelocytes may be seen. Persistent sepsis may be associated with anemia, which is multifactorial. Decreased secretion of erythropoietin in the presence of renal dysfunction or marrow resistance to the effects of erythropoietin may occur with the development of a normochromic, normocytic anemia and an inappropriately low reticulocyte count. Blood loss, due to a combination of venipuncture, invasive vascular procedures, stress ulceration, and coagulopathy, is common.

Thrombocytopenia is common and is also multifactorial. Marrow production is usually adequate in this regard, and peripheral consumption may be associated with infection, antiplatelet antibodies (e.g., secondary to prolonged heparin administration), or drug induction (especially antibiotics and H_2 blockers).

A coagulopathy may develop. Decreased production of clotting factors may occur because of liver failure, but more commonly, peripheral consumption of clotting factors may occur and progress to disseminated intravascular coagulation in which thrombocytopenia may be profound and concomitant fibrinolysis may result in bleeding from many sites. In addition, drug administration such as that of certain cephalosporins, can adversely affect prothrombin times (6, 92).

MANAGEMENT

The management of sepsis and septic shock (Table 5.4) consists of ameliorating the immediate effects of shock while evaluating the source of sepsis and commencing appropriate therapy. Despite the failure of

Table 5.4
Management of Septic Shock

	Early	Intermediate	Late
INVESTIGATIONS	Panculture		Repeat panculture
	Invasive monitoring	Assess oxygen utilization	
	Screen for noninfective causes	Consider further studies to rule out infection including bronchoscopy with brush and lavage, endoscopy, CT scan, other radiological studies as appropriate, radionuclide imaging, tissue biopsy, and diagnostic laparotomy	
	Daily serum and urine biochemistry, complete blood count, differential white cell count and platelet count, frequent prothrombin and partial thromboplastin times with formal coagulation screen if disseminated intravascular coagulopathy is suspected		
TREATMENT *Infection Control*	Broad-spectrum antibiotics	Ensure adequate antibiotic levels	Adjust antibiotic choice to culture results and clinical progress
	Selective decontamination of the digestive tract	Surgical débridement as indicated	Change invasive catheters with respect to time or suspicion of nosocomial infection
System Support Cardiovascular	Intravenous fluids Vasopressors/inotropes *Low dose dopamine* *Dopamine* *Norepinephrine* *Dobutamine*	Minimize oxygen debt *Increase delivery* (by use of fluids, inotropes, supplemental oxygen, and blood transfusions) *Reduce consumption* (by use of sedatives, muscle relaxants and antipyretics (if hyperpyrexial))	
Pulmonary	Supplemental oxygen	Mechanical intubation Positive end-expiratory pressure	Minimize airway pressures and supplemental oxygen if possible
Renal/metabolic	Intravenous fluids	Low dose dopamine Correct gross electrolyte and acid-base disturbances	Loop diuretics Hemofiltration Hemodialysis
Gastrointestinal	Nasogastric tube Stress ulceration prophylaxis	Parenteral nutrition	Enteral nutrition
Other		Replace with clotting factors as indicated	

these therapies (described below) to reduce mortality, the omission of effective resuscitative therapies in septic shock will hasten death. In sepsis syndrome, prompt intervention with invasive monitoring, intravenous fluids, and vasopressors, as necessary, may forestall the expression of full clinical shock. Since septic shock carries a worse prognosis than sepsis without shock, this prompt intervention may improve survival. Furthermore, early suspicion of an infective source and commencement of broad-spectrum antibiotics until the results of cultures are available are also likely to be of therapeutic benefit. Once frank shock develops, management consists of immediate resuscitation, postresuscitation, and long-term care. At each stage, consideration of a multisystems approach is recommended.

Respiratory Support

A compromised respiratory state is often the initial manifestation of sepsis, with a widened alveolar-arterial oxygen gradient progressing to frank arterial hypoxemia. This is associated with decreased lung compliance and increased lung edema, both interstitial and alveolar. Early intervention with supplemental oxygen is essential. While oxygenation may be improved by the addition of continuous positive airway pressure (without mechanical ventilation), the markedly increased work of breathing and the consequent increase in oxygen consumption by the respiratory muscles in septic shock favors early intervention with intubation, mechanical ventilation, and the addition of PEEP.

Cardiovascular Support

The early stages of sepsis may be associated with a profound vasodilatation, with a marked increase in venous capacitance and decrease in venous tone, resulting in decreased venous return. A compounding factor is arterial dilatation (so-called vasomotor paralysis), which results in an altered distribution of blood flow to high capacitance circuits and leads to a further decrease in venous return. Thus the early clinical findings may reflect hypovolemic

shock owing to an increase in intravascular unstressed volume.

The initial phase of circulatory resuscitation is characterized by volume repletion (often "massive"). The early use of invasive monitoring as clinical judgement of adequate volume resuscitation and central filling pressures is notoriously inaccurate. The optimal fluid for resuscitation remains in dispute (26, 34, 50). Certainly, in most settings, crystalloid solutions are adequate (90). In the setting of hypoalbuminemia (e.g., end-stage liver disease), the use of colloid solutions may be preferable with the goal of minimizing extravascular sequestration as edema or ascites. The major advantage of a colloid (e.g., 5% albumin, dextran or hetastarch) is that only one quarter of the volume, compared with a crystalloid, is required to effect a change in hemodynamics (74). Colloids may also favorably affect the oxygen supply and consumption relationship by increasing the oxygen consumption for a given delivery, lending support to the notion that colloids improve microcirculatory flow (44, 74, 77). Nevertheless, colloid solutions are expensive and dextran and hetastarch may alter coagulation (most likely a function of hemodilution) and induce a qualitative platelet defect. The issue of macromolecular aggregation within the macrophage system and the potential impairment of reticuloendothelial function remains unresolved. Transfusion with packed red blood cells to increase the hematocrit to at least 30% is also warranted, although both higher and lower values may be appropriate in certain settings.

On occasion, severe hypotension, end-organ dysfunction and hyperlactemia persist despite volume resuscitation sufficient to optimize cardiac output. While the restoration of blood pressure may not be the primary goal, it is critical to recall that end-organ perfusion is dependent on perfusion pressure. Thus the addition of a vasopressor following fluid resuscitation is often necessary. In the setting of inadequate cardiac output, the solution may be to add an inotrope such as dobutamine or amrinone to improve cardiac output. Likewise, if cardiac function is compromised by ischemia, treatment with nitrates and/or calcium channel blockade may be of benefit. However, in the majority of cases the cardiac output will appear adequate and the choice of a vasopressor is guided by the degree of vasodilatation and the potential for increased afterload to further decrease cardiac output. Thus, dopamine in low dose is often given initially since it should stimulate dopaminergic receptors and increase mesenteric, hepatic, and renal arterial blood flows (1, 38, 42, 56, 78–80, 86, 87). The dopamine is then increased into the range at which it exerts α effects. The beneficial effects of intermediate to higher infusion rates of dopamine (>10 mg/kg/hr) as compared to norepinephrine have not been shown.

If the vasodilatation is sufficiently profound that dopamine titrated to 10–20 μg/kg/min does not generate an adequate blood pressure response, then the substitution of norepinephrine for dopamine should be considered. However, norepinephrine increases the critical closing pressure for a capillary bed that, in severe hypotensive states, may exceed its effect on organ perfusion pressure, thus further compromising regional circulation at a given pressure. In clinical practice, the effects of norepinephrine on oxygen consumption, lactate, and end-organ function are monitored. If these variables suggest impaired cardiac function or reduced oxygen consumption, then a more potent β-adrenergic agent such as dobutamine (or epinephrine if hypotension is profound) can be added.

The goals of the initial resuscitative effort are, at a minimum, the restoration of adequate organ perfusion. Clinically, this is manifested as improved end-organ function with warm extremities, improved mentation, increased urine output, etc. Often this occurs before the restoration of "normal" blood pressure. In recent years, with the increased use of central pressure and hemodynamic monitoring (including systemic oxygen transport and delivery), the degree of adequacy of resuscitation from shock has been questioned (33, 83). In patients who appear to have evidence of restoration of organ function in the immediate post-resuscitation phase, those with a vasodilated hyperdynamic circulatory state appear to fare better than those with a lower cardiac index. Similarly, patients with a falling lactate level after resuscitation have a better outcome (4). A reasonable but aggressive approach to the patient in septic shock would be to institute an initial volume resuscitation until the cardiac output is optimized, with the addition of inotropes and/or vasopressors to increase oxygen transport until oxygen consumption increases no further (plateau) and lactate begins to decrease. Although theoretically attractive, this goal is often unattainable and may be associated with significant side effects of aggressive therapy (e.g., pulmonary edema, tachyarrhythmia).

The optimization of respiratory care in patients with acute lung injury (e.g., the increase in PEEP necessary to improve arterial oxygenation) may compromise cardiac output. In the initial resuscitation, the balance favors maintaining a hyperdynamic circulation and minimizing the negative effect of increased intrathoracic pressure on venous return. Another therapeutic consideration is to reduce the consumption side of the oxygen supply-consumption equation. Sedatives and narcotics may be administered and, if necessary, muscle relaxants, with the goal of decreased oxygen consumption. Hypothermia will also further reduce oxygen consumption; however, this beneficial effect may be counterbalanced by the immunosuppressive, circulatory, and thrombotic effects of hypothermia. Except in the setting of a profound compromise of oxygen transport, we favor limiting the thermoregulation intervention to control of hyperpyrexia.

Renal Support

Electrolyte abnormalities are common in this setting and may become severe as fluid shifts accompany the resuscitative efforts. The blood urea nitrogen and serum creatinine are routinely obtained but may be within the normal range in the early stages of renal failure. The urinalysis may be abnormal, not only when the urinary tract is the source of sepsis, but when the kidney is involved in the failure of multiple organ systems. Urine electrolytes and specific gravity may be helpful in defining the isosthenuric stage that precedes frank acute tubular necrosis. Once the clinical state has stabilized, the glomerular filtration rate may be estimated by a 24-hr creatinine clearance.

In the presence of renal dysfunction, volume overload may be precipitated by transfusion of blood products, infusions of medications, and nutritional supplementation. If loop diuretics such as furosemide are insufficient, in maintaining diuresis one may intervene early with hemofiltration using a venovenous system with a roller pump continuous venovenous hemofiltration or an arterial-venous system with continuous arteriovenous hemofiltration (39, 66, 94). Countercurrent infusion of dialysate during hemofiltration enables effective dialysis without the hemodynamic instability associated with formal hemodialysis in the critically ill patient.

Gastrointestinal Support

Liver function tests are valuable, as marked abnormalities of canalicular enzymes may point to a biliary source of sepsis. More commonly, cholestasis with minimal elevation of transaminases or canalicular enzymes is associated with the septic state. A depressed serum albumin is initially suggestive of chronic disease, but often the resuscitative effort (which may include infusion of albumin-containing products) and the shock state (which may lower the serum albumin) make the serum albumin levels uninterpretable. Coagulation defects documented by the prothrombin time and partial thromboplastin time should be sought. Significant abnormalities, when associated with thrombocytopenia, may reflect disseminated intravascular coagulation, and a more complete assessment of the coagulation state, including factor levels and markers of fibrinolysis (such as low fibrinogen, elevated fibrin degradation products, shortened euglobulin lysis times, and elevation of d-dimers), is indicated. The thromboelastograph can be used to rapidly assess the clinical effect of the coagulopathy and to guide blood product replacement.

Clinical Investigations

Once the initial resuscitation is under way, the focus must shift to defining the etiology of the septic state. The major sources of infection in decreasing frequency are the urinary tract, lung, and gut. While various diagnostic studies are obtained, body fluids, including blood, must be cultured for bacteria and fungi, and empiric antibiotic therapy initiated. A source of sepsis should be actively sought. In addition to a thorough physical examination, where attention is directed to the level of consciousness (and presence of neurologic abnormalities), the chest, the abdomen, and pelvis, laboratory studies should be obtained, both to help confirm the source and to define the extent of multisystem involvement.

The complete blood count may demonstrate a leukocytosis and shift toward immature forms which supports an infectious etiology of the septic state. Leukopenia, associated with the initial stages of sepsis, is a marker of decreased survival. A low hematocrit with normal red cell indices in the absence of apparent blood loss is suggestive of an underlying chronic disease process. The peripheral smear may also show signs of severe hemolysis and thrombocytopenia, which may reflect a disseminated intravascular coagulation or even extend the differential diagnosis to include thrombotic thrombocytopenic purpura.

Radiographic studies are performed as indicated. A chest radiograph should be routinely obtained to evaluate the lungs as a primary source of sepsis and to evaluate the lung in light of multiple systems organ failure. When the source of sepsis remains unclear, computerized tomography of the abdomen is indicated and this study has virtually replaced the "diagnostic" laparotomy in this setting.

As noted above, shock associated with a hyperdynamic hemodynamic profile, but not clearly infectious in etiology, may be seen after severe burn injury, multiple trauma, severe pancreatitis, end-stage liver disease, and acute cellular rejection of a transplanted organ. The initial evaluation must also consider these possibilities. The sepsis syndrome may also occur with viremia, and appropriate serology and viral cultures should be obtained. However, since untreated infectious etiologies of sepsis are uniformly fatal, never assume the sepsis syndrome is due to a noninfectious etiology in the initial stages of support.

Postresuscitation Support

Once appropriate resuscitative and diagnostic efforts have been initiated, the next stage begins. With support the patient may recover. However, some patients have only a partial recovery and 3–5 days after the initial insult have persistent hypotension secondary to arterial vasodilatation, a hyperdynamic cardiac profile, and progressive multisystem organ dysfunction with an increasing serum lactate suggestive of tissue ischemia. This represents a downward spiral that in many cases results in death. Intervention at this stage requires the same vigilance that was directed toward the initial management. Foci of active infection must be sought. Surgical débridement of necrotic tissue and drainage of abscesses are a mainstay of therapy. Pulmonary infection (both secondary and primary superinfection) should be considered with early use of diagnostic bronchoscopy with quantitative culture of lavage fluid and of a protected brush specimen.

The invasive catheter represents another violation of the host's protective defenses and is a portal for bacterial and fungal infection (57). The optimal duration of placement for an invasive catheter is unclear. Some have speculated that routine catheter changes are unjustified (64). However, catheter infection and subsequent sepsis may further insult an already compromised host. Factors to be considered are: the immunocompetence of the patient, the degree of catheter manipulation (most for multilumen catheters, least for dedicated, single lumen, total parenteral nutrition (TPN) catheters and hemo-

dialysis catheters), local catheter care, and the duration of placement of the catheter (58). Thus, while the hemodialysis catheter placed in the polytrauma patient with pigment-induced, acute renal tubular necrosis may not require exchange without suggestive clinical findings, the triple lumen catheter used for TPN, antibiotics, and blood products in a patient, status post liver transplant, should probably be changed within 5–7 days.

Antibiotic Therapy

The choice of antimicrobial agents depends on the source of infection, the severity of the insult, the most likely etiologic agents, and the spectrum of antimicrobial sensitivity of organisms isolated in a particular hospital. Thus while the patient with a community-acquired pneumonia and sputum Gram's stain characteristic of *Streptococcus pneumoniae* may be managed with penicillin alone, the hospitalized patient with a dehisced colonic anastomosis should be treated with a much broader spectrum of antibiotics.

In the setting of a defined, closed space infection, such as an abscess or empyema, adequate surgical drainage and débridement is the mainstay of therapy. Antimicrobials alone in such a setting are doomed to failure.

In the setting of septic shock of unclear etiology, broad-spectrum antimicrobial therapy should be initiated until culture results are available. At such time, the antimicrobial regimen can be tailored to address the pathogenic organisms. Empiric therapy must address the local sensitivity patterns for bacterial and fungal isolates. In many instances, a combination of a ureidopenicillin (such as piperacillin) with an aminoglycoside and vancomycin are appropriate initial agents. Appropriate antibiotic coverage with therapeutic levels are an essential part of the resuscitative effort and clearly influence outcome (52).

In patients at high risk for fungal overgrowth and subsequent infection, the early use of amphotericin B is advised. Fungal infections are more common in those patients who are older, who have undergone major surgery, who have multiple invasive catheters, and who are managed with parenteral nutrition (15). All of these characteristics are present in many intensive care unit patients. The role of newer imidazoles (ketoconazole, miconazole, fluconazole, itraconazole), used for prophylaxis and for treatment of established fungal infection in this setting, is under investigation (96). In immunocompromised hosts, such as those with the acquired immunodeficiency syndrome or those receiving immunosuppression (e.g., transplant recipients), the empiric antimicrobials selected should cover opportunistic organisms including *Pneumocystis carinii* and *Legionella pneumophila*. In such patients cytomegalovirus infection may also be present and should be treated with ganciclovir (dihydroxyproproxymethylguanine) (35).

Selective Decontamination of the Digestive Tract

The realization that nosocomial infection, particularly secondary respiratory infection, is caused by pathogenic organisms that have become integrated into the microbial flora of the patient has prompted investigations of selective decontamination of the digestive tract (76). Typical regimens include six hourly administrations of a solution containing tobramycin (or gentamicin), polymyxin E, and amphotericin B (or nystatin). In intubated patients, a paste containing the same antimicrobials may be applied to the nasopharynx. In several studies, cefotaxime has been coadministered for the first 96 hr until the effects of selective decontamination of the digestive tract are realized. While a systematic decrease in mortality has not been demonstrated, a decreased incidence of respiratory tract infections is evident (88).

Hemodynamic Management

The optimization of hemodynamics in this setting is also controversial. Interventions designed to increase oxygen consumption by increasing oxygen delivery may not be clearly beneficial. Indeed the oxygen supply dependent characterization of some

disease states, including sepsis and ARDS, has recently been questioned (54, 81). Increasing the hematocrit, the easiest way of increasing oxygen transport, may not be associated with increased oxygen consumption. The addition of inotropes, such as dobutamine, may be complicated by tachyarrhythmias and hypotension. One may follow both the serum lactate and oxygen consumption as well as the trend toward multiple systems organ failure as a monitor for the efficacy of intervention. A reasonable course would be to transfuse anemic patients to a hematocrit of 30 - 30% and, once adequate preload is assured, use dobutamine at a dose of 5–10 μg/kg/min. If no "improvement" is documented or if severe complications ensue, the inotrope is discontinued.

In summary, this secondary phase of sepsis is associated with multiple systems organ failure and often progresses inexorably to death. Aggressive intervention and support for organ failure (e.g., dialysis for acute renal failure) is indicated. In the setting where a septic focus cannot be determined, the gut should be considered the source. This may be particularly true once hepatocellular (and Kupffer cell) function has been compromised. It remains to be proven that selective decontamination of the digestive tract, which has been shown to reduce the incidence of nosocomial pneumonia, will also reduce the incidence of the secondary septic state.

FUTURE CONSIDERATIONS

It is clear that the current focus upon an infectious etiology and aggressive resuscitation for the management of both the initial and subsequent phases of the sepsis syndrome has only marginally altered outcome. In part this appears to be related to the inexorable progression of the sepsis syndrome mediated by unchecked host defenses and evolving into the multiple organ failure syndrome. Early trials with antiendotoxin antibodies are particularly encouraging with a significant reduction in mortality in culture positive Gram-negative rod septic shock demonstrated with a human monoclonal antiendotoxin (100). The potential for intervention at other stages in the cytokine cascade, such as with anti-tumor necrosis factor antibodies, is under active investigation (2, 37, 46). Thus, the future management of the sepsis syndrome will incorporate strategies directed at modulating the host's response to infection in addition to the resuscitative efforts outlined above.

Acknowledgments. The authors wish to thank Wendy Bouton, Celeste Misho, and Gretchen Winstein for their continuous help and Michael R. Pinsky for his invaluable advice.

References

1. Angehn W, Schmid E, Althaus, et al. Effect of dopamine on hepatosplanchnic blood flow. J Cardiovasc Pharmacol 1980;2:257–265.
2. Bahrami S, Redl H, Leichfried G, et al. Beneficial effects of anti-TNF monoclonal antibody (mAb) in endotoxin induced coagulation disorder in rats. Circ Shock 1991;34:167.
3. Baker JW, Deitch EA, Li M, Bert RD, Specian RD. Hemorrhagic shock induces bacterial translocation from the gut. J Trauma 1988;28(7):896–906.
4. Bakker J, Coffernils M, Leon M, et al. Blood lactate levels are superior to oxygen-derived variables in predicting outcome in human septic shock. Chest 1991;99:956–962.
5. Balk RA, Bone RC. The septic syndrome: definition and clinical implications. Crit Care Clin 1989;5(1):1–8.
6. Bank NU, Kammer RB. Hematologic complications associated with beta-lactam antibiotics. Rev Infect Dis 1983;5(suppl 2):S380.
7. Banks OG, Foulis AK, Ledingham IMcA, Mac-Sween RNM. Liver function in septic shock. J Clin Pathol 1982;35:1249–1252.
8. Barton R, Cerra FB. The hypermetabolism multiple organ failure syndrome. Chest 1989;96:1153–1160.
9. Bone RC. Sepsis, the sepsis syndrome, multiorgan failure: a plea for comparable definitions [Editorial]. Ann Inter Med 1991;114:332–333.
10. Bone RC. The pathogenesis of sepsis. Ann Intern Med 1991;115:457–469.
11. Bone RC, Fisher CJ, Clemmer TP, et al. Sepsis syndrome: a valid clinical entity. Crit Care Med 1989;17(5):389–393.
12. Bowton DL, Bertels NH, Prough DS, Stump DA. Cerebral blood flow is reduced in patients with sepsis syndrome. Crit Care Med 1989;17:399–403.
13. Bradfield JWB. Control of spillover: the importance of Kupffer cell function in clinical medicine. Lancet 1974;2:883–886.
14. Brezis M, Rosen S, Silva P, Epstein FH. Renal ischemia: a new perspective. Kidney Int 1984;26:375–383.
15. Bross J, Talbot GH, Maislin G, et al. Risk factors for nosocomial candidemia: a case control study in adults without leukemia. Am J Med 1989;87:614–620.
16. Cain S. Oxygen delivery and uptake in dogs during anemic and hypoxic hypoxia. J Appl Physiol 1977;42:228–234.
17. Cain SM. Peripheral oxygen uptake and the delivery in health and disease. Clin Chest Med 1983;4:139.
18. Carli A, Auclair MC, Benassayag C. Evidence for an elderly lipid soluble cardiodepressant factor in rat serum after a sublethal dose of endotoxin. Circ Shock 1981;8:301–312.
19. Carrico CJ, Meakins JL, Marshall JC, et al. Multiorgan-failure syndrome. Arch Surg 1986;121:196–200.
20. Centers for Disease Control. Increase in national hospital discharge survey rates for septicemia—United States, 1979–1987. MMWR 1990;39(2):31–34.
21. Christy JH. Treatment of Gram negative shock. Am J Med 1971;50:77.
22. Claypool JG, Delp M, Lin TK. Hemodynamic studies in patients with Laennec's cirrhosis. Am J Med Sci 1957;234:48.
23. Cunnion RE, Schaer GL, Parker MM, Natanson C, Parrillo JE. The coronary circulation in human septic shock. Circulation 1986;73:637–644.
24. Danek SJ, Lynch JP, Weg JG, Dantzker DR. The dependence of oxygen uptake on oxygen delivery in the adult respiratory distress syndrome. Am Rev Respir Dis 1980;122:387–395.
25. Danner RL, Elin RJ, Hosseini JM, et al. Endotoxemia in human septic shock. Chest 1991;99:169–175.
26. Dawidson I, Ottosson J, Reisch J. Colloid solution therapy of experimental ischemic intestinal shock in rats. Crit Care Med 1985;13:709–714.
27. Decamp MM, Demling RH. Posttraumatic multisystem organ failure. JAMA 1988;260:530–534.
28. Deitch EA, Berg R, Specian R. Endotoxin promotes the translocation of bacteria from the gut. Arch Surg 1987;122:185–190.
29. Deitch EA, Winterton J, Bey R. The gut as the portal of entry for bacteremia. Ann Surg 1987;205:681–692.
30. Dhainaut JF, Huyghebaert MF, Monsallier JF, Lefevre G, Dall'Ava-Santucci J, Brunet F, et al. Coronary hemodynamics and myocardial extraction of lactate, free fatty acids, glucose and ketones in patients with septic shock. Circulation 1987;75:533–541.
31. Doyle HR, Marino I, Miro A, et al. Adult respiratory distress syndrome secondary to end stage liver disease: successful outcome following liver transplantation. Transplantation (in press).
32. Edes TE, Walk BE, Austin JL. Diarrhea in tube fed patients: feeding formula not necessarily the cause. Am J Med 1990;88:91–94.
33. Edwards JD, Brown GCS, Nightingale P, et al. Use of survivors' cardiorespiratory values as therapeutic goals in septic shock. Crit Care Med 1989;17:1098.
34. Falk JL, Rackow EC, Astiz M, Weil MH. Fluid resuscitation in shock. J Cardiothoracic Vascular Anesth 1988;2:33–38.
35. Faulds D, Heel RC. Ganciclovir: a review of its antiviral activity, pharmacokinetic properties and

therapeutic efficacy in cytomegalovirus infections. Drugs 1990;39:597–638.

36. Filkins JP. Cytokines, mediators of the septic syndrome and septic shock. In: Taylor RW, Shoemaker WC, eds. Critical care state of the art. Vol 12. Fullerton, CA: Society of Critical Care Medicine, 1991;351–370.

37. Fisher CJ, Opal SM, Dhainaut JF, et al. Anti-TNF IgG monoclonal antibody (CB0006) in sepsis syndrome: pharmacokinetics, safety and role of pretreatment IL-6 as a predictor of time of survival. Circ Shock 1991;34:167–168.

38. Goldberg LI. Cardiovascular and renal actions of dopamine: potential clinical applications. Pharmacol Rev 1972;24:1–29.

39. Golper TA. Continuous arteriovenous hemofiltration in acute renal failure. Am J Kidney Dis 1985;6:373–386.

40. Grene LJ, Shapanka R, Glenn TM, Lefer AM. Isolation of myocardial depressant factor from plasma of dogs in hemorrhagic shock. Biochim Biophys Acta 1977;491:275–285.

41. Hasselgren PO, Fischer JE. Septic encephalopathy: etiology and management. Intensive Care Med 1986;12:13–16.

42. Hasselgren PO, Biber B, Fornander J. Improved blood flow and protein synthesis in the postischemic liver following infusion of dopamine. J Surg Res 1982;34:44–52.

43. Haupt MT, Gilbert EM, Carlson RW. Fluid loading increases oxygen consumption in septic patients with lactic acidosis. Am Rev Respir Dis 1985;131:912–916.

44. Hauser CJ, Shoemaker WC, Turpin I, et al. Oxygen transport responses to colloid and crystalloid in critically ill surgical patients. Surg Gynecol Obstet 1980;150:611.

45. Jacobs RF, Tabor DR. Immune cellular interactions during sepsis and septic injury. Crit Care Clin 1989;5(9):9–26.

46. Jesmok G, Lindsey D, Fournel M, Emerson T. Possible mechanisms of protection afforded by TNF-alpha monoclonal antibody (TNF MAB) in *E. coli* challenged pigs. Circ Shock 1991;34:167.

47. Johnson EE, Hedley-Whyte J. Continuous positive-pressure ventilation and portal flow in dogs with pulmonary edema. J Appl Physiol 1972;33:385–389.

48. Katz S, Grosfeld JL, Gross K. Impaired bacterial clearance and trapping in obstructive jaundice. Ann Surg 1984;199:14–20.

49. Kowalski HJ, Abelmann WH. The cardiac output at rest in Laennec's cirrhosis. J Clin Invest 1953;32:1025.

50. Kramer GC, Perron PR, Lindsey C, et al. Small volume resuscitation with hypertonic saline dextran solution. Surgery 1986;100:239–247.

51. Kreger BE, Craven DE, Carling PC, McCabe WR. Gram-negative bacteremia. III. Reassessment of etiology, epidemiology and ecology in 612 patients. Am J Med 1980;68:332–343.

52. Kreger BE, Craven DE, McCabe WR. Gram-negative bacteremia. IV. Reevaluation of clinical features and treatment in 612 patients. Am J Med 1980;68:344–355.

53. Lefer AM. Interaction between myocardial depressant factor and vasoactive mediators with ischemia and shock. Am J Physiol 1987;252:R193–R205.

54. Lorente JA, Renes E, Gomez-Aquinaga MA, et al. Oxygen delivery-dependent oxygen consumption in acute respiratory failure. Crit Care Med 1981;19:770–775.

55. Madoff RD, Sharpe SM, Fath JJ, et al. Prolonged surgical intensive care. Arch Surg 1986;120:698.

56. Maestracci P, Grimaud D, Livrelli N, et al. Increase in hepatic blood flow and cardiac output during dopamine infusion in man. Crit Care Med 1981;9:14–16.

57. Maki D. Infections associated with intravascular lines. In: Remington, JS, Swartz, MN, eds. Current clinical topics in infectious disease. Vol 3. New York: McGraw-Hill, 1982.

58. Maki DG. Risk factors for nosocomial infection in intensive care "devices vs nature" and goals for the next decade. Arch Intern Med 1989;149:30–35.

59. Matuschak GM, Rinaldo JE, Pinsky MR, et al. Effect of end-stage liver failure on the incidence of resolution of the adult respiratory distress syndrome. J Crit Care 1987;2:162–173.

60. Miller PD, Krebs RA, Neal BJ, McIntyre DO. Polyuric prerenal failure. Arch Intern Med 1980;140:907–909.

61. Mohsenifar Z, Goldbacxh P, Tashkin DP, Campisi DJ. Relationship between O_2 delivery and O_2 consumption in the adult respiratory distress syndrome. Chest 1983;84:267–271.

62. Montgomery AB, Stager MA, Carrico CJ, Hudson LD. Causes of mortality in patients with the acute respiratory distress syndrome. Am Rev Respir Dis 1985;132:485–489.

63. Murray JF, Dawson AM, Sherlock S. Circulatory changes in chronic liver disease. Am J Med 1957;24:358.

64. Norwood S, Ruby A, Civetta J, et al. Catheter-related infections and associated septicemia. Chest 1991;99:968–975.

65. Norwood SH, Civetta JM. Evaluating sepsis in critically ill patients. Chest 1987;92:137–144.

66. Ossenkoppele GJ, van der Meulen J, Bronsveld W, Thijs LG. Continuous arteriovenous hemofiltration as an adjunctive therapy for septic shock. Crit Care Med 1985;13:102–104.

67. Parker MM, Parrillo JE. Myocardial function in septic shock. J Crit Care 1990;5(1):47–61.

68. Parker MM, Suffredini AF, Natanson C, et al. Responses of left ventricular function in survivors and non-survivors of septic shock. J Crit Care 1989;4:19–25.

69. Parrillo JE. Management of septic shock: present and future [Editorial]. Ann Intern Med 1991;115(6):491–493.

70. Parrillo JE, Burch C, Shelhamer JH, et al. A circulating myocardial depressant substance in humans with septic shock. J Clin Invest 1985;76:1539–1553.

71. Parrillo JE, Parker MM, Natanson C, et al. NIH Conference. Septic shock in humans; advances in the understanding of pathogenesis, cardiovascular dysfunction, and therapy. Ann Intern Med 1990;113:227–242.

72. Pinsky MR, Matuschak GM. Multiple systems organ failure. Crit Care Clin 1989;5(2):199–220.
73. Pinsky MR, Schlichtig B. Defining the hypoxic threshold. Crit Care Med 1991;19(2):147–149.
74. Rackow EC, Falk JL, Fein IA, et al. Fluid resuscitation in circulatory shock: a comparison of the cardiorespiratory effects of albumin, hetastarch and saline solutions in patients with hypovolemic and septic shock. Crit Care Med 1983;11:839–850.
75. Ravin HA, Rowley D, Jenkins C, Fine J. On the absorption of bacterial endotoxin from the gastrointestinal tract of the normal and shocked animal. J Exp Med 1960;112:783–792.
76. Reidy JJ, Ramsay G. Clinical trials of selective decontamination of the digestive tract: review. Crit Care Med 1990;18:1449–1456.
77. Rhodes GR, Newell JC, Shah D, et al. Increased oxygen consumption accompanying increased oxygen delivery with hypertonic mannitol in adult respiratory distress syndrome. Surgery 1978;84:490–497.
78. Richardson PDI, Withrington PG. Responses of the canine hepatic arterial and portal venous vascular beds to dopamine. Eur J Pharmacol 1978;48:337–349.
79. Richardson PDI, Withrington PG. Liver blood flow. I. Intrinsic and nervous control of liver blood flow. Gastroenterology 1981;81:159–173.
80. Richardson PDI, Withrington PG. Liver blood flow. II. Effects of drugs and hormones on liver blood flow. Gastroenterology 1981;81:356–375.
81. Ronco JL, Phang PT, Walley KR, et al. Oxygen consumption is independent of changes in oxygen delivery in severe adult respiratory distress syndrome. Am Rev Respir Dis 1991;143:1267–1273.
82. Saba TM. Physiology and pathophysiology of the reticuloendothelial system. Arch Intern Med 1970;126:1031–1052.
83. Shoemaker WC, Appel PL, Kram HB. Prospective trial of supernormal values of survivors as therapeutic goals in high-risk surgical patients. Chest 1988;94:1176.
84. Snell RJ, Parrillo JE. Cardiovascular dysfunction in septic shock. Chest 1991;99:1000–1009.
85. Stathopoulos G, Chang EB. Diarrhea in the intensive care unit. In: Rippe JM, Irvin RS, Alpert JS, Fink MP, eds. Intensive care medicine. Boston: Little, Brown & Co, 1991.
86. Townsend MC, Schirmer WJ, Schirmer JM, Fry DE. Low dose dopamine improves effective hepatic blood flow in murine peritonitis. Circ Shock 1987;21:149–153.
87. Trachte GJ, Lefer AM. Influence of dopamine on liver dynamics in hemorrhagic shock. Circ Shock 1977;4:305–315.
88. Vandenbroucke-Grauls CMJE, Vandebroucke JP. Effect of selective decontamination of the digestive tract in respiratory tract infections and mortality in the intensive care unit. Lancet 1991;338:859–862.
89. Villar J, Slutsky AS, Hew E, Aberman A. Oxygen transport and oxygen consumption in critically ill patients. Chest 1990;98:687–692.
90. Virgilio RW, Ric CL, Smith DE, et al. Crystalloid vs colloid resuscitation: is one better? Surgery 1979;85:129–139.
91. Webster's medical desk dictionary. Springfield, MA: Merriam Webster, 1986:648.
92. Weitekamp MR, Aber RC. Prolonged bleeding times and bleeding diathesis associated with moxalactam administration. JAMA 1983;249:69.
93. Wells CL, Maddaus MA, Simmons RL. Proposed mechanisms for the translocation of intestinal bacteria. Rev Infect Dis 1988;10(5):958–979.
94. Wendon J, Smithies M, Sheppard M, et al. Continuous high volume venous-venous haemofiltration in acute renal failure. Intensive Care Med 1989;15:358–363.
95. Wilson RF. Special problems in the diagnosis and treatment of surgical sepsis. Surg Clin North Am 1985;65:965–989.
96. Wingard JR, Vaughan WP, Braine HG, et al. Prevention of fungal sepsis in patients with prolonged neutropenia: a randomized, double-blind, placebo-controlled trial of intravenous miconazole. Am J Med 1987;83:1103–1109.
97. Witt NJ, Zochodne DW, Bolton CF, et al. Peripheral nerve function in sepsis and multiple organ failure. Chest 1991;99:176–184.
98. Yokoyama I, Todo S, Miyata T, et al. Endotoxemia and human liver transplantation. Transplant Proc 1989;21:3833.
99. Young LS. Gram-negative sepsis. In: Mandell GL, Douglas RG Jr, Bennett JE, eds. Principles and practice of infectious diseases. 3rd ed. New York: Churchill Livingstone, 1990.
100. Ziegler EJ, Fisher CJ, Sprung CL, et al. Treatment of Gram-negative bacteremia and septic shock with HA-1A human monoclonal antibody against endotoxin. A randomized, double-blind, placebo-controlled trial. N Engl J Med 1991;324:429–436.
101. Zochodne DW, Bolton CF, Wells GA, et al. Critical illness polyneuropathy: a complication of sepsis and multiple organ failure. Brain 1987;110:819–842.

6

Physiologic Regulation of Systemic Blood Flow

Paul T. Schumacker

The cells that comprise body tissues perform many physiological functions, including growth, biosynthesis, contraction, membrane transport, and other metabolic processes, all of which require energy expenditure. The energetic needs for these obligatory and facultative functions are met by oxidative metabolism, leading to the formation of high energy compounds such as ATP. In most cells, ATP formation is accomplished primarily by the electron transport system, which transfers reducing equivalents to molecular oxygen. Under ideal conditions, the rate of oxygen consumption by cells should depend upon the level of metabolic activity, rather than on the availability of oxygen. In this situation, the mitochondrial oxygen concentration is present in excess, and electron transport is limited by the availability of ADP and reducing equivalents. When metabolic rates are increased during periods of stimulated cellular activity, ADP and NADH concentrations increase, and ATP production rises as electron transport rates are increased (11, 12). Despite wide changes in metabolic demand and tissue oxygen availability, mitochondrial oxygen supply is normally not a rate-limiting factor. Under conditions of maximal oxygen consumption in muscle, or situations where oxygen transport to a tissue becomes significantly impaired, supply-dependent oxygen uptake can occur (31). Acutely, this tissue hypoxia elicits many cellular responses, including an increase in anaerobic glycolysis. When the hypoxia is more sustained, tissue damage can develop. A major function of the cardiovascular system is to maintain tissue O_2 availability, thereby preventing or minimizing the development of supply-dependent O_2 uptake states.

Note that the range of metabolic activity within a single tissue may change by more than 10-fold, and the variation in metabolic rate among tissues can differ by nearly 50-fold in the extreme. To sustain this normal range of metabolic activities the cardiovascular system must be capable of achieving large increases in the rate of oxygen transport, defined as the product of blood flow and arterial oxygen content. Moreover, in the face of such diversity of potential needs, it must also be capable of distributing this transport among regions in accordance with their local oxygen demands. To achieve this optimization, oxygen transport is normally restricted in regions with low oxygen demand and augmented in regions with high demand, by redistributing blood flow within and among tissues (16). In addition, vascular changes within some metabolically active tissues lead to improvements in the ability of tissues to extract oxygen, by augmenting the arteriovenous oxygen content difference. Collectively, these adjustments help to prevent supply dependence of oxygen uptake, defined as the limitation to tissue metabolism caused by inadequate availability of oxygen and subsequent lack of adequate ATP availability.

The focus of this chapter is to review briefly the mechanisms contributing to the regulation of the distribution of oxygen transport, and the effects of vasoactive drugs on this regulation. We begin with a brief review of the factors determining cardiac output itself.

REGULATION OF CARDIAC OUTPUT

In steady state, cardiac output is normally limited by venous return (17). At the simplest level this certainly must be true, since the heart cannot pump out more blood than it receives. However, the reasons become clearer if one considers the sequence of events that occurs immediately after the heart is stopped. When this occurs, cardiac output stops and the pressures throughout the systemic vascular compartment fall rapidly, equilibrating at the *mean circulatory filling pressure* or *mean systemic pressure*. This static pressure is normally about 12–15 mm Hg and is determined entirely by the *volume of blood* in the vascular compartment (unstressed volume) and the *overall compliance* of the systemic vessels. Obviously, when the pressures are the same throughout the vascular system, no flow can occur because no pressure gradients exist between the aorta and periphery, or between the periphery and the right atrium. Consider the events that occur at the instant the heart is restarted. At that instant, the first heartbeat transfers blood from the venous compartment to the arterial compartment, causing the pressure at the aortic root to increase and the right atrial pressure to fall. Blood flow toward the peripheral tissues then begins because the aortic pressure is now higher than the mean circulatory filling pressure that still exists out in the microcirculation. Likewise, venous return from the microcirculation toward the heart begins, because right atrial pressure has now fallen below the mean circulatory filling pressure, which is still present out in the systemic vessels. With subsequent heartbeats, pressure in the aortic root increases further

as volume is moved from the (relatively compliant) venous vessels to the (less compliant) arterial vessels. As this occurs, blood flow toward the periphery increases because the gradient from the aorta to the microcirculation increases. Simultaneously, venous return to the heart increases as the right atrial pressure falls further, relative to the mean circulatory filling pressure.

What happens to mean circulatory filling pressure as all of this is happening? The answer is that mean circulatory filling pressure, which is set by vascular volume and overall vascular compliance, remains unchanged. To better understand this, consider what intravascular pressures would be encountered during a journey from the aorta to the right atrium via the microcirculation. Obviously, the mean pressure would be highest in the aorta and would decrease little until the major sites of vascular resistance (arterioles) were reached. In the microcirculation, intravascular pressure would decrease steeply in the arterioles and less so in the capillaries and venules. Finally, the pressure decrease from venules to the right atrium would be small, relative to the overall decrease in pressure across the system. Along this journey, a pressure equal to the mean circulatory filling pressure would be encountered somewhere in the microcirculation. (This must be true, since aortic and right atrial pressures are greater and less than mean systemic pressure, respectively.) By definition, the pressure at this location is no different from what it would be while the heart is stopped. Therefore, it can be said that all of the additional pressure in the aorta (generated by the heart) has been dissipated at that location, due to the flow resistance in the arterial circuit. If the aortic pressure head generated by the heart has been dissipated at that point, then blood flow from that point back to the right atrium will occur only by virtue of the fact that the heart lowers right atrial pressure as it raises aortic pressure. It follows that the only factors influencing venous return to the heart (from that location) are the mean circulatory filling pressure, right atrial pressure, and the resistance offered by the vessels in between.

Thus, it is said that venous return is determined by the relationship

$$\text{venous return} = \text{cardiac output} = \frac{\text{Pms} - \text{Pra}}{\text{Rvr}}$$

where Pms is the mean circulatory filling pressure, Pra is the mean right atrial pressure, and Rvr is the lumped vascular resistance encountered in vessels located between the microvascular location where Pms is encountered and the right atrium (13).

From the above, it should be clear that the heart functions both by raising aortic pressure and by lowering right atrial pressure. From a design standpoint, this may be beneficial for the microcirculation because it results in lower microvascular pressures than would occur if right atrial pressure remained constant while aortic pressure rose. Lower microvascular pressures will, in turn, tend to reduce the fluid filtration in the peripheral circulation while still allowing the capillaries to remain relatively permeable to solutes. From a functional standpoint, this means that factors that influence the difference between mean systemic pressure and right atrial pressure will tend to directly influence venous return, and thus cardiac output.

REGULATION OF ARTERIAL PRESSURE

Mean aortic pressure reflects a balance between cardiac output and the overall systemic vascular resistance. In steady state, systemic vascular resistance is regulated by neural and hormonal systems to maintain arterial pressure within normal limits. In response to acute changes in venous return caused by posture adjustments, clinical interventions, or voluntary maneuvers, the arterial baroreceptors signal changes in arterial pressure to the vasomotor center located in the medulla oblongata, which adjusts sympathetic and parasympathetic nervous system tone to adjust vascular tone accordingly (1). These adjustments include changes in the caliber of arteriolar resistance vessels, as well as changes in the tone of venous vessels. Changes in the former tend to maintain arterial pressure in the face of acute changes

in venous return and cardiac output, by adjusting vascular resistance in specific tissues. Changes in the latter tend to alter the capacitance of venous vessels. This alters the mean circulatory filling pressure, which is a primary determinant of venous return.

CONTROL OF TISSUE BLOOD FLOW

The organ systems of the body constitute a set of parallel vascular channels, among which the cardiac output is distributed. Factors that contribute to the regulation of blood flow distribution among tissues include (extrinsic) neural and humoral control systems and (intrinsic) metabolic and vascular control mechanisms, which are local to the tissue (10). The relative dominance among these influences varies markedly among tissues, leading to a diversity in the balance between extrinsic and intrinsic factors in vascular control. For example, the cerebral circulation exhibits extensive intrinsic autoregulatory (23) ability, yet its flow resistance is relatively insensitive to changes in sympathetic neural tone. By contrast, skin exhibits broad changes in blood flow in response to changes in sympathetic and parasympathetic tone, while its autoregulatory response is less evident. Vascular resistance in the intestine demonstrates a high sensitivity to changes in sympathetic and parasympathetic tone, but also demonstrates clear evidence of intrinsic control mechanisms (19, 22).

The local mechanisms controlling blood flow and flow distribution within tissues are incompletely understood and appear to vary widely among tissues. Among the primary mechanisms, local metabolic control and local vascular reflexes (myogenic) are known to play important roles. The myogenic theory of blood flow control (24) arises from the observation that vascular smooth muscle cells contract in response to increases in wall stress. Hence, increases in intravascular pressure evoke increases in constrictor tone, thereby regulating local blood flow. The "metabolic theory" of microvascular control explains local vascular adjustments based on the feedback of metabolic products on sites of vascular control (14, 15, 24). According to this theory, local adjustments in capillary recruitment and vascular resistance are linked to the ratio of oxygen supply to oxygen demand (27, 28). Under basal conditions, tissue oxygen supply greatly exceeds demand, and relatively few capillaries may receive blood flow. When tissue metabolic activity is stimulated, the ratio of oxygen supply to demand decreases, and accumulating metabolic by-products act to relax precapillary control sites, thereby increasing the density of perfused capillaries (29). The improved capillary recruitment is assumed to permit greater arteriovenous O_2 extraction and lower end-capillary O_2 tensions without introducing diffusion as a factor limiting transport. If the ratio of supply to demand is decreased further, metabolic products can accumulate further, dilating the larger, flow-controlling vessels and improving local oxygen supply.

While the metabolic theory provides a useful model that is generally consistent with much experimental data, its applicability to any specific tissue is limited. For example, while it generally explains the increases in perfused capillary density and reductions in resistance seen in skeletal muscle during exercise, its applicability to the same tissue under resting conditions when the supply of oxygen is reduced progressively is more questionable. Moreover, some investigators have argued that the partial pressure of oxygen in the tissue, which also varies with the supply-to-demand ratio, is a more likely stimulus, since no single metabolic vasodilator has been identified to explain the magnitude of the observed responses. Finally, no single vasodilator metabolite has been identified that can explain the magnitude of the hyperemic response seen, for example, in exercise. Hence, generalized models are useful starting points in understanding how local vascular control may act in a specific tissue, but not especially useful in describing any particular tissue.

Local intrinsic control of tissue blood flow frequently competes with systemic responses, especially in situations where the relationship between systemic oxygen supply and tissue oxygen demand is stressed (5). An excellent example of this competition among control systems is seen in muscular exercise. In exercise, the oxygen demand of specific muscle groups is significantly increased, while other tissues maintain only resting needs. Increases in sympathetic nervous system activation are systemic, and so tend to reduced blood flow in all vascular beds where neural control plays a significant role in regulating flow. In working muscles, local metabolic vasodilation overrides the neural vasoconstrictor stimulus, thereby augmenting blood flow preferentially in those vessels supplying working muscle groups. Simultaneously, a restriction of blood flow in nonworking muscle beds, skin, and the splanchnic circulation (and in some species, the kidney) help to preserve perfusion pressure for the working muscles and "vital" tissues such as cerebral and coronary beds. During severe exercise in a warm, humid environment, heat loss soon becomes a major problem, and neurally mediated decreases in the vascular resistance of skin vessels lead to a "vascular steal" of blood flow toward skin vessels mediating heat loss. The ensuing redistribution of blood flow away from working muscle groups is enough to significantly reduce maximal exercise capacity in subjects working in thermally stressful environments (25).

Another example of the diversity of vascular control mechanisms is seen in states where cardiac output is severely reduced, such as during hemorrhage. Removal of blood volume lowers mean circulatory filling pressure. This lowers venous return by reducing the vascular pressure gradient between the periphery and the right atrium, causing cardiac output to decrease. As cardiac output decreases, initial decreases in systemic arterial pressure lead to baroreceptor-mediated increases in sympathetic neural tone and decreases in parasympathetic tone. These autonomic responses lead to: (*a*) increases in venous vessel tone, thereby decreasing venous capacitance and initially limiting the fall in mean circulatory filling pressure; (*b*) increases in arteriolar smooth muscle tone, thereby increasing systemic vascular resistance to help maintain arterial pressure in the face of a falling cardiac output; (c) augmented cardiac contractility and heart rate; and (d) stimulated hormonal responses including catecholamine release from the adrenal medulla, stimulation of the renin-angiotensin system, and stimulation of other hormonal systems (1). Collectively, these mechanisms minimize the fall in systemic arterial pressure until blood loss becomes severe.

When the restriction of blood flow and oxygen delivery to "nonvital" tissues becomes severe, local metabolic responses within some tissues can override sympathetic-mediated increases in vascular resistance in a phenomenon known as autoregulatory escape (15). The onset of autoregulatory escape within tissues appears to coincide with the onset of supply-dependent O_2 uptake. For example, during progressive hemorrhage the intestine appears to become O_2 supply-dependent at about the same systemic O_2 delivery as whole body (22). This mechanism may prevent certain organs with strong neurally mediated limitations in blood flow from sustaining hypoxic cell injury in states where other organs are still adequately perfused. During severe reductions in cardiac output, local autoregulatory escape can significantly reduce systemic vascular resistance, leading to acute vascular collapse (30) as the perfusion pressure for the coronary and cerebral circulations is lost.

Some understanding of the roles of α and β receptors on vascular control has emerged from studies of the effects of pharmacologic blockade on whole body and tissue responses to hypoxia. During ventilation with low oxygen tensions, peripheral chemoreceptor stimulation mediates the increase in sympathetic activity seen. In anesthetized dogs challenged with 9.1% O_2, whole body O_2 extraction increased progressively with time during hypoxia, reaching nearly 90% at the end of the hypoxic period (4). In the same study, α blockade with phenoxybenzamine attenuated the increase in O_2 extraction, demonstrating that α-adrenergic vasoconstriction promotes the improvements in extraction during hypoxia. This effect is likely due to contribution of α-adrenergic

vasoconstriction to the redistribution of blood flow among organ systems during hypoxia. In a later study (7), it was shown that phenoxybenzamine limited the increase in whole body O_2 extraction during hypoxia, yet it did not attenuate the increase in extraction seen in the isolated hindlimb (primarily skeletal muscle). These findings suggest that adrenergic vasoconstriction is more critical for interorgan blood flow redistribution than for local microvascular responses mediating the increases in O_2 extraction during hypoxia. However, other studies have shown that the redistribution of blood flow to brain, heart, and respiratory muscles can still occur in the presence of combined α- and β-adrenergic blockade (9). Thus, local metabolic vasodilation is likely to be the dominant mechanism mediating redistribution.

The role of β-adrenergic receptors in peripheral blood flow responses to systemic hypoxia have also been the focus of study. Cain (3) found no effect of β-adrenergic blockade with propranolol on the critical oxygen delivery in anesthetized dogs during anemic or hypoxic hypoxia. In a study of hindlimb responses to transient periods of hypoxia, Cain and Chapler (6) reported that β-adrenergic blockade attenuated the fall in skeletal muscle resistance seen during hypoxia, which suggested that β receptors might play a role in mediating vasodilation during severe hypoxia. However, a clearer explanation for these findings was later offered by Bredle et al. (2) who suggested that circulating catecholamines released during hypoxia might also augment metabolic activity in skeletal muscle through a calorigenic action. By stimulating metabolism, this effect would presumably augment the metabolic vasodilation seen in the limb during systemic hypoxia, as well as through the effects of catecholamines on β_2 vascular receptors. This question was explored by measuring responses to systemic hypoxia in an isolated hindlimb kept normoxic by use of a membrane oxygenator. Catecholamines released from the adrenal medulla in response to the systemic hypoxia significantly increased O_2 demand in the normoxic hind limb. Moreover, selective β_2 inhibition prevented this increase in O_2

demand and augmented the increase in limb vascular resistance during the hypoxic challenge (2). These results suggest that during systemic hypoxia, circulating catecholamines can augment oxygen demands in some tissues, including skeletal muscle, and may also attenuate the α-adrenergic vasoconstriction by acting on vascular β_2-receptors mediating vasodilation.

EFFECTS OF VASOACTIVE DRUGS

Through their effects on vascular resistance and compliance, vasoactive drugs have the potential to disrupt the distribution of blood flow within and among organ systems. By competing with the physiologic regulation of regional and microvascular blood flow distribution, vasoactive substances could interfere with the ability of tissues to regulate regional blood flows in accord with local metabolic demands. If this were the case, then administration of vasoactive drugs could potentialy initiate O_2 supply dependency in some tissues, by selectively reducing their blood flow and confounding local microvascular responses such as adjustments in perfused capillary density. For example, one might expect the infusion of an α-agonist to increase vascular resistance preferentially in vascular beds with a high density of α receptors, such as skeletal muscle and the splanchnic circulation (18), leading to the induction of supply-dependent O_2 uptake in those beds as a consequence of their lowered blood flow.

Surprisingly, a number of studies have failed to demonstrate a clear impairment in tissue oxygen extraction ability in response to infusions of vasoactive drugs. For example, sodium nitroprusside infusion (5–15 μg/min/kg) in a canine model of progressive hypovolemia reduced mean blood pressure significantly, but did not initiate O_2 supply dependency at a significantly higher systemic O_2 delivery (26). This suggests that nitroprusside-induced relaxation in arteriolar tone did not occur preferentially in tissues with low or high O_2 extractions. Higher doses of nitroprusside could have different results, however, due to the loss in coronary and cerebral

perfusion pressure that would occur at lower blood pressures.

In a canine study of norepinephrine and dobutamine infusions, Lewis et al. (21) found that neither norepinephrine nor dobutamine infusion (10 μg/kg/min) caused a significant deterioration in the whole body critical oxygen extraction at the onset of O_2 supply dependency. These results suggest that local metabolic vasodilation can compete successfully with pharmacologic-induced alterations in vascular tone, thereby preserving the ability of tissues to regulate oxygen extraction in response to changes in oxygen delivery. However, this contrasts with the findings of Coburn and Pendleton (8), who concluded that high doses of norepinephrine might interfere with capillary recruitment mechanisms in resting skeletal muscle.

In a study of hypoxic hypoxia, King and Cain (20) used methoxamine infusions to test whether preferential vasoconstriction in specific tissue beds led to an increase in the O_2 deficit or repayment arising from a period of hypoxic ventilation. Their study found no such effect, suggesting that local vasodilation was sufficient to compete with the pharmacologic vasoconstriction. In the same study, isoproteranol infusion during hypoxia reduced the O_2 deficit, but this effect was probably mediated by its augmentation of cardiac output and overall oxygen transport during hypoxia, as opposed to a specific beneficial effect on blood flow distributions.

In summary, the pharmacological manipulation of α- and β-adrenergic receptors may affect the regional distribution of blood flow under conditions where overall oxygen supply is adequate. When vasoactive drugs are administered under conditions where O_2 uptake in some regions approaches supply dependency, local metabolic vasodilator responses appear to compete successfully with the vasoactive substance to preserve a relatively normal distribution of oxygen delivery among organs. Of course, overall oxygen supply may be reduced by α-adrenergic agonists that lower cardiac output via increases in left ventricular afterload. However, little evidence supporting the concept of a preferential oxygen supply reduction in tissues with a high density of α-adrenergic receptors has been reported. A secondary effect of vasoactive drugs with β_2 agonist activity arises due to a calorigenic stimulation of metabolic activity in some tissues. Under conditions where overall O_2 supply is limited, this effect may worsen the consequences of hypoxia by increasing the demand for an already limited supply of oxygen.

References

1. Berne RM, Levy MN. Cardiovascular physiology, 5th ed. St. Louis: CV Mosby, 1986.
2. Bredle DL, Chapler CK, Cain SM. Metabolic and circulatory responses of normoxic skeletal muscle to whole-body hypoxia. J Appl Physiol 1988; 65:2063–2068.
3. Cain SM. Oxygen delivery and uptake in dogs during anemic and hypoxic hypoxia. J Appl Physiol 1977;42:228–234.
4. Cain SM. Effects of time and vasoconstrictor tone on O_2 extraction during hypoxic hypoxia. J Appl Physiol 1978;45:219–224.
5. Cain SM. Gas exchange in hypoxia, apnea, and hyperoxia. In: Handbook of physiology: the respiratory system IV. Bethesda, MD: American Physiological Society, 1987:403–420.
6. Cain SM, Chapler CK. Oxygen extraction by canine hindlimb during hypoxic hypoxia. J Appl Physiol 1979;46:1023–1028.
7. Cain SM, Chapler CK. O_2 extraction by canine hindlimb during alpha-adrenergic blockade and hypoxic hypoxia. J Appl Physiol 1980;48:630–635.
8. Coburn RF, Pendleton M. Effects of norepinephrine on oxygenation of resting skeletal muscle. Am J Physiol 1979;236:H307–H313.
9. Doherty JU, Liang CS. Arterial hypoxemia in awake dogs. Role of the sympathetic nervous system in mediating the systemic hemodynamic and regional blood flow responses. J Lab Clin Med 1984;104:665–667.
10. Duling BR. Local control of microvascular function: role in tissue oxygen supply. Annu Rev Physiol 1980;42:373–382.
11. Forman NG, Wilson DF. Energetics and stoichiometry of oxidative phosphorylation from NADH to cytochrome c in isolated rat liver mitochondria. J Biol Chem 1982;257:12908–12915.
12. Forman NG, Wilson DF. Dependence of mitochondrial oxidative phosphorylation on activity of the adenine nucleotide translocase. J Biol Chem 1983;258:8649–8655.
13. Goldberg HS, Rabson J. Control of cardiac output by systemic vessels. Am J Cardiol 1991;47:696–702.
14. Granger HJ, Goodman AH, Cook BK. Metabolic models of microcirculatory regulation. Fed Proc 1975;34:2025–2030.
15. Granger HJ, Goodman AH, Granger DN. Role of resistance and exchange vessels in local microvascular control of skeletal muscle oxygenation in the dog. Circ Res 1976;38:379–385.
16. Granger HJ, Shepherd AP. Intrinsic microvascular control of tissue oxygen delivery. Microvasc Res 1973;5:49–72.
17. Guyton AC, Jones CE, Coleman TG. Circulatory physiology: cardiac output and its regulation. Philadelphia: WB Saunders, 1973:310–311.
18. Heyndrickx GR, Boettcher DH, Vatner SF. Effects of angiotensin, vasopressin, and methoxamine on cardiac function and blood flow distribution in conscious dogs. Am J Physiol 1976;231:1579–1587.
19. Johnson PC. Autoregulation of intestinal blood flow. Am J Physiol 1960;199:311–318.
20. King CE, Cain SM. Adrenergic and local control of O_2 uptake during and after severe hypoxia. J Appl Physiol 1986;61:1920–1927.
21. Lewis T, Samsel RW, Sanders WM, Caps MT, Wood LDH, Schumacker PT. The effect of adrenergic agents on oxygen delivery and consumption [Abstract]. Am Rev Respir Dis 1989;139:A311.
22. Nelson DP, King CE, Dodd SL, Schumacker PT, Cain SM. Systemic and intestinal limits of O_2 extraction in the dog. J Appl Physiol 1987;63:387–394.
23. Rapela CE, Green HD. Autoregulation of canine cerebral blood flow. Circ Res 1964;14(suppl):I-205–I-211.
24. Renkin EM. Volume IV, Microcirculation, Part 2; Control of microcirculation and blood-tissue exchange. In: Renkin EM, Michel CC, eds. Handbook of physiology: the cardiovascular system. Bethesda, MD: American Physiological Society, 1984:627–687.
25. Rowell LB. Human cardiovascular adjustments to exercise and thermal stress. Physiol Rev 1974;54:75–159.
26. Schumacker PT, Wood LDH. Effects of sodium nitroprusside infusion on the relationship between oxygen delivery (QO_2) and uptake (VO_2) in the dog [Abstract]. Am Rev Respir Dis 1985; 131 (part 2):A140.
27. Shepherd AP. Local control of intestinal oxygenation and blood flow. Annu Rev Physiol 1982;44:13–27.
28. Shepherd AP. Metabolic control of intestinal oxygenation and blood flow. Fed Proc 1982;41:2084–2089.
29. Shepherd AP. Role of capillary recruitment in the regulation of intestinal oxygenation. Am J Physiol 1982;242:G435–G441.
30. Walley KR, Becker CJ, Hogan RA, Teplinsky K, Wood LDH. Progressive hypoxemia limits left ventricular oxygen consumption and contractility. Circ Res 1988;63:849–859.
31. Wilson DF, Erecinska M. Effect of oxygen concentration on cellular metabolism. Chest 1985; 88:229S–232S.

7

O_2 Uptake, Critical O_2 Delivery, and Tissue Wellness

Robert Schlichtig

The cardiovascular system must provide tissues with a continuous supply of nutrients to sustain life. Fuel and oxygen are pivotally important, in part because mitochondria must generate ATP continuously to sustain vital forces such as membrane electrochemical gradients, cardiac contractions, and complex macromolecular synthesis. O_2 deprivation may cause tissue damage directly, owing to exhaustion of ATP and other high energy intermediates needed to maintain cellular structural integrity. For example, cells in isolation (65) and in some organs (5, 17) disintegrate within relatively short periods of time when deprived of oxygen. In addition, O_2 deprivation may cause damage indirectly during reperfusion, when adenine nucleotides and other cellular metabolites, transformed during dysoxia into producers of free radical species, are then provided with substrate during reperfusion (16).

Although these concepts are generally well accepted, it is not entirely clear how clinicians can use them to ensure adequate O_2 availability in patients. Many suspect that multiple organ failure encountered in the critical care setting is dysoxic in origin, because afflicted patients are usually hemodynamically unstable, and therefore seemingly vulnerable to tissue O_2 deprivation. For this reason, increasingly intensive and sophisticated resources are appropriately directed toward maintaining tissue O_2 delivery ($\dot{D}o_2$). However, a clinically useful definition of critical O_2 delivery ($\dot{D}o_2c$), linking hemodynamically oriented interventions to patient wellness, is lacking. Indeed many clinicians are painfully aware of their limited ability to determine when resuscitation should commence, or when further resuscitation is no longer needed. While few definitive statements can yet be made, a brief review of the relationship between O_2 transport parameters and tissue wellness will be of interest to those who routinely treat shock states.

DEFINITION OF TERMS

The vocabulary used to describe O_2 transport and utilization phenomena is potentially ambiguous, such that subtle differences among related parameters can be potentially confusing. It is therefore useful to conceptually separate macrovascular parameters from microvascular parameters of tissue oxygenation. Macrovascular parameters assess the oxygenation of whole organs, but are relatively insensitive measures of early dysoxic changes that may occur in the most vulnerable cell populations of these organs (i.e., those cells most distant from well-oxygenated capillary blood supply). Conversely, microvascular parameters measure oxygenation at the cellular level, but may provide incomplete information about whole organs, since only small populations of cells can be assayed at any one time.

Macrovascular parameters commonly used in clinical practice are O_2 uptake ($\dot{V}o_2$), $\dot{D}o_2$, and O_2 extraction ratio. $\dot{V}o_2$ is the quantity of O_2 consumed by a given tissue per unit time and is relatively easy to measure in whole animals and in many whole organs as the difference between the quantity of O_2 that enters and that which leaves a given vascular bed, i.e., flow times arteriovenous O_2 content difference,

$$\dot{V}o_2 = flow \cdot (Cao_2 - Cvo_2) \qquad (1)$$

where Cao_2 and Cvo_2 are the O_2 content of arterial and venous blood, respectively. Blood O_2 content (Cbo_2) is calculated as

$$Cbo_2 = (1.34 \cdot Hb \cdot Sbo_2) + (0.0031 \cdot Pbo_2) \qquad (2)$$

where Hb is hemoglobin concentration, and Sbo_2 and Pbo_2 are blood O_2 saturation and partial pressure, respectively. Because $\dot{V}o_2$ is primarily coupled to oxidative phosphorylation in mitochondria, it serves as a relatively sensitive, if nonspecific, measure of energy production and utilization. However, the accuracy with which $\dot{V}o_2$ measures oxidative phosphorylation can be variable, because approximately 14% of $\dot{V}o_2$ is cyanide-resistant in lung and liver. Cyanide-resistant $\dot{V}o_2$ is thought to represent extramitochondrial $\dot{V}o_2$ by O_2 transferases, by electron transfer oxidases unrelated to oxidative phosphorylation, and by mixed function oxidases (19). Potential variability of the extramitochondrial contribution to $\dot{V}o_2$ may be exemplified by lung, wherein $\dot{V}o_2$, presumably of partially extramitochondrial origin, can increase to an extraordinary degree during pneumonia (45).

$\dot{D}o_2$ is the bulk quantity of O_2 flowing into a given tissue and is calculated as flow times the blood O_2 content of feeding vessels.

$$\dot{D}o_2 = flow \cdot Cbo_2 \qquad (3)$$

Of course, only a fraction of $\dot{D}o_2$ normally diffuses into cells, and the remainder is carried away in the venous effluent. The fraction of $\dot{D}o_2$ that diffuses from capillaries into cells, expressed as the percent of total, is termed O_2 *extraction ratio* and is calculated as $\dot{V}o_2/\dot{D}o_2$. When flow is factored out of this equation, O_2 extraction ratio is calculated as

$$O_2 \text{ extraction ratio} = (Cao_2 - Cvo_2)/Cao_2 \qquad (4)$$

If one ignores the O_2 content of plasma, which accounts for only a small proportion of blood O_2 content (assuming normal hematocrit), the O_2 extraction ratio equation can be estimated as

$$O_2 \text{ extraction ratio} \approx (Sao_2 - S\bar{v}o_2)/Sao_2 \qquad (5)$$

where Sao_2 and Svo_2 are O_2 saturation of arterial and venous blood, respectively.

Microvascular parameters of O_2 utilization are generally impractical for use in clinical practice, but should be understood so as to facilitate understanding of the limitations of macrovascular parameters. Tissue Po_2, in contrast to $\dot{D}o_2$, provides a direct measure of cellular oxygenation in the cell population measured. However, within any given organ, tissue Po_2 varies considerably, with some cells appearing quite hypoxemic, and others well oxygenated, so that Po_2 histograms have been employed to gain further understanding (31, 32). The final determinant of mitochondrial oxidative phosphorylation is mitochondrial Po_2. The minimum driving pressure of oxygen needed to support oxidative phosphorylation in mitochondria is less than 0.5 torr (19) and is dependent both on O_2 convection (i.e., $\dot{D}o_2$) and O_2 diffusion from capillary to cell. However, the mean tissue Po_2 associated with tissue dysoxia is approximately 15 torr, owing to the Po_2 gradient needed to drive O_2 from tissue to mitochondria (31).

Estimates of tissue redox state, such as lactate/pyruvate ratio, β-hydroxybutyrate/acetoacetate ratio, and cytochrome a,a_3 reduction may serve as either macrovascular or microvascular parameters depending on the method of measurement and are discussed later in this chapter.

Dysoxia is a term recently advocated to describe curtailment of oxidative phosphorylation by insufficient O_2 and should be used when describing an O_2 deficiency suspected to cause tissue dysfunction. "Hypoxia" more correctly refers to inspired Po_2 less than normal, and "hypoxemia," to Pao_2 less than normal (11).

THE BIPHASIC $\dot{V}o_2$-$\dot{D}o_2$ MODEL

A sensitive and clinically definitive method to detect incipient dysoxia in ICU patients, using the above parameters, has yet to be developed. However, because clinicians can manipulate only whole body $\dot{D}o_2$ and (to a very limited extent, as during intraaortic balloon counterpulsation) organ $\dot{D}o_2$, the

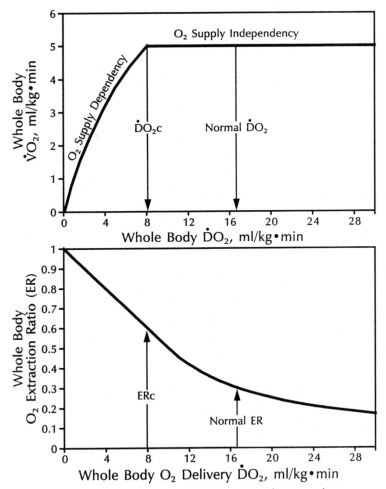

Figure 7.1. The biphasic $\dot{V}O_2$-$\dot{D}O_2$ model. Relation between $\dot{V}O_2$ and $\dot{D}O_2$ is shown on the *top panel*, and the corresponding relation between O_2 extraction ratio *(ER)* and $\dot{D}O_2$ is shown on the *bottom panel*. O_2 demand is assumed to be constant. $\dot{D}O_2$ is normally about twice the critical $\dot{D}O_2$ value ($\dot{D}O_2c$), and the critical ER(ERc) is normally about 30%.

biphasic $\dot{V}O_2$-$\dot{D}O_2$ model (Fig. 7.1) provides the best frame of reference from which to begin approaching the concept of adequate oxygenation in patients.

The $\dot{V}O_2$-$\dot{D}O_2$ model is based on laboratory observations of anesthetized animals in which $\dot{D}O_2$ is gradually lowered until death and simulates a condition of decreasing $\dot{D}O_2$ in a patient (Fig. 7.1). Using this approach, it has been shown that most mammalian tissues maintain $\dot{V}O_2$ reasonably constant as $\dot{D}O_2$ varies over a wide range, extracting only as much O_2 from the blood as appears needed to maintain vital metabolism. The phenomenon of

stable $\dot{V}O_2$ at variable $\dot{D}O_2$ is referred to as *O_2 supply independency* (8), and the active process is referred to as *O_2 regulation* (91). Stable $\dot{V}O_2$ during O_2 supply independency is thought to signify tissue wellness, because it appears that oxidative metabolism is maintained despite variation of $\dot{D}O_2$. Normally, $\dot{D}O_2$ at rest is roughly twice the minimum $\dot{D}O_2$ value needed to sustain supply-independent oxidative metabolism, and O_2 extraction ratio is approximately 30%.

When $\dot{D}O_2$ declines to a critical threshold value, $\dot{V}O_2$ can no longer be maintained constant, because the ability of tissues to maintain O_2 supply-independent metabolism by O_2 extraction is limited, presumably because the driving pressure of O_2 from capillary blood to the most distal mitochondria becomes inadequate. Therefore, below $\dot{D}o_2c$, $\dot{V}o_2$ declines in direct proportion to $\dot{D}o_2$, a phenomenon referred to as O_2 *supply dependency*. The O_2 extraction ratio associated with $\dot{D}o_2c$ in animals (8, 55, 67, 71) and in humans with end-stage congestive heart failure (68) is generally approximately 70%. However, because the relation between $\dot{D}o_2$ and O_2 extraction ratio is relatively linear in this region (Fig. 7.1, *bottom*), and because critical O_2 extraction ratio may vary among physiological conditions, the $\dot{V}o_2$-$\dot{D}o_2$ inflection provides a more reliable estimate of critical $\dot{D}o_2$. For the purposes of the present discussion, O_2 supply dependency will tentatively be taken as evidence of tissue dysoxia, because it appears that vital metabolism has then been curtailed because of inadequate $\dot{D}o_2$.

The biphasic behavior of $\dot{V}o_2$ as $\dot{D}o_2$ varies has been documented in many organs/organ systems, including whole body (8, 55, 65, 71), liver (46, 54, 67, 71), intestine (46, 55, 71), and skeletal muscle (66). Furthermore, this behavior has been demonstrated in a number of different laboratories and has been observed in a number of different mammalian species. Indeed it appears very likely that further laboratory investigation of this behavior will lead to essential understanding of the consequences of decreasing tissue O_2 delivery. Unfortunately, however, it appears very unlikely that direct application of the biphasic $\dot{V}o_2$-$\dot{D}o_2$ model will prove to be a useful clinical tool, because several assumptions (Table 7.1) must be made, at least some of which are usually incorrect in ICU patients. The following discussion

Table 7.1
Assumptions of the $\dot{V}o_2$-$\dot{D}o_2$ Model

O_2 demand is constant at all $\dot{D}o_2$ values
Whole body measurements accurately reflect oxygenation of all organs
All $\dot{D}o_2$ is equal for all physiologic conditions
All $\dot{V}o_2 - \dot{D}o_2$ covariation signifies dysoxia

explores a number of potentially incorrect assumptions that could lead to erroneous interpretation of $\dot{V}o_2$ and $\dot{D}o_2$ data analysis in patients by strict interpretation of the biphasic $\dot{V}o_2$-$\dot{D}o_2$ model as defined above.

Variable Muscular O_2 Demand

The most important potentially incorrect assumption encountered in *clinical* settings is that muscular $\dot{V}o_2$ demand is constant. In fact, inability to verify this assumption effectively invalidates a direct application of the $\dot{V}o_2$-$\dot{D}o_2$ model in the majority of ICU settings. Constant muscular $\dot{V}o_2$ demand is essential in $\dot{V}o_2$-$\dot{D}o_2$ data interpretation because the biphasic model assumes that covariation of $\dot{V}o_2$ and $\dot{D}o_2$ represents inadequate $\dot{D}o_2$ to support metabolism (Fig. 7.1). In this regard, it is important to note that laboratory demonstrations of biphasic whole body $\dot{V}o_2$-$\dot{D}o_2$ relations have usually been made during anesthesia and chemical muscular paralysis. In contrast, muscular $\dot{V}o_2$ demand of patients varies widely, by as much as severalfold of the resting whole body $\dot{V}o_2$ value. This variability is effectively unpreventable in the clinical setting, because the muscular paralysis and deep sedation that would be needed to abolish the variable work of breathing, rate of thermogenesis, and degree of agitation are rarely clinically indicated. The degree of variability of $\dot{V}o_2$ demand can be at least 30%, even in a chemically unrestrained patient who might appear to be resting (87, 88) and can be greater than 900% in vigorous individuals during exercise (58)!

Variable muscular $\dot{V}o_2$ demand creates two problems with respect to strict application of the $\dot{V}o_2$-$\dot{D}o_2$ model. First, the value of $\dot{D}o_2c$ varies directly with the change of $\dot{V}o_2$ demand. For example, assuming a critical O_2 extraction ratio of 70%, a doubling of $\dot{V}o_2$ demand from 5 to 10 ml/kg/min would cause critical $\dot{D}o_2$ to increase from 7.1 to 14.2 ml/kg/min. A variation of the biphasic concept could still be employed by using critical O_2 extraction ratio, if one could reasonably infer impending O_2 supply limitation by detection of the critical O_2 extraction ratio value. This principle serves as the basis for continuous mixed venous oximetry, a very useful monitoring tool in patients who are deeply sedated and paralyzed as, for example, early postoperative cardiac surgical patients. When arterial O_2 saturation is kept near 95% (the result of normal ICU interventions), venous O_2 saturation is a reasonable reflector of O_2 extraction ratio (equation 5). However, when muscular O_2 demand is permitted to vary, O_2 extraction ratio very close to critical O_2 extraction ratio is commonly reached during vigor-

ous exercise in healthy individuals (22) and in agitated patients with limited myocardial reserve (personal observations), neither of whom appear to be at risk of dysoxic injury. Thus, only low O_2 extraction ratios, observed during continuous mixed venous oximetry in anesthetized/ sedated patients, can be taken as evidence that shock is necessarily imminent (Fig. 7.2, *bottom panel*). This is not to say that continuous monitoring of mixed venous O_2 saturation is not helpful, but rather that

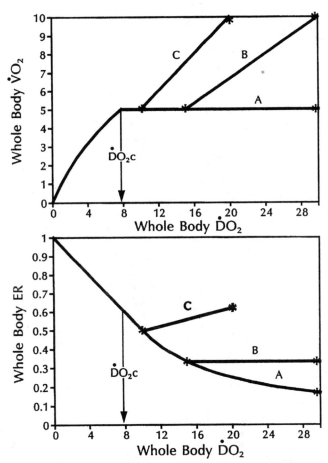

Figure 7.2. O_2 demand dependency. The relation between $\dot{V}o_2$ and $\dot{D}o_2$ is shown on the *top panel*, and the corresponding relation between ER and $\dot{D}o_2$ is shown on the *bottom panel*. *Curves A,* O_2 demand is constant between all *asterisks* on these curves, and $\dot{D}O_2$ varies with intravascular volume status. *Curves B,* $\dot{V}o_2$ demand is varying between the *asterisks* on these curves *(top)*, and $\dot{D}o_2$ responds normally, maintaining O_2 extraction ratio near 30% *(bottom)*. *Curves C,* $\dot{V}o_2$ demand varies by the same magnitude as *curves B;* however, myocardial reserve is deficient, so that $\dot{V}o_2$ and O_2 extraction ratio increase to a greater extent at equal $\dot{D}o_2$ values. Although $\dot{V}o_2$ and $\dot{D}o_2$ covary between *asterisks* of *curves B* and *C*, these conditions do not signify O_2 supply dependency, but rather O_2 demand dependency.

it does not provide a definitive indication of tissue dysoxia, and that it must be interpreted within the clinical context.

A second and much more important obstacle to clinical application of the $\dot{V}O_2$-$\dot{D}O_2$ model, imposed by variable muscular $\dot{V}O_2$ demand, is the fact that increased $\dot{V}O_2$ due to increased O_2 demand is normally supported not by an increase of O_2 extraction ratio, but rather by an increase of $\dot{D}O_2$. Though only recently recognized by those interested in $\dot{V}O_2$-$\dot{D}O_2$ relations in ICU patients, this statement must be correct. Assuming a normal O_2 extraction ratio of 30% and maximum O_2 extraction ratio of 70%, a "normal" value of cardiac output could support only slightly more than a twofold (i.e., 0.7 divided by 0.3) increase of $\dot{V}O_2$, or two metabolic equivalent system units (METS) (58). This would be barely adequate to support the increased $\dot{V}O_2$ observed during a bed bath (42)! Thus, when O_2 demand is permitted to vary, the normal relation between $\dot{V}O_2$ and $\dot{D}O_2$ is no longer biphasic, but linear (Fig. 7.2). This covariation of $\dot{V}O_2$ and $\dot{D}O_2$ does not represent "O_2 supply dependency," but rather "O_2 demand dependency" (62, 83, 87).

Recent clinical observations indicate that O_2 demand dependency routinely characterizes the $\dot{V}O_2$-$\dot{D}O_2$ relations of ICU patients. The relation between $\dot{V}O_2$ and $\dot{D}O_2$ in patients without apparent hemodynamic compromise covaried when these individuals were permitted normal ICU activities, with O_2 extraction ratio maintained near 30% as $\dot{V}O_2$ varied as much as twofold (84, 88). While this phenomenon is incompletely understood, one might speculate that the cardiovascular system normally provides tissues with twice the critical value of $\dot{D}O_2$ needed to support O_2 supply-independent metabolism. However, during more strenuous muscular activity, muscular O_2 demand begins to exceed the ability of the cardiovascular system to maintain basal $\dot{D}O_2$ to all organs (18), and O_2 extraction ratio only then increases appreciably.

The clearest clinical demonstrations of *biphasic* $\dot{V}O_2$-$\dot{D}O_2$ human behavior have been made in patients undergoing cardiac surgery, who are deeply anesthetized (21, 39, 76). Human demonstrations of O_2 supply-independent behavior have also been made in the absence of anesthesia, presumably because measurements were made in carefully controlled quiescent states and/or by measures that did not increase O_2 demand in the patients studies (1, 10, 23, 36, 85). However, a number of other investigators have failed to observe O_2 supply-independent behavior, but instead noted covariation of $\dot{V}O_2$ and $\dot{D}O_2$, with O_2 extraction ratios often near 30% (12, 13, 43, 61, 78, 79). Some of these observations may actually have signified O_2 supply-dependent metabolism, with a very low critical O_2 extraction ratio. However, because it is not clear that O_2 demand was kept constant with the interventions used, at least some of these studies may actually have been demonstrations of O_2 demand dependency (Fig. 7.2).

Thus, $\dot{V}O_2$-$\dot{D}O_2$ covariation does not necessarily indicate dysoxia in awake patients, but rather the normal response of $\dot{D}O_2$ to $\dot{V}O_2$ demand in the clinical setting. Clear discrimination of O_2 supply dependency from O_2 demand dependency then becomes a matter of crucial importance that could be overcome only by paralysis and deep sedation, which in most instances would be clinically inappropriate.

A similar problem of artifactual $\dot{V}O_2$-$\dot{D}O_2$ covariation, unrelated to skeletal muscle O_2 demand, is that $\dot{V}O_2$ and $\dot{D}O_2$ may covary a priori when thermodilution cardiac output is used to calculate both variables, because of errors inherent in these measurements ("mathematical coupling"). Thus, cardiac output and O_2 extraction ratio might actually be identical during two separate measurements in the same patient. However if, say, 10% over- and underestimates of cardiac output are made during these two measurements, then $\dot{V}O_2$ and $\dot{D}O_2$ will both appear to increase by 20%, leading to the false impression of $\dot{V}O_2$-$\dot{D}O_2$ covariation (81, 83). This problem will likely be exacerbated when ICU staff routinely discard values that appear to be outliers, but that actually represent true values of cardiac output that vary with the respiratory cycle. Biphasic demonstrations of $\dot{V}O_2$ and $\dot{D}O_2$ have been well demonstrated in animal models using thermodilution cardiac output; however, a much larger number of determinations were made than would be practical in the ICU setting, and the cardiac output values obtained encompassed the full range between the well-perfused state and terminal dysoxia (71, 72).

Critical $\dot{D}O_2$ of Whole Body versus Individual Organs

A second potentially incorrect assumption that limits direct application of the $\dot{V}O_2$-$\dot{D}O_2$ model to patient care is that the $\dot{V}O_2$-$\dot{D}O_2$ relation of whole body accurately reflects phenomena occurring in individual organs (Fig. 7.3). This presents a problem to application of whole body $\dot{V}O_2$-$\dot{D}O_2$ relations to clinicians, because it cannot be assumed that individual organ $\dot{V}O_2$—even of paralyzed, sedated individuals—behaves in a parallel manner with whole body $\dot{V}O_2$.

Although sufficient hard data are currently lacking, it is difficult to argue that O_2 supply dependency of isolated vascular beds—each of which accounts for only a

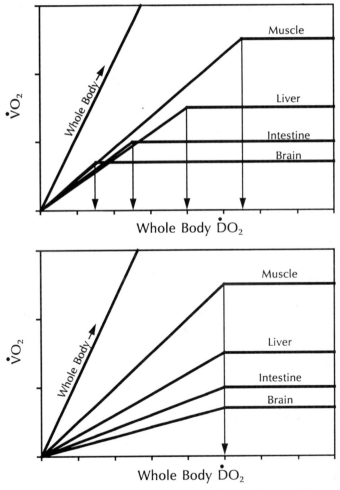

Figure 7.3. Potential hierarchies of organ dysoxia. *Top,* Organs become O_2 supply dependent in a hierarchical fashion, i.e., at different whole body $\dot{D}O_2$ values. *Bottom,* All organs become O_2 supply dependent at the same whole body $\dot{D}O_2$ value. In each instance, whole body $\dot{V}O_2$ is the sum of organ $\dot{V}O_2$ shown. Although laboratory animal demonstrations generally support the phenomena depicted in the *bottom panel,* those depicted in the *top* panel may represent critically ill patients receiving mechanical ventilation and/or pressor agents.

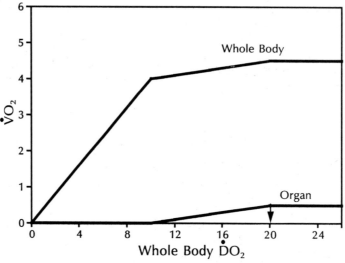

Figure 7.4. A hypothetical $\dot{V}o_2$–$\dot{D}o_2$ relationship of whole body and organ supplied by critically stenosed vessels. Blood pressure is varying exponentially with whole body $\dot{D}o_2$ and approaches critical closing pressure for the organ at a higher than normal whole body $\dot{D}o_2$ value. The resulting response of whole body $\dot{V}o_2$ is barely perceptible, however, and could not easily be detected by whole body clinical measurements.

small fraction of whole body $\dot{V}o_2$—could be obscured in a whole body $\dot{V}o_2$ measurement (Fig. 7.4). Several groups have noted that O_2 supply dependency of individual organs does commence at slightly different whole body $\dot{D}o_2$ values (56, 71). Under carefully controlled laboratory conditions wherein whole body $\dot{D}o_2$ is gradually and progressively lowered during anesthesia and paralysis, these differences appear of minor clinical significance. However, the conditions of these experiments may not be representative of critically ill patients, many of whom receive intense mechanical and pharmacological support that could alter the distribution of whole body $\dot{D}o_2$ among organs. For example, mechanical ventilation with high end-expiratory pressure (PEEP) may decrease hepatic blood flow (48, 50), and pressor agents are generally suspected to alter the distribution of whole body $\dot{D}o_2$ among organs (58). Similarly, patients who are profoundly septic routinely manifest cardiac index values (and therefore $\dot{D}o_2$ values) that are two to three times the normal resting value, but nevertheless may develop organ failure and severe lactic acidosis.

A number of common clinical examples illustrate the wisdom of assuming that all organs *do not* become O_2 supply-dependent simultaneously in the ICU setting (Fig. 7.4). These involve primarily instances wherein one or more organs are supplied by vessels that are partially obstructed. For example, vessels distal to critical arterial stenoses are presumably already maximally vasodilated, so that additional vasodilation cannot produce increased flow. Perfusion of these tissues is dependent not on whole body $\dot{D}o_2$, but rather on arterial blood pressure! For example, brain perfusion of a patient with subarachnoid hemorrhage and vasospasm is not likely to improve simply by increasing whole body $\dot{D}o_2$, unless blood pressure also increases. Alternatively, brain perfusion may improve by increasing blood pressure, which *may not increase whole body* $\dot{D}o_2$ (38, 44). Similarly, patients with bleeding esophageal varices who receive high dose infusion of vasopressin may experience intestinal ischemia, even though whole body $\dot{D}o_2$ of these individuals is generally several times higher than the normal value (24). Thus, it is essential that clinicians temper their understanding of the $\dot{V}o_2$-$\dot{D}o_2$ relation with the understanding that limited inferences may be drawn from whole body data with respect to individual organ wellness.

Diffusion versus Convection Limitation of O₂ Uptake

A third assumption made by the biphasic $\dot{V}o_2$-$\dot{D}o_2$ model is that all $\dot{D}o_2$ (i.e., $\dot{D}o_2$ provided in any form) is equal in all clinical conditions (Fig. 7.5). While it cannot be argued that $\dot{D}o_2$ is unnecessary, it is certainly possible that factors other than simple macrovascular $\dot{D}o_2$ ("convective" O₂ delivery) may determine whether it is sufficient. Using the biphasic model as a frame of reference, one extreme viewpoint would be that the same $\dot{D}o_2c$ value exists for all conditions, and the opposing viewpoint would be that $\dot{D}o_2c$ values are so widely divergent among conditions as to render $\dot{D}o_2$ useless as a general-purpose physiologic parameter of tissue wellness.

A clinical example that might illustrate this concern is the observation that the minimum value of whole body $\dot{D}o_2$ needed to sustain adequate tissue function in compensated congestive heart failure (68) is considerably lower than that required dur-

ing stress (77). As noted above, this phenomenon could represent maldistribution of whole body $\dot{D}o_2$ among organs, with overperfusion of some, and underperfusion of others. However, if all other assumptions are correct (Table 7.1), then this discrepancy might alternatively represent an inability of O₂ to diffuse from the circulation to tissues (Fig. 7.5). Indeed, some suspect that the apparent differences in critical $\dot{D}o_2$ are due to differences in barriers that can potentially retard O₂ diffusion from capillary to mitochondria. These diffusive barriers can potentially include normal structural barriers, such as erythrocyte membrane or plasma; abnormal structural barriers, such as arteriovenous shunts or capillary embolization; and physical/chemical barriers, such as increased erythrocyte transit time or increased hemoglobin affinity for O₂ (31). Each "barrier" may effectively reduce availability of capillary-borne O₂ to cells.

In nonseptic conditions, all available laboratory evidence indicates that convection is, for all practical purposes, the most important $\dot{V}o_2$-limiting variable. In fact, there is little argument that $\dot{D}o_2c$ values are indistinguishable when $\dot{D}o_2$ is progres-

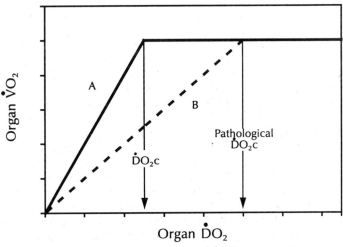

Figure 7.5. Convection versus diffusion limitation of $\dot{V}o_2$, viewed from the perspective of the biphasic $\dot{V}o_2$-$\dot{D}o_2$ model. *Model A,* Barriers to O₂ diffusion are normal, and the tissues can maintain O₂ supply-independent metabolism by extracting up to 60–70% of $\dot{D}o_2$. *Model B,* Barriers to O₂ diffusion are increased; $\dot{D}o_2$ remains an essential determinant of $\dot{V}o_2$, but the $\dot{D}o_2c$ value is increased, because the tissues cannot extract as much of the available $\dot{D}o_2$. *Models A* and *B* cannot be addressed by whole body data, because *model B* could represent maldistribution of whole body $\dot{D}o_2$ among organs.

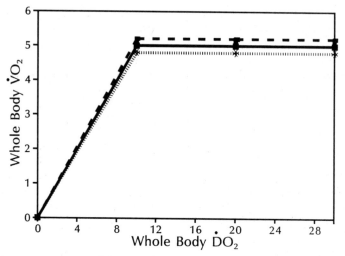

Figure 7.6. The relationship of $\dot{V}o_2$ and $\dot{D}o_2$ when $\dot{D}o_2$ is lowered by progressive anemia, hypoxemia, or flow stagnation. The $\dot{D}o_2c$ value is identical in each instance; however, the end-capillary venous $\dot{P}o_2$ observed at the $\dot{D}o_2c$ value is different in each instance.

sively reduced by incremental hemorrhage, anemia, or hypoxemia (7, 31, 74) (Fig. 7.6). However, at each $\dot{D}o_2$ value, these conditions differ substantially with respect to arterial O_2 content and end-capillary Po_2. These data could be interpreted as indicating that only bulk $\dot{D}o_2$ is rate-limiting, because $\dot{D}o_2$ appears a better predictor of O_2 supply limitation than does the diffusion gradient from capillary to mitochondria. In further support of this hypothesis, $\dot{D}o_2c$ values during progressive hemorrhage were not different when conditions of normal and increased hemoglobin O_2 affinity were compared, in spite of the fact that the two conditions should magnify any existing barrier to O_2 diffusion (73). However, in several investigations, wherein diffusion barriers were stressed by combination of two dysoxic stresses simultaneously (progressive stagnation and hypoxemia, at different rates), $\dot{V}o_2$ limitation has appeared somewhat better related to end-capillary Po_2 than to $\dot{D}o_2$, suggesting that barriers to O_2 diffusion from erythrocytes to mitochondria may actually determine $\dot{V}o_2$ limitation, thereby supporting different $\dot{V}o_2$ values at equal $\dot{D}o_2$ values in these conditions (28).

In recent studies, mean tissue Po_2 and dispersion of Po_2 values about the mean have been studied to further elucidate the relation between convection and diffusion limitation of oxidative metabolism. Dispersion of tissue Po_2 values about the mean provides an index of microcirculatory mismatch between capillary O_2 transport and tissue demand, with greater dispersion indicating greater microcirculatory mismatching of O_2 supply to O_2 demand. For the conditions of anemia and hypoxemia, mean tissue Po_2, Po_2 dispersion about the mean, and $\dot{D}o_2c$ values were similar. However, end-capillary Po_2 was different, so that the gradient between end-capillary Po_2 and mean tissue Po_2 was quite different, and yet convective $\dot{D}o_2$ still appeared to be the rate-limiting variable, because $\dot{D}o_2c$ values were indistinguishable. One explanation is that differences of diffusion barriers imposed by these conditions may balance out in such a manner that mean tissue Po_2 at the onset of O_2 supply limitation is identical despite different end-capillary Po_2 (31).

While the convection versus diffusion controversy is far from settled, several clinically relevant observations of nonseptic conditions are worth noting. First, while diffusion from capillary to cell may be more rate-limiting in some conditions than in others, it cannot occur without convection. Therefore, the controversy should not be taken as an argument that convection is anything less than an essential physiologic variable. For example, if normal resting $\dot{V}O_2$ demand is 150 ml/m²/min, and critical O_2 extraction ratio is, say, 60%, then a bare minimum $\dot{D}O_2$ value of 250 ml/m²/min (or cardiac index of approximately 2.1 liters/min, assuming normal hemoglobin and oxyhemoglobin concentrations) must be maintained to prevent dysoxia (20). Thus, while pulmonary artery catheterization has not been shown to alter mortality in patients with irritable and/or unsalvageable myocardium (25, 92), it is an essential tool for the care of other groups of hemodynamically unstable patients. These patients' lives can be saved when $\dot{D}O_2$ is improved by blood transfusion, volume loading, or other artificial means, provided that the information supplied by the catheter is promptly and appropriately used. Second, since clinicians currently can effectively manipulate $\dot{D}O_2$ but not O_2 diffusing capacity, $\dot{D}O_2$ is the only clinically relevant determinant of $\dot{V}O_2$. Third, it is difficult to argue that $\dot{D}O_2$ has proven anything less than an extremely powerful, albeit not always the best, predictor of $\dot{V}O_2$ among all the conditions studied. Therefore, of the methods available to manipulate $\dot{D}O_2$ (hemoglobin, flow, and hemoglobin O_2 saturation) all currently appear to be associated with very similar quantitative effects on oxidative metabolism. Finally, it is important to note that most clinicians painstakingly maintain hemoglobin concentration and hemoglobin O_2 saturation well within the normal range in critically ill patients, so that factors that may disturb O_2 diffusion generally involve flow, rather than blood O_2 content.

Although O_2 diffusion appears to assume only a minor role in $\dot{V}O_2$ limitation during nonseptic conditions, many suspect that conditions exist wherein O_2 diffusion barriers cause $\dot{D}O_2c$ values to be higher than normal. *Pathologic O_2 supply dependency* is a term used to describe this condition (9). Covariation of $\dot{V}O_2$ and $\dot{D}O_2$ at pathologically high values of $\dot{D}O_2$ was initially thought to characterize only critically ill patients with sepsis and/or multiple organ failure, and it was therefore thought that pathological macrovascular and/or microvascular O_2 diffusion ac-

counted for the observed covariation of $\dot{V}O_2$ and $\dot{D}O_2$. However, as noted above, it is possible that at least some of these observations may have partly reflected O_2 demand dependency (Fig. 7.2). In addition, it has been noted that whole body pathologic O_2 supply dependency could also result from "macrovascular" maldistribution of whole body $\dot{D}O_2$ among organs, with overperfusion of some and underperfusion of others, in the absence of O_2 diffusive barriers at the organ level (71). Nevertheless, the hypothesis that significant alterations of microcirculatory O_2 diffusive barriers may occur in some patients seems likely, because the value of $\dot{D}O_2c$ can be altered in individual organs by microembolization with microspheres (75) or by administering endotoxin (55) or live bacteria (57).

Variable Nonmuscular O₂ Demand

A final assumption made by the biphasic $\dot{V}O_2$-$\dot{D}O_2$ model, similar to the assumption of constant muscular O_2 demand, is the assumption that nonmuscular O_2 demand is also constant. For example, the $\dot{V}O_2$ versus $\dot{D}O_2$ relation of isolated, arterial-perfused liver was recently observed to be biphasic when $\dot{D}O_2$ was progressively decreased by decreasing flow (67). That the $\dot{D}O_2c$ inflection truly signified the threshold of dysoxia was suggested by the observation that lactate extraction was constant above the $\dot{D}O_2c$ value and decreased precipitously below the $\dot{D}O_2c$ value. However, liver $\dot{V}O_2$ decreased by 0–30% in the range of $\dot{D}O_2$ higher than the $\dot{D}O_2c$ inflection. These investigators hypothesized that covariation of $\dot{V}O_2$ and $\dot{D}O_2$ at values higher than the $\dot{D}O_2c$ inflection may have represented decreasing metabolic demand rather than dysoxia, because hepatic O_2 demand may vary with inflowing hepatic substrate and/or demand for extramitochondrial oxidative metabolism.

A striking example of $\dot{V}O_2$-$\dot{D}O_2$ covariation that more clearly represents variable nonmuscular O_2 demand (as opposed to dysoxia) is provided by intact mammalian kidney. Kidney blood flow, like most organs (excepting brain and heart), varies in direct proportion to cardiac output in anesthetized animals (71) as well as in awake humans (18), so that a reduction of cardiac output by one half will produce a similar reduction of renal blood flow (Fig. 7.7, *top*). However, in contrast to other organs, kidney $\dot{V}O_2$ decreases dramatically as kidney $\dot{D}O_2$ decreases, including all values of kidney $\dot{D}O_2$ within the physiological range of well-being (37, 72). Recently an inflection of the kidney $\dot{V}O_2$-$\dot{D}O_2$ relation, possibly representing kidney $\dot{D}O_2c$ (Fig. 7.7, *bottom*), was observed; however, kidney $\dot{V}O_2$ decreased by two thirds from the baseline $\dot{D}O_2$ value to the $\dot{D}O_2c$ value (72). As in the example of liver noted above, a strict interpretation of the biphasic $\dot{V}O_2$-$\dot{D}O_2$ model would identify this degree of covariation as "O_2 supply dependency," and could be taken as evidence of kidney dysoxia. However, this is unlikely because kidneys very effectively reclaim NaCl during congestive heart failure, wherein renal blood flow is markedly curtailed (18). More

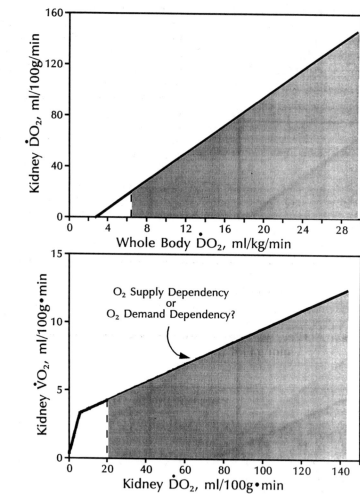

Figure 7.7. The response of intact mammalian kidney to progressive flow stagnation. The response of kidney $\dot{D}O_2$ to decreasing whole body $\dot{D}O_2$ (identical to the response of kidney blood flow to decreasing cardiac output) is shown by the *top panel*. The corresponding relation between kidney $\dot{V}O_2$ and kidney $\dot{D}O_2$ is shown by the *bottom panel*. Like most other organs, $\dot{D}O_2$ of kidney varies directly with whole body $\dot{D}O_2$. Unlike most organs, however, kidney $\dot{V}O_2$ decreases with decreasing kidney $\dot{D}O_2$ at all $\dot{D}O_2$ values, including all those associated with the physiologic range of well-being. $\dot{D}O_2$ associated with whole body $\dot{D}O_2$ greater than whole body $\dot{D}O_2c$ is shown by the *shaded areas*.

likely, decreasing kidney $\dot{V}o_2$ with decreasing kidney $\dot{D}o_2$ in the physiologically "normal" range represents decreasing demand to reabsorb NaCl from glomerular filtrate. (Recall that glomerular filtration decreases in direct proportion to renal blood flow, and that NaCl reabsorption accounts for approximately two thirds of renal $\dot{V}o_2$ under basal conditions.) Thus, it appears that the $\dot{V}o_2$-$\dot{D}o_2$ covariation of mammalian kidney, at least within the normal physiologic range, does not represent dysoxia, but rather O_2 demand dependency (Fig. 7.2), or *extrinsic O_2 conformity* (72).

ENHANCEMENT OF O_2 TRANSPORT PARAMETERS BY ESTIMATION OF TISSUE REDOX STATE

Of the inadequacies of the biphasic $\dot{V}o_2$-$\dot{D}o_2$ model discussed above, most disturbing is that covariation of $\dot{V}o_2$ and $\dot{D}o_2$ may signify dysoxia in some circumstances but not in others. In the cases of variable muscular O_2 demand (Fig. 7.2) and variable kidney resorptive O_2 demand (Fig. 7.7)

discussed above, $\dot{V}o_2$-$\dot{D}o_2$ covariation can reasonably be ascribed to variable O_2 demand. However, these observations raise the concern that covariation of $\dot{V}o_2$ and $\dot{D}o_2$ during O_2 supply dependency of other organs similarly may not signify dysoxia (Fig. 7.8). In other words, O_2 supply dependency could truly represent exhaustion of oxidative metabolism and tissue dysoxia, but might also represent O_2 *conformity*, a term that describes shutdown of nonessential metabolism when O_2 supply becomes inadequate (Fig. 7.8). In this manner, tissues might utilize available O_2 only to maintain metabolism that is immediately vital for survival, and thereby avoid dysoxic tissue damage (40). This phenomenon has been described in ectothermic animals, and could conceivably explain at least some portion of mammalian O_2 supply dependency. Thus, it appears that some estimation of tissue O_2 demand is also needed when interpreting covariation of $\dot{V}o_2$ and $\dot{D}o_2$.

That tissue O_2 demand is an important determinant of dysoxic injury is well demonstrated in clinical and laboratory settings. For example, the heart rarely devel-

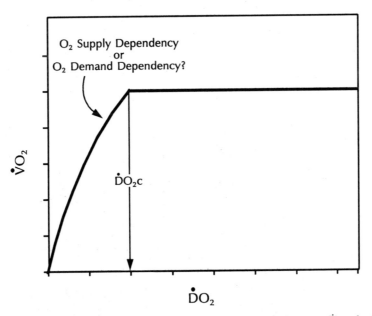

Figure 7.8. The biphasic $\dot{V}o_2$-$\dot{D}o_2$ model as a detector of tissue dysoxia. $\dot{V}o_2$ during the right-hand phase of O_2 supply dependency may signify dysoxia, but could also represent shutdown of nonessential metabolism and preservation of metabolism immediately needed to sustain life.

ops dysoxic injury of clinical consequence during cardiac bypass when cold cardioplegia is used to obliterate myocardial O_2 demand, despite the fact that it receives no blood supply during this period. Conversely, when myocardial O_2 demand remains intact, acute coronary obstruction produces myocardial injury within minutes. The same principle has been elegantly demonstrated in the laboratory. Renal tubular cells swell and burst within 30 minutes when perfused in a hypoxic medium, but remain intact when subjected to furosemide, which suppresses tubular demand to resorb sodium chloride (5). Similarly, cultured brain hippocampal cells quickly die and disintegrate when rendered hypoxic, but remain intact when energy-consuming spontaneous depolarizations are suppressed by addition of magnesium chloride (65). Using the same principle, intensivists are inclined to chemically paralyze and/or mechanically ventilate patients who are in shock, so as to reduce unnecessary O_2 demand, because they suspect that muscular $\dot{V}O_2$ may "rob" vital organs of essential $\dot{D}O_2$.

Unfortunately, to the frustration of many, the O_2 supply/demand ratio is difficult to measure. It may be best reflected by cellular redox state, which estimates the degree to which carriers of potential energy—scavenged from fuel—are oxidized. The primary carrier of potential energy in the cytoplasm is nicotine adenine dinucleotide (NAD), which can transfer its potential energy to mitochondria via the malate shuttle. In the mitochondria, energy carriers comprising the electron transport chain may be assayed to estimate redox state, particularly NAD and cytochrome a,a_3. Viewed simplistically, the reduced form of energy carrier, for example NADH, may be considered to reflect the need for energy supply, because fuel degradation is very tightly regulated by energy availability. During dysoxia, the available NAD pool becomes saturated (i.e., converted to NADH), and further fuel degradation is largely shut off. The oxidized form of energy carrier (NAD), on the other hand, depends on the adequacy of O_2 (Fig. 7.9). The ratio of reduced to oxidized energy carrier, for example NADH/NAD, may then

be thought of as an indicator of the O_2 supply-to-demand ratio.

Unfortunately, it appears that no single value of cellular redox state (like no single value of mixed venous O_2 saturation) can be yet taken as evidence of tissue dysoxia (11). For example, while it is thought that cytochrome a,a_3 is normally nearly completely oxidized, cytochrome a,a_3 has been found to be substantially reduced in brain (3, 34, 64) and kidney (2, 14) at normal Do_2 values. In addition, brain cytochrome a,a_3, like O_2 extraction ratio (Fig. 7.1), becomes progressively reduced in a linear fashion as Pao_2 decreases, including Pao_2 within the normal physiologic range, making it difficult to identify a critical cytochrome a,a_3 value (34). Further complicating matters, reduction of cellular redox state may be a normal compensatory response to decreasing mitochondrial Po_2; it has been shown that accumulation of NADH can actually drive oxidative phosphorylation toward ATP synthesis when mitochondrial Po_2 is very marginal, thereby maintaining $\dot{V}o_2$ by driving oxidative phosphorylation toward completion (91). Indeed it is believed by many that measures of cellular redox state alone cannot be used to identify the inception of dysoxia (11).

In spite of the limitations of both cellular redox state and $\dot{V}o_2$ as isolated measures of dysoxia, it may be possible to detect dysoxia by combining $\dot{V}o_2$-$\dot{D}o_2$ assessments with redox assessments (Fig. 7.10) (11). For example, muscle phosphocreatine-to-phosphorus ratio, a measure of muscle ATP depletion, has been found to be stable when $\dot{V}o_2$ is O_2 supply independent, and decreased when $\dot{V}o_2$ is O_2 supply dependent (30). Similarly, muscle cytochrome a,a_3 reduction varies directly with muscle $\dot{V}o_2$ when muscle $\dot{V}o_2$ is decreased by $\dot{D}o_2$ stagnation (33). These data suggest, as do complex theoretical considerations (11), that dysoxia may be detected when decreasing $\dot{V}o_2$ is associated with decreasing cellular redox state (Fig. 7.10). While these simultaneous analyses should presently be confined to the laboratory setting, it is worth exploring a few crude measures of redox state that may be used in the patient care.

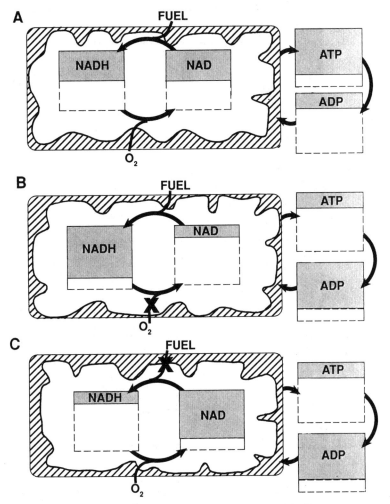

Figure 7.9. Three mitochondria. *A,* Fuel and O_2 are abundant. NADH and NAD appear in balanced proportions, and cytoplasmic ATP is adequate to support cellular metabolism. *B,* Fuel is adequate, but O_2 is not. The NADH pool is increased, the NAD pool is decreased, and ATP synthesis is inadequate to support cellular metabolism. *C,* Fuel supply is inadequate, and O_2 is abundant. The NADH pool is decreased, the NAD pool is increased, and ATP synthesis is inadequate to support cellular metabolism.

Blood Lactate

Except in several relatively unusual disease states, elevated blood lactate is accepted by many clinicians as evidence of tissue dysoxia (51). During states of O_2 unavailability, pyruvate cannot enter the Krebs cycle because pyruvate dehydrogenase is inhibited by NADH and acetyl-CoA, which cannot release their potential energy, owing to absence of the final electron acceptor, oxygen (82). Consequently lac-

tate accumulates in the blood. Lactate may also be viewed as an estimate of cytoplasmic NADH/NAD ratio, which is more correctly given as the lactate/pyruvate ratio (90). In early studies, arterial lactate was found to correlate closely with lactate/pyruvate ratio in critically ill humans (86).

Of particular interest is the finding that blood lactate is constant during whole body O_2 supply independency in experimental animals, and that blood lactate rises in a linear fashion during O_2 supply depen-

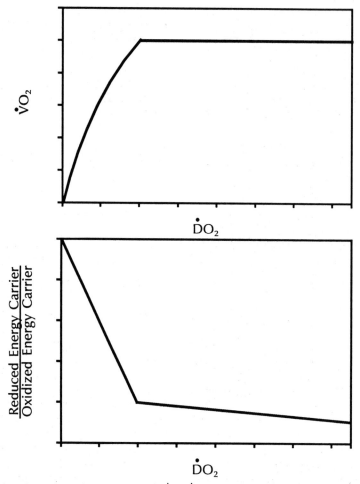

Figure 7.10. Combination of the biphasic $\dot{V}o_2$-$\dot{D}o_2$ model *(top)* and concurrent tissue redox assessment *(bottom)* to detect dysoxia, when PaO_2 is kept constant. Though incompletely investigated, current evidence suggests that cellular redox state is relatively constant during O_2 supply independency, but becomes progressively reduced during O_2 supply dependency.

dency (Fig. 7.10) (6, 15, 57). These data support the hypothesis that whole body O_2 supply dependency does indeed represent exhaustion of oxidative metabolism, rather than O_2 conformity. However, blood lactate, like $\dot{V}o_2$, is a "macrovascular" parameter of tissue wellness and gives no indication of the source of lactate production. In addition, because liver and myocardium are generally believed to be avid lactate scavengers, it is conceivable that anaerobiasis could commence in one or more vascular beds during O_2 supply dependency and not be detected by a blood lactate measurement. For example, lactic

acidosis is rarely detected during conditions of focal ischemia, as during myocardial ischemia, transient brain ischemic attack, or ischemia of an extremity. Conversely, lactate deriving from the Cori cycle (41, 69) may accumulate in the blood in the absence of anaerobiasis owing to defective clearance, as during the anhepatic and early postoperative phases of liver transplantation (52). Thus, lactic acidosis appears usually to be a good global indicator of tissue dysoxia; however, normal blood lactate does not necessarily indicate the absence of dysoxia in individual vascular beds.

Several groups of investigators have recently studied arterio-mixed venous pH difference (A-V pH). In patients with normal to marginal cardiac output, A-V pH was found to be narrow, while patients with cardiac arrest or severely reduced cardiac output manifested widened A-V pH (51). Similar observations have been made in animals, which have manifested very slowly increasing A-V pH during O_2 supply independency, and very steeply increasing A-V pH difference during O_2 supply dependency (4). These findings are of interest, because lactic acid per se should not theoretically be acidifying, but rather hydroxysis of ATP (51). Thus, whereas lactate may represent cumulative O_2 debt, A-V pH may provide an instantaneous measure of hydrogen ion production that is indirectly related to lactic acid accumulation.

A recent measurement, related to A-V pH, is monitoring of intestinal intramucosal pH. This method uses a saline-filled balloon placed in the GI tract. Because CO_2 easily diffuses across all tissues and membranes (including the balloon), CO_2 measured in the balloon gives an approximation of intestinal tissue acidity (35). Using this method, intramucosal pH has been reported to reflect blood loss during hemorrhage (35). Of interest, intramucosal pH, like A-V pH measurements of whole body, has been found to be relatively constant during intestinal O_2 supply independency, and increased during O_2 supply dependency (26).

β-Hydroxybutyrate/Acetoacetate Ratio

Another potential method to detect dysoxia by redox state is the β-hydroxybutyrate/acectoacetate ratio (βOHB/AcAc). Unlike lactate-to-pyruvate ratio, which assesses cytoplasmic redox state, βOHB/AcAc is thought to reflect mitochondrial NAD redox state. However, β-hydroxybutyrate dehydrogenase, the enzyme that catalyzes interconversion of the ketone body species, is primarily confined to the liver. Therefore, a number of investigators have used blood βOHB/AcAc to detect liver dy-

soxia (59) and to detect graft failure following liver transplantation (27, 52).

Very recently, hepatic venous βOHB/AcAc was examined during O_2 supply independency and during O_2 supply dependency of the liver. βOHB/AcAc was constant during O_2 supply independency, but increased in a linear fashion during O_2 supply dependency (70). Although hepatic venous βOHB/AcAc is an indirect measure of liver NADH/NAD, these data (like hepatic lactate extraction discussed earlier) suggest that decreasing $\dot{V}o_2$ during O_2 supply dependency of the liver does in fact indicate liver dysoxia.

IS ONLY O_2 RATE-LIMITING DURING SHOCK?

It is generally assumed that oxygen is the only clinically relevant blood nutrient. Though not intensively studied, currently available evidence suggests that this assumption is correct. While prolonged hypoglycemic coma, terminal beriberi, and other unusual nutritional disturbances may be associated with potentially lethal energy deficiency, no commonly encountered clinical form of shock appears to be characterized by an abundance of cellular O_2 and lack of usable cellular fuel (Fig. 7.10). In support of this hypothesis, forms of shock routinely treated by the intensivist are associated with elevated lactate-to-pyruvate ratio (86), and/or reduced aceto-acetate-to-β-hydroxybutyrate ratio (or elevated βOHB/AcAc ratio) (59), suggesting an abundance of potential energy, but deficiency of O_2. Though not intensively studied, shock has not been associated with normal values of these parameters, suggesting that O_2 delivery is indeed the relevant clinical variable. This would make sense teleologically, because the body contains no reservoir of O_2, but usually contains vast stores of potential fuel, as well as highly sensitive mechanisms for making this fuel available when needed (see Chapter 2, "Substrate Metabolism and Resting Energy Expenditure").

Although O_2 appears to be the only $\dot{V}O_2$-limiting nutrient in most circumstances, it should be noted that fuel deficits have been hypothesized in certain critically ill patients. For example, critically ill patients with terminal sepsis and multiple organ failure consumed branched-chain amino acids (BCAA) more readily than other amino acids, suggesting that BCAA may be more effectively used as fuel owing to metabolic blockades (60). Similarly, glutamine may be an obligate intestinal fuel source (80) that could be rate-limiting with respect to $\dot{V}O_2$ to a greater extent than O_2 during marginal intestinal perfusion (see Chapter 2). Dextrose and insulin have also been reported to restore the circulation during myocardial infarction, possibly because the myocardium needs less O_2 to sustain oxidative phosphorylation when glucose (as opposed to free fatty acids) is provided (49, 50, 63, 89). While data are incomplete, it is possible that intravenous infusion of certain foodstuffs may one day prove to enhance oxidative metabolism in a manner analogous to $\dot{D}O_2$

TIME AS AN INDEPENDENT VARIABLE

It is important to note that time is an important determinant of dysoxic injury. For example, vascular surgeons occasionally need to cross-clamp the aorta above the renal arteries during repair of abdominal aortic aneurysms, leaving distal organs without $\dot{D}O_2$ for 30–45 min. However, renal dysfunction of clinical consequence is unusual, possibly because renal O_2 demand is decreased by infusion of mannitol (53) and because renal O_2 demand decreases with decreasing $\dot{D}O_2$ (72). Similarly, cardiothoracic surgeons must cross-clamp the thoracic aorta during repair of descending thoracic aortic aneurysms for similar periods of time; however, intestinal, renal, or hepatic dysfunction of clinical consequence is rarely seen (personal observations). Thus, while dysoxia unquestionably will produce cell death eventually, it is important to remember that the duration of dysoxia needed to produce damage is highly variable among organs. For example, brain tolerates no more that 5 min of total ischemia, but myocardium can survive 15 min (47), liver 2–3 hr (17), and skeletal muscle 8 hr! Rea-

sons for these differences are not completely known, but could represent differences in the severity of dysoxia owing to variability of O_2 demand among these tissues, variability of phosphocreatine concentration, or variable ability to reduce unnecessary oxidative metabolism. Thus the expediency with which tissue $\dot{D}O_2$ must be restored varies within many clinical contexts.

SUMMARY: DEFINING THE DYSOXIC THRESHOLD

If only O_2 limitation can preclude sustenance of vital life forces, then it is essential to define the limits of O_2 adequacy. In experimental animal studies, measurement of $\dot{V}O_2$ during progressive $\dot{D}O_2$ reduction has revealed a biphasic pattern of $\dot{V}O_2$ response, with $\dot{V}O_2$ decreasing precipitously below a critical threshold $\dot{D}O_2$ value. These investigations confirm, as expected, that bulk tissue oxygen delivery (i.e., $\dot{D}O_2$) is an extremely powerful determinant of oxidative metabolism. Diffusion barriers may also play a role, however critical $\dot{D}O_2$ provided in virtually any form has proven an extremely sensitive indicator of the dysoxic threshold when subjects have been studied under identical physiological conditions. Unfortunately, to the disappointment of many, $\dot{V}O_2$ and $\dot{D}O_2$ have frequently been found to covary in patients who are seemingly well. Analysis of available literature suggests that the biphasic $\dot{V}O_2$-$\dot{D}O_2$ model is not a generally incorrect representation of human physiology, but rather that it is difficult to apply in the clinical setting, because assumptions are required that are difficult to verify in patients. The most important of these assumptions is that $\dot{V}O_2$ demand is constant, and that O_2 supply dependency commences simultaneously in all organs. Whole body measurements such as lactate and A-V pH, and whole organ measurements such as $\beta OHB/AcAc$ generally support the biphasic $\dot{V}O_2$-$\dot{D}O_2$ model as a detector of dysoxia in laboratory settings. Because $\dot{V}O_2$ demand of ICU patients is so highly variable, these measurements may enhance $\dot{D}O_2$ measurements, providing a more reliable independent variable than $\dot{V}O_2$. Combined with clinical acumen and a basic understanding of oxidative metabolism, these clinical variables may assist the clinician in detection and treatment of dysoxia during variation of $\dot{D}O_2$.

References

1. Annat G, Viale J-P, Percival C, Roment M, Motin J. Oxygen delivery and uptake in the adult respiratory distress syndrome. Am Rev Respir Dis 1986;133:999–1001.
2. Balaban RS, Sylvia AL. Spectrophotometric monitoring of O_2 delivery to the exposed rat kidney. Am J Physiol 1981;241:F257–F262.
3. Bashford CL, Barlow CH, Chance B, Haselgrove J. The oxidation-reduction state of cytochrome oxidase in freeze trapped gerbil brains. FEBS Lett 1980;113:78–80.
4. Bowles, SA, Schlichtig R, Klions HA, Kramer DJ. A-V pH and A-V PCO_2 during progressive hemorrhage. Am Rev Respir Dis 1990;141:A585.
5. Brezis M, Rosen S, Silva P, Epstein FH. Transport activity modifies thick ascending limb damage in the isolated perfused kidney. J Clin Invest 1984;73:182–190.
6. Cain SM. Arterial lactate responses in dogs made apneic or breathing nitrogen. J Appl Physiol 1977;42:39–43.
7. Cain SM. Oxygen delivery and uptake in dogs during anemic and hypoxic hypoxia. J Appl Physiol 1977;42:228–234.
8. Cain SM. Peripheral oxygen uptake and delivery in health and disease. Clin Chest Med 1983;4:139–148.
9. Cain SM. Supply dependency of oxygen uptake in ARDS: myth or reality? Am J Med Sci 1984;288:119–124.
10. Carlile PV, Gray BA. Effect of opposite changes in cardiac output and arterial PO_2 on the relationship between mixed venous PO_2 and oxygen transport. Am Rev Respir Dis 1989;140:891–898.
11. Connett RJ, Honig CR, Gayeski TEJ, Brooks GA. Defining hypoxia: a systems view of VO_2, glycolysis, energetics, and intracellular PO_2. J Appl Physiol 1990;68:833–842.
12. Danek SJ, Lynch JP, Weg JG, Dantzker DR. The dependence of oxygen uptake on oxygen delivery in the adult respiratory distress syndrome. Am Rev Respir Dis 1980;122:387–395.
13. Dorinsky PM, Costello JL, Gadek JE. Relationships of oxygen uptake and oxygen delivery in respiratory failure not due to the adult respiratory distress syndrome. Chest 1988;93:1013–1030.
14. Epstein FH, Balaban RS, Ross BD. Redox state of cytochrome a,a_3 in isolated perfused rat kidney. Am J Physiol 1982;243:F356–F363.
15. Fahey JT, Lister G. Postnatal changes in critical cardiac output and oxygen transport in conscious lambs. Am J Physiol 1989;66:561–566.
16. Fantone JC. Pathogenesis of ischemia-reperfusion injury: an overview. In: D'Alecy LG, et al. eds. Clinical ischemic syndromes. St. Louis: CV Mosby, 1990.
17. Farber JL, Chien KR, Mittnacht S. The pathogenesis of irreversible cell injury in ischemia. Am J Pathol 1981;102:271–281.
18. Finch CA, Lenfant C. Oxygen transport in man. N Engl J Med 1972;286:407–415.
19. Fisher AB, Forman HJ. Oxygen utilization and toxicity in the lungs. In: Handbook of physiology. The respiratory system, circulation and nonrespiratory functions. Section 3, vol I. Bethesda, MD: American Physiological Society, 1985:231–254.
20. Forrester JS, Diamond G, Chatterjee K, Swan HJC. Medical therapy of acute myocardial infarction by application of hemodynamic subsets (first of two parts). N Engl J Med 1976;295:1356–1362.
21. Fox LS, Blackstone EH, Kirklin JW, Stewart RW, Samuelson PN. Relationship of whole body oxygen consumption to perfusion flow rate during hypothermic cardiopulmonary bypass. J Thorac Cardiovasc Surg 1982;83:239–248.
22. Frommer PL, Ross J, Mason T, Gault JH, Braunwald E. Clinical applications of an improved, rapidly responding fiberoptic catheter. Am J Cardiol 1965;15:672–679.
23. Gibert EM, Haupt MT, Mandanas RY, Huaringa AJ, Carlson RW. The effect of fluid loading, blood transfusion, and catecholamine infusion on oxygen delivery and consumption in patients with sepsis. Am Rev Respir Dis 1986;134:873–878.
24. Gimson AE, Westaby D, Hegarty J, Watson A, Williams R. A randomized trial of vasopressin and vasopressin plus nitroglycerin in the control of acute variceal hemorrhage. Hepatology 1986;6:410–413.
25. Gore JM, Goldberg RJ, Spodick DH, Alpert JS, Dalen JE. A community-wide assessment of the use of pulmonary artery catheters in patients with acute myocardial infarction. Chest 1987;92:721–731.
26. Grum CM, Fiddian-Green RG, Pittenger GL, Grant BJB, Rothman ED, Dantzker DR. Adequacy of tissue oxygenation in intact dog intestine. J Appl Physiol 1984;56:1065–1069.
27. Gubernatis G, Bornscheuer A, Taki Y, Farie M, Lubbe N, Yamaoka Y, Beneking M, Burdeiski M, Oellerich M. Total oxygen consumption, ketone body ratio and a special score as early indicators of irreversible liver allograft dysfunction. Transplant Proc 1989;21:2279–2281.
28. Gutierrez G, Pohil RJ, Strong R. Effect of flow on O_2 consumption during progressive hypoxemia. J Appl Physiol 1988;65:601–607.
29. Gutierrez G, Andry JM. Increased hemoglobin O_2 affinity does not improve O_2 consumption in hypoxemia. J Appl Physiol 1989;66:837–843.
30. Gutierrez G, Pohil RJ, Narayana P. Skeletal muscle O_2 consumption and energy metabolism during hypoxemia. J Appl Physiol 1989;66:2117–2123.
31. Gutierrez G, Marini C, Acero AL, Lund N. Skeletal muscle Po_2 during hypoxemia and isovolemic anemia. J Appl Physiol 1990;68:2047–2053.
32. Gutierrez G, Lund N, Palizas F. Rabbit skeletal muscle Po_2 during hypodynamic sepsis. Chest 1991;99:224–229.
33. Hampson PA, Piantadosi CA. Skeletal muscle cytochrome a,a_3 oxidation level varies as a func-

tion of systemic oxygen consumption during controlled hemorrhage in cats. Am Rev Respir Dis 1986;133:A37.

34. Hampson NB, Camporesi EM, Stolp W, Moon RE, Shook JE, Griebel JA, Piantadosi CA. Cerebral oxygen availability by NIR spectroscopy during transient hypoxia in humans. J Appl Physiol 1990;69:907–913.

35. Hartman M, Montgomery A, Jonsson K, Haglund U. Tissue oxygenation in hemorrhagic shock measured as transcutaneous oxygen tension, subcutaneous oxygen tension, and gastrointestinal pH in pigs. Crit Care Med 1991;19:205–210.

36. Haupt MT, Gilbert EM, Carlson RW. Fluid loading increases oxygen consumption in septic patients with lactic acidosis. Am Rev Respir Dis 1985;131:912–916.

37. Hayman JM, Schmidt CF. The gaseous metabolism of the dog's kidney. Am J Physiol 1928;83:502–512.

38. Heros RC, Zervas N, Varos V. Cerebral vasospasm after subarachnoid hemorrhage: an update. Ann Neurol 1983;14:599–608.

39. Hickley RF, Hoar PF. Whole body oxygen consumption during low-flow hypothermic cardiopulmonary bypass. J Thorac Cardiovasc Surg 1983;86:903–906.

40. Hochachka PW. Defense strategies against hypoxia and hypothermia. Science 1986;213:14–24.

41. Hoffer LJ. Cori cycle contribution to plasma glucose appearance in man. JPEN 1990;14:646–648.

42. Johnston BL, Watt EW, Fletcher GF. Oxygen consumption and hemodynamic and electrocardiographic responses to bathing in recent postmyocardial infarction patients. Heart Lung 1981;10:666–671.

43. Kaufman BS, Rackow EC. The relationship between oxygen delivery and consumption during fluid resuscitation of hypovolemic and septic shock. Chest 1984;85:336–340.

44. Kosnik EJ, Hunt WE. Postoperative hypertension in the management of patients with intracranial arterial aneurysms. J Neurosurg 1976;45:148–154.

45. Light BR. Intrapulmonary oxygen consumption in experimental pneumococcal pneumonia. J Appl Physiol 1988;64:2490–2495.

46. Lutz J, Henrich H, Bauereisen E. Oxygen supply and uptake in the liver and intestine. Pflugers Arch 1975;360:7–15.

47. Mager A, Sclarovsky S, Wurtzel M, Menkes H, Strasberg B, Rechavia E. Ischemia and reperfusion during intermittent coronary occlusion in man. Studies of electrocardiographic and CPK release. Chest 1991;99:386–392.

48. Manny J, Justice R, Hechtman HB. Abnormalities in organ blood flow and its distribution during positive end-expiratory pressure. Surgery 1979;85:425–432.

49. Maroko PR, Libby P, Sobel BE. Effect of glucose-insulin-potassium infusion on myocardial infarction following experimental coronary artery occlusion. Circulation 1972;65:1160–1175.

50. Matuschak GM, Pinsky MR, Rogers RM. Effects

of positive end-expiratory pressure on hepatic blood flow and performance. J Appl Physiol 1987;62:1377–1383.

51. Mizock BA. Lactic acidosis. Dis Mon 1989;35:237–300.

52. Morimoto T, Taki UT, Koizumi K, Tokoo N, Tanaka A, Noguchi M, Yamamoto S, Nitta N, Kamiyama Y, Tamaoka Y, Ozawa K. Changes in energy metabolism of allografts after liver transplantation. Eur Surg Res 1988;20:120–127.

53. Myers BD, Miller C, Mehigan JT, Olcott C, Golbetz H, Robertson CR, Derby G, Spencer R, Friedman S. Nature of the renal injury following total renal ischemia in man. J Clin Invest 1984;73:329–341.

54. Nagano K, Gelman S, Parks DA, Bradley EL. Hepatic oxygen-supply-uptake relationship and metabolism during anesthesia in miniature pigs. Anesthesiology 1990;72:902–910.

55. Nelson DP, Samsel RW, Wood LDH, Schumacker PT. Pathological supply dependency of systemic and intestinal O$_2$ uptake during endotoxemia. J Appl Physiol 1988;64:2410–2419.

56. Nelson DP, Beyer C, Samsel RW, Wood LDH, Schumacker PT, Cain SM. Systemic and intestinal limits of O$_2$ extraction in the dog. J Appl Physiol 1987;63:387–394.

57. Nelson DP, Beyer C, Samsel RW, Wood LDH, Schumacker PT. Pathological supply dependence of O$_2$ uptake during bacteremia in dogs. J Appl Physiol 1987;63:1487–1492.

58. Oberman A. Rehabilitation of patients with coronary artery disease. In: Braunwald E, ed. Heart disease. A textbook of cardiovascular medicine. Philadelphia: WB Saunders, 1988.

59. Ozawa K, Aoyama H, Yasuda K, Shimahara Y, Nakatani T, Tanaka J, Yamamoto M, Kamiyama Y, Tobe T. Metabolic abnormalities associated with postoperative organ failure. A redox theory. Arch Surg 1983;118:1245–1251.

60. Pittiruti M, Siegel JH, Sganga G, et al. Increased dependence of leucine in post-traumatic sepsis: leucine/tyrosine clearance ratio as an indicator of hepatic impairment in septic multiple organ failure syndrome. Surgery 1985;98:378–386.

61. Powers SR, Mannal R, Neclerio M, English BS, Marr C, Leather R, Ueda H, Williams G, Custead W, Dutton R. Physiologic consequences of positive end-expiratory pressure (PEEP) ventilation. Ann Surg 1971;178:265–272.

62. Quinn TJ, Weissman C, Kemper M. Continual trending of Fick variables in the critically ill patient. Chest 1991;99:703–707.

63. Rogers WJ, Stanley AW, Breinig JB. Reduction of hospital mortality rate of acute myocardial infarction with glucose-insulin-potassium infusion. Am Heart J 1976;92:441–454.

64. Rosenthal MJ, LaManna JC, Jobsis FF, Lavasseur JE, Kontos HA, Patterson JL. Effects of respiratory gases on cytochrome *a* in intact cerebral cortex: is there a critical PO$_2$? Brain Res 1976;108:143–153.

65. Rothman SM. Synaptic activity mediates death of hypoxic neurons. Science 1983;220:536–537.

66. Samsei RW, Nelson DP, Sanders WM, et al.

"hyperdynamic" cardiovascular state consisting of an elevated cardiac index with reduced systemic vascular resistance index has been associated with severe sepsis. Arterial pressure may be high, normal, or low, often correlating poorly with the adequacy of tissue perfusion. This state forms one of the defining criteria for sepsis syndrome (4, 9, 11, 55, 64, 82). However, both prior to and following volume resuscitation to treat initial hypotension, ventricular preload is frequently depressed secondary to three mechanisms occurring singly or in combination. First, inadequate venous return owing to loss of venomotor tone and resultant splanchnic blood pooling produces commensurate reductions in left ventricular (LV) stroke volume (42, 107). Second, relative intravascular volume depletion derives from decreases in peripheral vasomotor tone, which affect the upstream driving pressure for venous return—mean systemic pressure—in the circulatory model proposed by Guyton et al. (45). In this regard, Dhainaut et al. (31) found that survivors of septic shock increased right ventricular (RV) preload by utilizing the Frank-Starling mechanism to maintain stroke volume (118), thereby preventing RV pump failure. Third, generalized increases in microvascular permeability permit enhanced transendothelial loss of protein-rich plasma, which reduces the circulating blood volume and mean systemic pressure (2, 45). Interacting effects of sepsis, baseline abnormalities in cardiac function, and fluid resuscitation modulate the expression of these changes, irrespective of the taxonomic class of the infecting organism (143, 146). In experimental models, the hyperdynamic state with tachycardia is commonly elicited by rapid intravenous infusions of purified lipopolysaccharide endotoxin, in contrast to a hypodynamic state with depressed cardiac output and elevated systemic vascular resistance, which evolves more slowly following bacterial peritonitis (1, 145). In the latter case, flow reductions may be partially offset by concomitant reductions in arterial pressure as an afterload to the ejecting LV. Guntheroth et al. demonstrated that LV contractility is depressed during Gram-negative endotoxic shock, but

postulated that this effect is masked by decreases in LV afterload consequent to arterial hypotension and frequency-dependent LV filling owing to tachycardia (43). The vigor of fluid resuscitation further modulates systemic blood flow and O_2 delivery (18, 62) by augmenting both ventricular filling and diastolic coronary perfusion. However, intrinsic myocardial depression plays a pivotal role in the genesis of septic shock and MSOF, evolving with progression of the septic inflammatory response to produce time-dependent alterations in cardiac performance (1, 103).

Determination of changes in cardiac performance during sepsis assumes an ability to obtain reliable estimates of the ventricular pressure-volume relationship to establish adequacy of ventricular filling. Inherent limitations of both clinical examination and right atrial pressure or pulmonary artery occlusion pressure monitoring for this purpose have been established (19, 112). For instance, Reuse et al. found no significant correlation between the RV end-diastolic volume index and right atrial pressure in critically ill patients during fluid challenge, and only weak correlations between the RV end-systolic index and pulmonary artery pressure (112). To permit inferences regarding myocardial contractile function during invasive hemodynamic monitoring, estimates should ideally be independent of ventricular loading conditions. Nevertheless, bedside measurement of cardiac output by thermodilution and ventricular function indices derived from it are highly load- or heart rate-dependent (130). The ventricular ejection fraction varies inversely with heart rate and afterload and, to a lesser extent, directly with preload (31, 112). Conversely, the ratio of peak systolic pressure to end-systolic volume index derived from ejection fraction measurements and the end-systolic pressure-diameter relationship permit determination of ventricular systolic function independent of load (116, 132).

Data obtained from animal models of sepsis indicate that, in spite of the hyperdynamic state, myocardial function is depressed to varying degrees (1, 79, 96). Central to the proper interpretation of such studies is an appreciation of the dynamic nature of pathophysiologic changes. Time-dependent changes may arise and resolve rapidly or over days, so that discussion of "characteristic" alterations requires temporal qualification. As alluded to above, fluid loading modulates this state by supporting blood volume, arterial pressure, and preload reserve as exemplified in a primate model of Gram-negative bacteremia (18).

Why is myocardial function depressed? One potential explanation is that Gram-negative bacterial endotoxin itself exerts a direct depressant effect on contractility. There is little data to support this possibility (1, 97). Studies using ex vivo contractility of neonatal rat myocytes incubated with endotoxin have furthermore not been confirmatory (102). Coronary hypoperfusion is another mechanism that might impair pump function, but there is no strong evidence in favor of this as a primary mechanism (1). In a canine model of acute *Escherichia coli* endotoxemia (107), arterial hypotension occurred within minutes of Gram-negative endotoxemia, a time course too rapid to implicate cytokine-dependent effects (48, 57, 141). Although depression of stroke volume might be responsible, there were no accompanying changes in ventricular function curves or the slope of the arterial pressure-flow relation representing arterial resistance (107). After 30 min, arterial pressure fell further while cardiac output increased during unchanging conditions of blood volume and arterial resistance. In other studies, depression of endocardial calcium (Ca^{2+}) transport by the sarcoplasmic reticulum has been implicated, and myocardial adenosinetriphosphatase (ATPase) and norepinephrine stores may be depleted, depending on the timing of their measurement (1, 56, 95). However, the myocardial dysfunction of hyperdynamic sepsis seems to be due to factors other than Ca^{2+} availability for contraction as assessed in isolated, perfused rat hearts, since ATPase blockade with oubain and Ca^{2+} channel blockade with verapamil only mildly changed ventricular function curves (79).

In a conscious canine model, Natanson et al. induced peritoneal infection with sustained bacteremia, which simulated the cardiovascular pattern of human septic shock (84, 85). Arterial and pulmonary arterial catheterizations, combined with radionuclide cineangiography, permitted analysis of systolic and diastolic ventricular performance, ventricular volumes, and pressure/volume relationships. Despite evolution of hyperdynamic cardiovascular indices after *E. coli* bacteremia, the LV ejection fraction was depressed. Ventricular dilation, confirmed by increases in end-systolic and end-diastolic volumes and evidence of increased LV compliance, was a reproducible cardiovascular response (84, 85). The underlying mechanism appears to be related to host production of myocardial depressant factor(s). Parrillo et al. demonstrated a circulating myocardial depressant factor by an in vitro neonatal rat cardiac myocyte model in which rhythmic contractions were variably suppressed by incubation with serum samples from septic patients (102). Although similar cardiovascular changes are elicited after infusions of purified endotoxin without Gram-negative organisms (88), indistinguishable changes develop after *Staphylococcus aureus* sepsis (87), demonstrating that endotoxemia per se is not a prerequisite. Two further points are relevant. First, intravenous infusions of endotoxin-free recombinant tumor necrosis factor-α (TNF-α) into a similar conscious canine model lead to equivalent cardiovascular findings (88). Second, similar to Gram-negative bacteremia, Gram-positive bacteremia also results in production of TNF-α and interleukin-1β (IL-1β) (50, 143). Although no in vitro myocardial depressant factor-like activity has been found after exposure of myocytes to endotoxin, IL-1β, or IL-2, reductions in contractility result following incubation with recombinant TNF-α (60).

To what extent can changes in ventricular systolic and diastolic function be implicated in cardiac depression during human endotoxemia? Experimentally, the pattern of cardiovascular changes prior to volume loading indicate systolic dysfunction evolving within 3 hr after endotoxin interacts with host cells. The cardiac index and heart rate increased by 53 and 36%, respectively, while the systemic vascular resistance decreased by 46% following an infusion of 4 ng/kg of *E. coli* endotoxin into normal humans (131). Load-independent LV performance, determined as the ratio of peak systolic pressure to the end-systolic volume index, was depressed relative to baseline without changes in the ionized serum Ca^{2+} concentration. Prospective hemodynamic analyses in critically ill patients combining pulmonary artery thermodilution catheter-derived data with radionuclide ventriculography and selective coronary sinus catheterization extend these findings while refining prognostication of survivorship or mortality in septic shock (93, 98–101, 111). Myocardial depression occurs in survivors with decreases in the ejection fraction (mean, 0.32) despite normal or elevated cardiac indices (98, 100). This demonstrates maintenance of stroke volume by acute cardiac dilation by intrinsic contractile dysfunction. Thereafter, hemodynamics normalize between days 6 and 14. Conversely, nonsurvivors had a preserved ejection fraction (mean, 0.55) over 48–72 hr and died within 5 days (98, 100). As in animal models, the mechanism of the depression of myocardial contractility does not appear to be decreased coronary blood flow (22), but is rather secondary to intrinsic reductions in contractility as assessed by joint determinations of biventricular ejection fractions. Moreover, the increases in ventricular end-systolic volume correlate with levels of myocardial depressant factor (111). Further analysis of myocardial depression in nonsurvivors has distinguished two subsets of patients. In the first, lack of compensatory decreases in the ejection fraction reflects an inappropriate Starling response despite fluid resuscitation (31, 100, 111). In the other, LV stroke volume is maintained by compensatory increases in end-diastolic volume despite reductions in the ejection fraction, but there are predominant decreases in the systemic vascular resistance. In either case, accompanying changes in ventricular compliance owing to myocardial edema (14) can cause variability in the end-diastolic volume at any level of pulmonary artery occlusion pressure following fluid loading (103). These sepsis-induced abnormalities, collectively

Table 10.1
Comparison of Changes in Cardiovascular Parameters in Survivors and Nonsurvivors of Septic Shock

Parameter	Survivors	Non-survivors
Cardiac index	nl or ↑	nl or ↑
SVRI[a]	↓	↓
Heart rate	↑	↑ ↑
Left ventricle		
LV stroke volume	nl or ↑	↓ or nl
LV end-systolic volume	↑ ↑	↑
LV end-diastolic volume	↑ ↑	nl or ↓
LV ejection fraction	↓	nl or ↑
Right ventricle		
RV stroke volume	nl or ↑	↓ or nl
RV end-systolic volume	↑ ↑	↑
RV end-diastolic volume	↑ ↑	nl or ↓
RV ejection fraction	↓	nl or ↑

[a]SVRI, systemic vascular resistance index; nl, normal.

summarized in Table 10.1, affect LV and RV function equally (31, 93, 101, 112). For the left heart, the effects of septic myocardial depression are partially counterbalanced by reductions in LV afterload associated with sepsis-related decreases in the systemic vascular resistance. Nonetheless, LV stroke volume and, consequently, cardiac output are inadequate unless accompanied by compensatory chamber dilatation. Finally, it must be noted that patients who are not adequately volume resuscitated may have coronary flow reductions that independently alter diastolic compliance, complicating interpretation of the pulmonary artery occlusion pressure.

Peripheral Vasomotor Tone

Vasomotor tone may be defined as the inward-acting transmural force responsible for the x (pressure)-axis intercept observed at zero flow on vascular pressure-flow plots. The pressure within a vessel with tone when flow is zero is the critical closing pressure. Under joint control by central autonomic mechanisms and local metabolic autoregulation, dysregulation of vasomotor tone during sepsis syndrome and septic shock is central to the genesis of hypotension and distributive blood flow abnormalities. The balance between central and local control systems regulates tone at discrete loci within the vasculature, and transmural vascular pressure is derived from their net interaction. The distribution of vascular smooth muscle and autonomic innervation is nonuniform (40); vasomotor tone likewise varies. The relation of the transmural distending pressure to blood volume, the vascular compliance, is significantly changed in both the arterial and venous circuits during severe sepsis. Two factors are important: (*a*) the arterial pressure-flow relationship; and (*b*) the distribution of closing pressures within organs. Arterial flow (Q) is the product of the reciprocal of arterial resistance (R) and the pressure gradient driving flow, or $Q = 1/R$ (Pi − Po), where Pi is the input pressure and Po the outflow pressure (40, 104). Increases in vasomotor tone within small arterial vessels shift the curve to the right while decreases in tone shift it to the left (Fig. 10.1). Since resistance is defined as a pressure drop divided by flow, the lumped-parameter model of the circulatory system described by the systemic vascular resistance calculation assumes right atrial pressure to be an arterial back pressure. However, since the diameter of small collapsible vessels can be affected by both intramural

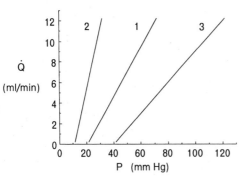

Figure 10.1. Relationship between arterial pressure *(P)* and flow *(Q̇)* within small vessels that function analogously to Starling resistors, with inward-acting vasomotor tone constituting an equivalent of a surrounding pressure. Schematic P-Q plots are shown for three conditions: *1*, the normal P-Q relation; *2*, decreases in vasomotor tone as occurring during sepsis; and *3*, increases in tone as might be seen following infusion of α-adrenergic agonists. The x-axis intercept at zero flow represents the critical closing pressure.

events (e.g., hypovolemia) and extramural forces (e.g., tissue edema), the distribution of intraorgan closing pressures ultimately determines the volumetric input into the capillary network, or tissue oxygen delivery. Because intra- and interorgan distributive resistances are not taken into account by the systemic vascular resistance calculation, one cannot equate systemic vascular resistance values with vasomotor tone itself. While valuable as an estimation of LV afterload for therapy to augment failing LV ejection, global systemic vascular resistance bears little relation to critical closing pressure during tissue hypoxia (135) and should therefore not be used to infer dysfunction or recovery of the distribution of systemic blood flow during sepsis.

The abnormal reductions in peripheral vasomotor tone during sepsis (leftward shift of the arterial pressure-flow relation) have been likened to a form of peripheral vasomotor "paralysis." Examination of early changes following acute endotoxemia is instructive. In a canine model, the hemodynamic response is biphasic: within minutes an early, disproportionate reduction in venous return is followed within 30 min by arterial hypotension and an increased systemic vascular capacitance (107). Where is the predominant site of loss of vasomotor tone that results in arterial hypotension? As outlined above, Permutt and Riley postulated that decreases in the total peripheral vascular resistance develop if the ratio of input pressure to output pressure decreases or critical closing pressure falls (104). Accordingly, changes in critical closing pressure at the level of the arterioles and precapillary sphincters resulting from sepsis and its treatment produce loss of vasomotor tone independent of changes in the large-vessel arterial resistance.

Microvascular Consequences

The effects of peripheral vasomotor paralysis on the production of shock and impaired regional organ perfusion during sepsis are amplified by corresponding microvascular changes owing to four factors: (*a*) activation and adherence of polymorphonuclear leukocytes to vascular endothelium (34, 125); (*b*) O_2 free radical-mediated injury to endothelial and parenchymal cells (78, 144); (*c*) thrombotic obstruction secondary to cytokine-mediated endothelial changes favoring a prothrombotic state (7, 90); and (*d*) increases in permeability resulting from oxidant injury and activation of endogenous lipid and peptide mediators (29, 30, 32, 48, 57, 68, 78, 141). Collectively, these events alter the balance of Starling forces to produce parenchymal cell injury and tissue edema. The resultant microvascular occlusion can reduce tissue O_2 extraction by interfering with capillary recruitment and increasing diffusion distances (47). Such events should not be viewed as deleterious in a one-dimensional sense, since a principal function is to localize bacteria and their products until resolution of the inflammatory focus occurs concomitant with tissue remodeling by proliferation of mesenchymal cells. When orchestration among these mechanisms becomes lost, tissue hypoperfusion results owing to mismatching of perfusion with cellular metabolic activity. Because of the distributive nature of septic shock, tissues with high O_2 requirements such as the intestine may have suboptimal DO_2 while those with low O_2 requirements are overperfused (91). Although the significance of pathologic supply dependence of systemic O_2 uptake (VO_2) on DO_2 has not been fully resolved secondary to regional differences in VO_2/DO_2 kinetics, lactic acidosis is the best marker of the severity of microvascular changes leading to tissue hypoperfusion (124). This arises from augmented tissue O_2 demands during hypermetabolic sepsis in the setting of microvascular obstruction and resultant derecruitment of capillary perfusion. Since O_2 extraction is a dual function of the distribution of flow to organs with varying metabolic rates and diffusional flux of O_2 from hemoglobin to mitochondria (120), the combination of persistently suboptimal DO_2 and impaired O_2 extraction leads to anaerobic glycolysis. Peripheral edema is a consequence of endothelial injury, since cell junction abnormalities reduce σ, the protein reflection coefficient in Starling's equation. Because of the associated enhanced transvascular escape rate of plasma protein, large-volume crystalloid resuscitation may augment tissue edema, which if unchecked, can increase the distribution of intraorgan closing pressures.

ENDOGENOUS INFLAMMATORY MEDIATORS: THE CYTOKINE-EICOSANOID NETWORK

Intercellular communication and its moment-to-moment modulation during infection and trauma is critical to maintaining systemic homeostasis. Recent studies have demonstrated the complex immunophysiology of cytokines during infection and trauma (32, 33, 48, 49, 52, 57, 117, 141). By the cooperative or antagonistic actions of these elements within a network (Table 10.2), the spectrum of cellular and cardiovascular responses is determined that typifies the septic response. This conception has analogy to neuronal networks in which integration of multiple excitatory and inhibitory stimuli modulate neuronal firing. The following general characteristics of cytokines summarize their activities: (*a*) *pleiotropic actions*, by which multiple activities are expressed on an array of cell types (Table 10.2); (*b*) *bidirectional effects*, or the capacity of individual cytokines such as TNF-α or IL-1 to serve as a proinflammatory mediator and yet demonstrate protective effects in other models of sepsis (35, 117, 123); (*c*) *overlapping actions*, in which additive or synergistic effects amplify inflammation (In this manner, shock, cardiac output depression, and organ injury are augmented during coadministration of recombinant TNF-α and recombinant IL-1 to anesthetized rabbits, compared to either agent alone (94).); and (*d*) *interaction with noncytokine-dependent pathways* of inflammation. For example, monoclonal antisera directed against the leukocyte intercellular adhesion molecule (ICAM-1) modulates the stimulated production of TNF-α, interferon-γ, and IL-1 (37). In other studies, therapy with protein C or a monoclonal antibody-to-tissue factor improves survival and organ system function in a primate model of Gram-negative bacteremia

Table 10.2
Selected Properties of Certain Cytokines and Their Interactions: Modulators and Antagonists

Cytokine	Cellular Source	Effects	Inducing Agents	Modulators
TNF-α	Mononuclear phagocytes, PMNs[a]	Hypotension; shock; PMN activation; pro-thrombotic state; induction of IL-1, IL-6, IL-8, IL-9 + MIP; cyclooxy-genase and acute-phase gene expression; fever; resistance to infection	Gram-negative and Gram-positive bacteria; LPS; *Legionella*; viruses; parasites; hypoxia-ischemia	*Gene expression:* ($-$) IL-6, IL-10, TGF-β, PGE$_2$, cAMP (PTX) ($+$) GM-CSF; IL-1, PGE$_2$ *Circulating levels:* soluble TNF-α receptors; acute-phase protein binding (α_2-macroglob-ulin); liver function
IL-1	Mononuclear phagocytes, endothelial cells, fibro-blasts B and T cells	Hypotension; shock; en-dothelial cell activation; induction of IL-6, IL-8, IL-9 + MIP; cyclooxy-genase and acute-phase gene expression; fever; resistance to infection	Gram-negative and Gram-positive bacteria; LPS; *Legionella*	*Gene expression:* ($-$) IL-10; TGF-β; PGE$_2$ ($+$) TNF-α; GM-CSF; lipoxygen-ase metabolites *Circulating levels:* soluble IL-1 receptors; IL-1 re-ceptor antagonist
IL-6	Mononuclear phagocytes, endothelial cells, fibro-blasts B and T cells	?Shock; B-cell differentia-tion; T-cell activation; stimulation of hemato-poietic precursors	Same as for TNF-α and IL-1; TNF-α; IL-1	Indirect via determinants of TNF-α and IL-1 pro-duction
IL-8, IL-9, MIP	Endothelial cells	PMN activation; PMN, monocyte, + lympho-cyte chemotaxis; inhibi-tion of PMN; endothe-lial interactions	LPS, TNF-α, IL-1	Indirect via determinants of TNF-α and IL-1 pro-duction

[a]PMNs, polymorphonuclear leukocytes; LPS, lipopolysaccharide; MIP, macrophage inhibitory proteins; GM-CSF, granulocyte-macro-phage colony stimulating factor; PTX, pheumothorax.

(136, 137). Thus, an inflammatory: coagu-lation axis exists during sepsis in which cellular injury can result from activation by one of several parallel molecular path-ways.

EPIDEMIOLOGY AND DEFINITIONS

Sepsis syndrome is the presence of micro-organisms or their products in the circu-lation plus the resultant acute cardiovas-cular, inflammatory, and metabolic responses (9, 11, 55). Between 70,000 and 300,000 cases of sepsis occur yearly in the United States (9, 103), although this is likely an underestimation. When accom-panied by reductions in arterial pressure of <90 mm Hg that are unresponsive to volume challenge or necessitate vasopres-sor therapy, *septic shock* is present. A va-riety of organisms serve as triggers, in-cluding viruses, rickettsiae, Gram-positive and Gram-negative bacteria, mycobac-teria, *Legionella*, fungi, and intracellular parasites. Most critically ill septic patients are infected with either aerobic or anaer-obic Gram-negative bacteria, *E. coli, Kleb-siella pneumoniae, Enterobacter, Pseudomonas aeruginosa, Staphylococcus,* or *Candida* (71, 103). That structurally different organisms generate stereotypic host responses such as fever, hypothermia, hypotension, met-abolic acidosis, and changes in circulating polymorphonuclear leukocytes has led to the belief that the magnitude and kinetics of mediators transducing these changes are similar. Although a large body of data supports this for TNF-α and IL-1 (38), le-thal shock and organ injury during exper-imental candidemia with acute disseminated candidiasis are not dependent on TNF-α (76).

When sepsis syndrome is severe, *MSOF* may supervene, even without antecedent shock. A number of important questions concerning MSOF are unresolved. What type, severity, and duration of organ system dysfunction constitutes MSOF? What features differentiate organ system dysfunction from organ "failure"? And finally, how does one categorize dysfunction in organ systems that are not readily accessible at the bedside, such as the liver and the gastrointestinal tract? Although a uniformly accepted definition is lacking, MSOF can be defined as a constellation of severe physiologic dysfunctions occurring in multiple (at least two) organ systems either sequentially or concomitantly after infection, major operation, or injury, which lasts for a minimum period of 24–48 hr. By these criteria and categorization of patients by APACHE II scoring, MSOF develops in 7–15% of patients requiring ICU admission (51, 64, 65). Two factors are especially predictive of mortality during MSOF: age of >65 years (64, 106) and the number of organ system failures (4, 38, 82). Meta-analysis of retrospective and prospective studies of MSOF occurring in both medical and surgical critical illness (4, 38, 64, 82, 89, 106) reveals a consistent progression: one organ system failure results in an approximate 33% mortality rate, whereas failure of two and three or more organ systems yields corresponding values of 66 and 90%, respectively. Although data are limited to determine whether dysfunction in specific organ systems predisposes to septic shock and MSOF and/or impairs their resolution, several lines of evidence suggest that the liver is a pivotal organ in this regard (73). Acquired liver dysfunction is proportionately greater in nonsurvivors of adult respiratory distress syndrome (ARDS) compared with survivors (121). Preexisting end-stage liver failure predisposes to ARDS, which is irreversible despite ventilatory support (74). Further evidence for a liver-lung axis of cardiopulmonary homeostasis are data obtained after induction of acute hepatocytic injury by the selective hepatotoxin D-galactosamine, in which mortality, lung vascular permeability, and neutrophilic alveolitis were augmented following *E. coli* endotoxemia (75).

PATHOGENESIS

Pertinent factors include the bacterial density of contamination and the underlying immune status. With normal immune function, containment of inocula of 10^5 colony-forming units (cfu)/ml of urine or 10^5 cfu/g of tissue can be achieved. More virulent organisms trigger a systemic inflammatory response or compromise local defenses at lower bacterial densities, especially with underlying disease. Mortality rates during Gram-negative bacteremia are >90% in septic patients with "rapidly fatal" diseases (e.g., acute leukemia, burns of >70% body surface area), 66% with "ultimately fatal" diseases (e.g., cirrhosis, chronic renal failure), and 10% with "nonfatal" diseases (e.g., diabetes mellitus, alcoholism) (77). The pathogenesis of the sepsis syndrome can be viewed as a series of progressive events: (*a*) failure of local integumentary, mucosal, or respiratory defenses to contain invading organisms; (*b*) "centrifugal" recruitment of regional host defenses mediated by activation of tissue-based macrophages such as aveolar macrophages and Kupffer cells and chemotactically driven neutrophilic influx; (*c*) oxidant and protease-mediated injury to endothelial and parenchymal cells by primed and activated polymorphonuclear leukocytes (34, 78, 125, 144); (*d*) loss of host regulatory control at transcriptional, posttranscriptional, and posttranslational levels of the production of TNF-α, IL-1, and IL-6 (32, 33, 48, 49, 52, 57, 141) or impairment of metabolic inactivation of cytokines or their eicosanoid second messengers (50, 69, 75); (*e*) complement activation within the intravascular compartment and inactivation of anti-proteases such as α_1-antiproteinase at the polymorphonuclear leukocyte:endothelial interface and within organs (30, 141); (*f*) generation of endothelium-derived relaxing factor and nitric oxide via arginine metabolism by activated leukocytes, which alters microvascular tone (23); and (*g*) generation of myocardial depressant factor-like compounds, which depress cardiac function and systemic O_2 delivery.

PATHOPHYSIOLOGY

To implicate causality in infectious disease, Koch postulated that three conditions were to be met: (a) a pathogenic organism must be present in all cases of the disease, (b) inoculation of the organism must cause disease, and (c) the organism must be recovered from inoculated animals and propagated again in culture. In like manner, a variety of mediators suspected of causing sepsis-related inflammation have been studied. Koch's postulates as applied to potential septic mediators can be restated: (a) a proposed mediator should be detectable during septic periods, (b) challenge with the mediator should result in pathophysiologic changes reproducing the septic state, and (c) specific inactivation of the proposed mediator should lead to measurable decreases in morbidity and mortality. Both exogenous and endogenous mediators fulfill these criteria.

Exogenous Mediators

During Gram-negative infection, the principal microbial toxin implicated in the sepsis syndrome with septic shock and MSOF is endotoxin. Experimentally, endotoxemia reproduces hemodynamic, inflammatory, and metabolic sequelae observed in septic humans (103). During severe Gram-negative infections, endotoxin is intermittently detectable, but bactericidal antimicrobial therapy does not consistently increase levels (13). The strongest indications of its central role in Gram-negative sepsis are results of clinical trials in which immunotherapy with polyclonal immune serum or HA-1A or E5 monoclonal IgM antibodies raised against the lipid A structures of the J5 mutant of *E. coli* blunt toxicity and increase survival (3, 41, 148, 149). Whether endotoxemia of enteric origin as an "endogenous" mediator (36), alone or combined with bacterial translocation across an intact gastrointestinal mucosal barrier (27, 28), plays a codominant role with endotoxin from localized sources such as pneumonia is unclear. Multiple

factors promote bacterial translocation: (a) systemic trauma, (b) thermal injury, (c) hemorrhagic shock, (d) deficient T-cell immunity, (e) endotoxemia itself, (f) intraabdominal abscess, (g) endotoxemia during malnutrition, and (h) intestinal obstruction (26, 27). Common factors are luminal bacterial overgrowth and increased gut microvascular permeability. Endotoxemia and endotoxin-induced mediators do not account for all observed changes in the septic shock syndrome. Lethal sepsis frequently complicates non-Gram-negative infections (50, 76, 87, 143, 146) and occurs in endotoxin-hyporesponder C3/HeJ mice with decreased capacity for TNF-α production (117). Gram-negative bacterial exotoxins, Gram-positive exotoxins, staphylococcal enterotoxins, pyrogenic staphylococcal and streptococcal exotoxins, and fungal enzymes may be other factors triggering the septic response.

Endogenous Mediators

The exact mechanisms by which microbial toxins provoke an inflammatory response are incompletely defined. Intermediary steps include receptor and nonreceptor-mediated interactions between toxins and the cell membrane, subreceptor signal transduction involving G proteins, and activation of relevant promotor sequences for genetic transcription of lipid and peptide mediators (32, 33, 48, 61). Activation of phagocytic cells including monocytes and resident macrophages leads to synthesis of an array of mediators. These can be categorized as acting "proximally" and "distally" with respect to shock and inflammation, although given their connotation of a one-way cascade, "early" and "late" are more accurate descriptions in view of the network model. Major endogenous mediators inducing immunophysiologic changes in septic states include cytokines, eicosanoids, platelet-activating factor (PAF), endorphins, and products of the complement, coagulation, fibrinolytic, and kinin pathways.

The autocrine, paracrine, and endocrine functions of cytokines are under several mechanisms of host regulation: (a) post-transcriptional control of the $t_{1/2}$ of messenger (m) RNA (The mRNA of TNF-α, IL-1, and other cytokines share a common nucleotide sequence in the 3'-untranslated region composed of a thymidine- and adenosine-rich sequence (the TTATTTAT element), which with flanking elements regulates message degradation and translation (17, 53).); *(b)* membrane shedding of receptors into the circulation in soluble form that, by ligand binding, prevents cytokine binding to cellular receptors (46); *(c)* naturally occurring substances that inhibit cytokine action either by competitive receptor antagonism as described for IL-1 (32) or nonreceptor-mediated binding as shown for α_2-macroglobulin (67); and *(d)* feedback inhibition of TNF-α gene expression by IL-6, PGE_2, and transforming growth factor-β (TGF-β) (33, 61, 128).

TNF-α is a 157-residue polypeptide produced by mononuclear and granulocytic leukocytes that is pivotal early during bacterial sepsis due to its microbiologic, immunologic, hemodynamic, biochemical, and metabolic effects (33, 48, 57, 61, 90, 94, 114, 141). After endotoxin stimulation, levels characteristically increase and peak within 1–2 hr, followed by a rapid return to baseline within 3–4 hr irrespective of subsequent shock. Infusions of recombinant TNF-α reproduce pathophysiologic changes seen in septic shock (138). Moreover, passive immunization is protective during otherwise lethal Gram-negative endotoxemia and bacteremia (6, 59, 139). In septic patients, divergent results have been reported with respect to serum TNF-α levels. Increased levels have been associated with increased mortality (16, 114) whereas in other reports, transition from sepsis syndrome to septic shock was not accompanied by secondary elevations (92). For example, plasma TNF-α concentrations in normal volunteers with experimental endotoxemia exhibit higher TNF-α levels (> 500 pg/ml) than in patients with shock (100–150 pg/ml) (16, 80, 92). These findings may reflect either downregulation of production or increased intravascular binding by soluble TNF-α receptors, which circulate at high concentrations even in normal individuals (1–4 ng/ml), or binding by plasma proteins (46, 67). Since endotoxic shock does not evolve until several hours after endotoxemia, TNF-α most likely induces the biosynthesis of coprimary mediators such as IL-1 and secondary mediators such as the eicosanoids and PAF (39, 80, 83).

The interleukins are a group of at least 11 polypeptides synthesized by monocytes/macrophages, endothelial cells, fibroblasts, and B and T cells (21, 32, 33, 81, 128). IL-1, IL-6, and IL-8 are of central importance during sepsis. IL-1 exists in two forms (IL-1_α and IL-1_β), which bind to the same receptor (32). After endotoxemia or Gram-positive bacteremia, circulating IL-1_β increases over 3 hr and, like *TNF-α*, remains elevated in nonsurvivors (16). Recent discovery of a naturally occurring receptor antagonist for IL-1 has shown that IL-1 receptor blockade is protective during otherwise lethal endotoxemia, independent of circulating levels of TNF-α (32). IL-6, a group of peptides synthesized by similar cells as for IL-1, is elevated in the blood of patients after trauma and during sepsis syndrome or septic shock (49, 52). It is unclear under which circumstances IL-6 is an "alarm" hormone signalling cell damage, a proinflammatory mediator, or an antiinflammatory substance (33). As in the case of TNF-α and IL-1, antibodies to IL-6 are protective during endotoxemia and recombinant TNF-α infusions (128). IL-8 is a neutrophil chemotactic factor that is elaborated by endothelial cells after induction by endotoxin, TNF-α, and IL-1, which regulates polymorphonuclear leukocyte influx into tissues following infection or injury (72, 81).

Phospholipase A_2 is the rate-limiting enzyme in the generation of arachidonic acid from membrane phospholipids after infection, ischemia, or trauma (127, 140). Subsequent metabolism of arachidonic acid via cyclooxygenase or lipooxygenase pathways yields several classes of vasoactive and immunoregulatory eicosanoids (105, 126). The cyclooxygenase products prostacyclin (PGI_2) and related prostaglandins have opposing hemodynamic and hematologic effects from thromboxane A_2 (105). PGI_2 and PGE_3 are vasodilators, whereas thromboxane A_2 and PGF-2a have vasoconstrictor properties, and while PGI_2 inhibits platelet aggregation, thromboxane

A_2 is proaggregatory. Lipooxygenase products include two classes of leukotrienes, leukotriene B_4 (LTB_4) and the sulfidopeptides LTC_4, LTD_4, and LTE_4 (126). LTB_4 is a potent chemotaxin for polymorphonuclear leukocytes and is present in the bronchoalveolar lavage fluid of patients with ARDS and at high risk for ARDS (129). LTC_4-LTE_4 are vasoconstrictors/bronchoconstrictors, which also increase microvascular permeability (126). Eicosanoids of both classes are involved in sepsis based on the following: *(a)* increased concentrations are found in blood and bronchoalveolar lavage fluid or lung lymph during sepsis; *(b)* shock and plasma extravasation follow their administration; and *(c)* receptor antagonists and inhibitors attenuate endotoxic shock (75, 126). PAF is a phospholipid that is rapidly synthesized following activation of phospholipase A_2 after trauma or stimulation by endotoxin or TNF-α (66, 68). All of the criteria for validation of a shock mediator have been fulfilled for PAF. Concentrations are elevated during shock. Synthetic PAF has a variety of actions that mimic those observed during sepsis, including cardiodepression, hypotension, altered microvascular permeability, bronchoconstriction, and platelet aggregation (68). Moreover, PAF receptor antagonists attenuate the severity of shock. Leukotrienes mediate several of the cellular actions of PAF, including induction of GI mucosal necrosis subsequent to endotoxemia (66).

The action of TNF-α, interleukins, eicosanoids, and PAF in the intravascular compartment may be complemented by cell-bound forms critical in local cell-cell communication (32, 63, 66). Once generated during infection, they may perpetuate tissue injury via the network of cytokine-eicosanoid interactions in conjunction with products of activated polymorphonuclear leukocytes and mononuclear cells. Dysregulation of these interactions can result in the malignant vascular inflammation that characterizes MSOF.

MANAGEMENT

Appropriate antimicrobial therapy to prevent progressive infection and metastatic abscesses and, where indicated, operative débridement and drainage are crucial to the resolution of sepsis. These measures address the microbiologic component of sepsis. Modulation of the inflammatory response comprising the sepsis syndrome, septic shock, and MSOF requires support of vital organ function, which the ICU environment provides (113).

Cardiovascular support requires restoration of the intravascular volume by fluid resuscitation to maintain ventricular preload. Limitations of clinical estimations of central hemodynamics during sepsis indicate that patients with hypotension refractory to initial volume infusions benefit from invasive hemodynamic monitoring (19). Refractory hypotension, especially when combined with respiratory failure or renal dysfunction, necessitates pulmonary artery catheterization to optimize LV filling pressure along with assessment of O_2 kinetics. Because of abnormal ventricular compliance during shock (103), conservative endpoints for initial fluid resuscitation are useful (e.g., pulmonary capillary wedge pressure = 12–15 mm Hg). If refractory hypotension persists despite pulmonary artery catheter-guided volume loading, dopamine infusions (5–10 μg/kg/min) can increase the pressure gradient for venous return by increasing the upstream mean systemic pressure.

Shock refractory to volume loading and dopamine in high doses (>15–20 μg/kg/min) are indications for norepinephrine, since dopamine's action is partly mediated by enzymatic conversion to norepinephrine and the efficiency of this conversion may be compromised (24). Initial doses are 0.05–0.1 μg/kg/min with rapid titration to maintain a mean arterial blood pressure of $\geq$65 mm Hg, in conjunction with other signs of improved perfusion such as better mentation, a urinary output of >30 ml/kg/hr, and resolution of ongoing lactic acidosis. Once achieved, infusion rates are reduced (1–2 μg/kg/min) to prevent excessive renal and splanchnic vasoconstriction (24, 122).

During this phase of resuscitation, repeated fluid boluses are usually required to maintain blood pressure, which enables construction of a modified ventricular function curve using the pulmonary capillary wedge pressure to estimate preload versus LV stroke volume index or stroke work index. The ideal resuscitation fluid remains controversial. Crystalloid alone, combinations of crystalloid and colloid solutions, and colloids alone have all been used (25, 109). Selection depends in part on the goals of resuscitation. Resuscitation of the intravascular space with crystalloid has several advantages: availability, lower blood viscosity, lack of infectious risk, and low cost. These may be dose dependently offset by rapid egress of crystalloid from the circulation in the setting of increased vascular permeability, necessitating a large volume resuscitation with resultant tissue edema. Colloid solutions have improved survival during experimental sepsis (109), but definitive answers await clinical trials. Since clearcut advantages of colloid resuscitation have not been demonstrated, initial fluid therapy is with isotonic crystalloid solutions. Albumin-containing solutions are generally reserved for hypoalbuminemic patients or those requiring fluids in excess of 50% total body water.

Other catecholamines employed include dobutamine and epinephrine. Dobutamine exerts strong inotropic effects with dose-dependent β_2 stimulation resulting in vasodilation at doses of >10 mg/kg/min. A dose of 5 μg/kg/min was prospectively studied during septic shock in patients initially stabilized with fluids, followed by addition of dopamine or norepinephrine for refractory hypotension (142). Adjuvant treatment with dobutamine was well tolerated but lactate levels were not obtained and outcome was not significantly altered. The hemodynamic effects of epinephrine at a dose range of 0.5–1.0 μg/kg/min during septic shock refractory to fluid loading and administration of dopamine at >15 μg/kg/min may yield short-term improvement in mean arterial pressure and LV stroke work index (8). However, it has not been demonstrated to alter overall outcome. Thus, dopamine is indicated when decreased vasomotor tone is the principal abnormality, norepinephrine when refractoriness to it is established, dobutamine with underlying systolic heart failure, and epinephrine when

patients become refractory to combinations of dopamine and norepinephrine. In patients developing supraventricular tachyarrythmias with these catecholamines, phenylephrine may be substituted to support arterial pressure (12).

The exact role of therapeutic manipulations to increase DO_2 and VO_2 has not been fully defined. During lactic acidosis, a critical DO_2 threshold level has been reached and DO_2 should accordingly be increased. An ability to match VO_2 deficits by increasing DO_2 may compensate for increased metabolic demands, improving survival (44). Although red cell transfusions will increase DO_2, they do not reproducibly increase VO_2. However, septic patients with O_2 extraction ratios of <24% and hemoglobin levels of <10 g/dl demonstrate increases in VO_2 after transfusion and may benefit more than patients with normal O_2 extraction (20).

Investigational interventions have been aimed at reducing and/or blocking the inflammatory response by removal of inflammatory stimuli, immunologic modulation, and antagonism of early and late endogenous mediators. Empiric laparotomy is based on the hypothesis that septic patients with occult etiologies for MSOF prove to have an intraabdominal source of infection (38, 106). This hypothesis has received little support in patients with medical illnesses (82). Present practice includes localization of an intraabdominal abscess by computed tomography and/or ultrasound, with radionuclide labeled white blood cell scanning in equivocal cases.

Plasmapheresis has been advocated in the management of patients with sepsis to facilitate removal of activated complement, clotting factors, lysosomal enzymes, cytokines, and arachidonic acid metabolites. However, preliminary data in an experimental canine model demonstrate increased mortality and worsened hemodynamics in pheresis-treated animals (86). Given the lack of definitive data, plasmapheresis is not presently recommended as adjunctive therapy. Conceivably, agents that absorb endotoxin such as polymyxin B during plasmapheresis with subsequent reinfusion of plasma may prove to be beneficial, as improved survival was obtained by this technique in a murine model of sepsis (15). This suggests that selective removal of only those mediators that initiate the septic response might be warranted.

Suppression of the immune response has been attempted by corticosteroid administration. Pretreatment of cells prevents production of TNF-α after endotoxin stimulation and prevents activation of phospholipase A_2 (48). However, two multicenter prospective trials found no indication for high-dose corticosteroid treatment of patients with sepsis syndrome and septic shock (10, 58). Such therapy furthermore does not influence the development of ARDS or its severity (70). Thus, the use of corticosteroids is not indicated except for documented adrenal insufficiency.

Antagonism of exogenous and endogenous shock mediators has been studied using passive immunization with polyclonal or monoclonal antibodies directed against the mediator or its receptor. Ziegler et al. showed reductions in mortality from 56 to 33% in patients with Gram-negative bacteremia and septic shock after treatment with a single intravenous infusion of HA-1A, a human monoclonal IgM antibody binding to the lipid A domain of endotoxin (148). There was no benefit in septic patients without Gram-negative bacteremia. Greenman et al. demonstrated comparable reductions in mortality only in patients with Gram-negative sepsis who were not in shock after two infusions of E5, a murine monoclonal IgM antibody (41). There was also improved resolution of organ failures. Whether multiple doses of either agent might offer greater benefit and whether earlier identification of endotoxemia by the *Limulus* amebocyte assay might assist in selecting patients likely to benefit await further study. Digestive tract decontamination to prevent absorption of gut-derived endotoxin and bacteria has shown promising results (110), but further trials are needed to define its exact role in the management of patients with sepsis or at enhanced risk for sepsis. Inhibition of IL-1 binding by an IL-1 receptor antagonist and an anti-IL-1 receptor monoclonal antibody modulate acute inflammation including IL-6 levels in vivo in a murine model (32). IL-1 receptor antagonism also dose dependently improves survival in murine models of endotoxemia. Multicenter clinical trials are now in progress to establish the effects of IL-1 and TNF-α antagonism.

Several animal studies have shown an ability of methylxanthine derivatives to attenuate inflammation during Gram-negative sepsis. Pentoxifylline, used clinically to treat peripheral vascular disease, has several pharmacologic effects of potential benefit: *(a)* elevation of intracellular 3'5'-c-AMP levels via phosphodiesterase inhibition; *(b)* attenuation of polymorphonuclear leukocyte and monocyte activation; *(c)* reduction of O_2 free radicals and lysosomal enzyme release from activated polymorphonuclear leukocytes; *(d)* dose-dependent inhibition of polymorphonuclear leukocyte activation and migration through the endothelium; and *(e)* inhibition of TNF-α mRNA synthesis (54, 119, 133). Aminophylline and pentoxifylline decrease extravasation of albumin during *E. coli* sepsis in a guinea pig model (54). Since hemodynamic measurements were unchanged, albumin leakage was considered secondary to capillary endothelial damage. Aminophylline but not pentoxifylline was associated with significant hypotension due to reductions in the systemic vascular resistance. Pentoxifylline has also improved survival during murine endotoxic shock when given within 4 hr after endotoxin administration (119).

Naloxone, an opiate antagonist, reverses experimental endotoxin-induced shock, but survival results are variable. High doses have been associated with adverse side effects including pulmonary edema and grand mal seizures. In a randomized, controlled study of naloxone in septic shock, patients were given naloxone as a 30 μg/kg loading dose followed by infusion of 60 μg/kg over 1 hr (115). There was no overall difference in survival compared with placebo. However, patients receiving naloxone within 7 hr of shock onset had improved hemodynamics and 100% survival, while those receiving it >10 hr after shock failed to respond and ultimately died. Definitive recommendations await further investigation. Clearly, such mechanism-oriented treatments of sepsis as defined above must dovetail with comprehensive, titrated care of the critically ill based on defined immunophysiologic principles.

SUMMARY

The acute inflammatory response is normally regulated at multiple hierarchic levels: genetic, cellular, organ-specific, and systemically within the intravascular space. Demarcating when this response is beneficial by upregulating defense mechanisms and when it is destructive by escape from host regulatory control is complex, a function of a dynamically changing balance among hemodynamic, humoral, and cellular elements. Failure of local defenses to contain invading organisms and their exogenous mediators is important in progression to the sepsis syndrome and to shock and MSOF. However, multiple branch points exist wherein this progression may be successfully blunted to bring the system back into an equilibrium state. Criteria for the sepsis syndrome enable early identification of the septic patient and should prompt aggressive clinical interventions. These include identification and removal of the septic stimulus, correction of metabolic derangements, support of dysfunctional organ systems leading to maintenance of overall tissue perfusion, and prevention of MSOF.

Acknowledgment. This work was supported in part by National Institutes of Health Grant RO1-43513 from the National Institute of General Medical Sciences.

References

1. Abel FI. Myocardial function in sepsis and endotoxic shock. Am J Physiol 1989;257:R1265–R1281.
2. Avila A, Warshawski F, Sibbald WJ, et al. Peripheral lymph flow in sheep with bacterial peritonitis: evidence for increased microvascular permeability accompanying sepsis. Surgery 1985;97:685–695.
3. Baumgartner JD, McCutchan DA, van Melle G, et al. Prevention of Gram-negative shock and death in surgical patients by antibody to endotoxin core glycolipid. Lancet 1985;2:59–63.
4. Bell RC, Coalson JJ, Smith JD, et al. Multiple organ system failure and infection in adult respiratory distress syndrome. Ann Intern Med 1983;99:293–298.
5. Bersten A, Sibbald WJ. Circulatory disturbances in multiple systems organ failure. Crit Care Clin 1989;5:233–254.
6. Beutler B, Milsark IW, Cerami AC. Passive immunization against cachectin/tumor necrosis factor protects mice from lethal effect of endotoxin. Science 1985;229:869–871.
7. Bevilacqua MP, Pober JS, Majeau GR, et al. Recombinant tumor necrosis factor induces procoagulant activity in cultured human vascular endothelium: characterization and comparison with the actions of interleukin 1. Proc Natl Acad Sci USA 1986;83:4533–4537.
8. Bollaert PE, Bauer P, Audibert G, et al. Effects of epinephrine on hemodynamics and oxygen metabolism in dopamine-dependent septic shock. Chest 1990;98:949–953.
9. Bone RC. Let's agree on terminology: definitions of sepsis. Crit Care Med 1991;19:973–976.
10. Bone RC, Fisher CJ, Clemmer TP, et al. A controlled trial of high-dose methylprednisolone in the treatment of severe sepsis and septic shock. N Engl J Med 1987;317:653–658.
11. Bone RC, Fisher CJ, Clemmer TP, et al. Sepsis syndrome: a valid clinical entity. Crit Care Med 1989;17:389–393.
12. Bonfiglio MF, Dasta JF, Gregory JS, et al. High-dose phenylephrine infusion in the hemodynamic support of septic shock. Drug Intell Clin Pharm 1990;24:936–939.
13. Brandtzaeg P, Kierulf P, Gustad P, et al. Plasma endotoxin as a predictor of multiple organ failure and death in systemic meningococcal disease. J Infect Dis 1989;159:195–203.
14. Bronsveld W, van Lambalgen AA, van den Bos GC, et al. Effects of glucose-insulin-potassium (GIK) on myocardial blood flow and metabolism in canine endotoxic shock. Circ Shock 1984;13:315–324.
15. Bysani GK, Shenep JL, Hildner WK, et al. Detoxification of plasma containing lipopolysaccharide by adsorption. Crit Care Med 1990;18:67–71.
16. Calandra T, Baumgartner JD, Grau GE, et al. Prognostic values of tumor necrosis factor/cachectin, interleukin-1, interferon-α, and interferon-gamma in the serum of patients with septic shock. J Infect Dis 1990;161:982–987.
17. Caput D, Beutler B, Hartog S, et al. Identification of a common nucleotide sequence in the 3'-untranslated region of mRNA molecules specifying inflammatory mediators. Proc Natl Acad Sci USA 1986;83:1670–1678.
18. Carroll GC, Snyder JV. Hyperdynamic severe intravascular sepsis depends on fluid administration in cynomolgus monkey. Am J Physiol 1982;243:R131–R141.
19. Connors AF Jr, McCaffree DR, Gray BA. Evaluation of right heart catheterization in the critically ill patient without acute myocardial infarction. N Engl J Med 1983;308:263–267.
20. Conrad SA, Rietrich KA, Herbert CA, et al. Effect of red cell transfusion on oxygen consumption

following fluid resuscitation in septic shock. Circ Shock 1990;31:419–429.

21. Creasey AA, Stevens P, Kenny J, et al. Endotoxin and cytokine profile in plasma of baboons challenges with lethal and sublethal *Escherichia coli*. Circ Shock 1991;33:84–91.

22. Cunnion RE, Schaer GL, Parker MM, et al. The coronary circulation in human septic shock. Circulation 1986;73:637–644.

23. Daniel TO, Ives HE. Endothelial control of vascular function. News Physiol Sci 1989;4:139–142.

24. Dasta JF. Norepinephrine in septic shock: renewed interest in an old drug. Drug Intell Clin Pharm 1990;24:153–156.

25. Davidson I, Ottoson J, Reisch J. Infusion volumes of Ringer's lactate and 3% albumin as they relate to survival after resuscitation from a lethal intestinal ischemic shock. Circ Shock 1986;18:277–287.

26. Deitch EA. Gut failure: its role in the multiple organ failure syndome. In: Deitch EA, ed. Multiple organ failure. New York: Thieme, 1990:40–59.

27. Deitch EA, Berg R. Endotoxin but not malnutrition promotes bacterial translocation from the gut in burned mice. J Trauma 1987;27:161–170.

28. Deitch EA, Berg R, Specian R. Endotoxin promotes the translocation of bacteria from the gut. Arch Surg 1987;122:185–192.

29. Deitch EA, Specian RD, Berg RD. Endotoxin-induced bacterial translocation and mucosal permeability: role of xanthine oxidase, complement activation, and macrophage products. Crit Care Med 1991;19:785–791.

30. Demling RH. The role of mediators in human ARDS. J Crit Care 1988;3:56–72.

31. Dhainaut JF, Lanore JJ, de Gournay JM, et al. Right ventricular dysfunction in patients with septic shock. Intensive Care Med 1988;14:488–491.

32. Dinarello CA. Interleukin-1 and interleukin-1 antagonism. Blood 1991;77:1627–1652.

33. Dinarello CA. The proinflammatory cytokines interleukin-1 and tumor necrosis factor and treatment of the septic shock syndrome. J Infect Dis 1991;163:1177–1184.

34. Dobrina A, Schwartz BR, Carlos TM, et al. CD11/CD18-independent neutrophil adherence to inducible endothelial-leukocyte adhesion molecules (E-LAM) in vitro. Immunol 1989;67:502–508.

35. Echtenacher B, Falk W, Manmel DN, et al. Requirement of endogenous tumor necrosis factor/cachectin for recovery from experimental peritonitis. J Immunol 1990;145:3762–3766.

36. Gathiram P, Wells MT, Brocke-Utne JG, et al. Oral administered nonabsorbable antibiotics prevent endotoxemia in primates following intestinal ischemia. J Surg Res 1988;45:187–195.

37. Geissler D, Gaggl S, Most J, et al. A monoclonal antibody directed against the human intercellular adhesion molecule (ICAM-1) modulates the release of tumor necrosis factor, interferon-gamma, and interleukin-1. Eur J Immunol 1990;20:2591–2596.

38. Goris RJA, te Boekhorst TPA, Nuytinck JKS, et al. Multiple-organ failure: generalized autodes-tructive inflammation? Arch Surg 1985;120:1109–1115.

39. Goto F, Wanatabe E, Maruyama N, et al. Prevention of the toxic action of tumor necrosis factor by cyclooxygenase inhibition and neutropenia. Circ Shock 1989;29:175–180.

40. Green JF. Circulatory mechanics. In: Green JF. Fundamental cardiovascular and pulmonary physiology. 2nd ed. Philadelphia: Lea & Febiger, 1987:59–95.

41. Greenman RL, Schein RMH, Martin MA, et al. A controlled clinical trial of E5 murine monoclonal IgM antibody to endotoxin in the treatment of Gram-negative sepsis. JAMA 1991;266:1097–1102.

42. Guntheroth WC, Kowabori I. The contribution of splanchnic pooling to endotoxic shock in the dog. Circ Res 1977;41:467–472.

43. Guntheroth WG, Jacky JP, Kawabori I, et al. Left ventricular performance in endotoxin shock in dogs. Am J Physiol 1982;242:H172–H176.

44. Gutierrez G, Pohil RJ. Oxygen consumption is linearly related to O_2 supply in critically ill patients. J Crit Care 1986;1:45–53.

45. Guyton AC, Jones CE, Coleman TC. Circulatory physiology: cardiac output and its regulation. Philadelphia: WB Saunders, 1973:237–262.

46. Fernandez-Botran R. Soluble cytokine receptors: their role in immunoregulation. FASEB J 1991;5:2567–2574.

47. Fletcher JE. Mathematical modelling of the microcirculation. Math Biosci 1978;38:159–202.

48. Fong Y, Lowry SF. Tumor necrosis factor in the pathophysiology of infection and sepsis. Clin Immunol Immunopathol 1990;55:157–170.

49. Fong Y, Moldawer LL, Marano M, et al. Endotoxemia elicits increased circulating beta 2-IFN/IL-6 in man. J Immunol 1989;142:2321–2324.

50. Freudenberg MA, Galanos C. Tumor necrosis factor alpha mediates lethal activity of killed Gram-negative and Gram-positive bacteria in D-galactosamine-treated mice. Infect Immun 1991;59:2110–2115.

51. Fry DE, Pearlstein L, Fulton RL, et al. Multiple organ failure: the role of uncontrolled infection. Arch Surg 1980;115:136–142.

52. Hack CE, de Groot ER, Felt-Bersma RJF, et al. Increased plasma levels of interleukin-6 in sepsis. Blood 1989;74:1704–1709.

53. Han J, Brown T, Beutler B. Endotoxin-responsive sequences control cachectin/tumor necrosis factor biosynthesis at the translational level. J Exp Med 1990;171:465–475.

54. Harada H, Ishizaka A, Yonemura H, et al. The effects of aminophylline and pentoxifylline on multiple organ damage after *Escherichia coli* sepsis. Am Rev Respir Dis 1989;140:974–980.

55. Harris RL, Musher DM, Bloom K, et al. Manifestations of sepsis. Arch Intern Med 1987;147:1895–1906.

56. Hess ML, Krause SM, Komwatana P. Myocardial failure and excitation-contraction coupling in canine endotoxin shock: role of histamine and sarcoplasmic reticulum. Circ Shock 1980;7:277–287.

57. Hesse DG, Tracey KJ, Fong Y, et al. Cytokine appearance in human endotoxemia and primate

bacteremia. Surg Gynecol Obstet 1988;166:147–153.

58. Hinshaw L, Reduzzi P, Young E, et al. Effect of high-dose glucocorticoid therapy on mortality in patients with clinical signs of systemic sepsis. N Engl J Med 1987;317:659–665.

59. Hinshaw L, Tekamp-Olson P, Chang ACK, et al. Survival of primates in LD$_{100}$ septic shock following therapy with antibody to tumor necrosis factor (TNFa). Circ Shock 1990;30:279–292.

60. Hollenberg SM, Cunnion RE, Lawrence M, et al. Tumor necrosis factor depresses myocardial cell function: results using an *in vitro* assay of myocyte performance [Abstract]. Clin Res 1989;37:528A.

61. Jaattela M. Biological activities and mechanisms of action of tumor necrosis factor-α/cachectin. Lab Invest 1991;64:724–742.

62. Kaufman BS, Rackow EC, Falk JL. The relationship between oxygen delivery and consumption during fluid resuscitation of hypovolemic and septic shock. Chest 1984;85:336–340.

63. Keogh C, Fong Y, Marisma MA, et al. Identification of a novel tumor necrosis factor-α/cachectin from the livers of burned and infected rats. Arch Surg 1990;125:79–85.

64. Knaus W, Draper E, Wagner D, et al. Prognosis in acute organ-system failure. Ann Surg 1985;202:685–693.

65. Knaus WA, Wagner DP. Multiple systems organ failure: epidemiology and prognosis. Crit Care Clin 1989;5:221–232.

66. Kriegler M, Perez C, DeFay K, et al. A novel form of TNF/cachectin is a cell surface cytostatic transmembrane protein: ramifications for the complex physiology of TNF. Cell 1988;53:45–53.

67. Lamarre J, Wollenberg GK, Gonias SL, et al. Cytokine binding and clearance properties of proteinase-activated α_2-macroglobulin. Lab Invest 1991;65:3–14.

68. Lefer AM. Induction of tissue injury and altered cardiovascular performance by platelet-activating factor: relevance to multiple systems organ failure. Crit Care Clin 1989;5:331–352.

69. Lehmann V, Freudenberg MA, Galanos C. Lethal toxicity of lipopolysaccharide and tumor necrosis factor in normal and D-galactosamine-treated mice. J Exp Med 1987;165:657–662.

70. Luce JM, Montgomery AB, Marks JD, et al. Ineffectiveness of high-dose methylprednisolone in preventing parenchymal lung injury and improving mortality in patients with septic shock. Am Rev Respir Dis 1988;138:62–70.

71. Marshall J, Sweeney D. Microbial infection and the septic response in critical surgical illness: sepsis, not infection determines outcome. Arch Surg 1990;125:17–23.

72. Martich GD, Danner RL, Ceska M, et al. Detection of interleukin 8 and tumor necrosis factor in normal humans after intravenous endotoxin: the effect of antiinflammatory agents. J Exp Med 1991;173:1021–1024.

73. Matuschak GM, Rinaldo JE. Organ interactions in the adult respiratory distress syndrome: role of the liver in host defense. Chest 1988;94:400–408.

74. Matuschak GM, Rinaldo JE, Pinsky MR, et al. Effect of end-stage liver failure on the incidence and resolution of the adult respiratory distress syndrome. J Crit Care 1987;2:162–173.

75. Matuschak GM, Pinsky MR, Klein EC, et al. Effects of D-galactosamine-induced acute liver injury on mortality and pulmonary responses to *E. Coli* lipopolysaccharide: modulation by arachidonic acid metabolites. Am Rev Respir Dis 1990;141:1296–1306.

76. Matuschak GM, Tredway TL, Klein CA, et al. Transduction of fungal septic shock is independent of tumor necrosis factor-alpha: cardiopulmonary changes in conscious rats and differential taxonomic response from *E. Coli* [Abstract]. Am Rev Respir Dis 1990;143:A804.

77. McCabe WR, Jackson GG. Gram-negative bacteremia, I: etiology and ecology. Arch Intern Med 1962;110:847–855.

78. McCord JM. Oxygen-derived free radicals in postischemic tissue injury. N Engl J Med 1985;312:159–163.

79. McDonough KH, Lang CH, Spitzer JJ. Effect of cardiotropic agents on the myocardial dysfunction of hyperdynamic sepsis. Circ Shock 1985;17:1–19.

80. Michie HR, Manogie KR, Spriggs M. Detection of circulating tumor necrosis factor after endotoxin administration. N Engl J Med 1988;318:1481–1487.

81. Moldawer LL. IL-8 in septic shock, endotoxemia, and after IL-1 administration. J Immunol 1991;146:3478–3482.

82. Montgomery AB, Stager MH, Carrico CJ et al. Causes of mortality in adult respiratory distress syndrome. Am Rev Respir Dis 1985;132:485–489.

83. Mozes T, Zijlatra FJ, Heiligers PC, et al. Sequential release of eicosanoids during endotoxin-mediated shock in anesthetized pigs. Prostaglandins Leukot Essent Fatty Acids 1991;42:209–215.

84. Natanson C, Fink MP, Ballantyne HK, et al. Gram-negative bacteremia produces both severe systolic and diastolic cardiac dysfunction in a canine model that simulates human septic shock. J Clin Invest 1986;78:259–270.

85. Natanson C, Danner RL, Fink MP, et al. Cardiovascular performance with *E. Coli* challenges in a canine model of human sepsis. Am J Physiol 1988;254:H558–H569.

86. Natanson C, Hoffman WD, Danner RL, et al. A controlled trial of plasmapheresis fails to improve outcome in an antibiotic treated canine model of human septic shock. Clin Res 1989;37:346A.

87. Natanson C, Danner RL, Elin RJ, et al. Role of endotoxemia in cardiovascular dysfunction and mortality: *E. coli* and *S. aureus* challenges in a canine model of human septic shock. J Clin Invest 1989;83:243–251.

88. Natanson C, Eichenholz PW, Danner RL, et al. Endotoxin and tumor necrosis factor challenges in dogs simulate the cardiovascular profile of human septic shock. J Exp Med 1989;169:823–832.

89. National Heart, Lung, and Blood Institute, Division of Lung Diseases. Extracorporeal support

for respiratory insufficiency: a collaborative study. Bethesda MD:NIH, 1979.

90. Nawroth PP, Stern DM. Modulation of endothelial cell hemostatic properties by tumor necrosis factor. J Exp Med 1986;163:740–745.

91. Nelson DP, Samsel RW, Wood LDH. Pathological supply dependence of systemic and intestinal O_2 uptake during endotoxemia. J Appl Physiol 1988;64:2410–2418.

92. Offner F, Phillipe J, Vogelaers D, et al. Serum tumor necrosis factor levels in patients with infectious disease and septic shock. J Lab Clin Med 1990;116:100–105.

93. Ognibene FP, Parker MM, Natanson C, et al. Depressed left ventricular performance: response to volume infusion in patients with sepsis and septic shock. Chest 1988;93:903–910.

94. Okusawa S, Gelfand JA, Ikejima T, et al. Interleukin 1 induces a shock-like state in rabbits: synergism with tumor necrosis factor and the effect of cyclooxygenase inhibition. J Clin Invest 1988;81:1162–1169.

95. Onji T, Liu MS. Shock-induced changes in the sodium-potassium adenosine triphosphate enzyme system in dog hearts. J Surg Res 1981;31:232–239.

96. Papadakis EJ, Abel FL. Left ventricular performance in canine endotoxic shock. Circ Shock 1988;24:123–131.

97. Parker JL, Adams HR. Myocardial effects of endotoxin shock: characterization of an isolated heart muscle model. Adv Shock Res 1979;2:163–175.

98. Parker MM, Shelhammer JH, Bacarach SL, et al. Profound but reversible myocardial depression in patients with septic shock. Ann Intern Med 1984;100:483–490.

99. Parker MM, Shelhammer JH, Natanson C, et al. Serial cardiovascular variables in survivors and nonsurvivors of human septic shock: heart rate as an early predictor of prognosis. Crit Care Med 1987;15:923–929.

100. Parker MM, Suffredini AF, Natanson C, et al. Responses of left ventricular function in survivors and nonsurvivors of septic shock. J Crit Care 1989;4:19–25.

101. Parker MM, McCarthy KE, Ognibene FP, et al. Right ventricular dysfunction and dilatation, similar to left ventricular changes, characterize the cardiac depression of septic shock in humans. Chest 1990;97:126–132.

102. Parrillo JE, Burch C, Shelhammer JH, et al. A circulating myocardial depressant substance in humans with septic shock. J Clin Invest 1985;76:1539–1553.

103. Parrillo JE, Parker MM, Natanson C, et al. Septic shock in humans: advances in the understanding of pathogenesis, cardiovascular dysfunction, and therapy. Ann Intern Med 1990;113:227–242.

104. Permutt S, Riley RL. Hemodynamics of collapsible vessels with tone: the vascular waterfall. J Appl Physiol 1963;18:924–929.

105. Petrak RA, Balk RA, Bone RC. Prostaglandins, cyclo-oxygenase inhibitors, and thromboxane synthetase inhibition in the pathogenesis of multiple systems organ failure. Crit Care Clin 1989;5:303–314.

106. Pine RW, Wertz ML, Lennard ES, et al. Determinants of organ malfunction or death in patients with intra-abdominal sepsis. Arch Surg 1983;118:242–249.

107. Pinsky MR, Matuschak GM. Cardiovascular determinants of the hemodynamic response to acute endotoxemia in the dog. J Crit Care 1986;1:18–31.

108. Pinsky MR, Matuschak GM. Multiple systems organ failure: failure of host defense homeostasis. Crit Care Clin 1989;5:199–220.

109. Rackow EC, Falk JL, Fein IA, et al. Fluid resuscitation in circulatory shock: a comparison of the cardiorespiratory effects of albumin, hetastarch, and saline solutions in patients with hypovolemic and septic shock. Crit Care Med 1983;11:839–850.

110. Reidy JJ, Ramsay G. Clinical trials of selective decontamination of the digestive tract [Review]. Crit Care Med 1990;18:1449–1456.

111. Reilly JM, Cunnion RE, Burch-Whitman C, et al. A circulating myocardial depressant substance is associated with cardiac dysfunction and peripheral hypoperfusion (lactic acidemia) in patients with septic shock. Chest 1989;95:1072–1080.

112. Reuse C, Vincent J-L, Pinsky MR. Measurements of right ventricular volumes during fluid challenge. Chest 1990;98:1450–1454.

113. Reynolds HN, Haupt MT, Thill-Bahorazian H, et al. Impact of critical care physicians staffing on patients with septic shock in a university hospital medical intensive care unit. JAMA 1988;260:3446–3450.

114. Roten R, Markert M, Feihl F, et al. Plasma levels of tumor necrosis factor in the adult respiratory distress syndrome. Am Rev Respir Dis 1991;143:590–592.

115. Safani M, Blair J, Ross D, et al. Prospective, controlled randomized trial of naloxone in early hyperdynamic septic shock. Crit Care Med 1989;17:1004–1009.

116. Sagawa K. The ventricular pressure-volume diagram revisited. Circ Res 1978;43:677–687.

117. Sanchez-Cantu L, Rode HN, Yun YJ, et al. Tumor necrosis factor alone does not explain the lethal effect of lipopolysaccharide. Arch Surg 1991;126:231–235.

118. Sarnoff SJ. Myocardial contractility as described by ventricular function curves: observations on Starling's law of the heart. Physiol Rev 1955;35:107–122.

119. Schade UF. Pentoxifylline increases survival in murine endotoxic shock and decreases production of tumor necrosis factor. Circ Shock 1990;131:171–181.

120. Schumacker PT, Samsel RW. Oxygen delivery and uptake by peripheral tissues: physiology and pathophysiology. Crit Care Clin 1989;5:255–269.

121. Schwarts DB, Bone RC, Balk RA, et al. Hepatic dysfunction in the adult respiratory distress syndrome. Chest 1989;95:871–877.

122. Shaer GL, Fink MP, Parillo JE. Norepinephrine

alone versus norepinephrine plus low-dose dopamine: enhanced renal blood flow with combination pressor therapy. Crit Care Med 1985;13:492–495.

123. Sheppard BC, Norton JA. Tumor necrosis factor and interleukin-1 protect against the lethal effects of tumor necrosis factor. Surgery 1991;109:698–705.

124. Shoemaker WC, Appel PL, Kram HB. Role of oxygen transport patterns on the pathophysiology, prediction of outcome, and therapy of shock. In: Bryan-Brown CW, Ayres SM, eds. New horizons: oxygen transport and utilization. Vol 2. Fullerton, CA: Society of Critical Care Medicine, 1987:65–92.

125. Smedley LA, Tonnesen MG, Sandhaus RA, et al. Neutrophil-mediated injury to endothelial cells: enhancement by endotoxin and essential role of neutrophil elastase. J Clin Invest 1986;77:1233–1243.

126. Sprague RS, Stephenson AH, Dahms TE, et al. Proposed role for leukotrienes in the pathophysiology of multiple systems organ failure. Crit Care Clin 1989;5:315–329.

127. Spriggs DR, Sherman ML, Imamura K, et al. Phospholipase A_2 activation and autoinduction of tumor necrosis factor gene expression by tumor necrosis factor. Cancer Res 1990;50:7101–7107.

128. Starnes HF, Pearce MK, Tewari A, et al. Anti-IL-6 monoclonal antibodies protect against lethal *Escherichia coli* infection and lethal tumor necrosis factor-α challenge in mice. J Immunol 1990;145:4185–4191.

129. Stephenson AH, Lonigro AJ, Hyers TM et al. Increased concentrations of leukotrienes in bronchoalveolar lavage fluid of patients with ARDS or at risk for ARDS. Am Rev Respir Dis 1985;138:714–719.

130. Stetz CW, Miller RG, Kelly GE, et al. Reliability of the thermodilution method in the determination of cardiac output in clinical practice. Am Rev Respir Dis 1982;126:1001–1006.

131. Suffredini AF, Fromm RE, Parker MM, et al. The cardiovascular response of normal humans to the administration of endotoxin. N Engl J Med 1989;321:280–287.

132. Suga H, Sagawa K. Instantaneous pressure volume relationship and their ratio in the excised, supported canine left ventricle. Circ Res 1974;45:117–126.

133. Sullivan GWE, Carper HT, Novick WJ Jr, et al. Inhibition of the inflammatory action of interleukin-1 and tumor necrosis factor (alpha) on neutrophil function by pentoxifylline. Infect Immun 1988;56:1722–1729.

134. Sun X-M, Hseuh W. Bowel necrosis induced by tumor necrosis factor in rats is mediated by platelet-activating factor. J Clin Invest 1988;81:1328–1331.

135. Sylvester JT, Gilbert RD, Traystman RJ, et al.

Effects of hypoxia on the closing pressure of the canine systemic arterial circulation. Circ Res 1981;49:980–987.

136. Taylor FB Jr, Chang A, Esmon CT, et al. Protein C prevents the coagulopathic and lethal effects of *E. coli* infusion in the baboon. J Clin Invest 1987;75:918–925.

137. Taylor FB Jr, Chang A, Ruf W, et al. Lethal *E. coli* septic shock is prevented by blocking tissue factor with monoclonal antibody. Circ Shock 1991;33:127–134.

138. Tracey KJ, Beutler B, Lowry SF, et al. Shock and tissue injury induced by recombinant human cachectin. Science 1986;234:470–474.

139. Tracey KJ, Fong Y, Hesse DG, et al. Anti-cachectin/TNF monoclonal antibodies prevent septic shock during lethal bacteremia. Nature 1987;330:662–664.

140. Vadas P, Pruzanski W, Stefanski E, et al. Pathogenesis of hypotension in septic shock: correlation of circulating phospholipase A_2 levels with circulatory collapse. Crit Care Med 1988;16:1–7.

141. van Deventer SJH, Buller HR, ten Cote JW, et al. Experimental endotoxemia in humans: analysis of cytokine release and coagulation, fibrinolytic, and complement pathways. Blood 1990;76:2520–2526.

142. Vincent J-L, Roman A, Kajn RJ. Dobutamine administration in septic shock: addition to a standard protocol. Crit Care Med 1990;18:689–693.

143. Wakabayashi GA, Gelfand JA, Jung WK, et al. *Staphylococcus epidermidis* induces complement activation, tumor necrosis factor, and interleukin-1: a shock-like state and tissue injury in rabbits without endotoxemia. J Clin Invest 1991;87:1925–1935.

144. Ward PA, Warren JS, Johnson KJ. Oxygen radicals, inflammation, and tissue injury. Free Radic Biol Med 1988;5:403–408.

145. Weisul JP, O'Donnell JF Jr, Stone MA, et al. Myocardial performance in clinical septic shock: effects of isoproterenol and glucose potassium insulin. J Surg Res 1975;18:357–363.

146. Wiles JB, Cerra FB, Siegal JH, et al. The systemic septic response: does the organism matter? Crit Care Med 1980;8:55–59.

147. Wilson RF, Thal AP, Kindling PH et al. Hemodynamic measurements in septic shock. Arch Surg 1965;91:121–129.

148. Ziegler EJ, Fisher CJ Jr, Sprung CL, et al. Treatment of Gram-negative bacteremia and septic shock with HA-1A human monoclonal antibody against endotoxin. N Engl J Med 1991;324:429–436.

149. Ziegler EJ, McCutchan JA, Fierer J, et al. Treatment of Gram-negative bacteremia and shock with human antiserum to a mutant *Escherichia coli*. N Engl J Med 1982;307:1225–1230.

11

Brain Death, Donor Management, and Withdrawal of Life Support

Lakshmipathi Chelluri

Advances in medical technology have occurred at a rapid pace in the last few decades, creating a multitude of ethical and moral problems in the treatment of critically ill patients. Patients can be kept alive for prolonged periods with the help of modern technology, which sometimes only increases their suffering and financial burden. The guiding principles of medical ethics are beneficence, nonmalfeasance, autonomy, and disclosure. In brief, these principles mandate that the physician act at all times for the patient's good, doing no harm, respecting the patient's right to decide, and informing the patient of his or her condition. These principles form the basis of the physician-patient relationship (9).

The physician-patient relationship can be well maintained with good communication between the physician and the patient. In critical illness, however, this is not always possible, and the decision-making process becomes difficult. The physician in the intensive care unit often must reach decisions about withholding or withdrawing life-sustaining therapy. Such decisions must take into account both the needs of the individual patient and family and the need to allocate the finite resources available. This chapter discusses three aspects of intensive care medicine

that involve issues of ethics and cost benefit: determination of brain death in adults, care of an organ donor with brain death, and decisions to forego life-sustaining therapy.

BRAIN DEATH IN ADULTS

In the past few decades, advances in cardiopulmonary resuscitation have resulted in effective support of the heart and lungs in severely brain-injured persons. This created confusion with regard to the definition of death. Cessation of cardiac function, which previously was used to define death, became invalid.

Definition of Brain Death

In 1968, Harvard Medical School published its criteria for determining death (1), and in 1981, the President's Commission for the Study of Ethical Problems in Medicine and Biomedical and Behavioral Research published its criteria (17). Since publication of the Harvard criteria, it has generally been accepted in the United States that irreversible and complete loss of brain function is recognized as death. The President's Commission defines death as "1. Irreversible cessation of circulatory and respiratory functions, or 2. Irreversible cessation of all functions of the entire brain including the brain stem" (17). This definition also states that death must be determined in accordance with accepted medical standards. The criteria used to determine death vary among different institutions, but the common goals are to eliminate mistakes in diagnosis and to be adaptable such that the criteria can be applied to various clinical situations.

Criteria for Brain Death

The critical elements needed to declare brain death are the cessation of function in all areas of the brain, including the brainstem, and its irreversibility. The determination of brain death usually involves general criteria, a clinical examination, and confirmatory tests. Criteria for brain death are summarized in Table 11.1.

The major goal of clinical examination (supplemented by laboratory tests) is to confirm cessation of brain function. In general, it is recommended that two physicians examine the patient at recommended intervals during a 2–72 hr time period. Brainstem function is evaluated by examination of cranial nerve and motor

Table 11.1
Criteria for Brain Death

General criteria
  Determination of the cause of coma
  Exclusion of potentially correctable
    hypothermia (body temperature <32°C),
    hypotension, hypoxemia, hypovolemia,
    severe electrolyte abnormalities, and
    intoxication from cerebral depressant
    drugs such as alcohol or barbiturates
Specific criteria
  Clinical examination to confirm absence of
    brain function including in the brainstem
  Deep coma without response
  Absence of brainstem function as
    indicated by apnea and absence of
    motor or cranial nerve activity
Confirmatory tests
  Absence of electrical activity on
    electroencephalogram
  Absence of cerebral blood flow as
    indicated by four-vessel cerebral
    arteriogram or cerebral blood flow
    determination by computed
    tomography technique (14)

activity and the presence of apnea (14). Decorticate or decerebrate posturing and shivering, which indicates temperature regulation by the hypothalamus, should be absent. However, complex movements associated with spinal cord reflexes are reported occasionally (6). Pupillary, corneal, oculocephalic, vestibuloocular, and oropharyngeal reflexes should be absent.

The absence of respiratory muscle movement after an adequate stimulus is very important. A number of techniques for testing apnea have been described (2, 10), but the main principles involve adequate oxygenation during the test (except in patients requiring hypoxic drive, in whom Pao_2 should be approximately 50 mm Hg) and an increase in $Paco_2$ to 55–60 mm Hg at the end of the test to stimulate respiratory effort.

These criteria for brain death are accepted in most of the Western Hemisphere. It is critical on the part of the clinician to follow the guidelines carefully to avoid mistakes, which are occasionally reported (7).

CARE OF ORGAN DONORS WITH BRAIN DEATH

Organ transplantation became a viable therapy for end-stage organ disease when advances in surgical techniques, preoperative and postoperative management, and immunosuppressive therapy improved graft and patient survival. However, a major limitation to organ transplantation is the availability of organs. The critical factor in maintaining an adequate organ supply is the appropriate management of organ donors so that their organs remain viable. Because most of these patients are treated in intensive care units, the intensivist should be familiar with the principles of their treatment (4, 8, 13, 22).

All patients with significant neurologic injury are potential organ donors. Infection, malignancy, significant damage to the organ to be donated, and old age usually exclude the patient from being an organ donor; nevertheless, skin, bone, and corneas can be obtained from most donors. The regional transplant center should be contacted about every potential organ donor to verify the criteria for donor eligibility. Once the potential organ donor has been identified, the previously described criteria for verifying brain death should be followed. In the United States, the consent for organ donation must be obtained from the immediate family; in some European countries, the principle of presumed consent is used.

Proper management of the potential organ donor should provide adequate perfusion to the individual donor organs. This includes the maintenance of hemodynamic variables, fluid and electrolyte balance, and ventilatory support, and the prevention of complications.

Hemodynamic Monitoring

Maintenance of adequate tissue perfusion is crucial for the viability of donor organs. Cardiovascular instability (12, 28) is not unusual, and monitoring with arterial and pulmonary artery catheters may be necessary. Hypertension from surgical stimulus during removal of organs is not uncommon and can be controlled with short-acting β-adrenergic blocking agents such as esmolol. Bradyarrhythmia should be controlled by infusion of an adrenergic agent, such as isoproterenol or epinephrine. Atropine is not useful because hypothalamic activity is absent. Hypotension resulting from cardiac dysfunction and vasodilation is common and can usually be managed with volume replacement to maintain central venous pressure at 8–10 mm Hg and systolic blood pressure at 90–120 mm Hg. After adequate volume expansion, vasopressors may be necessary. Dopamine is usually preferred because of its presumed mesenteric and renal vasodilating effects. A continuous intravenous infusion of dopamine at 2 μg/kg/min is recommended to maintain adequate renal perfusion.

Ventilatory Support

Adequate oxygenation (arterial oxygen saturation >95%) and physiologic pH are the major aims of ventilatory support. High concentrations of inspired oxygen are usually avoided to reduce pulmonary oxygen toxicity in lung donors. High levels of positive end-expiratory pressure (>10 cm H_2O) should also be avoided because its potential detrimental effect on cardiac output may result in renal and hepatic hypoperfusion. Sodium bicarbonate is used to treat metabolic acidosis and to decrease ventilatory requirements, as increased mean intrathoracic pressure associated with large tidal volume ventilation has deleterious hemodynamic effects on global blood flow.

Fluid and Electrolytes

Adequate volume replacement should maintain urine output at 100 ml/hr in a 70-kg donor. Sodium, calcium, potassium, magnesium, and phosphate levels should be closely monitored because abnormal levels might occur and will result in hemodynamic instability. Central diabetes insipidus is not uncommon in these patients and requires replacement of appropriate fluids and close monitoring of urine output. If urine output is excessive (greater than 250 ml/hr), a vasopressin preparation should be given to reduce urine output to 100–250 ml/hr.

Hormonal Changes

Serum levels of thyroxine, thyroid-stimulating hormone, cortisol, and insulin were recently studied in organ donors by Powner et al. (16). The changes in thyroid hormones were consistent with the sick euthyroid syndrome. Cortisol and insulin levels were normal or high. Hormone replacement therapy in this group of patients is controversial.

As stated earlier, the major limitation of transplantation is the unavailability of organs. Early identification of potential organ donors and meticulous care of the donor before and after declaration of brain death should increase the number of usable organs and improve their chances of organ survival following transplantation.

WITHHOLDING OR WITHDRAWING LIFE-SUSTAINING THERAPY

In the past few decades, an increasing number of critically ill patients have been brought to the hospital for treatment with improved life-support techniques and intensive care. Sometimes, however, this advanced technology serves only to prolong life with minimal benefit to the patient. In 1983, the President's Commission for the Study of Ethical Problems in Medicine and Biomedical and Behavioral Research published guidelines concerning the decision to forego life-sustaining therapy (18). The commission states that there is no ethically relevant distinction between withholding and withdrawing therapy. Withholding therapy refers to refraining from the use of certain life-sustaining therapies after prospective discussion between the patient and physician. On the other hand, withdrawing therapy refers to discontinuing therapy after it has been initiated. Withdrawal of therapy, the more common occurrence in the intensive care unit, requires a complete diagnostic and prognostic evaluation and discussion with the patient (if possible) and the family.

The issues involved in decisions to withhold or withdraw life-sustaining therapy have been reviewed by many authors (11, 19, 25, 26). The basic ethical principle supporting such decisions is patient autonomy, which is the right of an informed individual to accept or refuse treatment. The physician has the responsibility to inform the patient of his or her diagnosis, treatment options, and prognosis so that the patient can made a decision based on his or her needs and goals. (There are some exceptions to disclosure of information, although these situations are uncommon and should be avoided if possible.) The decision-making process is also a collaborative effort among the patient, the physician, and the patient's family. Patients and families should be encouraged to ask questions, and patients should be given the flexibility to change their decision according to the availability of new information. The patient cannot force a physician to withhold therapy if the physician disagrees on ethical grounds. Under these circumstances, the physician should transfer the patient's care to another physician.

As stated before, there is no ethical distinction between withholding and withdrawal of care. Although, emotionally, the decision to withdraw therapy might be more difficult than the decision not to start therapy in the first place. A detailed discussion should be held with the patient regarding the types of treatment to be withheld so that there is no confusion later among the individuals taking care of the patient. Terms such as "ordinary" and "extraordinary" should be avoided because they are highly subjective. Artificial alimentation and hydration, particularly the former, are usually considered routine treatment, but can be refused by patients for a variety of reasons. This has been supported by many court decisions (23, 27).

Mechanical ventilation is one mode of therapy that is difficult to withdraw because of the physical and psychological discomfort withdrawal could cause. Nevertheless, withdrawal of mechanical ventilation should be handled similarly to other therapies, and administration of narcotics to prevent discomfort during terminal weaning is recommended (20). Other treatments, such as dialysis, antibiotic therapy, and chemotherapy can also be withheld or withdrawn after discussion with and consent of the involved individuals.

In incompetent patients, informed consent cannot be obtained and the principle of substituted judgment is commonly applied. It is the responsibility of the physician to determine the patient's competence in making decisions. A family member, a friend, or person with the power of attorney can serve as a surrogate decision-maker. Discussion with a surrogate should focus on the patient's preference for various therapeutic options, keeping in mind that the surrogate's own views should be distinguished from the patient's view. In the absence of a surrogate, the principle of beneficence can be used, and the hospital's ethics committee may be involved in difficult decisions.

Advance directives, which are accepted in many states, can serve to document a person's wishes before a critical illness occurs. Advance directives are particularly useful when there is a disagreement between the surrogate and the patient's physicians.

Although a decision to withhold life-sustaining therapy may be made, the care of a patient should never stop. The critically ill person should always be provided with adequate nursing care and comfort.

The medical advances of the past decade have made it possible to sustain life for a prolonged period when recovery is virtually impossible. Some have questioned whether life-sustaining technology such as cardiopulmonary resuscitation should be offered when it is futile (3, 15). Because judgments of futility are subjective, no consensus has been reached on this issue, and attempts are being made to develop criteria for futility (21, 24, 29). In view of the escalating costs and finite resources of medical care, acceptable criteria leading to the avoidance of futile therapy are an important goal.

Despite the increasing knowledge of ethical principles among health care providers, communication between patients, families, and physicians is not always optimal (5). Intensivists, because of their central role in coordinating the care of critically ill patients, should be leaders in the decision-making process.

References

1. Beecher HK, Adams RD, Barger AC, Curran WJ, Denny-Brown D. A definition of irreversible coma. JAMA 1968;205:337–340.
2. Belsh JM, Blatt R, Schiffman PL. Apnea testing in brain death. Arch Intern Med 1986;146:2385–2388.
3. Blackhall LJ. Must we always use CPR? N Engl J Med 1987;317:1281–1284.
4. Darby JM, Stein K, Grenvik A, Stuart SA. Approach to management of the heartbeating "brain dead" organ donor. JAMA 1989;261:2222–2228.
5. Hechinger FM. They tortured my mother. Patronizing doctors, agonizing care. New York Times, January 24, 1991.
6. Ivan LP. Spinal reflexes in cerebral death. Neurology 1973;23:650–652.
7. Jastremski M, Powner D, Snyder J, Smith J, Grenvik A. Problems in brain death determination. Forensic Sci 1978;11:201–212.
8. Jordan CA, Snyder JV. Intensive care and intraoperative management of the brain-dead organ donor. Transplant Proc 1987;19:21–25.
9. Luce JM. Ethical principles in critical care. JAMA 1990;263:696–700.
10. Marks SJ, Zisfein J. Apneic oxygenation in apnea tests for brain death. A controlled trial. Arch Neurol 1990;47:1066–1068.
11. Meisel A, Grenvik A, Pinkus RL, Snyder JV. Hospital guidelines for deciding about life-sustaining treatment. Dealing with health "limbo." Crit Care Med 1986;14:239–246.
12. Nishimura N, Miyata Y. Cardiovascular changes in the terminal stage of disease. Resuscitation 1984;12:175–180.
13. Nygaard CE, Townsend RN, Diamond DL. Organ donor management and organ outcome: 6-year review from a level I trauma center. J Trauma 1990;30:728–732.
14. Pistoia F, Johnson DW, Darby JM, Horton JA, Applegate J, Yonas H. The role of xenon CT measurements of cerebral blood flow in the clinical determination of brain death. AJNR 1991;12:97–103.
15. Podrid PJ. Resuscitation in the elderly: a blessing or a curse? Ann Intern Med 1989;111:193–195.
16. Powner DJ, Hendrich A, Lagler RG, Ng RH, Madden RL. Hormonal changes in brain dead patients. Crit Care Med 1990;18:702–708.
17. President's Commission for the Study of Ethical Problems in Medicine and Biomedical and Behavioral Research. Guidelines for the determination of death. JAMA 1981;246:2184–2186.
18. President's Commission for the Study of Ethical Problems in Medicine and Biomedical and Behavioral Research. Deciding to forego life-sustaining treatment. Washington DC: US Government Printing Office, 1983.
19. Ruark JE, Raffin TA. Initiating and withdrawing life support. Principles and practice in adult medicine. N Engl J Med 1988;318:25–30.
20. Schneiderman LJ, Spragg RG. Ethical decisions in discontinuing mechanical ventilation. N Engl J Med 1988;318:984–988.
21. Schneiderman LJ, Jecker NS, Jonsen AR. Medical futility: its meaning and ethical implications. Ann Intern Med 1990;112:949–954.
22. Soifer B, Gelb AW. The multiple organ donor: identification and management. Ann Intern Med 1989;110:814–823.
23. Steinbrook R, Lo B. Artificial feeding—solid ground, not a slippery slope. N Engl J Med 1988;318:286–290.
24. Tomlinson T, Brody H. Futility and the ethics of resuscitation. JAMA 1990;264:1276–1280.
25. Wanzer SH, Adelstein SJ, Cranford RE, et al. The physician's responsibility toward hopelessly ill patients. N Engl J Med 1984;310:955–959.
26. Wanzer SH, Federman DD, Adelstein SJ, Cassel CK, Cassem EH, Cranford RE. The physician's responsibility toward hopelessly ill patients. A second look. N Engl J Med 1989;320:844–849.
27. Weir RF, Gostin L. Decisions to abate life-sustaining treatment for nonautonomous patients. Ethical standards and legal liability for physicians after Cruzan. JAMA 1990;264:1846–1853.
28. Wetzel RC, Setzer N, Stiff JL, Rogers MC. Hemodynamic responses in brain dead organ donor patients. Anesth Analg 1985;64:125–128.
29. Younger SJ. Who defines futility? JAMA 1988;260:2094–2095.

12

Paradigms in Management

Alan H. Morris

It is widely recognized by the medical, business, and government communities that both the quality and cost of medical care require serious reevaluation. This is a result of two major forces:

1. The increasing pressure to contain costs as a result of continued escalation of medical care expenditures in the face of a decreasing dollar supply, and
2. The recognition that much of the resource consumptive medical therapy delivered to patients is of unproved value (". . . it is still the case that *only about 15 percent* of all contemporary clinical interventions are supported by objective scientific evidence that they do more good than harm." (K. L. White, M.D., retired Deputy Director for Health Sciences, Rockefeller Foundation. In: Payer L, ed. Medicine and culture. New York: Henry Holt, 1988.))

The American health care system has lost the confidence of those it tries to serve. While most Americans are satisfied with their own health care interactions, they do not believe the health care industry routinely delivers effective, efficient care (21, 36). Health care costs, already consuming more that $650 billion per year, almost 12% of the total national economy, continue to increase at excessive rates. Improvement of community medical care through reformulation of medical policy is in large part dependent upon the analysis of patient outcomes. Unfortunately, because of ill-defined and nonstandardized care, much patient outcome data do not possess the level of credibility necessary to lead to changes in practice. Given these challenges, it is timely to examine the basic structure of medical decision making in critical care medicine. A discussion of the paradigm we teach and of the paradigm actually used in practice will be instructive

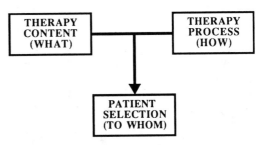

Figure 12.1. Clinical care elements.

and will focus attention on some basic limitations of critical care decision making and practice.

Clinical care can be conceptually viewed as a combination of three major elements: patient selection, therapy content, and therapy process (Fig. 12.1). Patient selection provides the object for care, the person "to whom" care is delivered. Therapy content comprises the procedures, drugs, interventions, etc. delivered to the patient. Therapy process comprises the delivery technique. While therapy content addresses "what" we do to patients (e.g., appendectomy or mechanical ventilation), therapy process addresses "how" we provide the care (e.g., the details of procedure including timing of the appendectomy or mechanical ventilation). Of the three major elements involved in clinical care and research, the content of clinical care, patient selection, and the process of clinical care (Fig. 12.1), only the content ("what" we do) is clearly defined. In most publications the drugs, mechanical interventions, or other therapeutic modalities used are usually clearly identified. Patient selection ("to whom" the "what" is delivered) is a more difficult issue. For example, there is still no uniformly accepted definition of adult respiratory distress syndrome (ARDS) and no accepted list of diseases that precipitate ARDS. Nevertheless, most publications contain useful information concerning patient selection. The process of medical care ("how" we deliver "what" "to whom") is, in contrast, almost never articulated. This is a serious shortcoming since it precludes achievement of the two most important goals of a scientific methods section (the provision of enough detail to both: (*a*) allow a reviewer to critically evaluate the results and its conclusions, and (*b*) allow the interested investigator to duplicate the work). This lack of precision seems to be generally accepted as a necessary limitation of the patient-physician encounter. Its consequence is the difficulty we all experience in comparing and interpreting the results of many clinical studies.

The value of medical care is best defined by the patient outcome. Once the patient has engaged the medical care delivery system, two major factors determine both the intensity of care to which the patient is subjected and the patient's outcome (Fig. 12.2). These two factors, the patient-disease complex and the clinical care team response to the patient-disease complex, interact and it is this interaction that determines the intensity of care and the patient's outcome. The three medical care elements (therapy content, patient selection, and therapy process) are related to these two major determinants of the intensity of care and of the ultimate patient outcome (the patient-disease complex and the response of the clinical care team) (Fig. 12.3). The clinical care team response varies from center to center, from unit to unit, and from physician to physician. Even individual physicians vary their responses over time. Response is influenced by training (e.g., internist versus surgeon), clinical setting (e.g., Veterans Administration versus private hospital), pharmacopoeia (e.g., United States versus Europe), available equipment (e.g., NMR scanner, two-dimensional echo, specialty representation), financial and community imperatives, and past experience. Clinical care team response varies not only with location but also with time. Recent experiences including exposure to conferences and publications may dramatically alter the decisions of physicians from one day to the next. Medical practice vogue or style frequently assumes widespread influence out of proportion to the observations or reports that initially stimulated the change.

Our focus in medicine for both clinical care and for clinical research is patient outcome, the most important of which is survival with resumption of a productive life. Unfortunately, the signal-to-noise ratio associated with outcome differences in clinical trials is frequently very low. The noise in the clinical environment is both random and nonrandom (bias). Random noise can be reduced by increasing the number of observations (or number of patients) made in a clinical trial. Since the

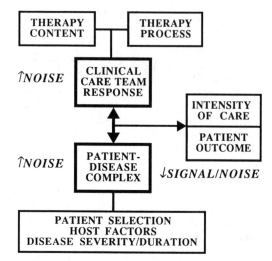

Figure 12.3. Relation of clinical care elements to the major determinants of intensity of care and patient outcome.

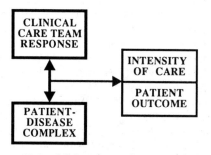

Figure 12.2. Major determinants of intensity of care and patient outcome.

signal-to-noise ratio for random noise is proportional to the square root of the number of observations, increasing the number of observations (or patients) 100-fold would increase the signal-to-noise ratio by 10. This is possible, but challenging in critical care medicine since the acquisition of large numbers of patients in clinical trials is not only difficult, but costly as well. In contrast, nonrandom noise (bias), quite common in clinical settings, is not influenced by increasing the number of observations (or patients) and therefore must be reduced by other means. The two major elements (the patient-disease complex and the clinical care team response) that determine the intensity of patient care and patient outcome (Figs. 12.2 and 12.3) are sources of both random noise and bias.

Noise is introduced in the *patient-disease complex* because of our inability to control host factors and the disease, its severity, and duration. Both random and nonrandom (bias) noise are included, since local factors will influence the probability of specific diseases and problems in the population being served. In addition, significant bias is introduced in patient selection, both in clinical care and, more pertinent to this discussion, in clinical trials. The patient identification and selection process is quite imperfect and incorporates much local bias due to the prejudices of individual clinical investigators and to the specific characteristics of their local clinical environments. The failure of the medical community to establish broadly accepted specific definitions of many diseases contributes significantly to this problem. Much work needs to be done and much improvement can be achieved in this regard. The other major element, the *clinical care team response* to the patient-disease complex, introduces both random noise and bias as well. Strong bias is injected into the response of the clinical care team as a result of many factors that play upon their behavior, including general and local cultural factors, local technical abilities, and experience—all of which affect the process of therapy. This process is usually poorly articulated and one frequently cannot uncover the rules behind decisions relating to important stages in the delivery of care.

For both clinical trials and case reports, this deficiency means it is not possible to define "how" the investigation is actually conducted.

PARADIGMS

Two paradigms play important roles in our interactions with patients. Although these two paradigms overlap and their clear separation may be difficult in many situations, their independent consideration herein will clarify important points. The scientific *therapy content* of medical practice is directed by a mechanistic cause and effect paradigm derived from Cartesian dualism and Newtonian determinism (8, 13). The *therapy process* of medical practice is directed by a paradigm based on the ethical principle of beneficence (19), the application of which requires individualization of the physician-patient encounter.

Content of Medical Practice

Isaac Newton developed a machine-like model of the universe in which predictable change in a system's output follows perturbation of its input. The output changes are determined by the characteristics of the particular system. Newtonian determinism produced the cause and effect model that forms the basis of modern science and that finds common application in routine daily life. René Descartes proposed the absolute separation between mind and body and established what became known as Cartesian dualism. According to Cartesian dualism, the body would, in the absence of the mind and its thoughts, behave exactly as it does (according to its corporeal, physical properties) when the mind is present and functioning. The body could be completely understood and described, according to this influential theory, independent of the presence, state, or function of the mind (note that the organic brain and its physiologic functions belong to the body, not to the mind). While thoughtful questions have been raised about this paradigm (8, 11), they have not shaken its basic structure. Newtonian determinism and Cartesian dualism established the basis for the common reductionist belief that the whole could be adequately understood through detailed mastery of its parts. The current emphasis on cell biological and biochemical reductionist research is the natural consequence of this framework. It fosters the view that when enough of the details are mastered, we will be able to control the problems that patients bring to our attention. This spawned an infatuation with the quick cure, the "magic bullet," the "answer," which when finally revealed makes the problem go away. This finds common expression in medical and nonmedical circles in statements like "if we can just keep him alive, maybe an effective drug will appear in the near future." This is not meant as a criticism, for this reductionist approach has resulted in a marvelous array of medicines and interventions that are the proud inheritance of modern physicians. It has unhappily fostered the belief that *all* of our complex problems will eventually yield to the search for "the cure." This seems unlikely (2, 8, 23) for many of the serious problems encountered in critical care medicine (e.g., septic shock, ARDS, severe burns) and for many chronic diseases as well.

The ability of this reductionist scientific model, based on dualism and determinism, to deal with the complex problems of medicine has recently been challenged (8, 13). It seems, however, premature to deem this traditional scientific medical model, or any other for that matter, inadequate. Current clinical patient outcome information is too incomplete for this purpose. This is especially true when applied to the critical care environment. It is widely accepted that patient outcome (survival generally being the most important) should be the major determinant of our medical care policy and actions. A major difficulty here surfaces because it is precisely this outcome data needed for important clinical decisions that is lacking. A low signal-to-noise ratio, for outcome results in critical care, figures prominently among the reasons for which we lack the necessary outcome data. Although randomized clinical trials, double blinded when possible, provide the most credible source of the required patient outcome data, they have special problems that derive from the human clinical environment itself. Random-

ized clinical trials are not only expensive (compared with basic laboratory research) but they are difficult to conduct.

Process of Medical Care

The process of medical care is based upon the ethical principle of beneficence (19). In general, the principle of beneficence establishes several clinical care imperatives, including: do good, be kind, act in the best interest of the patient, individualize the physician-patient encounter. It is critical for the development of the following arguments to establish whether the principle of beneficence is to be directed at *patient outcome* or at *physician intent*. If beneficence is defined as "the quality of charity or kindness" (17), it is synonymous with *benevolence* but is not necessarily linked to benefit. If beneficence is defined as "the doing of good" (32, 35), it is directly linked to *benefit* but is not necessarily associated with benevolence. When beneficence is defined as "the doing of good," benefit prevails and patient outcome is its natural object (physician benefit is not the goal of the patient-physician encounter). When beneficence is defined as "the quality of charity or kindness," benevolence prevails and physician intent is its natural object (kindness on the patient's part is not a determining factor in the patient-physician encounter). Benefit appears to be the overriding factor (19, pp. 14, 161) as it was for Hippocrates ("Be of benefit and do no harm.") (19, p. 11). Thus the ideal paradigm based upon the principle of beneficence defined as "the doing of good" requires the physician to come to a unique solution (therapy) that will do good, that is, that will favorably influence the patient's outcome (Fig. 12.4). This ideal paradigm, commonly taught to students, considers the patient as a unique individual psychobiologic unit (the corporeal side of Cartesian dualism) and challenges the physician to incorporate and evaluate all pertinent data.

Clinical decision making guided by the principle of beneficence is, unfortunately, confounded by both the uncertainty of medical scientific information and by the probabilistic nature of medical decision

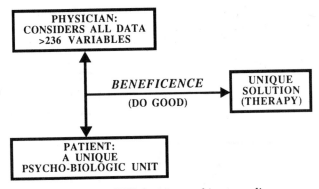

Figure 12.4. ICU decision making paradigm.

making. The problem is clear: The ideal paradigm based on the principle of beneficence defined as "the doing of good" implies patient benefit, but the outcome information necessary for the physician to be confident that patient benefit would follow the intervention is frequently missing! In addition, the effective application of this ideal paradigm is impeded by input information overload (22). In the past 30 years, there has been an explosion of information reflected in the proliferation of medical publications. It has found clear expression in the staggering amount of information produced by critical care patients. Recently, during morning rounds for one severe ARDS patient, 236 different variables in the patient's database were being evaluated by our medical staff. These 236 variables did not include all the patient's data since repeated (serial) measurements and physical examination, x-ray, special studies (e.g., CAT scans, ultrasound, angiography), physician consultation notes, nurse notes, respiratory therapist notes, physician progress notes, operating room notes, anesthesia notes, and pathologist reports were excluded. The 236 variables included variables in the following categories: hemodynamics (14), blood gases (15), ventilatory management (20), hemogram (20), urinalysis (20), ECG (11), blood chemistry (20), special blood chemistry (12), urine chemistry (4), bacteriology (10), bone marrow (17), nutritional balance (20), coagulation (7), temperature (1), weight (1), and medications (44). A mere mortal would not likely be able to effectively assimilate all these variables and

come to the "right clinical treatment decision." Even acknowledging that all variables are not necessary for every treatment decision and that all the data are not independent, it still seems likely that most physicians would have difficulty dealing systematically with this large mass of clinical data. In fact, as few as four adjustable variables seem to have prevented experienced pulmonary/critical care physicians from systematically managing a mechanical ventilator in the inverse ratio ventilation mode (see "Input Information Overload" below). The physician who attempts to integrate knowledge from the pertinent literature with all patient data, including results of the physical examination, frequently faces a nearly impossible task.

In actual practice, the paradigm used in critical care medicine decision making is usually based on the principle of beneficence defined as "the quality of charity or kindness." It is directed at physician intent (Fig. 12.5), rather than at patient outcome (Fig. 12.4). The physician usually chooses a few familiar and understood variables. The patient, while always viewed as an individual, is categorized on the basis of these few variables and an attempt to assign general outcome probabilities for different therapy options is made by drawing upon past experience (personal or published) with similar patients. Because of the complexity of the decisions frequently faced, the physician makes the therapeutic decision with the intent to do good, but usually without the outcome knowledge (from previously studied patients) that would enable the physician to draw a con-

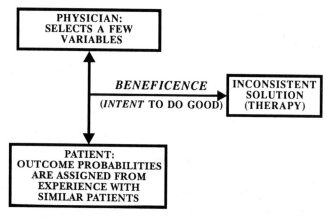

Figure 12.5.   Actual ICU decision making process.

clusion about benefit. This results in therapeutic decisions that are frequently inconsistent and difficult to reproduce.

REDUCING NOISE IN CLINICAL OUTCOME RESEARCH RESULTS

The ideal setting for the generation of highly credible clinical outcome research results would be a critical care environment that could function as a "human laboratory." A "human laboratory" is a site in which the two elements necessary for any laboratory (reliable data capture and control of therapy) are added to the requisite and expected delivery of good and ethical clinical care. My colleagues and I have taken advantage of a unique opportunity available to us because of the unusual hospital information/clinical decision support computer system at the LDS Hospital (the Health Evaluation through Logical Processing (HELP) hospital information system (14, 29–31) developed over a 25-year period) (Fig. 12.6). We have, as a result, made progress toward establishing a "human laboratory" in our ICU, by utilizing computerized protocols to generate therapy instructions that are displayed to clinical care team members in real time on bedside terminal screens.

The HELP protocols for management of arterial hypoxemia in patients with acute hypoxic pulmonary failure (ARDS) (7, 16, 25, 34) provide specific and detailed instruction to the clinical care team members. The protocols provide a standard therapeutic response to the arterial hypoxemia in mechanically ventilated patients with severe ARDS. These hypoxemia-focused protocols have been generated using the best information available in the published literature combined with that from local, national, and international experts. Physicians at our hospital agreed to abandon personal style and adopt a "standard" protocol therapy of arterial hypoxemia. The physician is free to decline to follow a protocol instruction, if he or she has a defensible reason. The protocols were developed by an iterative consensus generation technique illustrated in Figure 12.7 (7).

The protocol management of arterial hypoxemia is achieved primarily by manipulation of oxygen concentration and positive end-expiratory pressure during mechanical ventilator support of patients with severe pulmonary failure. This acceptance of protocol-controlled therapy has required a high level of collegiality and commitment from physicians, nurses, and respiratory therapists. Figure 12.8 illustrates a simplified and selected portion of one of approximately 30 pages of protocols used for the control of arterial oxygenation in these patients. Three sets of representative instructions generated during routine application in one patient are also shown.

The computerized versions of these protocols have been used for over 40,000

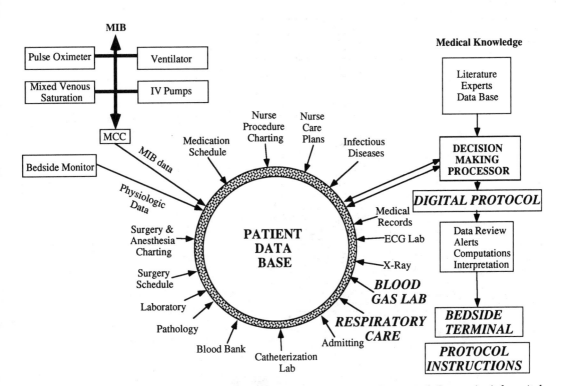

Figure 12.6. Overview of the HELP (Health Evaluation through Logical Processing) hospital information system (14, 29–31). The *stippled circle* represents interactions between the various sources of information stored in the single *Patient Data Base* file. *MIB* represents the Medical Information Bus, a standard electronic data acquisition route for direct access of data from medical devices such as the *Pulse Oximeter, Ventilator,* etc. Medical knowledge is stored, independently from the *Patient Data Base* and is obtained from the *Literature, Experts,* and from analysis of the *Data Base* of selected patient populations of LDS Hospital patients. The protocols were digitized and made part of the *Medical Knowledge* base and incorporated in the *Decision Making Processor.* The protocols are automatically run when new data, in real time, enter the *Patient Data Base* from the *Blood Gas Lab* and from bedside keyboard entry of ventilator data by members of the *Respiratory Care* department. *Protocol Instructions* (therapy instructions) are generated, in real time, and displayed to the members of the clinical care team on the patient's *Bedside Terminal.* The HELP system runs on a system of 12 Tandem Computer fault tolerant processors (the system is up 99.75% of the time). Eighteen Charles River Data Systems (CRDS), Unix-based minicomputers are interfaced to the Tandem. The CRDS machines serve as multiplexers and preprocessors for terminals and monitors on the hospital wards, in surgery, medical records, pulmonary division, and the medical informatics departments. A total of 1000 terminals and 200 line and laser printers are currently active throughout the hospital. All of the nursing units have terminals located at each patient bedside, at the nursing station, and at various hallway sites. The four intensive care units are fully computerized and have terminals at each bedside as well as at the nursing station. A fully functional Medical Information Bus *(MIB)* system links many of the medical devices in the ICUs directly to the HELP system. The MIB helps to assure accurate and timely patient data in the HELP system data base.

hr in routine care of over 125 ARDS patients around the clock (7, 16). The computerized protocols have proven to be more accurate than manually used bedside paper flow diagrams. Ninety-three percent of the computerized protocol instructions are followed and the computerized protocols control therapy of arterial hypoxemia in severe ARDS patients 94% of the day (23 of 24 hr) in our ICU (24, 26) (Fig. 12.9). In addition, they provide an audit trail that permits a detailed review of the perfor-

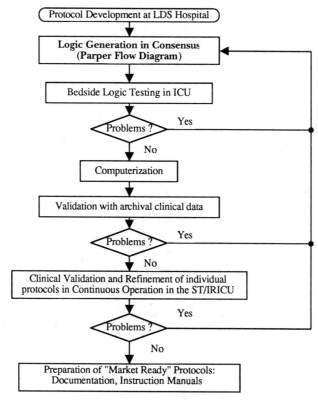

Figure 12.7. Overview of protocol development methods. *Logic Generation in the Consensus Group* initially produces paper-based flow diagrams similar to Figure 12.8. The *Consensus Group* initially consisted of a total of 14 physicians over a 2-year period. Pulmonary and Critical Care Medicine, and Anesthesiology (LDS Hospital and University of Utah) and Anesthesiology (University of Milan) members participated over the initial 2-year period (not all members simultaneously). Information from the expert group was joined with literature information for logic development. *ICU* and *ST/IRICU* both represent the Shock Trauma/Intermountain Respiratory ICU at the LDS Hospital. The final protocols were reviewed in detail and approved by a critical care department of the University of Paris (Cochin-Port-Royal Hospital) and by a critical care/anesthesia department of the University of Milan (Policlinico Hospital).

mance of the protocols in the clinical environment (16).

The complexity of the approximately 30 pages of flow diagrams used to control the different modes of ventilatory support stands in sharp contrast to the simplicity of the individual questions *(diamonds)* and instructions *(rectangles)* (Fig. 12.8). These hypoxemia management protocols are built upon the simplest approach that seemed reasonable, the use of Pao_2 as the arbiter of success or failure with regard to oxygenation. The protocols do not deal with heart-lung-blood interactions at all, in spite of the fact that we teach, like others, the importance of these interactions in tailor-ing therapeutic decisions to individual patient needs. Even though this approach has a simplistic air, it appears successful since the protocols perform satisfactorily in clinical practice (7, 16).

INPUT INFORMATION OVERLOAD

The result of application of an inverse ratio ventilation (IRV) protocol is particularly instructive because of its implication regarding the limited number of variables physicians are capable of managing (1, 6). Among the many publications that deal with IRV, there is no well-defined method,

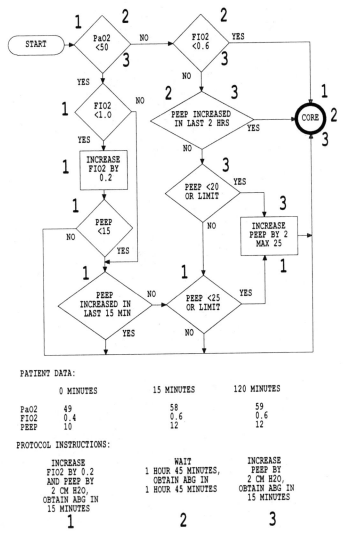

Figure 12.8. Illustrative simplified protocol. Selected questions *(diamonds)* and instructions *(rectangles)* taken from one of the continuous positive pressure ventilation protocol flow diagrams. 1–3 indicate three sequential paths through the protocol logic, with the associated *PATIENT DATA* that led to the *PROTOCOL INSTRUCTIONS* at the *bottom* of the figure.

and descriptions of the technique lack essential details (20). Information gained from domestic and international visits to medical centers has confirmed our local experience that IRV is usually applied by trial and error, with changes in ventilator settings based on pathophysiologic principles. The application of IRV is, therefore, neither systematic nor reproducible in the clinical setting.

Instructions from the HELP system protocols for therapy of arterial hypoxemia display the patient's desired end-expiratory alveolar pressure on the HELP system bedside terminal. This desired end-expiratory alveolar pressure is the new target value that is entered by keyboard into the IRV personal computer by the clinical staff. The IRV protocol operates in a dedicated personal computer linked to a mechanical ventilator (Fig. 12.10). Four simple adjustable ventilator variables (inspiratory/expiratory ratio, ventilatory rate, peak ventilator pressure, and positive end-expiratory

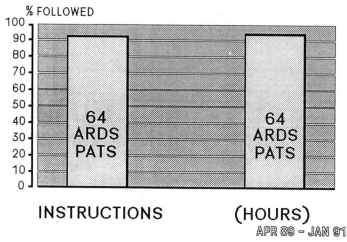

Figure 12.9. Computerized protocol application results for a recent subset of 64 severe ARDS patients at the Shock Trauma/Intermountain Respiratory ICU of the LDS Hospital. The computerized protocol was used for 21,955 hr, during which time 17,273 (therapy) instructions were generated and displayed on the patient's bedside terminal. Hours of use include all the time during which there was an attempt to apply the protocol, from the moment of initial application to the moment it was discontinued. All hours, including those during which the protocol could not be successfully applied, were counted. *Bars* represent the percent of 17,273 instructions actually followed by the clinical care team, and the percent of 21,955 hr during which the protocol controlled ventilator management.

pressure setting: I/E, VR, Ppeak, and setPEEP, respectively) determine the end-expiratory alveolar pressure (Fig. 12.9). "Controlled air trapping" (when end-expiratory alveolar pressure is >0) is achieved as the clinical staff regulate the four variables (I/E, VR, Ppeak, and setPEEP) according to the protocol instructions displayed on the IRV personal computer screen.

The computerized IRV protocol displays instructions for changing the four regulated variables (I/E, VR, Ppeak, and setPEEP) by small increments or decrements. Since the initial application of the computerized protocol in our ICU, IRV has been markedly simplified and is now considered a more systematic, predictable, and reproducible technique. This dramatic change in our perception of IRV performance was noted by physician, nurse, and respiratory therapist alike, and suggests that the four determining variables (I/E, VR, Ppeak, and setPEEP) were not managed systematically prior to computerized protocol control, even though IRV had been used by experienced pulmonary/critical care physicians within an academic training program. This suggests that, faced with the challenge of adjusting four apparently simple variables, experienced physicians were not able to develop a systematic response to ventilatory support problems. This inability of experienced physicians is probably an example of information input overload (22), and likely an example of a general limitation of our ability to manage clinical problems that have at least four variable determinants. While this may initially appear surprising, it seems to be a reasonable conclusion. It would be the rare individual who could, standing at the bedside without computational aids, solve in his or her head the four simultaneous equations necessary for a unique solution to a four-variable set. The rest of us wouldn't stand a chance. Within the more than 236 different variables noted in one of our ARDS patients (see "Process of Medical Care" above) there are a number of clinically important problems that require consideration of at least four adjustable variables. These include cardiac output (intracavitary pressures and pericardial or intrathoracic pressures on both the right and left sides of the heart, heart rate, elec-

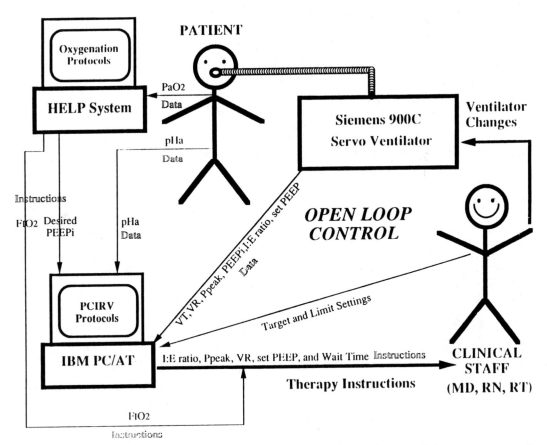

Figure 12.10. *OPEN LOOP CONTROL* schematic illustrating the application of the pressure control inverse ratio ventilation *(PCIRV)* protocol. The oxygenation protocols in the HELP hospital information system generate bedside terminal instructions for changes in fraction of inspired oxygen *(FIO2)* and desired intrinsic PEEP or end-expiratory alveolar pressure *(Desired PEEPi)* based upon measurement of the patient's Pao_2. The *Desired PEEPi* and the patient's measured *pHa* are then entered by keyboard by the clinical care team into the bedside *IBM PC/AT* (a second bedside computer independent of the HELP system) in which the PCIRV protocol resides. The IBM PC/AT protocol generates a new set of *Therapy Instructions* for inspiratory/expiratory time ratio, peak ventilator pressure, ventilatory rate, ventilator PEEP setting, and waiting time before the next therapy change (*I:E ratio, Ppeak, VR, set PEEP, and Wait Time,* respectively). The clinical care team members *(CLINICAL STAFF)* then carry out the instructions by changing the settings of the Siemens 900C Servo Ventilator. New Pao_2 and *pHa* data from the next arterial blood gas specimen examination drive the next cycle of this *OPEN LOOP CONTROL* scheme.

trical conduction and rhythm, arterial oxygenation, and medications), renal output (cardiac output, arterial oxygenation, venous pressure, abdominal pressure, intrathoracic pressure, and medications), and "tissue oxygenation" (cardiac output, arterial oxygen content, arterial oxygen pressure, oxygen consumption, bacteremia or infection, temperature, activity, and medications). It seems reasonable, therefore, to question our ability to come to the "right

therapeutic decision" when dealing with multivariate problems in severely ill patients.

IMPACT OF STANDARDIZING THE PROCESS OF MEDICAL CARE

It is clear that interpretations of clinical outcome results will remain difficult as long as the process of clinical care is poorly defined. Few studies have dealt with the impact of controlling the process of medical care. Although it is generally believed that detailed protocols will not be able to replace individual physician judgment (12, 27), the minute to minute management demands of severely ill ICU patients provide an unusually fertile field for application of detailed protocols. My colleagues and I have attempted to reduce the noise associated with the clinical care team's response by defining, with computerized protocols, the process of medical care associated with the management of arterial hypoxemia in a clinical trial of two therapies for ARDS (25, 26). It is now clear that this approach is feasible and, with the appropriate computer infrastructure, is practical (7, 16). Such computerized protocol control of the process of care does appear to control the intensity of care of severely ill patients (26). This use of computerized protocols to help physicians standardize care contrasts with the more common emphasis in medical informatics upon exploring how humans reason, and upon matching medical expert systems outputs to individual physician preferences (33). Whether our approach will be generalizable is currently unknown. If it is generalizable, it may allow the performance of clinical trials that have the potential of significantly decreasing the noise introduced by the response of the clinical care team and thus increasing the signal-to-noise ratio for outcomes. This will make a number of clinical studies very likely more credible and more definitive.

Before one can evaluate the outcome of a particular medical intervention, that intervention must be applied in a uniform manner to comparable patients (28). Practitioners can affect outcomes only through process steps. Outcome data are therefore most useful if they can be traced to specific treatment actions (5) in specific subsets of patients. Computerized protocols that control medical decision making reduce the noise introduced in the *clinical care team response* (Figs. 12.2 and 12.3) by standardizing care at a level of attention to detail that is unachievable without the computerized protocol decision-making support.

Unaided humans are not capable of providing the persistent commitment to detail and to decision-making logic (rules) necessary to effect a comparable level of standardization in general, and even less so in the hectic ICU environment.

There is already evidence that control of the process of medical care is beneficial (4, 37). Published work from the LDS Hospital indicates that computerized protocols have favorable impacts upon hospital pharmacy and infectious disease departments (9, 10, 15). The use of computerized protocols to control therapy for >40,000 hr in >125 ARDS patients was associated with a fourfold increase in survival (9–40%), suggesting that protocols may have a favorable impact on patient survival (24–26). There are definitive data, from randomized clinical trials using more general and manually applied protocols, that protocol controlled care favorably impacts the outcome of patients with thromboembolic disease (3, 18). In fact, a recent review of about 100 comparisons of decision accuracy of individual judgment compared with that obtained from well-defined rules indicates clear superiority of rule-based decisions (4). Rules were based either on clinical decision-making experience or on outcome data. Greater overall accuracy was achieved when clinicians relied on rule (protocol)-based conclusions and avoided independent judgments (4). The evidence to date, therefore, indicates that pursuit of protocol control of care is a desirable and productive medical research aim.

The standardization of therapy that can be achieved with computerized protocols may contribute to national medical policy formulation. Controlled randomized clinical trial outcome data that identify the therapies that lead to the best possible patient outcome at the lowest cost will likely be made more credible with protocols that standardize therapy. The higher the credibility of results from such trials, the greater the likelihood that they will eventually influence the formulation of medical policy. A cyclical process (Fig. 12.11) that generates new and credible outcome information is necessary and should be systematically supported.

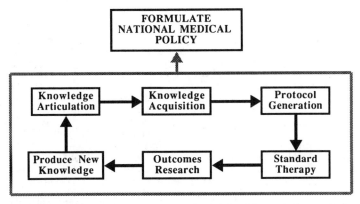

Figure 12.11. Overview of a scheme for using new medical knowledge to influence the formulation of national medical policy.

CONCLUSION

In conclusion, the personal, individualized, physician-patient encounter is the foundation stone of medical practice and must be protected and enhanced. Nevertheless, the ideal paradigm of the unaided knowledgeable physician applying all pertinent patient and published data to the unique psychobiologic unit represented by the patient (Fig. 12.4) has major shortcomings, especially in critical care medicine. A more realistic and actually used paradigm involves selection of a few pertinent pieces of information that are used in the context of patient outcome probabilities derived from past experience (Fig. 12.5). While this actually used paradigm defines beneficence as "the quality of charity or kindness," and has physician intent as its object (Fig. 12.5), this is only temporary. It will be superseded by application of the ideal paradigm based on beneficence defined as "the doing of good," with patient outcome as its object (Fig. 12.4), as soon as credible clinical outcome research data become available. Individualized patient care and protocol-directed care are not mutually exclusive. Standardization of care through protocol application based upon credible outcome results will likely simplify therapy, improve outcome, and enhance the physician-patient encounter. By contributing to credible outcome research results, it will likely permit the identification of ineffective therapy and thus set the stage for the elimination of resource consumptive interventions that do not contribute to favorable patient outcome. If the computerized protocol control technique proves generalizable and can be exported to other centers either in personal computers or in hospital information systems, or if the results of computerized protocol-controlled clinical trials are widely applicable in centers without computer support, we can expect additional benefits. All of these benefits seem likely to be realized. As physicians are relieved of routine tasks taken over by computerized protocols, time will be made available for more important issues and for dealing with higher order tasks.

References

1. Böhm SH, Peng L, East TD, Hoffmann BH, Weaver LK, Clemmer TP, Orme JF, Wallace CJ, Dean N, Morris AH. Computerized protocol management of pressure control inverse ratio ventilation [Abstract]. Chest 1990;98:77S.
2. Connett RJ, Honig CR, Gayeski TEJ, Brooks GA. Defining hypoxia: a systems view of Vo_2, glycolysis, energetics, and intracellular Po_2. J Appl Physiol 1990;68(3):833–842.
3. Cruikshank MK, Levine MH, Hirsh J, Roberts R, Siguenza M. A standard heparin normogram for the management of heparin therapy. Arch Intern Med 1991;151:333–338.
4. Dawes RB, Faust D, Meehl PE. Clinical versus actuarial judgement. Science 1989;243:1668–1674.
5. Donabedian A. The quality of care: how can it be assessed? JAMA 1988;260(12):1743–1748.
6. East TD, Böhm SH, Wallace CJ, Clemmer TP, Weaver LK, Orme JF Jr, Morris AH. A successful

computerized protocol for clinical management of pressure control inverse ratio ventilation in ARDS patients. Chest 1992;101:697–710.

7. East TD, Morris AH, Wallace CJ, Clemmer T, Orme JF Jr, Weaver LK, Henderson S, Sittig DF. A strategy for development of computerized critical care decision support systems. Int J Clin Monit Comput 1992;8:263–269.

8. Engel GL. The need for a new medical model: a challenge for biomedicine. Science 1977;196 (4286):129–136.

9. Evans RS, Burke JP, Pestotnik SL, Classen DC, Menlove RL, Gardner RM. Prediction of hospital infections and selection of antibiotics using an automated hospital database. Proceedings of the 14th Annual Symposium on Computer Applications in Medical Care. Los Alamitos, CA: IEEE Computer Society Press, 1990:663.

10. Evans RS, Pestotnik SL, Burke JP, Gardner RM, Larsen RA, Classen DC. Reducing the duration of prophylactic antibiotics use through computer monitoring of surgical patients. DICP, Ann Pharmacother 1990;24:351.

11. Feinstein A. An additional basic science for clinical medicine: I. The constraining fundamental paradigms. Ann Intern Med 1983;99:393–397.

12. Flanagin A, Lundberg GD. Clinical decision making: promoting the jump from theory to practice [Editorial]. JAMA 1990;263:279.

13. Foss L, Rothenberg K. The second medical revolution. Boston: New Science Library, Shambhala, 1988.

14. Gardner RM. Computerized management of intensive care patients. MD Computing 1986;3(1):36–51.

15. Gardner RM, Hulse RK, Larsen KG: Assessing the effectiveness of a computerized pharmacy system. Proceedings of the 14th Annual Symposium on Computer Applications in Medical Care. Los Alamitos, CA: IEEE Computer Society Press, 1990:668.

16. Henderson SE, Crapo RO, Wallace CJ, East TD, Morris AH, Gardner RM. Performance of computerized protocols for the management of arterial oxygenation in an intensive care unit. Int J Clin Monit Comput 1992;8:271–280.

17. The American heritage dictionary of the English language. Morris W, ed. Boston: Houghton Mifflin, 1979:123.

18. Hull RD, Raskob GE, Rosenbloom D. Heparin for 5 days as compared with 10 days in the initial treatment of proximal venous thrombosis. N Engl J Med 1990;322:1260–1264.

19. Jonsen AR, Siegler M, Winslade WJ. Clinical ethics. 2nd ed. New York: Macmillan, 1988.

20. Kaczmarek RM, Hess D. Pressure controlled inverse-ratio ventilation, panacea or auto-PEEP. Respir Care 1990;35:945.

21. Mayer D. U.S. likes its care, but not the cost. Healthweek News 1991;5(5):2,30 (March 11, 1991).

(Harvard Community Health Plan, Boston, MA; 1991 survey conducted by Louis Harris and Associates).

22. Miller JG. Living systems. New York: McGraw-Hill, 1978:121–202.

23. Miller JG, Miller JL. Introduction: the nature of living systems. Behav Sci 1990;35:157–163.

24. Morris AH, Wallace CJ, Beck E, Clemmer TP, Orme JF Jr, Butler S, Suchyta M, East T, Dean N, Sittig D, Henderson S. Protocols control respiratory therapy of ARDS [Abstract]. Clin Res 1990;38:138A.

25. Morris AH, Wallace CJ, Clemmer TP, Orme JF Jr, Weaver LK, Dean NC, Butler S, Suchyta MR, East TD, Sittig DF. Extracorporeal CO_2 removal therapy for adult respiratory distress syndrome patients. Respir Care 1990;35:224.

26. Morris AH, Wallace CJ, Clemmer TP, Orme JF Jr, Weaver LK, Dean NC, Butler S, Suchyta MR, East TD, Sittig DF. Extracorporeal CO_2 removal therapy for adult respiratory distress syndrome patients: a computerized protocol controlled trial. Réan Soins Intens Méd Urg 1990;6:485.

27. Petty T. Pulmonary perspectives: the use, abuse, and mystique of positive end-expiratory pressure. Am Rev Respir Dis 1988;138:475–478.

28. Pocock SJ. Clinical trials: a practical approach. New York: John Wiley & Sons, 1983.

29. Kuperman GJ, Gardner RM, Pryor TA. HELP: A dynamic hospital information system. New York: Springer-Verlag, 1991.

30. Pryor TA. The HELP medical record system. MD Computing 1988;5(5):22–33.

31. Pryor TA, Warner HR, Gardner RM, Clayton PD, Haug PJ. The HELP system development tools. In: Orthner H, Blum B, eds. Implementing health care information systems. New York: Springer-Verlag, 1989:365–383.

32. The Random House dictionary of the English language. 2nd ed. Flexner SB, ed. New York: Random House, 1987:193–194.

33. Rennels GD, Miller PL. Artificial intelligence research in anesthesia and intensive care. J Clin Monit 1988;4:274.

34. Sittig DF, Gardner RM, Pace NL, Morris AH, Beck E. Computerized management of patient care in a complex, controlled clinical trial in the intensive care unit. Comput Methods Programs Biomed 1989;30:77–84.

35. Webster's third international dictionary. Gove PA, ed. Springfield, MA: G & C Merriam, 1976:203.

36. Wildavsky A. Doing better and feeling: the political pathology of health policy. In: Knowles JH, ed. Doing better and feeling worse: health in the United States. New York: WW Norton, 1977.

37. Wirtschafter DD, Scalise M, Henke C, Gams RA. Do information systems improve the quality of clinical research? Results of a randomized trial in a cooperative multi-institutional cancer group. Comput Biomed Res 1981;14:78.

Section

2

ORGAN SYSTEM APPROACH TO THE MANAGEMENT OF THE CRITICALLY ILL

13

Determinants of Left Ventricular Performance

Alain Nitenberg

The task of the left ventricle is to transport arterial blood to organs. This goal is reached by ejecting a sufficient amount of blood at a given pressure against systemic arterial resistance. Thus, the function of the left ventricle is to transmit the energy of contraction into the flow of blood.

DEFINING THE LEFT VENTRICULAR PERFORMANCE

Pressure-Volume Loop and Ventricular Efficiency

The work produced by the cardiac muscle is determined by the force and the distance shortened. When left ventricular volume decreases from end-diastole to end-systole, an external mechanical work equal to the integration of the pressure-volume trajectory is produced. *The pressure-volume loop represents the external stroke work that the left ventricle delivers to the systemic circulation* (Fig. 13.1). It begins at the end-diastolic point of the pressure-volume relation that reflects the interplay between venous return and determinants of left ventricular passive properties. Ejection ends at a point located on the end-systolic pressure-volume relation that reflects both contractility and afterload. These two points are important determinants of left ventricular performance.

An area bound by the end-systolic and end-diastolic pressure-volume relationship curves and the relaxation line of the

pressure-volume loop is considered as a potential energy that can be partially used by the ventricle (19, 143) (Fig. 13.1). The total mechanical energy of the left ventricle is the sum of the external work and of the potential energy. It is represented by the pressure-volume area (Fig 13.1), which is highly correlated with the myocardial oxygen consumption per beat (143, 145).

The ventricular efficiency can be defined as the ratio between total mechanical work (pressure-volume area) and myocardial oxygen consumption. *The pump (or mechanical) efficiency can be defined as the ratio of external work (stroke work) and myocardial oxygen consumption (19). This ratio may be the better representation of left ventricular performance.*

BASIC DETERMINANTS OF LEFT VENTRICULAR PERFORMANCE

Myocardial fiber shortening is determined by preload, afterload, and contractility. In addition, left ventricular performance, both as a muscle and as a pump, is controlled by two interrelated mechanisms, which are the loading conditions (*preload and afterload*) and changes in *contractility.*

Left Ventricular Filling and Preload

Left ventricular end-diastolic volume determines the length of the sarcomeres be-

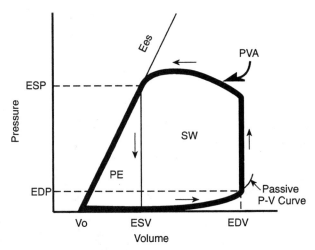

Figure 13.1. Schematic representation of the ventricular pressure-volume relationship. *EDP,* end-diastolic pressure; *EDV,* end-diastolic volume; *ESP,* end-systolic pressure; *ESV,* end-systolic volume; *Ees,* end-systolic elastance (slope of the end-systolic pressure-volume relationship); *Vo,* volume axis intercept of the end-systolic pressure-volume relationship; *PVA,* pressure-volume area is the sum of stroke work area *(SW)* and end-systolic potential energy *(PE).* (Redrawn from Suga H. Total mechanical energy of a ventricle model and cardiac oxygen consumption. Am J Physiol 1979;236:H494–H497.)

fore contraction, which represents the structural basis of the Frank-Starling law. End-diastolic volume depends on (46, 94): *(a)* the filling volume, which occurs during late relaxation (rapid filling), mid-diastole (passive filling), and end-diastole (atrial contraction) (It determines the intracavitary distending force.); and *(b)* forces that impede cavity dilation: myocardial elasticity and viscoelasticity, wall thickness, intramyocardial blood volume, mechanical interaction between ventricles and left and right atria within the pericardium, and pulmonary volume. The distending force is represented by the transmural diastolic pressure-volume curve that relates diastolic transmural pressure (difference between pericardial and intraventricular pressures) to muscle fiber length, which in turn determines the strength of the contraction according to the Frank-Starling mechanism. Transmural pressure cannot be estimated from intrapleural pressure, and either right ventricular end-diastolic pressure or mean right atrial pressure have been proposed as estimates of pericardial pressure (136). *Pressure-volume relation between aortic and mitral closure is governed by the continuous interplay between decaying con-*

tractile tension, passive properties of the ventricular chamber that depend on intrinsic myocardial stiffness, and extramyocardial determinants (17, 94).

Relaxation and Rapid Filling

Relaxation is the process by which the left ventricle returns to the precontractile configuration. Exact timing of the beginning and ending of relaxation are unknown. Myocardial relaxation depends on (Fig. 13.2): *(a)* the active energy-dependent removal of calcium by the sarcoplasmic reticulum *(inactivation system); (b)* calcium outflow from the cell; *(c)* sarcomere length (calcium affinity of troponin C decreases with shortening); and *(d)* force that faces the load, i.e., *load dependence of relaxation* (17, 46).

Relaxation load of the left ventricle has five components: *(a)* internal restoring load depending on cardiac fiber properties (138); *(b)* external restoring load produced by systolic deformation of musculoelastic structures (17); *(c)* hemodynamic load that is dependent on arterial input impedance; *(d)* load during isovolumic relaxation produced by rapid coronary filling (erectile effect) and ventricular remodeling; and *(e)*

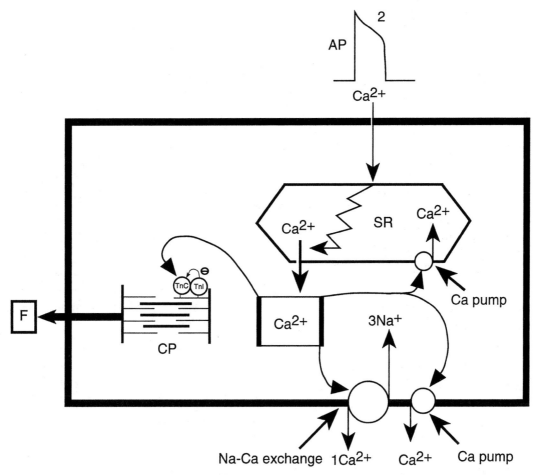

Figure 13.2. Diagrammatic representation of factors governing cardiac myocyte relaxation. *AP,* action potential; *CP,* contractile proteins; *F,* lengthening forces applied on the sarcomeres; *SR,* sarcoplasmic reticulum; *TnC,* troponin C; *TnI,* troponin I.

rapid ventricular filling after mitral valve opening. In addition, physiological non-uniformity of load distribution also determines the normal relaxation sequence (15) and is due to the electrical activation, which makes the transition from contraction to relaxation progressive, to different regional wall thicknesses, and to fiber orientation.

Among the mechanical functions of relaxation, active diastolic suction (153) is a major determinant of ventricular rapid filling. About 20% of filling occurs before minimum ventricular pressure (22). Transmitral flow rate, which is determined by the driving pressure and the impedance to flow, depends on *(a)* the rate of ventricular pressure fall, which is determined by the rate of relaxation, the end-systolic volume, and the viscoelastic properties of the myocardium *(elastic recoil)* because ventricular volume at the opening of the mitral valve is lower than the equilibrium volume (115) (Fig. 13.3); and *(b)* the magnitude of left atrial pressure, which depends on its mechanical properties, on its filling volume that is the stroke volume of the right ventricle, and on left ventricular end-diastolic pressure (72). Thus, ventricular filling in early diastole is an active process resulting in a positive pressure gradient between the left atrium and ventricle because atrial pressure decay is slower than in the ventricle (128). Relaxation is also involved in

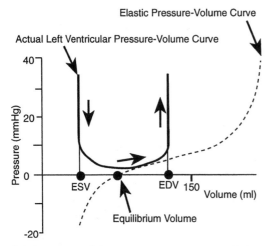

Figure 13.3. Schematic representation of the actual left ventricular pressure-volume curve and of the passive-elastic pressure-volume curve during end-relaxation and diastole. At end-systole, ventricular volume is lower than the equilibrium volume. End of relaxation and elastic recoil are two important determinants of early diastolic atrioventricular gradient. *EDV,* end-diastolic volume; *ESV,* end-systolic volume. (Redrawn from Gilbert JC, Glantz SA. Determinants of left ventricular filling and of the diastolic pressure-volume relation. Circ Res 1989;64:827–852.)

mitral valve opening because diameter increase occuring during isovolumic relaxation pulls the mitral valve by the papillary muscles attached to the ventricular wall (99, 151).

Ventricular relaxation can be evaluated by the time constant (τ) of an assumed exponential isovolumic pressure decline (158). The isovolumic relaxation time depends on the aortic pressure, the loading conditions of the ventricle, and the left atrial pressure, but it must be remembered that relaxation is still present during half of the filling period (108). Also, at the onset of filling, the relaxation load (13) may in turn alter the process of relaxation (108, 149).

Changes in loading conditions and/or in the inactivation process can alter left ventricular relaxation. Abrupt volume or pressure rise may delay relaxation (3, 121), but relaxation is not affected by modest changes in loading conditions in normal heart (140). Inactivation may be altered by metabolic control of the coronary circulation, neu-

rohumoral control, inotropic interventions, ions, drugs, and endocardium function (17).

Because inactivation is mainly controlled by metabolic mechanisms, alterations of myocardial metabolism may delay the decay of activation and decrease the physiological load dependence of relaxation. Hypoxia and ischemia suppress the reuptake of calcium by the sarcoplasmic reticulum (116), which impairs detachment of actin-myosin bridges. Relaxation becomes load independent and is slowed (157). Relaxation may also be prolonged by left ventricular hypertrophy (8, 68) due to pressure overload (54) or hypertrophic cardiomyopathy (137), aging (68, 87), hypothyroidism (18), myocardial diseases (58), hypothermia (148), posthypoxic reoxygenation (9), β-blockers, or phenylephrine. Conversely, volume overload hypertrophy does not alter relaxation (2).

Shortening of relaxation may be produced by catecholamines (74), dobutamine (72), hyperthyroidism (18), calcium, and vasodilators (13) that enhance inactivation directly through reuptake of calcium by the sarcoplasmic reticulum (77), or indirectly through increased shortening and length-dependence inactivation that facilitate dissociation of calcium from troponin C.

Alterations of relaxation may have important consequences on ventricular mechanics. When contractility is enhanced (70), reduction of end-systolic volume and enhancement of the rate of relaxation increase pressure gradient (72) and filling rate and maintain end-diastolic volume, i.e., end-diastolic sarcomere length (preload). Conversely, when relaxation becomes load independent, diastolic suction is absent (25) resulting in an impairment of left ventricular filling (162). However, early diastolic filling may be preserved by an increase in atrial pressure. In addition, depression of relaxation will result in incoordinate relaxation and may impede coronary diastolic inflow and delay mitral valve opening (22).

Although changes are generally not large enough to alter end-diastolic pressure and volume (46), enhancement or depression of myocardial relaxation may respectively result in a downward or upward shift of the passive pressure-volume relation that alters the left ventricular pressure-volume loop. In the former case, end-diastolic volume is increased for a lower end-diastolic pressure that potentially allows the ventricle to deliver a higher stroke volume if arterial elastance is not altered (Fig. 13.4*D*). In the latter case, end-diastolic volume is reduced for a higher end-diastolic pressure, which results in a reduction of stroke volume (Fig. 13.4*E*).

In summary, intrinsic properties of myocardial relaxation, i.e., *lusitropy*, may be modified either by physiological or pathological processes and by cardiovascular drugs (78). Alterations of myocardial lusitropic properties have important consequences on myocardial passive properties, ventricular filling and preload, and systolic performance. In respect to an integrated system, relaxation and rapid filling should be considered as a part of systole (15). A decrease in rapid filling rate may be due to a low atrial pressure and decreased atrial contraction energy, a slowing of left ventricular relaxation, an incomplete left ventricular relaxation, increased viscous properties, and diastolic passive stiffness.

Passive Properties of the Left Ventricle

Passive properties depend on myocardial relaxation, wall volume and thickness (59), and myocardial composition (11). They are also affected by external forces applied on the ventricle (relationships with other chambers within the pericardium, pulmonary volume), cavity size, and ventricular equilibrium volume (50). Passive properties can be assessed by evaluating myocardial stiffness and chamber stiffness (102).

Myocardial stiffness represents the resistance of myocardium to stretching. It depends on intrinsic properties that can be affected by extracellular collagen matrix (86), structures inside cardiac myocytes such as cytoskeletal filaments (98), myocardial metabolism, coronary circulation (blood flow and erectile properties), blood pH, temperature, circulating substances, and drugs. As seen above, passive properties of the myocardium participate in the dia-

stolic suction in a subtle interplay with the relaxation process. Because end-systolic volume is generally lower than the equilibrium volume (164)—that is, the volume corresponding to zero transmural pressure after relaxation has completed (49)—the elastic energy stored during contraction is released during relaxation resulting in an elastic recoil and in a rapid pressure drop that favors diastolic suction. *Thus, the difference between end-systolic volume and equilibrium volume is one of the determinants of the atrioventricular pressure gradient.*

Passive elastic stiffness of the myocardium can be described by a bilinear stiffness-strain relation with a greater stiffness constant in the higher than in the lower stress range (115). Increased myocardial collagen content and/or fibrosis increases the elastic quality of the heart (65) leading to higher diastolic pressures at any given volume. Thus, a higher pressure is needed for obtaining a given sarcomere length. Also, increase in coronary perfusion pressure results in increased stiffness due to erectile properties of the myocardium (155). In addition, diastolic pressure at a given volume increases as filling rate increases because myocardium is a viscoelastic material (48). Viscosity is operating during early diastole and during atrial systole (122).

Chamber stiffness is defined as a change in pressure relative to a change in volume. It assesses the ability of the ventricle to distend under pressure. Passive filling of the ventricle occurs only during diastasis. Diastasis is the most appropriate phase to evaluate passive properties of the myocardium when relaxation is completed and viscous properties are negligible (24). The pressure-volume relation has been described by a curvilinear relation between pressure and volume (110). The larger the volume, the larger is the pressure change for a given volume increase. This relation depends on operative stiffness of the myocardium (45). Isolated cardiac muscle is freely extensible in physiological conditions (no residual cross-bridges), but alterations of relaxation by hypoxia or ischemia may induce incomplete deactivation of myofilaments (1, 47, 132) and decrease passive distensibility resulting in elevation of diastolic pressures at any given volume.

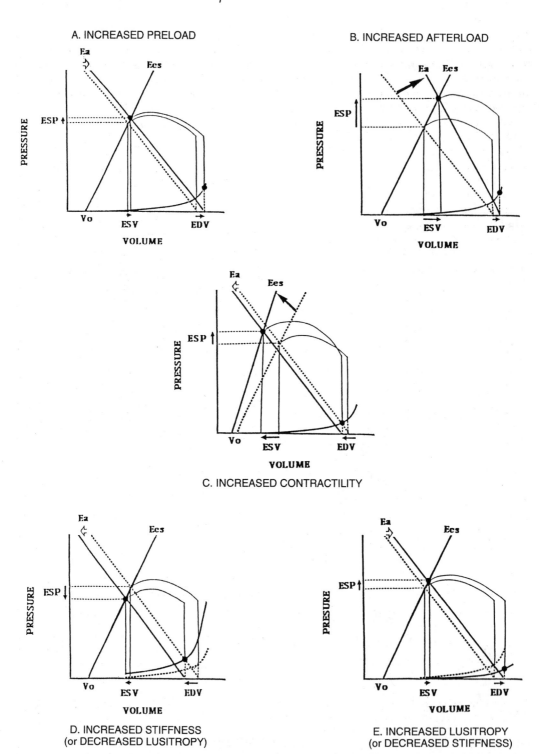

Figure 13.4. Representation of the potential effects of alterations of left ventricular loading conditions, contractility, and lusitropy on pressure-volume loop, stroke volume, and stroke work. *Ea,* effective arterial elastance; *Ees,* left ventricular end-systolic elastance; *EDV,* end-diastolic volume; *ESP,* end-systolic pressure; *ESV,* end-systolic volume; *Vo,* volume axis intercept of the

Thus, when end-systolic volume is increased and/or when relaxation is depressed, filling occurs on the steeper portion of the pressure-volume curve, and filling and stroke volume are reduced despite high end-diastolic pressure and volume (111) (Fig. 13.4E).

Ventricular hypertrophy with increased wall thickness results in an elevation of filling pressure for stretching normally the sarcomeres (93). Increased filling pressures are not necessarily due to increased myocardial stiffness (interstitial fibrosis or sarcomere projections from one cell to another (64)) *but to increased wall thickness* (64, 131). Conversely, myocardial infarction results in a leftward shift of the pressure-volume curve because scar fibrosis is stiffer than normal myocardium (26).

As the heart dilates chronically, the pressure-volume curve moves toward higher volumes and flattens (44). Thus, *(a)* a normal end-diastolic pressure may not stretch the sarcomeres to Lmax; and *(b)* a low variation of diastolic pressure corresponds to a large variation of volume (44).

Viscoelastic properties are dependent on stretch velocity and on the left ventricular volume at which rapid filling occurs (118). Deviations from the passive pressure-volume curve are present during early diastole and atrial contraction (118). However, viscosity is insignificantly small and does not influence ventricular filling (107). Viscous forces are enhanced in cardiac hypertrophy (64) and in cardiomyopathies, because fibrous tissue is increased (63), and by the decrease of temperature (148).

Atrial Contraction

More than 80% of ventricular filling occurs during rapid filling. The contribution of atrial contraction to ventricular filling depends on energy of atrial contraction (16), instantaneous ventricular volume, and ventricular compliance. The contribution is enhanced in diseases reducing rapid filling in order to maintain normal filling (and output). At heart rates higher than 180 beats/min, atrial contraction occurs during relaxation filling, increasing relaxation filling, but total filling, i.e., stroke volume, is reduced (22).

Diastolic Ventricular Interaction and the Pericardium

The pericardium is a fibrous structure stiffer than the myocardium that limits acute cardiac distension (24) and accentuates diastolic ventricular interaction (52). Its action appears when left ventricular dimensions increase above normal, that is, when filling pressure exceeds 10 mm Hg (73). Nonuniform deformation of the pericardium may contribute to atrioventricular mechanical coupling by facilitating atrial emptying and ventricular filling by additional elastic forces added to those of the atria (52, 97). The pericardium may have significant effect on ejection by storing energy during ventricular filling (52). Conversely, chronic cardiac dilation induces an increase in the size of the pericardium without any change in stiffness (41). When the pericardium is intact, intrapericardial pressure is higher than zero and transmural ventricular pressure is different from intracavitary pressure that affects relaxation and diastolic indices (40).

Direct Ventricular Interaction

An increase in right ventricular volume with an intact pericardium causes a leftward and upward shift of the passive pressure-volume curve of the left ventricle (10, 24). Left ventricular end-diastolic pressure is increased and end-diastolic volume (and preload) is reduced, which impairs systolic

---

end-systolic pressure-volume relationship. *A*, Increasing preload shift to the right arterial elastance without changing its slope. *B*, Increasing afterload reduces stroke volume, increasing end-systolic volume more than end-diastolic volume. *C*, Enhancement of contractility increases stroke volume and end-diastolic pressure by reducing end-systolic volume more than end-diastolic volume. Arterial elastance is displaced to the left without changing its slope. *D*, Increased chamber stiffness (or decreased lusitropy) results in a lower end-diastolic volume with a higher end-diastolic pressure and a reduction of stroke volume. *E*, Increased lusitropy (or reduced chamber stiffness) results in a higher end-diastolic volume with a lower end-diastolic pressure and an enhancement of stroke volume. In the two latter cases, slopes of ventricular and arterial elastances are not altered.

function (Fig. 13.4E). The interventricular septum shifts to the left, and left ventricular geometry is altered with a decreased septum-to-left ventricular free wall distance (82). Right ventricular loading is increased by acute elevation of pulmonary pressure (141), atrial septal defect (160), positive end-expiratory pressure ventilation (130), or right ventricular ischemia (53). Similarly, the left ventricular diastolic pressure-volume curve is displaced upward when left or right atrium volume is increased (62). Conversely, reduction of right ventricular volume produces a downward and leftward displacement of the left ventricular pressure-volume curve (95) (Fig. 13.4D).

Series Ventricular Interaction

Right ventricular output is the left ventricular input that determines the left ventricular preload (134). When right ventricular systolic dysfunction results in a decrease in right ventricular output, left ventricular filling is reduced, resulting in a lower end-diastolic volume and preload (53), which may be aggravated by a right ventricular enlargement and the direct ventricular interaction (51).

In summary, (a) the pericardium is a determinant of left ventricular preload and thus may affect the systolic performance through the Frank-Starling mechanism; (b) when the pericardium is intact, a right ventricular volume increase reduces left ventricle distensibility with concomitant elevation of diastolic pressures so that the end-diastolic pressure does not reflect left ventricular preload; and (c) by preserving end-diastolic volume when end-diastolic pressure is decreased by a downward shift of the pressure volume curve, diastolic ventricular interaction is an important mechanism maintaining left ventricular stroke volume (46).

Cardiac-Lung Interaction

Expansion of the lungs, by increasing external pressure, reduces transmural pressure resulting in a decrease in left ventricular end-diastolic volume and preload (126). Pulmonary inflation tends to increase right ventricular afterload and to decrease ve-

nous return. Thus, the effects on left ventricular preload depend (a) on the resulting right ventricular volume and output (left ventricular input), (b) on the operating level of the left ventricular pressure-volume curve, and (c) on the pulmonary volume that surround the heart (27).

Summary

Myocardial and chamber stiffnesses are two different determinants of the left ventricular diastolic pressure-volume relationship. Myocardial stiffness depends on intrinsic properties of the myocardium (64). Chamber stiffness depends on myocardial stiffness, extent of relaxation, viscoelastic forces, ventricular shape and wall thickness, coronary turgor, the pericardium, interaction with the other cardiac chambers within the pericardium, intrathoracic pressure, and lung volume (Table 13.1).

Because left ventricular filling is a function of transmural end-diastolic pressure, end-diastolic pressure, pulmonary artery wedge pressure, or left atrial pressure are inaccurate indexes of ventricular preload. End-diastolic volume that determines the end-diastolic sarcomere length is the major preload determinant of ventricular systolic performance independently of intraventricular pressure (112). *Thus, acute changes in the left ventricular diastolic pressure-volume relationship do not permit one to analyze ventricular function curves by plotting systolic performance against end-diastolic pressure. An*

Table 13.1
Factors That Affect Left Ventricular Filling

End-systolic volume
Loading conditions
Relaxation
  Velocity
  Extent
  Nonuniformity
Myocardial passive properties:
  Stiffness (collagen, fibrosis, passive properties of myocytes)
  Thickness
  Viscoelastic properties
Left atria mechanical passive properties
Atrial contraction
Ventricular interaction in the pericardium
Erectile effect of the coronary circulation

elevation or a decrease of end-diastolic pressure may correspond to the same, smaller, or higher left ventricular volume (24).

Myocardial Contractility and Left Ventricular Contraction

Basic Determinants of Myocyte Contractility

In mammals, ventricular myocyte activation and relaxation are due to the release and binding of calcium by the sarcoplasmic reticulum. Contraction is determined by the entry of calcium through the sarcolemma during the action potentials followed by the release of calcium by the sarcoplasmic reticulum, binding of calcium to troponin C, and formation and cycling of myosin cross-bridges with actin (21) that result in shortening generation, which develops force along the axis of shortening. Calcium binding to troponin facilitates cross-bridge binding to actin and, reciprocally, cross-bridge binding to actin facilitates calcium binding to troponin (37). This explains the deactivation effect of shortening because shortening reduces the number of attached cross-bridges (71). In addition, shortening reduces the force generated by each bridge (37). These effects are enhanced by the velocity of shortening (37).

Contractility of the myocardium is determined *(a)* by the number of cross-bridges activated (77), and *(b)* by the rate of cross-bridge cycling (69). Phosphorylation and dephosphorylation of myosin light chains may modulate cross-bridge kinetics (17). Myocardial contractility may also be modulated by the endothelium (14, 17) and several circulating substances.

Preload as a Positive Inotropic Factor

Traditional concepts of sarcomere mechanics suggest that the length-tension relation depends on overlap of the myofilaments (165) so that the inotropic state is not affected by changes in muscle length. However, diastolic volume and inotropic state are not independent regulators of cardiac performance (152) because intracellular calcium stores and troponin C calcium af-

finity are altered by muscle length (152).

In normal heart, the left ventricle works near the peak of its function curve, which corresponds to an end-diastolic pressure of 10 mm Hg in the supine position (114). As a pressure of 12 mm Hg has been demonstrated to correspond to a sarcomere length of 2.2 μm, a value associated with maximal tension generation (139), there is little reserve remaining in the Starling mechanism. However, performance may be enhanced by transmural recruitment and recruitment of unaligned fibers (165).

Left Ventricular Contraction

Ventricular contraction is a complex process that made the changes in performance due to increased contractility unable to be reflected by changes in indices derived from studies on isolated muscles (30). Since the mechanical behavior of the myocardium is greatly dependent on preload and on afterload, there is no simple method to evaluate the inotropic state of the left ventricle. In addition, heart rate, ventricular size, shape, and mass should also be considered (127).

End-systolic volume to which the ventricle contracts is a linearly increasing function of end-systolic ventricular pressure (146) (Fig. 13.1). The magnitude of slope of the end-systolic pressure-volume relation (volume elastance or end-systolic elastance) is representative of active stiffness of ventricular wall and is mainly determined by the contractile state. However, the end-systolic pressure-volume relationship is nonlinear and depends on afterload (43), chamber size (38, 144), and cavity shape (61). Nevertheless, providing a stable contractile state and a constant heart rate, maximal elastance is weakly affected by alterations in ventricular preload, afterload, or both (146). For clinical use, the end-systolic pressure-volume is probably the better way to assess myocardial contractility. For current practice, end-systolic stress-to-volume ratio may be particularly useful in that it takes into account pressure, cavity dimensions, and myocardial mass although this index is also size dependent in normal subjects (38).

Afterload and Ventriculoarterial Coupling

Arterial Impedance and Left Ventricular Afterload

Afterload determines both ejection pressure and the ability of the left ventricle to empty, and it influences myocardial oxygen consumption in that pressure work is energetically more costly than volume work (79). Systemic vascular resistance is not a reliable index of ventricular afterload, and discordant changes in ventricular afterload and systemic vascular resistance may occur during pharmacologic interventions (88). A better measure of ventricular afterload may be provided by end-systolic stress (124). Left ventricular afterload also can be appropriately represented by the integral of ventricular systolic wall stress over time. However, systolic stress that depends on the shape, dimensions, and wall thickness of the ventricle (57) does not entirely define the afterload because inertia and viscosity of the system (arterial and blood) are not taken into account.

Aorta and large arteries are distensible elastic elements that constitute a damping chamber transforming pulsatile blood flow generated by the left ventricular contraction into a near-constant flow for resistance vessels. *Thus, it appears that afterload should take into account all the factors that oppose ventricular ejection, i.e., aortic input impedance (101).*

The relation between pressure and flow in the systemic circulation is determined by the physical properties of the blood and the arterial wall (101). This relation is complicated by the sinusoidal characteristics of pressure and flow and their harmonics. The vascular impedance spectrum depends (a) on the characteristic impedance that is directly related to the vessel viscoelasticity and inversely related to its cross-sectional area, (b) on pressure and flow waves reflected from distal parts of the arterial tree, and (c) on viscosity and density of the blood. The aortic impedance spectrum (or input impedance of the systemic circulation) represents the hydraulic load presented to the ventricular ejection (101). It constitutes the more appropriate definition of afterload because it is dependent on vascular resistance, arterial compliance, and reflected waves. In addition it takes into account heart rate. Aortic impedance can be altered by physiological stimuli (autonomic nervous system, circulating substances), pharmacological agents (117), and pathological processes (atherosclerosis).

The arterial system can be represented by the three-element Windkessel model (159) composed of a characteristic impedance, a resistance, and a capacitance (or compliance). It has been demonstrated that, if the vascular parameters and systolic and diastolic times remain constant, end-systolic pressure increases linearly with stroke volume (147) (Fig. 13.5). The slope of the relation, named effective arterial elastance, is increased and stroke volume is reduced when arterial resistance rises. Conversely,

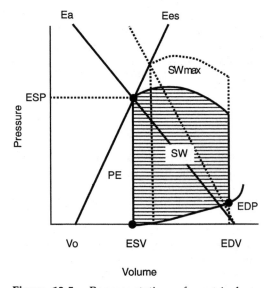

Figure 13.5. Representation of ventriculoarterial coupling. Physiological values of stroke work *(SW)*, end-diastolic pressure and volume *(EDP* and *EDV*, respectively), and end-systolic pressure and volume *(ESP* and *ESV*, respectively) are obtained when arterial elastance *(Ea)* is lower than left ventricular end-systolic elastance *(Ees)*. Maximal stroke work *(SWmax)* is produced when arterial elastance equals left ventricular elastance. *Vo*, volume axis intercept of the end-systolic pressure-volume relationship. (Redrawn from Asanoi H, Sasayama S, Kameyama T. Ventriculoarterial coupling in normal and failing heart in humans. Circ Res 1989;65:483–493.)

arterial compliance has little effect on the slope.

Ventriculoarterial Coupling

Matching between an energy source and its mechanical load is achieved when a maximal amount of energy is transferred from one to the other. This is realized when input impedance of the receptor equals output impedance of the energy source.

Left ventricular stroke work has been demonstrated to be maximal when ventricular end-systolic elastance, which represents the output impedance, equals effective arterial elastance (Fig. 13.5), which represents the input impedance (19). Superposition of the arterial pressure-volume relation on the ventricular pressure-volume relation in the same diagram so that the origin of the arterial relation falls on the end-diastolic volume point provides a graphic representation of the coupling between mechanical properties of the arterial system and the ventricle (147). Consequences of increasing end-diastolic volume, myocardial contractility, and arterial resistance can be predicted by this model (Fig. 13.4, C–E).

Mechanical Efficiency of the Left Ventricle

Physiological values of left ventricular end-diastolic and end-systolic volumes as well as end-systolic pressure are obtained when arterial impedance is approximatively one half the left ventricular impedance (19). In this situation, mechanical efficiency, that is the ratio of stroke work to myocardial oxygen consumption per beat or to pressure-volume area (111), is maximal but stroke work is lower than its maximal level (Fig. 13.5). Mechanical efficiency is rapidly reduced when stroke work is mildly altered by variations of arterial impedance. However, in vivo, acute elevation of vascular resistance or arterial impedance is followed by a progressive adaptation of preload (end-diastolic volume) and myocardial contractility, i.e., ventricular impedance (29). Enhancement of myocardial contractility produces an elevation of both arterial and ventricular impedances (111). When end-diastolic volume is reduced, stroke work approaches its maximal value relative to myocardial oxygen consumption, and mechanical efficiency is increased.

In cardiac failure, there is a progressive decrease in ventricular impedance and a progressive increase in arterial impedance and a mismatch occurs between the ventricle and the arterial load (5) (Fig. 13.6). *Stroke work and mechanical efficiency become more dependent on afterload alterations than in normal heart (19).* Reduction of afterload

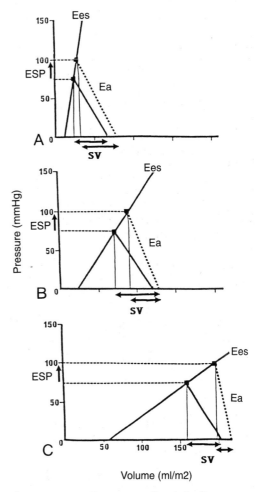

Figure 13.6. Representation of the consequences of increasing preload on ventriculoarterial coupling and stroke work. *A*, Patients with ejection fraction higher than 60%. *B*, Patients with ejection fraction between 40 and 59%. *C*, Patients with ejection fraction lower than 40%. *ESP*, end-systolic pressure; *SV*, stroke volume; *Ees*, left ventricular end-systolic elastance; *Ea*, arterial elastance. (Redrawn from Asanoi H, Sasayama S, Kameyama T. Ventriculoarterial coupling in normal and failing heart in humans. Circ Res 1989;65:483–493.)

has three major beneficial effects: *(a)* reduction of ventricular volume reduces the total energy expenditure; *(b)* ejection rate and stroke volume are enhanced with a decrease of energy expenditure due to the shorter fiber length; and *(c)* the efficiency of the myocardium is increased (36). Afterload reduction has other benefits due to decrease in diastolic pressure: it avoids pulmonary edema and it enhances the subendocardial perfusion (83).

Summary

The left ventricle can be represented as a power generator that delivers a fixed amount of total energy to arterial circulation. There is a permanent equilibrium between ventricular output and arterial flow. This ventriculoarterial coupling has the following properties (19): *(a)* stroke work is maximal when arterial impedance equals ventricular impedance; *(b)* afterload producing ventricular maximal stroke work is higher than afterload producing maximal mechanical efficiency; *(c)* mechanical efficiency is more sensitive to afterload alterations than is stroke work; *(d)* ventricular and arterial mechancial properties are matched in order to produce the higher mechanical efficiency rather than the higher stroke work making *ventriculoarterial coupling governed by the mechanical efficiency.* This optimal adaptation depends on end-diastolic volume, heart rate, and myocardial contractility.

The use of the entire pressure-volume loop for the characterization of left ventricular performance (a) allows separation of loading factors from ventricular properties, (b) clarifies the interrelationship between systolic and diastolic properties and (c) analyzes the coupling between ventricular and arterial mechanical properties enabling one to predict stroke volume and stroke work alterations produced by loading changes (75).

OTHER DETERMINANTS OF LEFT VENTRICULAR PERFORMANCE

Coronary Circulation and Myocardial Perfusion

Coronary circulation is an important determinant of left ventricular performance because an imbalance between myocardial oxygen demand and supply is rapidly followed by alterations of myocardial function that affect lusitropy, contractility, and passive properties of the myocardium. Major determinants of coronary blood supply are aortic pressure, myocardial extravascular compression, heart rate, and neural control through parasympathetic and sympathetic balance effects on coronary vasculature (32). Below the lower limit of coronary autoregulation (40–70 mm Hg), subendocardial ischemia may occur (20). Critical pressure may depend on the type of inhaled anesthetics (67) and heart rate (20). In addition, a mild coronary stenosis may become physiologically significant if a reduction of aortic pressure results in a distal coronary pressure below the critical pressure (20). Conversely, increased coronary flow per se enhances left ventricular contractility and myocardial oxygen consumption through Gregg's phenomenon (55, 100). It must be remembered that changes in intramyocardial blood volume during relaxation and diastole can affect diastolic properties of the left ventricle through an erectile effect (155).

Heart Rate

Apart from its effects on preload and afterload, heart rate must be considered because it alters performance per stroke and myocardial inotropic state (120). Heart rate represents a positive inotropic stimulus (42) even when end-diastolic and end-systolic volumes and ejection fraction decline (125). An increase in heart rate also increases the critical distal coronary pressure required for adequate subendocardial perfusion and reduces the diastolic coronary perfusion time (20).

Systolic Ventricular Interaction

Diastolic leftward displacement of the interventricular septum due to right ventricular loading persists during systole despite the higher left ventricular systolic pressure suggesting that diastolic events may alter systolic shape and function of the left ventricle (135). This shift enhances left ventricular stroke volume, slowed relaxation velocity, and increased inhomogeneity of relaxation for physiological range of right ventricular pressure (135). Right ventricular systolic hypertension (81) increases left ventricular stroke work and end-systolic elastance for a given end-diastolic volume, but reduces the actual left ventricular stroke work because preload is reduced (33).

Left Ventricular Hypertrophy

Hypertrophy is a physiologic adaptation occuring in response to chronic mechanical overload. Myocardial mass increase is due to myocyte enlargement, which increases the number of contractile elements per cell (161). Pressure overload results in concentric hypertrophy and volume overload results in eccentric hypertrophy. Myocardial hypertrophy of normal growth does not alter myocardial contractility. However, sustained cardiac overload is responsible for progressive deterioration of contractile properties, impaired relaxation (91) and passive stiffness of the myocardium (56). Degeneration of the myocytes is due to mechanical exhaustion and to alteration of coronary microcirculation, which produce a progressive increase of interstitial fibrosis (109).

Neurohormonal and Hormonal Interactions

Maintenance of circulatory homeostasis depends on various integrated actions on cardiac and vascular systems. Among them, actions of the autonomic nervous system, renin-angiotensin-aldosterone system, arginine-vasopressin, and atriopeptin are important.

Central Nervous System Release of Neurohormones

Neurohormones play an important role in systemic blood pressure, myocardial contractility, and renal function (113).

Autonomic Nervous System

Coordination between ventricular output and systemic vascular vessels (resistance and capacitance) depends on the autonomic nervous system (133). Afferent fibers, the central integrating system located in the brainstem, and efferent fibers form reflex arcs that elicit responses in the heart and blood vessels, which are directed to adapt the cardiovascular system to any disturbance of its equilibrium in order to maintain arterial pressure that provides satisfactory perfusion of heart and brain. The center receives input from arterial baro- and chemoreceptors, cardiopulmonary receptors, higher brain centers, and peripheral ergoreceptors and is connected to vagus and sympathetic nuclei. Cardiovascular responses are modulated by sympathetic and parasympathetic crosstalk that controls heart rate and vascular tone. Parasympathetic controls heart rate; sympathetic controls systemic vascular resistance (34). Dominant aortic action controls sympathetic nerve activity, and dominant carotid action controls heart rate (129).

Parasympathetic stimulation reduces ventricular performance (142). Duration of action potential is shortened (activation of potassium conductance), activated guanine nucleotide binding protein inhibits the adenylate cyclase activity (62), and the opening of calcium channels is inhibited (Fig. 13.7).

Sympathetic stimulation acts on α- and β-adrenergic receptors. α_1- and α_2-Receptors are sensitive mainly to norepinephrine released at nerve terminals. Stimulation of α_1-receptors mobilizes intracellular stores of calcium that results in contraction of smooth muscle cells (arterial and venous) and cardiac myocytes. However, α_1-receptor density is extremely low in the myocardium (12), where they increase the calcium affinity of troponin C and thus alter both contraction and relaxation (17) (Fig. 13.7). α_2-Receptor stimulation evokes an inhibition of adenylate cyclase (47) and inhibits the release of norepinephrine by terminal nerves (92). β_1-Receptors are located in the heart conducting system (increased heart rate and conduction). β_2 subtype evokes dilation of coronary microvessels, skeletal muscle resistance vessels, and cutaneous veins. Human ventricular myocardium contains a high proportion of β_2-receptors (12). β-Receptor stimulation activates adenylate cyclase (Fig. 13.7). By increasing cellular levels of cAMP, force and velocity of contraction are improved by increasing cross-bridge number and cycling rate (69), and rate of relaxation is enhanced (lusitropic effect) because of

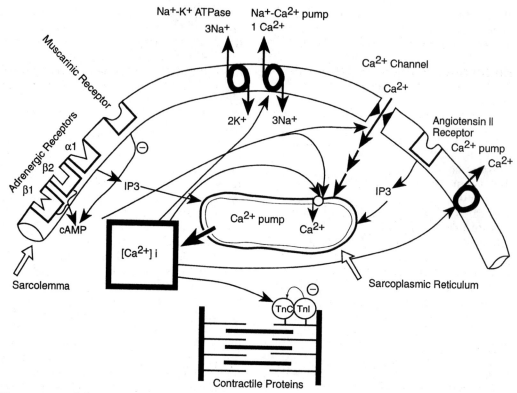

Figure 13.7. Schematic representation of the basic determinants of the cardiac myocyte. *[Ca²⁺]i*, intramyoplasmic calcium; *cAMP*, cyclic adenosine monophosphate; *IP3*, inositol triphosphate; *TnC*, troponin C; *TnI*, troponin I.

reuptake of calcium by the sarcoplasmic reticulum and by desensitization of troponin C due to phosphorylation of troponin I (17).

Arginine-vasopressin is a potent vasoconstrictor released by the posthypophysis (105). Arginine-vasopressin increases heart rate (6) and cardiac filling pressures by elevation of venous return (6). The effect of arginine-vasopressin on smooth muscle cells is mediated by a specific receptor (V2) different from the renal nephronic receptor (V1), which is responsible for water retention. Arginine-vasopressin also induces the release of atriopeptin probably by increasing atrial stretch (106).

Renin-Angiotension-Aldosterone System

The renin-angiotension system is a major component of circulatory regulation in health and disease. It is a classical endocrine system governed by the secretory activity of the juxtaglomerular apparatus in the kidney. β-Adrenergic stimulation or stimulation of sensory receptors in renal arterioles due to pressure reduction leads to release of renin and production of circulating angiotensin I. The preferential target of angiotensin II is the smooth muscle cell inducing contraction through a release of calcium by endoplasmic reticulum (60). Peripheral resistance is increased, arterial compliance is reduced, and aortic impedance (afterload) is increased. Membrane receptors for angiotensin II also have been demonstrated in human heart (154) (Fig. 13.7) and their stimulation induces a positive inotropic response (39, 104). In addition, through its action on aldosterone secretion, angiotension II induces salt and water retention that result in volume expansion (preload). Moreover, angiotensin

II enhances vasopressin secretion (119) and potentiates activation of the adrenergic system by a presynaptic action (80).

Endocrine, Autocrine, Paracrine, and Intracrine Functions of the Heart

Components of the renin-angiotensin system are evident in cardiac myocyte and non-myocyte cells (28). Renin is extracted from the plasma, and the other components of the system (angiotensinogen and converting enzyme) are synthetized locally (66). The cardiac renin-angiotensin system exerts endocrine, autocrine, paracrine, and intracrine functions (123) and probably interacts with locally generated catecholamines, calcitonin-related peptide, substance P, and other nonidentified substances that may alter myocardial contractility and coronary perfusion and induce hypertrophy. In addition, left ventricular performance can be altered by the action of the coronary vascular renin-angiotensin system.

Atriopeptin is synthesized and stored mainly in atrial cardiocytes. Its release is increased by elevation of atrial stretch (89) (congestive heart failure, atrial tachycardia (7)). Release of atriopeptin may also be due to acetylcholine, α- and β-receptor stimulation, vasopressin (150), and sodium ions (4). Atriopeptin has direct vasodilator effects on systemic circulation and on coronary circulation, which does not depend on the endothelium (23), and may have a direct depressor effect on the myocardium (84). In addition, atriopeptin exerts a sympathoinhibitory action through a direct central or a ganglionic action that results in hypotensive action (35) and antagonizes the action of other endogenous vasoconstrictor systems (renin-angiotensin, vasopressin) (90, 113). Vasodilator effects appear when vascular tone is elevated. Atriopeptin also alters renal function, and reduces aldosterone secretion (106). *Thus, the atriopeptin system functions as a cardiac endocrine system (106).*

Endothelin

Endothelin, a peptide produced by vascular endothelium (163), has vasoconstric-

tor action, modulatory effects on the renin-angiotensin-aldosterone system, and antinatriuretic effects (96). It has also been shown to induce positive chronotropic and inotropic effects in human hearts by direct effect on cardiac myocytes (103); however, its physiological role is questioned.

Hypoxia and Acidosis

Arterial hypoxemia results in an increased heart rate. As hypoxic stimulation of carotid bodies produces bradycardia (85), it appears that hypoxic tachycardia results from phasic pulmonary afferent feedback and is related to the strength of the Hering-Breuer reflex (76).

Acidosis has been demonstrated to depress myocardial contractility through a decrease in calcium sensitivity of myofilaments (31). Left ventricular performance is reduced although left ventricular stroke volume may be normal and cardiac output increased because end-diastolic volume is increased by enhancement of venous return, afterload is reduced by peripheral vasodilation, and heart rate is increased (156).

Reflex

Heart and blood vessel performance is mainly modulated by sympathetic and parasympathetic systems. However, numerous other reflexes have been depicted that act on the left ventricle.

Reflex Originating in the Heart

Mechanoreceptors or chemoreceptors located in atria and ventricular walls support various reflexes. Distension of walls, potassium ions, lactic acid, bradykinin, and prostaglandins may alter heart rate and/or systemic vascular resistance.

The Bainbridge reflex depends on venoatrial stretch receptors that signal cardiac filling through vagal afferents. It elicits tachycardia by increasing sympathetic outflow and diuresis.

The Bezold-Jarisch reflex resides within the activation of receptors located in the left ventricular wall (166). It results in peripheral vasodilation due to withdrawal of α-adrenergic tone and cholinergic stimulation, and bradycardia due to a vagal origin (166).

Reflexes Originating Elsewhere

Work receptors of skeletal muscles are activated by chemicals released (potassium and hydrogen ions) and tension in the muscle. They result in tachycardia, vasoconstriction, and positive inotropic effect. Somatic pain or visceral pain can evoke tachycardia and hypertension for the former, bradycardia and hypotension for the latter.

CONCLUSION

Because blood flows in a circle, stroke volume contributes to end-systolic volume, end-systolic volume contributes both to left ventricular relaxation that influences rapid filling and to end-diastolic volume, and end-diastolic volume is a major determinant of stroke volume so that systolic and diastolic functions are clearly interdependent.

Left ventricular performance results from the subtle interplay between three basic determinants: lusitropy, passive properties, and contractility of the myocardium. However, it must be remembered that left ventricular performance can be altered by heart rate and interactions with the other cardiac chambers within the pericardium (especially the right ventricle) and with lungs within the thorax. Furthermore, left ventricular function is submitted to numerous stimuli (through action of the autonomic nervous system and circulating factors) resulting from multiple interactions with systems implicated in body homeostasis. Importantly, heart can control its own function through autocrine, paracrine, and intracrine functions (Fig. 13.8).

References

1. Allen DG, Orchard CH. Myocardial contractile function during ischemia and hypoxia. Circ Res 1987;60:107–122.
2. Alvares RF, Shaver JA, Gamble WH, Goodwin JF. Isovolumic relaxation period in hypertrophic cardiomyopathy. J Am Coll Cardiol 1984;3:71–81.

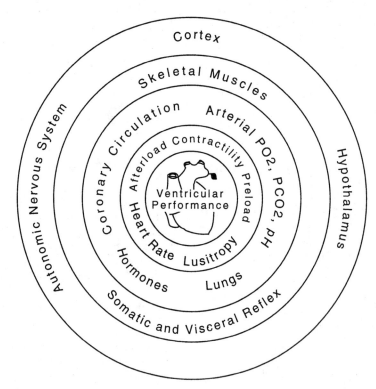

Figure 13.8. Diagrammatic representation of factors that are involved in the determination of left ventricular performance.

3. Ariel Y, Gaasch WH, Bogen DK, McMahon TA. Load-dependent relaxation with late systolic volume steps: servo-pump studies in the intact canine heart. Circulation 1987;75:1287–1294.
4. Arjamaa O, Vuolteenaho O. Sodium ions stimulate the release of atrial natriuretic peptide (ANP) from rat atria. Biochem Biophys Res Commun 1985;132:375–381.
5. Asanoi H, Sasayama S, Kameyama T. Ventriculoarterial coupling in normal and failing heart in humans. Circ Res 1989;65:483–493.
6. Aylward PE, Floras JS, Leimbach WN Jr, Abboud FM. Effects of vasopressin on the circulation and its baroreflex control in healthy men. Circulation 1986;73:1145–1154.
7. Bilder GE, Siegl PKS, Schofield TL, Friedman PA. Chronotropic stimulation: a primary effector for release of atrial natriuretic factor. Circ Res 1989;64:799–805.
8. Bing OHL, Matsushita S, Fanburg BL, Levine HJ. Mechanical properties of rat cardiac muscle during experimental hypertrophy. Circ Res 1971;28:234–245.
9. Blaustein AS, Gaasch WH. Myocardial relaxation. III. Reoxygenation mechanics in the intact dog heart. Circ Res 1981;49:633–639.
10. Bove AA, Santamore WP. Ventricular interdependence. Prog Cardiovasc Dis 1981;23:365–388.
11. Bristow JD, Van Zee B, Judkins MP. Systolic and diastolic abnormalities of the left ventricle in coronary artery disease. Circulation 1970;42:219–228.
12. Bristow MR, Ginsburg R, Umans V, Fowler M, Minobe W, Rasmussen R, Zera P, Menlove R, Shah P, Jamieson S, Stinson EB. β_1- and β_2-adrenergic-receptor subpopulations in nonfailing and failing human ventricular myocardium: coupling of both receptor subtypes to muscle contraction and selective β_1-receptor down-regulation in heart failure. Circ Res 1986;59:297–309.
13. Brutsaert DL, Housmans PR, Goethals MA. Dual control of relaxation. Its role in the ventricular function in the mammalian heart. Circ Res 1980;47:637–652.
14. Brutsaert DL, Meulemans AL, Sipido AR, Sys SU. Effects of damaging the endocardial surface on the mechanical performance of isolated cardiac muscle. Circ Res 1988;62:358–366.
15. Brutsaert DL, Rademakers FE, Sys SU. Triple control of relaxation: implications in cardiac disease. Circulation 1984;69:190–196.
16. Brutsaert DL, Rademakers FE, Sys SU, Gillebert TC, Housmans PR. Analysis of relaxation in the evaluation of ventricular function of the heart. Prog Cardiovasc Dis 1985;28:143–163.
17. Brutsaert DL, Sys SU. Relaxation and diastole of the heart. Physiol Rev 1989;69:1298–1315.
18. Buccino RA, Spann JF Jr, Pool PE, Sonnenblick EH, Braunwald E. Influence of the thyroid state on the intrinsic contractile properties and energy stores of the myocardium. J Clin Invest 1967;46:1669–1682.
19. Burkhoff D, Sagawa K. Ventricular efficiency predicted by an analytical model. Am J Physiol 1986;250:R1021–R1027.
20. Canty JM Jr, Giglia J, Kandath D. Effect of tachycardia on regional function and transmural myocardial perfusion during graded coronary pressure reduction in conscious dogs. Circ Res 1990;82:1815–1825.
21. Chapman RA, Excitation-contraction coupling in cardiac muscle. Prog Biophys Mol Biol 1979;35:1–52.
22. Cheng CP, Freeman GL, Santamore WP, Constantinescu MS, Little WC. Effect of loading conditions, contractile state, and heart rate on early diastolic left ventricular filling in conscious dogs. Circ Res 1990;66:814–823.
23. Chu A, Morris KG, Kuehl WD, Kusma J, Navetta F, Cobb FR. Effects of atrial natriuretic peptide on the coronary arterial vasculature in humans. Circulation 1989;80:1627–1635.
24. Courtois M, Kovacs SJ Jr, Ludbrook PA. Transmitral pressure-flow velocity relation. Importance of regional gradients in the left ventricle during diastole. Circulation 1988;78:661–671.
25. Courtois M, Kovacs SJ, Ludbrook PA. Physiological early diastolic intraventricular pressure gradient is lost during acute myocardial ischemia. Circulation 1990;81:1688–1696.
26. Diamond G, Forrester JS. Effect of coronary artery disease and acute myocardial infarction on left ventricular compliance in man. Circulation 1972;45:11–19.
27. Ditchey RV. Volume-dependent effects of positive airway pressure on intracavitary left ventricular end-diastolic pressure. Circulation 1984;69:815–821.
28. Dzau VJ, Re RN. Evidence for the existence of renin in the heart. Circulation 1987;75(suppl I):I-134–I-136.
29. Elzinga G, Westerhof N. Pressure and flow generated by the left ventricle against different impedances. Circ Res 1973;32:178–186.
30. Elzinga G, Westerhof N. How to quantify pump function of the heart. The value of variables derived from measurements on isolated muscle. Circ Res 1979;43:303–308.
31. Fabiato A, Fabiato FJ. Effects of pH on the myofilaments and the sarcoplasmic reticulum of skinned cells from cardiac and skeletal muscles. J Physiol (Lond) 1978;276:233–255.
32. Feigl EO. Coronary physiology. Physiol Rev 1983;63:1–205.
33. Feneley MP, Olsen CO, Glower DD, Rankin JS. Effect of acutely increased right ventricular afterload on work output from the left ventricle in conscious dogs. Systolic ventricular interaction. Circ Res 1989;65:135–145.
34. Ferguson DW, Abboud FM, Mark AL. Relative contribution of aortic and carotid baroreflexes to heart rate control in man during steady state and dynamic increases in arterial pressure. J Clin Invest 1985:76:2265–2274.
35. Floras JS. Sympathoinhibitory effects of atrial natriuretic factor in normal humans. Circulation 1990;81:1860–1873.
36. Ford LE Effect of afterload reduction on myocardial energetics. Circ Res 1980;46:16–166.
37. Ford LE. Mechanical manifestations of activation in cardiac muscle. Circ Res 1991;68:621–637.
38. Foult JM, Loiseau A, Nitenberg A. Size dependence of end-systolic stress/volume ratio in hu-

mans: implications for the evaluation of myocardial contractile performance in pressure and volume overload. J Am Coll Cardiol 1990;16:124–129.

39. Foult JM, Tavolaro O, Antony I, Nitenberg A. Direct myocardial and coronary effects of enalaprilat in patients with dilated cardiomyopathy: assessment by a bilateral intracoronary technique. Circulation 1988;77:337–344.

40. Frais MA, Bergman DW, Kingma I, Smiseth OA, Smith ER, Tyberg JV. The dependence of time constant of left ventricular isovolumic relaxation (τ) on pericardial pressure. Circulation 1990; 81:1071–1080.

41. Freeman GL, LeWinter MM. Pericardial adaptations during chronic cardiac dilation in dogs. Circ Res. 1984;54:294–300.

42. Freeman GL, Little WC, O'Rourke RA. Influence of heart rate on left ventricular performance in dogs. Circ Res 1987;61:455–464.

43. Freeman GL, Little WC, O'Rourke RA. The effects of vasoactive agents on the left ventricular end-systolic pressure-volume relation in closed-chest dogs. Circulation 1986;74:1107–1113.

44. Gaasch WH, Cole JS, Quinones MA, Alexander JK. Dynamic determinants of left ventricular diastolic pressure-volume relations in man. Circulation 1975;51:317–323.

45. Gaasch WH, Levine HJ, Quinones MA, Alexander J. Left ventricular compliance: mechanisms and clinical implications. Am J Cardiol 1976;38:645–653.

46. Gilbert JC, Glantz SA. Determinants of left ventricular filling and of the diastolic pressure-volume relation. Circ Res 1989;64:827–852.

47. Gilman AG. G proteins and dual control of adenylate cyclase. Cell 1984;36:577–579.

48. Glantz SA. A constitutive equation for the passive properties of the muscle. J Biochem 1974; 7:137–145.

49. Glantz SA, Kernoff RS. Muscle stiffness determined from canine left ventricular pressure-volume curves. Circ Res 1975;37:787–794.

50. Glantz SA, Parmley WW. Factors which affect the diastolic pressure-volume curve. Circ Res 1978;42:171–180.

51. Goldstein JA, Vlahakes GJ, Verrier ED, Schiller NB, Tyberg JV, Ports TA, Parmley WW, Chatterjee A. The role of right ventricular systolic dysfunction and elevated intrapericardial pressure in the genesis of low output in experimental right ventricular infarction. Circulation 1982;65:513–522.

52. Goto Y, LeWinter MM. Nonuniform regional deformation of the pericardium during the cardiac cycle in dogs. Circ Res 1990;67:1107–1114.

53. Goto Y, Yamamoto J, Saito M, Haze K, Sumiyoshi T, Fukami K, Hiramori K. Effects of right ventricular ischemia on left ventricular geometry and the end-diastolic pressure-volume relationship in the dog. Circulation 1985;72:1104–1114.

54. Granger CH, Karimeddini MK, Smith VE, Shapiro HR, Katz AM, Riba AL. Rapid ventricular filling in left ventricular hypertrophy. J Am Coll Cardiol 1985;5:862–868.

55. Gregg DE. Regulation of the collateral and coronary circulation of the heart. In: Mitchell J, ed. Circulation Proceedings of the Harvey Tercentenary Congress. Oxford: Blackwell, 1958:163–186.

56. Grossman W. Cardiac hypertrophy: useful adaptation or pathologic process. Am J Med 1980;69:576–584.

57. Grossman W, Jones D, McLaurin LP. Wall stress and patterns of hypertrophy in human left ventricle. J Clin Invest 1975;56:56–64.

58. Grossman W, McLaurin LP, Rolett EL. Alterations of left ventricular relaxation and diastolic compliance in congestive cardiomyopathy. Cardiovasc Res 1979;13:514–522.

59. Grossman W, Stefadouros MA, McLaurin LP, Rolett EL, Young DT. The quantitative assessment of left ventricular diastolic stiffness in man. Circulation 1973;47:567–574.

60. Guillemette G, Balla T, Baukal AJ, Spät A, Catt K. Intracellular receptors for inositol 1,4,5-triphosphate in angiotensin II target tissue. J Biol Chem 1987;262:1010–1015.

61. Hansen DE, Cahill PD, DeCampli WM, Harrison DC, Derby GC, Mitchell RS, Miller DC. Valvular-ventricular interaction: importance of mitral apparatus in canine left ventricular systolic performance. Circulation 1986;73:1310–1320.

62. Hescheler J, Kameyama M, Trautwein W. On the mechanism of muscarinic inhibition of the cardiac calcium current. Eur J Physiol 1986;407:182–189.

63. Hess OM, Grimm J, Krayenbuehl HP. Diastolic simple elastic and viscoelastic properties of the left ventricle in man. Circulation 1979;59:1178–1187.

64. Hess OM, Ritter M, Schneider J, Grimm J, Turina M, Krayenbuehl HP. Diastolic stiffness and myocardial structure in aortic valve disease before and after valve replacement. Circulation 1984;69:855–865.

65. Hess OM, Schneider J, Koch R, Bamert C, Grimm J, Krayenbuehl HP. Diastolic function and myocardial structure in patients with myocardial hypertrophy: special reference to normalized viscoelastic data. Circulation 1981;63:360–371.

66. Hial V, Gimbrone MA, Peyton MP, Wilcox CM, Pisano JJ. Angiotensin metabolism by cultured human vascular endothelial and smooth muscle cells. Microvasc Res 1979;17:314–329.

67. Hickey RF, Sybert PE, Verrier ED, Cason BA. Effects of halothane, enflurane, and isoflurane on coronary blood flow autoregulation and coronary vascular reserve in the canine heart. Anesthesiology 1988;68:21–30.

68. Hirota Y. A clinical study of left ventricular relaxation. Circulation 1980;62:756–763.

69. Hoh JFY, Rossmanith GH, Kwan LJ, Hamilton AM. Adrenaline increases the rate of cycling of crossbridges in rat cardiac muscle as measured by pseudo-random binary noise-modulated perturbation analysis. Circ Res 1988;62:452–461.

70. Hori M, Yellin EL, Sonnenblick EH. Left ventricular diastolic suction as a mechanism of ventricular filling. Jpn Circ J 1982;46:124–129.

71. Huxley AF. Muscle structure and theories of contraction. Prog Biophys Biophys Chem 1957;7:255–318.

72. Ishida Y, Meisner JS, Tsujioka K, Gallo JI, Yoran C, Frater RWM, Yellin EL. Left ventricular filling dynamics: influence of left ventricular relaxation

and left atrial pressure. Circulation 1986;74:187–196.

73. Janicki JS, Weber KT. The pericardium and ventricular interaction, distensibility and function. Am J Physiol 1980;238:H494–H503.

74. Karliner JS, LeWinter MM, Mahler F, Engler R, O'Rourke RA. Pharmacologic and hemodynamic influences on the rate of isovolumic left ventricular relaxation in the normal conscious dog. J Clin Invest 1977;60:511–521.

75. Kass DA, Maughan WL. From 'Emax' to pressure-volume relation: a broader view. Circulation 1988;77:1203–1212.

76. Kato H, Menon AS, Slutsky AS. Mechanisms mediating the heart rate response to hypoxemia. Circulation 1988;77:407–414.

77. Katz AM. Role of the contractile proteins and sarcoplasmic reticulum in the response of the heart to catecholamines: an historical review. Adv Cyclic Nucleotide Protein Phosphorylation Res 1979;11:303–343.

78. Katz AM. Influence of altered inotropy and lusitropy on ventricular pressure-volume loops. J Am Coll Cardiol 1988;11:438–445.

79. Katz LN, Katz AM, Williams FL. Metabolic adjustments to alterations of cardiac work in hypoxemia. Am J Physiol 1955;181:539–549.

80. Khairallah PA. Action of angiotensin on adrenergic nerve endings: inhibition of norepinephrine uptake. Fed Proc 1972;31:1351–1357.

81. King ME, Braun H, Goldblatt A, Liberthson R, Weyman AE. Interventricular septal configuration as a predictor of right ventricular systolic hypertension in children: a cross-sectional echocardiographic study. Circulation 1983;68:68–75.

82. Kingma I, Tyberg JV, Smith ER. Effects of diastolic transseptal pressure gradient on ventricular septal position and motion. Circulation 1983;68:1304–1314.

83. Kirk ES, LeJemtel TH, Nelson GR, Sonnenblick EH. Mechanisms of beneficial effect of vasodilatation and inotropic stimulation in the experimental feline ischemic heart. Am J Med 1978;65:189–196.

84. Kleinert HD, Volpe M, Odell G, Marion D, Atlas SA, Camargo MJ, Laragh JH, Maack T. Cardiovascular effects of atrial natriuretic factor in anesthetized and conscious dogs. Hypertension 1986;8:312–316.

85. Krasney JA, Koehler RC. Neural control of the circulation during hypoxia. In: Hughes MJ, Barnes CD, eds. Neural control of circulation. New York: Academic Press, 1980:123–147.

86. Krueger JW. Fundamental mechanisms that govern cardiac function: a short review of cardiac sarcomere mechanics. Heart Failure 1988;4:137–153.

87. Lakatta EG, Gerstenblith G, Angell CS, Shock NW, Weisfeldt ML. Prolonged contraction duration in aged myocardium. J Clin Invest 1975;55:61–68.

88. Lang RM, Borow KM, Neumann A, Janzen D. Systemic vascular resistance: an unreliable index of left ventricular afterload. Circulation 1986;74:1114–1123.

89. Lang RE, Thölken H, Ganten D, Luft FC, Ruskoaho H, Unger T. Atrial natriuretic factor—a circulating hormone stimulated by volume loading. Nature 1985;314:264–266.

90. Laragh JH. Atrial natriuretic hormone, the renin-angiotensin axis, and blood pressure-electrolyte homeostasis. N Engl J Med 1985;313:1330–1340.

91. Lecarpentier YC, Martin JL, Gastineau P, Hatt PY. Load dependence of mammalian heart relaxation during cardiac hypertrophy and heart failure. Am J Physiol 1982;242:H855–H861.

92. Leier CV, Binkley PF, Code RJ. α-Adrenergic component of the sympathetic nervous system in congestive heart failure. Circulation 1990;82(suppl I):I-68–I-76.

93. Levine HJ. Compliance of the left ventricle [Editorial]. Circulation 1972;46:423–426.

94. Lew WYW. Evaluation of left ventricular diastolic function. Circulation 1989;79:1393–1397.

95. Ludbrook PA, Byrne JD, McKnight RC. Influence of right ventricular hemodynamics on left ventricular diastolic pressure-volume relations in man. Circulation 1979;59:21–31.

96. Margulies KB, Hildebrand FL Jr, Lerman A, Perrella MA, Burnett JC Jr. Increased endothelin in experimental heart failure. Circulation 1990;82:2226–2230.

97. Maruyama Y, Ashikawa K, Isoyama S, Kanatsuka H, Ino-Oka E, Takishima T. Mechanical interactions between four heart chambers with and without the pericardium in canine hearts. Circ Res 1982;50:86–100.

98. Maruyama K, Kimura S, Juroda M, Handa S. Connectin, an elastic protein of muscle. Its abundance in cardiac muscle. J Biochem 1977;82:347–350.

99. Marzilli M, Sabbah HN, Lee T, Stein PD. Role of the papillary muscle in opening and closure of the mitral valve. Am J Physiol 1980;238:H348–H354.

100. Miller WP, Shimamoto N, Nellis SH, Liedtke AJ. Coronary hyperfusion and myocardial metabolism in isolated and intact hearts. Am J Physiol 1987;253:H1271–H1278.

101. Milnor WR. Arterial impedance as ventricular afterload. Circ Res 1975;36:565–570.

102. Mirsky I. Assessment of diastolic function: suggested methods and future consideration. Circulation 1984;69:836–841.

103. Moody CJ, Dashwood MR, Sykes RM, Chester M, Jones SM, Yacoub MH, Harding SE. Functional and autoradiographic evidence for endothelin 1 receptors on human and cardiac myocytes. Comparison with single smooth muscle cells. Circ Res 1990;67:764–769.

104. Moravec CS, Schluchter MD, Paranandi L, Czerska B, Stewart RW, Rosenkranz E, Bond M. Inotropic effects of angiotensin II on human cardiac muscle in vitro. Circulation 1990;82:1973–1984.

105. Morton JJ, Padfield PL, Forsling ML. A radioimmunoassay for plasma arginine-vasopressin in man and dog: application to physiological and pathological states. J Endocrinol 1975;65:411–424.

106. Needleman P, Greenwald JE. Atriopeptin: a cardiac hormone intimately involved in fluid, elec-

trolyte, and blood-pressure homeostasis. N Engl
J Med 1986;314:828–834.

107. Nikolic SD, Tamura K, Dahm M, Frater RWM,
Yellin EL. Diastolic viscous properties of the
intact canine left ventricle. Circ Res 1990;67:352–
359.

108. Nikolic S, Yellin EL, Tamura K, Frater RWM.
Effect of early diastolic loading on myocardial
relaxation in the intact canine left ventricle. Circ
Res 1990;66:1217–1226.

109. Nitenberg A, Foult JM. The coronary circulation:
clinical data. In: Swynghedauw B, ed. Cardiac
hypertrophy and failure. Paris: Les Editions IN-
SERM, 1990:591–612.

110. Noble MIM, Milne ENC, Goerke RJ, Carlsson
E, Domenech RJ, Saunders KB, Hoffman JIE.
Left ventricular filling and diastolic pressure-
volume relations in the conscious dog. Circ Res
1969;24:269–283.

111. Nozawa T, Yasumura Y, Futaki S, Tanaka N,
Uenishi M, Suga H. Efficiency of energy transfer
from pressure-volume area to external mechanical work increases with contractile state and
decreases with afterload in the ventricle of anesthetized closed-chest dog. Circulation 1988;
77:1116–1124.

112. Olsen CO, Tyberg GS, Maier GW, Spratt JA,
Davis JW, Rankin JS. Dynamic ventricular interaction in the conscious dog. Circ Res 1983;
52:85–104.

113. Packer M. Neurohormonal interactions and adaptations in congestive heart failure. Circulation
1988;77:721–730.

114. Parker JO, Case RB. Normal left ventricular
function. Circulation 1979;60:4–12.

115. Pasipoularides A, Mirsky I, Hess OM, Grimm
J, Krayenbuehl HP. Myocardial relaxation and
passive diastolic properties in man. Circulation
1986;74:991–1001.

116. Paulus W, Serizawa T, Grossman W. Altered
left ventricular diastolic properties during pacing-induced ischemia in dogs with coronary
stenoses. Potentiation by caffeine. Circ Res
1982;50:218–227.

117. Pouleur H, Covell JW, Ross J Jr. Effects of alterations in aortic input impedance on the force-
velocity-length relationship in the intact canine
heart. Circ Res 1979;45:126–135.

118. Pouleur H, Karliner JS, LeWinter MM, Covell
JW. Diastolic viscous properties of the intact
canine left ventricle. Circ Res 1979;45:410–419.

119. Printiz M, Philips MI, Ganten D. The brain
renin-angiotensin system (minireview). In: Ganten D, Printiz M, Philips MI, eds. The renin-
angiotensin system in the brain. New York:
Springer-Verlag, 1982:3–10.

120. Quinones MA, Gaasch WH, Alexander JK. Influence of acute changes in preload, afterload,
contractile state and heart rate on ejection and
isovolumic indices of myocardial contractility in
man. Circulation 1976;53:293–302.

121. Raff GL, Glantz SA. Volume loading slows left
ventricular isovolumic relaxation rate: evidence
of load-dependent relaxation in the intact dog
heart. Circ Res 1981;48:813–824.

122. Rankin JS, Arentzen CE, McHale FA, Ling D,

Anderson RW. Viscoelastic properties of the
diastolic left ventricle in the conscious dog. Circ
Res 1977;41:37–45.

123. Re R, Rovigatti U. New approaches to the study
of the cellular biology of the cardiovascular system. Circulation 1988;77(suppl I):I-14–I-17.

124. Reichek N, Wilson J, St John Sutton M, Plappert
TA, Goldberg S, Hirshfeld JW. Non-invasive
determination of left ventricular end-systolic
stress: validation of the method and initial application. Circulation 1981;65:99–108.

125. Ricci D, Orlick A, Alderman E, Ingels N,
Daughters C, Kusnick C, Reitz B, Stinson E.
Role of tachycardia as an inotropic stimulus in
man. J Clin Invest 1979;63:695–703.

126. Robotham JL, Rabson J, Permutt S, Bromberger-
Barnea B. Left ventricular hemodynamics during respiration. J Appl Physiol 1979;47:1295–
1303.

127. Ross J Jr, Peterson KL. On the assessment of
cardiac inotropic state. Circulation 1973;47:435–
438.

128. Sabbah HN, Stein PD. Pressure-diameter relations during early diastole in dogs. Incompatibility with the concept of passive left ventricular
filling. Circ Res 1981;45:357–365.

129. Sanders JS, Ferguson DW, Mark AL. Arterial
baroreflex control of sympathetic nerve activity
during elevation of blood pressure in normal
man: dominance of aortic baroreflexes. Circulation 1988;77:279–288.

130. Scharf SM, Brown R, Saunders N, Green LH,
Ingram RH. Changes in canine left ventricular
size and configuration with positive end-expiratory pressure. Circ Res 1979;44:672–678.

131. Schwarz F, Flameng W, Schaper J, Herhlein F.
Correlation between myocardial structure and
diastolic properties of the heart in chronic aortic
valve disease. Am J Cardiol 1978;42:895–903.

132. Serizawa T, Vogel WM, Apstein CS, Grossman
W. Comparison of acute alterations of left ventricular relaxation and diastolic chamber stiffness induced by hypoxia and ischemia. J Clin
Invest 1981;68:91–102.

133. Shepherd JT. Circulatory response to exercise
in health. Circulation 1987;76(suppl VI):VI-3–VI-
10.

134. Slinker BK, Glantz SA. End-systolic and end-
diastolic ventricular interaction. Am J Physiol
1986;251:H1062–H1075.

135. Slinker BK, Goto Y, LeWinter MM. Systolic direct ventricular interaction affects left ventricular contraction and relaxation in the intact dog
circulation. Circ Res 1989;65:307–315.

136. Smiseth OA, Frais MA, Kingma I, Smith ER,
Tyberg JV. Assessment of pericardial constraint
in dogs. Circulation 1985;71:158–164.

137. Smith VE, Schulman P, Karimeddini MK, White
WB, Merran MK, Katz AM. Rapid ventricular
filling in left ventricular hypertrophy. II. Pathologic hypertrophy. J Am Coll Cardiol 1985;5:869–
874.

138. Sonnenblick EH. The structural basis and importance of restoring forces and elastic recoil for
the filling of the heart. Eur Heart J 1980;1(suppl
8):423–431.

139. Spotnitz HM, Sonnenblick EH, Spiro D. Relation of ultrastructure to function in the intact heart. Sarcomere structure relative to pressure-volume curves of intact left ventricle of dog and cat. Circ Res 1966;18:49–66.

140. Starling MR, Montgomery DG, Mancini J, Walsh RA. Load independence of rate of isovolumic relaxation in man. Circulation 1987;76:1274–1281.

141. Stool EW, Mullins CB, Leshin SJ, Mitchell JH. Dimensional changes of the left ventricle during acute pulmonary arterial hypertension in dogs. Am J Cardiol 1974;33:868–875.

142. Stratton JR, Pfeifer MA, Halter JB. The hemodynamic effects of sympathetic stimulation combined with parasympathetic blockade in man. Circulation 1987;75:922–929.

143. Suga H. Total mechanical energy of a ventricle model and cardiac oxygen consumption. Am J Physiol. 1979;236:H494–H497.

144. Suga H, Hisano R, Goto Y, Yamada O. Normalization of end-systolic pressure-volume relation and Emax of different sized hearts. Jpn Circ J 1984;48:136–143.

145. Suga H, Hisano R, Goto Y, Yamada O, Igarashi Y. Effect of positive inotropic agents on the relation between oxygen consumption and systolic pressure-volume area in canine left ventricle. Circ Res 1983;53:306–318.

146. Suga H, Sagawa K. Instantaneous pressure-volume relationships and their ratio in the excised, supported canine left ventricle. Circ Res 1974;35:117–126.

147. Sunagawa K, Maughan WL, Burkhoff D, Sagawa K. Left ventricular interaction with arterial load studied in isolated canine ventricle. Am J Physiol 1983;245:H773–H780.

148. Templeton GH, Wildenthal K, Willerson JT, Reardon WC. Influence of temperature on the mechanical properties of cardiac muscle. Circ Res 1974;34:624–634.

149. ter Keurs HEDJ, Rijusburger WH, van Heuningen R, Nagelsmit MJ. Tension development and sarcomere length in rat cardiac trabeculae: evidence of length-dependence activation. Circ Res 1990;46:703–714.

150. Toth M, Ruskoaho H, Lang RE. Regulation of atrial natriuretic peptide secretion. J Hypertens 1986;4(suppl 6):s538–s541.

151. Tsakiris AG, Gordon DA, Padiyar R, Frechette D. Relation of mitral valve opening and closure to left atrial and ventricular pressures in the intact dog. Am J Physiol 1978;234:H146–H151.

152. Tucci PJF, Bregagnollo EA, Spadaro J, Cicogna AC, Ribeiro MCL. Length dependence of activation studied in the isovolumic blood-perfused dog heart. Circ Res 1984;55:59–66.

153. Tyberg JV, Keon WJ, Sonnenblick EH, Urschel CW. Mechanics of ventricular diastole. Cardiovasc Res 1970;4:423–428.

154. Urata H, Healy B, Stewart RW, Bumpus FM, Husain A. Angiotensin II receptors in normal and failing human heart myocytes. J Clin Endocrinol Metab 1989;69:54–66.

155. Vogel WM, Apstein CS, Briggs LL, Gaasch WH, Ahn J. Acute alterations in left ventricular diastolic chamber stiffness: role of the "erectile" effect arterial pressure and flow in normal and damaged heart. Circ Res 1982;51:465–478.

156. Walley KR, Lewis TH, Wood LDH. Acute respiratory acidosis decreases left ventricular contractility but increases cardiac output in dogs. Circ Res 1990;67:628–635.

157. Weisfeldt ML, Armstrong P, Scully HE, Sanders CA, Daggett WM. Incomplete relaxation between beats after myocardial hypoxia and ischemia. J Clin Invest 1974;53:1626–1636.

158. Weiss JL, Frederiksen JW, Weisfeldt ML. Hemodynamic determinants of the time-course of fall in canine left ventricular pressure. J Clin Invest 1976;58:751–760.

159. Westerhof K, Elzinga G, Sipkema P. An artificial arterial system for pumping hearts. J Appl Physiol 1971;31:776–781.

160. Weyman AE, Wann S, Feigenbaum H, Dillon JC. Mechanism of abnormal septal motion in patients with right ventricular volume overload. A cross-sectional echocardiography study. Circulation 1976;54:179–186.

161. Wikman-Coffelt J, Parmley WW, Mason DT. The cardiac hypertrophy process. Analysis of factors determining pathological vs. physiological development. Circ Res 1979;45:697–707.

162. Yamagishi T, Ozaki M, Kumada T, Ikezono T, Shimizu T, Furutani Y, Yamaoka H, Ogawa H, Matsuzaki M, Arima A, Kusukawa R. Asynchronous left ventricular diastolic filling in patients with isolated disease of the left anterior descending coronary artery: assessment with radionuclide ventriculography. Circulation 1984;69:933–942.

163. Yanagisawa M, Kurihara H, Kimura S, Tomobe Y, Kobayashi M, Mitsui Y, Yazaki Y, Goto K, Masaki T. A novel vasoconstrictor peptide produced by vascular endothelial cells. Nature 1988;332:411–415.

164. Yellin EL, Hori M, Yoran C, Sonnenblick EH, Gabbay S, Frater RWM. Left ventricular relaxation in the filling and nonfilling canine heart. Am J Physiol 1986;250:H620–H629.

165. Yoran C, Covell JW, Ross J. Structural basis of the ascending limb of the left ventricular function. Circ Res 1973;32:297–303.

166. Zucker IH, Cornish KG. The Bezold-Jarisch reflex in the conscious dog. Circ Res 1981;49:940–948.

14

Acute Left Ventricular Failure

Didier M. Payen
Sadek Beloucif

According to the considered pathophysiologic concepts, heart failure might correspond to different definitions. In critical care, heart failure is frequently defined as an alteration of cardiac pumping preventing an adequate systemic oxygen delivery at a rate commensurate with aerobic requirements of the metabolizing tissues. Many factors can result in the heart failing as a pump, and the complexity of these factors requires that one be able to distinguish changes in the contractile behavior of the myocardium from those due to altered hydraulic loading. Once the pathophysiology of heart failure has been ascertained, more rational therapeutic strategies can then be recommended.

DEFINITIONS AND CONCEPTS

Heart failure may be defined physiologically as the circumstances in which the heart does not deliver a sufficient cardiac output to maintain oxygen delivery to the tissues at a rate in keeping with their oxygen requirements. In the most advanced stage, i.e., circulatory failure, this energetic imbalance exists at rest. Clinically, heart failure can also be defined as congestive heart failure, which consists of a constellation of symptoms that arises from congested organs to hypoperfused tissues. At the initial compensated stage, compensatory changes allow resting stroke volume to remain normal. However, because of a reduction in cardiac reserve, its capacity to rise in response to several stimuli such as muscular activity, fever, pain, and sepsis is impaired as the severity of cardiac failure is more pronounced.

Many factors and processes can result

in heart failure. If one were to define heart failure etiologies based on cardiac processes, then four large categories can be considered. These are disturbances in rhythm, primary impairment in myocardial contractility, valvular dysfunction, and tamponade (Table 14.1). The most common etiologies for heart failure in the in-

Table 14.1
Pathophysiologic Classification of Heart Failure Etiologies

Abnormal electric conduction
  Bradyarrhythmias
    Sinus
    A-V blockade
  Tachyarrhythmias
    Sinus
    Supraventricular
    Ventricular
  Intraventricular conduction defects
    Ventricular paced beats (rare)
    Idioventricular
    Fascicular blockade
Primary myocardial dysfunction
  Ischemia and infarction
  Electrolyte imbalance
    Hypocalcemia
    Hypophosphatemia
  Dilated and infiltrative cardiomyopathies
    Viral
    Idiopathic
  Asymmetrical septal hypertrophy
  Toxic dysfunction
    Septicemia
    Drug-induced
    Toxemia (rare)
Valvular dysfunction
  Aortic
    Stenosis
    Insufficiency
      Acute
      Chronic

Table 14.1 (Continued)

Mitral
  Stenosis
  Insufficiency
    Acute
    Chronic
Pulmonic
  Stenosis
  Insufficiency
    Acute
    Chronic
Tricuspid[a]
  Stenosis
  Insufficiency
    Acute
    Chronic
Tamponade
  Pericardial constriction
    Acute (fluid)
    Chronic (fibrosis and thickening)
  Extrapericardial cardiac and vascular constriction
    Acute (clot)
    Chronic (tumor)
  Mediastinal fossa constriction
    Hyperinflation
    Excessive levels of PEEP
    Tension pneumothorax

[a]Tricuspid valvular dysfunction is rarely an isolated cause of heart failure, but a very common co-morbid factor in heart failure associated with increased pulmonary vascular resistance.

tensive care unit are ischemic myocardial dysfunction and myocardial infarction due to atherosclerotic coronary artery disease, acute and chronic aortic and mitral valvular disease, and hypotensive-hypoxemic myocardial dysfunction secondary to shock and arterial hypoxemia. If the inability of the myocardium to contract is long-standing, then volume and/or pressure overload will occur leading to either hypertrophy or dilation of the ventricles.

The venous and arterial factors determining cardiac output are discussed, and the importance of the mechanical coupling between the ventricle and the arterial circulation is emphasized. We do not discuss further the additional factors listed in Table 14.1 that may precipitate or worsen an acute circulatory failure, like hypovolemia, difficulty in breathing, an acute disturbance of cardiac rate and rhythm, or a surgically accessible cardiac defect that

should be recognized and treated early in the management of such patients.

The presentation of acute heart failure may differ from the classic signs of chronic heart failure. Although the right ventricular failure may be isolated, left ventricular (LV) failure is more common with only secondary impaired right heart function. Two separate but frequently related syndromes are usually observed: (*a*) "backward failure" associated with signs of back up of blood upstream from the LV, characterized by acute pulmonary edema in cases of high left atrial pressure or with signs suggesting the presence of an acute right heart failure with congestive hepatomegaly and possible jugular venous distension; and (*b*) "forward failure" associated with signs of an inability to deliver blood downstream from the LV. The dominant clinical manifestations of this acute circulatory failure with systemic hypotension include cyanosis, oliguria, and possible signs of decreased cerebral perfusion. Some patients may present with an association of both syndromes, which indicates a grave prognosis.

Finally, the frequent hypercapnia associated with a metabolic acidosis and a reduced lung compliance due to pulmonary congestion increases the work of breathing and then the whole body oxygen consumption is preferentially devoted to the respiratory muscles. The mismatching between oxygen demand and supply for respiratory muscles will lead to fatigue, which is one of the main causes of mortality justifying positive pressure ventilation.

A PATHOPHYSIOLOGIC RATIONALE FOR THE TREATMENT OF HEART FAILURE

Ventricular Performance

Compared to the adaptation seen in chronic congestive heart failure with cardiac hypertrophy or dilation secondary to pressure or volume overload, the compensatory mechanisms in acute heart failure are mainly the consequences of sympathetic stimulation that change myocardial metabolism (12, 23). This adaptation might induce arrythmias, peripheral vasoconstriction increasing LV afterload, and myocardial oxygen consumption. This can also modify the determinants of the ventriculoarterial coupling and of ventricular performance. In addition to heart rate, ventricular performance is determined by preload, afterload, and contractility. These parameters are examined in relation to their influence in the pathophysiology of heart failure, both as initial compensatory mechanisms and sites for specific therapeutic interventions.

Ventricular Diastolic Function

Ventricular diastolic function is commonly described as the relation between ventricular diastolic pressure and volume, which defines the diastolic compliance curve. Since diastole begins in conjunction with aortic valve closure and continues until the myocardial depolarization, impairment of diastolic properties also concerns ventricular relaxation. Ventricular relaxation is an active, energy consuming phenomenon that involves calcium uptake from troponin to sarcoplasmic reticulum. Abnormalities in diastolic properties observed in cardiomyopathy, for example, may have a biochemical and a structural basis (5). Impaired relaxation is commonly seen during ischemia and may elevate diastolic filling pressure without changing end-diastolic volume (LV diastolic dysfunction with reduced compliance). This dissociation between filling pressure and volume should be kept in mind whenever ventricular filling pressures are measured as an estimate of preload volume.

Preload is one of the simplest factors in which one can intervene to enhance global ventricular function in acute heart failure. In contrast to the classic ventricular function curve of Starling's law of the heart, Guyton et al. plotted right atrial pressure, the dependent variable on the x axis, and venous return, the independent variable on the y axis (9). The format of Guyton et al.'s venous return curve therefore describes how right atrial pressure is influenced by venous return, rather than how right atrial pressure influences cardiac output (Starling curve). In the former, right atrial pressure is viewed as the back pressure for venous return, whereas in the latter, right atrial pressure is taken as an estimate of preload. Since cardiac output equals venous return in the steady state, the relationships between right atrial pressure and cardiac output or venous return are coupled, a given hemodynamic condition being characterized by a single value of cardiac output and right atrial pressure. According to this framework, cardiac output and venous return can be represented on the ordinate and right atrial pressure on the abscissa of the same diagram. Such a representation may be extremely useful to represent various hemodynamic situations. Figure 14.1 shows the effects of an

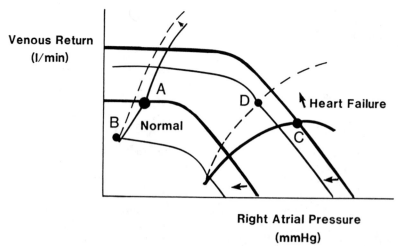

Figure 14.1. Guyton's venous return curve in normal and failing hearts.

infusion of nitroprusside in a normal heart and in the presence of a left ventricular failure. In the normal heart, the value of cardiac output is determined by the intersection of systemic venous return and right ventricular cardiac output curve *(point A)*. The administration of nitroprusside will decrease the vascular tone and shift the venous return curve left and downward (30). Despite a slight enhancement of the cardiac output curve *(dotted line)* induced by the decreased afterload, cardiac output will fall because of a predominant effect on venous return, and the new equilibrium *(point B)* will be characterized by decreased cardiac output and right atrial pressure. In contrast, during heart failure the cardiac output curve is depressed and the venous return curve is shifted to the right because of neurohormonal reflex vasoconstriction and water and salt retention, with an increase in mean systemic pressure *(point C)*. In this case, the infusion of nitroprusside may not change the venous return curve because a shift of blood from the central to the peripheral circulation tends to counteract the venodilating effects of the drug. Compared to a normal heart, the failing heart is relatively preload independent. However, being relatively afterload dependent (6), the cardiac output function curve *(dotted line)* will be displaced leftward and upward when afterload is reduced, thus resulting in a higher cardiac output and a lower right atrial pressure (30) *(point D)*.

Systolic Ventricular Elastance

Using an isolated beating heart preparation, Suga and coworkers have described an intrinsic contractile property of the ventricle that they termed "ventricular elastance" (35, 36). Elastance is a quantitative description of the dependence of ventricular pressure on chamber volume and time throughout systole (35). Ventricular elastance reflects the underlying process of active contraction (stiffening) that is time-dependent. Thus, elastance increases during systole, peaks at end-systole, and then returns to baseline after end-ejection (Fig. 14.2). It has been shown that ventricular elastance, especially at end-systole, is relatively independent of preload and afterload. Accordingly, end-systolic elastance fulfills the criteria for a descriptor of myocardial ventricular contractility (35). Ventricular pressure is also dependent on instantaneous flow from the ventricle so that elastance in the ejecting ventricle overestimates true ventricular pressure. This flow-dependent property of the ventricle is termed "resistance." Since at end-diastole and end-systole there is no flow, resistive behavior is unimportant at these phases of the cardiac cycle. Elastance is determined not only by the properties of the myocardium, but also by chamber geometry and mass. Comparison between patients should then imply a normalization of pressure and volume. This normalization should minimize the influence of ventricular mass,

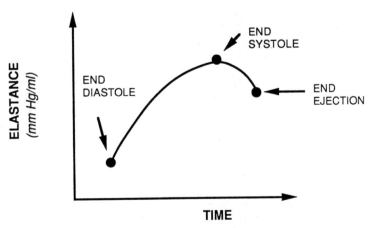

Figure 14.2. Instantaneous elastance plotted against time. Note that the maximum elastance occurs at end-systole and not at end-ejection.

size, and shape on elastance, and pressure-volume data can be converted for this purpose to a stress-volume relationship (39).

From these notions, the heart is viewed as a chamber with a time-varying elastance, with a maximum elastance (Emax) found near end-systole and an end-systolic elastance, both of which are used as measures of ventricular contractility. Emax can be estimated from the slope of the end-systolic pressure-volume relationship (35). The ventricular pressure-volume loop is a measure of instantaneous ventricular pressure and volume throughout the cardiac cycle (Fig. 14.3). In the clinical setting, this loop can be obtained by the simultaneous measurement of instantaneous ventricular pressure from a high fidelity catheter and instantaneous chamber volume measured with a conductance catheter (16). Estimates of chamber volume can be derived from measures of chamber cross-sectional area using two-dimensional echocardiographic techniques. Filling pressure and volume can be modified in humans, without changing the contractile state, by transient occlusions of the inferior vena cava with an inflatable balloon. A series of pressure-volume loops for different loading conditions can be constructed, and the end-systolic pressure-volume relationship can be determined.

This relationship is approximately linear, with a slope approximating Emax (35). Since flow is almost zero at end-systole, resistive behavior of the ventricle at its end-systolic volume approximates peak isovolumetric pressure in a nonejecting beat for the same volume at the onset of contraction. Like Emax, the end-systolic pressure-volume relationship is relatively insensitive to loading conditions and reflects changes in the myocardial contractile state (Fig. 14.3).

Afterload and Aortic Input Impedance

For given contractility and preload conditions, afterload is an important determinant of cardiac output. The magnitude of myocardial fiber shortening (and the corresponding stroke volume ejected by the ventricle) is inversely related to ventricular afterload. This relationship is influenced by the inotropic state, with a steeper relation in the presence of heart failure, i.e., a greater decrease in stroke volume will be observed for a given afterload in patients with heart failure (6). A family of "ventricular function curves" may then be described considering the afterload and stroke volume, similar to Sarnoff's ventricular function curves between preload and stroke volume. The greater sensitivity

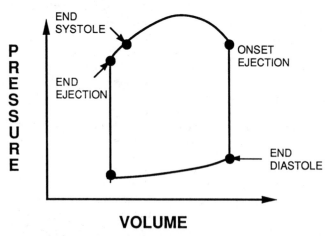

Figure 14.3. The ventricular pressure-volume loop. At end-systole corresponding to maximum elastance, the ventricle begins to relax although ejection continues briefly until the ventricular pressure falls below aortic pressure and the aortic valve closes.

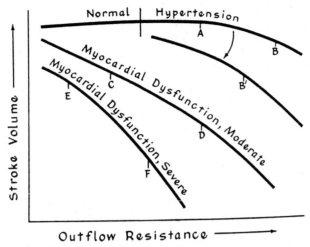

Figure 14.4. Cardiac output modifications following changes in afterload in normal and failing hearts. (From Cohn J, Franciosa J. Vasodilator therapy of cardiac failure. N Engl J Med 1977;297:27–31,254–258.)

of a failing heart to an increased afterload explains the usual hemodynamic benefit observed with an arterial vasodilatory therapy in these patients. Considering Figure 14.4, for a similar decrease in afterload, the improvement in stroke volume is critically dependent on the baseline ventricular function. In normal subjects, the administration of an arterial vasodilator will decrease afterload and lower the arterial pressure since cardiac output will also decrease (Fig. 14.4). In contrast during heart failure, afterload becomes an important determinant of stroke volume, and the increased stroke volume obtained with an arterial vasodilator counteracts a potential decrease in blood pressure, resulting in an increased cardiac output at an unchanged blood pressure.

The essential function of the heart is to transform chemical energy into mechanical energy to insure sufficient nutrient flow for peripheral tissues. The external work of the heart represents only 10–15% of the energy consumed by the myocardium during contraction. The remaining 85–90% (internal work of the ventricle) are dissipated as heat.

The energy transfer between the ventricle and the aorta is associated with an important work loss since pulsatile flow pumps generally have low mechanical ef-ficiencies. At the aortic root during systole, blood velocity rapidly changes with time from 0 to 100 or 120 cm/sec in 50 msec. This implies an acceleration of several "*g*" with turbulences and energy loss. However, measurements of different indexes of left ventricular external mechanical work reveal that the energy coupling between the heart and the arteries is remarkably efficient (15). This is the consequence of the geometry and the mechanical properties of the arterial bed (18, 20).

Aortic input impedance, a combination of elastance, resistance, and inductance parameters, needs to be addressed in conjunction with the corresponding arterial pressure in defining the afterload system for the LV. Considering the LV in isolated terms is too simplistic and neglects the behavior of the vasculature. Thus, one misses half the story. The aorta and arterial circulation represent the external load imposed on the ventricle (28) and the hydraulic load facing the LV is more than resistance alone. Aortic input impedance describes the relationship between instantaneous aortic pressure and flow and is a more complete description that incorporates both the pulsatile and the nonpulsatile load. The input impedance is calculated by decomposing pressure and flow waves into their sinusoidal components (harmonics) by Fourier analysis (15, 19–21). The pulsatile load is determined by: (a) the compliance of the large arteries; (b) the phenomenon of wave propagation with finite wave velocity; and (c) wave reflections (18). The input impedance is not a simple quotient of pressure and flow waveforms but an "impedance spectrum" consisting in the quotients for each harmonic between pressure and flows (modulus ratio and phase delay) (Fig. 14.5). During heart failure, arterioles constrict and peripheral resistance is increased in relation with activation of the neurohormonal system and to structural changes within the vessels, but little is known about the alterations in pulsatile load that occur in such patients and the available data are conflicting.

Ventriculoarterial Coupling

The left ventricle and the arterial circulation are joined together during ejection to form a coupled biological system, the behavior of which is determined by the mechanical properties of each unit, i.e., elastance and resistance for the ventricle, and aortic input impedance for the arterial system. Thus, left ventricle ejection performance is influenced by resistance, compliance, and inductance of the arterial system. To analyze the coupling between the heart and the arterial circulation, the mechanical properties of each unit are described in terms of pressure, volume, flow, and time allowing one to determine an equilibrium point. In most clinical circumstances, mean values of pressure and flow are sufficient

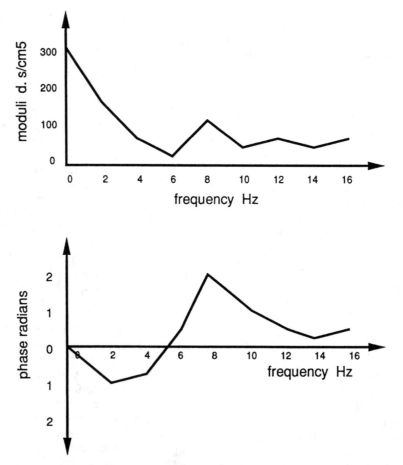

Figure 14.5. Representative aortic input impedance spectrum (moduli shown on *top* and phase angles on *bottom*). Note the marked oscillation of moduli of impedance consistent with important wave reflection. Phase delay is negative (difference between pressure and flow phase angles).

to predict the response of the coupled equilibrium point to a pharmacologic intervention or fluid resuscitation. However, if the impact of reflective pressure waves from the periphery back on the ejecting LV needs to be examined, then a coupling analysis using instantaneous values for both the LV and arterial current will then be needed (33).

By analogy to the coupling between cardiac output and venous return curves, a given hemodynamic situation may be seen as the result of an interaction between ventricular and arterial parameters. Sunagawa et al. have presented a conceptual framework that illustrates this concept (37). In the ventricular pressure-volume relationship format, the end-systolic pressure (Pes) is taken as an estimate of the ventricular afterload for given preload and inotropic level (represented respectively by the end-diastolic volume and the ventricular and systolic elastance, or slope of the end-systolic pressure-volume relationship). On the other hand, seen from the arterial circulation, Pes also increases linearly as stroke volume increases, this relationship being dependent on the mechanical properties of the arterial system. The slope of this vascular pressure-volume relationship represents the elastance of the arterial system. By including this relationship in the ventricular end-systolic pressure-volume relationship format, a single couple of values of stroke volume and Pes for a given hemodynamic situation can be defined. As proposed by the authors (37), the slope of the arterial elastance can be rearranged so that its origin on the volume axis lies at end-diastolic volume. This allows one to present on a single diagram the ventricular end-systolic pressure-volume relationship and the arterial elastance. The intersection of arterial and end-systolic elastance is represented by the Pes (Fig. 14.6). The application of this method of graphic analysis is useful in explaining particularities observed when a vasodilator therapy is given to a patient in heart failure. A venous vasodilator will lead to a decrease in stroke volume from SV to SV' at constant inotropic state (Fig. 14.6). If a similar decrease in Pes is achieved by the use of a pure arteriolar vasodilator,

this induces a pure afterload reduction as shown by a decrease in the slope of the arterial elastance from Ea to Ea'. At a constant preload, stroke volume increases from SV to SV'. In clinical practice, the reductions in preload and afterload are often linked after the use of a vasodilating drug because of their frequent balanced effects or because of an interaction between the modifications in preload and afterload.

This format is helpful to analyze the relationships between preload and afterload. The failing ventricle is relatively preload independent, since it operates on the flat portion of its Starling curve and is very sensitive to alterations in afterload. The analysis of the effects of nitrate therapy may help illustrate this point. Even if nitroglycerin is predominantly a venodilator, the increase in cardiac output observed during heart failure seems to be secondary to a reduction of the arteriolar tone. In patients with a normal heart function, the administration of nitroglycerin decreases preload without significant modifications in arterial resistances. If a decrease in preload of similar magnitude is obtained this time by mechanical maneuvers, a vasoconstrictive reaction is observed, with an increase in systemic vascular resistance (29). This suggests that during nitroglycerin therapy an arterial vasodilator effect was present and abolished by the arteriolar vasoconstriction induced by the decrease in preload (22, 29). In contrast, heart failure is characterized by an important vasoconstrictive reaction trying to maintain arterial pressure at the expense of cardiac performance. However, the reflex vasoconstriction during a baroreflex activation is attenuated (10, 25). This will lead to marked differences in the effect of nitroglycerin therapy compared to normal subjects: the mechanical maneuvers that decrease preload will not induce an increase in systemic vascular resistance, whereas the administration of nitroglycerin will, for a similar reduction in preload, decrease systemic vascular resistance (8). This vasodilating effect is beneficial in congestive heart failure patients, the arterial pressure being maintained by a corresponding increase in cardiac output.

The coupling concept between left ven-

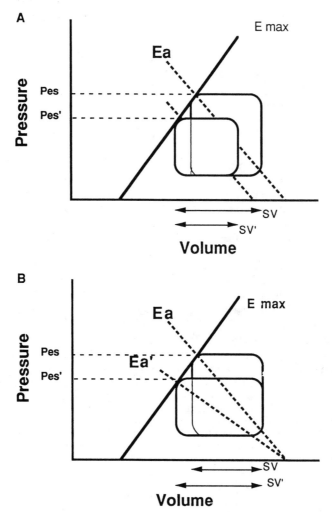

Figure 14.6. Schematic representation of pressure-volume loop with figuration of end-systolic ventricular elastance and the elastance of the arterial system *(Ea* and *Ea').* *Pes* is the end-systolic pressure; *SV* is the stroke volume before and SV', after hemodynamic modifications. *A* illustrates the impact of preload reduction induced by nitrates. The absence of any arteriolar effect implies that the slope of Ea remains constant and the observed Pes decrease results only from preload reduction. *B* illustrates the impact of a similar decrease in Pes *(Pes')* induced by a pure afterload reduction. Note the decrease in Ea *(Ea')* marked by the decrease in the Ea slope.

tricle and arterial circulation can be illustrated and applied to patients with heart failure using mean values of pressure and flow (Fig. 14.7) (32). The inverse relationship between end-systolic pressure and stroke volume *(line AP)* is used to describe the mechanical properties of the failing left ventricle. The slope of this relationship is an index of contractility. The depression of this slope compared to the normal slope *(line BP)* implies a myocardial depression.

The relationship between end-systolic pressure-stroke volume as illustrated in Figure 14.7 *(line OX)* describes the arterial elastance, an index of arterial impedance. In heart failure, this relation is steeper *(line OX)* than normal *(line OY)* due to vasoconstriction. Both mechanical properties defined an equilibrium point in *position 1.* When a pure inotropic agent is infused, the slope of the ventricular relation is increased *(line CP)* whereas there is no effect

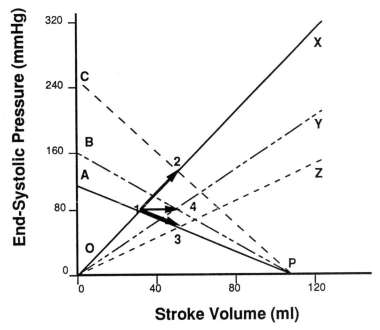

Figure 14.7. *Lines* between *P* and *A*, *B*, and *C* describe the end-systolic pressure-stroke volume relations for the left ventricle. *Lines* between *O* and *X*, *Y*, and *Z* depict the same relation but for the arterial circulation. The baseline equilibrium point in a patient with heart failure is *point 1*. A pure inotropic agent will change only the ventricular relation and moves the equilibrium point to *position 2* along the *slope OX*. A pure arteriolar vasodilator moves the equilibrium point to *position 3* along *line PA* changing only the slope arterial elastance to *line OZ*. A combination of arteriolar vasodilation and inotropic stimulation shift the equilibrium point to *position 4*. (Adapted from Shroff SG, Weber KT, Janicki JS. Coupling of the left ventricle with the arterial circulation. In: Nichols WW, O'Rourke MF, McDonald DA, eds. Blood flow in arteries. 3rd ed. London: Edward Arnold (in press).)

on arterial elastance *(line OX)*. The equilibrium point is now in *position 2*. If a pure arteriolar vasodilator is used, only the slope of arterial elastance is decreased *(line OZ)* allowing a new equilibrium point *(point 3)*. The use of an inovasodilator shifts the equilibrium point toward normal *(point 4)*.

TREATMENT

General Considerations

The alteration of myocardial contractility characterizing heart failure implies an impairment of myocardial ability to shorten and develop force. The extent of shortening and force developed are dependent on several factors: *(a)* the initial fiber length or preload, *(b)* the force that must be sustained during contraction or afterload, *(c)* the frequency of stimulation or heart rate,

and *(d)* the contractility. All these variables influence ventricular function in patients suffering from heart failure. Accordingly, an ideal clinical measure of contractility must change in an appropriate manner when interventions known to either increase or decrease contractility are administered, and it must be independent of the other factors such as preload and afterload. Clinical assessment of the alteration of myocardial contractility remains difficult because of methodological limitations. Recent developments in noninvasive Doppler methods authorize the instantaneous clinical measurement of maximum acceleration of the blood in the ascending aorta (27, 33). This parameter will provide an early and sensitive assessment of the contractile property of the heart (3, 14, 18, 27). It will be then possible to differentiate alterations in ventricular performance due to a reduction in contractility from abnormal hydraulic loading.

In addition, recent efforts in two-dimensional echocardiography have attempted to measure chamber contractility as the relationship between end-systolic meridional stress and fiber shortening (4). This approach has the potential to be useful in assessing contractility among patients with heart failure if several problems are properly addressed: (a) in patients with heart failure the ratio between circumferential and meridional stress may not be fixed because of changes in shape of the heart; (b) an intervention may cause change in shape, making the use of meridional wall stress even more questionable; and (c) noninvasive determination of end-systolic pressure from carotid pulse tracing could be inaccurate.

In routine clinical practice, these sophisticated measurements of ventricular and arterial mechanics are feasible, and the evaluation of the severity of heart failure is based on usual clinical parameters, invasive and/or noninvasive measurement of resting ventricular function. Furthermore, it might be essential to evaluate the ability of the heart to augment cardiac output in response to physiological stress like an increase in oxygen demand. Such an approach may provide information about the severity of heart failure and the compensatory mechanisms operating to maintain stroke volume, cardiac output, and arterial pressure to ensure an adequate oxygen supply. The recent progress in ultrasound and computer technologies (33) associated with the development of a fiberoptic Swan-Ganz catheter will provide relatively complete data assessing: (a) the resting adaptation of oxygen supply to oxygen demand; (b) the left ventricular mechanical behavior by transthoracic or transesophageal two-dimensional echocardiography; and (c) instantaneous outflow from the left ventricle and the derived parameters of myocardial function and arterial mechanics from Doppler measurements.

In critically ill patients, especially if they are mechanically ventilated, these methods might be difficult to use with sufficient accuracy and sensitivity. However, the consequences of severe heart failure for peripheral tissues can be easily limited by the reduction in respiratory work (intubation and mechanical ventilation), the reduction in whole body oxygen demand (deep sedation), and the use of appropriate methods to monitor the effects of different therapeutic strategies.

Specific Therapeutics

The therapeutic interventions should restore myocardial contractility, increase peripheral organ delivery with an adequate peripheral tissular oxygenation, and suppress the signs of pulmonary vascular engorgement, without any deleterious effect on cardiac rate or rhythm and ideally with a reduction of myocardial oxygen consumption. If it is difficult in clinical practice to reach all of these goals, a better knowledge of the pathophysiologic mechanisms involved in heart failure may help determine which specific therapeutic intervention needs to be established for a given condition.

Volume Loading

In patients with acute heart failure, the early detection and treatment of an associated hypovolemia is mandatory before starting a more aggressive therapy with inotropic or vasodilating drugs. According to the Frank-Starling relation, volume replacement is especially important in cases of acute heart failure since the acutely failing heart may be relatively preload sensitive, i.e., a marked decreased in cardiac output can be observed when cardiac filling pressures are not elevated. This condition is suspected in the following circumstances: acute heart failure in an otherwise normal individual, inappropriate diuretic therapy, excessive use of vasodilators, or vomiting. In patients with severe circulatory impairment, this will be recognized when only modest signs of congestion of the pulmonary vascular bed are present and diagnosed by a pulmonary artery occlusion pressure lower than 15 mm Hg. Rapid infusions of 50–100 ml of fluid are then warranted under strict monitoring of pulmonary artery occlusion pressure and cardiac output values. If pulmonary artery occlusion pressure rises by >5–8 mm Hg to >20 mm Hg without an increase in cardiac output, then that heart is not responsive to volume loading and alternative therapies must be given to increase cardiac output.

Inotropes

Dobutamine is a synthetic catecholamine that has predominant β_1-adrenergic agonist properties. It also has slight α-adrenergic effects that are partially clinically offset by a peripheral β_2 vasodilating action, the net effect of dobutamine infusion being a marked stimulation of cardiac β_1-adrenergic receptors resulting in an enhanced inotropic effect. Dobutamine is usually the drug of choice when an increase in contractility is needed since it has usually minimum effects on heart rate and rhythm. Blood pressure is maintained, suggesting that the increased cardiac output observed is balanced by a peripheral vasodilating effect. This absence of deleterious effects on blood pressure and heart rate may explain the beneficial effects of dobutamine on the balance between myocardial oxygen consumption and myocardial oxygen supply (coronary blood flow).

Dopamine is a natural catecholamine, a precursor of epinephrine and norepinephrine. Like dobutamine, dopamine has potent β_1-adrenergic effects inducing an increased contractility, but unlike dobutamine, this drug has potent vasoconstrictive effects via a stimulation of peripheral α_1-adrenergic receptors, both directly and indirectly by stimulation of the release of endogenous norepinephrine. Dopamine also has venoconstrictive effects that can reduce systemic venous compliance and further increase ventricular filling pressures when the vasoconstrictive properties of dopamine override the beneficial inotropic effects. Thus, despite its inotropic action, dopamine is rarely used as a sole agent for the treatment of acute heart failure because of these vasopressor effects that may precipitate a myocardial energetic imbalance. The distinct pharmacologic feature of dopamine over the other sympathomimetic drugs in fact is the stimulation of dopaminergic-specific receptors resulting in direct renal and mesenteric vasodilation for doses of 2–3 μg/kg/min. At these low doses, mesenteric and renal blood flows are increased, with a beneficial effect on glomerular filtration rate and sodium excretion. Great care should be used clinically when seeking these "dopaminergic" doses of dopamine since the α-adrenergic vasoconstriction that offsets the dopaminergic mesenteric and renal effects can appear for doses as low as 5 μg/kg/min.

Norepinephrine is the endogenous catecholamine, mediator of the sympathetic nervous system. Compared to epinephrine, norepinephrine has similar effects on β_1 cardiac receptors, but on the peripheral level, norepinephrine is devoided of β_2 peripheral vasodilating activity. It therefore has a predominant α vasoconstrictive action. Its main indication is thus a "peripheral failure" with low blood pressure as in vasoplegic/septic shock. In acute heart failure complicating a septic shock, the doses of norepinephrine used should be carefully titrated to maintain coronary perfusion pressure without deleterious effects on cardiac output, since the intense peripheral vasoconstriction observed after norepinephrine administration may adversely affect organ perfusion while increasing cardiac work and perpetuating myocardial ischemia.

Epinephrine is the prototypical endogenous catecholamine. In addition to the stimulation of cardiac β_1-receptors, epinephrine has potent effects on β_2 and α peripheral adrenergic receptors. The pharmacologic effects of epinephrine should be considered according to the dose administered. At low doses (1–2 μg/min), the dominant effect is a stimulation of β_1- and β_2-receptors, with an enhanced contractility and a systemic vasodilation increasing cardiac output. From 2 to 10 μg/min, stimulation of the peripheral α receptors becomes marked, inducing a vasoconstriction although the stimulation of the β_1 cardiac receptors is still present. At higher doses (10–20 μg/min), an intense vasoconstrictive reaction is observed secondary to a marked stimulation of peripheral α-receptors that may override the cardiac β_1

effects. Epinephrine is proposed for the treatment of acute heart failure, "peripheral failure" as in septic shock, and during anaphylaxis. Epinephrine is also used after cardiac surgery for weaning of bypass and was proposed to be more frequently effective in this indication than dopamine or dobutamine (34). Finally, in cases of severe right ventricular failure due to intense pulmonary hypertension after cardiac valvular surgery, the vasoconstrictive properties of epinephrine can be used during a systemic infusion through a left atrial pressure catheter to counteract the systemic vasodilation observed after the infusion of a pulmonary vasodilator (such as isoproterenol or a prostaglandin such as PGE_1) administered in the right atrium.

Isoproterenol is a synthetic catecholamine with essentially β_1 and β_2 activity. It is therefore an inotropic drug, but the marked vasodilation observed after administration of isoproterenol can induce a decrease in arterial pressure. Because of these actions, associated with a marked chronotropic effect, isoproterenol is seldom used during acute heart failure because of the fear of precipitating a myocardial energetic imbalance as coronary perfusion pressure is reduced, whereas the tachycardia and the increased inotropic stimulation might induce a deleterious increase in myocardial oxygen consumption. Isoproterenol has been proposed to reverse the effects of β-blockers, or to pharmacologically treat the effects of an atrioventricular heart block such as after cardiac transplantation. Finally, isoproterenol has been proposed as a treatment of acute right ventricular failure secondary to acute pulmonary hypertension (7) since the observed decrease in pulmonary vascular resistances seems to be slightly more pronounced than the decrease of systemic vascular resistances.

Vasodilators

Although vasodilators are usually classified according to their principle site of action (predominantly "arterial" or predominantly "venous"), the actually commercially available vasodilators have usually both arterial and venous vasodilating

effects (24). Furthermore, the hemodynamic consequences of the administration of a vasodilator will vary according to the initial level of myocardial performance and to the interplay between preload and afterload modifications during the physiologic adaptation to a situation of acute heart failure (17, 31).

Nitroprusside is a very potent vasodilator inducing an arterial and venous vasodilation (17, 24). Because nitroprusside is a short-acting drug, it can be easily titrated in order to relieve the signs and symptoms of acute heart failure via a decrease in afterload (see above) and avoid the occurrence of a systemic hypotension that might decrease coronary perfusion pressure. Thiocyanate toxicity may develop in cases of infusions lasting longer than 2 days, but the particular hemodynamic profile of nitroprusside makes it an extremely useful agent for ICU patients in association with a continuous invasive hemodynamic monitoring (26).

Among the therapeutic agents suggested for the treatment of cardiac failure, a new class of agents has recently been proposed—the phosphodiesterase inhibitors (amrinone and enoximone)—that combine inotropic and vasodilating properties. The inotropic action of endogenous and synthetic catecholamines is secondary to a stimulation of adenylate cyclase via the β_1 cardiac receptors. Cyclic AMP (cAMP) will then be produced from intracellular ATP and will lead to an increase in intracellular calcium concentration, leading to an increase in contractility. The phosphodiesterase inhibitors act selectively on the phosphodiesterase enzymes that usually metabolize cAMP. Such a treatment induces an increase in intracellular cAMP levels in the cardiac muscle and the peripheral vascular smooth muscle, thus explaining its inotropic and vasodilating properties, independently of a catecholamine receptor stimulation. This dual action seems beneficial for the treatment of acute heart failure. Compared to dobutamine, the phosphodiesterase inhibitor enoximone induces a similar increase in cardiac index, but with a greater decrease in pulmonary artery occlusion pressure, without any deleterious increase in heart rate (11), whereas compared to sodium nitroprusside, for a similar decrease in pulmonary artery occlusion pressure and systemic vascular resistances, cardiac index and mean arterial pressure are higher after intravenous enoximone administrations (1). The effects of enoximone on left ventricular performance seem secondary to these inotropic and vasodilating properties, but enoximone also improves ventricular relaxation: pulmonary artery occlusion pressure is decreased at a constant end-diastolic volume, suggesting an increased left ventricular diastolic compliance (13).

Several disadvantages, however, exist with this new therapeutic class. In addition to increased mortality, initially described in patients receiving a prolonged treatment with milrinone (2), even though the functional signs of chronic heart failure were reduced, other disadvantages are: *(a)* in acute heart failure, the long-lasting action of these drugs compared to dobutamine, epinephrine, or sodium nitroprusside can become a disadvantage in potentially rapidly changing situations; *(b)* the vasodilating effect of phosphodiesterase inhibitors may be a handicap in hypovolemic patients and preload needs to be regularly controlled and optimized if needed by fluid loading; and *(c)* finally, these drugs can increase intrapulmonary shunt, a potentially deleterious effect in already hypoxemic patients before treatment if the increase in cardiac output after phosphodiesterase inhibitor treatment is not accompanied by a marked increase in mixed venous saturation that would counteract the effect of the increased venous admixture (38).

Acknowledgments. This work was partially sponsored by grants from the Delegation a la Recherche Clinique de l'AP-HP de Paris and the Direction de la Recherche et de l'Enseignement Doctoral 1990–1991.

References

1. Amin D, Shah P, Hulse S, Shellock F. Comparative acute hemodynamic effects of intravenous sodium nitroprusside and MDL-17,043, a new inotropic drug with vasodilator effects, in refractory congestive heart failure. Am Heart J 1985;109:1006–1012.

2. Baim D, Colucci W, Monrad E, Smith H, Wright R, Lanoue A, Gauthier D, Ransil B, Grossman W, Braunwald E. Survival of patients with severe congestive heart failure treated with oral milrinone. J Am Coll Cardiol 1986;7:661–670.

3. Bennett E, Barclay S, Davis A, Mannering D, Mehta N. Ascending aortic blood velocity and acceleration using Doppler ultrasound in the assessment of the left ventricular function. Cardiovasc Res 1984;18:632–638.

4. Borow K, Green L, Grossman W, et al. Left ventricular end-systolic stress shortening and stress-length relations in humans: normal values and sensitivity to inotropic state. Am J Cardiol 1982;50:1301–1309.

5. Brutsaert D, Paulus W. Loading and performance of the heart as muscle and pump. Cardiovasc Res 1977;11:1–16.

6. Cohn J, Franciosa J. Vasodilator therapy of cardiac failure. N Engl J Med 1977;297:27–31, 254–258.

7. Daoud F, Reeves J, Kelly D. Isoproterenol as a potential pulmonary vasodilator in primary pulmonary hypertension. Am J Cardiol 1978;42:817–822.

8. Franciosa J, Blank R, Cohn J. Nitrate effects on cardiac output and left ventricular outflow resistance in chronic congestive heart failure. Am J Med 1978;64:207–213.

9. Guyton A, Jones C, Coleman T. Circulatory physiology: cardiac output and its regulation. Philadelphia: WB Saunders, 1973.

10. Higgins C, Vatner S, Eckberg D, Braunwald E. Alterations in the baroreceptor reflex in conscious dogs with heart failure. J Clin Invest 1972;51:715–724.

11. Installe E, Gonzalez M, Jacquemart J, Collard P, Roulette F, Pourbaix S, Tremouroux J. Comparative effects on hemodynamics of enoximone (MDL-17,043), dobutamine and nitroprusside in severe congestive heart failure. Am J Cardiol 1987;60:46C–52C.

12. Katz A. Cardiomyopathy of overload. A major determinant of prognosis in congestive heart failure. N Engl J Med 1990;322:100–110.

13. Kereiakes D, Viquerat C, Lanzer P, Botvinick E, Spangenberg R, Buckingham M, Parmley W, Chatterjee K. Mechanisms of improved left ventricular function following intravenous MDL-17,043 in patients with severe chronic heart failure. Am Heart J 1984;108:1278–1284.

14. Laskey W, Kussmaul W, Martin J, Kleaveland J, Hirshfeld J, Shroff S. Characteristics of vascular hydraulic load in patients with heart failure. Circulation 1985;72:61–71.

15. McDonald D. Blood flow in arteries. London: Edward Arnold, 1974.

16. McKay R, Miller M, Ferguson J, et al. Assessment of left ventricular end-systolic pressure-volume relations with an impedance catheter and transient inferior vena cava occlusion: use of this system in the evaluation of the cardiotonic effects of dobutamine, milrinone, posicor and epinephrine. J Am Coll Cardiol 1986;8:1152–1161.

17. Miller R, Fennell W, Young J, Palomo A, Quinones M. Differential systemic arterial and ve-

nous actions and consequent cardiac effects of vasodilator drugs. Prog Cardiovasc Dis 1982;24:353–374.

18. Milnor W. Hemodynamics. Baltimore: Williams & Wilkins, 1982.

19. Nichols W, Pepine C, Geiser E, Conti C. Vascular load defined by the aortic input impedance spectrum. Fed Proc 1980;39:196–201.

20. O'Rourke M. Arterial function in health and disease. New York: Churchill Livingstone, 1982.

21. O'Rourke M, Taylor M. Input impedance of the systemic circulation. Circ Res 1967;20:365–380.

22. Packer M. Mechanisms of nitrate action in patients with severe left ventricular failure: conceptual problems with the theory of venosequestration. Am Heart J 1985;110:259–264.

23. Packer M. Role of the sympathetic nervous system in chronic heart failure. A historical and philosophical perspective. Circulation 1990; 82 (suppl I):I-1–I-6.

24. Packer M, LeJemtel T. Physiologic and pharmacologic determinants of vasodilator response: a conceptual framework for rational drug therapy for chronic heart failure. Prog Cardiovasc Dis 1982;24:275–292.

25. Packer M, Meller J, Medina N, Yushak M, Gorlin R. Determinants of drug response in severe chronic heart failure. 1. Activation of vasoconstrictor forces during vasodilator therapy. Circulation 1981;64:506–514.

26. Parillo J. Vasodilator therapy. In: Chernow B, et al, eds. The pharmacologic approach to the critically ill patient. 2nd ed. Baltimore: Williams & Wilkins, 1988:346–364.

27. Payen D, Fratacci M, Dupuy P, Laborde F. Evaluation of left ventricular performance based on peak flow velocity and maximal acceleration of the blood with aortic implantable pulsed Doppler probes [Abstract]. Circulation 1988;78(suppl II):2190.

28. Pepine C, Nichols W. Aortic input impedance in cardiovascular disease. Prog Cardiovasc Dis 1982;24:307–318.

29. Petrovitch L, Smith G, Quinones M, Adyanthaya A, Alexander J. Hemodynamic effects of nitroglycerin vs pure preload reduction: masked arteriolar dilatory effect [Abstract]. Circulation 1978;57 & 58(suppl II):II223.

30. Pouleur H, Covell J, Ross J. Effect of nitroprusside on venous return and central blood volume in the absence and presence of acute heart failure. Circulation 1980;61:328–337.

31. Ross J. Afterload mismatch and preload reserve. Prog Cardiovasc Dis 1976;18:255–270.

32. Nichols WW, O'Rourke MF, McDonald DA, eds. Coupling of the left ventricle with the arterial circulation. In: Blood flow in arteries. 3rd ed. London: Edward Arnold, 1990:363–960.

33. Spencer K, Lang R, Neumann A, Borow K, Scroff S. Doppler and electromagnetic comparison of instantaneous aortic flow characteristic in primates. Circ Res 1991;68:1369–1377.

34. Steen P, Tinker J, Pluth J, et al. Efficiency of dopamine, dobutamine, and epinephrine during emergence from cardiopulmonary bypass in man. Circulation 1978;57:378–384.

35. Suga H, Sagawa K. Instantaneous pressure-volume relationships and their ratio in the excised, supported canine left ventricle. Circ Res 1974;35:117–126.

36. Suga H, Sagawa K, Shoukas A. Load impedance of instantaneous pressure-volume ratio of the canine left ventricle and effects of epinephrine and heart rate on the ratio. Circ Res 1973;32:314–322.

37. Sunagawa K, Maughan W, Burkhoff D, Sagawa K. Left ventricular interaction with arterial load studied in isolated canine ventricle. Am J Physiol 1983;245:H773–H780.

38. Vincent J, Carlier E, Berre J, Armistead C, Kahn R, Coussaert E, Cantraine F. Administration of enoximone in cardiogenic shock. Am J Cardiol 1988;62:419–423.

39. Weber K, Janicki J, Hunter W, et al. The contractile behavior of the heart and its functional coupling to the circulation. Prog Cardiovasc Dis 1982;24:375–400.

15

Acute Myocardial Ischemia

Claude Perret

Acute myocardial ischemia generates a variety of clinical syndromes sharing a similar pathogenesis and a high risk for life-threatening complications, justifying admission of patients to specialized intensive care units. Two broad categories are usually considered: unstable angina and acute myocardial infarction.

UNSTABLE ANGINA

Definition

Unstable angina designates under a single term several clinical syndromes reflecting acute myocardial ischemia. In fact, it encompasses several clinical entities that correspond to different pathophysiological mechanisms, prognosis, and responsiveness to therapy. Until recently, there was a lack of agreement on the precise definition of unstable angina and this was the source of confusion. A new classification based on historical features and electrocardiographic (ECG) changes has been proposed defining severity (18).

Class I

a. *New onset* (<2 months in duration), severe or frequent (> three episodes a day) exertional angina pectoris.
b. *Accelerated angina* to designate the development in patients with chronic stable angina of a crescendo pattern (as attested by an increase in frequency, severity, duration of angina; or brought on by distinctly less exertion than previously) but without a history of pain at rest during the preceding 2 months.

Class II

Angina at rest, subacute. Patients report one or more episodes of angina at rest but not within the preceding 48 hr.

Class III

Angina at rest, acute. Patients with one or more episodes of angina at rest within the preceding 48 hr.

Class II and Class III patients with angina at rest are those admitted to the coronary care unit because of the high risk involved of developing acute myocardial infarction or life-threatening arrhythmias.

A further distinction is made according to the clinical circumstances in which unstable angina occurs.

Class A

Secondary unstable angina designating those patients in whom angina appears to be related to a clearly identified condition known to reduce myocardial oxygen supply (e.g., anemia, carbon monoxide intoxication, hypoxemia, hypotension) or increase myocardial oxygen demand (e.g., fever, infection, uncontrolled hypertension, tachycardia, stress, thyrotoxicosis).

Class B

Primary unstable angina, designating patients who develop unstable angina in the absence of an extracardiac condition that has intensified ischemia.

Class C

Postinfarction (within the first 2 weeks) unstable angina.

Diagnosis

History is by far the most important feature in the diagnosis of unstable angina. It is usually associated with transient changes in the ECG characterized by depression or elevation of the ST segment, frequently associated with T wave inversion. In the absence of ECG changes, the diagnosis should be reasonably maintained in the presence of a typical history and previously documented coronary artery disease. It should be discarded if the pain described is not characteristic in a patient without previously known coronary disease. As a rule, ECG changes are transient; if persistent (>6 hr), they usually indicate the development of non-Q wave infarction, as attested by a slight and temporary increase in cardiac enzymes (total CPK and MB fraction).

In unstable angina, cardiac enzymes are classically in the normal range. This does not exclude, however, the presence of small areas of myocardial necrosis, as demonstrated by the use of sensitive markers of myocardial cell damage (71). These results suggest that occult ischemic myocardial damage can supervene in the absence of the classical ECG and enzymatic criteria. They also tend to demonstrate that there is no clear-cut qualitative distinction between unstable angina and myocardial infarction.

Pathogenesis

Acute myocardial ischemia may be related to a sudden reduction of coronary flow leading to a critical myocardial oxygen delivery or to an excessive increase in oxygen demand in the presence of a limited coronary flow reserve. This latter mechanism is principally involved in conditions such as exercise- or, stress-induced angina in which the combination of hypertension, tachycardia, and/or increased contractility augments myocardial oxygen needs without appropriate coronary vasodilation. On the other hand, in unstable angina at rest, as well as in acute myocardial infarction and ischemic sudden death, the principle mechanism involved appears to be an impaired antegrade coronary flow. The subsequent clinical syndome largely depends on the extent and duration of myocardial ischemia and on the effectiveness of collateral blood flow. On the basis of pathologic, angiographic, and angioscopic data, there is now growing evidence to support the concept of a common pathogenic mechanism in the development of acute

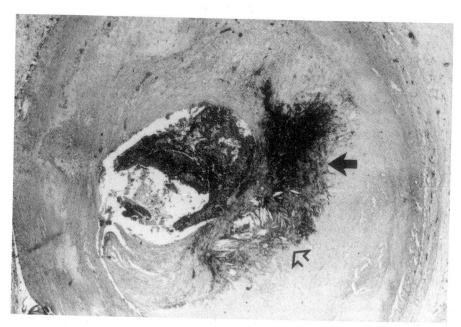

Figure 15.1. Cross-section of a coronary artery (low power photomicrograph). Severe atherosclerotic thickening of intima (plaque) with needle-like cholesterol crystals *(open arrow)* and recent intramural hemorrhage *(solid arrow)*. The lumen is partially obstructed by an organized *(lower part)* and a recent *(upper part)* thrombus.

coronary syndromes. Sudden plaque rupture or fissuring appears to be the primary phenomenon in the occlusive process (5, 31, 38, 126). This leads to the exposure of subintimal thrombogenic material (fibrillar collagen) with subsequent activation of platelet metabolism (39, 52) and release of numerous potent factors such as ADP, thromboxane A_2, platelet factor 3, von Willebrand factor, and serotonin. Platelet

CONCENTRIC LESIONS

ECCENTRIC LESIONS

Type I

or

Type II

or

MULTIPLE IRREGULARITIES

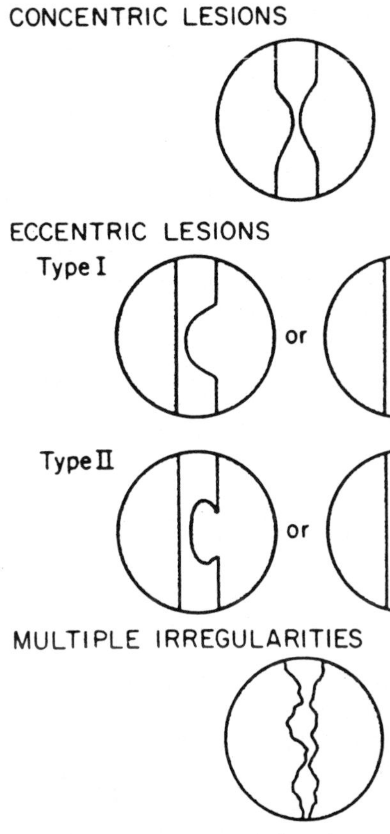

Figure 15.2. Schematic drawings of the morphology findings in coronary artery disease. Concentric lesions are symmetric and usually smooth. Type I eccentric lesions are asymmetric and smooth. Most Type I lesions are like those depicted on the *right* of the diagram. Type II eccentric lesions either are smooth with a narrow neck *(left)* or have irregular borders *(right)*. Multiple irregularities include vessels with serial lesions or severe diffuse disease. (From Ambrose JA et al. Coronary angiographic morphology in myocardial infarction: a link between the pathogenesis of unstable angina and myocardial infarction. J Am Coll Cardiol 1985;6:1233–1238.)

adhesion and aggregation trigger the coagulation system via both intrinsic and extrinsic pathways. In unstable angina, intracoronary thrombi may be present although not as frequently as in myocardial infarction (Fig. 15.1). Occlusion is usually partial and transient but sufficient to reduce temporarily the coronary flow to a critical level.

Angiographic findings have been of particular interest for demonstrating a similar mechanism in the development of acute coronary syndromes (Fig. 15.2). Asymmetric or eccentric stenoses with irregular borders (Fig. 15.3) are present in the ma-

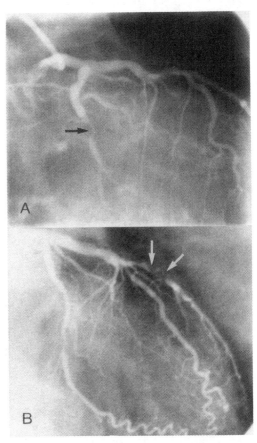

Figure 15.3. Coronary arteriogram of the left coronary artery in the right anterior oblique projection. In *A*, there is a smooth, eccentric (Type IIa), midcircumflex severe stenosis in a patient with unstable angina. In *B*, note the presence of several radiolucent filling defects consistent with intraluminal thrombi causing a near-total occlusion of the left anterior descending artery.

jority of patients with unstable angina (3, 42) and correspond to plaque rupture with secondary thrombus. In such conditions, episodes of angina appear to be related to intermittent coronary occlusion due to either superimposed vasoconstriction or thrombus formation with spontaneous lysis.

Acute ischemia produced by sudden reduction in oxygen delivery induces profound metabolic changes, as demonstrated noninvasively by positron emission tomography (21, 25). Due to an impairment in oxidation of fatty acids (120), glycolysis is enhanced leading to rapid consumption of glycogen stores and subsequently to anaerobic glycolysis. Local accumulation of lactate and protons supervenes as a consequence of an insufficient removal by reduced coronary flow. Tissue acidosis develops, leading to secondary inhibition of glycolysis and energy production. Ultimately, cell machinery is impaired, and cell membranes are disrupted, leading to tissue necrosis.

Intervention Strategies

Considering the different mechanisms involved in the development of acute myocardial ischemia, one can distinguish schematically several pathways of therapy. The aim can be:

1. To reduce myocardial oxygen needs and thus decrease metabolic imbalance (nitrates, β-blockers, and calcium antagonists).
2. To relieve a coronary spasm and thus increase coronary flow and oxygen delivery (calcium antagonists, nitrates).
3. To inhibit platelet activation and thrombus formation on vascular injury following plaque fissuring (aspirin, heparin).
4. To obtain early reperfusion in the presence of acute thrombotic coronary occlusion in order to prevent or limit myocardial damage (thrombolysis, emergency percutaneous transluminal coronary angioplasty (PTCA), emergency surgical revascularization).

Pharmacological Approach

Nitrates

Nitrates represent the basic drug therapy. They produce a nonselective vasodilation by a direct relaxation of vascular smooth muscle. Their predominant effect on venous capacitance vessels leads to a decrease in both right and left ventricular preload with subsequent reduction of ventricular wall stress and myocardial oxygen demand. At high dosage, nitrates reduce afterload by systemic vasodilation. Furthermore, nitrates relieve coronary spasm and local vasoconstriction superimposed on organic stenosis (16, 23). They improve collateral flow and redistribute blood flow from epicardial to endocardial areas (64) by decreasing left ventricular end-diastolic pressure. They stimulate prostacyclin synthesis by endothelial cells (78) and inhibit platelet recruitment and deposition on arterial wall injury (75).

Nitroglycerin (NTG) and isosorbide dinitrate are the most frequently used. The intravenous route appears much more effective than the oral or topical routes. The initial starting doses (5–10 μg/min of NTG; 2.0–3.0 mg/hr of isosorbide dinitrate) can be progressively titrated up to 500 μg/min or even higher for NTG, up to 8–10 mg/hr for isosorbide dinitrate, with the advantage of a rapid reversal if adverse effects occur. Therapy is maintained for 48–72 hr in order to prevent the development of myocardial infarction. The development of tolerance may be responsible for the recurrence of angina in some patients with intravenous nitrate therapy. At high doses, particular attention should be given to the monitoring of blood pressure. Excessive unloading of the heart leading to a fall in cardiac output with hypotension and tachycardia may counterbalance the beneficial effects of nitrate therapy.

In unstable angina, nitrate therapy is usually associated with the administration of calcium antagonists and β-blockers. This use is based on the belief that the combination of different drugs with various pharmacological impacts may have complementary actions and can prevent reflex therapeutic actions, which limit the effectiveness of a given drug on myocardial ischemia.

β-Blockers and Calcium Antagonists

The beneficial effects of β-blockers on myocardial ischemia are classically related to a decrease in oxygen demand due to several factors: a reduction of blood pressure and heart rate, a decrease in contractility, and an increase in diastolic perfusion time.

Among the calcium antagonists, nifedipine and diltiazem are the most widely used. They produce a potent peripheral arteriolar and coronary vasodilation by blocking slow calcium channels; they relieve myocardial ischemia without significant dromotropic or cardiodepressant effects at usual doses (60–80 mg daily and 120–360 mg in four daily doses, respectively). Nifedipine and diltiazem are of particular interest in patients with contraindication to β-blockers (asthma, left ventricular failure, bradycardia, peripheral vascular disease). In patients with persistent tachycardia, diltiazem has the advantage of an inhibitory effect on the sinus node activity.

Combination of β-blockers with calcium antagonists has been recommended on the theoretical basis of a synergistic antianginal effect: the potential risk of producing or enhancing coronary vasoconstriction would be balanced by calcium-entry blockers through a direct dilating effect on the coronary vasculature. In fact, recent observations suggest that this traditional view may not be entirely correct. Combined treatment might favor the development of more adverse effects than the use of a single antianginal drug (105). A trial (58) suggests a detrimental effect of nifedipine when added to metoprolol in patients not already on β-blockade. The response appears to be different in patients chronically treated with β-blockers in which the association of nifedipine reduces the incidence of recurrent ishemia and myocardial infarction within 48 hr (92). Overviews of several clinical trials demonstrate the complexity of interpreting and analyzing the effectiveness of traditionally accepted therapies (56, 155) and the difficulty of predicting the individual response to therapy.

Heparin and Aspirin

The determinant role of platelet activation and thrombus formation in the development of unstable angina non-Q wave and Q wave myocardial infarction has been demonstrated only recently, but early clin-ical studies had already suggested a beneficial role of anticoagulant agents in acute myocardial ischemia (90, 154). Heparin is the most effective agent, possessing, besides its anticoagulant properties, a number of physiological effects on platelet activity, endothelial function, the complement, and the fibrinolytic systems. Aspirin irreversibly inhibits cyclooxygenase and thus interrupts prostanoid production from platelets recruited at the site of endothelial injury and especially thromboxane A_2 release, a potent platelet activator and vasoconstrictor.

A recent trial (133) has demonstrated that administration of heparin in the acute phase of unstable angina significantly reduced the incidence of refractory angina, myocardial infarction, and death. The same was true for aspirin or the combination of heparin and aspirin, with a trend favoring heparin first.

Thrombolysis

The incidence of intracoronary thrombus angiographically detected in patients with unstable angina varies widely (30, 41). This is due to different factors: the lack of standardized strict criteria for defining intracoronary thrombus, the largely variable delay between the onset of symptoms and coronary angiography, and finally the overlap between unstable angina and myocardial infarction.

In spite of numerous studies trying to demonstrate the value of thrombolysis in unstable angina, no definitive conclusion can be drawn (4, 34, 43, 46, 113, 140, 141, 147). Angiographic improvement is not regularly associated with clinical stabilization and the incidence of myocardial infarction is not negligible (34). Large randomized double-blind trials are in progress (TIMI III and UNASEM trials) with the aim of assessing the effectiveness of thrombolytics to improve myocardial perfusion and determining the optimal initial and follow-up management strategy (9, 116).

There is presently no clear evidence about the advantages provided by the combination of the different drugs available. Nevertheless, as a rule, nitrates associated with heparin or aspirin have been shown to be useful in reducing the frequency of attacks, the incidence of myocardial infarction, and the possible mortality rate (157). Additional β-blockers in patients who were not treated as such is probably justified in the absence of contraindication. Combination with nifedipine should presently be reserved for patients who become or remain unstable despite β-blockade (80).

Emergency Angioplasty and Bypass Surgery

Ideally, angioplasty should be performed after stabilization of the situation, but for a small proportion of patients in whom drug therapy fails, angioplasty must be done in emergency.

It appears to be nearly as effective as in stable angina with an initial success rate of approximatively 80–90% (32, 87, 108, 123, 128, 129, 137) but with a significantly higher incidence of complications and especially of acute coronary occlusions due to thrombosis or vasospasm. This higher complication rate is related to the cascade of factors triggered by endothelial injury leading to platelet aggregation and formation of a labile thrombus at the site of dilatation (37, 39). Nevertheless, the method has demonstrated its value in providing an effective way to rapidly relieve critical ischemia (88, 153).

There are mainly two conditions in which surgery must be preferred to emergency angioplasty: (*a*) severe left ventricular dysfunction, and (*b*) multivessel disease or significant stenosis on the left main artery. By-pass surgery compared to angioplasty has the advantage of a lower recurrence rate of stenosis, but it has a larger early mortality rate (93, 106, 111).

MYOCARDIAL INFARCTION

Most commonly, acute myocardial infarction is secondary to intracoronary occlusion by development of a thrombus on the site of an atherosclerotic plaque disruption or fissuring. Less frequently, it is the consequence of a prolonged vasospasm (149), a coronary embolism complicating endocarditis or left-sided thrombi, a primary (traumatic) or secondary coronary dissection due to the extension of an aortic root-dissecting hematoma.

According to the presence or absence of a Q wave on a 12-lead ECG, two patterns can be distinguished: Q wave and non-Q wave myocardial infarction. Q wave infarction does not necessarily correspond to a transmural necrosis, but it usually implies a more extended myocardial damage due to the total occlusion of a coronary artery with insufficient collateral flow.

Non-Q wave infarction represents the intermediary syndrome between unstable angina and Q wave infarction, with a slight and usually transient increase in cardiac enzymes, attesting to a lesser damage. By different invasive and noninvasive techniques, it is possible to demonstrate that the diagnosis of non-Q wave myocardial infarction can be missed when using a conventional serum enzymatic approach (27). The in-hospital mortality of non-Q wave infarction is lower than that with Q wave infarction, but total mortalities at 1 year are similar (96, 99). Anatomically, non-Q wave infarction does not correspond necessarily to a subendocardial necrosis. Pathogenically, it may be the consequence of a rapid spontaneous reperfusion of an occluded coronary artery, of a persistent occlusion in the presence of well-developed collaterals or of an acute decrease of coronary flow subsequent to a transient reduction in perfusion pressure.

As a rule, infarct size not only depends on the limitation of coronary flow but also on the myocardial oxygen demand at the time of coronary occlusion. Factors that enhance myocardial oxygen needs may exaggerate the extent of myocardial injury. By the same way, the rapid release of catecholamines at the early stages of myocardial infarction may play a deleterious role by stimulating inotropism, increasing heart rate and blood pressure. Similarly, the persistence of physical activity might explain the extended necrosis frequently observed in symptomless patients.

Functional Impairment

Normal left ventricular (LV) function implies an adequate balance beteen myocardial oxygen supply and demand. In the presence of transient myocardial ischemia, the initial hemodynamic impairment observed is a reversible increase in LV end-diastolic pressure (48), which is related both to a decreased LV distensibility and to an impaired contractility leading to increased LV end-diastolic volume (118). This results in an upward and rightward shift of the LV diastolic pressure/volume curve.

Experimental models have been extensively used to investigate the functional impairment induced by ischemia (54, 68, 130), but sudden coronary occlusion in experimental animals does not reproduce the conditions observed in patients with long-standing coronary stenosis and variably developed collateral flow.

In human studies, LV function has been evaluated during provocative tests such as pacing (35, 85, 117), isometric and dynamic exercise (98, 107), or catecholamine infusion (146). These conditions reproduce those of exercise-induced angina, by increasing myocardial oxygen demand, and may not apply to unstable angina at rest for which sudden reduction in coronary flow is the primary determinant of ischemia.

From a metabolic point of view, supply ischemia differs from demand ischemia by the simultaneous development of a mitochondrial oxygen deprivation leading to a decreased ATP availability and the tissue accumulation of metabolites consecutive to the drop in coronary flow (102). This results in rapid increase in cellular concentrations of protons, inorganic phosphate, and lactate, which subsequently interfere with the contractile process.

Intracellular acidosis due to both CO_2 retention and organic acids has been proposed as the main mechanism for impaired systolic function (29, 72), but this has not been entirely confirmed (63).

The study of myocardial function during percutaneous transluminal coronary angioplasty provides a unique opportunity to evaluate the acute reversible coronary occlusion and to determine the sequence of functional disturbances produced by ischemia. Myocardial relaxation is affected in the first seconds of occlusion, characterized by a sudden fall in peak negative dP/dt associated with a marked prolongation of the isovolumic relaxation time. Systolic function impairment follows as shown by a linear fall of positive dP/dtmax accompanied by an increase in the isovolumic contraction time, a decrease in ejection fraction, and a progressive increase in left ventricular filling pressures (127). Furthermore, there is an early alteration in filling dynamics due to diastolic asynchrony between ischemic and nonischemic segments (121).

Intervention Strategies to Minimize Myocardial Injury

As functional impairment and prognosis are directly related to the extent of myocardial injury, the primary objective of therapy is to improve the balance between myocardial oxygen demand and coronary oxygen supply. On a theoretical basis, this can be obtained in two ways: optimizing loading conditions with appropriate pharmacological intervention or restoring blood flow with the aim of salvaging the myocardium at risk of necrosis. This latter objective has been made possible with the use of thrombolytic agents and the development of percutaneous transluminal coronary angioplasty.

The benefit from thrombolytic therapy has been clearly shown by a number of well-conducted convincing clinical trials demonstrating that survival rate was increased (2, 49, 62, 151) and left ventricular function was improved (51, 60, 104, 150). This approach is evidently superior to all prior pharmacological interventions. However, due to the application of strict selection criteria, the proportion of patients that can presently benefit from thrombolytic therapy is less than 50%. This implies that nowadays the majority of patients at the early stage of myocardial infarction are still managed according to a common pharmacological approach that has demonstrated significant, although less dramatic, beneficial effects.

Myocardial-Specific Pharmacological Intervention

Nitrates

Experimentally, early nitrate intravenous therapy has been shown effective in limiting infarct size (64, 65), in reducing the incidence of both infarct extension and cardiogenic shock, and finally in improving survival rate. To be effective, therapy should be initiated within the first hours of the onset of symptoms and the dose cautiously titrated to obtain a significant decrease in systemic or mean blood pressure without inducing hypotension or tachycardia. In patients with suspected right ventricular infarction, nitrate administration should be avoided because of the risk of decreasing right ventricular preload with a subsequent drop in cardiac output.

β-Blockers

By reducing heart rate, contractility, and blood pressure, β-blockers are expected to improve the metabolic balance of the ischemic myocardium. However, the experimental demonstration of a limiting effect on myocardial injury is still lacking (55, 74, 82). In patients with acute evolving myocardial infarction, early administration of intravenous β-blockers reduces significantly enzyme release and presumably infarct size; the incidence of recurrent ischemic events is also decreased and early survival rate improves (61, 66, 89, 97, 131, 156). A number of mechanisms have been invoked to account for the decreased mortality rate, among which is a reduction in the incidence of cardiac rupture, related to a decreased shearing stress on the necrotic tissue. If confirmed, this finding would also be of interest in patients treated by thrombolysis in whom an unexpected higher mortality has been reported during the 24 hr following the onset of symptoms (49), a phenomenon that has been related to early cardiac rupture. Retrospective analysis of clinical trials suggests that in diabetics benefit from β-blockers is of a larger magnitude (81).

Calcium Antagonists

A number of experimental and clinical investigations have been carried out to evaluate the potentially protective effects of calcium antagonists on myocardial ischemic injury. By improving coronary flow and decreasing coronary oxygen demand, calcium antagonists were assumed to reduce infarct size as well as reinfarction and mortality rates. However, no definitive

conclusions could be drawn from the meta-analysis of the available studies grouping thousands of patients (56).

Thrombolysis

The benefits of early administration of thrombolytics have become evident with the demonstration that prompt reperfusion of occluded coronary arteries preserved LV function and improved mortality rate in patients with myocardial infarction (2, 49, 60, 62, 76, 151). The intravenous route provides evident advantages over the intracoronary administration such as reduced delay and cost, greater safety, and wider applicability.

The currently available thrombolytic agents can be distinguished in two categories according to their fibrin selectivity, designating their relative capacity to achieve local activation of the fibrin-plasminogen complex. Selective agents include tissue-type plasminogen activator (t-PA) and single-chain urokinase plasminogen activator (scu-PA). They provide a more rapid reperfusion with a less extensive fibrinogen breakdown and a reduced dependency on the delay of administration. Nonselective agents, including streptokinase (SK), urokinase, and anisoylated plasminogen streptokinase activator complex (APSAC), activate circulating and fibrin-bound plasminogen and thus produce an extensive fibrinogenolysis with higher titers of fibrinogen split products. This results in a marked platelet-inhibitory function (11, 134), which could account for a lower incidence of rethrombosis.

Streptokinase

Considering the pooled results of a total of 17 clinical trials using high dose intravenous SK, Topol (139) reports a mean reperfusion rate (defined by angiographic demonstration of successful recanalization of an occluded artery) of 42% and a mean patency rate (defined as an "open" vessel at an arbitrary point in time after initiation of therapy) of 51%. Overall mortality reduction is around 20% (49, 62, 84), the benefit being clearly dependent on the delay for applying therapy after the onset of symptoms (49).

Anisoylated Plasminogen Streptokinase Activator Complex

APSAC is a derivative of SK and contains acyl groups at the active site, which prevents plasminogen activation in the circulation. Its theoretical advantages over SK are related to a higher clot specificity and a prolonged half-life due to its slow deacylation; as a consequence, it can be administered as a bolus. Its main disadvantages include, as does streptokinase, hypotension and possible allergic reactions in a small proportion of patients. There is also a potential risk of viral component transmission due to the mode of preparation of the agent.

Regarding the proportion of recanalization (6, 17, 138) and patency (20, 69) APSAC appears more effective than SK, but this has not been confirmed in all studies (7, 148). It seems that the induction of a systemic lytic state demonstrated by a low plasma fibrinogen concentration is a prerequisite for the efficacy of the thrombolytic agent (24). Mortality rate is markedly reduced (47% at 30 days) in APSAC versus placebo group patients (2, 86).

Urokinase

Urokinase has also the advantage of a bolus administration. Being not antigenic, it has a considerably lower incidence of adverse effects. The patency rate appears to be very similar to that of t-PA (83, 94). Its main disadvantage is its cost.

Prourokinase (scu-PA)

Prourokinase is relatively fibrin selective with a half-life similar to that of urokinase. Preliminary data indicate a patency rate comparable to that obtained with SK (70, 79, 110).

Tissue Plasminogen Activator (t-PA)

The development of recombinant techniques has allowed the clinical use of this endothelium-derived protease enzyme. Extensive clinical investigation has confirmed the effectiveness of t-PA: survival rate is significantly increased (151, 152) and LV function is improved (8, 51). Col-

lecting data from a total of 19 clinical trials representing more than 1750 patients, Topol reports a 69% recanalization rate and a 76% patency rate (139). The relative clot selectivity of t-PA accounts for a less marked decrease in circulating fibrinogen (112, 141), but the incidence of bleeding complications is similar when compared to nonselective agents (45). There is still no agreement on the optimal dosage and regimen of administration (95) that will obtain the maximal efficacy and decrease the risk of reocclusion without enhancing the incidence of bleeding complications. At the present time, it appears important that the dose be large enough in the first 4 hr (28, 142, 143) in order to achieve reperfusion with a limited total duration to prevent bleeding complications. Another strategy proposes to combine t-PA with a non-clot-selective thrombolytic agent such as SK, in order to avoid coronary reocclusion by an adequate reduction in plasma fibrinogen (47, 144). Recurrent unstable ischemia in patients with acute myocardial infarction, treated by t-PA, may be successfully resolved by a second infusion without serious bleeding complications (10).

Adjunctive Pharmacological Therapy during and after Thrombolysis

The rationale for adjunctive antithrombotic and antiplatelet therapy during and after thrombolysis is based on a better knowledge of different factors involved in the process of reocclusion. Marked platelet activation is induced by thrombolysis and leads to the generation of thromboxane A_2 and serotonin, which favor platelet recruitment and vasoconstriction on the site of a high-grade stenosis. Combination of a low dose of aspirin with SK reduces the incidence of reinfarction and improves short- and long-term survival rates, without significant increase in major bleeding complications (62). Thrombin generation by activation of the coagulation cascade is attested by elevated levels of fibrinopeptide A during thrombolysis (36). Heparin was assumed to be useful in preventing recurrent thrombosis. However, in spite of several clinical trials, the question of whether heparin therapy is indicated remains unresolved (44). Heparin administration after thrombolysis could improve infarct-related vessel patency (59, 62, 145) and survival rate (119) at the cost of a possible increased incidence of minor bleeding (15).

Combination of early intravenous β-blockers with thrombolysis leads to a significant reduction in recurrent ischemia and reinfarction (114, 135). It might also contribute to decrease the incidence of early death due to cardiac rupture (61). Nitrates might be theoretically effective in preventing reocclusion by reducing preload and alleviating vasoconstriction at the site of coronary stenosis; an additive beneficial effect could be expected from their antiplatelet activity as demonstrated experimentally. To date, no definitive clinical benefit has been reported regarding the use of nitrates in this setting. In contrast, the early administration of angiotensin-converting enzyme inhibitors prevents progressive LV dilatation after anterior myocardial infarction (109).

In patients at high risk for reocclusion or at high risk for hemodynamic deterioration because of an extended myocardial infarction, intraaortic balloon counterpulsation might be of interest after thrombolytic therapy (100).

At the present time, in the absence of contraindications, the combination of intravenous thrombolysis with early low dose aspirin and early intravenous β-blockers constitutes the adequate approach for reperfusion and prevention of reocclusion of the infarct-related vessel. The benefit seems to be directly related to the extent of the infarct and possibly to its site (anterior rather than inferior); in the elderly patient, the potential bleeding risk increases and the efficacy of thrombolytic therapy, although likely, is not yet established.

Comparison of the respective effectiveness on reperfusion, LV function, and mortality rate of the different thrombolytics with or without adjunctive antithrombotic and antiplatelet therapy represents a formidable task. To date, two large multicenter randomized open trials have evaluated the relative merits of SK and t-PA (50, 132). Their effectiveness and safety for use in routine conditions of care appear similar (50, 132). There is no apparent benefit provided by the addition of heparin (12,500 units subcutaneously twice daily, starting 12 hr after beginning the t-PA or SK infusion) to the treatment of aspirin. The incidence of major bleeding increases in the SK- and heparin-treated group (50, 132), whereas the overall incidence of strokes appears to be higher with t-PA than with SK (1.3 versus 1%) (132).

Reperfusion Injury

Restitution of coronary blood flow on a previously ischemic myocardium may induce a sequence of biochemical and structural events responsible for the development of severe arrhythmias and prolonged LV dysfunction (stunned myocardium) (19). This may be associated with extensive microvascular injury leading to the no-reflow phenomenon.

Arrhythmia in humans is not as common as in experimental animals. The mechanisms involved are still debated. Generation of highly reactive oxygen species combined with cytosolic calcium overload are supposed to cause membrane damage and relative calcium insensitivity of the contractile mechanism (103). Local activation of neutrophils probably plays an important role in this process: by releasing chemotactic factors, vasoactive agents, and cytokines at reperfusion, neutrophils can produce an endothelial injury, which may ultimately result in mechanical obstruction and irreversible cell damage (26, 57).

Emergency PTCA and Surgical Revascularization

Primary coronary angioplasty in myocardial infarction has been proposed as a strategy to achieve reperfusion more rapidly than with intravenous thrombolytic therapy (12, 53, 67, 91, 115). Although effective, this method has major drawbacks: it implies exceptional logistic facilities, it enhances the risks of vascular damage with subsequent reocclusion, and it favors the development of severe arrhythmias.

This strategy must be considered in two conditions: (*a*) in patients with extensive anterior infarction suggesting a proximal occlusion of the left anterior descending artery, in whom thrombolysis cannot be performed because of major contraindications; and *(b)* in patients with cardiogenic shock or severe LV dysfunction who do not respond to conventional pharmacological therapy. Recent data strongly suggest that successful emergency coronary angioplasty improves prognosis in cardiogenic shock with a survival rate of more than 50% (22, 77, 101, 122) as compared with the 80% mortality rate usually reported when drug therapy is used (73, 124, 136). In such conditions, recanalization may produce a dramatic and sustained improvement in LV performance as attested by a marked increase in cardiac output with a reduction in LV filling pressure (14). This response can probably be attributed to a prompt relief of critical ischemia in an extended myocardial mass with subsequent limitation of infarct size. This concept is corroborated by experimental data that demonstrate that recanalization achieved with angioplasty significantly reduces the extent of myocardial injury (40).

An apparent benefit from early bypass surgery for cardiogenic shock has been reported (13, 33). Surgical myocardial revascularization is likely to improve survival when performed within the first hours of the onset of shock, but it requires exceptional logistic facilities, which considerably limit its application. Nowadays, the indications for emergency bypass surgery in the early phase of myocardial infarction remain essentially persistent pain or hemodynamic instability after a failed angioplasty and the development of postinfarct angina when coronary angioplasty is contraindicated. In patients with irreversible myocardial damage and shock, an LV assist device, if available, should be considered while waiting for heart transplantation.

Prospective randomized studies are urgently needed to define the indications and limitations of invasive therapy in patients with cardiogenic shock. Until more experience is gained, immediate angioplasty should be considered in those patients with poor prognosis who usually do not benefit from thrombolytic therapy (49)

and for whom intraaortic balloon counterpulsation represents essentially a temporary support for achieving hemodynamic stability (125).

CONCLUSIONS

At the present time, the rationale for thrombolytic treatment is clearly established and the assumption that early reperfusion of an occluded artery could save jeopardized myocardium is correct. There is also strong evidence that the combination of oral aspirin and SK is effective and safe. Further addition of heparin is theoretically attractive considering the risk of thrombus formation after successful thrombolysis, but the benefit is not demonstrated and the incidence of bleeding complications appears to be enhanced.

Many questions are still unresolved. Which among the available thrombolytic agents provides the best risk-to-benefit ratio? What are the limitations of thrombolysis in the different subsets of patients and, notably, in the group of elderly patients? What is the ultimate delay after onset of symptoms for instituting reperfusion therapy? In which conditions should primary angioplasty be preferred to thrombolysis?

A recent report of the American College of Cardiology and the American Heart Association establishes current guidelines for treatment of acute myocardial infarction, with the aim of defining the indications for diagnostic procedures and therapeutic interventions (1). This important publication will serve every clinician who must cope with the management of acute myocardial infarction.

References

1. ACC/AHA guidelines for the early management of patients with acute myocardial infarction. Circulation 1990;82:664–707.
2. AIMS Trial Study Group: Effect of intravenous APSAC on mortality after acute myocardial infarction: preliminary report of a placebo-controlled clinical trial. Lancet 1988;1:545–549.
3. Ambrose JA et al. Coronary angiographic morphology in myocardial infarction: a link between the pathogenesis of unstable angina and myocardial infarction. J Am Coll Cardiol 1985;6:1233–1238.
4. Ambrose JA, Hjemdahl-Monsen C, Borrico S et

al. Quantiative and qualitative effects of intracoronary streptokinase in unstable angina and non Q-wave infarction. J Am Coll Cardiol 1987;9:1156–1165.

5. Ambrose JA, Winters SL, Arora RR, et al. Angiographic evolution of coronary artery morphology in unstable angina. J Am Coll Cardiol 1986;7:472–478.

6. Anderson JL, Rothbard RI, Hackwoerthy RA, et al. Multicenter reperfusion trial of intravenous anisoylated plasminogen streptokinase activator complex (APSAC) in acute myocardial infarction: controlled comparison with intracoronary streptokinase. J Am Coll Cardiol 1988;11:1153–1163.

7. Anderson JL, Sorensen SG, Moreno FL, et al. Multicenter patency trial of intravenous anistreplase compared with streptokinase in acute myocardial infarction. The TEAM-2 Study Investigators. Circulation 1991;83:126–140.

8. Armstrong PW, Baigrie RS, Daly PA, et al. Tissue plasminogen activator Toronto (TPAT): randomized trial in myocardial infarction. J Am Coll Cardiol 1989;13:1469–1476.

9. Bär FW. Thrombolysis in patients with unstable angina. In: Bleifeld W, et al, eds. Unstable angina. Berlin: Springer-Verlag, 1990:225–234.

10. Barbash GI, Hod H, Roth A, et al. Repeat infusions of recombinant tissue-type plasminogen activator in patients with acute myocardial infarction and early recurrent myocardial ischemia. J Am Coll Cardiol 1990;16:779–783.

11. Barnhart MI, Cress DC, Henry RL, Riddle JM. Influence of fibrinogen split products on platelets. Thromb Diath Haemorrh 1967;17:78–98.

12. Beauchamp GD, Vacek JL, Robuck W. Management comparison for acute myocardial infarction: direct angioplasty versus sequential thrombolysis-angioplasty. Am Heart J 1990;120:237–242.

13. Berg R, Selinger SL, Leonard JL, et al. Immediate coronary artery bypass for acute evolving myocardial infarction. J Thorac Cardiovasc Surg 1981;81:493–497.

14. Seydoux C, Goy JJ, Beuret P, et al. Effectiveness of percutaneous transluminal coronary angioplasty in cardiogenic shock during acute myocardial infarction. Am J Cardiol 1992;69:968–969.

15. Bleich SD, Nichols TC, Schumacher RR, et al. Effect of heparin on coronary arterial patency after thrombolysis with tissue plasminogen activator in acute myocardial infarction. Am J Cardiol 1990;66:1412–1417.

16. Bleifeld W. Unstable angina: pathophysiology and drug therapy. Eur J Clin Pharmacol 1990;38(suppl 1):S73–76.

17. Bonnier HJRM, Visser RF, Klomps HC, Hoffmann HJML, and the Dutch Invasive Reperfusion Study Group. Comparison of intravenous anisoylated plasminogen streptokinase activator complex and intracoronary streptokinase in acute myocardial infarction. Am J Cardiol 1988;62:25–30.

18. Braunwald E. Unstable angina: a classification. Circulation 1989;80:410–414.

19. Braunwald E, Kloner RA. The stunned myocardium: prolonged, postischemic ventricular dysfunction. Circulation 1982;66:1146–1149.

20. Brochier ML, Quillet L, Kulbertus H, et al. Intravenous APSAC versus intravenous streptokinase in evolving myocardial infarction. Drugs 1987;33(suppl 3):140–145.

21. Brown MA, Myears DW, Bergmann SR. Noninvasive assessment of canine myocardial oxidative metabolism with ^{11}C-acetate and positron emission tomography. J Am Coll Cardiol 1988;12:1054–1063.

22. Brown TM, Ianonne LA, Gordon DF, et al. Percutaneous myocardial reperfusion (PMR) reduces mortality in acute myocardial infarction (MI) complicated by cardiogenic shock. Circulation 1985;72:III-309.

23. Brown BG, Bolson E, Petersen RB et al. The mechanism of nitroglycerin action: stenosis vasodilation as a major component of dosing response. Circulation 1981;64:1089–1097.

24. Brugemann J, van der Meer J, Takens BH, Hillege H, Lie KI. A systemic non-lytic state and local thrombolytic failure of anistreplase (anisoylated plasminogen streptokinase activator complex, APSAC) in acute myocardial infarction. Br Heart J 1990;64:355–358.

25. Buxton DB, Nienaber CA, Luxen A, Ratib O, Hansen H, Phelps ME, Schelbert HR. Noninvasive quantitation of regional myocardial oxygen consumption in vivo with [L-^{11}C]acetate and dynamic positron emission tomography. Circulation 1989;79:134–142.

26. Carp H, Janoff A. In vitro suppression serum elastase-inhibitory capacity by reactive oxygen species generated by phagocytosing polymorphonuclear leukocytes. J Clin Invest 1979;63:793–797.

27. Carpeggiani C, L'Abbate A, Marzullo P, et al. Multiparametric approach to diagnosis of non-Q-wave acute myocardial infarction. Am J Cardiol 1989;63:404–408.

28. Clozel J, Tschopp T, Luedin E, Holvoet P. Time course of thrombolysis induced by intravenous bolus or infusion of tissue plasminogen activator in a rabbit jugular vein thrombosis model. Circulation 1989;79:125–133.

29. Cobbe SM, Poole-Wilson PA. The time of onset and severity of acidosis in myocardial ischemia. J Mol Cell Cardiol 1980;12:745–760.

30. Cowley MJ, DiSciascio G, Rehr RB, Vetrovec GW. Angiographic observations and clinical relevance of coronary thrombus in unstable angina pectoris. Am J Cardiol 1989;63:108E–113E.

31. Davies MJ, Thomas AC. Plaque fissuring—the cause of acute myocardial infarction, sudden ischemic death, and crescendo angina. Br Heart J 1985;53:363–373.

32. de Feyter PJ, Serruys PW, van den Brand M, et al. Emergency coronary angioplasty in refractory unstable angina. N Engl J Med 1985;313:342–347.

33. de Wood MA, Spores J, Berg R, et al. Acute myocardial infarction: a decade of experience with surgical reperfusion in 701 patients. Circulation 1983;68(suppl II):8.

34. de Zwaan CH, Bär FW, Janssen J, et al. Effects of thrombolytic therapy in unstable angina: clinical and angiographic results. J Am Coll Cardiol 1988;12:301–309.

35. Dwyer EM. Left ventricular pressure-volume alterations and regional disorders of contraction during myocardial ischemia induced by atrial pacing. Circulation 1970;42:1111–1122.
36. Eisenberg PR, Sherman LA, Jaffe AS. Paradoxic elevation of fibrinopeptide A after streptokinase: evidence for continued thrombosis despite intense fibrinolysis. J Am Coll Cardiol 1987;10:527–529.
37. Falk E. Unstable angina with fatal outcome: dynamic coronary thrombosis leading to infarction and/or sudden death. Circulation 1985;71:699–708.
38. Falk E. Plaque rupture with severe pre-existing stenosis precipitating coronary thrombosis. Characteristics of coronary arterosclerotic plaques underlying fatal occlusive thrombi. Br Heart J 1983;50:127–134.
39. Fitzgerald DJ, Roy L, Catella F, FitzGerald GA. Platelet activation in unstable coronary disease. N Engl J Med 1986;315:983–989.
40. Force T, Kemper A, Leavitt M, Parisi AF. Acute reduction in functional infarct expansion with late coronary reperfusion: Assessment with quantitative two-dimensional echocardiography. J Am Coll Cardiol 1988;11:192–200.
41. Freeman MR, Williams AE, Chisholm RJ, Armstrong PW. Intracoronary thrombus and complex morphology in unstable angina. Relation to timing of angiography and in-hospital cardiac events. Circulation 1989;80:17–23.
42. Fuster V, Badimon L, Cohen M, Ambrose JA, Badimon JJ. Insights into the pathogenesis of acute ischemic syndromes. Circulation 1988;77:1213–1220.
43. Gold HK, Johns JA, Leinbach RC, et al. A randomized, blinded placebo-controlled trial of recombinant human tissue-type plasminogen activator in patients with unstable angina pectoris. Circulation 1987;75:1192–1199.
44. Gold HK, Leinbach RC, Garabedian HD, et al. Acute coronary reocclusion after thrombolysis with recombinant human tissue-type plasminogen activator: prevention by a maintenance infusion. Circulation 1986;73:347–352.
45. Gore JM, Sloan M, Price TR, Randall AM, et al. Intracerebral hemorrhage, cerebral infarction, and subdural hematoma after acute myocardial infarction and thrombolytic therapy in the Thrombolysis in Myocardial Infarction Study. Thrombolysis in Myocardial Infarction, Phase II, pilot and clinical trial. Circulation 1991;83:448–459.
46. Gotoh K, Minamino T, Katoh O, et al. The role of intracoronary thrombus in unstable angina: angiographic assessment and thrombolytic therapy during ongoing anginal attacks. Circulation 1988;77:526–534.
47. Grines CL, Nissen SE, Booth DC, et al. A new thrombolytic regimen for acute myocardial infarction using combination half dose tissue-type plasminogen activator with full dose streptokinase: a pilot study. J Am Coll Cardiol 1989;14:573–580.
48. Grossmann W. Why is the left ventricular diastolic pressure increased during angina pectoris? J Am Coll Cardiol 1985;5:607–608.
49. Gruppo Italiano per lo Studio della Streptochinasi nell'Infarto Miocardico (GISSI). Effectiveness of intravenous thrombolytic treatment in acute myocardial infarction. Lancet 1986;1:397–401.
50. Gruppo Italiano per lo Studio della Sopravvivenza nell'Infarto Miocardico (GISSI-2). A factorial randomised trial of alteplase versus streptokinase and heparin versus non heparin among 12490 patients with acute myocardial infarction. Lancet 1990;336:65–71.
51. Guerci AD, Gerstenblith G, Brinker JA, et al. A randomized trial of intravenous tissue plasminogen activator for acute myocardial infarction with subsequent randomization to elective coronary angioplasty. N Engl J Med 1987;317:1613–1618.
52. Hamm CW, Lorenz R, Bleifeld W, Kupper W, Wober W, Weber PC. Biochemical evidence of platelet activation in patients with persistent unstable angina. J Am Coll Cardiol 1987;10:998–1004.
53. Hartzler GO, Rutherford BD, McConahay DR. Percutaneous transluminal coronary angioplasty: Application for acute myocardial infarction. Am J Cardiol 1984;53:117C–121C.
54. Hearse DJ. Oxygen deprivation and early myocardial contractile failure: a reassessment of the possible role of adenosine triphosphate. Am J Cardiol 1979;44:1115–1121.
55. Hearse DJ, Yellon DM, Downey JM: Can betablockers limit myocardial infarct size? Eur Heart J 1986;7:925–930.
56. Held PH, Yusuff S, Furberg D. Calcium channel blockers in acute myocardial infarction and unstable angina: an overview. Br Med J 1989;299:1187–1192.
57. Hoffstein ST, Friedman RS, Weissmann G. Degranulation, membrane addition and shape change during chemotactic factor-induced aggregation of human neutrophils. J Cell Biol 1982;95:234–241.
58. Holland Interuniversity Nifedipine/Metoprolol Trial (HINT) Research Group. Early treatment of unstable angina in the coronary care unit. A randomised, double blind, placebo controlled comparison of recurrent ischemia in patients treated with nifedipine or metoprolol or both. Br Heart J 1986;56:400–413.
59. Hsia J, Hamilton WP, Kleiman N, et al. A comparison between heparin and low-dose aspirin as adjunctive therapy with tissue plasminogen activator for acute myocardial infarction. Heparin-Aspirin Reperfusion Trial (HART) Investigators. N Engl J Med 1990;323:1433–1437.
60. ISAM Study Group. A prospective trial of intravenous streptokinase in acute myocardial infarction (ISAM). N Engl J Med 1986;314:1465–1471.
61. ISIS-I Collaborative Group. Randomized trial of intravenous atenolol among 16,027 cases of suspected acute myocardial infarction: ISIS-I. Lancet 1986;2:57–66.
62. ISIS-2 Collaborative Group. Randomized trial of intravenous streptokinase, oral aspirin, both, or neither among 17,187 cases of suspected acute myocardial infarction: ISIS-2. Lancet 1988;2:349–360.
63. Jacobus WE, Pores IH, Lucas SK, et al. Intracel-

lular acidosis and contractility in the normal and ischemic heart as examined by ^{31}P NMR. J Mol Cell Cardiol 1982;14(suppl 3):13–20.

64. Jugdutt BI, Becker LC, Hutchins GM, et al. Effect of intravenous nitroglycerin on collateral flow and infarct size in the conscious dog. Circulation 1981;63:17–28.

65. Jugdutt BI, Warnica JW. Intravenous nitroglycerin therapy to limit myocardial infarct size, expansion, and its complications: effect of timing, dosage, and infarct location. Circulation 1988;78:906–916.

66. Jurgensen JH, Frederiksen J, Hansen DA, et al. Limitation of myocardial infarct size in patients less than 66 years treated with alprenolol. Br Heart J 1981;45:583–588.

67. Kander NH, O'Neil WW, Mileski R, Topol EJ, Ellis SG. Two-year post-discharge survival after emergency coronary angioplasty for myocardial infarction: importance of the timing and success of angioplasty. J Am Coll Cardiol 1989;13:193A.

68. Karliner JS, Le Winter MM, Mahler F, Engler R, O'Rurke RA. Pharmacologic and hemodynamic influences on the rate of isovolumic left ventricular relaxation in the normal conscious dog. J Clin Invest 1977;60:511–521.

69. Kasper W, Meinertz T, Wollschlager H, et al. Early clinical evaluation of the intravenous treatment of acute myocardial infarction with anisoylated plasminogen streptokinase activator complex. Drugs 1987;33:112–116.

70. Kasper W, Hohnloser SH, Engler H, et al. Coronary reperfusion studies with pro-urokinase in acute myocardial infarction: evidence for synergism of low dose urokinase. J Am Coll Cardiol 1990;16:733–738.

71. Katus HA, Diederich KW, Hoberg E, et al. Circulating cardiac myosin light chains in patients with angina at rest: identification of a high risk subgroup. J Am Coll Cardiol 1988;3:487–493.

72. Katz AM, Hecht HH. The early "pump" failure of the ischemic heart. Am J Med 1969;47:497–502.

73. Killip T, Kimball JT. Treatment of myocardial infarction in a coronary care unit. A two year experience with 250 patients. Am J Cardiol 1967;20:457–464.

74. Kudoh Y, Maxwell MP, Hearse DJ, et al. Failure of metoprolol to limit infarct size during 24 hours of coronary artery occlusion in a closed chest dog. J Cardiovasc Pharmacol 1984;6:1201–1209.

75. Lam JYT, Chesebro JH, Fuster V. Platelets, vasoconstriction and nitroglycerin during arterial wall injury: a new antithrombotic role for an old drug. Circulation 1988;78:712–716.

76. Lavie CJ, O'Keefe JH, Chesebro JH, Clements IP, Gibbons RJ. Prevention of late ventricular dilatation after acute myocardial infarction by successful thrombolytic reperfusion. Am J Cardiol 1990;66:31–36.

77. Lee L, Bates ER, Pitt B, et al. Percutaneous transluminal coronary angioplasty improves survival in acute myocardial infarction complicated by cardiogenic shock. Circulation 1988;78:1345–1351.

78. Levin RI, Jaffe EA, Weksler BB, et al. Nitroglycerin stimulates synthesis of prostacyclin by cul-

tured human endothelial cells. J Clin Invest 1981;67:762–780.

79. Loscalzo J, Wharton TP, Kirshenbaum JM, et al. Relative clot-selective coronary thrombolysis with prourokinase. Circulation 1989;79:776–782.

80. Lubsen J. Calcium antagonists and beta-blockers in the treatment of unstable angina. In: Bleifeld W, et al, eds. Unstable angina. Berlin: Springer-Verlag, 1990:177–187.

81. Malmberg K, Herlitz J, Hjalmarson A, et al. The effects of metoprolol on mortality and late infarction in diabetics with suspected acute myocardial infarction: retrospective data from two large studies. Eur Heart J 1989;10:423–428.

82. Maroko PR, Kjekshus JK, Sobel BE, et al. Factors influencing infarct size following experimental coronary artery occlusion. Circulation 1971;4:67–82.

83. Mathey DG, Schofer J, Sheehan FH, et al. Intravenous urokinase in acute myocardial infarction. Am J Cardiol 1985;55:878–882.

84. Mauri F, DeBiase AM, Franzosi MG, et al. GISSI: analisi delle cause di morte intraospedaliera. G Ital Cardiol 1987;17:37–44.

85. McLaurin LP, Rolett EL, Grossmann W. Impaired left ventricular relaxation during pacing-induced ischemia. Am J Cardiol 1973;32:751–757.

86. Meinertz T, Kasper W, Schumacher M, Just H. The German multicenter trial of anisoylated plasminogen streptokinase activator complex versus heparin for acute myocardial infarction. Am J Cardiol 1988;62:347–351.

87. Meyer J, Schmitz HJ, Kiesslich R, et al. Percutaneous transluminal coronary angioplasty in patients with stable and unstable angina pectoris. Analysis of early and late results. Am Heart J 1983;106:973–980.

88. Meyer J, Böcker B, Erbel R, et al. Treatment of unstable angina with percutaneous transluminal coronary angioplasty. Circulation 1980;62:III-160.

89. MIAMI Trial Research Group: Metoprolol in acute myocardial infarction (MIAMI): a randomized placebo controlled international trial. Eur Heart J 1985;6:199–226.

90. Michaels L. Heparin administration in acute coronary insufficiency. JAMA 1972;221:1235–1239.

91. Miller PF, Brodie BR, Weintraub RA, et al. Emergency coronary angioplasty for acute myocardial infarction: results from a community hospital. Arch Intern Med 1987;147:1565–1570.

92. Muller JE, Turi ZG, Pearle DL, et al. Nifedipine and conventional therapy for unstable angina. A randomized, double-blind comparison. Circulation 1984;69:728–739.

93. Naunheim KS, Fiore AC, Arango DC, et al. Coronary artery bypass grafting for unstable angina pectoris: risk analysis. Ann Thorac Surg 1989;47:569–574.

94. Neuhaus KL for the G.A.U.S. study group. Thrombolysis in acute myocardial infarction: results of the German-Activator-Urokinase-Study (G.A.U.S.). Eur Heart J 1987;8:49.

95. Neuhaus KL, Feuerer W, Jeep-Tebbe W, Vogt A, Tebbe U. Improved thrombolysis with a modified dose regimen of recombinant tissue-type plas-

minogen activator. J Am Coll Cardiol 1989;14:1566–1569.

96. Nicod P, Gilpin E, Dittrich H, et al. Short- and long-term clinical outcome after Q wave and non-Q wave myocardial infarction in a large patient population. Circulation 1989;79:528–536.

97. Norris RM, Clarke ED, Sammel NL, et al. Protective effect of propranolol in threatened myocardial infarction. Lancet 1978;2:907–909.

98. O'Brien KP, Higgs LM, Glancy DL, Epstein SE. Hemodynamic accompaniments of angina: a comparison during angina induced by exercise and by atrial pacing. Circulation 1969;39:735–743.

99. O'Brien TX, Ross J. Non-Q wave myocardial infarction: incidence, pathophysiology, and clinical course compared with Q-wave infarction. Clin Cardiol. 1989;12(7 suppl 3):1113–1119.

100. Ohman EM, Califf RM, George BS, et al. The use of intraaortic balloon pumping as an adjunct to reperfusion therapy in acute myocardial infarction. The Thrombolysis and Angioplasty in Myocardial Infarction (TAMI) Study Group. Am Heart J 1991;121:895–901.

101. O'Neill W, Erbel R, Laufer N, et al. Coronary angioplasty therapy of cardiogenic shock complicating acute myocardial infarction. Circulation 1985;72:III–309.

102. Opie LH. Lack of oxygen: ischemia and angina. In: The heart, physiology and metabolism. New York: Raven Press, 1991:425–450.

103. Opie LH. Reperfusion injury and its pharmacological modification. Circulation 1989;80:1049–1062.

104. O'Rourke M, Baron D, Keogh A, et al. Limitation of myocardial infarction by early infusion of recombinant tissue-type plasminogen activator. Circulation 1988;77:1311–1315.

105. Packer M. Drug therapy. Combined beta-adrenergic and calcium-entry blockade in angina pectoris. N Engl J Med 1989;320:709–718.

106. Parisi AF, Khrui S, Deupree R, Sharma GV, Scott S, Luchi R. Medical compared with surgical management for unstable angina. Circulation 1989;80:1176–1189.

107. Parker JD, DiGiogi S, West RO. A hemodynamic study of acute coronary insufficiency precipitated by exercise: with observations on the effect of nitroglycerin. Am J Cardiol 1966;17:470–483.

108. Perry RA, Seth A, Hunt A, Shiu MF. Coronary angioplasty in unstable angina and stable angina: a comparison of success and complications. Br Heart J 1988;60:367–372.

109. Pfeffer MA, Lamas GA, Vaughan DE, et al. Effect of captopril on progressive ventricular dilatation after anterior myocardial infarction. N Engl J Med 1988;319:80–86.

110. PRIMI Trial Study Group. Randomized double-blind trial of recombinant pro-urokinase against streptokinase in acute myocardial infarction. Lancet 1989;2:863–868.

111. Rahimtoola SH, Nunley D, Grunkemeier G, Tepley J, Lambert L, Starr A. Ten-year survival after coronary bypass surgery for unstable angina. N Engl J Med 1983;308:676–681.

112. Rao AK, Pratt C, Berke A, et al. Thrombolysis

in Myocardial Infarction (TIMI) Trial–Phase I: Hemorrhagic manifestations and changes in plasma fibrinogen and the fibrinolytic system in patients treated with recombinant tissue plasminogen activator and streptokinase. J Am Coll Cardiol 1988;11:1–11.

113. Rentrop P, Blanke H, Karsch KR, et al. Selective intracoronary thrombolysis in acute myocardial infarction and unstable angina pectoris. Circulation 1981;63:307–317.

114. Roberts R, Rogers WJ, Mueller HS, et al. Immediate versus differed beta-blockade following thrombolytic therapy in patients with acute myocardial infarction. Results of the Thrombolysis in Myocardial Infarction (TIMI) II-B Study. Circulation 1991;83:422–437.

115. Rothbaum DA, Linnemeier TJ, Landin RJ, et al. Emergency percutaneous transluminal coronary angioplasty in acute myocardial infarction: a 3 year experience. J Am Coll Cardiol 1987;10:264–272.

116. Rutherford JD. Unstable angina and thrombolysis. Chest 1990;97(4 suppl):156S–160S.

117. Rutishauser W, Amende J, Mehmel H. Comparison of left ventricular dynamics in normals and patients with ischemic heart disease at rest, during pacing and exercise. Eur J Clin Invest 1972;2:304.

118. Sasayama S, Nonogi H, Miyazaki S, et al. Changes of diastolic properties of the regional myocardium during pacing-induced ischemia in human subjects. J Am Coll Cardiol 1985;5:599–606.

119. SCATI (Studio sulla Calciparina nell'Angina e nella Trombosi Ventricolare nell'Infarto) Group. Randomized controlled trial of subcutaneous calcium-heparin in acute myocardial infarction. Lancet 1989;2:182–186.

120. Schelbert HR, Henze E, Schön HR, Najafi A, Hansen H, Huang SC, Barrio JR, Phelps ME. C-II palmitic acid for the noninvasive evaluation of regional myocardial fatty acid metabolism with positron computed tomography. IV. In vivo demonstration of impaired fatty acid oxidation in acute myocardial ischemia. Am Heart J 1983;106:736–750.

121. Serruys PW, Wijns W, Piscione F, de Feyter P, Hugenholtz PG. Ejection, filling and diastasis during transluminal occlusion in man: consideration on global and regional left ventricular function. In: Grossman W, et al. Diastolic relaxation of the heart. Pasadena, CA: Beverly Foundation, 1987:255–279.

122. Shani J, Rivera M, Greengart A, et al. Percutaneous transluminal coronary angioplasty in cardiogenic shock. J Am Coll Cardiol 1986;7:149A.

123. Sharma B, Wyeth RP, Kolath GS, Gimenez HJ, Franciosa JA. Percutaneous transluminal coronary angioplasty of one vessel for refractory unstable angina pectoris: efficacy in single and multivessel disease. Br Heart J 1988;59:280–286.

124. Sheidt S, Ascherian R, Killip T. Shock after acute myocardial infarction. A clinical and hemodynamic profile. Am J Cardiol 1970;26:556–564.

125. Sheidt S, Wilner G, Mueller H, et al. Intra-aortic

counterpulsation in cardiogenic shock. Report of a co-operative clinical trial. N Engl J Med 1973;288:979–984.

126. Sherman CT, Litvack F, Grundfest W, et al. Coronary angioscopy in patients with unstable angina pectoris. N Engl J Med 1986;315:913–919.

127. Sigwart U, Grbic M, Payot M, et al. Ischemic events during coronary artery balloon obstruction. In: Rutishauser W, ed. Silent ischemia. Berlin: Springer-Verlag, 1985:29–36.

128. Steffenino G, Meier B, Finci L, Rutishauser W. Follow-up results of treatment of unstable angina by coronary angioplasty. Br Heart J 1987;57:416–419.

129. Suryapranata H, deFeyter PJ, Serruys PW. Coronary angioplasty in patients with unstable angina pectoris: is there a role for thrombolysis? J Am Coll Cardiol 1988;12(suppl A):69A–77A.

130. Tennant R, Wiggers CJ. The effect of coronary occlusion on myocardial contraction. Am J Physiol 1935;112:351–361.

131. The International Collaborative Study Group. Reduction of infarct size with the early use of timolol in acute myocardial infarction. N Engl J Med 1984;310:9–15.

132. The International Study Group. In-hospital mortality and clinical course of 20 891 patients with suspected acute myocardial infarction randomised between alteplase and streptokinase with or without heparin. Lancet 1990;336:71–75.

133. Théroux P, Ouimet H, McCans J, et al. Aspirin, heparin, or both to treat acute unstable angina. N Engl J Med 1988;319:1105–1111.

134. Thorsen LI, Brosstad F, Gogstad G, Sletten K, Solum NO. Competitions between fibrinogen with its degradation products for interactions with the platelet-fibrinogen receptor. Thromb Res 1986;44:611–623.

135. TIMI Study Group. Comparison of invasive and conservative strategies after treatment with intravenous tissue plasminogen activator in acute myocardial infarction. N Engl J Med 1989;320:618–628.

136. Timmis AD, Fowler MB, Chamberlain DA. Comparison of hemodynamic response to dopamine and salbutamol in severe cardiogenic shock complicating acute myocardial infarction. Br Med J 1981;282:7–9.

137. Timmis AD, Griffin B, Crick JCP, Sowton E. Early percutaneous transluminal coronary angioplasty in the management of unstable angina. Int J Cardiol 1987;14:25–31.

138. Timmis AD, Griffin B, Crick JCP, Sowton FE. Anisoylated plasminogen streptokinase activator complex in acute myocardial infarction: a placebo-controlled arteriographic coronary recanalization study. J Am Coll Cardiol 1987;10:205–210.

139. Topol EJ. Thrombolytic intervention. In: Topol EJ, ed. Textbook of interventional cardiology. Philadelphia: WB Saunders, 1990:76–120.

140. Topol EJ, Nicklas JM, Kander NH, et al. Coronary revascularization after intravenous tissue plasminogen activator for unstable angina pec-

toris: results of a randomized double-blind, placebo-controlled trial. Am J Cardiol 1988;62:368–371.

141. Topol EJ, Bell WR, Weisfeldt ML. Coronary thrombolysis with recombinant tissue-type plasminogen activator: hematologic and pharmacologic study. Ann Intern Med 1985;103:837–843.

142. Topol EJ, George BS, Kereiakes DJ, et al. Comparison of two dose regimens of intravenous tissue plasminogen activator for acute myocardial infarction. Am J Cardiol 1988;61:723–728.

143. Topol EJ, Ellis SG, Califf RM, et al. Combined tissue-type plasminogen activator and prostacyclin therapy for acute myocardial infarction. J Am Coll Cardiol 1989;14:877–884.

144. Topol EJ, Califf RM, George BS, et al. Coronary arterial thrombolysis with combined infusion of recombinant tissue-type plasminogen activator and urokinase in patients with acute myocardial infarction. Circulation 1988;77:1100–1107.

145. Topol EJ, George BS, Kereiakes DJ, et al. A randomized controlled trial of intravenous tissue plasminogen activator and early intravenous heparin in acute myocardial infarction. Circulation 1989;79:281–286.

146. Vatner SF, Millard RV, Patrick TA, Heyndrickx FR. Effect of isoproterenol on regional myocardial function, electrocardiograms and blood flow in conscious dogs with myocardial ischemia. J Clin Invest 1976;57:1261.

147. Vetrovec GW, Leinbach RC, Gold HK, Cowley MJ. Intracoronary thrombolysis in syndromes of unstable ischemia: angiographic and clinical results. Am Heart J 1982;104:946–952.

148. Vogt P, Schaller MD, Monnier P, Kaufmann U, et al. Systemic thrombolysis in acute myocardial infarction: bolus injection of APSAC versus infusion of streptokinase. Eur Heart J 1988;9(suppl A):213.

149. Wei JY, Genecin A, Greene HL, Achuff SC: Coronary artery spasm with ventricular fibrillation during thyrotoxicosis: response to attaining euthyroid state. Am J Cardiol 1979;43:335–339.

150. White HD, Norris RM, Brown MA, et al. Effect of intravenous streptokinase on left ventricular function and early survival after acute myocardial infarction. N Engl J Med 1987;317:850–855.

151. Wilcox RG, von der Lippe G, Olsson CG, et al. Trial of tissue plasminogen activator for mortality reduction in acute myocardial infarction. Lancet 1988;2:525–530.

152. Wilcox RG, van der Lippe G, Olsson CG, et al. Effects of alteplase in acute myocardial infarction: 6-month results from the ASSET study. Anglo-Scandinavian Study of Early Thrombolysis. Lancet 1990;335:1175–1178.

153. Williams DO, Riley RS, Singh AK, Gewirtz H, Most AS. Evaluation of the role of coronary angioplasty in patients with unstable angina pectoris. Am Heart J 1981;102:1–9.

154. Wood P. Acute and subacute coronary insufficiency. Br Med J 1961;13:215–216.

155. Yusuf S, Wittes J, Friedman L. Overview of

results of randomized clinical trials in heart disease. II. Unstable angina, heart failure, primary prevention with aspirin, and risk factor modification. JAMA 1988;260:2259–2263.

156. Yusuf S, Sleight P, Rossi P, et al. Reduction in infarct size, arrhythmias and chest pain by early intravenous beta blockade in suspected acute myocardial infarction. Circulation 1983;67:32–41.

157. Yusuf S, Collins R, MacMahon S, et al. Effect of intravenous nitrates on mortality in acute myocardial infarction: an overview of the randomized trial. Lancet 1988;1:1088–1092.

16

Acute Left-Sided Valvular Regurgitation

Jean-Pierre Belot

BEDSIDE ASSESSMENT AND ADVANCED STUDIES

Clinical Examination

Clinical examination is the keystone of diagnosis and management of acute mitral and aortic regurgitant lesions, which, in most cases, require a rapid surgical correction. Physical examination provides not only a rapid means of diagnosis, but also an immediate estimation of severity.

Making the Diagnosis

Symptoms manifested by patients with either acute mitral regurgitation or acute aortic regurgitation depend upon etiology and are related to the development of an abrupt left ventricular volume overloading (4, 23, 50, 80).

Clinical findings are nonspecific: tachycardia, dyspnea related to pulmonary hypertension or pulmonary edema, cyanosis, chest pain, fever, and even neurological event or cardiac tamponade (9, 23, 24, 80).

Acute Mitral Regurgitation

Whatever the cause of an acute mitral regurgitation, the auscultation findings are usually holosystolic murmur heard at the apex, radiating to the base of the heart or to the axilla (9, 50). However, especially in patients with a normally sized left atrium and a normal compliance, the pressure gradient between the left ventricle and atrium declines at the end of systole and the murmur may be decrescendo, ending

before A2 and usually softer than that heard in chronic mitral regurgitation (9). Moreover, an associated ejection systolic murmur, or a loud holosystolic murmur following rupture of the interventricular septum, may be confusing. Occasionally, and not only in the presence of a very low cardiac output, the systolic murmur may indeed be absent (50).

Acute Aortic Insufficiency

As opposed to chronic aortic regurgitation, peripheral signs of aortic regurgitation are generally mild or absent. The aortic pulse is decreased and the early diastolic murmur of acute aortic insufficiency is lower pitched and shorter than that of chronic regurgitation. S1 may be soft or absent because of the premature closure of the mitral valve. However, this closure may be incomplete and diastolic regurgitation may occur (9). Because of the combined effects of increased myocardial oxygen demand and reduced coronary blood flow, patients are at high risk of developing myocardial ischemia (23).

Once mitral or aortic regurgitations have been identified, a careful clinical examination may point towards an etiology:

An infective endocarditis will be highly suggestive with a prior history of rheumatic heart disease or valve replacement, fever, change in the character of a known murmur, pallor of the skin, neurological complication, or presence of Osler nodes in a patient who was recently well (66, 99).

An acute partial rupture of a papillary muscle, complicating myocardial infarction, will be suggested in a setting of chest pain with

Table 16.1
Main Causes of Acute Valvular Regurgitation

Acute mitral regurgitation
  Infective endocarditis (native valve or
    prosthetic valve)
  Ischemia, acute myocardial infarction, left
    ventricle aneurysm
  Trauma
  Iatrogenic causes
    Percutaneous mitral balloon valvotomy
    Early complications of valve repair or
      replacement
  Miscellaneous causes
    Acute rheumatic fever
    Amyloidosis, sarcoidosis
    Systemic lupus erythematosus
    Left atrial myxoma
    "Spontaneous" causes (rupture of
      chordae tendineae, myxomatous valve,
      Marfan's syndrome)
Acute aortic insufficiency
  Infective endocarditis (native valve or
    prosthetic valve)
  Dissection of the aorta
  Trauma
  Iatrogenic causes
    Percutaneous balloon valvotomy
    Early complications of valve repair or
      replacement
  Miscellaneous causes
    Takayashu's arteritis, Behçet's syndrome
    Systemic lupus erythematosus
    "Spontaneous" rupture (bicuspid valve,
      Marfan's syndrome, myxomatous
      valve)

characteristic ECG findings, followed by rapid development of severe pulmonary edema or indeed shock, with a harsh apical systolic murmur (69, 80).
A diagnosis of acute dissection of the proximal aorta may be easily argued with a history of chest pain radiating to the back, in a hypertensive patient with a diastolic murmur heard at the left side of the sternum, a pulse deficit, neurological manifestations, and ECG usually showing the absence of signs of myocardial ischemia or infarction (24).

However, one should bear in mind the frequent occurrence of very complex and confusing clinical pictures that require a thorough investigation in order to make an accurate diagnosis.

Main causes of acute mitral regurgitation and acute aortic insufficiency are shown in Table 16.1.

Assessing the Severity of Symptoms

The severity of symptoms is, in most cases, closely linked to the extent of heart failure, which is related to the effects of the sudden volume overloading on a left ventricle or a left atrium with normal compliance (4, 80).

A broad spectrum of clinical status may be observed, from a well-tolerated valvular insufficiency that requires a standard medical management, to a poorly tolerated state that demands emergency institution of both noninvasive and invasive monitoring as well as inotropic and ventilatory support. In all events, a close cooperation between medical and surgical staffs is essential (32).

Laboratory Investigations of Immediate Urgency: The "Emergency Room Trilogy"

The assessment of both the etiology and the severity of acute valvular regurgitation is supported by systematic laboratory investigations.

Electrocardiogram

In most cases of acute valvular insufficiency, the usual electrocardiographic finding is sinus tachycardia, a normal left ventricular voltage, and minor repolarization abnormalities. One possible confounding feature may occur when an acute mitral regurgitation complicates a chronic mitral regurgitation, where the rhythm classically is atrial fibrillation (80).

Arterial Blood Sampling

This investigation is useful for assessment of the initial respiratory tolerance of heart failure, especially in the case of an apparently well-tolerated ventilatory status associated with a severe hypoxemia.

Chest Roentgenogram

If an acute valvular regurgitation occurs in a previously "normal" heart, the cardiac silhouette is normal or mildly increased (except for aortic dissection), and a broad spectrum of findings, linked to pulmonary hypertension, may be observed (9, 17, 80).

On the other hand, if an acute valvular regurgitation occurs in the case of existing heart disease, the chest radiograph may show enlargement of the left ventricle, left atrium, and possibly the ascending aorta (23, 50).

M-Mode, Two-Dimensional, and Doppler Echocardiography: The "Noninvasive" Approach

Rapid advances in transthoracic echocardiography, as a noninvasive technique of assessment of valvulopathies, has led to a progressive decrease in the use of invasive techniques (i.e., left-sided cardiac catheterization), which carry potentially deleterious effects (67, 76, 77, 87). Subsequently, in infective endocarditis, both M-mode and two-dimensional echocardiography have been widely evaluated and proved to play a major role in the diagnosis and the detection of complications (8, 21, 45, 53, 62, 75).

The transthoracic approach has also been helpful in cases of acute mitral regurgitation complicating acute mitral infarction, rupture of chordae tendineae, and acute aortic dissection (24, 59, 65). However, such a technique requires a skilled operator, its complexity being related to the complex reconstruction of three-dimensional structures from two-dimensional imaging.

The usual echocardiographic "screening" to perform in acute mitral regurgitation and acute aortic insufficiency, when using M-mode and two-dimensional echocardiography, is summarized in Figure 16.1.

Transesophageal Approach for Mitral Valve Disorders

In well-tolerated lesions or, alternatively, in mechanically ventilated patients, transesophageal echocardiography is now accepted to be more sensitive than the transthoracic approach, especially in mitral valve disease, providing striking views of the left atrium and the mitral apparatus (37, 58, 70, 89). As previously emphasized by Erbel et al. (25), then by Mügge et al. (62), the transesophageal approach has proved to be of great relevance in infective endocarditis in improving the sensitivity

of detection of vegetations. Moreover, for patients with mitral valve endocarditis, a vegetation diameter larger than 10 mm has been shown to be highly sensitive in identifying patients at risk of embolic events (62). In other mitral valve diseases such as mitral valve prolapse, with or without a flail mitral leaflet (42, 44), mitral prosthetic valve dysfunction (64, 93), and ischemic rupture of a papillary muscle as well (85), this technique has proved to be a very sensitive and reliable tool.

Transesophageal Approach for Aortic Valve Disorders

Erbel et al. demonstrated the relevance of transesophageal echocardiography in the preoperative assessment of aortic dissection (26, 70, 85) with a better sensitivity than computed tomography and angiography. Daniel et al. have also recently reported the usefulness of this technique in the diagnosis of aortic root abscesses (21). With prosthetic aortic valves, the transesophageal approach can detect a flail porcine cusp and vegetations. However, the anterior attachment of the aortic valve prosthesis and its internal structure may be masked by shadowing from the posterior side of the prosthesis, because of the short-axis plane interrogation of the aortic ring (51).

Being able to perform these techniques portably and within a confined space is highly convenient for use in the intensive care unit. Conventional Doppler echocardiography has been shown extensively to have both good sensitivity and specificity in detecting left-sided valvular regurgitation and thereby provides an optimization of the diagnosis of valvular diseases (40, 78, 91, 98). The emergence of color Doppler has made possible the real-time visualization of the jets within cardiac structures (46, 60, 68, 81). More recently, transesophageal echocardiography represents a further advance as a "new window to the heart," especially in the assessment of mitral valve diseases, as there is a very close relationship between the esophagus and left atrium (14, 18, 20, 48, 49, 64, 84, 85). Moreover, this noninvasive approach of the entire left ventricular chamber may be of invaluable help in both perioperative and postoperative cardiac monitoring (10,

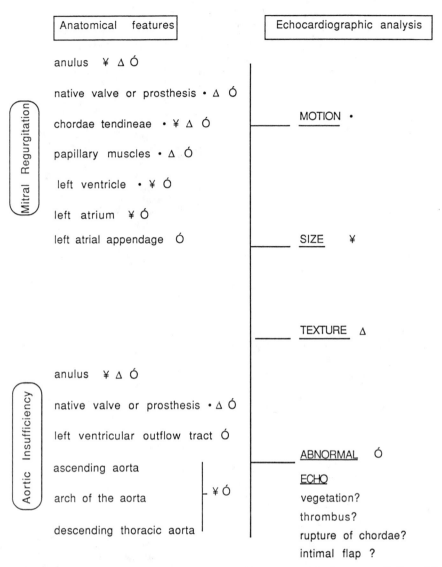

Figure 16.1. Echocardiographic diagnostic "screening" in acute valvular regurgitation. M-mode and two-dimensional echocardiography transthoracic and transesophageal approaches.

55, 56, 82). This technique initially allowed a monoplane approach to the heart, and, more recently, even a biplane approach (63, 85, 86).

Noninvasive Assessment of Both Valvular Disorder and Leak: Diagnostic Information

The next step toward confirmation of the diagnosis and correct management of the patient is to compare these with echocardiographically obtained information, which ideally should be collected at the bedside.

Identification of Mitral and Aortic Valve Disorders: M-Mode and Two-Dimensional Echocardiography

Transthoracic Approach. M-mode and two-dimensional echocardiography are both able to provide a morphological and a functional analysis.

These two modes are essential and must be used prior to Doppler echocardiography: M-mode allows a functional analysis of the valve by assessing its motion as a function of time. This was formerly reported to be of great relevance in describing features of mitral valve prolapse (39). Initially, in the acute aortic insufficiency setting, and especially from infective endocarditis, premature closure of the mitral valve resulting from the rapid rise in left ventricular pressure was shown to be an accurate index of the severity of the leak, leading to urgent surgical correction (17, 38). Moreover, as emphasized by Daniel et al., the detection of aortic insufficiency was not formally demonstrated to be improved by transesophageal studies (20). Nevertheless, the use of multiple plane probes in the near future should permit a three-dimensional analysis of cardiac structures (28, 57, 63, 86).

Identification of Mitral and Aortic Leaks: Doppler Echocardiography

Transthoracic Approach. Doppler echocardiography has been widely shown to be the procedure of choice for identifying any valvular leak (73, 78, 94, 98).

Pulsed-wave Doppler, defined by a given pulse repetition frequency, allows an accurate localization of blood velocities within the heart chambers or great vessels, but is limited by its inability to record high velocities.

Continuous-wave Doppler is able to record high blood velocities but is unable to detect the origin of backscattered signals along the entire path of the ultrasound beam (40, 76, 77). Using a transthoracic apical view, a mitral regurgitant jet will be visualized as a negative waveform (Fig. 16.2). Conversely, an aortic regurgitant jet will be recorded as a positive waveform, using the same view (Fig. 16.3).

Color-flow mapping (i.e., color Doppler), a more recent development, allows real-time visualization of the regurgitant jets, either in the left atrium in acute mitral regurgitation or in the left ventricular outflow tract in acute aortic insufficiency (46). This acoustic procedure, derived from pulsed-wave Doppler, is based on specific color encoding of velocities within a sector scan. The flow direction toward the transducer is expressed in red, and away from the transducer in blue. With regard to the velocity variance, green is added to each color in proportion to the extent of turbu-

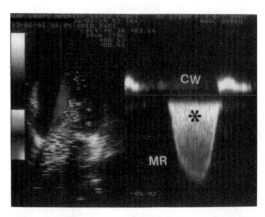

Figure 16.2. Continuous-wave (*CW*) Doppler recording from a patient with mitral regurgitation (*MR*) displayed as a negative waveform (*star*). Transthoracic approach (four-chamber plane).

lence (68, 81). This technique allows a relatively sensitive analysis of the origin, direction, morphology, eccentricity, and expansion of regurgitant jets (46, 48, 71). In most cases of severe acute mitral or aortic regurgitations, high velocities and turbulences are coded as a "mosaic" pattern of blue, red, and green mixed colors (60). Quite good correlations were reported by Miyatake et al., then by Perry et al., when comparing color Doppler grading to angiographic grading according

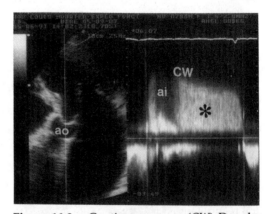

Figure 16.3. Continuous-wave (*CW*) Doppler recording from a patient with aortic insufficiency (*ai*) displayed as a positive waveform (*star*) and simultaneous two-dimensional imaging. *ao,* aortic root. Transthoracic approach (four-chamber plane).

to the classification of Sellers, especially in mild or in severe regurgitation (61, 72).

Thus, as recently emphasized by Shah, insofar as color Doppler provides an accurate semiquantitative assessment of valvular regurgitations, this should limit the indications for the systematic use of invasive procedures (87).

Transesophageal Approach. As already stated above, transesophageal Doppler echocardiography is the approach of choice in ventilated patients and in case of indeterminate transthoracic findings (14).

As shown in Figures 16.4–16.6 color flow mapping of a severe mitral regurgitant jet is obviously displayed in a mosaic pattern (related to the high kinetic energy level of the jet). As with two-dimensional echocardiography, the Doppler mode during a transesophageal procedure has been widely shown to provide more accurate information concerning the patterns of the jets (71, 73, 89). A valvular aortic leak detected by both pulsed-wave and color Doppler is shown in Figure 16.7. A schematic overview of these patterns, in both acute mitral regurgitation and acute aortic insufficiency by transesophageal echocardiography is summarized in Figure 16.8.

The diagnostic improvement provided by the transesophageal approach when

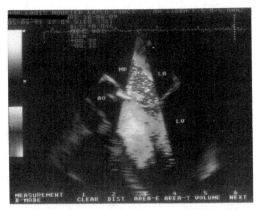

Figure 16.5. Severe mitral regurgitation (*MR*). Color Doppler; transesophageal approach (four-chamber plane). *LA*, left atrium; *LV*, left ventricle; *AO*, aortic root.

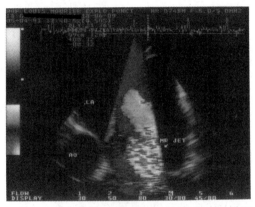

Figure 16.6. Aliased mitral regurgitant (*MR*) jet in a mosaic color pattern (color Doppler). Transesophageal approach (four-chamber plane). *LA*, left atrium; *AO*, aortic root.

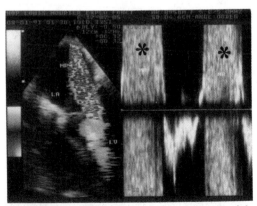

Figure 16.4. Severe mitral regurgitation following rupture of chordae tendineae. The mitral regurgitant jet (*MR*) is directed toward the free wall of the left atrium (*LA*), emerging from the anterior mitral leaflet (counterclockwise motion) (color Doppler). The simultaneous pulsed-Doppler recording (*stars*) is displayed. Transesophageal approach (four-chamber plane). *LV*, left ventricle.

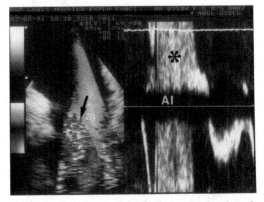

Figure 16.7. Aortic insufficiency (*ai*) displayed using color Doppler (*arrow*) and simultaneous pulsed-Doppler recording (*AI-star*). Transesophageal approach (four-chamber plane).

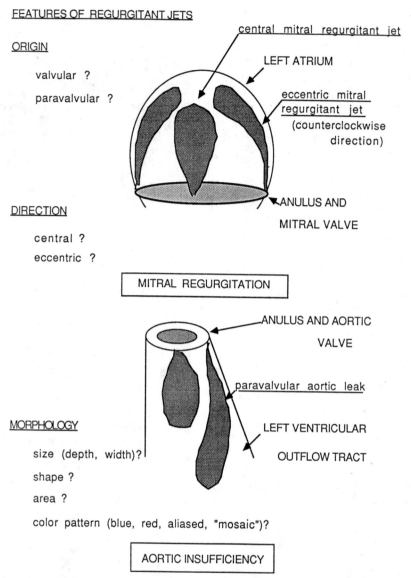

Figure 16.8. Color flow mapping in acute valvular regurgitation (transesophageal approach).

compared to transthoracic echocardiography is summarized in Table 16.2.

Noninvasive Assessment of Both Regurgitant Volume and Left Ventricular Performance: Prognostic Information

Two major components of prognosis in the preoperative assessment of acute valvular regurgitation are the appraisal of the *regurgitant volume* and *left ventricular function*.

Doppler Assessment of Regurgitant Volume: Quantification of Regurgitation

State of the Art. Numerous methods to evaluate the severity of valvular insufficiencies have been reported. To date, none allows an accurate quantitation of regurgitant volume (22).

Pulsed-wave Doppler echocardiography was initially used to estimate regurgitant jet extension in the left atrium (mitral regurgitation) or in the left ventricle

Table 16.2
Diagnostic Improvement by Transesophageal Echocardiography

Acute mitral regurgitation
 Diagnosis of mitral valve prolapse and flail
  mitral leaflet (rupture of chordae
  tendineae)
 Accurate analysis of both texture and
  motion of the mitral leaflets
 Visualization of valvular vegetation and
  abscess
 Assessment of mitral prosthetic valve
  dysfunction
 Identification of mitral regurgitant jet and
  distinction between valvular and
  paravalvular leak
 Identification of mass (i.e., thrombus or
  vegetation) within the left atrium or the
  left atrial appendage
Acute aortic insufficiency
 Accurate diagnosis of aortic root abscess
  and Valsalva aneurysm
 Accurate diagnosis of dissection of the aorta
 Assessment of bioprosthetic valve
  dysfunction
 Distinction between valvular and
  paravalvular leak
 Visualization of valvular vegetation

(aortic insufficiency) in native and prosthetic valve dysfunction by velocity mapping (78, 94, 98). Regurgitant fraction has been estimated, using either pulsed- or continuous-wave Doppler, in patients with isolated mitral or aortic regurgitation, from the difference between total and forward stroke volumes (16, 76, 77). Continuous-wave Doppler has been also used to assess the severity of aortic leak, employing the Doppler half-time technique (54). Numerous publications have emphasized the relevance of color Doppler for quantitation of regurgitation in native and prosthetic valves.

In *mitral regurgitation*, the length, width, and planimetry of the regurgitant jet area in the left atrium, or the ratio of the jet area to left atrium area, have been proposed by several authors using either transthoracic or transesophageal approaches. Quite good correlations against angiographic grading were reported, especially in mild, and even in severe, leaks (33, 41, 61, 64, 92, 93).

In *aortic regurgitation,* the maximal length and area of the regurgitant jet used by several authors were proved to be poorly predictive of the angiographic grade of regurgitation (94). Nevertheless, the thickness of the regurgitant beam at its origin relative to the size of the left outflow tract seems to be a better predictor of the severity of aortic insufficiency (2, 72).

Pitfalls. However, in spite of some good correlations with angiographic grading, all these methods do not provide a real estimation of the regurgitant volume and remain semiquantitative (22, 41, 61). Such a liablity also applies to angiography, often considered as a gold standard, but also unable to provide a precise quantitative measurement of regurgitant volume (6, 19, 22).

Several essential points should be borne in mind when considering the noninvasive quantitation of a regurgitant volume, the main point being that *the echo-Doppler imaging displayed is related to the analysis of a complex pathophysiological phenomenon through complex and sophisticated technology.*

Physiological considerations. Regurgitant volume is conditioned by several linked factors such as heart rate, loading conditions of both left atrium and left ventricle, geometry and compliance of the aorta and the heart chambers, inotropic state of the left ventricle, and day-to-day variability of hemodynamic status (6, 7). Furthermore, the complexity of the regurgitant jets must be emphasized such as the three-dimensional moving shape of the jets, spatial and temporal expansion of the jets in a more or less confined receiving chamber, mixing of the jets in the receiving chambers (e.g., pulmonary venous flow in the left atrium, transmitral forward flow in the left ventricle), problems of jet boundary delineation, adherence effect to the walls, and swirling and reflection of the jets along both atrial and ventricle walls (6, 12, 15, 43, 79).

Technological considerations. The influence of several factors, especially on color display, must be pointed out, namely, gain setting, axial and lateral resolution, filtering, pixel encoding algorithms, frame rate, pulse repetition frequency, transducer frequency, signal-to-noise ratio, methods of transferring color Doppler image data, and operator dependency (3, 6, 68, 79, 88, 90, 96).

Thus, as strongly emphasized by numerous authors, the information provided by Doppler echocardiography, especially relative to mild to moderate valvular regurgitation, must be cautiously interpreted and systematically compared to the clinical status of the patient, and eventually to other techniques such as angiography, in order to improve the accuracy of decision making (6, 22, 30, 31). Nevertheless, in the setting of fulminant acute valvular regurgitation, a properly executed echo-Doppler evaluation by a skilled operator allows, in most cases, recognition of a severe leak, even though the true regurgitant volume cannot be assessed. However, it must be emphasized that an acute valvular regurgitation *does not* systematically imply that the leak is severe, but it may also be mild or moderate. Furthermore, decisions about the advisabilty and timing of surgery are based more on symptoms and hemodynamic and ventilatory stability than on an accurate regurgitant volume.

Hopes. The use of both in vitro models and experimental in vivo models has allowed the development of several promising methods of quantitation of regurgitant flow. Four of them will be successively met. One attractive method makes use of in vitro Doppler flow mapping energy measurements. These appear to be linearly related to delivered *kinetic energy* by fluid jets. This method, well described by Bolger et al., was proved to be unaffected by orifice area (origin of the jet), gain setting, or compliance of the receiving chamber, in contrast to color flow mapping area measurements (5).

Another method, reported by Cape et al., employs the fluid-dynamics law that states the *axial momentum* of free turbulent jets is conserved (in models of mitral regurgitation). Flow rate is described as a function of maximal jet velocity and a distal centerline jet velocity assessed at a known distance downstream from the regurgitant orifice (11, 95). Thus, regurgitant volume is determined from the product of orifice area and the continuous-wave Doppler time-velocity integral of maximal jet

velocity (11). Another approach, emphasized by Utsunomiya et al., considers the *proximal isovelocity area* of aliasing due to the flow acceleration proximal to an orifice. This phenomenon ("flow convergence") is based on the acceleration of fluid from a high pressure chamber through an orifice, toward a low pressure chamber. Regurgitant flow is assumed to be the product of the known isovelocity at which aliasing occurs (defined as the Nyquist limit) multiplied by the surface area of the aliasing (easily identified blue-red interface) (97). Another possible approach of mitral regurgitation is based on the Doppler echocardiographic analysis of *pulmonary venous flow* using the transesophageal approach (47).

Echocardiographic Assessment of Left Ventricular Function

Beside semiquantitative estimation of regurgitant volume, noninvasive assessment of both myocardial performance and right-heart pressures form part of the preoperative evaluation of the patient and must be considered as an essential prognostic factor. As a rule of thumb, the assessment of ventricular function must be performed at the same time as both morphological and functional analyses of the valves, using either a transthoracic or transesophageal approach, depending on the clinical status of the patient.

Assessment of Myocardial Performance. Myocardial performance can be assessed by M-mode and two-dimensional echocardiography or Doppler echocardiography in addition. These two complementary techniques should be jointly interpreted when assessing left ventricular function.

The exhaustive description of all these echo-Doppler techniques would be outside the scope of this chapter, however, it must be remembered that they are schematically based upon two types of data: *(a) morphological data,* i.e., assessment of both end-diastolic and end-systolic left ventricular diameters, surfaces, or volumes, by M-mode and two-dimensional echocardiography (27, 29, 82); and *(b) velocimetric data,* i.e., assessment of aortic, mitral, or pulmonary flows, and indices derived from velocity curves such as ejection duration, acceleration, deceleration, peak velocities, velocity-time integrals, and so forth, by Doppler echocardiography (1, 29, 40).

In the setting of acute valvular insufficiency, the questions to be answered are:

1. Is the left ventricle dilated or not? (assessment of both the end-diastolic and the end-systolic diameters).
2. Is there a left ventricular hypertrophy or not? (assessment of the wall thickness and of the left ventricular mass).
3. Is there a regional left ventricular dysfunction or not? (identification of regional contraction abnormalities using a standard nomenclature for degree of asynergy by two-dimensional echocardiography).
4. Is there a global left ventricular dysfunction or not? (assessment of the end-diastolic and the end-systolic volumes and ejection fraction) (27, 29).

However, in most cases of acute mitral or aortic valvular regurgitation: *the left ventricle appears neither dilated nor thickened and left ventricular function is considered to be normal with a marked enhancement of global left ventricular wall motion* (4, 9, 17, 23, 39).

Nevertheless, these usual findings are not observed in the following cases:

1. Acute myocardial infarction associated with acute mitral leak, where wall motion abnormalities are observed;
2. Previous mitral or aortic valvulopathies, where both left atrium and left ventricle can be dilated with prior impairment of left ventricular function;
3. Acute prosthetic valve dysfunction with preoperative impairment of ·left ventricular function.

Assessment of Intracardiac Pressures. From the peak systole velocity of a tricuspid regurgitation, the modified Bernoulli equation allows accurate calculation of the peak pressure difference between the right ventricle and right atrium (i.e., the systolic pulmonary artery pressure), by applying the formula, $\Delta P = 4V2$, where ΔP is systolic right ventricular pressure minus right atrium pressure (empirically estimated at 5–10 mm Hg) and V is peak systolic velocity of tricuspid regurgitation (83).

Cardiac Catheterization: The "Invasive" Approach

Right-Sided Cardiac Catheterization

Indication

In patients in whom a severe and rapidly life-threatening heart failure occurs, requiring emergency management in the intensive care unit, the indication for right-heart catheterization appears reasonable.

Findings

In acute mitral regurgitation, besides an increase in pulmonary pressures, the major finding is a giant V wave related to a nondilated left atrium operating on the steepest portion of its pressure-volume curve (9).

Classically, V waves greater than twice the mean pulmonary wedge pressure are suggestive of severe mitral regurgitation and the diagnosis is strongly suggested when the height of the V waves is three times that of the mean wedge pressure (35, 50). However, such giant waves can be seen in the absence of mitral regurgitation when pulmonary blood flow is increased (e.g., in acute ventricular septal defect complicating myocardial infarction). Moreover, *the absence of a giant V wave does not rule out severe mitral regurgitation* in the case of an acute event complicating a chronic mitral valvulopathy where the left atrium is enlarged and therefore operating on the less steep part of its pressure-volume curve.

In acute aortic regurgitation associated with severe heart failure, pulmonary pressures are, as in acute mitral regurgitation, markedly increased, without any giant V wave in this case (4, 23).

Left-Sided Heart Catheterization

Indications

The indication for such an invasive procedure now tends to be limited to individual cases where a noninvasive procedure is expected to be less informative.

Left heart catheterization, selective left ventricular angiocardiography, and coronary arteriography are schematically indicated in the following states:

1. Discrepancies between clinical and echo-Doppler findings in order to confirm both the diagnosis and severity of the leak;
2. Assessment of the status of coronary arteries in populations supposed to be at high risk of coronary artery disease in order to evaluate the advisability of a coronary artery bypass grafting combined with valve repair;
3. Complementary assessment of acute aortic dissection patterns.

However, it should be borne in mind that the use of such invasive techniques:

1. May be seriously deleterious (e.g., bleeding, arrythmias, conduction disturbances, infections, systemic embolizations of vegetations, aggravation of an unstable hemodynamic state or indeed death) (34);
2. Do have serious limitations in the quantitation of regurgitant volume and remain obviously a semiquantitative technique (19).

Findings in Acute Mitral Regurgitation

Mitral regurgitation implies a double outlet to the left ventricle; therefore, the impedance to ventricular emptying is reduced. The volume of mitral regurgitant flow depends on several linked factors: size of the regurgitant orifice, pressure gradient between the left ventricle and left atrium (depending on left atrial compliance, pulmonary venous flow, inotropy, and geometry of the left ventricle), duration of systole, aortic impedance to ejection (afterload), and forward stroke volume that is conditioned by aortoventricular coupling (9, 35, 100).

Thus, in acute mitral regurgitation, left ventricular contractility has been shown to be usually preserved in both experimental and clinical studies, with preload being mildly increased or unchanged, afterload markedly decreased, and ejection fraction markedly increased (100). Furthermore, left-atrial compliance is generally normal, thus, left atrial pressure will be expected to be acutely and markedly increased as the left atrial pressure-volume relationship is operating on its steepest part (9, 74).

Findings in Acute Aortic Regurgitation

In the case of experimental acute aortic insufficiency, a marked rise in preload, wall tension, and myocardial oxygen consumption has been demonstrated (9). The regurgitant volume fills, in addition to diastolic inflow from the left atrium, a left ventricle generally of normal size, which is unable to adapt to this acute volume overloading. Such a situation contrasts with that observed in acute mitral regurgitation and also in chronic aortic regurgitation (4, 9). Thus, the left ventricle operates on the steep portion of its diastolic pressure-volume curve (4). The elevation in left ventricular end-diastolic pressure is dramatic, but there is only a small increase in total stroke volume, because end-diastolic volume increases very little (4). The noncompliant myocardium and possibly the pericardium are the factors limiting the increase in left ventricular end-diastolic volume in response to acute severe aortic regurgitation (4). Moreover, hemodynamic findings in acute severe aortic insufficiency (such as infective endocarditis) compared with chronic aortic regurgitation showed a significant reduction of the mean aortic pressure and forward stroke volume (4, 52). Furthermore, left ventricular pressure was shown to exceed left atrial pressure in late diastole ("diastasis"). This serves as a transitory means of reducing diastolic reflux and maintaining forward stroke volume (23, 52). Diastasis leads to a premature closure of mitral valve, which protects the pulmonary venous system from backward transmission of the markedly increased end-diastolic pressure (52).

PREDICTING RESPONSE TO MEDICAL THERAPY: FACTORS OF PROGNOSIS

Thus, the predictive response to medical therapy will be conditioned by the following four major prognostic factors:

1. The *clinical status* prior to the acute valvular event: age, history of prior ischemic heart disease or valvulopathy, coexistent pulmonary disease, and so forth;
2. The *volume of regurgitation*: assessed by clinical examination, echocardiography, or angiography;

3. The *left ventricular function:* assessed by clinical examination, echocardiography, and catheterization;
4. The *underlying etiology:* assessed by both clinical examination and echocardiography in most cases (4, 23, 38, 39, 50, 80).

A broad spectrum of cases may be considered, from a mild acute valvular regurgitation to a life-threatening fulminant acute valvular insufficiency. Thus, one can schematically consider two possible opposite conditions: good tolerance state and poor tolerance state.

Good Tolerance State

The clinical status may be initially encouraging with no signs of heart failure. A diagnosis of acute valvular regurgitation will be highly suggested by clinical examination, ECG, and chest radiograph. Patients should be rapidly referred for transesophageal echocardiography, to allow definite confirmation of the diagnosis.

The aim of medical therapy will be to reduce the left ventricle diastolic overloading and to avoid massive pulmonary edema. Vasodilating agents such as intravenous nitroprusside, hydralazine, or calcium blockers are the drugs of choice in this setting. These drugs lower impedance to ejection and therefore increase forward stroke volume and diminish regurgitant volume (80). They may also improve ventricular relaxation and diastolic compliance. As left ventricular volume decreases, the size of the mitral anulus and the area of the regurgitant orifice also decline (50, 80). Intravenous diuretics may also be instituted in order to reduce left ventricular volume. Furosemide rapidly lowers ventricular filling pressures, related to its acute venodilatory effect that increases venous capacitance (4, 80). While waiting for imminent surgical correction within a matter of days, patients will be carefully monitored in the intensive care unit for signs of either clinical improvement or deterioration under medical therapy.

Poor Tolerance State

The clinical status may be initially worrying, with signs of severe congestive heart failure, pulmonary edema, or shock. Critically ill patients will usually be referred for emergency cardiac catherization. In acute severe mitral regurgitation, urgent insertion of an intraaortic balloon pump must be performed under inotropic support with catecholamines. This procedure will decrease the impedance to ventricular outflow still further and will allow safer left-heart catheterization and anesthesia induction (50, 80). In severe acute aortic regurgitation, intraaortic counterpulsation is a well-known contraindication. This condition requires a still more urgent aortic valve replacement (4, 23). In the case of an initial acute respiratory distress or a cardiogenic shock, mechanical ventilation should be promptly initiated that allows transesophageal echocardiography and catherization to be performed with relative safety. If, as expected, the valvular leak is shown to be severe, it is unlikely that acute valvular regurgitation will be responsive to medical therapy, and an emergent surgical procedure should be proposed after rapid estimation of the benefit-to-risk ratio.

A rational approach of diagnosis and management in acute valvular regurgitation is proposed in Figure 16.9.

TIMING OF SURGICAL REPAIR

In most cases of acute valvular regurgitation, the timing of surgical repair is usually a matter of hours or days and is based on the four main prognostic factors aforementioned.

Acute Mitral Regurgitation

It is important to remember that, in acute mitral regurgitation regardless of etiology, the patient may appear well compensated under medical therapy until left ventricular failure occurs. Once the left ventricular impairment happens, such a patient may have a fatal outcome in a matter of minutes to hours (50, 80).

Infective Endocarditis

The objectives of surgery are to debride all infected tissue (if possible), to repair or replace damaged valves, and to correct any other acquired defect such as septal perforation or abscess.

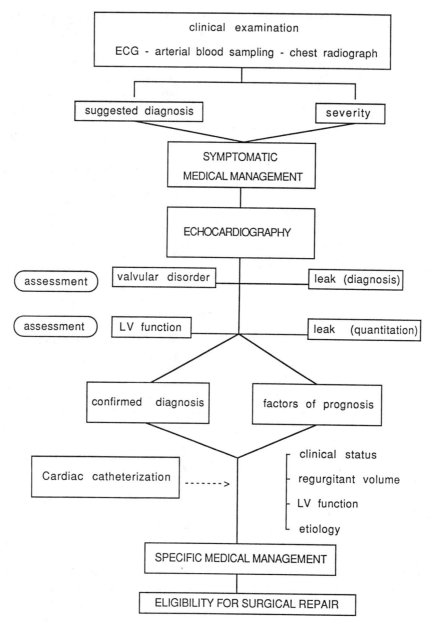

Figure 16.9. A rational approach to acute valvular regurgitation.

Congestive heart failure represents a major risk factor and one half of patients with heart failure will die without surgery in spite of active medical treatment (66). Furthermore, two additional factors must lead to an imperative and urgent surgical correction: fungal endocarditis, or persisting bacteremia or relapse after adequate antibiotherapy, suggesting an abscess.

Thus, whatever the type of mitral valve (i.e., native or prosthetic), a surgical procedure should obviously be contemplated in most cases within a matter of hours or days, ideally before the aggravation of congestive heart failure. In rare cases of acute mitral regurgitation with a mild leak and particularly good clinical tolerance following medical therapy, surgical repair may be postponed. However, it should be borne in mind that:

1. A complete antimicrobial course is not required in this setting;
2. Mitral regurgitation begets mitral regurgitation;
3. A sudden deterioration of the hemodynamic status may occur at any time during medical management leading to a refractory heart failure state (9, 99).

Ischemic Heart Disease

As recently recommended by the American College of Cardiology/American Heart Association Task Force report (36), surgical intervention in acute myocardial infarction is usually indicated as an emergency in cases of papillary muscle rupture and is considered urgent in cases of acute mitral regurgitation with intractable cardiac failure. In cases of severe acute mitral regurgitation with controlled failure, cardiac repair appears acceptable and urgent. In the other cases, it may be preferable to stabilize the patient and defer surgery for at least 2 weeks following myocardial infarction (80).

Mitral Valve Prolapse and Miscellaneous Causes

In the case of rupture of chordae tendineae complicating a mitral valve prolapse and in the case of spontaneous rupture, or less common etiologies, indications for surgical repair should be contemplated as soon as possible (50, 80). In all events, the surgical repair should be determined by the degree of heart failure and the underlying cause and performed in a matter of hours, days, or even weeks in particularly well-stabilized patients.

It is noteworthy that patients should be referred for conservative surgical management of the mitral valve as much as possible, as extensively reported by Carpentier (13).

Acute Aortic Insufficiency

The timing of surgical repair in acute aortic insufficiency appears much clearer than in the setting of chronic aortic regurgitation (4, 23).

Infective Endocarditis

In infective endocarditis, the involvement of the aortic valve is more often the cause of intractable cardiac failure than in the case of mitral valve. However, it has become clear that the presence of active infection is not a contraindication to cardiac surgery in patients whose valves have been seriously injured by infection (99). Thus, a full course therapy is no longer needed prior to surgical repair in the acute setting (23). It appears, as in acute mitral regurgitation, that even in active infective endocarditis, rapid surgical intervention must be undertaken. Moreover, as aforementioned, mitral valve involvement carries a better prognosis than aortic involvement, justifying a still faster surgical procedure for the latter (23).

Acute Aortic Dissection

Agreement is generally unanimous on the necessity of urgent surgical repair in aortic regurgitation associated with either acute proximal dissection or even acute distal dissection. In the former presentation, whose progression can lead to potentially devastating consequences such as aortic regurgitation or cardiac tamponade, immediate repair tends to a better outcome. It is noteworthy to emphasize that aortic regurgitation occurs in over 50% of patients with proximal dissection in most series. Moreover, heart failure, in this case, is almost always due to the sudden onset of severe acute aortic insufficiency (24). In the latter presentation, concerning aortic regurgitation complicating an acute distal dissection, patients are for the most part older and have a particularly high surgical risk. However, if medical therapy is generally the rule in uncomplicated distal dissection, surgical repair must be indicated in case of associated aortic regurgitation (4, 23, 24).

Most surgical teams have become more aggressive about replacing the aortic valve with a prosthesis, even if a mild aortic regurgitation remains present after the leaflets are decompressed (4, 24).

Miscellaneous Causes

In cases when the source of acute aortic valvular incompetence is noninfective (i.e., inflammatory diseases, trauma, iatrogenic causes), aortic surgery must be also undertaken, ideally before congestive heart failure occurs, because these patients are at high risk of sudden deterioration (4, 32).

Finally, we mention studies reported by Schiller and Maurer and coworkers, which have emphasized the utility of intraoperative echocardiography in the assessment of both cardiac function and mitral or aortic valve repair (48, 56, 82). As extensively shown in the preoperative period, these noninvasive techniques provide an invaluable help during cardiac surgery and should be expanded in the future, through specific training involving cardiologists, intensivists, and anesthetists, in order to improve the accuracy of decision making in the intensive care setting and in the operating room.

Acknowledgment. The author is indebted to Mervyn Singer, M.D., M.R.C.P., for his friendly help during the preparation of this manuscript.

References

1. Appleton CP, Hatle LK, Popp RL. Relation of transmitral flow velocity patterns to left diastolic function: new insights from a combined hemodynamic and Doppler echocardiographic study. J Am Coll Cardiol 1988;12:426–440.
2. Baumgartner H, Kratzer H, Helmreich G, Kühn P. Quantitation of aortic regurgitation by colour coded cross-sectional Doppler echocardiography. Eur Heart J 1988;9:380–387.
3. Baumgartner H, Schima H, Kühn P. Value and limitations of proximal jet dimensions for the quantitation of valvular regurgitation: an in vitro study using Doppler flow mapping. J Am Soc Echo 1991;4:57–66.
4. Benotti JR. Acute aortic insufficiency. In: Dalen JE, Alpert JS, eds. Valvular heart disease. 2nd ed. Boston: Little, Brown, 1987:319–351.
5. Bolger AF, Eigler HL, Pfaff M, Resser KJ, Maurer G. Computer analysis of Doppler color flow mapping images for quantitative assessment of in vitro fluid jets. J Am Coll Cardiol 1988;12:450–457.
6. Bolger AF, Eigler NL, Maurer G. Quantifying valvular regurgitation. Limitations and inherent assumptions of Doppler techniques. Circulation 1988;78:1316–1318.
7. Borow KB, Marcus RH. Aortic regurgitation: the need for an integrated physiologic approach. J Am Coll Cardiol 1991;17:898–900.
8. Buda AJ, Zotz RJ, LeMire MS, Bach DS. Prog-

nostic significance of vegetations detected by two-dimensional echocardiography in infective endocarditis. Am Heart J 1986;112:1291–1296.
9. Braunwald E. Valvular heart disease. In: Braunwald E, ed. Heart disease: a textbook of cardiovascular medicine. 3rd ed. Philadelphia: WB Saunders, 1988:1034–1068.
10. Cahalan MK, Litt L, Botvinick EH, Schiller NB. Advances in noninvasive cardiovascular imaging: implications for the anesthesiologist. Anesthesiology 1987;66:356–372.
11. Cape EG, Skoufis EG, Weyman AE, et al. A new model for noninvasive quantification of valvular regurgitation based on conservation of momentum. In vitro validation. Circulation 1989;79:1343–1353.
12. Cape EG, Yoganathan AP, Weyman AE, Levine RA. Adjacent solid boundaries alter the size of regurgitant jets on Doppler color flow maps. J Am Coll Cardiol 1991;17:1094–1102.
13. Carpentier A. Cardiac valve surgery—the "French correction." J Thorac Cardiovasc Surg 1983;86:323–337.
14. Chandrasekaran K, Bansal RC, Mintz GS, Ross JJ, Shah PM. Impact of transesophageal color flow Doppler echocardiography in current cardiology practice. Echocardiography 1990;7:125–145.
15. Chen C, Flachskampf FA, Anconina J, Weyman AE, Thomas JD. Three-dimensional shape of wall jets and free jets: implication for quantitation of valvular regurgitation by color Doppler imaging [Abstract]. J Am Coll Cardiol 1990;15:89A.
16. Ciobanu M, Abbasi AS, Allen M, Hermer A, Spellberg R. Pulsed Doppler echocardiography in the diagnosis and estimation of severity of aortic insufficiency. Am J Cardiol 1987;49:339–343.
17. Cohn LH, Birjiniuk V. Therapy of acute aortic regurgitation. In: Carabello BA, ed. Cardiology clinics. Valvular heart disease. Philadelphia: WB Saunders, 1991:339–352.
18. Cormier B, Bertrand S, Roger V, Enriquez L, Acar J. Transesophageal echocardiography for the detection of prosthetic complications [Abstract]. Circulation 1990;82(suppl. III):67.
19. Croft CH, Lipscomb K, Mathis K, et al. Limitations of qualitative angiographic grading in aortic or mitral regurgitation. Am J Cardiol 1984;53:1593–1598.
20. Daniel LB, Grigg LE, Weisel RD, Rakowski H. Comparison of transthoracic and transesophageal assessment of prosthetic valve dysfunction. Echocardiography 1990;7:83–95.
21. Daniel W, Mügge A, Martin R, et al. Improvement in the diagnosis of abscesses associated with endocarditis by transesophageal echocardiography. N Engl J Med 1991;324:795–800.
22. DeMaria AN, Smith MD, Harrison MR. Clinical significance of in vitro and in vivo experimental findings regarding Doppler flow velocity recordings. J Am Coll Cardiol 1989;13:1682–1685.
23. Dervan J, Goldberg S. Acute aortic regurgitation: pathophysiology and management. In: Frankl WS, Brest AN, eds. Cardiovascular clinics. Valvular heart disease: comprehensive evaluation and

management. Philadelphia: FA Davis, 1986:281–288.

24. Eagle KA, De Sanctis RW. Diseases of the aorta: aortic dissection. In: Braunwald E, ed. Heart disease: a textbook of cardiovascular medicine. Philadelphia: WB Saunders, 1988:1554–1561.

25. Erbel R, Rohmann S, Drexler M, et al. Improved diagnostic value of echocardiography in patients with infective endocarditis by transesophageal approach. A prospective study. Eur Heart J 1988;9:43–53.

26. Erbel R, Renollet H, Engberding R, et al. Transesophageal imaging of the thoracic aorta in aortic dissection. In: Erbel R, Khandheria BK, Brennecke R, Meyer J, Seward JB, Tajik AJ, eds. Transesophageal echocardiography. A new window to the heart. Berlin: Springer-Verlag, 1989:131–145.

27. Feigenbaum H. Echocardiography. In: Braunwald E, ed. Heart disease: a textbook of cardiovascular medicine. 3rd ed. Philadelphia: WB Saunders, 1988:83–139.

28. Flachskampf FA, Hoffmann R, Hanrath P. Experience with a transesophageal echo transducer allowing full rotation of the viewing plane: the omniplane probe [Abstract]. J Am Coll Cardiol 1991;17:34A.

29. Force TL, Folland ED, Aebischer N, Sharma S, Parisi AF. Echocardiographic assessment of ventricular function. In: Marcus ML, Schelbert HR, Skorton DJ, Wolf GL, eds. Cardiac imaging: a companion to *Braunwald's Heart Disease*. Philadelphia: WB Saunders, 1991:374–401.

30. Goldberg SJ. A perspective on color-coded Doppler echocardiography: utility or just another pretty picture? J Am Coll Cardiol 1989;14:977–978.

31. Goldman ME. Real-time two-dimensional flow imaging: a word of caution [Editorial]. J Am Coll Cardiol 1988;7:89–90.

32. Greenberg BH. Medical therapy for patients with aortic insufficiency. In: Carabello BA, ed. Cardiology clinics. Valvular heart disease. Philadelphia: WB Saunders, 1991:255–270.

33. Grigg LE, Fulop J, Daniel L, Weisel R, Rakowski H. Doppler echocardiography assessment of prosthetic heart valves. Echocardiography 1990;7:97–113.

34. Grossman W. Complications of cardiac catheterization: incidence, causes, and prevention. In: Grossman W, ed. Cardiac catherization and angiography. 3rd ed. Philadelphia: Lea & Febiger, 1986:30–42.

35. Grossman W. Profiles in valvular heart disease. In: Grossman W, ed. Cardiac catheterization and angiography. 3rd ed. Philadelphia: Lea & Febiger, 1986:359–381.

36. Gunnar RM, Bourdillon PD, Dixon DW, et al. ACC/AHA Task Force Report: guidelines for the early management of patients with acute myocardial infarction. J Am Coll Cardiol 1990;16:249–292.

37. Gussenhoven EJ, Taams MA, Roelandt JR, et al. Transesophageal two-dimensional echocardiography: its role in solving clinical problems. J Am Coll Cardiol 1986;8:975–979.

38. Hall RJC, Julian DG. Aortic regurgitation. In: Hall RJC, Julian DG, eds. Diseases of the cardiac valves. Edinburgh: Churchill Livingstone, 1989:120–141.

39. Hall RJC, Julian DG. Non-rheumatic mitral valve disease. In: Hall RJC, Julian DG, eds. Diseases of the cardiac valves. Edinburgh: Churchill Livingstone, 1989:161–175.

40. Hatle L, Angelsen B. Doppler ultrasound in cardiology. Philadelphia: Lea & Febiger, 1985.

41. Helmcke F, Nanda NC, Hsiung MC, et al. Color Doppler assessment of mitral regurgitation with orthogonal planes. Circulation 1987;75:175–183.

42. Himelman RB, Kusumoto F, Oken K, et al. The flail mitral valve: echocardiographic findings by precordial and transesophageal imaging and Doppler color flow mapping. J Am Coll Cardiol 1991;17:272–279.

43. Hoit BD, Jones M, Eidbo EE, Elias W, Sahn DJ. Sources of variabilty for Doppler color flow mapping of regurgitant jets in an animal model of mitral regurgitation. J Am Coll Cardiol 1989;13:1631–1636.

44. Hozumi T, Yoshikawa J, Yoshida K, Yamaura Y, Akasaka T, Shakudo M. Direct visualization of ruptured chordae tendineae by transesophageal two-dimensional echocardiography. J Am Coll Cardiol 1990;16:1315–1319.

45. Jaffe WM, Morgan DE, Pearlman AS, Otto CM. Infective endocarditis, 1983–1988: Echocardiographic findings and factors influencing morbidity and mortality. J Am Coll Cardiol 1990;15:1227–1233.

46. Kisslo J, Adams DB, Belkin RN, eds. Doppler color flow imaging. New York: Churchill Livingstone, 1988.

47. Klein AL, Cohen GI, Davison MB, et al. Importance of sampling both pulmonary veins in the transesophageal assessment of severity of mitral regurgitation [Abstract]. J Am Coll Cardiol 1991;17:199A.

48. Kleinman JP, Maurer G. Transesophageal echocardiography and color flow mapping. In: Maurer G, Mohl W, eds. Echocardiography and Doppler in cardiac surgery. New York: Igaku-Shoin, 1989:171–202.

49. Kuecherer HF, Lee E, Schiller NB. Role of transesophageal echocardiography in diagnosis and management of cardiovascular disease. In: Schiller NB, ed. Cardiology clinics. Doppler echocardiography. Philadelphia: WB Saunders, 1990:377–388.

50. Kusiak V, Brest A. Acute mitral regurgitation: pathophysiology and management. In: Frankl WS, Brest AN, eds. Cardiovascular clinics. Valvular heart disease: comprehensive evaluation and management. Philadelphia: FA Davis, 1986:257–280.

51. Lee E, Schiller NB. Transesophageal echocardiography in clinical cardiology. In: Marcus ML, Schelbert HR, Skorton DJ, Wolf GL, eds. Cardiac imaging: a companion to *Braunwald's Heart Disease*. Philadelphia: WB Saunders, 1991:605–617.

52. Mann T, McLaurin L, Grossman W, Craige E. Assessing the hemodynamic severity of acute aortic regurgitation due to infective endocarditis. N Engl J Med 1975;293:108–113.

53. Martin RP, Meltzer RS, Chia BL, Stinson EB,

Rakowski H, Popp RL. Clinical utility of two dimensional echocardiography in infective endocarditis. Am J Cardiol 1980;46:379–385.

54. Masuyama T, Kodama K, Kitabatake A, et al. Noninvasive evaluation of aortic regurgitation by continuous-wave Doppler echocardiography. Circulation 1986;73:460–466.

55. Matsumoto M, Oka Y, Strom J, et al. Application of transesophageal echocardiography to continuous intraoperative monitoring of left ventricular performance. Am J Cardiol 1980;46:95–105.

56. Maurer G, Czer LSC, Chaux A, et al. Intraoperative Doppler color flow mapping for assessment of valve repair for mitral regurgitation. Am J Cardiol 1987;60:333–337.

57. Meerbaum S. Quantitative two- and three-dimensional echocardiography. In: Maurer G, Mohl W, eds. Echocardiography and Doppler in cardiac surgery. New York: Igaku-Shoin, 1989:21–48.

58. Mills TJ, Talierco CP, Bailey KR, et al. Transthoracic versus transesophageal two-dimensional echo/Doppler flow imaging in surgical patients with mitral regurgitation [Abstract]. J Am Coll Cardiol 1989;13:68A.

59. Mintz GS, Kotler MN, Segal BL, Parry WR. Two-dimensional echocardiographic recognition of ruptured chordae tendineae. Circulation 1978;57:244–250.

60. Miyatake U, Okamoto M, Kinoshita N, et al. Clinical applications of a new type of real-time two-dimensional Doppler flow imaging system. Am J Cardiol 1984;54:857–868.

61. Miyatake K, Izumi S, Okamoto M, et al. Semiquantitative grading of severity of mitral regurgitation by real-time two-dimensional Doppler flow imaging technique. J Am Coll Cardiol 1986;6:82–88.

62. Mügge A, Daniel WG, Frank G, Lichtlen PR. Echocardiography in infective endocarditis: reassessment of prognostic implications of vegetation size determined by the transthoracic and the transesophageal approach. J Am Coll Cardiol 1989;14:634–638.

63. Nanda NC, Pinheiro L, Sanyal R, Storey O. Transesophageal biplane echocardiographic imaging: technique, planes, and clinical usefulness. Echocardiography 1990;7:771–787.

64. Nellessen U, Schnittger I, Appleton CP, et al. Transesophageal two-dimensional echocardiography and color Doppler flow velocity mapping in the evaluation of cardiac valve prostheses. Circulation 1988;78:848–855.

65. Nishimura RA, Schaff HV, Shub C, Gersh BJ, Edwards WD, Tajik AJ. Papillary muscle rupture complicating acute myocardial infarction: analysis of 17 patients. Am J Cardiol 1983;51:373–377.

66. Oikawa JH, Kaye D. Endocarditis: epidemiology, pathophysiology, management and prophylaxis. In: Frankl WS, Brest AN, eds. Cardiovascular clinics. Valvular heart disease: comprehensive evaluation and management. Philadelphia: FA Davis, 1986:335–357.

67. Olson LJ, Tajik AJ. Echocardiographic evaluation of valvular heart disease. In: Marcus ML, Schelbert HR, Skorton DJ, Wolf GL, eds. Cardiac imaging: a companion to *Braunwald's Heart Disease.* Philadelphia: WB Saunders, 1991:419–448.

68. Omoto R, Kondo Y. Basic principles of color flow mapping technique. In: Maurer G, Mohl W, eds. Echocardiography and Doppler in cardiac surgery. New York: Igaku-Shoin, 1989:9–19.

69. Pasternak R, Braunwald E, Sobel BE. Acute myocardial infarction. In: Braunwald E, ed. Heart disease: a textbook of cardiovascular medicine. 3rd ed. Philadelphia: WB Saunders, 1988:1281–1284.

70. Pearlman AS. Transesophageal echocardiography—sound diagnostic technique or two-edged sword? N Engl J Med 1991;324:841–843.

71. Pearson AC, Vrain JS, Mrosek D, Labovitz AJ. Color Doppler echocardiographic evaluation of patients with a flail mitral leaflet. J Am Coll Cardiol 1990;16:232–239.

72. Perry GJ, Helmcke F, Nanda NC, Byard C, Soto B. Evaluation of aortic insufficiency by Doppler color flow mapping. J Am Coll Cardiol 1987;9:952–959.

73. Perry GJ, Bouchard A. Doppler echocardiographic evaluation of mitral regurgitation. In: Schiller NB, ed. Cardiology clinics. Doppler echocardiography. Philadelphia: WB Saunders, 1990:265–275.

74. Pierpont GL, Talley RC. Pathophysiology of valvar heart disease. The dynamic nature of mitral valve regurgitation. Arch Intern Med 1982;142:998–1001.

75. Pollak SJ, Felner JM. Echocardiographic identification of an aortic valve ring abscess. J Am Coll Cardiol 1986;7:1167–1173.

76. Popp RL. Medical progress: echocardiography (first of two parts). N Engl J Med 1990;323:101–109.

77. Popp RL. Medical progress: echocardiography (second of two parts). N Engl J Med 1990;323:165–172.

78. Quinones MA, Young JB, Waggoner AD, Ostojic MC, Ribeiro LG, Miller RR. Assessment of pulsed Doppler echocardiography in detection and quantification of aortic and mitral regurgitation. Br Heart J 1980;44:612–620.

79. Ram Rao S, Richardson SG, Simonetti J, Katz SE, Caldeira M, Pandian NG. Problems and pitfalls in the performance and interpretation of color Doppler flow imaging: observations based on the influences of technical and physiological factors on the color Doppler examination of mitral regurgitation. Echocardiography 1990;7:747–769.

80. Rippe JM, Howe JP. Acute mitral regurgitation. In: Dalen JE, Alpert JS, eds. Valvular heart disease. 2nd ed. Boston: Little, Brown, 1987:151–176.

81. Sahn DJ. Real-time two-dimensional Doppler echocardiographic flow mapping. Circulation 1985;71:849–853.

82. Schiller NG, Cahalan MK, Lee E. Intraoperative monitoring of left ventricular function by transesophageal echocardiography. In: Maurer G, Mohl W, eds. Echocardiography and Doppler in cardiac surgery. New York. Igaku-Shoin, 1989:203–209.

83. Schiller NB. Pulmonary artery pressure estima-

tion by Doppler and two-dimensional echocardiography. In: Schiller NB, ed. Cardiology clinics. Doppler echocardiography. Philadelphia: WB Saunders, 1990:277–287.

84. Schlüter M, Hinrichs A, Thier W, et al. Transesophageal two-dimensional echocardiography: comparison of ultrasonic and anatomic sections. Am J Cardiol 1984;53:1173–1178.

85. Seward JB, Khanderia BK, Oh JK, et al. Transesophageal echocardiography: technique, anatomic correlations, implementation, and clinical applications. Mayo Clin Proc 1988;63:649–680.

86. Seward JB, Khanderia BK, Edwards WD, Oh JK, Freeman WK, Tajik AJ. Biplanar transesophageal echocardiography: anatomic correlations, image orientation, and clinical applications. Mayo Clin Proc 1990;65:1193–1213.

87. Shah PM. Cardiac surgery without or with limited cardiac catheterization. In: Maurer G, Mohl W, eds. Echocardiography and Doppler in cardiac surgery. New York: Igaku-Shoin, 1989:153–170.

88. Shandas BS, Belot J-P, Cali G, Moïses V, Sahn DJ. Comparison of analog and digital methods of transferring color Doppler image data for off-line analysis [Abstract]. J Am Coll Cardiol 1990;15:88A.

89. Sheikh KH, De Bruijn NP, Rankin JS, et al. The utility of transesophageal echocardiography and Doppler color flow imaging in patients undergoing cardiac valve surgery. J Am Coll Cardiol 1990;15:363–372.

90. Smith MD, Grayburn PA, Spain MG, DeMaria AN. Observer variability in the quantitation of Doppler color flow jet areas for mitral and aortic regurgitation. J Am Coll Cardiol 1988;11:579–584.

91. Smith MD. Evaluation of valvular regurgitation by Doppler echocardiography. In: Carabello BA, ed. Cardiology clinics. Valvular heart disease. Philadelphia: WB Saunders, 1991:193–228.

92. Spain MG, Smith MD, Grayburn PA, Harlamert EA, DeMaria AN. Quantitative assessment of mitral regurgitation by Doppler color flow imaging: angiographic and hemodynamic correlations. J Am Coll Cardiol 1989;13:585–590.

93. Taams MA, Gussenhoven EJ, Cahalan MK, et al. Transesophageal Doppler color flow imaging in the detection of native and Björk-Shiley mitral valve regurgitation. J Am Coll Cardiol 1989;13:95–99.

94. Teague SM. Doppler echocardiographic evaluation of aortic regurgitation. In: Schiller NB, ed. Cardiology clinics. Doppler echocardiography. Philadelphia: WB Saunders, 1990:249–263.

95. Thomas JD, Cape EG, Thoreau DH, Levine RA, Yoganathan A, Weyman AE. Automated jet momentum calculation from digital Doppler flow maps [Abstract]. J Am Coll Cardiol 1991;17:149A.

96. Utsunomiya T, Ogawa T, King SW, et al. Pitfalls in the display of color Doppler jet areas: combined variability due to Doppler angle, frame rate, and scanning direction. Echocardiography 1990;7:739–745.

97. Utsunomiya T, Ogawa T, Doshi R, et al. Doppler color flow "proximal isovelocity surface area" method for estimating volume flow rate: effects of orifice shape and machine factors. J Am Coll Cardiol 1991;17:1103–1111.

98. Veyrat C, Witchitz S, Lessana A, Ameur A, Abitbol G, Kalmanson D. Valvar prosthetic dysfunction. Localisation and evaluation of the dysfunction using the Doppler technique. Br Heart J 1985;54:273–284.

99. Weinstein L. Infective endocarditis. In: Braunwald E, ed. Heart disease: a textbook of cardiovascular medicine. 3rd ed. Philadelphia: WB Saunders, 1988:1093–1134.

100. Wisenbaugh T, Berk M, Essop R, Middlemost S, Sareli P. Effect of abrupt mitral regurgitation after balloon valvuloplasty on myocardial load and performance. J Am Coll Cardiol 1991;17:872–878.

17

Determinants of Right Ventricular Performance

Michael R. Pinsky

The role of the right ventricle (RV) in the maintenance of normal cardiovascular homeostasis is not clear. Numerous conflicting studies have been published in the clinical literature. Several authors have demonstrated that severe impairment of the RV free wall, as occurs with inferior wall myocardial infarction, has minimal effects on baseline cardiovascular status and does not prevent a good outcome. Whereas other studies have shown that RV failure is one of the most common causes of mortality and morbidity in critically ill patients with acute respiratory failure, as well as one of the most difficult dysfunctions to correct. The reasons for this dichotomy relate to several factors, all of which interact in the critically ill patient.

DIFFERENCES BETWEEN DETERMINANTS OF RIGHT AND LEFT VENTRICULAR PERFORMANCE

Our knowledge of RV function is rudimentary at best. This is in contrast to our understanding of left ventricular (LV) function. The reason for this lack of understanding relates to our inability to both model the RV and accurately measure RV hemodynamics. Furthermore, if one were to examine RV function relative to parameters used to monitor LV function, it is clear that similar factors have disproportional effects on the two ventricles. These differences relate, in large part, to the structural differences between the two ventricles and to the interdependence that each may show the other during both diastole and systole. The factors that determine LV performance can be grouped into those factors that alter myocardial contrac-

tility, preload, and afterload. Although discussed in greater detail in the following chapter, specific observations will be mentioned here.

Myocardial Contractility

Myocardial contractility is a function of intrinsic myocardial function, sympathetic tone, and coronary blood flow. Since the RV free wall mass is small, other factors that determine RV contractility, such as changing level of sympathetic stimulation and coronary blood flow will have a proportionally greater effect on RV function than on LV function, although the absolute magnitude of the response should be much greater for the LV. RV myocardial blood flow characteristics are also different from LV and septal blood flow characteristics. The blood supply to the RV myocardium is delivered both in systole and diastole, unlike the LV, which receives most of its blood supply only during diastole. Thus, RV myocardial perfusion pressure is best estimated at systemic arterial pressure minus pulmonary arterial pressure (9). Accordingly, increases in pulmonary arterial pressure will decrease RV myocardial blood flow as much as decreases in systemic arterial pressure. Thus, acute increases in pulmonary arterial pressure may induce ischemic RV dysfunction, independent of any specific effects of pulmonary arterial pressure on RV afterload.

Preload

The RV is a large thin-walled muscular structure that shares a common thick muscular intraventricular septum with the LV. Being a thin-walled structure, the RV is

280

much more distensible than the LV. Furthermore, it is dependent more on pericardial interactions to determine its diastolic compliance than is the LV (4). In fact, no clinical study has yet been able to define a linear relation between RV end-diastolic volume and pressure. This can be the case only if the ability to measure RV pressures and volume are inaccurate or if the RV is highly compliant. What is clear, however, is that there is little if any relation between right atrial pressure and RV (5). Extending this observation further, increases in lung volume, as may occur at end-inspiration or with the application of positive end-expiratory pressure (PEEP), will initially decrease RV more than it will LV (1).

Complicating matters further, it is also not clear if changes in RV alter RV contractility by the Frank-Starling mechanism in the same way as changes in LV alter LV ejection. The RV is thin-walled and highly compliant relative to the left ventricle. Increases in RV may reflect conformational changes in the RV or minimal changes in end-diastolic wall stress, such that ejection performance is relatively unaffected by changing RV. Whether this explanation is correct or not is not known. What is known, however, is that changes in RV may bear little relation to changes in RV systolic function under most clinical conditions.

Afterload

Right ventricular ejection is more complex than is LV ejection. Furthermore, RV afterload may not change in a similar fashion to changes in ejection pressure as does LV afterload. The RV musculature contracts during systole in a peristaltic fashion, starting with the inflow tract and proceeding antegrade through apex to infundibulum (1). Although this peristaltic wave does not push blood out of the heart, in a fashion similar to peristalsis in the bowel, it does decrease the mechanical efficiency of the RV by making RV myocardial fiber shortening less synchronous. Furthermore, it is difficult to accurately define RV end-systole because RV ejection continues long after peak pulmonary artery pressure. The reasons for this may relate to systolic coupling of contraction forces from

left to right through the common ventricular septum and interdigitating free wall fibers as well as the remarkable ability of the pulmonary circulation to handle large increases in flow with only minimal changes in pressure.

Like the LV, the RV changes shape during contraction to approximate more of a sphere. Since the RV starts off in a more irregular shape than the LV, this conformational change for the RV probably reduces the radius of curvature of its free wall, more than for the LV free wall. Since, by Laplace's law, wall stress of a sphere is a function of the radius of curvature and the transmural pressure, decreasing RV free wall radius should actually reduce RV systolic wall stress.

In the opposite direction, however, if the RV becomes overdistended it may acutely fail, because the increase in wall stress will exceed the myocardium's ability to counteract it. Sudden increases in RV ejection pressure, as occur in association with acute massive pulmonary embolism, will induce RV dilation and acute cor pulmonale. More gradual increases in ejection pressure, as occur with chronic pulmonary hypertension, can be surprisingly well tolerated because the RV free wall hypertrophies, becoming more like the LV. Increasing lung volume or hyperinflation will also increase pulmonary vascular resistance. However, the effect that hyperinflation will have on RV ejection is variable. Since increasing lung volume will compress the RV, RV may actually decrease. Thus, acute RV dilation may not be seen with acute respiratory failure in patients with chronic airflow obstruction because of both chronic RV hypertrophy and decreased RV. These points are addressed further in a subsequent chapter on pulmonary hypertension.

EFFECT OF RV PERFORMANCE ON CARDIOVASCULAR HOMEOSTASIS

Under conditions of normal pulmonary and systemic vascular tone and LV contractility, RV performance only minimally alters the cardiovascular response to moderate exercise (2). Even complete ablation of RV free wall contractile function is compatible with life (8). This remarkable observation relates, in part, to the interaction between the LV and the RV wherein LV contraction mechanically is coupled to RV-developed pressure. Accordingly, LV-developed pressure is transmitted into the RV chamber, such that RV pressure rises during systole, even if the RV free wall does not move (6).

Why then do patients die of RV failure? The answer to this question can be complex and appears to be related to coexistent LV dysfunction, valvular insufficiency, and associated increases in pulmonary vascular resistance. As described above, if acute volume or pressure overload increases RV wall stress, then the RV may fail. As the RV distends, it decreases LV diastolic compliance by shifting the septum into the LV and by restricting absolute biventricular pericardial volume. These points are discussed in greater detail in the chapter on heart-lung interactions. The bottom line is, however, that RV dilation will decrease LV filling, decreasing LV output and systemic arterial pressure. This results in a negative feedback loop of decreasing RV myocardial blood flow (decreased RV coronary perfusion pressure), RV ischemic dysfunction, further RV dilation, and its associated further decrease in LV diastolic compliance and LV preload.

The presentation of acute cor pulmonale will then be low output, systemic hypotension, pulmonary hypertension, and markedly elevated RV filling pressures. Whether LV filling pressures are elevated or not is variable. The treatment for this life-taking process is to rapidly decrease RV wall stress and increase RV myocardial blood flow. If pulmonary embolism induced an outflow obstruction, then measures that reduce this obstruction (such as thrombolytic therapy and embolectomy) should be used. If hyperinflation induced the RV failure, then measures aimed at reducing lung volume (prolonged expiratory time, bronchodilator therapy, etc.) should be used. It should be clear from the above scenario, however, that massive volume expansion plays a minor role in the management of acute cor pulmonale. Volume overexpansion may actually precipitate cor pulmonale in the setting of RV

ischemia, if it is not associated with a concomitant increase in cardiac output and arterial pressure. Measures aimed at maintaining coronary perfusion pressure are preferable to volume expansion in this setting. Accordingly, vasopressor therapy to maintain systemic arterial pressure is often required to help stabilize these patients while awaiting resolution of the clot via thrombolytic therapy (3, 7).

Under conditions in which the RV has seen chronically elevated ejection pressures, such as occur in patients with severe end-stage obstructive airway disease, interstitial fibrosis, and idiopathic pulmonary hypertension, the RV hypertrophies. This hypertrophic change alters both RV diastolic compliance and RV adaptation to further increases in ejection pressure. RV diastolic compliance decreases, such that greater pressures are necessary to distend the hypertrophied RV. Under these conditions the relation between RV and pressure becomes better defined and more like the LV in nature. The RV also does not dilate as much in response to increased pressure loads. In essence, the RV becomes a mirror image of the LV in all aspects except in its level of coronary blood flow, which cannot change.

SUMMARY

The effect that RV dysfunction will have on overall cardiovascular homeostasis will be dependent on the intrinsic level of RV performance, the intrathoracic factors limiting RV diastolic filling, the tone and impedance of the pulmonary arterial circuit to which the RV ejects, concomitant LV function, and effective RV myocardial blood flow.

References

1. Armour JA, Pace JB, Randall WC. Interrelationship between architecture and function of the right ventricle. Am J Physiol 1970;218:174–180.
2. Furey SA, Zieske HA, Levy MN. The essential function of the right ventricle. Am Heart J 1984;107:404–410.
3. Ghigonne M, Girley L, Prewitt RM. Volume expansion versus norepinephrine in treatment of a low cardiac output complicating an acute increase in right ventricular afterload in dogs. Anesthesiology 1984;60:132–135.
4. Goldstein JA, Vlahaker GJ, Verrier ED, Schiller

NB, et al. The role of right ventricular systolic dysfunction and elevated intra-pericardial pressure in the genesis of low output in experimental right ventricle infarction. Circulation 1982;65:513–522.

5. Pinsky MR. Assessment of the right ventricle in the critically ill: facts, fancy, and perspectives. In: Vincent JL, ed. Update in intensive care and emergency medicine. Berlin: Springer-Verlag 1989:518–523.

6. Santamore WP, Lynch PR, Heckman JL, Bove AA, Meier GD. Left ventricular effects on right developed pressure. J Appl Physiol 1976;41:925–932.

7. Sharf SM, Wraner KG, Josa M, Khuri SF, Brown R. Load tolerance of the right ventricle: effect of increased aortic pressure. J Crit Care 1986;3:163–173.

8. Starr I, Jeffers WA, Meade RH. The absence of conspicuous increment of venous pressure after severe damage to the right ventricle of the dog. Am Heart J 1943;26:291.

9. Urabe Y, Tomoike H, Ohzono K, Koyanoagi S, Nakamura M. Role of afterload in determining regional right ventricular performance during coronary underperfusion in dogs. Circ Res 1985;57:96–104.

18

Acute Right Ventricular Failure

Pierre Squara
Jean-François A. Dhainaut
Fabrice Brunet

In the early 20th century, the right ventricle (RV) was considered to be little more than a conduit for blood flow between the peripheral venous circulation and the pulmonary arterial tree (199), the "weak sister" of the left heart (71, 75, 79). The physiologic role of the RV systole has been reexamined, especially because of the observations of acute cor pulmonale and RV infarction, in which the RV failure may be responsible for a circulatory shock.

In 1979, Laver et al. (116) epitomized the clinical problem of acute RV overload. Indeed, some patients with acute pulmonary hypertension, such as pulmonary embolism, adult respiratory distress syndrome, acute thermal injury, asthma attack, and acute exacerbations of chronic obstructive pulmonary disease, develop a marked increase in RV afterload. This results in increased RV volumes, wall stress, and myocardial oxygen consumption. If severe enough, these changes may lead to a decline in cardiac output, which may limit survival in certain critically ill patients.

Because maintenance of cardiac output may depend on RV function during critical illness, the clinician needs to be able to discern the presence of RV dysfunction and whether it is due to decreased ventricular filling, increased RV afterload, decreased contractile state via a myocardial ischemia, or a combination of two or even three of these causes (96).

RIGHT VENTRICULAR ROLE IN OVERALL HEMODYNAMICS

Anatomic and Physiologic Background

In contrast to the systemic circulation, the main physical characteristic of the pulmonary circulation is low resistance to flow. After birth, RV anatomy is remodelled to work against low physical constraints. This remodelling explains the inability for the RV to face a sudden increase in pulmonary resistance such as may occur in pulmonary embolism or in acute respiratory failure. The RV wall is normally thinner (4–5 mm) than the left ventricular wall, but the adaptation to chronic pulmonary hypertension may induce a thickness that may nearly equal that of the left ventricle (LV). The RV chamber is anatomically composed of three walls: anterior, inferior, and posterolateral, i.e., the ventricular septum that bulges into the RV cavity under normal conditions. The normal contraction of the ventricular septum contributes essentially to decrease the diameter of the left ventricle. Nevertheless, the septum position is responsive to the transseptal gradient throughout the cardiac cycle. Then, marked displacement may occur depending on the respective left and right intrachamber pressure (190). In any case of increased RV intrachamber pressure, a leftward septal displacement is expected that further reduces the apparent compliance of the left ventricle and accounts for possible decrease in LV stroke output. Such a displacement is of less magnitude in systole than in diastole due to the different myocardial stiffness.

The RV and LV are mechanically coupled (70, 177). Experimental studies performed by electively cauterizing the RV free wall demonstrated that both the right atrial and pulmonary arterial pressures did not change (199). These studies illustrated most dramatically that this function is not significantly impaired by elective RV free wall destruction. By virtue of the anatomic continuity, tension that is developed during contraction of the intact LV is transmitted to the damaged RV wall, thus preserving the RV pump function (177). In contrast, it has been shown, in a hemodynamic model of exclusion of the RV developed by Furey et al. (79), that acute elimination of RV function usually leads to a significant decrease in cardiac output. When the fluid volume was increased sufficiently, cardiac output was restored to the control level, but central venous pressure markedly increased. Thus, the normal role of the RV seems to be maintenance of a low systemic venous pressure.

The RV is crescent-shaped with an angle when seen in horizontal cross-section of 60°. It is embryologically, anatomically, and functionally divided into sinus (*inflow*) and conus (*outflow*) regions (204). The sinus extends from the tricuspid valve to the crista supraventricularis that arches from the anterior wall to the septum over the anterior leaflet of the tricuspid valve. The sinus is limited externally by the inferior and anterior walls; the internal aspect shows the trabecular muscles acting as chords during the RV contraction. RV sinus also contains the major part of the three tricuspid papillary muscles inserted in each RV wall. The conus extends to the pulmonary valve and differs from the sinus by the presence of the circumvascular muscles derived the embryologic bulbus cordis, from which also derives the aortic root.

During *systole*, the greatest relative motion occurs in the tricuspid valve plane and the least in the anterior and inferior segments. The motion of the tricuspid valve annulus may be compared to the mitral annulus motion and suggests a sphincter-like action (87, 192). In resting normal subjects, the reduction of the tricuspid annulus is 33% (212). Even in the absence of tricuspid annulus dilatation, a slight tricuspid regurgitation may be detected in half of the normal subjects by Doppler echocardiography (15). RV contraction proceeds sequentially from the sinus to the conus. During sinus contraction, the conus dilates concomitantly with the initial part of the pulmonary artery acting as a reservoir (156). Under physiologic conditions, the conus contracts 25 to 50 msec after the sinus and remains contracted when the inflow tract relaxation begins. This delay is shortened by stellate stimulation or epinephrine infusion (6). Rather than a booster, the RV contraction has been compared to a peristaltic movement, initiated by the atrial systole even, stricto sensu, this term is not consensual (135). When RV ejection is impeded by acute pulmonary hypertension, the functional difference between inflow and outflow tract persists (230). It may be assumed that this sinus-conus asynchronism is adequate to protect the sensitive pulmonary arteries from high peaks of pressure and to promote a continuous blood flow in the pulmonary vessels for optimal hematosis.

Since the RV ejects against a low resistance circuit, the blood ejection continues after peak pressure is developed within the RV. Consequently, the shape of the global pressure-volume loop differs from those of the LV. The more triangular shape makes end-systole more difficult to point out (130). In addition, it has been recently shown in a canine model of adult respiratory distress syndrome (ARDS) that the RV inflow tract and outflow tract may have different pressure-volume loops, making global RV function difficult to schematize (230). Although the end-systole is defined as the peak of the active contractile process, identified as the time of maximal elastance (176), most of the clinical studies concerning the RV end-systolic pressure-volume relation have used the ratio of pulmonary artery dicrotic notch pressure or peak RV pressure to minimum RV volume (end-ejection), because of their easy measurements. However, it has been demonstrated that the end-systolic pressure-volume relation defined by maximal elastance (max P/V-VO) is a more reliable index to assess RV function (28). Misjudging this point causes one to underestimate RV contractile function or response to inotropic medications. Nevertheless, when pulmonary hypertension occurs, both the inflow tract and outflow tract have more quadrangular pressure-volume loops and the ratio peak pressure:minimum volume becomes an acceptable variable to assess the active RV pressure volume relationship (28, 58, 230).

These considerations also account for a particular feature of the RV diastole. Diastole begins at the end of systole. Then, up to one-third of the stroke volume may be ejected during the active relaxation phase. This explains the very short isovolumic relaxation period. It is then impossible to calculate, as for the LV, a time constant of relaxation, except when pulmonary hypertension occurs. The relaxation is consequently investigated by the maximum negative dP/dt (202). The passive part of diastole is associated with ventricle filling. Even though the mechanism remains unknown (20, 24, 172), it is now accepted that filling is enhanced by a ventricle suction that may approximate −5 mm Hg (175, 202), and may be clinically relevant in ventricle filling in cases of tachycardia or tricuspid stenosis. Mention should be made of the atrioventricular synchronism in filling the ventricle in end-diastole because loss of the atrial systole may be responsible for a decrease in cardiac output up to 20% (97).

The RV is highly compliant during filling. This high compliance of the RV has two direct consequences: to allow low systemic venous pressure that favors tissue perfusion, and to prevent acute pulmonary edema in situations associated with LV dysfunction. The passive pressure-volume relationship of the normal RV is quite horizontal and linear inside its usual limits. Several factors make difficult and controversial the rigorous investigation of RV preload (152, 222). First, the measurement of RV end-diastolic volume appears to be critical, and the complex geometry of the RV explains the difficulties in modeling volume calculations from one or several measured dimensions. Second, since the RV is functioning below its unstressed volume, changes in volume do not result in measurable changes in pressure, but only changes in ventricular geometry. Therefore, since the RV distending pressure changes little during filling, it is clear that muscle length and tension must also not change greatly, i.e., under normal conditions RV preload may be poorly related to end-diastolic volume.

Finally, even the filling pressure could be an acceptable measure of the RV preload. When positioned on the ascending limb of the pressure-volume relationship, the heart fills, not as a function of absolute intrachamber pressure, but according to transmural pressure (intrachamber pressure minus juxtacardiac pressure). Changes in juxtacardiac pressure depend on pericardial capacity, changes in regional lung volume, and chest wall compliance. The pericardial stress-strain relationship is J-shaped. In most clinical circumstances, the pericardial cavity is unstressed and pericardectomy is uneventful (185). However, when the RV is markedly overextended, both ventricles compete inside the inextensible pericardial space, amplifying the ventricular interdependence. In addition, the lungs may directly compress the heart and induce an anterior heart rotation. In practice, measuring juxtacardiac pressure is complex and often underestimated when evaluated by the intraesophageal or pleural pressure, except when the subject is in the lateral position (126).

RV RESPONSES TO WALL STRESS AND DECREASED CONTRACTILITY

In isolated contracting intact heart models the effects of sudden changes in preload on RV performance may be studied separate from changes in afterload. In contrast, in the clinical setting, abnormalities in right ventricular preload and afterload often coexist in the same patient. For example, in a left-to-right shunt, the primary RV abnormality is volume overload. However, the high pulmonary blood volume is generally accompanied by an increase in pulmonary artery pressure. Both contribute to an abnormally high RV afterload. Conversely, in patients with primary pressure overload states, such as pulmonary embolism and obstructive lung disease, volume overload occurs as a consequence of the inability of the RV to sustain systolic performance. These interactions between RV preload and afterload should be considered when properly interpreting data derived from intact animal models and in clinical settings (112). Despite this interaction, we discuss the RV responses to volume and pressure overload, respectively, to simplify the understanding of this issue.

Structural and Functional Changes in Volume Overload

Sudden and chronic volume overload alter the architecture of the RV wall and cavity, as well as the pattern of systolic motion (11, 69, 110, 134). When the short axis of the RV is viewed in two-dimensional echocardiography the normal LV maintains a circular appearance, with the two minor axes approximately equal. In patients with RV volume overload the interventricular septum is flattened at end-diastole, displacing the septum into the LV domain resulting in inequality of the LV minor axes. This pattern of right ventricular motion closely resembles that of the LV with motion of free wall and septum toward a central axis (69, 150). Theoretically, in pure volume overloaded RV, the flattened end-diastolic septum must reassure its normal concave leftward configuration at end-systole since the normal transseptal systolic pressure gradient is conserved (174, 187, 191). Depending on the degree of diastolic leftward septal shift (and of frequent associated pressure overload), the right ventricular protosystolic motion may be paradoxic. This motion pattern should also be distinguished from one in which septal contractile function is decreased, which is characterized by a depressed septal systolic thickening.

The sudden effect of increased end-diastolic volume on ventricular systolic function may be expressed by the Starling relation when RV stressed volume is reached. Accordingly, the volume overload of the RV results in a marked increase in stroke volume, but may not be fully explained by an increased segment length (138). It could be possible that the more spheric RV end-diastolic shape induces a better mechanical effect of the contractile force. In addition, a quicker relaxation has been observed when diastolic fiber length is enlarged. This may contribute to RV filling (156). The existence of a true descending limb of the Starling curve in a clinical setting associated with excessive preload remains debated. An apparent descending limb may result from functional tricuspid regurgitation (112). The function of the tricuspid valve apparatus is more sensitive than that of the mitral valve to changes in annulus size or papillary muscle mechanics due to ventricular dilatation (212). The result is that the tricuspid regurgitating flow tends to negate the classic Starling effect during RV volume overload, and forward cardiac output may decrease.

Experimental chronic RV volume overload, in contrast to that of the LV has not been found to exhibit significant alteration of contractile function and energetics (41). In patients with left-to-right shunt, who provide acceptable models for RV volume overload, the RV rarely fails in the absence of significant pulmonary vascular obstructive disease. With surgical repair, the RV ejection fraction often falls, thus revealing systolic dysfunction that had been masked through the Starling mechanism (112). In addition, the return to normal pattern of septal motion is in part related to the duration of the volume overload prior to repair and often needs a long period of time to appear (150). These findings should be interpreted cautiously since cardiac surgery is followed by the appearance of paradoxic septal motion presumably related to an alteration in the geometry of the entire heart rather than altered right ventricular load.

Structural and Functional Changes in Pressure Overload

Specific configurational changes in the presence of RV pressure overload are less well described because of the constant coexistence of pressure and volume overload in such circumstances. The RV pressure increases, and may compete with the LV pressure to position the interventricular septum (138, 174, 187, 190). The systolic leftward septal shift optimizes the mechanical effect of the RV contraction (116).

Changes in the configuration of both ventricles have been observed during sudden RV pressure loading in dogs. Following acute pulmonary artery constriction, the LV septal-free wall dimension and shortening are reduced as well as its contribution to global LV systolic function (219), whereas in chronic RV pressure overload, the LV septal-free wall dimension and shortening are maintained (8). This leftward shift of the ventricular septum has at least two mechanisms: competition between both ventricles inside an inextensive pericardial cavity, and series interactions with a decreased LV filling due to a decreased RV stroke volume. Since the absence of pericardium has little influence in ventricular interdependence in a canine model, the series interactions may predominate when the RV is afterloaded (33).

To what degree the contractile state of the RV myocardium is altered by chronic pressure overload remains uncertain. Indeed, since the ventricular response to chronic pressure overload has been extensively studied in animals, the results of these investigations differ somewhat, and special attention must be given to the species utilized, the magnitude of hypertrophy produced, and the duration of pressure load produced (112). Usually, RV and LV hypertrophy was produced by constriction of the pulmonary artery and aorta, respectively. In the former, ventricle:body weight ratios increased 44–90%, while in reports of LV pressure overload, the hypertrophy was more modest (30–40%) (42, 43, 91, 93, 104, 194, 225). In most studies, the maximum active tension developed by hypertrophied papillary muscles, the time derivative of tension development, V_{max},

and the maximum measured velocity of shortening were observed to be reduced. Time to peak tension, a measure of the duration of active state, was found to be normal or, most frequently, prolonged. The rate at which the pressure load is applied to the ventricle does not appear to influence these mechanical abnormalities since the same findings are observed in models where the pressure load is gradual as when it is abrupt (43).

The long-term effects of chronic pressure overload were examined by Williams and Potter (225), who compared the mechanical characteristics of the RV of the hypertrophied cat at 6 and 24 weeks. The authors observed that maximum active tension, (dT/dt) and V_{max} were depressed and time to peak tension was prolonged at 6 weeks. In contrast, none of these abnormalities could be demonstrated at 24 weeks. The magnitude of hypertrophy was the same at both time points, as previously reported for the LV. Hoffmann and Covell (93) found depressed contractile indices 9 and 40 days after pulmonary artery constriction in the rabbit; the late group (96 days) manifested normal indices. Interestingly, ejection phase indices of systolic performance in the intact RV correlated poorly with the findings in isolated papillary muscles, suggesting that compensatory mechanisms in intact animals mask the intrinsic functional abnormalities of hypertrophied heart muscle.

In clinical studies of chronic RV pressure overload, decreased ejection fraction is frequently present, essentially due to the systolic load present at the time of study, but abnormalities in RV contractility are generally absent (201, 227).

Finally, the early response to pressure overload of the RV is a reduction in the intrinsic velocity of the contractile apparatus, associated with a compensatory prolonged duration of force development. In the intact organism, these defects may be masked by neurohumoral effects and are not easily detected by clinical indices of systolic pump function. With sustained pressure overload, these mechanical abnormalities may revert toward normal. However, further depression of contractile function during prolonged and severe pressure overload is demonstrated in isolated heart muscle (194).

Response of Right Coronary Circulation to RV Overload

The RV is mainly perfused by the right coronary artery. It has been shown that volume work requires less energy than pressure work (68). Relative to the myocardial mass, the subendocardial coronary vasculature of the RV is less developed than in the LV. However, the RV coronary perfusion is maintained during both systole and diastole since the driving pressure (intracoronary pressure-right myocardial tissue pressure) remains always positive. The intracoronary pressure equals the aortic pressure, and the RV myocardial tissue pressure can be estimated by the intracavity pressure (46). As for the LV, the right ventricular myocardial oxygen extraction is almost maximum (venous Po_2 ranges from 18–20 mm Hg) (89). Then, an increase in the RV oxygen requirement must be mainly met by an increase in coronary blood flow, mostly obtained by a vasodilatation mediated by several metabolic factors, one of which is AMP (17, 33). The total RV amount of high-energy phosphate is lower than in the LV. This could explain a particular sensitivity to hypoxia. In patients undergoing elective coronary artery bypass, a threefold increase has been shown in the ratio ADP/ATP and a 100-fold increase in the ratio AMP/ATP for the right as compared to the LV after cold cardioplegic arrest (37). Consequently, the recovery of the RV after cardioplegic arrest may take longer than for the LV.

For the LV a close relation has been shown between myocardial oxygen consumption and the total pressure volume area determined by both systolic and diastolic pressure volume lines and the portion of the pressure volume loop from end-diastole to end-systole (206). Thus, increased afterload increases LV oxygen consumption. Since RV oxygen consumption is difficult to measure, no clinical data are available for the RV. However, Calvin and Quinn (34) argue, on the basis of experimental studies, for the hypothesis of an increased RV myocardium oxygen demand in acute pressure overload. In many other pathologic circumstances, a RV ischemia has been hypothesized, even in the absence of significant coronary disease, when the systolic coronary perfusion driving pressure is decreased. This is likely to occur and consequently to induce a decreased contractility when an acute pulmonary hypertension coexists with a reduced systemic pressure (34, 216, 220). Furthermore, Scharf et al. (180) have shown an increased RV performance when increasing aortic pressure in canine studies where two models of pulmonary hypertension have been performed (82, 180). The precise mechanism was not fully demonstrated, a global decreased RV ischemia was not found, but the authors have speculated that there is an increased perfusion of the deeper layers of the RV myocardium (180). However, the last study shows that RV ischemia is not necessary for RV failure to occur in acute pulmonary hypertension. Therefore, in patients without coronary disease, a decrease in contractility due to a RV ischemia may be only advocated in extreme situations.

Hypertrophied hearts (125) may have a particular sensitivity to hypoxia that could be clinically relevant (113). If the coronary blood flow per unit weight of muscle is normal in hypertrophied hearts, coronary vascular resistance is higher in hypertrophied than in normal myocardium (147), and a greater proportion of the total vasodilation reserve is used to maintain resting flow in hypertrophy situations (142). An important expression of this defect has been the finding of a disproportionate decrease in the endocardial:epicardial flow ratio in hypertrophy during the stress of pacing (142) and during exercise (143). While most of these studies have involved models of LV hypertrophy, reduced vasodilator response has been observed in dogs with RV hypertrophy (143) and in the RV of patients with atrial septal defects and pulmonary hypertension (65).

RV Response to Decreased Contractile State

There has been little published on the investigation of specific RV response to elective contractile impairment. The reason for this is the lack of a valid model. When studying global cardiomyopathy or inferior LV-associated RV infarction, the RV response accounts for both ventricular interdependence and postcapillary RV pressure overload. The RV free wall infarction may be considered a better model, but several associated factors such as modified ventricular coupling, geometric consequences of infarction, or postischemic relaxation impairment may have important additional but nonvaluable effects. Furthermore, the constraining effect of the pericardium seems to be a major contributor to hemodynamic consequences of impaired RV contractility.

With the pericardium intact, Goldstein et al. (84) showed that the experimental RV free wall infarction was followed by a fall in cardiac output, an increase in both RV filling pressure and size, and a decrease in LV end-diastolic dimension and pressure, leading to the classic diastolic pressures equalization (40). However, in accordance with other studies in open chest models (9, 103, 211), when the pericardium is open, right and left dimensions increase as do cardiac output and both right and left stroke work indices; RV pressure decreases and diastolic equalization resolves. Therefore, when faced with a decreased contractile state, at least three factors may preserve ejection and cardiac output: ventricular coupling, RV dilation due to an increased postsystolic residue that increases the contractile force via a Starling effect (and may additionally increase the mechanical effect of a given contractile force via geometric modification as rightward systolic septal motion, even below the unstressed volume) (9), and, as evidenced in pulmonary hypertension, a slower RV relaxation that may favor ejection (156). In such circumstances the pericardium decreases the apparent ventricle compliance, promotes ventricular interference, and acts as a limiting factor for both RV dilatation and ejection force (86).

In summary, to maintain RV stroke volume (hence, end-systolic pressure remains constant) a decreased E_{max} should be balanced by an increased RV end-diastolic volume in the same proportion. Therefore,

the respective levels of (1) maximum diastolic volume (according to extramural: pleural, pericardial, right atrial and LV constraints), (2) pulmonary resistance, and (3) minimum forward stroke volume to maintain adequate cardiac output are the determinants of a given decreased contactility-induced RV failure. Since natural life includes exercise and various situations of increased oxygen demand (i.e., increased pulmonary resistance and increased needed cardiac output), RV performance may become an important limiting factor to cardiac output and may be of great prognostic value in global cardiomyopathy with comparable LV performance (154).

The Heart as an Endocrine Organ

The right atrium contains granules of an immunoreactive peptide, the atrial natriuretic factor (52). To date, vasodilatation, diuresis, natriuresis, inhibition of angiotensin II, release of aldosterone, relaxation of smooth muscles, and negative inotropic power on the myocardium have been shown (137). Both experimental and clinical studies (10) have shown that the release of atrial natriuretic factor depends on atrial stretching as it may occur during RV acute failure (161). During right ventricular infarction, a significant increase in the atrial natriuretic factor has been shown. However, whether this release could be a specific marker of the RV infarction is currently unlikely and the question needs further investigation (167). Nevertheless, the increased levels of natriuretic factor observed during the RV infarction may contribute to the hemodynamic pattern (167).

RV FAILURE IN CRITICAL ILLNESS: IMPLICATIONS FOR THERAPY

The right ventricle is affected by critical illness through aberrations of the elementary actions that have been described in the preceding section. In this section, we will describe several of the more common critical situations and give their main pathophysiologic findings that support treatment of the RV dysfunction.

To face various grade of increased afterload and/or decreased contractile state with or without coronary impairment, these critical situations have in common the need for optimal filling. Optimal RV filling is the maximum forward stroke volume as described by the Starling mechanism without overdilation-induced severe tricuspid regurgitation, impaired LV filling, and pulmonary edema. However, rehabilitation of critical illness does not depend on a single approach since several elementary pathologic effects are usually involved. It is the role of the clinician to determine for each given patient what is predominant and what is minor.

Adult Respiratory Distress Syndrome (ARDS)

In ARDS, lung injury is associated with various degrees of intrapulmonary vessels destruction, thrombosis, and vasoconstriction (229) mediated by inflammation and/or hypoxemia (12). High-inspired oxygen fraction (FIo_2) may also injure pulmonary vessels (45). Thus, in conjunction with the initial etiology, such as sepsis, multiple organ failure or other causes of decreased myocardial contractility, ARDS, in relation to the RV, is mainly a sudden pressure load challenge (229).

In response to the increased load to the RV, cardiac output is preserved by an increased stroke work and RV dilation, until RV failure occurs, leading to a decline in LV performance as judged by the Starling mechanism (32). This load challenge is the major hemodynamic problem; aside from the ARDS etiology, afterload indices have been shown to be the related factors (30, 59). Additional ischemic alterations of the contractile state, presumably caused by both overload-induced increased myocardial oxygen demand (34) and impaired myocardial driving pressure (18), have also been found. However, this is debatable (180) depending on the ARDS model, the associated disease, and the method for contractile state assessment. Another challenge of the RV is to increase systemic oxygen delivery to meet the demands of increased tissue oxygen demand and decreased tissue oxygen extraction seen in ARDS and sepsis. This seems to be related to specific etiologies (such as sepsis) since oxygen-related variables are of poor prognostic value in some other cases (such as trauma) and in overall ARDS (59).

A cornerstone of treatment for ARDS is mechanical ventilation allowing continuous positive airway pressure. Several modes of ventilation are available, all having the purpose of maintaining a normal hematosis by alveoli recruitment with minimum barotraumatism (1, 66, 135). All these modes of mechanical ventilation may limit venous return (Fig. 18.1) and additionally impede the RV. Limitation of ventricular filling is mediated by a peripheral translocation of the thoracic blood volume (22, 44, 73, 158, 184). The precise mechanism of this fluid translocation has been recently restudied by Fessler et al. (72). Because the mean systemic pressure is also increased, the gradient pressure for venous return (i.e., right atrial pressure − mean systemic pressure) remains unchanged. An increase in venous resistance and a PEEP-induced right atrium waterfall upstream have been hypothesized. In addition, filling in both ventricles may be limited by ventricular interdependence and the direct heart compression by hyperinflated lungs (209). This may occur even in the absence of excessive PEEP, as in the case of inhomogeneous pulmonary disease (80) or in bullous dystrophic evolution (117).

There is a close relationship between lung volume and pulmonary vascular resistance that is inversely parabolic with a minimum (nadir) functional residual capacity (189). PEEP, when applied with the goal of restoring normal functional residual capacity, may help to optimally decrease the right ventricular afterload (56, 207). At low pulmonary volumes, pulmonary vascular resistance is essentially due to hypoxic vasoconstriction of extraalveolar vessels and vascular endothelial injury. In contrast, when higher pulmonary volumes are reached by using a gradual increase of PEEP, pulmonary vascular resistance exponentially increases with volume through further intraalveolar vessel compression (zone II enlargement at the expense of zone III). This may be dramatic in the case of excessive PEEP (18, 102, 183).

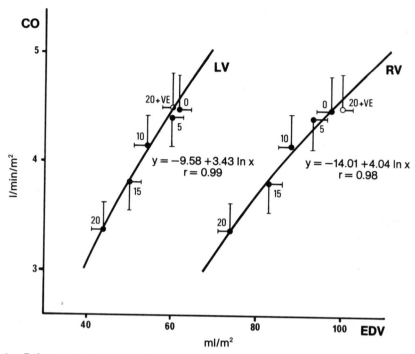

Figure 18.1. Relationship between the cardiac output (CO) and the end-diastolic volume (EDV) of the right ventricular (RV) *(right curve)* and the left ventricular (LV) *(left curve)* as airway pressure was progressively increased from 0 (upper right data point) to 20 cm H_2O (lower left data point). Each value represents the mean ± SEM. VE = volume expansion. (From Dhainaut JF, Devaux JY, Monsallier JF, Brunet F, Villemant D, Huyghebaert MF. Mechanisms of decreased left ventricular preload during continuous positive pressure ventilation in ARDS. Chest 1986;90:74–80.)

In addition, pulmonary injury is often inhomogeneous and a given level of PEEP may have no distending effects on noncompliant lung units and, conversely, promote hyperinflation of the others, increasing right ventricular afterload (63). From functional residual capacity, pulmonary vascular resistance is further increased by the inspiratory lung inflation. It has been shown that optimal RV stroke volume and ejection fraction were obtained when this additional peak inspiratory volume (and/or pressure) is minimized by using low tidal volumes, inverted inspiratory/expiratory (I/E) ratio (1, 115), or spontaneous inspiration with or without pressure support. Extracorporeal CO_2 removal may provide an adequate response if more simple technology were available (81).

Hence, the physiologic basis for *treatment* may follow these steps. First, pulmonary output impedance must be minimized. This is done not only by treating the specific cause of ARDS, but also by relentless efforts to search for methods that may contribute significantly to maintaining afterload in an acceptable range. Among these methods are sedation and curarization, if needed, hypoxemia control without deleterious F_{IO_2}, and pulmonary volume control by finding the best level of PEEP (207) and the best mode of ventilation. To further decrease pulmonary vascular resistance, several reports emphasize the need for hemodilution to decrease blood viscosity (4, 157) and of antiaggregant or anticoagulant drugs to improve intrapulmonary vessel obstruction (98). The use of pulmonary vasodilation, although improving RV function, has adverse effects, decreasing hypoxic vasoconstriction on nonventilated area. The improvement of RV function and cardiac output is counterbalanced by an increased intrapulmonary shunt. Therefore, if vasodilators are tested, oxygen delivery and tissue oxygen consumption should be carefully evaluated in order to determine whether positive or negative effects are predominant (133, 165, 193).

Second RV filling must be preserved by decreasing the back pressure to venous return by lowering the intrathoracic pressure. Changes in intrathoracic pressure induced by positive-pressure ventilation will also decrease pulmonary blood volume. This may be counterbalanced by fluid infusion (88), or eventually by reducing venous capacitance with small doses of dopamine (92). However, increasing RV filling must be performed cautiously as excessive RV filling induces tricuspid regurgitation and a further decrease in forward cardiac output.

Last, inotropic medication such as dobutamine (217) should be used if RV ejection fraction declines rapidly or if cardiac output cannot be maintained at a sufficient level to meet metabolic needs. Obviously, low systemic arterial pressure must be avoided. No threshold value could be proposed, but a marked fall in RV stroke volume or ejection fraction concomitant to a fall in systemic arterial pressure may theoretically indicate an ischemia-induced fall in contractility and should be treated by restoring adequate coronary perfusion pressure.

When specifically treating ARDS-induced RV failure, infusion of vasoactive drugs such as dopamine or epinephrine should be carefully evaluated since the usual effect is a further increase in pulmonary hypertension and a dramatic fall in cardiac output (166, 215). Although difficult to apply to ARDS, an original approach has been proposed that uses a combination of venous vasodilator infusion to decrease pulmonary pressure and arterial vasoconstrictor via a left atrial catheter to increase right coronary artery filling pressure (49).

Chronic Obstructive Pulmonary Disease (COPD)

Although the acronym of COPD includes a group of clinical entities characterized by an increase in airway resistance, a wide range of pathophysiologic events is in-

volved, which results in marked differences in bronchial obstruction, reversibility of airflow obstruction, grade of emphysema, loss of capillaries (140), lungs volume, respiratory muscles activity, and metabolic needs (16, 224). Where there is bronchial obstruction, transpulmonary pressure increases, intrinsic PEEP occurs, functional residual capacity increases, and lungs become hyperinflated depending on the expiratory time constant and the respiratory rate. Emphysema contributes to increase expiratory time constant through an increase in lung compliance that favors air trapping and lung inflation. Conversely, the capillary loss increases pulmonary vascular resistance but, in contrast, provides protection against intrapulmonary shunt. Bronchodilatator treatment tends to improve alveolar ventilation and hypoxemia, but, in the case of nonreversible small airway obstruction, increases the ventilation/perfusion (Va/Q) mismatching through an increased volume in the nonrespiratory airway. This may decrease oxygen delivery and, consequently, diaphragmatic efficiency. This example explains that the close and nonlinear relations between hypoxemia, pulmonary hypertenson, RV performance, cardiac output, alveolar ventilation, Va/Q mismatching, oxygen delivery, tissue oxygen oxygenation, and metabolic needs may be shifted in an unpredictable manner by any additional event, such as therapeutic intervention.

In stable COPD, pulmonary hypertension is a common occurrence, but remains mild for a long period of time. It may be reversed by correction of hypoxemia (19, 223) and other contributing factors such as pulmonary inflation, hypercarbia, acidosis, increased cardiac output (226), polycythemia (4). It is also frequently associated with diseases such as LV dysfunction or pulmonary embolism. Muscularization of normally nonmuscular pulmonary arteries over a long period of time may also correct the condition (163). The usual RV response is both dilatation and hypertrophy, which may sustain a high pulmonary pressure for a long time without the development of RV failure. These structural and functional adaptations to COPD are commonly referred to as cor pulmonale. However, advanced COPD may lead to congestive heart failure with water and sodium retention, leading to peripheral edema (74). However, low cardiac output is a rare event in cor pulmonale and the sodium retention seems predominantly due to associated LV failure. This could explain why both digoxin (29) and diuretics (127) have beneficial effects only in cases of associated LV dysfunction. (The clinical use of the experimentally demonstrated positive effect of digitalis on diaphragmatic contractility (7) remains to be evaluated.) Since high cardiac output is a common finding in stable patients with COPD, a low mixed venous Po_2 carries a poor prognosis (106, 213). Thus, an important hemodynamic objective in COPD is to maintain adequate cardiac output to cover the metabolic needs of the heart, brain, and other vital organs (224). In such circumstances, RV performance may act as a limiting factor that has to be optimized.

The major determinants of pulmonary hypertension are air flow-dependent. Thus, elective treatment of RV performance in COPD fits well with the bronchodilating treatment. A decrease in pulmonary hypertension and improvement in survival are closely related to oxygen therapy (131, 146). Intermittent oxygen therapy is usually chosen when Sao_2 remains close to 0.80–0.85 at rest. Specific treatment of cor pulmonale via treatment of pulmonary hypertension has been proposed. Pulmonary vasodilators such as hydralazine (108) nifedipine (140), urapidil (3), and prostacyclin (144) have proved effective in treating pulmonary hypertension, RV performance, and cardiac output (171, 224). However, the immediate response should be carefully evaluated because there is a constant decrease in Pao_2, which may lead to hazardous hypoxemia, and the long-term results remain controversial. The promising effects of almitrine on hypoxemia, via an enhancement of hypoxic vasoconstriction, may increase oxygen delivery. However, there are substantial arguments that this is mediated by an adverse increase in pulmonary hypertension (122). Phlebotomy is recommended to decrease blood viscosity only when hemato-

crit exceeds 55%, even after smoking cessation and oxygen supplementation (35).

During acute exacerbation of COPD caused by air flow obstruction, the increased inspiratory transpulmonary pressure is paralleled by an increase in both the pulmonary volume and large abdominopleural pressure respiratory swings that are close to the pathophysiologic findings in acute asthma (Fig. 18.2) (57). The specific treatment for optimal RV performance is also similar. Even though chronic pressure load-induced ventricular modifications may improve the ability of the right heart to face an acute pulmonary hypertension, it has been argued that RV hypertrophy may increase the occurrence of RV infarction (113). In case of a decline in the contractile state requiring inotropic support, decompensated COPDs are more likely to be associated with other diseases, such as LV failure from coronary insufficiency (200), acute pulmonary embolism, or infectious pneumonitis that may require important variations in treatment. In such circumstances, concomitant diagnosis of associated diseases and precipitating factors, evaluation of the RV function and its consequences on global cardiac performance, and attention to oxygen delivery and oxygen consumption are required to sort major therapeutic priorities.

During adapted mechanical ventilation, hypoxemia often improves, large changes in pleural pressure are corrected, and oxygen requirements parallel the decreased activity of the respiratory muscles. Since forced expiration often leads to increased airway collapse (55), the pulmonary hyperinflation may improve when adequate mechanical ventilation is applied. Special attention should be given to the ventilatory mode, since excessive tidal volume and insufficient expiratory time may have adverse effects on intrinsic PEEP, pulmonary overinflation, and vascular resistance (66, 151). Pressure support may decrease intrinsic PEEP and therefore, pulmonary hyperinflation. However, the expected beneficial effect on RV performance needs to be shown.

Hence, when adequately applied, mechanical ventilation may partly correct pulmonary hypertension. Nevertheless, nor-

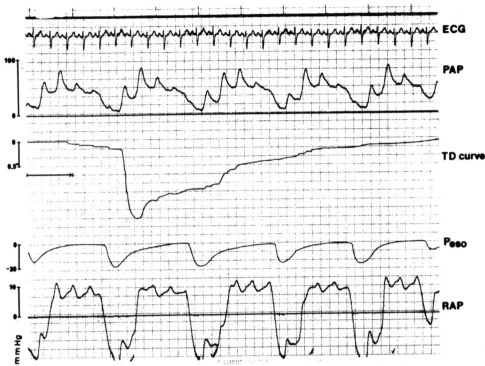

ECG

PAP

TD curve

Peso

RAP

Figure 18.2. Tracing of a simultaneous recording of ECG, pulmonary artery pressure (PAP), thermal curve (TD curve), esophageal pressure (P_{eso}), and right atrial pressure (RAP) from a patient during an acute exacerbation of chronic obstructive pulmonary disease. A cold bolus was injected over the time marked by the arrow. This patient exhibited cyclic changes of RV ejection fraction as assessed by beat-to-beat plateau analysis. Throughout the respiratory cycle: RV ejection fraction was minimal (18%) during inspiration and coincided with minimum pulmonary pulse pressure; conversely, the RV ejection fraction was maximal (36%) two beats after the onset of expiration and coincided with maximum pulmonary pulse pressure. From Dhainaut JF, Brunet F. Phasic changes of right ventricular ejection fraction in patients with acute exacerbations of COPD. Intensive Care Med 1987;12:214–215.

mal RV function could be adversely affected by two pathophysiologic effects: (1) the remaining pulmonary hypertension, hyperinflation, hypoxemia, and viscosity have to be optimally corrected, and (2) the remaining intrinsic PEEP alters the optimal adaptation of the ventilation pattern. In order to avoid inotropic support in this situation where associated coronary disease is a common occurrence, optimal RV filling is a key factor. Intrinsic PEEP may act as external PEEP on systemic venous return. Since lung compliance is normal or increased in COPD, a given level of PEEP would decrease the intrathoracic blood volume in larger amounts than required for ARDS. Accordingly, the filling of both ventricles could be underestimated if eval-

uated by the intrachamber pressure (151). In other words, filling would be better evaluated by studying the ventricle volume or by transmural pressure.

Asthma

The physiologic challenge for patients who have acute asthma is to open the constricted airway and move enough tidal air to allow for gas exchange. Obviously, in practice this is done by increased transpulmonary pressure throughout the respiratory cycle (inspiratory and expiratory) and subsequently by a chest distension mediated by a marked increase in contraction of respiratory muscles, particularly those in the diaphragm. An important effect is an inspiratory fall in pleural pressure that may reach −40 mm Hg and a concomitant increase in abdominal pressure. In contrast, during expiration the very long time constant for exhalation prevents the return to normal functional residual capacity and induces an intrinsic PEEP or hyperinflation that increases the intrathoracic pressure. Moreover, the difference of time constraints for relaxation between distended chest wall and obstructed lungs promotes a positive expiratory pleural pressure. Both pleural pressure and intrinsic PEEP may also be increased if a "panic" forced expiratory effort occurs. Thus, spontaneously breathing in the setting of acute bronchospasm is associated with marked phasic changes in both pleural and abdominal pressures.

The influence of these changes on cardiac performance is well known because clinical indicators such as paradoxic pulse or respiratory variation in jugular vein distension may be easily detected (64, 111, 162). The precise mechanism of the inspiratory decline in arterial pulse (i.e., the paradoxic pulse) has been studied for a long time by workers at the Johns Hopkins University in Baltimore. Several of the following mechanisms have been invoked: increased impedance to LV ejection (149, 169, 170, 173, 178), mechanical impairment of LV filling by ventricular interdependence (26), decreased pulmonary venous return (31, 179).

A major contribution to our understanding of these interactions has been provided by clinical studies from Jardin et al. (100, 101), using both hemodynamic and echocardiographic assessment of the cardiac performance. They showed that a pulmonary pressure variation precedes that of the LV by one beat. Both pulmonary systolic and pulse pressure were minimal at end-inspiration, maximum at early-expiration, and then slowly decreased. Various factors known to increase pulmonary vascular resistance have been experienced during asthma; these include pulmonary hyperinflation, hypoxia, hypercapnia, and acidosis. During inspiration, the RV is additionally afterloaded by the negative pleural pressure because transpulmonary pressure that surrounds intrapulmonary

vessels is high (100, 101). In contrast, RV filling should be enhanced by the negative swings in pleural pressure during inspiration. However, several limiting factors for RV filling have been clearly identified: first, it is limited by pericardial capacity; second, there is an inspiratory collapse of the vena cava (100, 101) at the thorax entrance when major inspiratory efforts are tried that corresponds to the concept of a vascular waterfall (210); and last, hypovolemia is frequently associated with acute asthma (205). Thus, the inspiratory fall in RV ejection may be caused mainly by an important afterload that is inadequately compensated by limited filling (196). In the setting of hypovolemia, inspiration promotes a decrease in the RV ejection fraction and also in the stroke volume. LV preload is consequently reduced at end-inspiration via a series phenomenon. Ventricular interdependency (100) and a possible pulmonary venous pooling (27) may further contribute to a marked decrease in LV filling. However, a decrease in the paradoxic pulse with increasing RV filling (196) has been reported; in such circumstances, a series phenomenon may predominate. The marked negative swings in intrathoracic pressure seen with spontaneous inspiratory efforts in acute asthma also markedly increase LV afterload impairing LV ejection.

During early expiration, both decreased pulmonary volume and increased pleural pressure cause an improved RV ejection and a decrease in RV volume followed by an increase in LV stroke volume and arterial pressure (100, 101). At end-expiration, progressive positive intrathoracic pressure leads to a decrease in the systemic venous return and a limit in the RV performance. Then, except for early expiration, the RV is unfavorably loaded throughout the respiratory cycle. This may be the cause of inadequate cardiac output in hypoxemia and increased metabolic needs (5, 100).

It has also been hypothesized that coronary insufficiency may occur during severe asthma (94), but this has not been substantiated in the literature. Theoretically, RV coronary perfusion may be phasically inadequate with increased oxygen demand because of pressure overload. In pleural pressure, inspiratory RV intra-chamber systolic pressure increases while systemic arterial pressure decreases because of the decreased stroke volume (101); hence, the systolic component of the coronary perfusion may decrease during inspiration.

Accordingly, therapeutic modalities that have been tested have been done in accordance with this physiologic model (94, 203). When such a person breathes spontaneously, the hemodynamic support should maintain RV filling. This is obtained by fluid infusion or transient MAST inflation (196). The risk for pulmonary edema in this situation seems low and has been rarely reported (197). The marked negative pleural pressure may produce a strong pressure gradient between the capillary bed and the LV, promoting venous return rather than interstitial extravasation. Further hemodynamic improvement could be made by lowering both transpulmonary pressure and phasic changes in both abdominal and pleural pressures. This is likely to occur when bronchospasm is resolved and when patients are ventilated using CPAP to levels equal to intrinsic PEEP.

When patients are mechanically ventilated, sudden phasic pressure changes disappear. There remain, however, problems of both pulmonary hyperinflation and auto PEEP, effects that are comparable in COPD patients.

Pulmonary Embolism

Pulmonary embolism reduces the cross-sectional area of the pulmonary vascular bed. If severe enough, this reduction in vascular area results in an increment in pulmonary vascular resistance and pressure. If there is no existing cardiopulmonary disease, there is a close relationship between mild to moderate pulmonary vascular obstruction and pulmonary artery pressure (12). However, the normal reserve capacity of the pulmonary vascular bed is high, and a rather large obstruction may be tolerated with mild increase in pulmonary pressure. In these instances, pulmonary pressure rarely exceeds 40 mm Hg in the absence of prior cardiopulmo-

nary diseases; such a pulmonary pressure is related to a 50% vascular obstruction (121). Typically, cardiac index is normal to elevated in hypoxemia. As the obstruction exceeds 50%, the RV afterload increases sharply (48). In massive embolism, pulmonary pressure can no longer be considered representative of the pulmonary obstruction because cardiac output consequently falls and pulmonary pressure may be paradoxically normalized (141). Fitzpatrick and Grant (76) have shown, in a canine model of pulmonary embolism, that the forward hydrolic power of the RV ejection may lose two-thirds of its energy because of pulmonary wave reflection. This is probably generated by the waves impinging on fragments of clots lying in the vascular arterial tree. If this may be extrapolated to human settings, the distinctive effect of pulmonary embolism in afterloading the RV may have specific therapeutic implications.

Pulmonary embolism, then, is a RV pressure overload situation. Regardless of associated cardiopulmonary diseases, the hemodynamic compromise depends on two additional factors, filling status and contractile state. In the absence of associated bronchial disease, the usual respiratory response to acute embolism is an increase in ventilation through polypnea. Thus, contrary to obstructive pulmonary diseases, no intrathoracic pressure swings phasically impede the RV and the systemic venous return.

Massive embolism is one situation in which the optimal filling status may be difficult to determine because of the over-distended state of the RV. A fluid bolus may induce hemodynamic collapse (82, 139), tricuspid regurgitation, and the opening of a patent foramen ovale (51). RV overload-induced coronary insufficiency is also strongly suspected, even though it is not totally clinically demonstrated when systemic hypotension occurs (53, 141).

Hemodynamic management may be schematized as follows:

1. Clot removal obviously improves RV afterload. In extreme situations external cardiac massage may help to fragment clots, as well as thrombolysis, transvenous catheter

embolectomy, or embolectomy under extracorporeal circulation (53).

2. Fluid resuscitation permits optimal filling. This should be controlled by assessing RV volume or monitoring central venous pressure, prohibiting any additional filling to prevent a large increase in central venous pressure.

3. Inotropic medications, even though only supported by anecdotal clinical studies, may be of theoretical interest through various mechanisms. Isoproterenol, a bronchodilatator and vasodilatator inotropic drug, has been successfully tested in pulmonary embolism with no systemic hypotension and may help to close a patent foramen ovale and to restore sufficient systemic oxygen delivery (139). Dobutamine may increase cardiac output and maintain blood pressure. Inotropic drugs with vasopressor effects should be considered in cases of systemic hypotension in order to break a "vicious circle" initialized through an overload-induced coronary insufficiency. The proposed mechanism of vasopressor-induced improvement in RV functions includes an increase in both cardiac output and peripheral vascular resistance allowing restoration of a systolodiastolic pressure gradient for right myocardial tissue perfusion. Additionally, a stiffening of proximal pulmonary arteries occurs. In the case of pulmonary embolism, this may have a decreasing afterload effect because a lack of increased vascular tone (67) and an increase in pulmonary characteristic impedance may strongly reduce wave reflection (76).

4. Vasodilatators are usually not recommended in cases of massive embolism because a reduction in systemic vascular resistance is not paralleled by an equivalent increase in cardiac output; hence, blood pressure falls. The administration of ketanserin had promising experimental effects, but has inconstant results in humans, exposing them to hypotension (95). Vasodilatators may have more interesting results in cases of cor pulmonale following obliterative pulmonary hypertension (50).

Septic Shock

In cases of sepsis, there is an unquestionable dilemma of a marked increase in metabolic demand, a decrease in maximum tissue oxygen extraction, and, hence, the need for a high cardiac output. The RV challenge in sepsis is to deliver to the LV the high flow that allows for high cardiac output. Unfortunately, several factors act to limit meeting these objectives. Their cumulative effects may precipitate into hypoxia and septic shock in the septic patient.

Severe sepsis is accompanied by various grades of intrapulmonary vessel congestion and the invasion and margination of leucocytes and microthrombi. The usual consequence is diffuse alveolar collapse, interstitial edema, and consequently a reduction in ventilation/perfusion ratio and hypoxemia that further increases the load of the RV and the corresponding need for high cardiac output to maintain oxygen delivery (39). Although moderate in its early stage, a systolic pulmonary hypertension up to 45 mm Hg has been found in septic patients without chest X-ray evidence of pulmonary edema and without sufficient hypoxemia to be included in an ARDS group (38). Such a pulmonary hypertension is commonly associated with low cardiac output and poor prognosis (62, 188).

Another well-established hemodynamic consequence of severe sepsis is peripheral vasodilatation. This will decrease the LV ejection pressure and may increase cardiac output (148). Conversely, in the venous site, the vasodilatation provokes a marked increase in venous capacity that tends to decrease the back pressure for venous return. Generalized capillary leak additionally decreases the venous return. It has also been hypothesized that an impairment in RV compliance and/or relaxation occurs in sepsis since diastolic pressure volume curves are displaced leftward (62, 109). All these mechanisms act to greatly decrease the needed RV preload to face the increased afterload.

Lastly an impairment in the RV contractile state is recognized in the early stages of sepsis (Fig. 18.3) because a decrease in the mean pulmonary pressure/ejection fraction relationship and a rightward shift in the systolic pressure volume relationship has been shown in both experimental and clinical studies (62, 109, 148, 181). The precise mechanism is not fully known but myocardial depressing factors have been isolated and seem to play a major role (57).

	SV	HR	LVEF	LVEDV	RVEF	RVEDV
Control pts (n = 10)	50	70	0,60	83	0,52	96
SS (all) (n = 20)	42*	115*	0,48*	87	0,39*	108*
Survivors (n = 9)	40	110	0,45	89	0,36	111
Non-surv. (n = 11)	44	122	0,50	87	0,42	105

Figure 18.3. Comparison between the LV and RV performance parameters in 20 patients with septic shock (SS) and 10 control patients. SV = stroke volume (ml/m²), HR = heart rate, EF = ejection fraction, EDV = end-diastolic volume (ml/m₂), * = p<0.01 patients with septic shock versus control group. Reproduced with permission from J. F. Dhainaut (unpublished data).

No proof of coronary hypoperfusion has been given (61), but, as in other causes of RV failure, systemic hypotension may result in a decline in myocardial tissue perfusion (2) and myocardial oxygen extraction may also be impaired through sepsis-induced myocardial edema (155). The LV myocardial contractile depression (148) may also cause a decrease in ventricular coupling, thus decreasing the mechanical effect of the RV ejection. Then, if one considers that few guidelines for treatment may be given for decreased RV afterload, they should emphasize the role of optimal preload and inotropic drugs. Optimal preload may be difficult to attain because capillary leak may divert volume infusion from the expected intravascular bed. In addition, risk of acute respiratory failure makes volume expansion hazardous. Hence, when fluid resuscitation has been sufficiently tested with regards to Pao₂, cardiac output, oxygen delivery and consumption, inotropic drugs should be used. Inotropic drugs with strong vasoconstricting effects have been widely used in such circumstances, but they should be used only when uncontrolled systemic hypotension occurs despite conventional treatment (182).

RV Infarction

RV infarction was considerably underestimated until the first report on its specific hemodynamic profiles was published by Cohn et al. (40). Right atrial and end-diastolic ventricular pressures were found

to be elevated both in absolute levels and relative to LV pressures. Since this report, numerous studies have investigated RV infarction secondary to coronary artery occlusion. RV infarction with normal coronary arteries is a rare event (113).

Obviously, there is a decrease in the RV contractile state in the early phase of the infarction. However, many observations emphasized the role of superimposed factors as there was no correlation between the infarction size and the hemodynamic consequences. First, there has been report of stunned myocardium adjacent to the infarction that seems to be due to coronary insufficiency (23). Second, except in rare cases (168), RV infarction is associated with extensive LV infarction, involving the septum and the posteroinferior left ventricular wall. Although not proven, this may greatly decrease the mechanical effect of ventricular coupling as well as stiffness of the infarcted RV. In addition, LV dysfunction may increase pulmonary vascular resistance and impede RV ejection.

The normal RV response to acute infarction is a ventricular dilatation. There are strong arguments that the ventricular diastolic function is also adversely affected because a severe noncompliant pattern has been shown to be a sensitive hemodynamic feature of RV infarction, including diastolic pressure equalization and "dip-plateau" configuration consistent with diastolic stiffening (159). The major reason for these findings seems to be that the marked RV dilatation extends heart volume to maximum pericardial capacity (84). Accordingly, hemodynamic features of tamponade, including paradoxic pulse and Kussmaul sign, have been reported as frequent evidences in RV infarction (119). An additional argument is the experimental improvement of this hemodynamic profile when the pericardium is open (84, 211). The beneficial Starling effect accompanying RV dilatation is also frequently adversely affected by additional complications observed in this setting, such as tricuspid regurgitation that limits cardiac output, and heart block that causes a loss in the atrial systole; even RV pacing restores the normal heart rate. This is also observed in cases of tachyarrhythmia (97).

Consequently, the systolic performance of the RV may dramatically fall (84).

In clinical practice, extensive RV infarction is usually followed by a severe RV failure, including a low cardiac output, a pronounced rise in systemic venous pressure, and a systemic hypotension. The possible role of the atrial natriuretic factor in the occurrence of this syndrome has been hypothesized, although not yet proven, by Robalino et al. (167). However, cardiogenic shock due to RV infarction seems a better prognosis than when due to elective LV infarction (124, 186).

Apart from coronary recanalization following thromobolysis (21) and/or transluminal angioplasty, guidelines for treatment may be listed as follows:

1. Optimalization of the LV function that decreases right ventricular afterload, decreases ventricular interdependence, and restores ventricular coupling. This may lead to use of vasodilators if needed and if allowed by a normal systemic arterial pressure. Selective arterial·vasodilators should be prescribed rather than mixed vasodilators because impairment of the venous return to the RV may have strong deleterious effects. Inotropic medications or, eventually, intraaortic counterpulsation may also be considered as potent interventions to improve LV function.

2. Optimalization of blood volume status. When faced with a compromised hemodynamic status, as when clinical signs of tamponade or tricuspid regurgitation are present, clinical studies confirm that increased preload is unlikely to be able to compensate the decreased contractile state (54, 60, 186). In contrast, in other circumstances, fluid therapy has been efficiently used alone to restore low cardiac output (40, 118). Finally, inotropic medications that have moderate effects in increasing myocardial oxygen demand, such as dobutamine, may have an amplifying effect because an increase in both ventricular contractile forces (54, 60) may have additional positive mechanical consequences such as decreased ventricular interdependence and increased ventricular coupling that may interrupt a vicious cycle of increased myocardial O_2 demand decreased coronary blood flow. Tricuspid regurgitation seems more difficult to treat since a mechanical dysfunction due to ischemia may occur in addition to annulus dilatation. Accordingly, inotropic medications have little

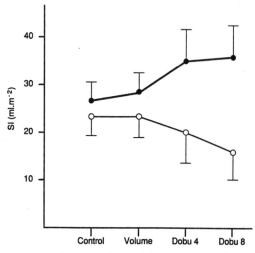

Figure 18.4. Variations of stroke index (SI) in response to therapy in the group with (*open circle*) and without (*solid circle*) tricuspid regurgitation in patients with RV infarction associated with low cardiac output syndrome. Intergroup differences and variations are all statistically significant ($p < 0.001$). (From Dhainaut JF, Ghannad E, Brunet F, Villemant D, Devaux JY, Shremmer B, Squara P, Weber S, Monsallier JF. The role of tricuspid regurgitation and left ventricular damage in the treatment of right ventricular infarction-induced cardiogenic shock. Am J Cardiol 1989;66:289–295.

effect on the forward stroke volume (Fig. 18.4) (60). In anecdotal cases, tricuspid valve replacement has been proposed for prolonged and severe tricuspid regurgitation (114) and a pulmonary artery counterpulsation for a severe postoperative RV infarction (136).

Cardiac Surgery

In contrast to early observation (199), it is recognized that a right ventricular dysfunction is a common feature after cardiac surgery although there is both increased afterload and decreased contractility (36, 160). Increased right ventrical afterload has been shown after extracorporeal circulation due to various mechanisms including microthrombi, complement and platelet activation, thromboxane release, hemolysis, endogenous catecholamine release, and eventually, pulmonary edema and hypoxia caused by volume overload or LV dysfunction.

It is known that the RV contractile state

is impaired within 24 hours postoperatively. Indeed, the RV is particularly sensitive to cardioplegia (85); a low amount of high-energy storage may play a role (37). Otherwise, rewarming of the RV is done more rapidly than the LV due to the warm systemic venous return to the right atrium, the noncoronary collateral blood flow, and the anterior position exposed to the operating room air and lights. Finally, right ventricular preload may be adversely affected by postoperative pericardial suffusion or frequent tachyarrhythmia or sinus blockage that removes the atrial systole and consequently decreases RV filling.

The cumulative effect of this three-step elementary phenomenon induces a usual decrease in the RV ejection fraction. However, the stroke volume is preserved and RV failure rarely occurs in the absence of other associated problems. Another common postoperative observation is a paradoxic systolic septal motion, although reasons for this are not convincingly demonstrated. The roles of RV afterloading, insufficient septal cardioplegia, and distortion of ventricle architecture through conduit placement have been described.

In addition to preventive therapy based on careful cardioplegia and rewarming, therapeutic objectives are simple: lowering right ventricular afterload by adequate mechanical ventilation and LV filling, optimizing RV filling with special attention to pleural space drainage, and using inotropic medications with low myocardial oxygen demand, such as dobutamine or phosphodiesterase inhibitors. In cases of elevated pulmonary vascular resistance without systemic hypotension, the associated inotropic and vasodilatator effects of isoproterenol may be used.

EVALUATION OF RV FUNCTION: LIMITATIONS AND PERSPECTIVES

Evaluating and monitoring RV performance is often necessary in ventilatory support and for intensive care. This proves the need for methods that are not only easy to use at the bedside, but are sensitive and reproducible both to diagnose and predict response to therapy. Nevertheless, more than the absolutely accurate measurement of the RV performance, the time-course evolution and the response to various events in daily practice are the major determinants of treatment.

What are useful variables in assessing RV performance? These were extensively debated in the last chapter. RV performance is determined by the heart rate, the loading conditions, and the contractile state. The RV preload has to be assessed by both RV end-diastolic volume and pressure (25). On the passive RV pressure-volume curve, the optimal RV filling is near the ascending limb of the pressure-volume relationship and one may take into consideration the time-course variation of both filling pressure or volume and stroke volume to appreciate in a continuous real-time evaluation the relative RV preload magnitude. RV afterload may be evaluated according to pulmonary artery pressure or pulmonary vascular resistance (128). RV contractility assessment is clinically difficult because of the marked influence of RV afterload in ejection phase indices. This illustrates the need to construct RV active pressure-volume relations as they seem minimally affected by the RV loading conditions (130). However, constructing these lines is time-consuming and needs almost 3 or 4 points that should be realized by a preload challenge (58, 164).

Hence, an accurate assessment of RV performance requires measurements of both RV volumes and transmural pressures to construct pressure-volume loops. Once these loops have been evaluated, one may validly investigate the real-time evolution of the RV performance by concomitant analysis of the following variables: heart rate, right atrial transmural pressure, stroke volume, mean pulmonary pressure, and RV ejection fraction. Several other variables may be added: analysis of the V_{3R}, V_{4R} ECG ST segments, and arterial and venous oxygen saturations, as RV takes its place in the circulatory system and should be analyzed in terms of two ratios, myocardial oxygen demand:supply and peripheral tissue oxygen demand:supply.

Contrast Angiography

Contrast ventriculography was the first method used to investigate RV function (77). Mathematical approximations are required to calculate volumes from the measured radiocontrast area. Several geometrical models have been proposed, all of which have in common their doubtful accuracy. This is mainly due to the difficulties to model the shape of the RV because of heavy trabeculations, right atrial overlap, and the complex geometry of the RV.

In addition, even digitalized, this method does not meet the previously defined requirements for monitoring. First, this is an invasive method that potentially carries the risk of cardiac catheterization. Also, radiographic contrast products have many cumulative side effects, such as excessive volume infusion and renal failure. Finally, cumulative x-ray exposure and the high cost should be considered. Accordingly, contrast ventriculography is no longer recommended for RV function monitoring, but only in diagnostic assessments of such conditions as pulmonary embolism or valvular disease.

Radionuclide Angiography

Radionuclide angiography using autologous erythrocytes labeled with technetium-99m pyrophosphate is the oldest method used to assess ventricular volumes and function in intensive care and has been extensively validated in a wide spectrum of RV conditions (123, 153). To date, this has been the reference method. Two distinct techniques have been proposed.

As in conventional angiography, in a "first-pass" study, sequential images are acquired as a marker bolus mixes in the central circulation and transits through the heart. Because the marker is radioactive, the changes in externally detected radioactive counts are proportional to changes in chamber volume, and the stroke count may be calculated by a computerized difference in activity between end-systole and end-diastole. This method has two advantages. (1) There is no assumption concerning the RV shape or pattern of contraction needed. (2) Underestimation due to overlaps between right atrium and RV can be minimized since the right atrial has peak activity prior to the RV activity. Nevertheless, the first-pass method is only based on three to four cardiac cycles and the low

count rates of the raw data may be a cause of error, especially when heart beat is irregular. This can be circumvented when the radioactive bolus is injected directly into the right atrium to assure a rapid and complete mixing with the blood stream. Since first-pass imaging requires a relatively large amount of radioactivity, serial measurements are often not possible except when very short half-time isotopes are used such as ^{191m}iridium or ^{81m}krypton. However, these isotopes are rarely available (145).

In the equilibrium-gated technique, the radioactive count is analyzed after the entire equilibrium of blood pool and intravascular blood labeling. With this technique, sequential images are acquired and gated to the R wave of the ECG. A major problem is the overlap between the right atrium and RV activity, which may cause systematic errors. A left anterior oblique position of the camera and accurate separation of both systolic and diastolic right atrium and RV areas are required to obtain reproducible results (123). Another disadvantage of the gated technique is the long duration. Each determination requires 2 to 8 minutes of imaging time and the patient must be in a steady state during this period. However, sequential measurements for up to 4 to 6 hours are possible after a single injection.

In conclusion, even as a reference method, radionuclide techniques are expensive, not easy to perform, and require bulky systems and a specialized personnel that are not always available at any moment. Except in special units, it is unlikely that these techniques could meet the requirements for daily monitoring of the RV performance.

Echocardiography

Because echocardiographic two-dimensional imaging allows measurement of area, but only to evaluate volume from the measured area and several mathematical models, echocardiography is not considered a reference method to establish pressure-volume loops. However, from several sequential plane examinations, both ventricle area and fractional area contraction measurements have been shown as acceptable assessments of, respectively, RV volume and ejection fraction in a wide range of clinical settings (101, 102, 105, 198, 221). Echocardiography has the considerable advantage of being easy to use at bedside, totally harmless (except for the transesophageal method), reproducible and inexpensive. Conclusions drawn by clinical studies using this method for RV function evaluation are widely accepted. In addition, numerous important data for critically ill patient diagnoses and monitoring may be provided from dynamic imaging, such as distinctive patterns of pressure and volume overload (26), myocardial wall thickness, valvular morphologies, diastolic function, and pericardial space investigation. The effect of many events such as mechanical ventilation, fluid infusion, or drug infusion could be instantaneously evaluated. When coupled with Doppler examination, pulmonary artery systolic pressure (228) may be calculated. However, since the method is based on the Bernoulli equation ($DP = 4 \times V^2$), there needs to be a tricuspid regurgitation and a right atrial pressure empirical evaluation (14, 90). Fortunately, tricuspid regurgitation is trivial and enhancement of the signal could be obtained by various methods of contrast injection (13). Evaluation of cardiac output has been studied (132) even though the reliability of the method is debatable for critically ill patients. Better evaluation of tricuspid regurgitation than contrast echocardiography alone (47) and better evaluation of diastolic function (78) have been also reported using Doppler-combined echocardiography.

Finally, echocardiographic evaluation of the RV at the bedside is becoming essential in most intensive care units. The method has been shown to be reproducible and sufficiently efficient. However, such efficiency requires a high level of training. In critically ill patients, correct imaging could be very difficult to obtain especially in patients with acute respiratory failure, in postoperative cases, and/or mechanically ventilated patients. In such instances, the subcostal short axis view may be the only possible assessment (100). Because this is a serious impediment to widespread rou-

tine use, important progress should be made in areas of material ease of use and personnel practice to peak interest in the use of echocardiography for RV performance monitoring. Transesophageal imaging has gained new responses to this concern, since higher quality imaging is expected. However, this method becomes invasive and has potent side effects.

Right Heart Catheterization

Right heart catheterization to determine RV function has been widely used for 20 years (208). Difficulty in interpretation of the usual hemodynamic variables as indicators of the RV function has been emphasized above. However, two new alternatives have shown successful results in RV function monitoring: RV ejection fraction as assessed by thermodilution technique, and continuous Svo_2 monitoring that may be combined with continuous monitoring of SaO_2 noninvasively. Obviously, these methods carry the usual risks of right heart catheterization (129).

The calculation of the RV ejection fraction by thermodilution is based on the conservation of energy as measured using a fast-response thermistor. Ventricular volumes are then derived using the stroke volume as usually assessed by dividing cardiac output by heart rate:

$$\underset{1}{(C \times T_1 \times ESV)} + \underset{2}{(C \times T_b \times SV)} = \underset{3}{(C \times T_2 \times EDV)}$$

1 represents the blood heat at the end of a given systole (C is a constant related to blood gravity and heat capacity, T_1 is the blood temperature). 2 represents the blood heat that enters the RV during the following diastole (C is the same constant, T_b is the baseline blood temperature). 3 represents the blood heat when 1 and 2 are mixed at the end of the diastole (C is the blood constant, T_2 is the blood temperature). Rearranging the equation results in:

$$ESV/EDV = (T_b - T_1)/(T_b - T_2)$$

and as $EF = 1 - ESV/EDV$,

$$EF = 1 - (T_b - T_1)/(T_b - T_2)$$

The RV volume calculations, as the ejection fraction calculation, have been shown to be reliable in a wide range of clinical situations (58, 107, 218). However, several limitations have appeared. When an irregular heart rate occurs, such as in the case of atrial fibrillation, at least five cold bolus injections should be averaged to calculate reliable mean RV ejection fraction values. Similarly, when large intrathoracic pressure swings occur, mean values between extreme values should be averaged. More difficult are the problems of tricuspid regurgitation (Fig. 18.5) and intracardiac shunts since the backward stroke output must be deducted from the global stroke volume to assess the forward stroke volume. Theoretic answers to this problem that strive to place another thermistor to measure regurgitant flow remain to be validated.

Direct continuous measurement of marked venous blood saturation is not specifically an aspect of RV monitoring. However, since the RV interacts with the global circulation, and since variations of both Sao_2 and Svo_2 parallel cardiac output variations (214), oxygen-related variables can no longer be ignored as powerful indicators of acute RV dysfunction in real-time continuous monitoring. No definite conclusion can be drawn from a given Sao_2 or Svo_2 variation; however, decreases in either represent urgent signs that demand further investigations.

Despite sometimes less than accurate measurements and less than complete results when compared to other methods such as echocardiography (99), right heart catheterization has the advantage of a continuous monitoring. Such real-time monitoring may lead in the future to continuous real-time diagnosis of cardiovascular instability (195).

CONCLUSION

Right ventricular function is complex and needs to be investigated in light of pulmonary mechanics and oxygen-related variables. Most critically ill patients have various grades of RV dysfunction that may eventuate in tissue hypoxia. No standard can be proposed to evaluate RV function. Depending on the particular patient status and associated diseases, either echocardiographic study or right heart catherization should be indicated. The former has superior diagnostic qualities, the latter is especially dedicated to monitoring. Careful investigation of pathophysiology will facilitate the therapeutic approach that has the same objectives it has had for half a century: decreasing afterload, optimizing preload, and increasing contractility sufficiently.

References

1. Abraham E, Yoshihara G. Cardiorespiratory effects of pressure controlled inverse ratio ventilation in severe respiratory failure. Chest 1989;96:1356–1359.
2. Adiseshiah M, Baird RJ. Correlation of the changes in diastolic myocardial tissue pressure and regional coronary blood flow in hemorrhagic and endotoxinic shock. J Surg Res 1978;24:20–25.
3. Adnot S, Andrivet P, Piquet J, et al. The effect of Urapidil therapy on hemodynamics and gas exchange in exercising patients with chronic obstructive pulmonary disease and pulmonary hypertension. Am Rev Respir Dis 1988;137:1068–1074.
4. Agarwal JB, Paltoo R, Palmer WH. Relative viscosity of blood at varying hematocrits in pulmonary circulation. J Appl Physiol 1970;29:866–871.

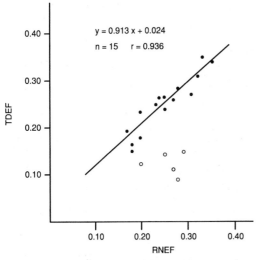

$$y = 0.913 x + 0.024$$
$$n = 15 \quad r = 0.936$$

Figure 18.5. Relationship between RV ejection fraction (EF) assessed by thermodilution technique (TD) and by radionuclide technique (RN). The relation was good in patients without tricuspid regurgitation *(solid circle)*, in contrast to the others with regurgitation *(open circle)*. Reproduced with permission from J. F. Dhainaut (unpublished data).

5. Appel D, Rubenstein Rm Schrager K, Williams MH. Lactic acidosis in severe asthma. Am J Med 1983;75:580–584.

6. Armour JA, Pace JB, Randall WC. Interrelationship between architecture and function of the right ventricle. Am J Physiol 1970;218:174–180.

7. Aubier M, Murciano D, Viires N, et al. Effects of digoxin on diaphragmatic strength generation in patients with chronic obstructive pulmonary disease during acute respiratory failure. Am Rev Resp Dis 1987;135:544–548.

8. Badke FR. Left ventricular dimensions and function during exercise in dogs with chronic right ventricular pressure overload. Am J Cardiol 1984;53:1187–1193.

9. Bakos AC. The question of the function of the right ventricle following extensive damage by cauterization. Circulation 1950;1:724–731.

10. Bates ER, Shenker Y, Grekin RJ. The relationship between plasma levels of immunoreactive atrial natriuretic hormone and hemodynamic function in man. 1986;73:1155–1161.

11. Bemis CE, Serur JR, Borkenhagen D, et al. Influence of right ventricle filling pressure on left ventricle pressure and dimension. Circ Res 1974;34:498–504.

12. Benumof JL. Hypoxic pulmonary vasoconstriction and infusion of sodium nitroprusside. Anesthesiology 1979;50:481–483.

13. Beppu S, Tanabe K, Shilmizu T, et al. Contrast enhancement of doppler signal by sonicated albumin for estimating right ventricle systolic pressure. Am J Cardiol 1991;67:1148–1149.

14. Berger M, Haimovitz A, Van Tosh A, et al. Quantitative assessment of pulmonary hypertension in patients with tricuspid regurgitation using continuous wave doppler ultrasound. 1985;6:359–365.

15. Berger M, Hecht SR, Van Tosh A, Lingam U. Pulsed and continuous wave doppler echocardiography assessment of valvular regurgitation in normal subjects. J Am Coll Cardiol 1989;13:1540–1545.

16. Bergofsky EH. Tissue oxygen delivery and cor pulmonale in chronic obstructive pulmonary disease. N Engl J Med 1983;308:1092–1094.

17. Berne RM. The role of adenosine in the regulation of the coronary blood flow. Circ Res 1980;47:807–816.

18. Biondi JW, Schulman DS, Souffer R, et al. The effect of incremental positive end expiratory pressure on right ventricle hemodynamics and ejection fraction. Anest Analg 1988;84:144–151.

19. Bishop JM, Cross KW. Use of other physiological variables to predict pulmonary arterial pressure in patients with various categories of chronic obstructive pulmonary disease: Multi center study. Eur Heart J 1981;2:509–517.

20. Bloom WL, Ferris EB. Elastic recoil of the heart as a factor of diastolic filling. Trans Assoc Am Physicians 1956;69:200–206.

21. Braat SH, Ramentol M, Halders S, et al. Reperfusion with streptokinase of an occluded right coronary artery: effects on early and late right and left ventricular ejection fraction. Am Heart J 1987;113:257–260.

22. Braunwald E, Binion JT, Morgan WL, et al. Alteration in central blood volume and cardiac output induced by positive pressure breathing and counteracted by metaraminol (Aramine). Circ Res 1957; 5:670–675.

23. Braunwald E, Kloner RA. The stunned myocardium-prolonged postischemic ventricular dysfunction. Circulation 1982;66:1146–1149.

24. Brecher GA. Critical review of recent work on ventricular diastolic suction. Circ Res 1958;6:554–565.

25. Brent BN, Berger HL, Matthay RA, et al. Physiologic correlates of right ventricular ejection fraction in chronic obstructive pulmonary disease. A combined radionuclide and hemodynamic study. Am J Cardiol 1982;50:255–262.

26. Brinker JA, Weiss JL, Lappe DL, Rabson JL, Summer WR, Permutt S, Weisfeld M. Leftward septal displacement during right ventricular loading in man. Circulation 1980;61:626–632.

27. Brower R, Wise RA, Hassapoyannes C, Bromberger-Barnea B, Permutt S. Effect of lung inflation on lung blood volume and pulmonary venous flow. J Appl Physiol 1985;58:954–963.

28. Brown KA, Ditchey RV. Human RV end-systolic pressure-volume relation defined by maximal elastance. Circulation 1988;78:81–91.

29. Brown SE, Pakron FJ, Milne N, et al. Effects of digoxin on exercise capacity and right ventricular function during exercise in chronic airflow obstruction. Chest 1984;85:187–191.

30. Brunet F, Dhainault JF, Devaux JY, Huyghebaert MF, Villemant D, Monsallier J. Right ventricular performance in patients with acute respiratory failure. Intensive Care Med 1988;14:474–477.

31. Buda AJ, Pinsky MR, Ingels NB, Daughters GT, Stinson EB, Alderman EL. Effects of intrathoracic pressure on left ventricular performance. N Engl J Med 1979;301:453–459.

32. Calvin JE, Baer RW, Glantz SA. Pulmonary injury depressed cardiac systolic function through the Starling mechanism. Am J Physiol 1986;251:H722–H733.

33. Calvin JE, Langlois S, Garneys G. Ventricular interaction in a canine model of acute pulmonary hypertension and its modulation by vasoactive drugs. J Crit Care 1988;3:43–55.

34. Calvin JE, Quinn B. Right ventricular pressure overload during acute lung injury: cardiac mechanics and the pathophysiology of right systolic dysfunction. J Crit Care 1989;4:251–265.

35. Chetty KG, Brown SE, Light RW. Improved exercise tolerance in the polycythemic lung patient following phlebotomy. Am J Med 1983;74:415–420.

36. Christakis GT, Fremes SE, Weisel RD, et al. Right ventricle dysfunction following cold potassioum cardioplegia. J Thorac Cardiovasc Surg 1985; 90:243–250.

37. Christakis GT, Weisel RD, Mickel DAG, Ivanov J, Tumiati LC, Zuech PE, Madonik MM, Liu P. Right ventricle function and metabolism. Circulation 1990;82:IV332–IV340.

38. Clowes GH, Farrington GH, Zuschneid W, et al. Circulating factors in the etiology of pulmonary insufficiency and right heart failure accompanying severe sepsis. Ann Surg 1970;171:663–679.

39. Clowes GH, Zuschnied W, Turner M, et al. Observation on the pathogenesis of pneumonitis associated with severe infection in other part of the body. Ann Surg 1968;167:630–640.

40. Cohn JN, Gwha NH, Broder MI, Limas CJ. Right ventricle infarction. Clinical and hemodynamic features. Am J Cardiol 1974;33:209–214.

41. Cooper G, Puga FJ, Zujko KJ, Harrison CE, Coleman HN. Normal myocardial function and energetics in volume-overload hypertrophy in the cat. Circ Res 1973;32:140–148.

42. Cooper G, Satava RM, Harrisson CE, Coleman HN. Mechanism for abnormal energetics of pressure-induced hypertrophy of cat myocardium. Circ Res 1973;33:213–223.

43. Cooper G, Tomanek RJ, Ehrhardt JC, Marcus ML. Chronic progressive pressure overload of the cat right ventricle. Circ Res 1981;48:488–497.

44. Cournand A, Motley HL, Werko L, et al. Physiological studies of the effects of intermittent positive breathing on cardiac output in man. Am J Physiol 1948;152:162–174.

45. Crapo JD, Barry BE, Foscue HA, et al. Structural and biochemical changes in rat lungs occurring during exposure of lethal and adaptative dose of oxygen. Am Rev Respir Dis 1980;122:123–130.

46. Cross CE. Right ventricular pressure and the coronary blood flow. Am J Physiol 1962.

47. Curtius JM, Thyssen M, Breuer HW, et al. Doppler versus contrast echocardiography for diagnosis of tricuspid regurgitation. Am J Cardiol 1985;56:333–336.

48. Dalen JE, Haynes FW, Hopper FG, et al. Cardiovascular responses to experimental pulmonary embolism. Am J Cardiol 1967;20:3–9.

49. D'Ambra MN, La Raia PJ, Philbin DM, et al. A new therapy for refractory right heart failure and pulmonary hypertension after mitral valve replacement. J Thorac Cardiovasc Surg 1985;89:567–577.

50. Dantzker DR, Bower JS. Partial reversibility of chronic pulmonary hypertension caused by pulmonary thromboembolism disease. Am Rev Respir Dis 1981;124:129–131.

51. Dantzker DR, Bower JS. Alteration in gas exchange following pulmonary thrombo embolism. Chest 1982;81:495–501.

52. De Bold AJ, Borenstein HB, Veress AT, Sonnenberg HA. A rapid and potent natriuretic response to intravenous injection of atrial myocardial extract in rats. Life Sci 1981;29:89–94.

53. Dehring DJ, Arens JF. Pulmonary thromboembolism: disease recognition and patient management. Anesthesiology 1990;73:146–164.

54. Dell'Italia LJ, Starling MR, Blumhardt R, et al. Comparative effects of volume loading, dobutamine, and nitroprusside in patients with predominant right ventricular infarction. Circulation 1985;72:1327–1335.

55. Derenne JP, Fleury B, Pariente R. Acute respiratory failure of chronic obstructive pulmonary disease. Am Rev Respir Dis 1988;1006–1033.

56. Dhainaut JF, Aouate P, Monsallier JF, et al. Improvement of right ventricle performance by continuous positive airway pressure in ARDS. J Crit Care 1987;15:15–21.

57. Dhainaut JF, Brunet F. Phasic changes of right ventricular ejection fraction in patients with acute exacerbations of COPD. Intensive Care Med 1987;12:214–215.

58. Dhainaut JF, Brunet F, Monsallier J, et al. Beside evaluation of RV performance using a rapid computerized thermodilution method. Crit Care Med 1987;15:148–154.

59. Dhainaut JF, Flandre P, Squara P. Hemodynamic profile during SDRA description and prognostic value. European collaborative ARDS study [Abstract]. Am Review Resp Dis 1989;139:A268.

60. Dhainaut JF, Ghannad E, Brunet F, Villemant D, Devaux JY, Shremmer B, Squara P, Weber S, Monsallier JF. The role of tricuspid regurgitation and left ventricular damage in the treatment of right ventricular infarction-induced cardiogenic shock. Am J Cardiol 1989;66:289–295.

61. Dhainaut JF, Huyghebaert MF, Monsallier JM, Lefevre G, Dall'ava-Santucci J, Brunet F, Villemant D, Carli A, Raichvarg D. Coronary hemodynamics and myocardial metabolism of lactate, free fatty acids, glucose and ketones in human septic shock. Circulation 1987;75:533–541.

62. Dhainaut JF, Lanore JJ, De Gournay JM, et al. Right ventricular dysfunction in patients with septic shock. Circ Shock 1987;21:335–336.

63. Dhainaut JF, Schlemmer B, Monsallier JF, Fourestié V, Carli A. Behavior of the right ventricle following PEEP in patients with mild and severe ARDS. Am Rev Respir Dis 1984;129:A99.

64. Dornhorst AC, Howard P, Leathart GL. Pulsus paradoxus. Lancet 1952;1:746–748.

65. Doty D, Wright C, Eastham C, Marcus M. Coronary reserve in atrial septal defect. Circulation 1980;62(suppl 3):III–115.

66. Dreyfuss D, Soler P, Basset G, Saumon G. High inflation pressure pulmonary edema. Am Rev Respir Dis 1988;137:1159–1164.

67. Ducas J, Girling L, Shick U, et al. Pulmonary vascular effects of hydralazine in a canine preparation of pulmonary thrombo-embolism. Circulation 1987;73:1050–1056.

68. Evans CL, Mutsuoka Y. The effect of various mechanical conditions on the gaseous metabolism and efficiency of the mammalian heart. J Physiol 1915;378:45.

69. Feneley MP, Gavaghan T. Paradoxical and pseudoparadoxical interventricular septal motion in patients with right ventricular volume overload. Circulation 1986;74:230–238.

70. Feneley MP, Gavaghan TP, Baron DW, Branson JA, Roy PR, Morgan JJ. Contribution of the left ventricular contraction to the generation of right ventricular systolic pressure in the human heart. Circulation 1985;71:473–480.

71. Ferlink J. Right ventricular function in adult cardiovascular disease. Cardiovasc Dis 1982;25:225–267.

72. Fessler HE, Brower RG, Wise RA, Permutt S. Effects of positive end expiratory pressure on the gradient for venous return. Am Rev Respir Dis 1991;143:19–24.

73. Fewell JE, Abendschein DR, Carlson CJ, et al. Mechanism of decreased right and left ventricular end diastolic volume during continuous positive ventilation. Circ Res 1980;47:467–472.

74. Fishman AP. Chronic cor pulmonale. Am Rev Respir Dis 1976;114:775–794.
75. Fisk RL. The right heart. Philadelphia: FA Davis, 1987.
76. Fitzpatrick JM, Grant JB. Effects of pulmonary vascular obstruction on right ventricle afterload. Am Rev Respir Dis 1990;141:944–952.
77. Freis ED, Rivara GL, Gilmonte BL. Estimation of residual and end-diastolic volumes of the right ventricle of men without heart disease, using the dye dilution method. Am Heart J 1960;60:898–904.
78. Fujii J, Yazaki Y, Sawada H, et al. Non invasive assessment of left and right ventricular filling in myocardial infarction with two-dimentional doppler echocardiographic method. J Am Coll Cardiol 1985;5:1150–1160.
79. Furey SA, Zieske HA, Levy MN. The essential function of the right ventricle. Am Heart J 1984;107:404–410.
80. Gattinoni L, Pesenti A, Bombono M, et al. Relationship between lung tomographic density, gas exchange, and PEEP in acute respiratory failure. Anesthesiology 1988;69:824–832.
81. Gattinoni L, Pesenti A, Rossi GP, et al. Treatment of acute respiratory failure with low frequency positive pressure ventilation and extra corporeal CO_2 removal. Lancet 1980;2:292–299.
82. Ghigonne M, Girley L, Prewitt RM. Volume expansion versus norepinephrine in treatment of a low cardiac output complicating an acute increase in right ventricular afterload in dogs. Anesthesiology 1984;60:132–135.
83. Gold FL, Bache RJ. Trans mural right ventricular blood flow during acute pulmonary hypertension in the sedated dog. Circ Res 1982;51:196.
84. Goldstein JA, Vlahaker GJ, Verrier ED, et al. The role of right ventricle systolic dysfunction and elevated intra-pericardial pressure in the genesis of low output in experimental right ventricle infarction. Circulation 1982;65:513–522.
85. Gonzales AC, Brandon TA, Fortune RL, et al. Acute right ventricular failure is caused by inadequate right ventricular hypothermia. J Thorac Cardiovasc Surg 1985;89:386–399.
86. Goto Y, Yamamoto J, Saito M, et al. Effects of right ventricular ischemia on left ventricle geometry and the end-diastolic pressure-volume relationship in dogs. Circulation 1985;72:1104–1114.
87. Grant RP, Downey FM, MacMahon H. The architecture of the right ventricle outflow tract in the normal heart and in the presence of ventricular septal defect. Circulation 1961;24:223–230.
88. Greenbaum D. Positive end expiratory pressure, constant positive airway pressure and cardiac performance. Chest 1979;76:248–249.
89. Gregg DE, ed. Coronary circulation. In: Health and diseases. Philadelphia: Lea & Febiger, 1950.
90. Hamer HP, Takens BL, Posma JL, Lie KI. Noninvasive measurement of RV systolic pressure by combined color-coded and continuous wave doppler ultrasound. Am J Cardiol 1988;61:668–671.
91. Hamrell BB, Alpert NR. The mechanical characteristics of hypertrophied rabbit cardiac muscle in the absence of congestive heart failure. Circ Res 1977;40:20–25.
92. Hemmer M, Suter PM. Treatment of cardiac and renal effects of PEEP with dopamine in patients with acute respiratory failure. Anesthesiology 1979;50:399–403.
93. Hoffmann H, Covell JW. Relationship between ejection phase indices of performance and myocardial functions during the development of pressure overload hypertrophy. Am Heart J 1984;107:738–744.
94. Hopewell PC, Miller RT. Pathophysiology and management of severe asthma. Clin Chest Med 1984;5:623–634.
95. Huet Y, Brun-Buisson C, Lemaire F, et al. Cardiopulmonary effects of Ketanserin infusion in human pulmonary embolism. Am Rev Respir Dis 1987;135:114–117.
96. Hurford WE, Zapol WM. The right ventricle and critical illness: a review of anatomy, physiology and clinical evaluation of function. Intensive Care Med 1988;14:448–457.
97. Isner JM, Fischer JP, DelNegro AA, et al. Right ventricular infarction with hemodynamic decompensation due to transient loss of active atrial augmentation: successful treatment with atrial pacing. Am Heart J 1981;102:792–794.
98. Jacob HS, Craddock PR, Hammerschmidt DE, Moldow CF. Complement induced granulocytes aggregation: an unsuspected mechanism of disease. N Engl J Med 1980;302:789–794.
99. Jardin F, Brun-Ney D, Hardy A, et al. Combined thermodilution and two dimentional echocardiographic evaluation of right ventricular function during respiratory support with PEEP. Chest 1991;99:162–168.
100. Jardin F, Dubourg O, Margairaz A, Bourdarias JP. Inspiratory impairment in right ventricular performance during acute asthma. Chest 1987;92:789–795.
101. Jardin F, Farcot JC, Boisante L, Prost JF, Guéret P, Bourdarias JP. Mechanism of paradoxic pulse in bronchial asthma. Circulation 1982;66:887–894.
102. Jardin F, Farcot JC, Gueret P, et al. Echographic evaluation of ventricles during continuous positive airway passage breathing. J Appl Physiol 1984;56:619–627.
103. Kagan A. Dynamic response of the right ventricle following extensive damage by cauterization. Circulation 1952;5:816–823.
104. Kaufmann RL, Homburger H, Wirth H. Disorder in excitation-contraction coupling of cardiac muscle from cats with experimentally produced right ventricular hypertrophy. Circ Res 1971;28:346–357.
105. Kaul S, Tei C, Hopkins JM, et al. Assessment of right ventricle function using two-dimensional echocardiography. Am Heart J 1984;107:526–531.
106. Kawakami Y, Kishi F, Yamamoto H, et al. Relation of oxygen delivery, mixed venous oxygenation and pulmonary hemodynamics to prognosis in chronic obstructive pulmonary disease. N Engl J Med 1983;308:1045–1049.
107. Kay HR, Afshari M, Barash P, et al. Measurement of ejection fraction by thermal dilution technique. J Surg Res 1983;34:337–346.
108. Keller CA, Shepard JW, Chun DS, et al. Effects

of hydralazine on hemodynamics, ventilation and gas exchange in patients with chronic obstructive pulmonary disease. Am Rev Respir Dis 1984;130:606–611.

109. Kimshi A, Ellrod AG, Berman DS, et al. Right ventricular performance in septic shock; a combined radionuclide and hemodynamic study. J Am Coll Cardiol 1984;4:945–951.

110. Kingma I, Tyberg JV, Smith ER. Effects of diastolic trans-septal pressure gradient on ventricular septal position and motion. Circulation 1983;68:1304–1314.

111. Knowles GK, Clark TJ. Pulsus paradoxus as a valuable sign indicating severity of asthma. Lancet 1973;2:1356–1359.

112. Konstram MA, Levin HJ. Effects of afterload and preload on right ventricular systolic performance. In: Konstram MA, Isner JM, eds. The right ventricle. Boston: Kluwer Academic Publishers, 1988:17–35.

113. Kopelman HA, Forman MB, Wilson BH, et al. Right ventricular myocardial infarction in patients with chronic lung disease; possible role of right ventricular hypertrophy. J Am Coll Cardiol 1985;5:1302–1307.

114. Korr KS, Levinson H, Bough EW, et al. Tricuspid valve replacement for cardiogenic shock after right ventricular infarction. JAMA 1980;244:1958–1960.

115. Lachmann B, Haendly H, Schultz H, Johnson B. Improved arterial oxygenation, CO_2 elimination, compliance and decrease barotrauma following changes in volume-generated PEEP ventilation with I/E ratio of 1/2 to pressure-generated ventilation with I/E ratio of 4/1 in patients with ARDS. Intensive Care Med 1980;6:64–70.

116. Laver MB, Strauss HW, Pohost GM. Right and left ventricular geometry: adjustments during acute respiratory failure. Crit Care Med 1979;7:509–519.

117. Lemaire F, Cerrina J, Lange F, Harf A, Carlet J, Binion J. PEEP induced airspace overdistension complicating paraquat lung. Chest 1982;81:654–657.

118. Lloyd EA, Gersh BJ, Kennedy BM. Hemodynamic spectrum of "dominant" right ventricle infarction in 19 patients. Am J Cardiol 1981;48:1016–1022.

119. Lorell B, Lienbach RC, Pohost GM, et al. Right ventricular infarction. Clinical diagnosis and differentiation from cardiac tamponade and pericardial constriction. Am J Cardiol 1979;43:465–471.

120. MacIntyre KM, Sasahara AA. The hemodynamic response to pulmonary embolism in patient without prior cardiopulmonary disease. Am J Cardiol 1971;28:288–294.

121. MacIntyre KM, Sasahara AA. Determinants of the right ventricular function and hemodynamics after pulmonary embolism. Chest 1974;65:534–543.

122. Mac Nee W, Connaughton JJ, Rhind GB, et al. A comparison of the effects of almitrine or oxygen breathing on pulmonary arterial pressure and right ventricular ejection fraction in hypoxic chronic bronchitis and emphysema. Am Rev Respir Dis 1986;134:559–565.

123. Maddahi J, Berman DS, Matsuoka DT, et al. A new technique for assessing right ventricular ejection fraction using a multiple gated equilibrium cardiac blood pool scintigraphy. Circulation 1979;50:581–590.

124. Marco MR, Aguilar LR, O'Callaghan AC, et al. Etude de l'etat de choc à pression capillaire normale par défaillance ventriculaire droite dans l'infarctus myocardique aigu. Arch Mal Coeur 1979;72:130–138.

125. Marcus ML, Mueller TM, Gascho JA, Kerber RE. Effects of cardiac hypertrophy secondary to hypertension on the coronary circulation. Am J Cardiol 1979;44:1023–1028.

126. Marini JJ, O'Quin R, Culver BH, Butler J. Estimation of transmural cardiac pressure during ventilation with PEEP. J Appl Physiol 1981;53:384–391.

127. Mathur PN, Pugsley SO, Powles P, et al. Effects of diuretics on cardiopulmonary performance in severe chronic airway obstruction. Arch Intern Med 1984;144:2154–2158.

128. Matthay RA, Berger HJ, Loke J. Effects of aminophilline upon right and left ventricle performance in chronic obstructive pulmonary disease: non invasive assessment by radionuclide angiography. Am J Med 1978;65:903–910.

129. Matthay RA, Chatterjee K. Bedside catheterization of the pulmonary artery: risks compared with benefits. Ann Intern Med 1988;109:826–34.

130. Maughan WL, Shoukas AA, Sagawa K, Weisfeldt ML. Instantaneous pressure-volume relationship of the canine right ventricle. Circ Res 1979;44:309–318.

131. Medical Research Council Working Party. Long term domiciliary oxygen therapy in chronic obstructive cor pulmonale complicating chronic bronchitis and emphysema. Lancet 1981;1:681–685.

132. Meijboom EJ, Horowitz S, Valdes-Cruz LM, et al. A doppler echocardiographic method for calculating volume flow across the tricuspid valve: correlative laboratory and clinical studies. Circulation 1985;71:551–556.

133. Melot C, Deschamps P, Hallemans R, et al. Enhancement of hypoxic pulmonary vasoconstriction by low dose almitrine bismesylate in normal humans. Am Rev Respir Dis 1989;139:111–119.

134. Meyer RA, Schwartz DC, Benzing G. Ventricular septum in right ventricular volume overload. Am J Cardiol 1972;30:349–353.

135. Midei MG, Maugham WL, Sugiura S, Oikawa RY. The right ventricular pressure volume relationship is independent of intraventricular flow direction—evidence against a peristaltic movement. Circulation 1986;74(suppl 2):290.

136. Miller DC, Moreno-Cabral RJ, Stinson EB, Shumway N. Pulmonary artery balloon counterpulsation for acute right ventricle failure. J Thorac Cardiovasc Surg 1980;80:760–763.

137. Mizgala HF. Atrial natriuretic factor: a new diagnostic marker for right ventricle infarction. J Am Coll Cardiol 1990;15:554–556.

138. Molaug M, Geiran O, Stockland O, et al. Dynamics of the interventricular septum free wall during blood volume expansion and selective right ventricular volume loading in dogs. Acta Physiol Scand 1982;116:245–256.
139. Molloy WD, Lee KY, Girling L, et al. Treatment of shock in a canine model of pulmonary embolism. Am Rev Respir Dis 1984;130:870–874.
140. Morisson NJ, Abboud RT, Miller NL, et al. Pulmonary capillary blood volume in emphysema. Am Rev Respir Dis 1990;141:141–153.
141. Moser KM. Venous thromboembolism. Am Rev Respir Dis 1990;141:235–249.
142. Mueller TM, Marcus ML, Kerber RE, Young JA, Barnes RW, Abboud FM. Effect of renal hypertension and left ventricular hypertrophy on the coronary circulation in the dog. Circ Res 1978;42:543–549.
143. Murray PA, Vatner SF. Reduction of maximum coronary vascular response to exercise in dogs with severe right ventricular hypertrophy. J Clin Invest 1981;67:1314–1323.
144. Naeije R, Melot C, Mols P, et al. Reduction in pulmonary hypertension by prostaglandin E_1 in chronic obstructive pulmonary disease. Am Rev Respir Dis 1982;125:1–5.
145. Niebader CA, Spielman RP, Wasmus G, Mathey DG, Montz R, Bleifeld WH. Clinical use of ultrashort lived radionuclide Krypton-81m for non invasive analysis of right ventricular performance in normal subjects and patient with t-right ventricular dysfunction. Eur Heart J 1985; 5:687–695.
146. Noctural Oxygen Therapy Trial Group. Continuous or noctural oxygen therapy in chronic obstructive lung diseases. Ann Intern Med 1980;93:391–398.
147. O'Keefe DD, Hoffman JI, Cheitlin R, O'Neill MJ, Allard JR, Shapkin E. Coronary blood flow in experimental canine left ventricular hypertrophy. Circ Res 1978;43:43–51.
148. Parker MP, Shelhamer JH, Bacharach SL, et al. Profound but reversible myocardial depression in patients with septic shock. Ann Intern Med 1984;100:483–490.
149. Parsons GH, Green JF. Mechanisms of pulsus paradoxus in upper airway obstruction. J Appl Physiol 1978;45:598–603.
150. Pearlman AS, Borer JS, Clark CE, Henry WL, Redwood DR, Morow AG, Epstein SE. Abnormal right ventricular size and ventricular septal motion after atrial septal defect closure. Am J Cardiol 1978;41:295–301.
151. Pepe PE, Marini JJ. Occult positive end expiratory pressure in mechanically ventilated patients with airflow obstruction. Am Rev Respir Dis 1982;126:166–170.
152. Pinsky MR. Assessment of the right ventricle in the critically ill: facts, fancy, and perspectives. In: Vincent J, ed. Update in intensive care and emergency medicine. Berlin: Springer-Verlag, 1989:518–523.
153. Pitt B, Strauss HW. Evaluation of ventricular function by radioisotopic techniques. N Engl J Med 1977;296:1097–1103.
154. Pollack JF, Holmann BL, Wynne J, Colucci WS.

Right ventricle ejection fraction: an indicator of increased mortality in patient with congestive heart failure associated with coronary artery disease. J Am Coll Cardiol 1983;2:217.
155. Postel J, Schloerb PR. Cardiac depression in bacteremia. Ann Surg 1977;186:74–82.
156. Pouleur H, Lefevre J, Van Mechelem H, Charlier AA. Free wall shortening and relaxation during ejection of the canine right ventricle. Am J Physiol 1980;239:H601.
157. Prewitt RM, Ghignone M. Treatment of right ventricular dysfunction in acute respiratory failure. Crit Care Med 1983;11:346–352.
158. Qvist J, Pontoppidan H, Wilson RS, et al. Hemodynamic response to mechanical ventilation with PEEP. The effect of hypervolemia. Anesthesiology 1975;42:45–55.
159. Raabe DS, Chester HA. Right ventricular infarction. Chest 1978;73:96–99.
160. Rabinovitch MA, Elstein J, Chiu R, et al. Selective right ventricular dysfunction after coronary artery bypass grafting. J Thorac Cardiovasc Surg 1983;86:444–450.
161. Raine AE, Erne P, Burgisser E, et al. Atrial natriuretic peptide and atrial pressure in patients with congestive heart failure. N Engl J Med 1986;315:533–537.
162. Rebuck AS, Pengelly LD. Development of pulsus paradoxus in the presence of airways obstruction. N Engl J Med 1973;288:66–69.
163. Reid LM. Structure and function in pulmonary hypertension: new perceptions. Chest 1986; 89:279–288.
164. Reuse C, Vincent JL, Pinsky MR. Measurements of right ventricular volumes during fluid challenge. Chest 1990;96:1450–1454.
165. Reyes A, Roca J, Rodriguez-Voisin R, et al. Effect of almitrine on ventilation-perfusion distribution in adult respiratory distress syndrome. Am Rev Respir Dir 1988;137:1062–1067.
166. Rich S, Gubin S, Hart K. The effect of phenylephrine on right ventricular performance in patients with pulmonary hypertension. Chest 1990;98:1102–1106.
167. Robalino BD, Petrella RW, Jubran MD, et al. Atrial natriuretic factor in patients with right ventricle infarction. J Am Coll Cardiol 1990; 15:546–553.
168. Roberts N, Harrison DG, Reimer KA, et al. Right ventricle infarction with shock but without significant left ventricular infarction: a new clinical syndrome. Am Heart J 1985;110:1047–1053.
169. Robotham JL, Lixfield W, Holland L, MacGregor D, Bryan CA, Rabson J. Effects of respiration on cardiac performance. J Appl Physiol 1978; 44:703–709.
170. Robotham JL, Mitzner W. A model of the effects of respiration on left ventricle performance. J Appl Physiol 1979;46:411–418.
171. Rubin LJ. Vasodilatator and pulmonary hypertension. Where do we go from here? Am Rev Respir Dis 1987;135:288–293.
172. Rushmer RF, Crystal DK, Wagner C. The functional anatomy of ventricle contraction. Circ Res 1953;1:162–170.
173. Ruskin J, Bache RJ, Rembert JC, Greenfield JC.

Effect of respiration on left ventricle stroke volume. Circulation 1973;48:79–85.

174. Ryan T, Petrovic O, Dillon JC, Feigenbaum H, Conley MJ, Armstrong WF. An echocardiographic index for separation of right ventricular volume and pressure overload. J Am Coll Cardiol 1985;5:918–924.

175. Sabbah HN, Stein PD. Negative diastolic pressure in the intact canine right ventricle. Evidence of a diastolic suction. Cir Res 1981;49:108–113.

176. Sagawa K, Suka H, Shoukas AA, Bakalar KM. End systolic pressure volume ratio. Am J Cardiol 1977;40:748–753.

177. Santamore WP, Lynch PR, Heckman JL, Bove AA, Meier GD. Left ventricular effects on right developed pressure. J Appl Physiol 1976;41:925–932.

178. Scharf SM, Brown R, Saunders N, Green LH. Effects of normal and loaded spontaneous inspiration on cardiovascular function. J Appl Physiol 1979;47:582–588.

179. Sharf SM, Brown R, Tow DE, Parisi AF. Cardiac effects of increased lung volume and decreased pleural pressure in man. J Appl Physiol 1979;47:257–262.

180. Sharf SM, Warner KG, Josa M, Khuri SF, Brown R. Load tolerance of the right ventricle: effect of increased aortic pressure. J Crit Care 1986;3:163–173.

181. Schneider AJ, Teule GJ, Kester AD, et al. Biventricular function during volume loading in porcine *E. coli* septic shock, with emphasis on right ventricular function. Circ Shock 1986;18:53–63.

182. Schreuder WO, Schneider AJ, Groeneveld AJ, Thijs LG. Effects of dopamine vs norepinephrine on hemodynamics in septic shock. Chest 1989;95:1282–1288.

183. Schulman DS, Biondi JW, Matthay RA, et al. Effect of positive end expiratory pressure on right ventricle performance. Am J Med 1988;84:57–67.

184. Seely RD. Dynamic effect of inspiration on the stroke volume of the right and left ventricles. Am J Physiol 1980;154:273–280.

185. Shabetai R. Pericardial influence on the right heart. In: Konstram MA, Isner JM, eds. The right ventricle. Boston: Kluwer Academic Publishers, 1988:55–70.

186. Shah PK, Maddahi J, Berman DS, et al. Scintigraphically detected predominant right ventricular dysfunction in acute myocardial infarction: clinical and hemodynamic correlates and implication for therapy and prognosis. J Am Coll Cardiol 1985;6:1264–1272.

187. Shimada R, Takeshita A, Nakamura M. Non invasive assessment of right ventricle systolic pressure in atrial defects: analysis of the end-systolic configuration of the ventricular septum by two dimentional echocardiography. Am J Cardiol 1984;53:117–1123.

188. Sibbald WJ, Paterson NA, Holliday RL, et al. Pulmonary hypertension in sepsis. Measurement by the pulmonary arterial diastolic-pulmonary wedge pressure gradient and the influ-

ence of passive and active factors. Chest 1978;73:583–591.

189. Simmons PH, Linder CM, Miller JR, et al. Relation of lung volume and pulmonary vascular resistance. Circ Res 1961;9:465–471.

190. Smith EF, Kingma I, Smiseth OA, et al. Ventricular response to acute constriction of the pulmonary artery in conscious dogs. Am Rev Respir Dis 1985;131:A57.

191. Smith ER, Tyberg JV. Ventricular interdependence. In: Konstram MA, Isner JM, eds. The right ventricle. Boston: Kluwer Academic Publishers, 1988:650–669.

192. Smith HL, Essex HE, Baldes EJ. A study of the movements of heart valves and heart sounds. Ann Intern Med 1950;33:1357–1362.

193. Snider MT, Rye MA, Lauer A, Zapol W, Reid L. Normoxic pulmonary vasoconstriction in ARDS. Detection by sodium nitroprusside and isoproterenol infusion. Am Rev Resp Dis 1980;121:191–195.

194. Spann JF, Buccino RA, Sonnenblick EH, Braunwald E. Contractile state of cardiac muscle obtained from cats with experimentally produced ventricular hypertrophy and heart failure. Circ Res 1967;21:341–354.

195. Squara P, Dhainaut JF, Lamy M, et al. Computer assistance for hemodynamic evaluation. J Crit Care 1989;4:273–282.

196. Squara P, Dhainault JF, Schremmer B, Sollet JP, Bleichner G. Decreased paradoxic pulse from increased venous return. Chest 1990;97:377–383.

197. Stalcup SA, Mellins RB. Mechanical forces producing pulmonary edema in acute asthma. N Engl J Med 1977;297:592–595.

198. Starling MR, Crawford MH, Sorensen SG, O'Rourke RA. A new two-dimensional echocardiographic technique for evaluating right ventrical size and performance with chronic obstructive lung disease. Circulation 1982;66:612–620.

199. Starr I, Jeffers WA, Meade RH. The absence of conspicuous increment of venous pressure after severe damage to the right ventricle of the dog. Am Heart 1943;26:291.

200. Steele P, Ellis JH, Vandyke D, et al. Left ventricular ejection fraction in severe chronic obstructive airway disease. Am J Med 1975;59:21–28.

201. Stein PD, Sabbah HN, Anbe DT, Marzilli M. Performance of the failing and nonfailing right ventricle of patients with pulmonary hypertension. Am J Cardiol 1979;44:1050–1055.

202. Stein PD, Sabbah HN, Mazilli M, Anbe DT. Effect of chronic pressure overload on the maximum rate of pressure fall of the right ventricle. Chest 1980;78:10–15.

203. Stempel DA, Mellon M. Management of acute severe asthma. Pediatr Clin North Am 1984;31:879–890.

204. Stool EW, Mullins CB, Leshin SJ, Mitchell JH. Dimensional changes of the left ventricle during acute pulmonary arterial hypertension in dogs. Am J Cardiol 1974;33:498–504.

205. Straub PW, Bühlman AA, Rossier PH. Hypovolemia in status asthmaticus. Lancet 1969;2:923–926.

206. Suga H, Hayashi T, Shirahata M. Ventricular systolic pressure volume area as a predictor of cardiac oxygen consumption. Am J Physiol 1981;240:H39–H44.
207. Suter P, Fairley H, Isenberg M. Optimum end expiratory airway pressure in acute respiratory failure. N Engl J Med 1975;292:284–289.
208. Swan HJ, Ganz W, Forrester J, et al. Catheterization of the heart in man with use of a flow directed balloon-tipped catheter. N Engl J Med 1970;283:447–451.
209. Takata M, Robotham JL. Ventricular external constraint by the lung and pericardium during positive end expiratory pressure. Am Rev Respir Dis 1991;143:872–875.
210. Takata M, Wise RA, Robotham JL. Effects of abdominal pressure on venous return: abdominal vascular zone conditions. J Appl Physiol 1991.
211. Tani M. Roles of the right ventricular free wall and ventricular septum in right ventricular performance and influence of the parietal pericardium during ventricular failure in dogs. Am J Cardiol 1983;52:195–202.
212. Tei C, Pilgrim JP, Shah PM, Ormiston JA, Wong M. The tricuspid valve annulus: study of size and motion in normal subjects and in patients with tricuspid regurgitation. Circulation 1982;66:665–671.
213. Tenney SM, Mithoefer JC. The relationship of mixed venous oxygenation to oxygen transport with special reference to adaptation to high altitude and pulmonary disease. Am Rev Respir Dis 1982;125:474–479.
214. Thys D, Cohen E, Eisenkrfat J. Mixed venous oxygen saturation during thoracic anesthesia. Anesthesiology 1988;69:1005–1009.
215. Turley K. The challenge of pulmonary hypertension. Chest 1990;99:6–7.
216. Urabe Y, Ohzono K, Koyanagi S, Nakamura M. Role of afterload in determining regional right ventricular performance during coronary underperfusion in dogs. Circ Res 1985;57:93–104.
217. Vincent JL, Reuse C, Kahn RJ. Effects on right ventricle function of a change from dopamine to dobutamine in critically ill patients. Crit Care Med 1988;16:659–663.
218. Vincent JL, Thirion M, Brimouille S, et al. Thermodilution measurement of right ventricle ejection fraction with a modified pulmonary artery catheter. Intensive Care Med 1986;12:33–38.
219. Visner MS, Arentzen CE, O'Conner MJ, Larson EV, Anderson RW. Alterations in left ventricular three-dimensional dynamic geometry and systolic function during acute right ventricular hypertension in the conscious dog. Circulation 1983;67:353–365.
220. Vlahakes GJ, Turkey K, Hoffman JIK. The pathophysiology of failure in right ventricular hypertension. Circulation 1981;63:87–95.
221. Watanabe T, Katsume H, Matsukubo H, et al. Estimation of right ventricular volume with two-dimensional echocardiography. Am J Cardiol 1982;44:1946–1953.
222. Weber KT, Janicki JS, Shroff SG, et al. The right ventricle: physiologic and pathophysiologic considerations. Crit Care Med 1983;11:323–328.
223. Weitzenblum E, Sautegeau A, Ehrhart M, et al. Long term course of pulmonary artery pressure in chronic obstructive pulmonary disease. Am Rev Respir Dis 1979;130:993–998.
224. Wiedemann HP, Matthay RA. Cor pulmonale in chronic obstructive pulmonary disease. Clin Chest Med 1990;11:523–545.
225. Williams JF, Potter RD. Normal contractile state of hypertrophied myocardium after pulmonary artery constriction in the cat. J Clin Invest 1974;54:1266–1272.
226. Wright JL, Lawson L, Pare PD, et al. The structure and function of the pulmonary vasculature in mild chronic obstructive disease. Am Rev Respir Dis 1983;128:702–707.
227. Wroblewski E, James F, Spann JF, Bove AA. Right ventricular performance in mitral stenosis. Am J Cardiol 1981;47:51–55.
228. Yock PG, Popp RL. Non invasive estimation of right ventricle systolic pressure by Doppler ultrasound in tricuspid regurgitation. Circulation 1984;70:657–662.
229. Zapol WM, Snider MT. Pulmonary hypertension in severe acute respiratory failure. N Engl J Med 1977;296:476–480.
230. Zwissler B, Forst H, Messmer K. Local and global function of the right ventricle in a canine model of pulmonary microembolism and oleic acid edema: influence of ventilation with PEEP. Anesthesiology 1990;79:964–975.

19

Acute Pulmonary Hypertension

Max Rattes
James E. Calvin

Acute pulmonary hypertension, defined as an increase in either the resting pulmonary artery systolic pressure above 30 mm Hg or the resting mean pressure above 20 mm Hg (45), is a commonly missed diagnosis. This is largely due to the lack of sensitivity and specificity of the symptoms and signs at initial examination of the patient. With few exceptions, severe acute pulmonary hypertension, when first diagnosed, is often irreversible and associated with a high mortality (65, 66). Treatment of this condition is most successful when it is diagnosed early and the inciting cause is identified and checked before irreversible damage has been done to the pulmonary vasculature. Patients with primary pulmonary hypertension, a chronic disorder, have an even worse prognosis (92). With the exception of a few cases of reports of patients in remission, about 20% of patients are alive after 5 years of initial diagnosis (37).

The incidence of acute pulmonary hypertension is difficult to estimate. However, pulmonary thromboembolism is the most common cause of acute pulmonary hypertension in hospitalized patients. It has been estimated that as many as 15% of all persons admitted to hospitals may have complications of pulmonary embolism. This represents a total incidence of 630,000 cases annually in the United States, with an annual mortality rate exceeding 200,000. In 67,000 cases, the patient presents as sudden cardiac death with survival of less than an hour (25).

THE NATURE OF THE PULMONARY CIRCULATION

The normal pulmonary circulation, in contrast to the systemic circulation, is a high-flow/low-pressure system (45). The resistance to blood flow across the normal pulmonary circulation is very low and equal to one tenth of the resistance across the systemic bed (45). The mean pressure in the pulmonary artery is only 12 ± 2 mm Hg. Since normal left atrial mean pressure is 6 ± 2 mm Hg, the pressure gradient across the normal pulmonary circulation is only 6 mm Hg. In contrast, for a normal cardiac output of 5 liters/min, the pressure gradient between the left ventricle and the right atrium is 80 to 100 mm Hg.

Passive Regulation of the Pulmonary Circulation

The Calculation of Pulmonary Vascular Resistance and Its Limitations

The calculation of resistance to flow through the pulmonary circulation represents only one element of the pulmonary vascular load. However, it is the easiest to assess at the bedside. Vascular properties such as compliance and wave reflections (6, 17, 50, 84) are not taken into account and these can only be calculated by measuring instantaneous pressure and flow and computing the pulmonary input impedance.

Steady flow conditions in the pulmonary vasculature can be described by Ohm's law:

$$PVR = \frac{(P_{inflow} - P_{outflow}) \times 80}{\dot{Q}} \, (\text{dynes} \cdot \text{second} \cdot \text{cm}^{-5})$$

Where PVR = pulmonary vascular resistance, P_{inflow} = the inflow pressure usually measured as the mean pulmonary artery pressure, $P_{outflow}$ = the effective outflow pressure, and $\dot{Q}$ = pulmonary blood flow.

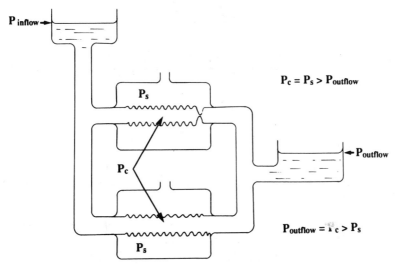

$$P_c = P_s > P_{outflow}$$

$$P_{outflow} = P_c > P_s$$

Figure 19.1. The pulmonary circulation modeled as a Starling resistor. The pulmonary circuit consists of two rigid tubes connected by a collapsible segment exposed to an external pressure (P_s). The critical outflow pressure (P_c) is the pressure distending the collapsible segment. When the external pressure (P_s) is $< P_{outflow}$ then P_c becomes the effective outflow pressure and the pressure gradient for blood flow is the difference between the inflow pressure (P_{inflow}) and P_c. When P_s is $< P_{outflow}$ the driving pressure is represented by the difference between P_{inflow} and $P_{outflow}$. In this case the $P_{outflow} = P_c$.

The usual clinical assumption is that $P_{outflow} = P_{La}$ (left atrial pressure). As we shall see, this assumption is not always valid. Hence, this frequently used calculation can be very misleading in terms of assessing pulmonary vasomotor tone.

The observation that the pulmonary circulation acts as a Starling resistor has special relevance in this discussion (70, 86, 123, 124). A Starling resistor circuit consists of two rigid, noncollapsible tubes connected by a segment that is thin-walled, collapsible, and exposed to an external pressure (P_s) (Fig. 19.1). The pressure inside the collapsible segment is designated as the critical outflow pressure (P_c). If P_s is greater than the $P_{outflow}$, flow varies directly with the difference between P_{inflow} and P_s. P_c represents a vascular waterfall in this case and is equal to P_s. If $P_{outflow}$ exceeds P_s, then no waterfall exists, $P_c = P_{outflow}$, and the pressure gradient for flow is the difference between P_{inflow} and $P_{outflow}$.

West and coworkers (123, 124) have used this concept to classify the pulmonary blood distribution into three zones that are governed by gravity, hydrostatic pressure gradients, and alveolar pressure. If the alveolar pressure of the lungs (P_A) is greater than the pulmonary artery pressure (P_a), then the vascular segment is collapsed and there is no flow (Fig. 19.2). This hypoperfused lung zone occurs at the top of the lungs (West's zone I). When P_a exceeds P_A the segment is open and flow is present. However when the P_v (pulmonary venous pressure) is subatmospheric (i.e., less than P_A), the pressure gradient for flow is the difference between P_a and P_A (West's zone II). The proportion of zone II can increase during positive pressure ventilation (increased P_A) or hypovolemia (decreased P_v). This zone represents a Starling resistor circuit. In the dependent portion of the lung, P_v exceeds P_A and the pressure gradient for flow is the difference between P_a and P_v (West's zone III). In this case, the collapsible segment is distended and no waterfall exists.

Theoretically, a fourth zone may exist where blood flow is decreased. This has been demonstrated in vertical lung preparations and in upright humans (55, 77). The mechanism for the existence of this fourth zone is believed to appear at residual volume when blood flow decreases

RESPIRATORY PHYSIOLOGY

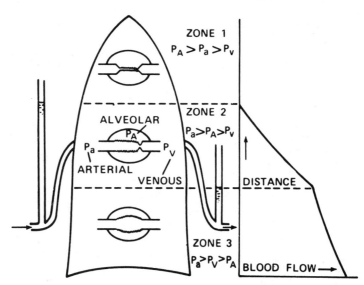

Figure 19.2. West's zones of the lung. P_a = pulmonary artery pressure, P_A = alveolar pressure, and P_v = pulmonary venous pressure. (From West JB, Dollery CT, Naimark A. Distribution of blood flow in isolated lung: relation to vascular and alveolar pressures. J Appl Physiol 1964;19:713.)

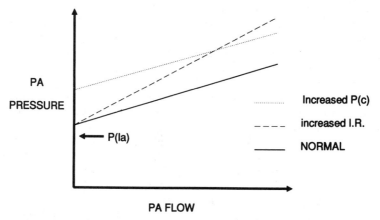

Figure 19.3. Pressure:flow relationships in acute pulmonary hypertension. Pulmonary artery (PA) pressure and flow relationships are plotted as pulmonary artery flow is systematically increased. P(c) represents the pressure intercepted at zero flow and is analogous to the critical outflow pressure. IR = the incremental resistance and represents the resistance upstream from P(c). Acute pulmonary hypertension can be represented by either a change in the incremental resistance or change in the critical outflow pressure.

during forced expiration, and has been attributed to either an increase in interstitial pressure at lung bases or to closure of small airways at low lung volumes.

Pressure Flow Relationships

Investigators concerned about the effects of inflation, collapsible capillaries, and hy-drostatic gradients have used pulmonary artery pressure/flow relationships (Fig. 19.3) to describe pulmonary vascular tone (12, 79, 123). The use of pressure/flow curves allows one to describe the pulmonary vascular tone in terms of some critical outflow pressure (P_c) represented by pressure intercept at zero flow and the incremental resistance (IR, 1/slope). This latter resistance term refers to the resistance localized upstream to the critical outflow pressure (P_c), which can be thought of as the pressure necessary to distend the Starling resistor.

Investigators have determined that lung inflation causes parallel shifts in the pressure/flow relationships (i.e., increased P_c) providing strong evidence that a Starling resistor model is appropriate. In this case, the alveolar pressure acts as P_c in the capillary Starling resistor (79).

A variety of models of pulmonary hypertension have also been studied using pressure/flow relationships in an attempt to determine whether the locus of increased resistance is at the level of the Starling resistor or upstream from it.

In a canine model of pulmonary thromboembolism, pulmonary artery pressure/flow relationships were measured before and after autologous clot embolism (30, 31). Critical outflow pressure increased dramatically after clot embolism with only a small increase in upstream resistance; hydralazine, in part, reversed these effects (30). Similar observations were reported in oleic acid pulmonary edema (12). These observations confirm the importance of Starling resistors in describing the pulmonary vasculature in pathologic states and, at least in these models, the locus for the increase in pulmonary vascular resistance is at the level of the Starling resistor.

A Dynamic View of the Pulmonary Circulation

Up to now, we have analyzed the pulmonary circulation under steady flow conditions. However, circulation is pulsatile. By computing the pulmonary input impedance spectra we can study the dynamic nature of circulation (78). Pulmonary input impedance is obtained by recording instantaneous pulmonary artery pressure and flow signals in the time domain and transforming these signals into the frequency domain by decomposing each into a complex series of sine and cosine waves. In this way, the amplitude and phase angle of the pressure/flow relation at each frequency can be calculated. The pressure/flow relation at 0 Hz is represented by the mean amplitude or modulus of pulmonary artery pressure divided by mean pulmonary artery flow and is called the input resistance; it depends on the cross-sectional area of the downstream pulmonary vascular bed. The average modulus of the pressure/flow relationship at high frequencies is called the characteristic impedance and represents the pulsatile component of the impedance. This latter impedance depends on the vascular wall compliance and the blood inertia. A pulmonary input impedance spectrum from a healthy dog is shown in Fig. 19.4. The normal input resistance in man is 245 ± 51 dynes·second·cm^{-5} and the normal characteristic impedance is 23 ± 3 dynes·second·cm^{-5}. In addition to the calculation of pulmonary input resistance and the characteristic impedance, oscillations of the impedance spectra are noted with minimum moduli between 2 and 4 Hz and maximum being measured between 6 and 8 Hz. The minima also corresponds to the point where the phase angle becomes positive and represents the frequency at which wave reflecting sites are one quarter wavelength away. The significance of these observations is that the site of increased resistance can be determined.

Vasoconstriction produced by serotonin has been shown to increase the input resistance and the amplitude of the oscillations of the higher frequency moduli (84) (Fig 19.5). These changes are likely on the basis that peripheral wave reflection factors are modified (i.e., the minima and maxima moduli are also shifted to the right because of an increase in the elastic modulus—stiffness of the vessel wall—and wave phase velocity). Vasodilators have the opposite effect (84).

A proximal pulmonary artery constriction increases both input resistance and characteristic impedance, the latter likely because of a reduction in the caliber of the main pulmonary artery (17). However, small glass emboli increase only input resistance, consistent with an isolated downstream injury where only the cross-sectional area of the distal bed is affected (17).

These observations illustrate how upstream and downstream effects can be differentiated experimentally and how changes in vasomotor tone can also be assessed.

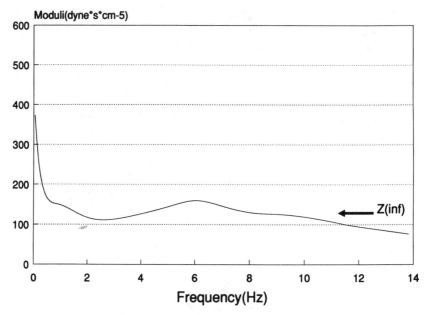

Figure 19.4. Pulmonary artery input impedance of the dog during baseline conditions. The modulus of the relationship of the pulmonary artery pressure:pulmonary artery flow relationship at 0 Hz is called the input resistance. The average value of the moduli at high frequencies is called the characteristic impedance and is designated Z(inf).

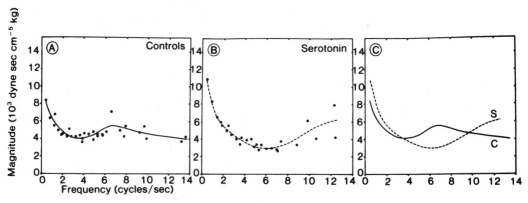

Figure 19.5. Pulmonary artery vascular impedance in a dog infused with serotonin. The vaso-constrictor effects of serotonin increase the frequency of the first minimal value and increase the magnitude of oscillation of the impedance moduli at high frequency. (From Bergel DH, Milnor WR. Pulmonary vascular impedance in the dog. Circ Res 1965;16:401–415.)

Active Regulation of the Pulmonary Circulation

Neurohumoral Influences

Although neurohumoral responses by pulmonary circulation can be demonstrated, their importance in regulating pulmonary vascular tone is unclear. Various mediators such as catecholamines (42, 53, 57, 72, 103), acetylcholine, prostaglandins, histamines, bradykinin, serotonin, and angiotensin, may be involved in regulation of vascular resistance, but the exact site of action of these agents is uncertain at present (49, 53, 56, 57).

Hypoxic Pulmonary Vasoconstriction

It is well known than alveolar hypoxia produces pulmonary vasoconstriction. Indeed, it may be one of the most potent stimuli for vasoconstriction yet identified. Acidemia has also been shown to modulate the response of hypoxia. In general, when the degree of oxygen saturation is quite low, pulmonary artery pressure is quite sensitive to the hydrogen ion concentration, whereas it is quite insensitive when the oxygen saturation is high (68, 71, 97). The major site of hypoxic pulmonary vasoconstriction is thought to be arterial, but there is good evidence that all segments of the vascular bed participate (11, 40, 44, 81).

The mechanism of hypoxic pulmonary vasoconstriction is still unclear (75, 76). The pulmonary vascular response to hypoxemia can be blunted by calcium-blocking agents, suggesting that increased cytosolic calcium in smooth muscle cells may represent a final common pathway (74, 104, 107, 111, 126). There is much speculation, however, as to how hypoxemia is sensed and pulmonary vasoconstriction is triggered. In general, there are two major hypotheses. First, mediators may be released from endothelial (24, 36), neuroepithelial (5), or mast cells (47), which stimulate vasoconstriction. The second hypothesis states that hypoxia has a direct effect on pulmonary vasomotor tone.

Possible mediators are listed in Table 19.1. Unfortunately, there is a great deal of conflicting data for any of these to be considered the prime mediator. In the case of histamine (47, 53, 112), angiotensin II (48, 88), and lipooxygenase products (3), specific inhibitors of these mediators fail

Table 19.1
Potential Mediators of Hypoxic Pulmonary Vasoconstriction

Histamine
Norepinephrine
Angiotensin II
Serotonin
Arachnidonic acid metabolites
Lipooxygenase products

to attenuate hypoxic pulmonary vasoconstriction. Norepinephrine release (42,103) has not been observed during hypoxic pulmonary vasoconstriction and serotonin appears to have little effect in man and cattle (52, 122). Paradoxically, inhibitors of cyclooxygenase products result in greater hypoxic pulmonary vasoconstriction (49, 115, 116, 120, 121).

Direct effects of alveolar hypoxia may be mediated by a reduction in the oxidative phosphorylation potential (93, 106). Studies have demonstrated that inhibitors of the tricarboxylic acid cycle increase pulmonary vasoconstriction (93, 106, 109). It is likely that the reduced [ATP]/{ADP} {P_1} ratio mediates mitochondrial release of calcium (74, 76, 104, 111).

CLASSIFICATION OF ACUTE PULMONARY HYPERTENSION

Determinants of Pulmonary Artery Pressure

As discussed earlier, arterial pressures in the pulmonary circulation are related to the hydraulic equivalent of Ohm's law. That is, resistance (R) equals the difference in inflow and outflow pressure divided by blood flow (Q). For the pulmonary circulation, the upstream pressure is represented by the mean pulmonary artery pressure (P_a) and the downstream pressure by the pulmonary venous pressure (P_v). Therefore,

$$R = (P_a - P_v) / Q \qquad (1)$$

and rearranging

$$P_a = (Q \times R) + P_v \qquad (2)$$

from Poiseuille's law resistance,

$$R = (8nL \div \pi r^4), \qquad (3)$$

where n = viscosity of fluid and L and r = length and radius of the vessel, respectively. Thus,

$$P_a = (8nL \div \pi r^4 \times Q) + P_v. \qquad (4)$$

From equation 2 it is clear that pulmonary artery pressure can be increased by increased resistance or increased flow. From equation 4 it can be seen that resistance can be increased by increased viscosity and decreased cross-sectional area of the pulmonary vascular bed (i.e., decreased *r*).

This analysis assumes that flow is steady and not pulsatile. This assumption fails to take into account the fact that pulsatile flow is also dependent on arterial compliance, blood inertia, and wave reflections. These factors have been demonstrated in animal models of pulmonary hypertension (6, 17, 84) and contribute significantly to vascular load, although the relevance to pathologic states in man is unclear.

Physiologic Classification of Acute Pulmonary Hypertension

Equation 4 does allow, however, for a physiologic basis for classifying pulmo-nary artery hypertension as described in Table 19.2.

Intracardiac left-to-right shunts are an uncommon cause of acute pulmonary hypertension, with the exception of ventricular septal defects after myocardial infarction. Left ventricular (LV) failure is the most common cause of elevated pulmonary venous pressure and acute pulmonary hypertension. Reduced LV distensibility secondary to myocardial ischemia can also elevate pulmonary venous pressures acutely. Left ventricular inflow tract obstruction from mitral stenosis or left atrial myxoma more commonly causes chronic pulmonary hypertension.

Pulmonary venous obstruction from tumor impingement, scarring, or venoocclu-

Table 19.2
Classification of Acute Pulmonary Hypertension

Physiologic Disturbance	Pathologic Entities
Increased pulmonary flow (Q)	Left-to-right intracardiac shunt (ASD, VSD, PDA)[a]
Increased outflow pressure (Pv)	LV failure
	Decreased LV compliance
	Mitral valve disease[a]
	Left atrial myxoma[a]
	Pulmonary venous obstruction[a]
	Pulmonary venoocclusive disease[a]
	Tumor impingement[a]
	Radiation fibrosis[a]
Anatomic decrease in pulmonary cross-sectional area (r) Intrinsic	
Large arteries	Pulmonary embolism
Small arteries	Peripheral pulmonary stenosis[a]
	Parenchymal lung diseases
	Eisenmenger's reaction[a]
	Primary pulmonary hypertension[a]
	Vasculitis[a]
	Pulmonary embolism
Extrinsic Large & small arteries	Tumor
	Fibrosis[a]
	Extensive pleural disease[a]
Small arteries	Increased airway pressure
Functional decrease in pulmonary cross-sectional area (r)	
Small arteries	Hypoxemia
Increased blood viscosity (n)	Vascular injuries
	Hemoglobinopathy[a]
	Polycythemia[a]

[a]More commonly a chronic cause.

sive disease is rare but can influence outflow pressure. Usually, this occurs over a long period of time.

Anatomic decreases in the pulmonary cross-sectional area can occur from both intrinsic and extrinsic lesions of small and large arteries. Intrinsic obstruction of a large pulmonary artery can occur secondary to pulmonary embolism or peripheral pulmonary stenosis (usually congenital). Extrinsic compression of larger arteries can occur secondary to chronic tumor compression or fibrosis. Anatomic intrinsic causes of obstruction to small arteries are most commonly secondary to parenchymal lung diseases, small pulmonary emboli, pulmonary vasculitis, or acute lung injuries (110).

Pulmonary hypertension is a common sequel of chronic obstructive lung disease. It used to be thought that the elevated pulmonary artery pressures in patients with emphysema resulted from obstruction of the pulmonary vascular bed. However, the extent of destruction of alveoli and the accompanying reductions in alveolar surface do not correlate closely with the degree of pulmonary hypertension. Therefore, the decrease in the pulmonary capillary bed in such patents plays a minor role in elevating pulmonary vascular resistance.

In patients with bullous emphysema, two mechanisms are implicated in the development of pulmonary hypertension. In addition to destruction of alveoli and decrease in the pulmonary vascular bed, physical compression of or encroachment on pulmonary capillary beds may play a role (35).

Extrinsic causes of obstruction to small arteries include parenchymal lung diseases, which compress and gradually obliterate the small pulmonary vessels from outside, causing increased resistance to blood flow with resultant pulmonary hypertension. Severe fibrosis, tumor compression, and increased airway pressure from mechanical ventilation are common causes.

Pulmonary hypertension occasionally may be due to extensive lung resection or fibrothorax. Normally, almost two thirds of the lungs have to be removed before pulmonary arterial pressures reach hypertensive levels. In an extensive fibrothorax from a traumatic hemothorax, tuberculous or nontuberculous empyema, or pleural effusion, chronic pulmonary hypertension may result from compression of normal underlying lung parenchyma and vessels.

Acute vascular injuries of the lung manifest themselves in two ways: increased permeability to water and protein, and increased pulmonary vascular resistance. This latter phenomena, when present in patients with acute lung injury, is associated with a poor prognosis (10, 102, 127). Both of these phenomena have been demonstrated in experimental models of sepsis, endotoxemia (10, 14, 28, 125), and microembolism (73). Demling and coworkers (28) demonstrated that infusion of endotoxin in sheep resulted in an early hypertensive phase during which plasma and lung lymph levels of thromboxane B_2 (TxB_2) and prostaglandin $F_{2\alpha}$ were elevated. The degree of pulmonary hypertension correlated well with the lymph level of TxB_2. Inhibitors of cyclooxygenase can blunt this phase both in endotoxin models (64, 82) and glass bead microembolism (19). It is likely that either pulmonary vascular endothelium or pulmonary macrophages are the source of these mediators.

This implication of arachidonic acid metabolites as mediators has resulted in two clinical studies investigating the efficacy of prostaglandin, a prostaglandin vasodilator, in treating patients with hypoxemic respiratory failure. The first study demonstrated improved survival in such patients (54). A second, a multicenter trial, showed lower pulmonary vascular resistance with prostaglandin E_1 treatment but mortality was not affected (13). At the present time, prostaglandin appears to be indicated only in patients with significant pulmonary hypertension.

Thrombi in the lungs of patients with acute lung injury have also been demonstrated and correlate with disease severity (43, 115) and presumably contribute to the pulmonary hypertension of acute lung injury as well.

An important cause of pulmonary hypertension in critical care patients is extrinsic compression of small arteries by increased airway pressure and/or changes in lung volume. Increasing lung volume or alveolar pressure has significant mechanical effects upon right ventricular afterload. As lung volume increases during a normal breath, alveolar vessels are compressed while extraalveolar vessels are dilated. However, as lung volume increases above functional residual capacity (FRC), the major effect is alveolar vessel compression and an increase in pulmonary vascular resistance. Remembering our discussion of Starling resistors, this increase in pulmonary vascular resistance really is best thought of as an increase in critical outflow pressure (P_c).

Positive pressure ventilation magnifies the effect of increasing lung volumes by compressing alveolar vessels. Both Smith et al. (105), looking at the effects of positive end expiratory pressure, and Calvin et al. (17), looking at the effects of lung hyperinflation, demonstrated increases in pulmonary input impedance (increased afterload) and decrease in right ventricular (RV) end-diastolic dimensions (decreased preload). Both of these studies were concerned with rather high lung volumes and/or airway pressures, however. Normal ventilation (17, 87) has not been shown to have major effects on PVR or RV systolic performance. Furthermore, if lung volumes are below FRC (causing extraalveolar vessels to collapse) and hypoxemia (causing pulmonary vasoconstriction) is present, artificial ventilation may actually cause PVR to fall.

If an elevated RV afterload is produced by lung hyperinflation, RV preload must increase to compensate for it. However, reduced preloads have been documented during continuous positive pressure vented action (33). Furthermore, increases in lung volumes have been shown to produce a direct contact pressure around the heart, limiting both RV and LV distensibility and end-diastolic volumes (17, 22, 69). In this case, there is a mismatch between afterload and preload. Right ventricular stroke volume falls to a greater degree than would be predicted by the change in afterload alone. Furthermore, filling pressure may have to be higher than expected to maintain stroke volume. This is illustrated using a force-velocity concept. An increase in the transmural pulmonary artery pressure should result in a decrease in stroke volume so long as preload is unchanged (Fig. 19.6, point A to B). If preload is reduced because lung inflation limits RV distensibility, stroke volume will fall further (Fig. 19.6, point C). For stroke volume to remain at the level prior to lung inflation (Fig. 19.6, point A), preload must be increased above the normal level (Fig. 19.6, point D).

Pulmonary hypertension may also result from an increased vascular resistance secondary to increased vasomotor tone. Acute hypoxia is the most important stimulus for vasoconstriction in the pulmonary vascular bed, and hypoxia-induced vasoconstriction probably plays a major role in producing pulmonary hypertension in those living at high altitudes and in patients with chronic obstructive lung disease.

CIRCULATORY CONSEQUENCES OF ACUTE PULMONARY ARTERY HYPERTENSION

The Impact of the Type of Vascular Bed Lesion Upon RV Function

The site of a vascular lesion causing pulmonary hypertension has significant impact upon RV function as well. Calvin et al. (17) demonstrated that glass bead microembolism resulted in a relative smaller proportion of RV hydraulic power being used to generate pulsations and a greater proportion being used to maintain steady flow compared to pulmonary artery constriction. In a follow-up paper, Calvin (16) also demonstrated, using RV segment length crystals to assess RV preload, that RV function was better preserved with glass bead microembolism than pulmonary artery constriction at matched levels of pulmonary artery pressure (Fig. 19.7). The reasons for this are unclear, but the preservation of hydraulic power to maintain steady flow with resultant less energy loss was demonstrated and may be important.

The effect of lung inflation upon RV afterload and preload

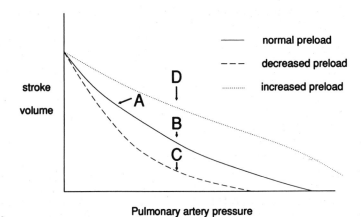

Figure 19.6. Relationship of stroke volume to the transmural pulmonary artery pressure during lung inflation. As the transmural pulmonary artery pressure is increased, stroke volume falls from point A to point B. By limiting or reducing RV preload, through surface contact, stroke volume falls even further (point C). In order to maintain stroke volume at baseline conditions, preload has to be increased over and above normal values (point D).

Effect of Increased Pulmonary Artery Pressure on Right and Left Heart Function

As discussed above, the pulmonary circulation is a high-flow, low-resistance circuit that is capable, under normal conditions, of accepting a maximum RV output at a pressure one fifth of that generated in the systemic arterial system. Fundamental differences also exist between the right and left ventricles. First, the left ventricle is a pressure generator pump, whereas the right ventricle more closely resembles a flow generator pump. The wall of the right ventricle is less than one half as thick as that of the left ventricle because of the low resistance of the pulmonary circulation. Second, LV failure generally results from conditions that directly affect myocardial structure and function. On the other hand, conditions that produce RV dysfunction generally preserve the structure or function of the myocardium. For instance, acute pulmonary embolism can cause a right ventricle pressure overload state and congenital disorders such as atrial or ventricular septal defects may cause volume overload

without directly depressing RV contractility. The third difference between the ventricles relates to the relationship between end-diastolic volume and ventricular end-diastolic pressure. This relationship is not identical for these two chambers. The right ventricle is a highly compliant chamber and considerable changes in end-diastolic volume may be accompanied by only small increments in end-diastolic pressure. Additionally RV output increases with increasing ventricular volume, even up to moderately elevated end-diastolic pressures if afterload is unchanged.

Mechanism of Low Output States Accompanying Acute Pulmonary Hypertension

The development of a low cardiac output state during acute pulmonary hypertension is a combination of RV afterload mismatch leading to both RV ischemia and failure, and complex mechanical interactions with the left ventricle. Earlier research confirmed that the right ventricle became ischemic in severe acute pulmonary hypertension in association with either

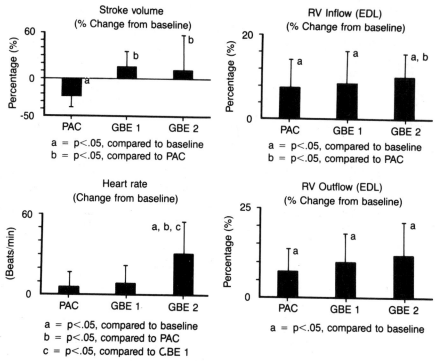

Figure 19.7. Representative hemodynamic changes during pulmonary artery constriction (PAC) and glass bead embolism (GBE) in dogs. The animal's pulmonary artery was constricted by a snare sufficiently to double the pulmonary artery systolic pressure. The glass beads were embolized into the pulmonary circulation sufficient to first match the mean pulmonary artery pressure observed during PAC (GBE1) and then to match the pulmonary artery systolic pressure during PAC (GBE2). The PAC resulted in a reduction in stroke volume with increases in the RV end-diastolic length of both inflow and outflow regions of the RV free wall surface. In contrast, GBE1 and GBE2 resulted in increases in stroke volume at relatively similar changes in RV end-diastolic segment lengths.

hypotension or severe reduction in cardiac output (41, 119). In both the study by Vlahakes et al. (119) and Gold and Bache (41), ischemia was found in the presence of decreased RV coronary blood flow. Also, increases in aortic pressure restored coronary perfusion presumably by increasing coronary perfusion pressure to a coronary vascular bed that was maximally vasodilated. These findings supported the hypothesis that RV ischemia and systolic dysfunction were major determinants in the pathogenesis of the low output state accompanying acute pulmonary hypertension. However, Gold and Bache and other studies (21, 34) also demonstrated increases in right coronary blood flow during acute pulmonary hypertension of less

severe degrees, especially if hypotension was not present (Fig. 19.8).

Until recently it was unknown whether cardiac output fell prior to the development of RV ischemia. A second hypothesis proposed by Calvin (19) was that cardiac output fell initially because of afterload mismatch. He demonstrated that tripling of the pulmonary artery pressure by glass bead embolism was well tolerated by the right ventricle, with cardiac output being maintained by both the heart rate (or chronotropic) response and the Frank-Starling mechanism (preload reserve). However, further increases in pulmonary artery pressure sufficient to decrease the cardiac output by 20% result in a disproportionate increase in end-systolic volume

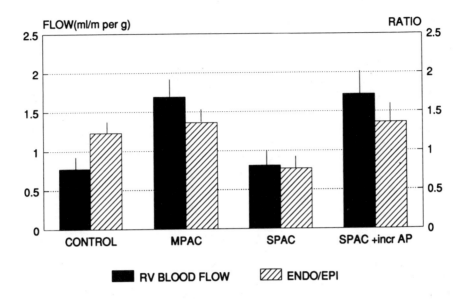

GOLD AND BACHE,1982

Figure 19.8. Right ventricular myocardial blood flow during acute pressure overload. A modest pulmonary artery constriction (MPAC) unassociated with hypotension results in increases in both total RV blood flow and the endocardial/epicardial ratio. Severe pulmonary constriction sufficient to produce hypotension (SPAC) decreases both RV blood flow and endocardial/epicardial ratios, suggesting myocardial ischemia. By increasing aortic pressure at this point (SPAC + incr AP), these changes can be reversed. (Adapted from Gold FL, Bache RJ. Transmural right ventricular blood flow during acute pulmonary artery hypertension in the sedated dog. Circ Res 1982;51:196–204.)

compared to end-diastolic volume (i.e., stroke volume and ejection fraction fall as a result). At this particular point, the right ventricle performs largely pressure work and very little flow work. The ATP and creatinine phosphate levels are normal. These phenomena are most consistent with afterload mismatch initiating a decrease in cardiac output during acute pulmonary hypertension not depressed contractility. To compensate, heart rate and RV end-diastolic volume increase. Unfortunately, these initial compensations are undermined by complex ventricular interactions that impair LV filling (4, 20, 39, 60, 61, 108, 118).

These interactions consist of a series interaction, whereby LV filling falls proportionate to the decrease in RV stroke output; a mechanical interaction mediated by the pericardium, whereby a dilated right ventricle occupies disproportionately more of the pericardial space than the left ven-

tricle thereby influencing its distensibility and filling; and a mechanical interaction mediated by the interventricular septum.

As we have mentioned above, an inverse relationship between the vascular load and stroke output has been previously demonstrated. Calvin et al. (17) demonstrated that RV stroke volume was inversely related to the pulmonary input resistance (a more precise measurement of vascular load) (Fig. 19.9).

The pericardium plays a significant role in mediating a direct interaction between right and left ventricles. As the right ventricle dilates within an intact pericardium (108), RV end-diastolic pressure increases. The first implication of this observation is that the intrapericardial pressure increases and this external pressure is exerted upon the left ventricle and affects its distensibility and further aggravates LV underfilling (20, 39). This is demonstrated in Figure 19.10. In an experimental model of acute

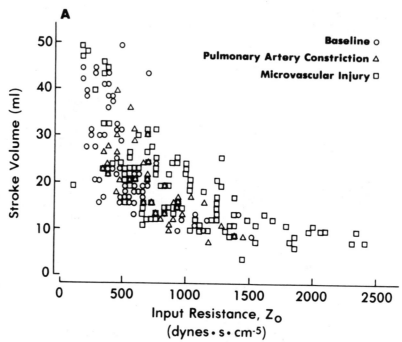

Figure 19.9. Inverse relationship between stroke volume and pulmonary artery input resistance (Z_0) in the dog. As input resistance is increased through pulmonary artery constriction or a microvascular injury induced by glass beads, stroke volume falls. (From Calvin JE, Baer RW, Glantz SA. Pulmonary artery constriction produces a greter right ventricular dynamic afterload than lung microvascular injury in the open chest dog. Circ Res 1985;56:40–56.)

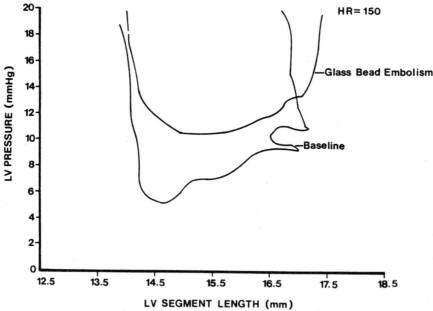

Figure 19.10. Ventricular diastolic function during acute pulmonary hypertension. Glass bead embolism sufficient to double the mean pulmonary artery pressure results in an upward shift in the LV diastolic pressure-segment length relationship, suggesting reduced distensibility. (From Calvin JE, Langlois S, Barneys B. Ventricular intervention in a canine model of acute pulmonary hypertension and its modulation by vasoactive drugs. J Crit Care 1988;3:43–55.

pulmonary hypertension produced by ventricular glass bead embolism, Calvin et al. (20) determined that LV diastolic pressure: segment length (measured by small piezoelectric crystals inserted into the ventricular muscle and measuring size change) relationship were shifted upward, indicating decreased distensibility. This effect was found to be independent of any heart rate change and was associated with reduced LV end-diastolic segment length (preload).

The second implication of these events is that the transseptal pressure gradient decreases or in fact reverses. As a result, the septum shifts leftward, further impairing LV filling (61). This is demonstrated in Figure 19.11, which illustrates the two-dimensional echo of a patient with acute pulmonary hypertension. The right ventricle is dilated and septal curvature (normally rightward) is flattened. Kingsma et al. (61) have clearly demonstrated the inverse relationship between the transseptal pressure gradient and the RV septal-free wall dimension and the direct relationship between the transseptal pressure gradient and the LV septal-free wall dimension.

All of these interactions undermine LV filling or preload. As a result LV stroke volume falls along with aortic pressure.

As RV pressure increases and the right ventricle dilates, the demand for oxygen increases. As discussed above, there is significant evidence to suggest that right coronary blood flow does initially increase to meet this demand (21, 34, 41). However, because of the inability to increase coronary blood further, an imbalance of RV oxygen supply and demand could develop before RV blood flow declines. Indeed, this imbalance has been demonstrated by measuring RV blood flow: tension time index ratios (Fig. 19.12) before and after acute pulmonary hypertension produced by glass bead embolism (21). The myocardial blood flow/tension time index falls before the development of acute RV failure and decreased RV coronary blood flow. Ischemia can develop as a result of this imbalance. Finally, as the RV coronary vascular bed maximally vasodilates to match the increased O_2 demand, O_2 supply becomes dependent upon RV coronary perfusion pressure. Right ventricular coronary perfusion pressure falls during shock states because of two factors. First, the downstream pressure (i.e., RV end-diastolic pressure) increases and second, the upstream pressure (aortic pressure) falls as a result of LV underfilling. These mechanisms are summarized in Figure 19.13, with the resulting effects on ventricular hemodynamics and geometry schematically depicted in Figure 19.14.

Pulmonary Blood Volume

The volume of blood within the lungs at any given moment has some important implications and may be influenced by pulmonary hypertension. It acts as a determinant of lung elasticity, is important for gas exchange, helps maintain adequate LV preload, may contribute to the pathogenesis of *cardiac* pulmonary edema by influencing hydrostatic forces, and may act as a stimulus to the sensation of dyspnea. It is influenced by the relative outputs of the two ventricles and by ventilation itself. Clearly, pulmonary blood volume can be increased by left-to-right shunts and elevated left-sided filling pressures. It may be diminished by a limitation of the cross-sectional area of the pulmonary vascular bed.

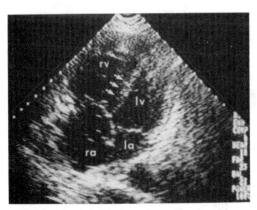

Figure 19.11. Two-dimensional echocardiogram in a patient with acute pulmonary hypertension. Both the right ventricle (rv) and right atrium (ra) are dilated, while left atrium (la) and left ventricle (lv) are smaller than normal. The normal septal configuration which is normally curved toward the right ventricle is flattened *(arrows)*.

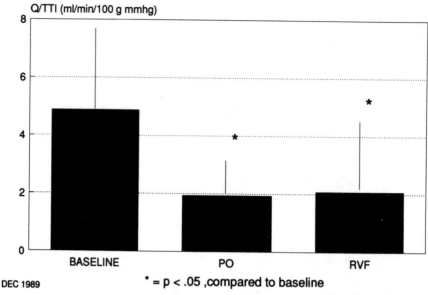

DEC 1989 * = p < .05 ,compared to baseline

Figure 19.12. Right ventricular myocardial supply:demand ratio measured by determination of RV myocardial blood flow (Q) derived from microsphere technique and the tension time index (TTI) measured by planimetry of the RV pressure tracings in the time domain. The ratio of these two measurements is performed under baseline conditions during acute RV pressure overload (PO) when the systolic pulmonary artery is tripled and during RV failure when cardiac output has been reduced by more than 30% (RVF). The ratio declines prior to the onset of RV failure. (Adapted from Calvin JE, Quinn B. Right ventricular pressure overload during acute lung injury: cardiac mechanics and the pathophysiology of right ventricular systolic dysfunction. J Crit Care 1989;4:251–265.)

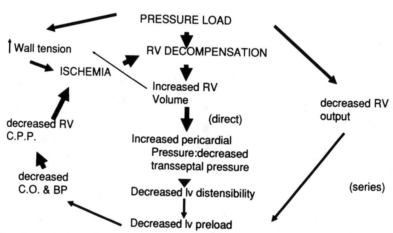

Figure 19.13. Summary of the pathophysiology of RV failure during acute pulmonary hypertension. As pulmonary artery pressure is increased, an increase in RV wall tension is observed and at the same time stroke output from the right ventricle falls. The right ventricle dilates, which exacerbates the increase in wall tension, increases pericardial pressure, and reduces the transseptal pressure gradient. These latter two observations result in reduced LV distensibility and a reduction in LV preload. The LV preload also falls because of the series interaction between both ventricles. As LV preload falls, LV cardiac output and blood pressure fall. This leads to reduced RV coronary perfusion pressure (C.P.P.). The combination of an increased wall tension leading to a reduction in myocardial oxygen supply:demand ratios and the reduced RV coronary perfusion pressure culminates in RV ischemia.

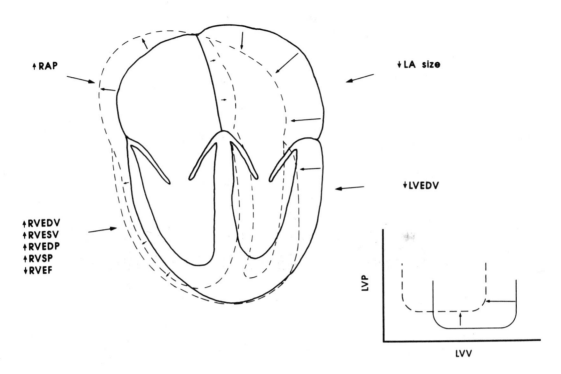

– – – – **Change induced by acute PH**

Figure 19.14. Schemata of the ventricular geometric and hemodynamic changes occurring during acute pulmonary hypertension. Right-sided pressures (RAP, RVEDP) increase along with increases in RV end-diastolic and end-systolic volumes (RVEDV and RVESV, respectively). Right ventricular ejection fraction (RVEF) falls. Right ventricular systolic pressure (RVSP) falls as a result of the reduction in RV stroke output. Both left atrial (LA) size and LV end-diastolic volume (LVEDV) fall in association with an upward and leftward shift in the LV diastolic pressure:volume relationship.

Implications for Gas Exchange

Normal blood gas exchange depends upon adequate matching of ventilation and blood flow within the various lung regions (26, 27). Three common problems observed with gas exchange are hypoventilation, intrapulmonary shunting, and impaired diffusion. When global hypoventilation occurs, $Paco_2$ rises in a predictable fashion. Intrapulmonary shunting occurs when perfusion occurs in nonventilated areas of lung. Impaired diffusion of oxygen across the pulmonary capillary can occur in a variety of pulmonary disorders.

Regional inequalities of ventilation and perfusion can also occur and can influence overall gas exchange leading to hypoxemia.

Pulmonary vascular diseases causing pulmonary hypertension such as pulmonary embolism and primary pulmonary hypertension are accompanied by regional ventilation perfusion abnormalities (26, 27). Hypoxemia occurs as a result of this abnormality and low cardiac output.

CLINICAL IDENTIFICATION OF INCREASED PULMONARY ARTERY PRESSURE

History and Physical Examination

The symptoms and signs of pulmonary hypertension are nonspecific and a high index of suspicion is needed to make the diagnosis. They may not be present until the resting pulmonary artery pressure is about two or more times normal. The symptoms most associated with the diagnosis of acute pulmonary hypertension include exertional dyspnea without orthopnea, fatigue, weakness, effort syncope, angina-like chest pain, palpitations, cough, hemoptysis, and hoarseness. They may be present alone or in any combination (113).

On examination, tachypnea is observed in over 80% of cases of acute pulmonary hypertension, with tachycardia more variable. Other physical findings to look for are a prominent "a" or "v" wave in the jugular venous pulse (Fig. 19.15), palpation of a sustained RV lift, a loud and palpable P2, an audible right-sided S4 and/or S3, a pulmonic-systolic ejection click, a high-pitched early diastolic murmur of pulmonic insufficiency or the holosystolic murmur of tricuspid regurgitation. The physical examination is more specific than the history and may also provide important information as to the etiology of the pulmonary hypertension (i.e., mitral stenosis, chronic lung disease, congenital heart disease, and collagen-vascular disease).

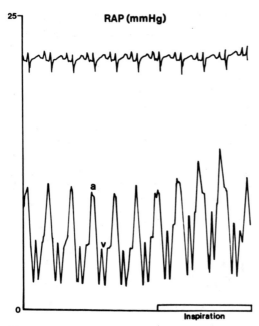

Figure 19.15. Right atrial pressure (RAP) tracings in a patient with pulmonary hypertension. Note the increase in the amplitude of the "a" wave and the increase in right atrial pressure during inspiration (Kussmaul's sign).

Ancillary Tests

Chest X-Ray

The chest x-ray is useful in the evaluation of a patient with suspected pulmonary hypertension because it may provide a clue to the etiology and severity of pulmonary hypertension. The estimation of the pulmonary artery pressure by chest x-ray is inaccurate because it depends on the measurement of the cardiothoracic ratio and the assessment of the degree of vascularity in the peripheral lung fields. The assessment of lung vascularity is difficult and the measurement of the heart size is, on the other hand, not very sensitive in predicting the degree of pulmonary hypertension. The most important radiographic signs of pulmonary hypertension are based on measurements of the diameter of the large pulmonary arteries (23). A commonly used measurement is the width of the descending branch of the right pulmonary artery. Its normal size ranges from 9 to 16 mm (58, 117).

ECG

The electrocardiogram is a rather insensitive test for the diagnosis of pulmonary hypertension, although is is quite specific. Patients with chronic pulmonary hypertension have ECG findings that reflect the high pressures in the right side of the heart. Right atrial hypertrophy is evidenced by a symmetrical and peaked P wave greater than 2.5 mm in amplitude in any lead. Right ventricular hypertrophy can be suspected when a QR is observed in V_1 (in the absence of myocardial infarction), the QRS axis in the frontal plan is $\geq110°$, there is delay of intrinsicoid deflection in V_1 or V_2 ≥0.035 seconds, the R/S ratio in V_1 is >1, or R/S ratio in V_6 is <1.

In patients presenting with acute pulmonary embolism, the ECG is diagnostic in about 25% of the cases. The most characteristic feature is the transient nature of the changes. Our best source of information comes from patients with acute pulmonary embolism (Table 19.3) (114). Rhythm disturbances, QRS abnormalities, and ST abnormalities were found to be present in a majority of cases (90%). The presence of atrial and ventricular premature beats are not common. Both right and

Table 19.3
Electrocardiographic Abnormalities in 131 Patients with Pulmonary Embolism[a]

Abnormalities	Percent of Patients
Rhythm Disturbances	
Premature beats	11
Atrial	3
Ventricular	9
Atrial fibrillation	3
QRS	65
Right axis	5
Left axis	12
Incomplete right bundle branch block	5
Complete right bundle branch block	11
Right ventricular hypertrophy	5
$S_1 S_2 S_3$ pattern	9
$S_1 Q_3 T_3$ pattern	11
ST-T	64
T-wave inversion	40
ST-T segment depression	33
ST-T segment depression	11

[a]From National Cooperative Study: Urokinase-Pulmonary Embolism Trial. Circulation 1973; 47(suppl II):1. By permission of the American Heart Association, Inc.

left axis abnormalities can be detected and right bundle branch block observed in some cases. The characteristic S_1, S_2, S_3 and S_1, Q_3, T_3 patterns are observed in approximately 10% of cases each (Fig. 19.16). T wave inversion and nonspecific ST segment depression also occur in over a third of the cases.

Noninvasive Means

Both scintigraphic and echocardiographic studies can be employed to determine RV function. First-past RV ejection fractions have been widely employed to estimate RV function. The normal RV ejection fraction is approximately 55% (7–9). Echocardiography represents a major advance and allows one to look at RV size, the configuration of the intraventricular septum, and contractility. Echo Doppler assessment allows one to estimate the pulmonary artery pressure with a great deal of accuracy (100).

Two measurements are necessary for calculation of the peak systolic pulmonary artery pressure. These are the mean right atrial pressure (MRAP), which is either measured clinically or assumed, and the peak systolic gradient (PSG) between the right ventricle and right atrium. This latter gradient can be estimated in the presence

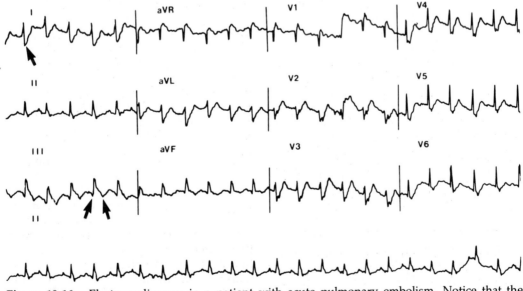

Figure 19.16. Electrocardiogram in a patient with acute pulmonary embolism. Notice that the right axis shows a prominent S_1, Q_3, T_3 pattern indicated by the *arrows*.

of tricuspid regurgitation by using the Bernoulli equation ($PSG = 4V^2$) to calculate the peak systolic gradient between the right ventricle and the right atrium. The peak regurgitant velocity (V) is obtained from continuous wave Doppler recordings.

The pulmonary artery systolic pressure (PASP) can then be calculated as

$$PASP = PSG + MRAP$$

Invasive Means

Contract ventriculography can be performed (40). However, the geometry of the right ventricle makes it difficult to compute volume (38). It is rarely used now and has been replaced by the noninvasive techniques. Hemodynamic monitoring, however, does remain the mainstay of managing the acutely ill patient with RV decompensation. The use of a Swan Ganz catheter allows the determination of right atrial, RV, and pulmonary artery pressures. Right heart pressure can confirm the elevated right atrial pressure, prominence of either "a" or "v" waves and "y" descents and the elevated pulmonary artery pressure. The RV pressure tracing may show a square root sign in its diastolic portion.

Cardiac output can also be measured by a thermodilution catheter. Pulmonary vascular resistance can thus be calculated by the following formulae:

$$PVR \text{ (dynes·second·cm}^{-5}) = \frac{\{(PAP - PCWP)\}}{\left\{ \dfrac{}{CO} \right\}} \cdot 80$$

where PAP = mean PA pressure, PCWP = pulmonary capillary pressure, and CO = cardiac output. The normal range of PVR is between 40 and 90 dynes·second·cm^{-5} (45).

Recently, the thermodilution technique has been refined, allowing for the determination of RV ejection fraction and volumes. This advance is based on the recent manufacture of a rapid-response thermistor allowing for beat-to-beat temperature variations (59). Although this is an exciting advance, the influence of a concomitant tricuspid regurgitation on the estimation of ejection fraction and volume still remains to be determined. Intepretation of the results should be made with caution.

MANAGEMENT OF ACUTE PULMONARY HYPERTENSION

A pathophysiologic approach to the treatment of pulmonary hypertension includes: (1) identification and removal of the inciting cause when it is possible, (2) decreasing resistance to pulmonary blood flow by using oxygen and other pulmonary arterial vasodilators, and (3) management of right heart failure.

It is essential that diagnostic effort be vigorously pursued in patients with acute pulmonary hypertension in order to prevent irreversible damage to the pulmonary vasculature. Pulmonary embolism should be excluded by means of pulmonary angiography and systemic anticoagulation started. Acidosis and hypercarbia should be corrected.

Reduction of Pulmonary Vascular Resistance

Vasodilators, as we shall see below, are commonly used to treat the elevated pulmonary vascular resistance observed in acute RV pressure overload (Table 19.4). However, their effects on the systemic circulation to lower aortic pressure can actually precipitate RV ischemia and shock (83). It is advisable to keep a close eye on the aortic diastolic pressure and pressor agents should be added to keep it from falling significantly.

Oxygen is a useful and safe vasodilator and relieves the pulmonary hypoxic vasoconstriction in chronic obstructive pulmonary disease (1), acute respiratory failure (2), and primary pulmonary hypertension (80). It has very little effect on systemic blood pressure.

A good pulmonary vasodilator is still yet to be found, although many have been tried (Table 19.3). There are a number of reports attesting to the utility of calcium blockers (91, 95), hydralazine (46, 96), diazoxide (62), isoproterenol (101), acetylcholine (51) and arachidonic acid metabolites (13, 46, 54, 94) in pulmonary hypertensive disorders. Although hydralazine can be used in such patients, it does have a potent effect on the systemic circulation and must be used with a great deal of caution. There appears to be little role for the use

Table 19.4
Pulmonary Vasodilators

Drug	Adverse Effect
Tolazoline (IV)	Gastrointestinal distress, systemic hypoxemia
Phentolamine (IV)	Further elevation of pulmonary artery pressure
Prazosin (p.o.)	Systemic hypotension
Acetylcholine (intrapulmonary artery)	Systemic hypoxemia
Isoproterenol (sublingual)	Pharmacologic tolerance palpitations, tremulousness, systemic hypoxemia, exacerbation of pulmonary hypertension, severe chest pain, dyspnea
Diazoxide (p.o., IV, intrapulmonary artery)	
Acute use	Marked reflex tachycardia, severe hypotension, asystole, nausea, vomiting, atrioventricular block, death
Long-term use	Exacerbation of pulmonary hypertension Hyperglycemia, fluid retention, nausea, vomiting, hirsutism, postural hypotension
Hydralazine	Tachycardia, hypotension, death, systemic hypoxemia, renal insufficiency, systemic lupus erythema, tosus, angina, dyspnea
Nitroglycerin (sublingual, topical)	Systemic hypoxemia, tachycardia, hypotension
Calcium-channel blockers	
Verapamil (intrapulmonary artery)	Deterioration in RV performance, cardiogenic shock, hypotension
Nifedipine (p.o.)	Systemic hypoxemia, hypotension, gastrointestinal disturbances, deterioration in RV performance, cardiogenic shock
Captopril (p.o.)	Profound hypotension, exacerbation of pulmonary hypertension
Prostaglandins (IV) PGI$_2$, PGE$_1$	Hypotension, flushing, headache, nausea, vomiting, epigastric pain, bradycardia
Amrinone	Tachycardia
Oxygen	System vasoconstriction, which may compromise renal function and limit natriuresis

of calcium blockers in patients with acute RV pressure overload, although in chronic primary pulmonary hypertension, they have been shown to be of benefit (91). The use of nitroglycerin and nitroprusside have not been demonstrated to have consistent beneficial effect in an experimental model of canine oleic acid pulmonary edema (85); indeed, hydralazine appeared to be superior to nitroprusside (67).

Prostaglandin E$_1$ has been used in a number of clinical situations with varying success. Initial enthusiasm was based on a clinical study by Holcroft et al. (54), which suggested reduced mortality in pa-tients with acute lung injury treated with prostaglandin E$_1$. Bone et al. (13) confirmed its ability to reduce pulmonary vascular resistance but showed no effect on mortality in patients with acute lung injury. Other studies in experimental models have shown minimal success with prostaglandin E$_1$ as a vasodilator (29, 90).

Once a diagnosis of acute pulmonary embolus is either established or highly suspected (on the basis of clinical presentation and noninvasive testing), therapy with intravenous heparin should be initiated. Heparin enhances the inhibitory effect of antithrombin III on thrombin and factor Xa. It should be continued for 7–10 days. Coumadin should be started between days 5 and 7 and eventually heparin discontinued. It suppresses production of vitamin K-dependent factors of coagulation (factors II, VII, IX, X). Treatment should continue for 3–6 months.

In patients with hemodynamic compromise or at least involvement of two lobar arteries complicating pulmonary embolism, thrombolytic agents such as streptokinase, urokinase, and tissue plasminogen activator (tPA) should be considered (113, 114). This therapy is, however, contraindicated in patients who have undergone either a surgical procedure, a thoracentesis, a paracentesis, or an intraarterial diagnostic procedure in the past 10 days. It is obviously contraindicated in patients with recent gastrointestinal bleeding, intracranial lesions, severe hypertension, allergies, or bleeding diathesis.

Surgical embolectomy is reserved for patients with ongoing hemodynamic compromise beyond the 1st hour (98) or in whom thrombolytic therapy is contraindicated.

Management of Right Heart Failure

Most authorities believe that RV preload must be optimized as an initial step in managing acute right heart failure. The optimal range of right-sided filling pressures in acute RV pressure overload is not known and treatment should be individualized. Work by Prewitt and Ghignore (89) has suggested that volume loading can indeed be deleterious. In their study, pulmonary hypertension in dogs was induced by glass bead embolism. Volume loading sufficient to raise the RV and LV end-diastolic pressures above 10 mm Hg resulted in a decrease in cardiac output. This observation is probably explained by the fact that if RV contractility is markedly depressed, the Frank-Starling curve is relatively flat. Increasing RV filling pressure in this situation will not increase stroke output but will increase RV end-diastolic pressure and intrapericardial pressure and will reverse the transseptal pressure gradient. These changes exacerbate the peri-

cardial and transseptal interactions we have alluded to above. The best guide is to manage each patient individually. Volume loading should be initiated when the central venous pressure is less than 10 mm Hg and the cardiac output should be followed closely. Further volume loading should be avoided when the right atrial pressure increases more than 3 mm Hg without an appreciable change in cardiac output.

The maintenance of aortic pressure is an important issue in managing such patients (41, 89, 99, 119). Agents that increase aortic pressure have been shown to reverse RV ischemia and actually improve RV function. Norepinephrine and dopamine are the drugs of choice.

The use of inotropic agents to increase RV contractility still remains an important tool. Isoproterenol, norepinephrine, dopamine, and dobutamine can all increase RV contractility. In an experimental model of glass bead embolism, norepinephrine (89) and dobutamine (15) have enhanced RV function and can be used in the clinical setting to manage such patients.

Amrinone has also been shown to be of benefit, partially because of its inotropic properties and partially because of its pulmonary vasodilator properties (63). However, the vasodilator properties of both dobutamine and amrinone can have potential deleterious effects upon RV preload and systemic pressure. They should be used cautiously in such patients, starting with low doses that are carefully titrated against physiologic end-points.

SUMMARY

Acute RV failure is an increasingly more common clinical entity and problem. A good understanding of pathophysiology is required to develop a treatment strategy. Principles of treatment, which are outlined, include optimizing RV preload, cautiously reducing RV afterload, and enhancing RV contractility.

References

1. Abraham AS, Cole RB, Bishop JM. Reversal of pulmonary hypertension by prolonged oxygen

administration to patients with chronic bronchitis. Circ Res 1968;23:147–157.

2. Abraham AS, Cole RB, Greene ID, Hedworth-Whitty RB, Clarke SW, Bishop JM. Factors contributing to the reversible pulmonary hypertension in patients with acute respiratory failure studied by serial observation during recovery. Circ Res 1969;24:51–60.

3. Ahmed T, Oliver W Jr. Does slow reacting substance of anaphylaxis mediate hypoxic pulmonary vasoconstriction? Am Rev Resp Dis 1983;127:566–571.

4. Bemis CE, Serur JR, Borkenhager D, Sonnonblick EH, Urschel CW. Influence of right ventricular filling pressure on left ventricular pressure and dimension. Circ Res 1974;34:498–504.

5. Benumof JL, Mathers JM, Wahrenbrock EA. The pulmonary interstitial compartment and the mediator of hypoxic pulmonary vasoconstriction. Microvasc Res 1978;15:69–75.

6. Bergel DH, Milnor WR. Pulmonary vascular impedance in the dog. Circ Res 1965;16:401–415.

7. Berger HJ, Matthay RA. Radionuclide right ventricular ejection fraction: applications in valvular heart disease. Chest 1981;79:497–498.

8. Berger HJ, Matthay RA. Noninvasive radiographic assessment of cardiovascular function in acute and chronic respiratory failure. Am J Cardiol 1981;47:950–962.

9. Berger HJ, Matthay, Loke J, Marshal RC, Gotschalk A, Zaret BL. Assessment of cardiac performance with quantitative radionuclide angiocardiography: right ventricular ejection fraction with reference to findings in chronic obstructive pulmonary disease. Am J Cardiol 1978;41:897–905.

10. Bernard GR, Brigham KL. Pulmonary edema. Chest 1986;89:594–600.

11. Bjertnaes LJ, Hauge A, Torgrinsen T. The pulmonary vasoconstrictor response to hypoxia. The hypoxia-sensitive site studied with a volatile inhibitor. Acta Physiol Scand 1980;109:447–462.

12. Boiteau P, Ducas J, Shick U, Girling L, Prewitt RM. Pulmonary vascular pressure-flow relationship in canine oleic acid pulmonary edema. Am J Physiol 1986;251:H1163–H1170.

13. Bone RC, Slotman G, Maunder R, et al. Randomized double blind multi-centre study of prostaglandin E_1 in patients with the adult respiratory distress syndrome. Chest 1989;96:114–119.

14. Brigham KL, Meyrick B. Endotoxin and lung injury. Am Rev Respir Dis 1986;33:913–927.

15. Calvin JE. Right ventricular afterload mismatch during acute pulmonary hypertension and its treatment with dobutamine: a pressure segment length analysis in a canine model. J Crit Care 1989;4:239–250.

16. Calvin JE. Pressure segment length analysis of right ventricular function: the influence of loading conditions. Am J Physiol 1991;29.

17. Calvin JE, Baer RW, Glantz SA. Pulmonary artery constriction produces a greater right ventricular dynamic afterload than lung microvascular injury in the open chest dog. Circ Res 1985;56:40–56.

18. Calvin JE, Baer RW, Glantz SA. Pulmonary injury depresses cardiac systolic function through

Starling mechanism. Am Physiol Soc 1986:H722–H733.

19. Calvin JE, Dervin G. Intravenous ibuprofen blocks the hypoxemia of pulmonary glass bead embolism in the dog. Crit Care Med 1988;16:852–853.

20. Calvin JE, Langlois SF, Garneys GG. Ventricular interaction in a canine model of pulmonary microvascular injury and its modulation by vasoactive drugs. J Crit Care 1988;3:43–55.

21. Calvin JE, Quinn B. Right ventricular pressure overload during acute lung injury: cardiac mechanics and the pathophysiology of right ventricular systolic dysfunction. J Crit Care 1989;4:251–265.

22. Cassidy SS, Mitchell JH, Johnson RL. Dimensional analysis of right and left ventricles during positive pressure ventilation in dogs. Am J Physiol 1982;242:H549–H556.

23. Change CH. The normal roentgenographic measurement of the right descending pulmonary artery in 1085 cases. Am J Roentgenol 1962;87:929–935.

24. Cherry PD, Furchgott RF, Zawadski JV, Jothianandan D. Role of endothelial cells in relaxation of isolated arteries by bradykinin. Proc Natl Acad Sci 1982;79:2106–2110.

25. Dale JE, Alpert JS. Natural history of pulmonary embolism. Prog Cardiovasc Dis 1975;17:259–270.

26. Dantzker DR, Bower JS. Mechanisms of gas exchange abnormality in patients with chronic obliterative pulmonary vascular disease. J Clin Invest 1979;64:1050–1979.

27. Dantzker DR, Wagner PD, Tornabene VW, Alazraki NP, West JB. Gas exchange after pulmonary thromboembolization in dogs. Circ Res 1978;42:92–102.

28. Demling RH, Smith M, Gunther R, et al. Pulmonary injury and prostaglandin production during endotoxemia in conscious sheep. Am J Physiol 1981;240:H348–H353.

29. Dervin G, Calvin JE. Role of prostaglandin E_1 in reducing pulmonary vascular resistancae in an experimental model of acute lung injury. Crit Care Med 1990;18:1129–1133.

30. Ducas J, Duval D, DaSilva H, Boiteau P, Prewitt RM. Treatment of canine pulmonary hypertension: effects of norepinephrine and isoproterenol on pulmonary vascular pressure-flow characteristics. Circulation 1977;75:235–242.

31. Ducas J, Girling L, Shick U, Prewitt RM. Pulmonary vascular effects of hydralazine in a canine preparation of pulmonary thromboembolism. Circulation 1986;73:1050–1057.

32. Ferlinz J. Right ventricular function in adult cardio-vascular disease. Prog Cardiovas Dis 1982;25:225–267.

33. Fewell JE, Abendschein DR, Carlson CJ, et al. Continuous positive-pressure ventilation does not alter ventricular pressure-volume relationship. Am J Physiol 1981;240:H821–H826.

34. Fixler DE, Archie JP, Ullyot DJ, et al. Effects of acute right ventricular systolic hypertension on regional myocardial blood flow in anesthesized dogs. Am Heart J 1973;85:491–500.

35. Foreman S, Weill H, Duke R, George R, Ziskind M. Bullous disease of the lung: physiologic im-

provement after surgery. Ann Intern Med 1980;93:391–398.

36. Furchgott RF, Zawadski JV. The obligatory role of endothelial cells in the relaxation of arterial smooth muscle by acetylcholine. Nature (Lond) 1980;288:373–376.

37. Fuster V, Steele PM, Edwards WD, Gersh BJ, McGoon MD, Frye RL. Primary pulmonary hypertension: natural history and the importance of thrombosis. Circulation 1984;70:580–587.

38. Gentzler R, Briselli J, Gault J. Angiographic estimation of right ventricular volume in man. Circulation 1974;50:324–330.

39. Glantz SA, Misbach GA, Moores WY, Mathey DG, Lekven J, Stowe DF, Parmley WW, Tyberg JV. The pericardium substantially affects the left ventricular diastolic pressure volume relationship in the dog. Circ Res 1978;42:433–441.

40. Glazier JB, Murray JF. Sites of pulmonary vasomotor reactivity in the dog during alveolar hypoxia and serotonin and histamine infusion. J Clin Invest 1971;50:2550–2580.

41. Gold FL, Bache RJ. Transmural right ventricular blood flow during acute pulmonary artery hypertension in the sedated dog. Circ Res 1982;51:196–204.

42. Goldring RA, Turino GM, Cohen G, Jameson AG, Bass BG, Fishman AP. The catecholamines in the pulmonary arterial pressor response to acute hypoxia. J Clin Invest 1964;41:1211–1220.

43. Greene R, Zapol WM, Snider MT, Reid L, Snow R, O'Connell RS, Novelline RA. Early bedside detection of pulmonary vascular occlusion during acute respiratory failure. Am Rev Respir Dis 1981;124:593–601.

44. Grimm DJ, Dawson CA, Hakin TS, Linehan JH. Pulmonary vasomotion and the distribution of vascular resistance in a dog lung lobe. J Appl Physiol 1978;45:545–550.

45. Grossman W, Braunwald E. Pulmonary hypertension in heart disease. In: Braunwald E, ed. A textbook of cardiovascular medicine. 3rd ed. Philadelphia: WB Saunders, 1988:793.

46. Groves BM, Rubin LJ, Frosolono MF, Cato AE, Reeves JT. A comparison of the acute hemodynamic effects of prostacyclin and hydralazine in primary pulmonary hypertension. Am Heart J 1985;110:1200–1204.

47. Hales CA, Kazemi H. Role of histamine in the hypoxic vascular response of the lung. Resp Physiol 1975;24:81–88.

48. Hales CA, Rouse ET, Kazemi H. Failure of saralasin acetate, a competitive inhibitor of angiotensin II, to diminish alveolar hypoxic vasoconstriction in the dog. Cardiovasc Res 1977;11:541–546.

49. Hales CA, Rouse ET, Slate JL. Influence of aspirin and indomethacin on variability of alveolar hypoxic vasoconstriction. J Appl Physiol 1978;45:33–39.

50. Hamman JW, Smith PK, McHale PA, Vanbenthuysen KM, Anderson RW. Analysis of pulsatile pulmonary artery blood flow in the unanesthetized dog. J Appl Physiol 1981;50:805–813.

51. Harris P. Influence of acetylcholine on the pulmonary arterial pressures. Br Heart J 1957;9:272–278.

52. Harris P, Fritts HW Jr, Cournand A. Some circulatory effects of 5-hydroxytryptamine in man. Circulation 1969;21:1134–1139.

53. Hauge A, Melmon KL. Role of histamine in hypoxic pulmonary hypertension in the rat. II. Depletion of histamine, serotonin and catecholamines. Circ Res 1968;22:385–392.

54. Holcroft JW, Vossar MJ, Weber CJ. Prostaglandin E_1 and survival in patients with the adult distress syndrome. Ann Surg 1986;203:371–380.

55. Hughes JMB. Pulmonary circulation and fluid balance. In: Widdicombe JG, ed. Respiratory physiology II. Baltimore: University Park Press, 1977:135–183.

56. Kadowitz PJ, Hyman AL. Differential effects of prostaglandins A_1 and A_2 on pulmonary vascular resistance in the dog. Proc Soc Exp Biol Med 1975;149:282–286.

57. Kadowitz PJ, Joiner PD, Hyman AL. Effect of sympathetic nerve stimulation on pulmonary vascular resistance in the intact spontaneously breathing dog. Proc Soc Exp Biol Med 1974;147:68–71.

58. Kanemoto N, Furunya H, Etoh T, Sasamoto H, Matsuyama S. Chest roentgenograms in primary pulmonary hypertension. Chest 1979;76:45–49.

59. Kay HR, Afshari M, Barash P, et al. Measurement of ejection fraction by thermal dilution techniques. J Surg Res 1983;38:337–346.

60. Kelly DT, Spotnitz HM, Beiser GD, Pierce JE, Epstein SE. Effects of chronic right ventricular volume and pressure loading on left ventricular performance. Circulation 1971;44:403–412.

61. Kingsma I, Tyberg JV, Smith ER. Effects of diastolic trans-septal pressure gradient on ventricular septal position and motion. Circulation 1983;68:1304–1314.

62. Klinke WP, Gilbert JAL. Diazoxide in primary pulmonary hypertension. N Engl J Med 1980;302:91–93.

63. Konstam MA, Cohen SR, Salem DN, Das D, Arnovitz MJ, Brockway BA. Effect of amrinone on right ventricular function: predominance of afterload reduction. Circulation 1986;74:359–366.

64. Kopolovic R, Thrailkile KM, Martin DT, et al. A critical comparison of the hematologic, cardiovascular and pulmonary response to steroids and non-steroid anti-inflammatory drugs in a model of sepsis and adult respiratory distress syndrome. Surgery 1986;100:679–688.

65. Kuida H. Pulmonary hypertension: mechanism and recognition in the heart. In: Hurst JW, ed. The heart. 6th ed. New York: McGraw-Hill, 1986:1091–1098.

66. Kuida, Hiroshi. Primary and secondary pulmonary hypertension: Pathophysiology, recognition and treatment. In: Hurst JW, ed. The heart. 7th ed. New York: McGraw-Hill, 1990:1196.

67. Lee KY, Molloy DW, Slykerman L, et al. Effects of hydralazine and nitroprusside on cardiopulmonary function when a decrease in cardiac output complicates a short-term increase in pulmonary vascular resistance. Circulation 1983;68:1299–1303.

68. Lloyd TC Jr. Influence of blood pH on hypoxic

pulmonary vasoconstriction. J Appl Physiol 1966;21:358–364.

69. Lloyd TC Jr. Respiratory system compliance as seen from the cardiac fossa. J Appl Physiol 1982:53:57–62.

70. Lopez-Muniz R, Stephens NL, Bromberger-Barnea B, Permutt S, Riley RL. Critical closure of pulmonary vessels analyzed in terms of Starling Resistor model. J Appl Physiol 1968;24:625–635.

71. Malik AB, Kidd BSL. Independent effects of changes in $H+$ and CO_2 concentrations on hypoxic pulmonary vasoconstriction. J Appl Physiol 1973;34:318–324.

72. Malik AB, Kidd BSL. Adrenergic blockade and the pulmonary vascular response to hypoxia. Res Physiol 1973;19:96–106.

73. Malik AB, Van der Zee H. Mechanism of pulmonary edema induced by microembolization in dogs. Circ Res 1978;43:72–79.

74. McMurtry IF, Davidson AB, Reeves JT, Grover RF. Inhibition of hypoxic pulmonary vasoconstriction by calcium antagonists in isolated rat lungs. Circ Res 1976;38:99–104.

75. McMurtry IF, Rounds S, Stanbrook HS. Studies of the mechansim of hypoxic pulmonary vasoconstriction. Adv Shock Res 1982;8:21–33.

76. McMurtry IF, Stanbrook HS, Rounds S. The mechanism of hypoxic pulmonary vasoconstriction: a working hypothesis. In: Loeppky JA, Riedesel ML, eds. Oxygen transport to human tissues. New York: Elsevier North Holland Inc, 1982:77–89.

77. Milic-Emili J, Siafakas NM. The nature of zone 4 in regional distribution of pulmonary blood flow. In: Cumming G, Bonsignoie G, eds. Pulmonary circulation in health and disease. New York: Plenum, 1980:211–224.

78. Milnor WR, Bergel DH, Bargainer CJD. Hydraulic power associated with pulmonary blood flow and its relation to heart rate. Circ Res 1966;19:467–480.

79. Mitzner W. Resistance of the pulmonary circulation in cardiovascular-pulmonary interaction in normal and diseased lungs. Clin Chest Med 1983;43:127–138.

80. Nagasaka Y, Akuisu H, Lee YS, Fugimoto S, Chikamori J. Longterm favourable effects of oxygen administration on a patient with primary pulmonary hypertension. Chest 1978;74:299–300.

81. Nagasaka Y, Bhattacharya J, Cgopper MA, Staub NC. Micropuncture measurement of lung microvascular pressure profile during hypoxia in cats. Fed Proc 1983;42:595.

82. Ogletree ML, Brigham KL. Effects of cyclooxygenase inhibitors on pulmonary vascular responses to endotoxin in unanaesthetized sheep. Prostaglandins Leukotrienes Med 1982;8:489–502.

83. Packer M. Vasodilator therapy for primary pulmonary hypertension. Ann Intern Med 1985;103:258–270.

84. Patel DJ, Defreitas FM, Fry DL. Hydraulic input impedance to aorta and pulmonary artery in dogs. J Appl Physiol 1963;18:134–146.

85. Pearl RG, Rosenthal MH, Ashton JPA. Pulmonary vasodilator effects of nitroglycerin and so-dium nitroprusside in canine oleic acid-induced pulmonary hypertension. Anesthesiology 1983;58:514–518.

86. Permutt S, Riley RL. Hemodynamics of collapsible vessels with tone: the vascular waterfall. J Appl Physiol 1963;18:924–932.

87. Pinsky MR. Determinants of pulmonary artery flow variation during respiration. J Appl Physiol 1984;56:1237–1245.

88. Prewitt RL, Leffler CW. Feline hypoxic pulmonary vasoconstriction is not blocked by the angiotensin I-converting enzyme inhibitor, captopril. Cardiovasc Pharmacol 1981;3:293–298.

89. Prewitt RM, Ghignone M. Treatment of right ventricular dysfunction in acute respiratory failure. Crit Care Med 1983;11:346–352.

90. Prielipp RC, Rosenthal MH, Pearl RG. Hemodynamic profiles of prostaglandin E_1, isoproterenol, prostacyclin, and nifedipine in vasoconstrictor pulmonary hypertension in sheep. Anesth Analg 1988;67:722–729.

91. Rich S, Brundage BH. High dose calcium channel-blocking therapy for primary pulmonary hypertension: evidence for long term reduction in pulmonary artery pressure and regression of right ventricular hypertrophy. Circulation 1987;76:135–141.

92. Rich S, Brundage BH, Levy PS. The effect of vasodilator therapy on the clinical outcome of patients with primary pulmonary hypertension. Circulation 1985;72:1191–1196.

93. Rounds S, McMurtry IF. Inhibitors of oxidative ATP production cause transient vasoconstriction and block subsequent pressor responses in rat lungs. Circ Res 1981;48:393–400.

94. Rubin LJ, Mendoza J, Hood M, et al. Treatment of primary pulmonary hypertension with continuous intravenous Prostacyclin. Ann Intern Med 1990;112:485–491.

95. Rubin LJ, Nicod P, Hills LD, Firth BG. Treatment of primary pulmonary hypertension with nifedipine. A hemodynamic and scintigraphic evaluation. Ann Intern Med 1983;99:433–438.

96. Rubin LJ, Peter RH. Oral hydralazine therapy for primary pulmonary hypertension. N Engl J Med 1980;302:69–73.

97. Rudolph AM, Yuan S. Response to the pulmonary vasculature to hypoxia and $H+$ ion concentration changes. J Clin Invest 1966;45:399–411.

98. Sautter RD, Myers WO, Ray JF III, Wenzel FJ. Pulmonary embolectomy. Review and Current Status. Prog Cardiovasc Dis 1975;17:371–389.

99. Scharf SM, Warner KG, Josa M, et al. Load tolerance of the right ventricle: effect of increased aortic pressure. J Crit Care 1986;3:163–173.

100. Schiller NB. Pulmonary artery pressure estimation by Doppler and two-dimensional echocardiography. Cardiology Clin 1990;8:277–288.

101. Shettigar VR, Hultgren HN, Specter M, Martin R, Davies DH. Primary hypertension: favourable effect of isoproterenol. N Engl J Med 1978;295:1414–1415.

102. Sibbald WJ, Paterson NA, Holliday RL, Anderson RA, Lobb TR, Duff JH. Pulmonary hypertension in sepsis: measurement by the pulmonary arterial diastolic-pulmonary wedge pressure

gradient and the influence of passive and active factors. Chest 1978;73:583–591.

103. Silove Ed, Grover RF. Effects of alpha adrenergic blockade and tissue catecholamine depletion on pulmonary vascular responses to hypoxia. J Clin Invest 1968;47:274–285.

104. Simonneau G, Escourrou P, Duroux P, Lockhart A. Inhibition of hypoxic pulmonary vasoconstruction by nifedipine. N Engl J Med 1981;304:1582–1585.

105. Smith PK, Tyson GS, Hammon JW, Olsen CO, Hopkins RA, Maier GW, Sabiston DC, Rankin JS. Cardiovascular effects of ventilation with positive end-expiratory pressure. Ann Surg 1982;95:121–131.

106. Stanbrook HS, McMurtry IF. Inhibition of glycolysis potentiates hypoxic vasoconstriction in rat lungs. J Appl Physiol 1983;55:1467–1473.

107. Stanbrook HS, Morris KG, McMurtry IF. Prevention and reversal of hypoxic pulmonary hypertension by calcium antagonists. Am Rev Respir Dis 1984;130:81–85.

108. Stool EW, Mullin CB, Leshin SJ, Mitchell JH. Dimensional changes of the left ventricle during acute pulmonary arterial hypertension in dogs. Am J Cardiol 1974;33:868–875.

109. Sylvester JT, McGowen C. The effects of agents that bind to cytochrome P-450 on hypoxic pulmonary vasoconstriction. Circ Res 1978;43:429–437.

110. Tomashefski JF, Davies P, Boggis C, et al. The pulmonary vascular lesions of the adult respiratory syndrome. Am J Pathol 1983;112:112–126.

111. Tucker A, McMurtry IF, Grover RF, Reeves JT. Attenuation of hypoxic pulmonary vasoconstriction by verapamil in intact dogs. Proc Soc Exp Biol Med 1976;151:611–614.

112. Tucker A, Weir EK, Reeves JT, Grover RF. Failure of histamine antagonists to prevent hypoxic pulmonary vasoconstriction in dogs. J Appl Physiol 1976;40:496–500.

113. Urokinase Pulmonary Embolism Trial. Circulation 1973;47(suppl 2):1.

114. Urokinase-Streptokinase Embolism Trial. Phase 2 results: a cooperative study. JAMA 1974;229:1606–1613.

115. Vaage J, Bjertnaes L, Hauge A. The pulmonary vasoconstrictor response to hypoxia: effects of inhibitors of prostaglandin biosynthesis. Acta Physiol Scand 1975;95:95–101.

116. Vaage J, Hauge A. Prostaglandins and the pulmonary vasconstrictor response to alveolar hypoxia. Science 1975;189:899–900.

117. Viamonte M, Parks RE, Barrera F. Roentgenographic prediction of pulmonary hypertension in mitral stenosis. Am J Roentgenol 1962;87:936–947.

118. Visner MS, Arentzen CE, O'Conner MJ, Larson EV, Anderson RW. Alterations in left ventricular three-dimensional dynamic geometry and systolic function during acute right ventricular hypertension in the conscious dog. Circulation 1983;67:353–365.

119. Vlahakes GJ, Turley K, Hoffman JIE, et al. The pathophysiology of failure in acute right ventricular hypertension. Hemodynamic and biochemical correlations. Circulation 1981;63:87–95.

120. Weir EK, McMurtry IF, Tucker A, Reeves JT, Grover RF. Prostaglandin synthetase inhibitors do not decrease hypoxic pulmonary vasoconstriction. J Appl Physiol 1976;41:714–718.

121. Weir EK, McMurtry IF, Tucker A, Reeves JT, Grover RF. Inhibition of prostaglandin synthesis or blockade of prostaglandin action increase the pulmonary pressor response to hypoxia. In: Samuelsson B, Paoletti R, eds. Advances in Prostaglandin and Thromboxane Research. Vol. 2. New York: Raven Press, 1976:914–915.

122. Weir EK, Will DH, Alexander AF, McMurtry IF, Looga R, Reeves JT, Grover RF. Vascular hypertrophy in cattle susceptible to hypoxic pulmonary hypertension. J Appl Physiol 1979;46:517–521.

123. West JB, Dollery CT. Distribution of blood flow and the pressure-flow relations of the whole lung. J Appl Physiol 1965;20:175–183.

124. West JB, Dollery CT, Naimark A. Distribution of blood flow in isolated lung: relation to vascular and alveolar pressures. J Appl Physiol 1964;19:713–724.

125. Winn R, Harlan J, Nadir B, et al. Thromboxane A_2 mediates lung vasoconstriction but not permeability after endotoxin. J Clin Invest 1983;72:911–918.

126. Young TE, Lundquist LJ, Chesler E, Weir EK. Comparative effects of nifedipine, verapamil and diltiazem on experimental pulmonary hypertension. Am J Cardiol 1983;51:195–200.

127. Zapol W, Snider MI. Pulmonary hypertension in severe acute respiratory failure. N Engl J Med 1977;296:476–480.

20

Cardiac Tamponade

William M. Davies
Martin LeWinter

ANATOMIC CONSIDERATIONS

The pericardium is a tough, fibrous sac that encloses the heart within a thin film of lubricating, serous fluid (Fig. 20.1) (1). The outer fibrous layer of the parietal pericardium is composed of interlacing collagen and elastin, rendering it relatively noncompliant. The inner layer of the parietal pericardium is a serous membrane lined with mesothelial cells, and is continuous with the serous visceral pericardium that overlies the epicardium.

The collagenous parietal pericardium blends with the adventitia of the great arteries, sealing the heart within its sac at the base. Two inner recesses or sinuses extend from the pericardial space within the pericardial sac. The oblique sinus extends behind the left atrium, and is bounded by the pulmonary veins and inferior vena cava. The transverse sinus extends between the anterior surface of the atria and posterior surface of the great arteries. There are ligamentous attachments of the pericardium to the sternum anteriorly and the diaphragm inferiorly. This architecture supports and confines the heart to the protected interior of the chest cavity (26).

There is normally up to 50 ml of fluid in the pericardial space, secreted by vis-

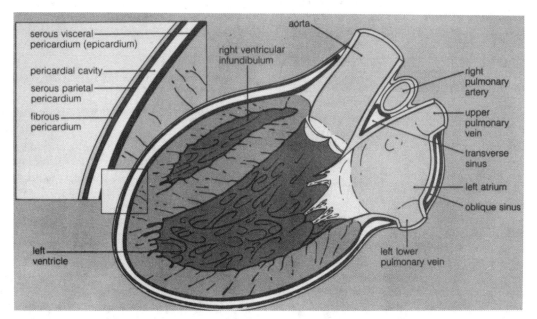

Figure 20.1. Anatomic aspects of the pericardiectomy and its relation to the heart and great vessels. (From Anderson RH, Wilcox BR, Becker AF. Anatomy of the normal heart. In: Hurst JW, ed. Atlas of the heart. New York: Gower Medical Publishing, 1988:1.2–1.20.

ceral pericardial cells. The fluid drains via the parietal layer to the thoracic lymph duct, and through the right pleural space to the right lymphatic duct (26).

NORMAL PERICARDIAL PHYSIOLOGY

The force distending the cardiac chambers is the transmural pressure. This force is the difference between intracavity pressure and pericardial pressure. In some prior investigations, the pericardial pressure was measured with open-ended, fluid-filled catheters. Under these conditions, the measured pressure is close to zero regardless of the cardiac volume, and essentially identical to the adjacent pleural pressure (48). More recently, however, it has become clear that the parietal pericardium exerts a significant radial stress on the surface of the heart, which is proportional to the volume of the heart (61). When this "contact pressure" is measured with flat balloons, which are more appropriate for this purpose than catheters, it is found to be significantly positive, which is consistent with the downward shifts of the intracavitary diastolic pressure-volume relations of both ventricles that are observed following pericardiectomy (55). In other words, the pericardium can significantly restrain the cardiac volume. Under normal physiologic conditions, the volume of the heart is most likely either less than or at the lower range of the stressed volume of the pericardium. Even under these conditions, the magnitude of the pericardial "contact pressure" may not be trivial in relation to the right heart filling pressure (21).

Under pathologic conditions, pericardial restraint can have several important consequences. Cardiac chamber compliance decreases dramatically once cardiac volume begins to exceed the nonstressed pericardial volume since further incremental increases in chamber volume must distend the tough pericardial sac. Cardiac chamber volume, therefore, is restricted to small increments above the nonstressed pericardial volume despite major increases in cavitary filling pressure (59). From a teleologic perspective, this pericardial limit

on cardiac volume expansion may prevent traumatic rupture, but it can result in high ventricular filling pressures in pathologic conditions associated with acute or subacute volume overload.

A second important consequence of pericardial restraint is augmentation of diastolic ventricular interaction. Ventricular interaction refers to the influence of one ventricle on the compliance and filling pressure of the other. This occurs, in part, because the ventricles share a common wall, the interventricular septum. In addition, the pericardial sac places an upper limit on total heart volume, and a large increase in the volume of one chamber may cause the total cardiac volume to exceed the nonstressed pericardial volume such that the compliance of the other chambers is decreased. In acute right ventricular infarction with right ventricular dilation, for example, right ventricular filling occurs at the expense of the left ventricle, resulting in decreased left ventricular chamber compliance (20). This diastolic competition between the ventricles is present even at normal filling volumes, but becomes progressively more important as filling volume increases (62). It is of major importance in the pathophysiology of cardiac tamponade due to compression of the cardiac chambers by the pericardial effusion.

PATHOPHYSIOLOGY AND HEMODYNAMICS OF "CLASSIC" CARDIAC TAMPONADE

Cardiac tamponade can be defined as pathologic restraint of cardiac filling due to increased pericardial pressure, caused by the accumulation of fluid in the pericardial space. By "classic" tamponade, we refer to the pathophysiologic changes seen when an otherwise normal heart is compressed by a circumferential pericardial effusion under uniform pressure.

The central element of tamponade pathophysiology is that as fluid accumulates in the pericardial space, the pericardial presure rises, resulting in a decrease in transmural pressure and, therefore, decreased chamber volumes. The increased pericardial pressure is transmitted to the cardiac chambers, resulting in increased intracavitary filling pressure despite the abnormally small chamber volumes. Despite a number of compensatory mechanisms, if the pericardial pressure continues to increase, the reduced diastolic chamber volume and consequent reduced utilization of the Frank-Starling mechanism eventually result in a decreased cardiac output (45) and, ultimately, progressive circulatory shock.

The pericardial pressure-volume relation plays a key role in the pathophysiology of tamponade. As shown in Figure 20.2, the relation is very flat at low volumes, but makes a relatively abrupt transition to a steep slope at higher volumes, reflecting a marked decrease in compliance. Since it is the pericardial pressure (not the volume) that influences cardiac filling, a certain amount of pericardial fluid is well tolerated, but small additional increments can cause large increases in pressure and rapid clinical deterioration.

The direct compressive effect of increased pericardial pressure is mainly exerted on the right heart chambers and caval vessels, while left heart performance is depressed primarily in a secondary fashion because it is underfilled by the right heart (11, 13). This is probably related to the higher right compared to left ventricular compliance, the fact that a portion of the left atrium is extrapericardial, and the

fact that the caval vessels have rather long intrapericardial segments.

During cardiac tamponade, a number of compensatory factors help maintain cardiac output and vital organ perfusion. The retarded filling of the right heart results in a shift of blood volume from the pulmonary to systemic circulation, which in turn elevates the mean systemic pressure and tends to restore right heart venous return toward normal. Baroreceptor and sympathetic activation lead to augmented heart rate and contractility and vasoconstriction to maintain cardiac output and systemic blood pressure. Renin and angiotensin release also contribute to vasoconstriction, and augmented aldosterone release enhances sodium and water retention. Atrial natriuretic peptide secretion is suppressed because chamber distention is decreased, which further facilitates sodium and water retention (27, 42). In cardiac tamponade, salt and water retention is useful because it tends to increase intravascular and cardiac chamber volume.

In addition to the rather unusual combination of small cardiac volume and high intracavitary filling pressures, there are a number of other notable pathophysiologic and hemodynamic features of cardiac tamponade. Normally, right heart filling pressures are lower than left heart filling pressures. As tamponade progresses, intracavitary filling pressure increases faster on the right than on the left side. Eventually, left- and right-sided intracavitary filling pressures become equal (typically 15–20 mm Hg) and virtually identical to the pericardial pressure, i.e., the transmural filling pressures approach zero (45, 52). Equalization of filling pressures is one of the hemodynamic hallmarks of tamponade. At some point, pericardial pressure actually begins to exceed intracavitary chamber pressure at certain times during the cardiac cycle, resulting in transient collapse of the right ventricle in diastole and invagination of the right atrium. The latter observations are consistent with the concept that compression is more pronounced in the right heart.

In tamponade, the restraining effects of the high pericardial pressure cause the total cardiac volume to become effectively

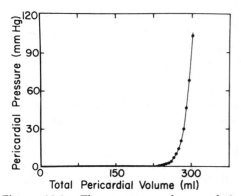

Figure 20.2. The pressure-volume relationship as fluid is injected into the pericardial space. (From Holt JP. The normal pericardium. Am J Cardiol 1970;26:455–465.)

fixed. As a result, blood can only enter the atria when it simultaneously exits the ventricles, i.e., during ejection. The hemodynamic counterpart of this effect is abbreviation and ultimately obliteration of the y descent of right atrial or jugular venous pressure waveform (58).

Respiratory variation in right heart filling is exaggerated in tamponade. The inspiratory decrease in pleural pressure greatly facilitates right heart filling under conditions of marginal chamber distension and elevated central venous pressure. As the right ventricle fills, the fixed total cardiac volume dictates that expansion of the right ventricle must occur at the expense of filling of the left ventricle (57). In addition, there is an inspiratory decrease in the pressure gradient driving left heart filling because the inspiratory decrease in pleural pressure is transmitted to the pulmonary veins, but less so to the pericardium and left heart chambers (3). Both of these effects result in an exaggeration of the normal reciprocal relationship between right and left ventricular performance during inspiration. This is especially prominent on the left, where stroke volume during inspiration is strikingly reduced during severe tamponade. The hemodynamic and clinical counterpart is the paradoxical pulse, a decrease of 12 mm Hg or more in systolic blood pressure during normal inspiration.

In summary, "classic" cardiac tamponade is marked by:

1. Elevated and equal diastolic chamber pressures that are approximately equal to the pericardial pressure.
2. Severely restricted diastolic filling such that (a) blood can only enter the atria during ventricular ejection, and (b) there is competition between the ventricles for diastolic filling that magnifies the small variation normally seen with respiration, and is manifested as pulsus paradoxus.
3. Decreased cardiac output with tachycardia, peripheral vasoconstriction, and increased sodium/water retention that may progress to frank shock.

DEVIATIONS FROM CLASSIC CARDIAC TAMPONADE PATHOPHYSIOLOGY

Several conditions that are commonly encountered in an intensive care unit setting may alter the pathophysiology of classic cardiac tamponade. The presence of preexisting structural heart disease is one example. If left ventricular diastolic pressure is severely elevated, critical right heart compression can occur before pericardial pressure approaches left ventricular filling pressure, and pulsus paradoxus may be absent. This has been described in patients with severe aortic regurgitation, and with left ventricular dysfunction and renal failure (22, 52). Conversely, if right ventricular diastolic pressure is severely elevated, left heart compression may occur before pericardial pressure approaches right-sided diastolic pressure, as has been described in the setting of severe primary pulmonary hypertension (15). If a large atrial septal defect is present, pulsus paradoxus may be absent because the inspiratory augmentation of systemic venous return may also be distributed to the left heart via right-to-left shunting (65). In severe aortic stenosis, increased respiratory variation of left ventricular systolic pressure may be present, but not transmitted to the aortic or arterial pressures (35). Patients with severe chest wall trauma or neuromuscular disease may fail to show pulsus paradoxus because they are unable to develop the normal changes in intrathoracic pressure with respiration. Positive pressure mechanical ventilation reverses the normal respiratory changes (33).

Regional tamponade may occur secondary to a localized intrapericardial hematoma or a loculated effusion, an especially important problem in postcardiac surgical patients. If tamponade is isolated to the right-sided chambers, right-sided diastolic pressure increases with pericardial pressure, but left atrial pressure decreases, associated with a decreased stroke volume and systemic blood pressure. If tamponade is isolated to the left-sided chambers, systemic blood pressure is usually relatively preserved, but stroke volume can drop in association with peripheral vasoconstriction. Left-sided filling pressure rises with pericardial pressure, but right atrial pressure does not. In both cases, diastolic equalization and pulsus paradoxus are absent (14).

Low-pressure tamponade refers to tamponade in the setting of modestly elevated or even normal filling pressures (2). In this situation, pericardial pressure is only modestly elevated, but transmural chamber distending pressures are very low because of relative intravascular volume depletion. Pulsus paradoxus may also be absent. This condition is typically seen in patients undergoing renal dialysis, and in patients with malignant or tuberculous effusions who may be dehydrated. A cautious fluid challenge will often unmask the more classic findings of tamponade as the intravascular volume returns to normal.

There are also substantial numbers of patients with a disease process producing both a hemodynamically significant effusion and constrictive pericarditis, the so-called subacute effusive-constrictive pericarditis. A complete description of these patients is beyond the scope of this chapter. The pathophysiology and resulting hemodynamics can be complex, but generally reflect tamponade physiology before pericardiocentesis. After drainage of the effusion and normalization of pericardial pressure, the hemodynamics reflect pericardial constriction (23).

ETIOLOGY OF CARDIAC TAMPONADE

Virtually any cause of pericarditis and/or pericardial effusion can cause tamponade (Table 20). Tamponade can also occur as the result of hemorrhage into the pericardial sac. The most frequently encountered causes in medical patients are malignancy, renal failure, and idiopathic/viral pericarditis (3, 38, 43).

Malignancies may extend locally to the pericardium, form nodular pericardial deposits via hematogenous or lymphatic dissemination, or infiltrate the pericardium, causing local or diffuse thickening. Adenocarcinomas of the lung and breast, lymphomas, and leukemias are the most common culprits (19). Tumors that invade superior mediastinal lymph nodes may cause pericardial effusion by impeding lymphatic drainage (44). Occasionally, a previously occult malignancy may be present with cardiac tamponade (24).

Idiopathic/viral pericarditis is responsible for approximately 20% of all pericarditis cases (3, 38, 43). Coxsackie virus group

Table 20.1
Etiology of Cardiac Tamponade

Medical illness
  Common
    Malignancy
    Renal failure
    Idiopathic/viral pericarditis
  Less common
    Postradiation therapy
    Rheumatoid arthritis
    Hypothyroidism
    Systemic lupus
    Myocardial infarction with ventricular
      rupture; with thrombolytic therapy
    Tuberculosis
    AIDS
    Anticoagulant therapy and coagulopathy
    Purulent pericarditis
Surgical/traumatic conditions
  Invasive cardiac procedures with perforation
  Cardiovascular surgery
  Postpericardiotomy syndrome
  Multitrauma
  Aortic dissection

B has been identified as a specific etiologic agent (5), but a variety of other viruses have been associated with pericarditis. It is believed that many cases of idiopathic pericarditis are in fact caused by undiagnosed viral infections.

Renal failure/uremia cause 10–12% of tamponade in medical patients (3, 38, 43). Uremic pericarditis results in a hemorrhagic, fibrinous exudate with little inflammatory cellular reaction. The precise cause of the pericarditis is not clear. Although uremic pericarditis has been viewed primarily as a complication of severe renal failure and tends to improve with institution or increased frequency of dialysis, there is not a good correlation between severity and the level of uremic metabolites, and progressive pericarditis and tamponade can occur despite intense dialysis. In contrast, low-pressure tamponade typically occurs in patients undergoing chronic dialysis who have low BUN/creatinine (53). Tamponade is also a well-recognized complication of AIDS-related heart disease (12, 63).

CLINICAL PRESENTATION

The clinical presentation of pericarditis is influenced by the underlying etiology, presence of other heart or lung disease, and especially by the rapidity of accumulation of the fluid. The normal, unstretched pericardium can accommodate rapid accumulation of 80–300 ml before the stressed pericardial volume is reached and pericardial pressure rises rapidly (48). Among the medical causes of tamponade, purulent (bacterial) pericarditis is notable for the rapidity with which tamponade can occur (56). If fluid accumulates slowly over weeks to months, much larger amounts can be accommodated. The mechanism of this accommodation is unclear, but may include actual growth of the pericardium (39).

With tamponade caused by acute, severe intrapericardial hemorrhage, the patient will present in severe shock with the triad of decreased systemic arterial pressure, elevated central venous pressure, and a small, quiet heart (4). If the pericardial fluid accumulates more slowly, as occurs with most medical etiologies of tamponade, the pericardial volume will enlarge, and there usually is sufficient compensation to produce a less critical hemodynamic condition. In this more common situation, a cardinal symptom of tamponade is dyspnea, usually with orthopnea (3). Indeed, patients with tamponade almost invariably prefer sitting forward because of the apparent orthopnea and/or because they may also have pericardial pain. To the extent that the cardiac output is impaired, patients will manifest a number of systemic symptoms and signs, including fatigue, a low-output syndrome and, ultimately, shock. The elevated central venous pressure may produce peripheral edema.

With a large pericardial effusion, there may be symptoms secondary to mechanical compression of adjacent structures. Lung compression and atelectasis cause dyspnea, bronchial and tracheal compression cause coughing, dysphagia may result from esophageal compression, while hiccoughs or hoarseness may be caused by pressure on the phrenic or recurrent laryngeal nerves. If pericarditis is present, chest pain may be a prominent complaint. Such pain is ordinarily variable in location and quality, but is almost always pleuritic and relieved by sitting forward. Radiation of chest pain to the trapezius ridge is virtually specific for pericarditis.

Physical findings usually include elevated jugular venous pressure, unless the patient is hypovolemic. The y descent of the jugular venous presure is diminished or absent. The majority of patients have tachycardia and tachypnea. Pulsus paradoxus is ordinarily present, but may be absent in the circumstances described previously (3, 43). There is a rough correlation between the magnitude of pulsus paradoxus and the severity of tamponade (10). The precordium is usually quiet and the point of maximal impulse is difficult or impossible to identify. Heart sounds are frequently reduced in intensity. A pericardial friction rub is present in only about one-third of patients with tamponade (3, 43). Depending on the degree of hemodynamic compromise, there may be overt peripheral vasoconstriction with coolness and pallor of the extremities, and peripheral cyanosis. Sympathetic nervous system activation may result in diaphoresis. Urine output may be diminished, and the sensorium may be clouded (43).

The chest x-ray often shows an enlarged cardiac silhouette, but change in heart size can be remarkably subtle with rapidly accumulating fluid. The lung fields typically are oligemic, consistent with a pulmonary-to-systemic blood volume shift, unless there is associated pulmonary disease or vascular congestion from coexisting heart disease. Electrocardiographic changes are nonspecific and include reduced voltage and electrical alternans. All of the changes of pericarditis can also be present (3, 43).

DIAGNOSIS

The differential diagnosis of a patient presenting with acute or subacute dyspnea, elevated venous pressure, and clear lung fields can be divided into cardiac etiologies, which include tamponade, constrictive pericarditis, right ventricular infarction, and restrictive cardiomyopathy, and pulmonary categories, which include pulmonary embolism, tension pneumothorax, and obstructive lung disease with cor pulmonale. When this constellation is present in conjunction with a paradoxic pulse and enlarged cardiac silhouette, tamponade should be the leading diagnosis (3, 43). If it is difficult to assess the venous pressure, or there is coexisting disease that has produced lung field opacities or infiltration, the differential diagnosis is much wider, and cardiac tamponade can easily be missed. Cardiac tamponade should always be considered as a possible etiology of unexplained hemodynamic deterioration, particularly in patients with renal failure, malignancy, chest trauma, or who have had recent cardiac surgery or invasive cardiac procedures.

The most useful noninvasive test to screen for and determine the severity of cardiac tamponade is echocardiography (33). This procedure can be performed rapidly at the bedside. With the advent of transesophageal echocardiography, excellent imaging can be obtained in virtually all patients, including the critically ill in whom transthoracic imaging may be severely limited. Echocardiography is gener ally quite sensitive for detecting pericardial effusion. Circumferential effusions are rarely missed, but pericardial hematomas or loculated hemorrhagic effusions may occur in the postcardiac surgery setting and are not as easily visualized. Blood that is static tends to appear echogenic, rather than echo free, and may result in underestimation of hemopericardium (40). Tamponading hematomas localized to an atrial chamber may be missed unless good images are obtained and the heart is carefully explored (17). Transesophageal echocardiography is especially helpful in postoperative situations in which sternal incisions and positive pressure mechanical ventilation place major limits on the quality of standard transthoracic studies. Computed axial tomography may accurately delineate localized pericardial hematomas, but is costly and less convenient. The specificity of echocardiography is quite high, particularly with the uniform use of two-dimensional imaging. Occasionally, subepicardial adipose tissue may mimic a localized anterior effusion (29). Pleural effusions can generally be differentiated from pericardial effusions with two-dimensional imaging in multiple planes.

The absence of a pericardial effusion is extremely helpful in excluding the diagnosis of cardiac tamponade. Although it is possible for an acute intrapericardial hemorrhage to cause tamponade in a patient with a previously thickened, restrictive pericardium without producing what is ordinarily reported as a significant effusion, this is very rare and the diagnostic approach should generally be shifted to other possibilities. The presence of a pericardial effusion does not prove the diagnosis of tamponade. Tamponade is a pathophysiologic and clinical diagnosis, not an anatomic one, since large volumes of pericardial fluid can accumulate slowly without causing an important elevation in pericardial pressure. Pericardial effusions are commonly observed in renal failure, postpericardiotomy snydrome, postmyocardial infarction, and after cardiac surgery, but the percentage that cause tamponade is small (16, 18, 28, 50, 64, 66).

Direct observation of right atrial or ventricular compression with echocardiography has been shown to be helpful in determining the hemodynamic significance of an effusion. Right atrial invagination tends to occur at a lower pericardial pressure than right ventricular collapse, possibly due to lower atrial wall stiffness. Left-sided chamber collapse is rare. The reported sensitivities of right atrial and right ventricular collapse for tamponade are 70–100% and 60–90%, respectively, with specificities of 80–100% (54). The diagnostic value of right ventricular invagination for tamponade appears superior to pulsus paradoxus (31, 60). Chamber invagination may be a key finding in the diagnosis of low-pressure tamponade (34). Since right heart chamber invagination is determined by both chamber and pericardial pressure, it may be absent or delayed if diastolic chamber pressure is significantly elevated (30). This may occur if the chamber is abnormally hypertrophied or noncompliant, or if intravascular volume is significantly increased (15). Localized left heart tamponade is not associated with right chamber collapse. Right heart chamber invagination may occur in the absence of frank tamponade, but this finding indicates that pericardial pressure is elevated relative to chamber pressure, and suggests a pretamponade condition with diminished stroke volume and cardiac output (37, 38).

The diameter of the inferior vena cava and the extent of constriction with deep inspiration have been found to correlate with right atrial and ventricular diastolic pressure (46, 47). The finding of inferior vena cava "plethora," defined as failure of the inferior vena cava to constrict at least 50% with deep inspiration, is a sensitive (>90%), but less specific (40%) sign of tamponade since it is present when central venous pressure is elevated for other reasons (25). Exaggerated inspiratory flow velocity profiles may be measurable with Doppler techniques. An 80% increase in tricuspid inflow velocity in association with a 30% reduction in mitral and aortic flow velocities reflect the physiology of pulsus paradoxus, and therefore suggest tamponade (36). Respiratory variation of the left ventricular inflow profile, isovolumic relaxation time, and hepatic vein flow reversal have also been described (3, 6).

Right heart catheterization with a balloon-tipped pulmonary artery catheter is helpful to confirm the diagnosis of tamponade if the clinical and echo findings are equivocal, and is extremely helpful in subsequent management. In classic tamponade, there is elevation and equalization of right atrial, right ventricular diastolic, pulmonary artery diastolic, and pulmonary capillary wedge pressures to within a few millimeters of mercury (22, 45). The right atrial pressure waveform loses the y descent, while the right ventricle-developed pressure is reduced, paralleling the small stroke volume. In contrast, in constrictive pericarditis, there is also elevation and equalization of filling pressures, but the y descent is exaggerated. Kussmaul's sign, an inspiratory rise in right atrial pressure, is also typical of constriction, but is not present in tamponade (58). Pulsus paradoxus can be quantitated by blood pressure cuff or an arterial pressure tracing. In addition to tamponade, it is observed in about one-third of patients with constrictive pericarditis and in a variety of noncardiac conditions associated with wide variation in intrapleural pressure, most commonly asthma and chronic obstructive lung disease. In the setting of nonclassic tamponade, however, many of these findings may be modified or absent. In this case, the diagnosis requires a high

index of suspicion, a sophisticated hemodynamic and echo-Doppler assessment, and the demonstration of elevated pressure in the pericardial space and clinical improvement following a drainage procedure.

TREATMENT

The only effective treatment of cardiac tamponade is drainage of the pericardial effusion or evacuation of the hematoma. The degree of hemodynamic impairment will dictate the level of urgency. In the setting of impending or ongoing cardiac arrest, prompt blind percutaneous pericardiocentesis via the subxiphoid approach at the bedside may be required to save the patient's life. If at all possible, it is best to perform the procedure with echocardiographic guidance so that the location and accessibility of the effusion can be assessed. The standard subxiphoid approach will be appropriate for many situations, but loculated, posterior effusions may not be accessible without significant risk of ventricular perforation or coronary laceration. Exploration with two-dimensional echocardiography will identify the shortest path to the effusion that avoids intervening lung, myocardium, or abdominal organs (8). Frequently, anterior axillary line (between the seventh and ninth intercostal spaces) or left parasternal approaches permit safe access to the pericardial effusion using a short 2–4 cm 18-gauge intracath needle (7). Once the route has been identified, continuous observation by echo is generally not helpful, but entry into the pericardial space can be confirmed by injection of agitated saline through the needle and visualizing the bubble contract by echocardiography (9). This is particularly helpful if sanguineous fluid is encountered and entry of the right ventricular cavity is suspected. If no safe access to the effusion is identified by echocardiography, surgical drainage may be indicated. Because of the potential for cardiac perforation, arrhythmia, pneumothorax, or coronary laceration, it is essential to proceed with caution, employing ECG and, frequently, hemodynamic monitoring in an intensive care unit or cardiac catheterization laboratory setting, with resuscitation equipment and skilled personnel available. It is also important to obtain a complete laboratory assessment of the pericardial fluid collected, including cultures and stains for bacteria, tuberculosis, and fungi, as well as cytology, cell counts, amylase, glucose, and protein.

In situations where cardiovascular collapse is not imminent, it is optimal to perform pericardiocentesis in the cardiac catheterization laboratory (41). Fluoroscopic guidance can be used to facilitate the placement of a 7 French pigtail catheter in the pericardial space for safer and more complete drainage, and simultaneous high-quality pressure tracings of pericardial and chamber pressures can be obtained to make a definitive diagnosis of tamponade. The pericardial catheter may be left in place for 24–72 hours. An indwelling catheter allows for the assessment of the rate of reaccumulation and the need for a definitive surgical procedure, and avoids repeat pericardiocentesis. Intermittent drainage and heparinized saline flushes have not been found to be effective, even when the catheter is left in place for more than 72 hours (32).

Medical therapy for tamponade is a temporizing measure at best and should not be substituted for or delay pericardiocentesis. Volume expansion should be considered to increase diastolic pressure and prevent chamber collapse. Positive end-expiratory pressure should be minimized to avoid further elevation of pericardial pressure. Inotropic support with isoproterenol or norepinephrine, while usually ineffective, can be attempted for short periods to increase cardiac output and maintain systemic blood pressure. If the patient is on anticoagulant medication, prompt discontinuation or reversal should be considered to minimize intrapericardial hemorrhage.

After initial drainage of the effusion and relief of tamponade, the long-term treatment will depend on the etiology. Pericarditis, postpericardiotomy syndrome, and connective tissue diseases will often respond to antiinflammatory or steroidal medication. Uremic pericarditis usually improves with intensification of hemodialysis. Intrapericardial infusion of chemotherapy or tetracycline has been advocated for malignant effusions, but the support for this approach consists of case reports; others emphasize intensification of systemic chemotherapy for responsive malignancies, complemented by pericardial surgery if necessary (51). Purulent pericarditis, cardiac perforation or rupture, and aortic dissection will require prompt surgical management.

In patients with recurrent, hemodynamically significant effusions, surgery may be necessary to provide long-term relief. Several types of procedures have been developed. A limited pericardiectomy with decompression and evacuation of the pericardial space may be performed from the subxiphoid approach. This technique has the advantage of avoiding a thoracotomy or sternotomy, and may be performed under local anesthesia if the patient is unstable. A more extensive pericardiectomy may be performed via a left thoracotomy approach.

Operative mortality is approximately 5–6% in patients with benign disease, but over 20% in patients with malignancy due to complications of disseminated malignant disease. Long-term success, defined as avoidance of both recurrent effusion or the development of constriction, is directly related to the amount of pericardium left behind. Subxiphoid approaches result in failure in 7–12% of patients, but this procedure is generally tolerated by even critically ill patients. Failure of complete pericardiectomy is very uncommon, but the procedure is more involved and requires a longer period of recuperation. Although there is controversy regarding the use of subxiphoid versus complete pericardiectomy, there is general agreement that in patients in whom long-term survival is expected and are in good overall medical condition, complete pericardiectomy is more effective at preventing symptomatic recurrence of pericardial disease. For patients with advanced malignancy, a bleak long-term prognosis, and poor overall condition in whom temporary palliation is desired, a limited subxiphoid pericardiectomy should be performed if percutaneous drainage fails (49).

References

1. Anderson RH, Wilcox BR, Becker AF. Anatomy of the normal heart. In: Hurst JW, ed. Atlas of the heart. New York: Gower Medical Publishing, 1988;1.2–1.20.

2. Antman EM, Cargill V, Grossman W. Low-pressure cardiac tamponade. Ann Int Med 1979;91:403–406.

3. Appleton CP, Hatle LK, Popp RL. Cardiac tamponade and pericardial effusion: respiratory variation in transvalvular flow velocities studied by Doppler echocardiography. J Am Coll Cardiol 1988;11:1020–1030.

4. Beck CS. Two cardiac compression triads. JAMA 1935;104:714–716.

5. Brodie HR, Marchessault V. Acute benign pericarditis caused by Coxsackie virus group B. N Engl J Med 1960;262:1278–1280.

6. Burstow DJ, On JK, Bailey KR, Seward JB, Tajik AJ. Cardiac tamponade: characteristic Doppler observations. Mayo Clin Proc 1989;64:312–324.

7. Callahan JA, Seward JB, Nishimura RA, Miller FA, Reeder GS, Shub C, Callahan MJ, Schattenberg TT, Tajik AJ. Two-dimensional echocardiographically guided pericardiocentesis in 117 consecutive patients. Am J Cardiol 1985;55:476–479.

8. Callahan JA, Seward JB, Tajik AJ, Holmes DR, Smith HC, Reeder GS, Miller FA. Pericardiocentesis assisted by two-dimensional echocardiography. J Thorac Cardiovasc Surg 1983;85:877–879.

9. Chandraratna PAN, Reid CL, Nimalasuriya A, Kawanishi D, Rahimtoola SH. Application of 2-dimensional contrast studies during pericardiocentesis. Am J Cardiol 1983;52:1120–1122.

10. Curtiss EI, Reddy PS, Uretsky BF, Cecchetti AA. Pulsus paradoxus: definition and relation to the severity of cardiac tamponade. Am Heart J 1988;115:391–398.

11. Ditchey RV, Engler R, LeWinter MM. The role of the right heart in acute cardiac tamponade in dogs. Circ Res 1981;48:701–710.

12. Fink L, Reichek N, St. John Sutton MG. Cardiac abnormalities in acquired immune deficiency syndrome. Am J Cardiol 1984;54:1161–1163.

13. Fowler NO, Gabel M. The hemodynamic effects of cardiac tamponade: mainly the result of atrial, not ventricular compression. Circulation 1985;71:154–157.

14. Fowler NO, Gabel M, Bancher CR. Cardiac tamponade: a comparison of right versus left heart compression. J Am Coll Cardiol 1988;12:187–193.

15. Frey MJ, Berko B, Palevsky H, Hirshfeld JW, Herrmann HC. Recognition of cardiac tamponade in the presence of severe pulmonary hypertension. Ann Int Med 1989;111:615–617.

16. Frommer JP, Young JB, Ayus JC. Asymptomatic pericardial effusion in uremic patients: effect of long-term dialysis. Nephron 1985;39:296–301.

17. Fyke FE, Tancredi RE, Shub C, Julsrud PR, Sheedy PF. Detection of intrapericardial hematoma after open heart surgery: the roles of echocardiography and computed tomography. J Am Coll Cardiol 1985;5:1496–1499.

18. Galve E, Garcia-Del-Castilllo H, Evangelista A, Batlle J, Permanyer-Miralda G, Soler-Soler J. Pericardial effusion in the course of myocardial infarction: incidence, natural history, and clinical relevance. Circulation 1986;73:294–299.

19. Gassman HS, Meadows R, Baker LA. Metastatic tumors of the heart. Am J Med 1955;19:357–365.

20. Goldstein JA, Vlahakes GH, Verrier ED, Schiller NB, Tyberg JV, Ports TA, Parmley WW, Chatterjee K. The role of right ventricular systolic dysfunction and elevated intrapericardial pressure in the genesis of low output in experimental right ventricular infarction. Circulation 1982;65:513–522.

21. Goto Y, LeWinter MM. Nonuniform regional deformation of the pericardium during the cardiac cycle in dogs. Circ Res 1990;67:1107–1114.

22. Guberman BA, Fowler NO, Engel PJ, Gueron M, Allen JM. Cardiac tamponade in medical patients. Circulation 1981;64:633–639.

23. Hancock EW. Subacute effusive-constrictive pericarditis. Circulation 1971;43:183–192.

24. Haskell RJ, French WJ. Cardiac tamponade as the initial presentation of malignancy. Chest 1985;88:70–73.

25. Himelman RB, Kircher B, Rockey DC, Schiller NB. Inferior vena cava plethora with blunted respiratory response: a sensitive echocardiographic sign of tamponade. J Am Coll Cardiol 1988;12:1470–1477.

26. Holt JP. The normal pericardium. Am J Cardiol 1970;26:455–465.

27. Hynynen M, Salmenpera M, Harjula ALS, Tikkanen I, Fyhrquist F, Heinonen J. Atrial pressure and hormonal and renal responses to acute cardiac tamponade. Ann Thorac Surg 1990;49:632–637.

28. Ikaheimo MJ, Heikki HV, Airaksinen KEJ, Korhonen UR, Linnaluoto MK, Tarkka MR, Takkunen JT. Pericardial effusion after cardiac surgery: incidence, relation to the type of surgery, antithrombotic therapy, and early coronary bypass graft patency. Am Heart J 1988;116:97–102.

29. Isner JM, Carter BL, Roberts WC, Bankoff MS. Subepicardial adipose tissue producing echocardiographic appearance of pericardial effusion. Documentation by computed tomography and necropsy. Am J Cardiol 1983;51:565–569.

30. Klopfenstein HS, Cogswell TL, Bernath GA, Wann LS, Tipton RK, Hoffmann RG, Brooks HL, Janzer DJ, Peterson DM. Alterations in intravascular volume affect the relation between right ventricular diastolic collapse and the hemodynamic severity of cardiac tamponade. J Am Coll Cardiol 1985;6:1057–1063.

31. Klopfenstein HS, Schuchard GH, Wann LS, Palmer TE, Hartz AJ, Gross CM, Singh S, Brooks HL. The relative merits of pulsus paradoxus and right ventricular diastolic collapse in the early detection of cardiac tamponade: an experimental echocardiographic study. Circulation 1985;71:829–833.

32. Kopecky SL, Callahan JA, Tajik AJ, Seward JB. Percutaneous pericardial catheter drainage: report of 42 consecutive cases. Am J Cardiol 1986;58:633–635.

33. Kronzan J, Cohen ML, Winer HE. Contribution of echocardiography to the understanding of the pathophysiology of cardiac tamponade. J Am Coll Cardiol 1983;1:1180–1182.

34. Labib SB, Udelson JE, Pandian NG. Echocardiography in low pressure cardiac tamponade. Am J Cardiol 1989;63:1156–1157.

35. Lange RL, Botticelli JT, Tsagaris TJ, Walter JA, Gani M, Bustamante RA. Diagnostic signs in compressive cardiac disorders. Constrictive peri-

carditis, pericardial effusion, and tamponade. Circulation 1966;33:763–777.

36. Leeman DE, Levine MJ, Come PC. Doppler echocardiography in cardiac tamponade: exaggerated respiratory variation in transvalvular blood flow velocity integrals. J Am Coll Cardiol 1988;11:572–578.

37. Leimgruber PP, Klopfenstein HS, Wann LS, Brooks HL. The hemodynamic derangement associated with right ventricular diastolic collapse in cardiac tamponade: an experimental echocardiographic study. Circulation 1983;68:612–620.

38. Levine MJ, Lorell BH, Diver DJ, Come PC. Implications of echocardiographically assisted diagnosis of pericardial tamponade in contemporary medical patients: detection before hemodynamic embarrassment. J Am Coll Cardiol 1991;17:59–65.

39. LeWinter MM, Pavelec R. Influence of the pericardium on left ventricular end-diastolic pressure-segment relations during early and later stages of experimental chronic volume overload in dogs. Circ Res 1982;50:501–509.

40. Lopez-Senden J, Garcia-Fernandez MA, Coma-Canella I, Silvestre J, deMiguel E, Jadraque LM. Identification of blood in the pericardial cavity in dogs by two-dimensional echocardiography. Am J Cardiol 1984;53:1194–1197.

41. Lorrell BH, Grossman W. Profiles in constrictive pericarditis, restrictive cardiomyopathy, and cardiac tamponade. In: Grossman W, ed. Cardiac catheterization and angiography. Philadelphia: Lea & Febiger, 1986.

42. Mancini GBJ, McGillem MJ, Bates ER, Weder AB, DeBoe SF, Grekin RJ. Hormonal responses to cardiac tamponade: inhibition of release of atrial natriuretic factor despite elevation of atrial pressures. Circulation 1987;76:884–890.

43. Markiewicz W., Borovik Z, Ecker S. Cardiac tamponade in medical patients: treatment and prognosis in the echocardiographic era. Am Heart J 1986;111:1138–1142.

44. Markiewicaz W, Gladstein E, London EJ, Popp RI. Echocardiographic detection of pericardial effusion and pericardial thickening in malignant lymphoma. Radiology 1977;123:161–164.

45. Metcalfe J, Woodbary JW, Richards V, Burwell CS. Studies in experimental pericardial tamponade. Effects on intravascular pressure and cardiac output. Circulation 1952;5:518–523.

46. Mintz GS, Kotler MN, Parry WR, Iskandran AS, Kane SA. Real-time inferior vena caval ultrasonography: normal and abnormal findings and its use in assessing right heart function. Circulation 1981;64:1018–1025.

47. Moreno FL, Hagan AD, Holman JR, Pryor TA, Strickland RD, Castle CH. Evaluation of size and dynamics of the inferior vena cava as an index of right-sided cardiac function. Am J Cardiol 1984;53:579–585.

48. Morgan BC, Guntheroth WC, Dillard, DH. The relationship of pericardial to pleural pressure during quiet respiration and cardiac tamponade. Circ Res 1965;16:493–498.

49. Piehler JM, Pluth JR, Schaff HV, Danielson GK, Orszulak TA, Puga FJ. Surgical management of effusive pericardial disease. Influence of extent of pericardial resection on clinical course. J Thorac Cardiovasc Surg 1985;90:506–516.

50. Pierard LA, Albert A, Henrard L, Lempereur P, Sprynger M, Carlier J. Incidence and significance of pericardial effusion in acute myocardial infarction as determined by two-dimensional echocardiography. J Am Coll Cardiol 1986;8:517–520.

51. Press OW, Livingston R. Management of malignant pericardial effusion and tamponade. JAMA 1987;257:1088–1092.

52. Reddy PS. Curtiss EI, O'Toole JD, Shaver JA. Cardiac tamponade: hemodynamic observations in man. Circulation 1978;58:265–272.

53. Renfrew R, Buselmeier TJ, Kjeilstrand CM. Pericarditis and renal failure. Annu Rev Med 1980;31:345–360.

54. Reydel B, Spodick DH. Frequency and significance of chamber collapse during cardiac tamponade. Am Heart J 1990;119:1160–1163.

55. Ringertz HG, Misbach GA, Tyberg JV. Effect of the normal pericardium on the left ventricular diastolic pressure-volume relationship. Acta Radiol 1981;22:529–534.

56. Rubin RH, Moellering RC. Clinical microbiologic and therapeutic aspects of purulent pericarditis. Am J Med 1975;59:68–78.

57. Shabetai R, Fowler NO, Fenton JC, Masangkay M. Pulsus paradoxus. J Clin Invest 1965;44:1882–1898.

58. Shabetai R, Fowler NO. Guntheroth WA. The hemodynamics of cardiac tamponade and constrictive pericarditis. Am J Cardiol 1970;26:480–489.

59. Shirato K, Shabetai R, Bhargave V, Franklin D, Ross J Jr. Alteration of the left ventricular diastolic pressure-segment length relation produced by the pericardium. Circulation 1978;57:1191–1197.

60. Singh S, Wann LS, Klopfenstein HS, Hartz A, Brooks HL. Usefulness of right ventricular diastolic collapse in diagnosing cardiac tamponade and comparison to pulsus paradoxus. Am J Cardiol 1986;57:652–656.

61. Smiseth OA, Frais MA, Kingma I, Smith ER, Tyberg JV. Assessment of pericardial constraint in dogs. Circulation 1985;71:158–164.

62. Spadaro JA, Bing OHL, Gaasch WH, Weintraub RM. Pericardial modulation of right and left ventricular diastolic interaction. Circ Res 1981;48:233–238.

63. Stotka JL, Good CB, Downer WR, Kapoor WN. Pericardial effusion and tamponade due to Kaposi's sarcoma in acquired immunodeficiency syndrome. Chest 1989;95:1359–1361.

64. Weitzman LB, Tinker WP, Kronzon J, Cohen ML, Glassman E, Spencer FC. The incidence and natural history of pericardial effusion after cardiac surgery—an echocardiographic study. Circulation 1984;69:506–511.

65. Winer HE, Kronzon I. Absence of paradoxical pulse in patients with cardiac tamponade and atrial septal defects. Am J Cardiol 1979;44:378–380.

66. Yoshida K, Skiina A, Asano Y, Hosoda S. Uremic pericardial effusion: detection and evaluation of uremic pericardial effusion by echocardiography. Clin Nephrol 1980;13:260–265.

21

Pharmacologic Cardiovascular Support

Simon Weber

When one prescribes cardiovascular medications to critically ill patients, the following considerations must be taken into account: *(a)* The high prevalence of metabolic and electrolytic disorders may alter the pharmacodynamic profile of the drug, decreasing its therapeutic effect and/or increasing its toxicity. *(b)* Cardiac, renal, and hepatic failure may profoundly alter drug pharmacokinetics, potentially requiring an adjustment in the dosage and monitoring of drug blood levels in selected patients. *(c)* Drug interaction is an unavoidable problem in the critically ill patient. *(d)* The hemodynamic status of the patient is often highly unstable and the need for a specific pharmacologic agent may fluctuate from moment to moment. *(e)* Prescription should therefore take into account classic pharmacologic data as well as an astute knowledge of drug-disease interaction. *(f)* Antiarrhythmics, vasodilators, and inotropic agents are the most commonly used compounds for the pharmacologic support of the failing heart.

ANTIARRHYTHMIC DRUGS

Arrhythmias, ventricular or supraventricular, are common in acutely ill patients with left ventricular (LV) failure. They may either be the cause of left ventricular decompensation or the consequence of myocardial failure or left atrial hypertension-dilation. They may be provoked or at least facilitated by hypoxia and metabolic and hydroelectrolytic (mainly hypokalemia) disorders. Whatever the mechanism of LV failure, maintenance of a normal sinus rhythm is highly desirable to allow atrioventricular synchronism and to benefit from

a normal atrial systolic contraction and an optimal left ventricular diastolic filling.

Management of arrhythmias includes conversion to normal sinus rhythm, which may be obtained by antiarrhythmic agents (2, 41, 42) as well as by electrical cardioversion or intracardiac temporary pacing. Maintenance of this normal rhythm involves the prescription of antiarrhythmic drugs as well as the treatment of associated metabolic disorders and of the underlying cardiac disease.

Classification and Pharmacology of the Principal Antiarrhythmic Agents

The prediction of the therapeutic effects of an antiarrhythmic agent by the analysis of its electrophysiologic effect at the cellular level is far from perfect. However, the classification by Vaughan-Williams is widely used and provides useful data for the choice of a drug in a given clinical situation (Tables 21.1 and 21.2).

Class I: antiarrhythmic agents that block the fast inward sodium channel during the phase 0 of the action potential. Class I is divided into three sub-classes according to differential electrophysiological specificities (Table 21.2) leading to different activity and toxicity profiles (42).

Class II: blockers of β-adrenergic receptor. All β-blockers have a marked negative inotropic effect and are therefore hazardous to prescribe in patients with LV dysfunction. β-blockers with an ultrashort half-life (<10 min) are now available and may be considered in selected "borderline" patients.

Table 21.1
Classification, Dosage, and Major Side Effects of the Main Antiarrhythmic Drugs[a]

Drug	Dosage	Adverse Effects
Class IA		
Procainamide	Oral: 800–4000 mg/kg in divided dosages (depending on preparation) IV: 10–15 mg/kg loading 2–4 mg/min maintenance	HF, GI, agranulocytosis, leukopenia, lupus-like syndrome, proarrhythmia, hypotension (IV)
Quinidine	Oral: 600–1600 mg/day in 2–4 divided doses (depending on preparation)	Diarrhea, thrombocytopenia, cinchonism, fever, hepatic rash, proarrhythmia
Disopyramide	Oral: 200–800 mg/day in 2 or 3 divided doses (depending on preparation)	HF, anticholinergic (dry mouth, urinary retention, blurred vision)
Class IB		
Lidocaine	IV: 1–2 mg/kg loading, 1–4 mg/min maintenance	CNS (including seizures, psychosis, apnea), GI
Mexiletine	Oral: 600–1000 mg/day in 3 or 4 divided doses (with food)	CNS (blurred vision), hepatic, blood dyscrasias, GI
Phenytoin	Oral: 14 mg/kg loading, then 200–400 mg/day in 1 or 2 divided doses IV: 20–100 mg every 5 min to maximum 1000 mg loading, 200–400 mg/day maintenance	CNS, blood dyscrasias hypotension (IV), fever, rash, hepatitis, gingivitis
Class IC		
Flecainide	Oral: 100–200 mg twice daily IV§: 1–2 mg/kg over 10–20 min	Blurred vision, CNS, GI, HF, proarrhythmia (+ + +)
Propafenone	Oral: 600–1200 mg/day in 2 or 3 divided doses	Bradycardia, dry mouth, CNS, nausea, proarrhythmia, HF
Encanide	Oral: 150–450 mg/day in 3 divided doses	CNS, GI, HF, proarrhythmia
Ethmozine	Oral: 300–900 mg/day in 3 divided doses	CNS, GI, proarrhythmia
Class II		
Propranolol	Oral: 40–240 mg/day in 3 or 4 divided doses IV: 0.5–1.0 mg every 5 min to maximum 0.2 mg/kg loading	HF, bradycardia, hypotension, bronchospasm, fatigue, CNS HF, bradycardia, hypotension, bronchospasm, fatigue, CNS
Esmolol	IV: 10–50 mg (maximum, 500 µg/kg) over 1 min loading, 1–20 mg (25–300 µg/kg)/min maintenance after titration in 1–5 min (25–50 µg/kg)/min steps	Hypotension, HF, bradycardia, bronchospasm
Sotalol§ (with mild class III action)	Oral: 160–240 mg/day in 2 divided doses	Bradycardia, HF, bronchospasm, hypotension, CNS, fatigue, proarrhythmia
Class III		
Amiodarone	Oral: Loading dose—30 mg/kg or 1200 mg/day × 5 days Maintenance—100–400 mg/day IV§: 5–10 mg/kg/20 min–2 hr; followed by 600 mg over next 24 hr	CNS, GI, thyroid, asymptomatic corneal microdeposits, skin, pulmonary fibrosis, hepatic fibrosis
Bretylium	IV: 5–10 mg/kg loading, 5–10 mg/kg every 6 hr or 0.5–4.0 mg/min	GI, orthostatic hypotension

Table 21.1 (*continued*)

Drug	Dosage	Adverse Effects
Class III	continuous infusion for maintenance	
Class IV		
Verapamil	Oral: 160–480 mg/day in divided doses IV: 3–10 mg bolus over 2 or 3 min, repeated in 30 min, if necessary; 0.125 mg/min maintenance infusion	Hypotension, HF, bradycardia, constipation

a HF, heart failure; IV, intravenous; GI, gastrointestinal; CNS, central nervous system. §, not available in U.S.

Table 21.2
Class I Antiarrhythmics: Differential Electrophysiologic Effects *a*

	1A	1B	1C
dV/dt	↓	= or ↓	↓ ↓
APD	↑	↓	=
ERP	↑	↓	↑
Automaticity	↓	↓	↓

a dV/dt, Rate of rise of action potential; APD, action potential duration; ERP, effective refractory period.

Class III: agents that prolong the action potential and the effective refractory period.

Class IV: calcium antagonists of the benzothiazepine (diltiazem) or phenyl-alkylamine (verapamil) type.

Prescription of these drugs should be done by taking into account their pharmacokinetic profile (30) as well as their modifications by heart, liver, or kidney failure (Table 21.3).

Treatment of Specific Arrhythmias

The precise electrocardiographic diagnosis of the type of tachyarrhythmia is only one of the parameters involved in the choice of the appropriate treatment. Three other factors must be taken into consideration. The first of these is knowledge of the underlying cardiac function. An altered left ventricular function and/or atrioventricular or intraventricular conduction disturbance may preclude the use of certain antiarrhythmics. Second, a metabolic or hydroelectrolytic disorder usually requires correction before considering a specific treatment of the arrhythmia. Third, the

hallmark of decision-making remains, however, the clinical and hemodynamic tolerance of the tachycardia. Evidence of acute coronary insufficiency, low cardiac output, or left ventricular failure requires immediate control of the arrhythmia. Direct current (DC) cardioversion is most frequently the best choice in this particular situation although it requires anesthesia, which may lead to temporary mechanical ventilation in critical patients.

If the arrhythmia is well tolerated, meaning that the patient has a stable blood pressure without evidence of myocardial ischemia, then pharmacologic treatment can be attempted. However, caution should be taken to not persist in case the antiarrhythmic agent fails. As time passes and as antiarrhythmic drugs are successively administered, the hemodynamic and coronary consequences of the arrhythmia worsen; cumulative toxicity of the antiarrhythmic agents may become a major concern. Electrical cardioversion should thus be reconsidered after each unsuccessful attempt of pharmacologic treatment.

Sinus Tachycardia

Sinus tachycardia is the usual response to cardiac failure, particularly left ventricular failure, or a noncardiac disorder such as hypovolemia, anemia, sepsis, fever, or hyperthyroidism. One must, of course, find the cause and treat it. The use of a negative chronotropic agent, such as propranolol, is useless and often deleterious since, in this situation, tachycardia is a truly compensatory mechanism.

Sinus nodal re-entrant tachycardia, indistinguishable from sinus tachycardia by

Table 21.3
Main Pharmacokinetic Characteristics of Major Antiarrhythmic Drugs

Drug	Time to Peak Plasma Concentration (hours) (per os)	Effective Plasma Concentration (μg/ml)	Protein Binding	Elimination Half-life (hour)	Bioavailability	Principal Route of Elimination
Quinidine	1.5–3	0.8–3	80	5–9	60–80	Liver
Disopyramide	1–2	2–7	40	8–9	80–90	Kidney
Lidocaine	—	1.5–6	60–70	1–2 (IV)[a]	50	Liver
Phenytoine	8–12	10–20	90	18–36	Variable	Liver
Mexiletine	2–4	0.8–2	70	9–12	85	Liver
Sotalol	1–3	0.1–0.3	<10	10–16	>90	Kidney
Propranolol	2–4	0.05–0.1	70–95	3–6	20–50	Liver
Amiodarone	4	(1–5?)		13–63 days	50	
Bretylium	—	0.5–1.5		8–14	25	Kidney
Verapamil	1–2	≈0.1–0.15	90	3–8	10–35	Liver
Flecainide	1.5–3	≈0.2–0.8	? (40 in vitro)	14–20	95	Liver
Propafenone	1–3	2	90	3–4	50–75	Liver

[a]Intravenous.

the surface ECG, is rare, usually well-tolerated, and responds to maneuvers which increase vagal tone. β-Adrenergic-blockers, verapamil or digoxin (if an underlying sick sinus syndrome is suspected), may be considered in refractory cases.

Atrial Fibrillation

The goals of therapy in recent onset atrial fibrillation are to control the ventricular rate, to avoid systemic embolism, and to restore sinus rhythm as soon as possible. Anticoagulation with intravenous heparin should be started immediately and continued until the normal sinus rhythm is restored. Rate control may be obtained by digoxin, intravenous verapamil, or a β-adrenergic blocker. These drugs may also be all that are necessary to restore the sinus rhythm within several hours. If atrial fibrillation persists, oral amiodarone (loading dose, 30 mg/kg body weight) is most frequently effective. Cardioversion should be considered if the arrhythmia is poorly tolerated or should the antiarrhythmic drugs fail. The need and the choice of maintenance therapy depend on the underlying cardiopathy.

Atrial Flutter

Atrial flutter requires therapeutic treatment similar to that of atrial fibrillation. In atrial flutter, however, intravenous drugs such as flecainide may be needed to restore sinus rhythm. Rapid atrial stimulation using a transvenous electrode catheter or a transesophagal pacing device is a reasonable alternative to cardioversion.

Atrioventricular Nodal Re-entrant Tachycardia

This type of tachycardia is usually well tolerated when there is no associated LV dysfunction. In critically ill patients, however, an episode of re-entrant tachycardia may be triggered by fever, an electrolyte imbalance, and the like, and be responsible for a worsening of their hemodynamic status. Maneuvers that increase vagal tone are often sufficient treatment. The intravenous bolus injection of the purine nucleotide, adenosine, is effective in most cases (>90%); its ultrashort half-life (10 seconds) precludes any sustained depressant effect. Intravenous verapamil is also highly efficient in this situation. Overdrive pacing or DC cardioversion are seldom required for this arrhythmia.

Ventricular Tachycardia

Episodes of ventricular tachycardia are frequently poorly tolerated (fast heartbeat, associated ischemic heart disease), and DC cardioversion is usually the first choice of therapy. Intravenous antiarrhythmics may be successful, but should be used with extreme caution because they may aggravate the ventricular tachycardia or even induce ventricular fibrillation. Lidocaine, disopyramide, and flecainide are the most commonly used drugs for this condition.

Torsade de Pointes

Torsade de pointes is a tachyarrhythmia characterized by the electrocardiographic appearance of QRS complexes of changing amplitudes and axes, twisting around the isoelectric line. The rate is usually above 200 beats/min. The episodes seldom last over 20–30 seconds, but their recurrence may lead to severe hemodynamic impairment. A prolonged QT interval on the ECG is necessary for the arrhythmia to be classified as "torsade de pointes." Its most frequent causes are hypokalemia, antiarrhythmic drugs such as quinidine or bepridil, and extreme bradycardia. Treatment includes correction of the triggering mechanism, intravenous isoprenaline, temporary ventricular pacing (90–100 beats/min), and intravenous magnesium sulfate.

INOTROPIC AGENTS

The most obvious approach in treating LV failure seems to be pharmacologic stimulation of myocardial contractility. Positive inotropic agents improve LV function as quantified by change in stroke work performed as filling pressure is increased. Available inotropic agents, from the centuries-old glycosides to the β-adrenergic agonist or phosphodiesterase inhibitors, are altogether disappointing in the long-term management of LV failure. They are, however, highly effective in the immediate and short-term treatment of acute LV dysfunction (8, 10).

Mechanisms of Inotropic Action at the Cellular Level

The interaction of the myocardial contractile proteins actin and myosin is an energy-dependent process, requiring adenosine triphosphate and controlled by a regulatory protein complex, tropomyosin. The catalytic activity of tropomyosin is, in turn,

dependent on the level of free cytosolic calcium. Contraction and relaxation of the heart are triggered by cyclic increases and decreases in free cytosolic "activator" calcium. The major source of cytosolic Ca^{++} is the sarcoplasmic reticulum, but exchanges of Ca^{++} between the cytoplasm and the sarcoplasmic reticulum are regulated by transmembrane influx of smaller amounts of Ca^{++} through voltage-dependent Ca^{++} channels.

All the available inotropic agents, i.e., digitalis glycosides, β-adrenergic agonists, and phosphodiesterase inhibitors, ultimately increase the level of free cytosolic "activator" Ca^{++}, stimulate the tropomyosin complex, and therefore increase the degree of interaction between actin and myosin (Fig. 21.1). The increase in contractility is necessarily followed by an increase in energy expenditure and in oxygen consumption, which represents the major limitation to the long-term use of positive inotropic agents. These phenomena may also be a major concern if the acute episode of left ventricular failure is provoked by coronary artery disease. New mechanisms of stimulation of myocardial contractility such as calcium channel agonists, sodium channel agonists, and calcium sensitizers of the tropomyosin system are currently under investigation.

Digitalis Glycosides

Three or four decades ago, glycosides were the only available treatment for heart failure. Their use is now limited to the management of acute left ventricular failure, and it is controversial in the long-term treatment of left ventricular dysfunction as long as sinus rhythm is maintained. The basis of their inotropic effect is an inhibition of a membrane Na-K-ATPase, which in turn stimulates Ca^{++} influx by way of an Na^+-Ca^{++} exchange. Their cardiac effects also include a negative chronotropic action on the sinus node, a decrease in atrioventricular conduction, and an increase in ventricular automaticity, which may lead to proarrhythmia. The main pharmacokinetic feature of digoxin is its long half-life (35 hours) and its elimination by the kidneys.

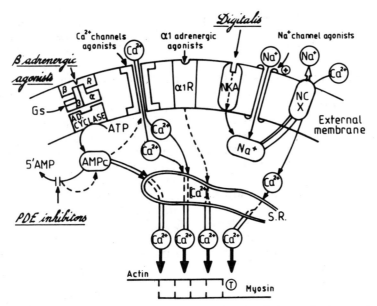

Figure 21.1. Mechanisms of action, at the cellular level, of the main inotropic agents. PDE, phosphodiesterase; GS, regulatory protein of the β-receptor; SR, sarcoplasmic reticulum; T, troponin-tropomyosin complex; NKA, $Na^+ - K^+$ ATPase; NCX, $Na^+ - Ca^{++}$ exchanger.

In severe acute left ventricular failure the magnitude of the inotropic effect of digoxin is insufficient. Digitalis toxicity is common in these circumstances (32) because toxicity is enhanced by hypoxia, hypokalemia, and renal insufficiency; the long half-life makes dosage difficult to adapt to the hemodynamic requirements. Newer, more powerful intravenous inotropic agents with short half-lives have replaced glycosides in the treatment of acute LV failure. Digitalis may remain useful if a supraventricular arrhythmia such as atrial fibrillation is associated with or responsible for the heart failure involved.

β-Adrenergic Agonists

β-Adrenergic agonists act on a membrane receptor coupled, through a G-protein, to adenylate cyclase. β-Receptor stimulation thus results in the production of cyclic adenosine monophosphate (cAMP), which increases the influx of Ca^{++} through voltage-dependent channels and stimulates inotropism (19). In the normal heart, the β_1-adrenergic receptor is largely predominant; however, β_2-adrenergic receptors represent 25% of the receptor sites, and

the inotropic effect of the stimulation of a single β-receptor is at least equivalent to the stimulation of a β_1-adrenergic-receptor site (1). In left ventricular failure, the myocardium is exposed to high levels of catecholamines as a consequence of reflex activation of the sympathetic system (3, 9, 15). This sustained exposure to a high concentration of agonists leads to β-adrenergic receptor down regulation, mainly through uncoupling of the receptor site from the regulatory G-protein (9); the failing myocardium becomes less sensitive to the inotropic effect of catecholamines. Exposure of the receptors to persistent stimulation by β-adrenergic agonist drugs may result in a further down regulation, which may be associated with a decrease or even a total loss of the hemodynamic response (tachyphylaxis). With the β_1-agonist dobutamine, approximately 50% of the initial inotropic effect is lost after 100 hours of continuous infusion. Down regulation is more profound on β_1- than on β_2-adrenergic receptor subtypes; thus, in severe heart failure, the proportion of the β_2-subtype may reach up to 40% of the total receptor sites. In this situation, β_2-adrenergic pharmacologic stimulation may be nearly as important as the "cardioselective" β_1 agonist effect.

The main pharmacologic characteristics of the available intravenous β-adrenergic agonists are summarized in Table 21.4. They all have a short half-life of several minutes, allowing immediate dosage adaptation to the hemodynamic requirements. They also have in common a β_1-adrenergic agonist effect. Their differences lie in the effect of their affinity for other receptor sites.

α-Adrenergic receptors induce arterial and arteriolar vasoconstriction; β_2-adrenergic receptors induce arterial vasodilation and additional inotropic effects (especially in acute episodes of chronic left ventricular failure); and dopaminergic receptors (DA1) induce renal vasodilation and have a diuretic effect (14).

The most commonly used inotropic agents of the β-agonist type are dobutamine and dopamine. *Dobutamine* (21, 22, 25, 33) acts predominantly by β_1 stimulation and does not trigger the release of intramyocardial norepinephrine at low to moderate doses. It does not induce direct vasodilation by β_2 stimulation, and its positive chronotropic and arrhythmogenic effects are mild. The usual optimal dosage is from 2.5–15 μg/kg/min; an occasional higher infusion rate up to 40 μg/kg/min may be considered.

The pharmacology of *dopamine* (14, 28, 34) is more complex. Its affinity for the various adrenergic receptor subtypes is dose-dependent. At low doses, dopamine acts predominantly on the dopaminergic DA1 receptors of the renal artery (vasodilation and natriuresis) with a much weaker effect on the DA2 receptor (presynaptic, pituitary gland, emetic center). At higher doses, it stimulates β_1 myocardial receptors directly and indirectly through myocardial norepinephrine release. It also stimulates vasoconstrictive arterial α_1-adrenergic receptors. The hemodynamic effects of dopamine are thus highly dependent on the infusion rate.

Several other adrenergic agonist agents may be of value in selected clinical situations.

Epinephrine

Epinephrine stimulates arterial α_1-adrenergic receptors and both β_1- and β_2-adrenergic receptors; epinephrine thus elicits an increase in cardiac output and arterial vasoconstriction. Epinephrine is given intravenously (or endotrachealy) in cardiac resuscitation, in anaphylactic shock, and in some cases of low-output states after cardiac surgery.

Norepinephrine

Norepinephrine stimulates α_1- and β_1-adrenergic receptors; its inotropic effect is associated with a marked arterial vasoconstriction. Its intravenous use, at low doses, may be warranted in cardiogenic shock (massive pulmonary embolism, myocardial infarction) with profound arterial hypotension.

Table 21.4
Pharmacodynamic Profile of Major Intravenous Adrenergic Agonists

Agent	Affinity for Adrenergic Receptor: Subtypes[a]				Hemodynamic Effects			
	β_1	β_2	α_1	DA$_1$	Positive Inotropism	Vasodilation	Vasoconstriction	Renal Dilation
Epinephrine	+	+	+		+		+	
Norepinephrine	+		+		+		+	
Isoprenaline	+	+			+	+		
Salbutamol		+			+	+		
Dobutamine	+				+			
Dopamine								
Low dose <1–4 μg/kg/min			+					+
High dose >5 μg/kg/min	+		+		+			+

[a]DA1, dopaminergic.

Isoproterenol

This agent stimulates both β_1- and β_2-adrenergic receptors. Its positive chronotropic and inotropic effects increase cardiac output, but arterial pressure usually decreases because of peripheral vasodilation and venous pooling. The main indication of isoproterenol is major, hemodynamically significant bradycardia that is unresponsive to atropine such as complete, infranodal, atrioventricular block. Isoproterenol should be initiated at a low (1–2 μg/min) infusion rate and titrated upward. Usually 5–15 μg/min are necessary to maintain heart rate around 60 beats/min. Isoproterenol may induce ventricular arrhythmias and may aggravate myocardial ischemia; therefore, cardioacceleration should be provided as soon as possible by a transvenous pacemaker and isoproterenol discontinued when electrical pacing is efficient.

Dopexamine

Dopexamine (4) predominantly stimulates cardiac β_2-adrenergic receptors and DA1 and DA2 dopaminergic receptors. Its intravenous administration causes a mild inotropic effect, an arterial vasodilation, and an increase in diuresis and natriuresis. Dopexamine may be considered for treatment of acute left ventricular failure with marked vasoconstriction and oliguria.

Phosphodiesterase Inhibitors

The inotropic phosphodiesterase inhibitors share a relative selectivity for phosphodiesterase III, the predominant cAMP-specific isoform in cardiac tissue; however, they exert a diffuse relaxant effect on smooth muscle cells and induce arterial vasodilation. The net hemodynamic effect is thus the result of the combination of the inotropic and the vasodilator action (7). Several compounds are now available for intravenous use.

Amrinone

Amrinone (13, 16, 20, 37–39) was the first available selective inhibitor of phophodiesterase III. Its arterial vasodilator effects are potent, whereas the magnitude of its direct inotropic effect in vivo remains controversial. Some authors (13, 39) claim that most of the observed increase in cardiac output is the consequence of afterload reduction rather than an enhancement of inotropism. Amrinone pharmacokinetics depend on the hemodynamic status: the plasma half-life is 2–3 hours in healthy volunteers and ranges from 3–10 hours in heart-failure patients. Patients can be either fast or slow acetylators of drugs based on individual patient genetic makeup. Acetylator status influences the mean plasma half-life, which is doubled in slow acetylators (20).

Thrombocytopenia is the major side effect, with an incidence of 2–3% after short-term infusion. In most cases, thrombocytopenia is moderate (50,000 to 100,000 per cubic millimeter) and rapidly reversible, but more severe cases have been reported. Gastrointestinal side effects such as nausea and vomiting are not uncommon. Treatment is usually initiated with a 0.5–0.75 μg/kg/min intravenous bolus followed by a continuous 5–10 μg/kg/min infusion. In patients with severe acute pulmonary edema and marked arterial vasoconstriction, an intravenous bolus of amrinone is frequently rapidly effective at augmenting cardiac function and may prevent the use of endotracheal intubation and mechanical ventilation for the treatment of these complications.

Milrinone

Milrinone (1, 17, 18) is very similar to amrinone, but its inhibitor effect on phosphodiesterase III is, at least in vitro, 30 to 50 times more potent. In vivo, its inotropism:vasodilation ratio seems to be higher and its side effect profile is more favorable than that of amrinone (11). The incidence of thrombocytopenia is much lower. Treatment is usually initiated with a 50 μg/kg body weight loading dose followed by a 0.3–0.8 μg/kg/min continuous intravenous infusion (31).

Enoximone

Enoximone (16, 25, 36) is an imidazole derivative with a potent inhibitor effect on phosphodiesterase III and a marked positive in vivo inotropic effect associated with arterial vasodilation and moderate tachycardia. Enoximone has a 6–8 hour plasma half-life in heart-failure patients; its main sulfoxide metabolite retains some of its inotropic potency and has a much longer half-life. Side effects include proarrhythmia, nausea, vomiting, and diarrhea. Some cases of moderate transient thrombocytopenia have been reported.

Treatment is usually initiated with a 0.5–1 mg/kg body weight loading dose administered over 5 minutes, followed by a 5–20 μg/kg/min continuous infusion. Oral enoximone (not commercially available) has been used during several weeks or months as a "pharmacologic bridge" to cardiac transplantation in patients with end-stage heart failure.

SYSTEMIC MODULATION WITH VASODILATORS

Although some of the most commonly used vasodilators such as nitrates have been known since the beginning of the century, the concept of pharmacologic modulation of the venous and arterial vasomotor tone as a treatment of chronic or acute left ventricular failure was not widely accepted until the early 1970s (6). Vasoconstriction, mainly secondary to the stimulation of sympathetic nerves and activation of the renin-angiotensin system, is a "compensatory" mechanism designed to maintain arterial pressure in the setting of reduced cardiac output in heart failure states (5). The degree of activation of this reflex, vasoconstriction, was thought to have been set at the optimal level by the "natural" compensatory mechanisms of left ventricular failure. In most cases of severe LV dysfunction, however, it appears that the degree of vasoconstriction is higher than what is needed to maintain an adequate systemic perfusion pressure, and that this "excess" vasoconstriction increases the burden of the failing left ventricle. Pharmacologic modulation of the venous and arterial tone to achieve the best compromise, in a given patient at a given moment, between the loading conditions of the left ventricle and the end-organ perfusion pressure is the goal of vasodilator therapy (23).

Mechanisms of Vasoregulation

Several physiologic systems are involved in the regulation of the vascular tone; the diameter of a vessel, the resistance of a regional circulation, is the net result of various vasoconstrictive and vasodilatory mechanisms (Fig. 21.2).

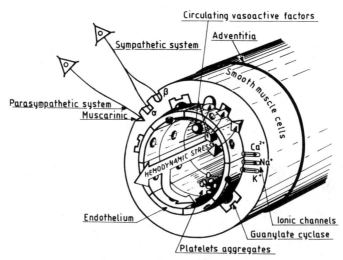

Figure 21.2. Regulatory mechanisms of vasomotion.

Neurogenic Vasoregulation

Arteries and veins are innervated by sympathetic and parasympathetic postganglionic nerve endings. Activation of the cholinergic muscarinic receptor elicits vasoconstriction, although, in vivo, intraarterial infusion of acetylcholine induces endothelium-mediated vasodilation. The effects of the sympathetic adrenergic system are more complex. Stimulation of the postsynaptic α_1-adrenergic receptor elicits vasoconstriction, whereas stimulation of the vascular β_2-adrenergic receptor elicits vasodilation. In the majority of the vascular beds α_1-adrenergic receptors are predominant and the net result of sympathetic stimulation is vasoconstriction.

Vasoactive Factors

Circulating factors such as angiotensin II and epinephrine, or products of local "metabolism" such as bradykinin and adenosine, act on specific receptors of the smooth muscle cell to elicit relaxation or constriction. A local increase in adenosine concentration is an indicator of high-energy adenosine triphosphate depletion and immediately induces a compensatory "metabolic" vasodilation.

Ionic Channels

Transmembrane Ca^{++} influx is a major vasoconstrictive mechanism. Calcium fluxes are modulated through either receptor- or voltage-dependent mechanisms and represent the final common pathway of numerous physiologic vasomotor stimuli.

Endothelial-dependent Vasodilation

The major physiologic role of the endothelium in the regulation of vasomotion has been clearly established in recent years. The endothelial cell produces a relaxing factor (endothelium-derived relaxing factor, EDRF) that stimulates guanylate cyclase of the underlying smooth muscle cells (11, 12). Elevation of intracellular cyclic guanosine monophosphate elicits relaxation by stimulating activator Ca^{++} extrusion and by direct inhibition of the contractile activity of smooth muscle myosin light chains. The EDRF is also produced at the luminal site of the endothelial cell and stimulates platelet guanylate cyclase and, hence, has a potent antiaggregant effect. The chemical structure of EDRF is nitric oxide (NO) or a more complex molecule with NO in its active site such as a nitrosocysteine (11, 24). L-Arginine is the metabolic precursor of NO. The NO half-life is extremely short (5–6 seconds) due to its destruction by interaction with hemoglobin and other oxygenated molecules. Another EDRF has recently been discovered (EDRF 2). Its relaxant vasodilator effect is mediated through smooth muscle cell membrane hyperpolarization; its chemical structure is still unknown.

Endothelial EDRF-mediated vasodilation is triggered by three types of stimuli:

1. Hemodynamic parietal stress, perpendicular and tangential to the vessel wall (shear stress)—any local increase in flux velocity is thus followed by endothelium-mediated vasodilation (27);
2. Circulating factors such as histamine and bradykinin;
3. Products of platelet aggregation such as serotonin ADP and thrombin.

Vasoconstrictive factors (such as polypeptide endothelin) are also produced by endothelium. Their physiologic importance is still controversial (40). If endothelial function is impaired, such as in atherosclerosis and most probably in chronic left ventricular failure and hypertension, the potency of endothelium-mediated vasodilation is markedly attenuated.

All the numerous above-mentioned vasoregulatory mechanisms can be evidenced in any part of the circulatory system—arterial, arteriolar, or venous. Their magnitude and thus their individual contribution to local vasoregulation varies considerably, however, from one regional circulation to the other. This variability accounts for most of the pharmacodynamic differences between the various vasodilators.

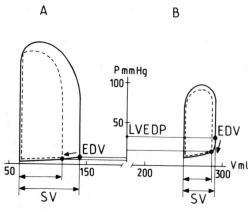

Figure 21.3. Hemodynamic effects of a venous vasodilator. *A,* normal left ventricle. *B,* failing left ventricle. In *A,* a small left ventricular end diastolic pressure *(LVEDP)* decrease results in a large stroke volume *(SV)* reduction. In *B,* a marked *LVEDP* decrease minimally reduces the *SV. EDV,* end diastolic volume.

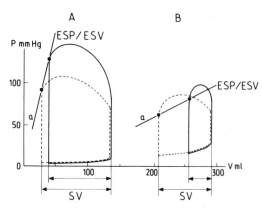

Figure 21.4. Hemodynamic effects of an arterial vasodilator. *A,* normal left ventricle. *B,* failing left ventricle. In *A,* marked decrease in arterial pressure is needed to induce a small increase in stroke volume *(SV).* In *B,* a small decrease in arterial pressure induces a marked improvement in *SV. ESP,* end systolic pressure; *ESV,* end systolic volume.

Hemodynamic Effects of Vasodilation

Venous Vasodilation

Venodilation induces peripheral blood pooling, namely in the dilated splanchnic and lower limbs areas (Fig. 21.3). The decrease in central venous pressure results in a concomitant decrease of LV end-diastolic pressure and volume. The consequences of the decrease in left ventricular end-diastolic pressure are markedly different, according to Starling's Law of the Heart and to the shape of the LV pressure-volume relationship, in the normal and in the failing left ventricle. If the LV end-diastolic pressure is normal, any decrease will result in a decrease in stroke volume. The decrease in stroke volume induces a reflex tachycardia in an attempt by the body to maintain cardiac output (29) (Fig. 21.3A). If LV end-diastolic pressure is elevated, as in LV failure, small decreases in end-diastolic volume will not significantly reduce stroke volume whereas symptoms of pulmonary and venous congestion may be markedly improved because of the associated decrease in pulmonary venous and systemic venous pressures, respectively (Fig. 21.3B).

Arterial Vasodilation

Arterial vasodilation involves large arteries (and even the aorta) as well as smaller arterioles. Consequences of arterial dilation also depend on the baseline hemodynamic status. A linear relationship between end-systolic pressure and end-systolic volume of the left ventricle was established in experimental as well as in clinical studies (35). Its slope is representative of the contractile state of the left ventricle: steep in the normal heart (Fig. 21.4A) and flat in the failing heart (Fig. 21.4B). In the normal heart, a marked decrease in arterial pressure is thus needed to produce a modest increase in stroke volume. Conversely, in heart-failure patients, a large increase in stroke volume may be obtained with a only minimal decrease in arterial pressure. The goal of an optimal pharmacologic arterial dilation is to simultaneously increase cardiac output and maintain arterial pressure. Moderate hypotension at baseline should not preclude the careful prescription of progressive doses of vasodilators.

Consequences of Systemic Dilation on Coronary Hemodynamics

Systemic vasodilation may have the opposite consequences on myocardial metabolism and coronary hemodynamics: The decrease in end-diastolic pressure and in arterial pressure reduces myocardial oxygen requirements, but an exaggerated fall in coronary perfusion pressure may compromise myocardial supply, especially in the presence of severe coronary stenosis. Reflex tachycardia decreases the length of diastole and thus decreases coronary perfusion while it increases myocardial oxygen consumption.

Careful titration of vasodilator doses is thus mandatory for an optimal effect on the coronary circulation. Optimal does improve myocardial energetics, while excessive doses may be deleterious.

Pharmacology of the Major Classes of Vasodilators

The pharmacodynamic effects of the available vasodilators depend on: (a) their differential effects on the various regional vascular beds—venous or arterial, coronary, mesenteric, renal; (b) their direct cardiac effect (if any)—chronotropic and/or inotropic; (c) the degree of activation of the compensatory mechanism, especially the baroreflex; and (d) their pharmacokinetic profile—an intravenous drug with a very short half-life is more adequate for the treatment of hemodynamically unstable patients.

It should be noted that in vitro experimental vasodilator effects and clinical results may be very different. A hemodynamic assessment of vasodilation, such as the calculation of arterial resistances, represents the sum of the direct vascular effect of the drug and the associated counter regulatory mechanisms it triggers. Furthermore, global indexes of vasodilation do not take into account the variability of the response of the various regional circulations (Table 21.5).

α-Adrenergic Blockers

α-Adrenergic blockers elicit a predominantly arterial vasodilation. Phentolamine is a nonselective α-adrenergic blocker. α_1-Postsynaptic blockade elicits a marked arterial vasodilation, but α_2-presynaptic blockade triggers norepinephrine release and thus tachycardia and attenuation of the hemodynamic effects. Intravenous phentolamine had been used in the treatment of severe acute left ventricular failure, but its therapeutic effects are limited by tachycardia and tachyphylaxia. Prazosin is a selective α_1-postsynaptic blocker. Its effects on heart rate are moderate. Its venous vasodilator effects are initially consistent, but rapidly dissipate with repeat dosing. Prazosin is not commercially available in its intravenous form.

Table 21.5
Hemodynamic Effects of Intravenous Vasodilators

Drug[a]	Arterial Dilation	Venous Dilation	Heart Rate	Ejection Fraction	Coronary Steal
Phentolamine (α blocker)	+ + +	+	+ +	+	?
Calcium antagonists					
Verapamil, DTZ	+ +	0	↓	↓	0
DHP	+ + +	0	+	+	±
Nitroprusside	+ + +	+	+	+ +	+ +
Low-dose nitrates					
NTG <50 μg/min or ISDN <75 μg/min	+	+ + +	+	0	0
High-dose nitrates					
NTG >50 μg/min or ISDN >75 μg/min	+ +	+ + +	+	+	0

[a]DTZ, diltiazem; DHP, dihydropyridine; NTG, nitroglycerin; ISDN, isosorbide dinitrate.

Calcium Antagonists

Calcium antagonists, with a significant negative inotropic effect such as diltiazem and verapamil should be avoided in heart-failure patients. Calcium antagonists of the dihydropyridine type have a minimal direct negative inotropic effect, which is counterbalanced by reflex sympathetic activation and unloading of the failing left ventricle. In most, but not all cases, their net effect is an increase in cardiac output. However, their use should be restricted to patients whose heart failure is secondary to hypertension and in some cases of coronary artery disease.

Nitrates and Nitroprusside

Nitrates and nitroprusside share a very similar mechanism of action. Their nitrosyl group, similar to the endothelial vasodilator mediator EDRF, stimulates the guanylate cyclase of the smooth muscle cell; the increased intracellular levels of cyclic guanosine monophosphate promote arterial and venous vasodilation. With nitroprusside, arterial vasodilation predominates at all infusion rates, whereas nitroglycerin is a predominant venous vasodilator at low doses. Its arterial dilator effect becomes significant at higher infusion rates (50 μg/min).

Nitroglycerin dilates epicardial coronary arteries and collateral vessels, it increases flow to the ischemic myocardium. Thus, it does not induce any coronary flow diversion away from ischemic myocardium (steal phenomenon). Nitroprusside may decrease perfusion of the ischemic myocardium and hence aggravate myocardial ischemia. Both drugs inhibit platelet aggregation, but the clinical significance of this phenomenon remains uncertain.

Nitroprusside (7) is the agent of choice in patients with severe hypertension and in heart-failure patients with a predominance of low cardiac output over congestion. Conversely, nitroglycerin should be used in coronary artery disease and heart-failure patients with a predominance of congestion. Prolonged nitroprusside administration is hampered by the risk of thiocyanate toxicity. Thiocyanate accumulates with prolonged administration (>72

hours), even at moderate infusion rates. This phenomenon is aggravated by hepatic and renal failure. Thiocyanate toxicity occurs with blood levels over 5 mg/100 ml. Its reactions include vomiting, tremors, convulsions, rigidity, and psychotic behavior.

Prolonged nitroglycerin administration is limited by the development of tolerance (tachyphylaxia) with attenuation of the hemodynamic and antiischemic effects of the drug (26). This phenomenon is the consequence of three mechanisms: (a) sodium and fluid retention, as with any vasodilator; (b) hemodilution due to selective dilation of the venous side of the capillary system inducing an extracellular fluid influx. The resultant increase in volemia attenuates the effects of nitroglycerin-induced venodilation; and (c) sulfhydryl radicals are necessary for the intracellular transformation of nitroglycerin to its active metabolite. Consumption-depletion of sulfhydryl radicals is probably the principal phenomenon involved in nitrate tolerance. The first two mechanisms can be controlled by an adequate diuretic prescription. Administration of the sulfhydryl group donor N-acetylcysteine has been proven to maintain or restore the hemodynamic effects of nitroglycerin after the development of tolerance by prolonged administration. However, experience with N-acetylcysteine in this situation remains limited.

Other vasodilators are also available for clinical use. Intravenous isosorbide dinitrate probably induces a lesser degree of tolerance than nitroglycerin but is less often used. Indications to angiotensin-converting enzyme inhibitors in the treatment of acute LV failure are limited. Their prolonged and sometimes unpredictable hemodynamic effects are not well suited for the variability of the hemodynamic status commonly seen in these patients.

Combination Therapy

Simultaneous modulation of inotropism, preload, and afterload is often necessary in cases of severe left ventricular dysfunction. Some drugs such as β_2-adrenoceptor agonists and phophodiasterase inhibitors

Table 21.6
Choice of Intravenous Drugs According to the Desired Hemodynamic Objective[a]

Hemodynamic Goal	Drug
Venous V/D	NTG, low dose
Arterial V/D	Nitroprusside; NTG, high dose; DHP
Renal V/D	DOPA, low dose
Inotropic	DOBU
Inotropic + arterial V/D	PDE inhibitors, salbutamol
	DOBU + nitroprusside
	DOBU + NTG, high dose
Inotropic + renal V/D	DOBU + DOPA, low dose
Inotropic + V/C	DOPA, high dose; norepinephrine

[a] V/D, vasodilation; NTG, nitroglycerin; DHP, dihydropyridine; DOPA, dopamine; DOBU, dobutamine; PDE, phosphodisterase; V/C, vasoconstriction.

have both vasodilator and positive inotropic effects. In selected clinical situations, as summarized in Table 21.6, a combination of inotropes and vasodilators may represent the optimal therapy.

References

1. Alousi AA, Stankus GP, Stuart JC, et al. Characterization of the cardiotonic effects of milrinone, a new and potent bipyridine, on isolated tissues from several species. J Cardiovasc Pharmacol 1983;5:804–811.
2. Boyden PA, Wit A. Pharmacology of the antiarrhythmic drugs. In: Rosen MR, Hoffman BF, eds. Cardiac therapy. The Hague: Martinus Nijhoff Publishers, 1983:171–234.
3. Bristow MR, Ginsberg R, Umans V, et al. Beta 1 and beta 2 adrenergic receptor subpopulations in non failing and failing human ventricular myocardium: coupling of both receptor subtypes to muscle contraction and selective beta down-regulation in heart failure. Circulation 1986;59:287–309.
4. Brown RA, Dixon J, Farmer JB, et al. Dopexamine: a novel agonist at peripheral dopamine receptors and beta 2-adrenoceptors. Br J Pharmacol 1985;85:599–605.
5. Burton, AC. Physical principles of circulatory phenomena: The physical equilibria of the heart and blood vessels. In: Handbook of Physiology. Circulation 1. Bethesda, MD, 1962:85–106.
6. Cohn J, Franciosa J. The role of vasodilator therapy in heart failure. New Engl J Med 1977;297:27–32.
7. Cohn JN, Burke LP. Nitroprusside. Ann Intern Med 1979;91:752–761.
8. Colucci WS, Wright RF, Braunwald E. New positive inotropic agents in the treatment of congestive heart failure. Mechanisms of action and recent clinical developments. New Engl J Med 1986;314:349–355.
9. Fowler MB, Laser JA, Hopkins GL, Minobe W, Bristow MR. Assessment of the beta adrenergic pathway in the intact failing human heart: progressive receptor down regulation and subsensitivity to agonist response. Circulation 1986;74:1290–1302.
10. Francis GS. The role of inotropic agents in the management of heart failure. In: Cohn J, ed. Drug treatment of heart failure. New York: Advanced Therapeutics Communications, 1983:121–151.
11. Furchgott RF, Khan MT, Jothianandan D, Kahn AS. Evidence that the endothelium-derived relaxing factor of rabbit aorta is nitric oxide. In: Bevan JA, Majewski H, Maxwell RA, Story DF, eds. Vascular neuroeffector mechanisms. Oxford: IRL Press, 1988:77–84.
12. Furchgott RF, Zawadzki JV. The obligatory role of endothelial cells in the relaxation of arterial smooth muscle by acetylcholine. Nature (Lond) 1980;299:373–376.
13. Goenen M, Pedemonte O, Baele P, et al. Amrinone in the management of low cardiac output after open heart surgery [Abstract]. Am J Cardiol 1986;53:33B.
14. Goldberg LI, Rajfer SI. Dopamine receptors: applications in clinical cardiology. Circulation 1985;72:245–253.
15. Golf S, Hansson V. Effects of beta blocking agents on the density of beta adrenoceptors and adenylate cyclase response in human myocardium: intrinsic sympathomimetic activity favours receptor up regulation. Cardiovasc Res 1986;20:637–644.
16. Hamilton RA, Kowalsky SF, Wright EM, et al.: Effects of acetylator phenotype on amrinone pharmacokinetics. Clin Pharmacol Ther 1986;40:615–621.
17. Kariya T, Willie LJ, Dage RC. Biochemical studies on the mechanism of cardiotonic activity of MDL 17,043. J Cardiovasc Pharmacol 1982;4:509–518.
18. Kubo SH, Cody RJ, Chatterjee K, et al. Acute dose range study of milrinone in congestive heart failure. Am J Cardiol 1985;55:726–732.
19. Lefkowitz R, Caron M, Stiles G. Mechanisms of membrane receptor regulation. New Engl J Med 1984;310:1570–1579.
20. Lejemtel TH, Keung E, Sonnenblick EH, et al. Amrinone: a new non-adrenergic cardiotonic agent effective in the treatment of intractable myocardial failure in man. Circulation 1979;59:1098–1103.
21. Leier CV, Unverferth DV. Dobutamine. Ann Intern Med 1983;99:490–497.
22. Liang C, Sherman LG, Doherty JU, et al. Sustained improvement of cardiac function in patients with congestive heart failure after short-term infusion of dobutamine. Circulation 1984;69:113–120.
23. Merillon JP, Motte G, Lecarpentier Y, Masquet C, Gourgon R. Le rapport pression-volume télésystolique ventriculaire gauche. Etude comparative lors de modifications de charge et d'inotropisme. Arch Mal Coeur 1977;70:1013–1024.

24. Myers PR, Minor RL Jr, Guerra R Jr, Bates JN, Harrison DG. Vasorelaxant properties of the endothelium-derived relaxing factor more closely resemble S-nitrosocystéine than nitric oxide. Nature (Lond) 1990;345:161–163.

25. Okerholm RA, Chan KY, Lang JF, et al. Biotransformation and pharmacokinetic overview of enoximone and its sulfoxide metabolite [Abstract]. Am J Cardiol 1987;60:21C.

26. Packer M, Lee WH, Kessler PD, et al. Prevention and reversal of nitrate tolerance in patients with congestive heart failure. New Engl J Med 1987;317:799–806.

27. Pohl TT, Holtz J, Busse R, et al. Crucial role of endothelium in the vasodilator response of increased flow in vivo. Hypertension 1986;8:37–44.

28. Robie NW, Goldberg LI. Comparative systemic and regional hemodynamic effects of dopamine and dobutamine. Am Heart J 1975;90:340–348.

29. Rowell LB. General principles of vascular control in human circulation. New York: Oxford University Press, 1986:8–43.

30. Shanks RG, Harrison DC. Pharmacokinetic principles in cardiac arrhythmias: a decade of progress. Boston: GK Hall, 1981:91–96.

31. Simonton CA, Chatterjee K, Cody RJ, et al. Milrinone in congestive heart failure: acute and chronic hemodynamics and clinical evaluation. J Am Coll Cardiol 1985;6:453–458.

32. Smith TW, Autman EM, Friedman PL, et al. Digitalis glycosides: mechanisms and manifestations of toxicity. Prog Cardiovasc Dis 1984;26:413–419.

33. Sonnenblick EH, Frishman WH, Lejemtel TH. Dobutamine: a new synthetic cardioactive sympathetic amine. New Engl J Med 1979;300:17–25.

34. Stoner JD, Balen JL, Harrison DC. Comparison of dobutamine and dopamine in treatment of severe heart failure. Br Heart J 1977;39:536–542.

35. Suga H, Sagawa K. Instantaneous pressure-volume relationship and their ratio in the excised supported left ventricle. Circ Res 1974;35:117–125.

36. Weber KT, Janicki JS, Jain MC. Enoximone (MDL 17,043) for stable, chronic heart failure secondary to ischemic or idiopathic cardiomyopathy. Am J Cardiol 1986;58:589–596.

37. Wilmshurst PT, Walker JM, Fry CH, et al. Inotropic and vasodilator effects of amrinone on isolated human tissue. Cardiovasc Res 1984;18:302–310.

38. Wilmshurst PT, Webb-Peploe MM. Side effects of amrinone therapy. Br Heart J 1983;49:447–554.

39. Wilmshurst PT, Thomson DS, Jenkins BS, et al. The hemodynamic effects of intravenous amrinone in patients with impaired left ventricular function. Br Heart J 1983;49:77–89.

40. Yanagisawa M, Kurihara H, Kimura S, et al. A novel potent vasoconstrictor peptide produced by vascular endothelial cells. Nature (Lond) 1988;332:411–415.

41. Zipes DP. Management of cardiac arrhythmias. In: Braunwald E, ed. Pharmacological, electrical and surgical techniques in heart disease. New York: WB Saunders, 1984:648–682.

42. Zipes DP, Troup PJ. New antiarrhythmic agents: amiodarone, aprindine, disopyramide, ethmozin, mexiletine, tocainide, verapamil. Am J Cardiol 1978;41:1005–1024.

22

Postoperative Care of the Cardiac Surgical Patient

Keith L. Stein

The principal goals in the early postoperative period following all cardiac surgery, as for other types of surgery, are to optimize the balance between cellular oxygen supply and demand, restore adequate perfusion pressure, and preserve visceral function. What complicates therapeutic intervention to varying degrees in patients of this particular group are the coincident alterations in myocardial oxygen supply and demand that follow cardiopulmonary bypass, revascularization (as in coronary artery bypass grafting), alterations in loading conditions (as in valve surgery or repair of intracardiac defects), or preservation and denervation (as in cardiac transplantation).

GENERAL PRINCIPLES OF ORGAN SYSTEM SUPPORT

Cardiovascular Support

The myocardial oxygen supply/demand relationship is different from that of the rest of the body in that the entirely aerobic myocardium functions constantly near its maximum oxygen extraction. Thus, at all levels of myocardial oxygen delivery, myocardial oxygen consumption is supply-dependent (21). Factors including preload, afterload, heart rate, and contractility all affect the level of oxygen consumption and compete with factors such as coronary arterial stenosis for an optimal match between supply and consumption (1). A decline in myocardial oxygen transport of as little as 10–20% (induced by anemia, hypoxemia, or a reduction in coronary blood flow) may result in notable myocardial dysfunction, the diagnosis of which may

be elusive using conventional measures such as ECG or pulmonary artery occlusion pressure tracings (38). As in all critically ill patients, the myocardium is straining to maintain its own integrity and to increase performance to meet the needs of the rest of the other vital viscera.

Cardiopulmonary bypass cellular oxygen demand is significantly depressed immediately as a result of residual hypothermia, anesthesia, and neuromuscular blockade. However, as rewarming occurs, shivering may ensue. This tremendous level of metabolic work often increases the total-body oxygen demand by 100% (55). Simultaneously, altered ventricular function evidenced by impaired systolic performance with decreased stroke volume and cardiac output may compromise cellular oxygen delivery (9, 64). In addition, oxygen consumption may become supply-dependent during this early postoperative phase, necessitating careful attention to the response to increased oxygen delivery and to serum lactate levels (40). Microcirculatory changes involving the redistribution of blood flow may also contribute to deficiencies in regional cellular oxygen delivery (3). Oxygen consumption can be limited with therapeutic neuromuscular blockade to inhibit shivering and concomitant efforts at central rewarming using heated humidified gases through the ventilator (Table 22.1).

Therapy for optimizing oxygen delivery is focused on manipulation of preload (by volume expansion), contractility (by inotropic pharmacotherapy), afterload (by vasodilation or intraaortic balloon counterpulsation), and arterial hemoglobin and

Table 22.1
Early Postoperative Changes in Cardiovascular Function and Oxygen Supply and Demand

Hypothermia
  Decreased cellular oxygen demand
  Initial elevation in the systemic vascular
    resistance index
  Decreased ventricular systolic function
  Decreased stroke volume and cardiac index
  Oxygen consumption supply dependent
Rewarming and shivering
  Vasodilation
  Increased venous capacitance
  Increased oxygen demand
  Regional redistribution of blood flow

Table 22.2
Cardiovascular Support

Goal
  Improved perfusion, renal function, lactic
    acidosis, Svo_2, oxygen consumption
  Preload: volume expansion with colloid,
    transfusion
  Afterload: vasodilators for hypertension
  Contractility: pharmacologic intervention
Heart rate
  Rate preservation, sinus rhythm or atrio-
    ventricular pacing
Other
  Correct hypophosphatemia, treat ischemia,
    maintain hemoglobin saturation

saturation. Such treatments are invasive by use of hemodynamic monitoring (using pulmonary and peripheral arterial catheters) and thermodilution cardiac output measurements. Successful therapeutic intervention is indicated by improved tissue perfusion as reflected in adequate renal function, absence or resolution of metabolic lactic acidosis, and acceptable levels of mixed venous hemoglobin saturation (Table 22.2). In addition, a plateau in oxygen consumption despite further increases in oxygen delivery suggests supply independence, a desirable state.

Although volume expansion may be accomplished with either crystalloids or colloids, the latter are more efficient because the immediate response to a small volume (e.g., 25% albumin) is greater and perhaps more sustained (39). Fluids are administered carefully according to the responses

of stroke volume and cardiac indices to changes in pulmonary artery occlusion. Interpretation of the pulmonary artery occlusion pressure is particularly difficult because of the changes in diastolic compliance (typically, depression) associated with rewarming from hypothermia. Nonetheless, rewarming usually reduces vasomotor tone with relative intravascular volume depletion, which requires replacement (36).

Anemia, particularly when accompanied by hypothermia, alkalosis, and low levels of 2,3-diphosphoglycerate (2,3-DPG), may significantly compromise cellular oxygen delivery. Although the ideal hematocrit has yet to be determined, convention dictates judicious use of transfusions to a level greater than 30%, at least for the most critically ill patients. In fact, some authors have reported that the highest survival rates occur in critically ill postsurgical patients with a hematocrit of approximately 33% (15). Hypophosphatemia may be associated with diminished 2,3-DPG levels, diminished myocardial performance (17, 52), platelet and leukocyte dysfunction, central nervous system impairment, and prolonged respiratory insufficiency (51) and should be corrected promptly by intravenous replacement of phosphates.

Augmentation of preload through volume expansion does not necessarily improve myocardial performance and oxygen delivery. In fact, myocardial function as reflected in ejection fraction may deteriorate, particularly when certain end-diastolic volume indices are exceeded (46). Newer monitoring techniques such as the measurement of right ventricular (RV) ejection fraction by use of a pulmonary artery catheter (8, 20) and transesophageal echocardiography (60) are being evaluated as adjuncts in determining the adequacy of volume expansion.

If oxygen delivery remains inadequate after volume repletion, inotropic intervention to increase contractility and stroke volume is applied. The synthetic catecholamine dobutamine has been particularly useful during low output states after cardiopulmonary bypass (59). As a result of its predominant effects on β_1- and β_2-adrenergic receptors, dobutamine typically induces inotropism and mild vasodilation, increasing stroke volume and cardiac index. The resulting pulmonary vasodilation may also improve RV performance. However, the chronotropic effects of dobutamine may result in tachyarrhythmias, and vasodilation may overcome hypoxic pulmonary vasoconstriction, exacerbating transpulmonary shunt and hypoxemia. Thus, careful attention must be paid to the mechanism of improved cardiac index (tachycardia versus increased stroke volume) and the overall effect on oxygen delivery. Alternative catecholamine (e.g., dopamine) and noncatecholamine (e.g., amrinone) pharmacologic interventions may be used according to their selective effects on cardiac and peripheral muscle function.

Ventricular afterload may also be manipulated to improve myocardial performance. Although left ventricular (LV) afterload is probably best indicated by systolic wall stress (42), this is not readily measured at the bedside. Instead, the calculated systemic vascular resistance index is used as a crude indicator of the contribution of peripheral vasomotor tone to LV afterload. Hypertension is common soon after cardiac surgery, occurring in as many as 40% of these patients (25). The deleterious effects of high blood pressure on LV systolic and diastolic function (62) are minimized with systemic vasodilators such as sodium nitroprusside, β-blockers such as labetolol (14), or selective calcium-channel blockers such as isradipine (10). As with inotropes, vasodilation (particularly by nitroprusside) may exacerbate hypoxemia. Hypotension with compromise of coronary perfusion pressure and resultant myocardial ischemia must be avoided.

Cardiac function depends on adequate heart rate and rhythm. Synchronized atrial contraction augments ventricular filling and, thus, preload-dependent cardiac output. Antiarrhythmic therapy is designed to establish normal sinus rhythm and ventricular dysrhythmias. Frequently used agents such as lidocaine and procainamide have important side effects. Lidocaine can accumulate to toxic levels associated with neurologic dysfunction and seizures and should be monitored, particularly in patients with poor systemic and hepatic perfusion. Negative inotropic properties have

been associated with procainamide, and the accumulation of its active metabolite, n-acetyl procainamide, may result in renal insufficiency (26). Bradyarrhythmias are treated with cardiac pacing through epicardial wires placed intraoperatively. Significant hemodynamic benefit may be achieved through sequential atrioventricular pacing (22).

In reviewing the postoperative ECG, careful attention should be paid to ischemic changes. If there is evidence of myocardial ischemia, intravenous nitroglycerin is administered and other therapies are adjusted to minimize myocardial oxygen demand. Immediate coronary and graft angiography may then be considered as a therapeutic action.

Pulmonary Support

Oxygen delivery is critically dependent on adequate oxygen resaturation of hemoglobin during the blood's transpulmonary transit (Table 22.3). Hypoxemia is particularly deleterious in these patients because the normal compensatory responses such as increased cardiac output (53) are absent in the early postoperative period. Postoperative ventilatory support should maximize arterial oxygen saturation while avoiding oxygen toxicity and the cardiovascular consequences of positive-pressure ventilation and positive end-expiratory pressure (PEEP). The fractional concentration of inspired oxygen (FIo_2) should be maintained at 0.5 as determined by digital pulse oximetry and intermittent

Table 22.3
Pulmonary Support

Postoperative changes
   Hypothermia: respiratory alkalosis, decreased CO_2 production
   Rewarming/shivering: marked increase in CO_2 production, respiratory acidosis possible
Goal
   Ensure arterial hemoglobin saturation
   Avoid deleterious effects of high FIo_2 and PEEP
   Titrate minute ventilation to normocarbia
   Wean FIo_2 to 0.5 or less with SAo_2 $\geq$95%

analysis of arterial blood gases. Noncardiogenic pulmonary edema may rarely occur after cardiopulmonary bypass. The precise mechanism remains elusive, although complement activation has been implicated (41). Treatment usually requires administration of increased levels of FIO_2 and PEEP (45). The application of PEEP at high levels is likely to compromise the utility of the pulmonary artery occlusion pressure as an accurate indicator of LV filling pressure (54) and thus complicate hemodynamic management. Moderate volume loading may be necessary to combat the usual decline in cardiac output that results from the inhibition of venous return induced by the increase in intrathoracic pressure by PEEP (29).

Hypercapnia is avoided through adjustment of minute ventilation (usually through changes in rate), as respiratory acidosis induces an elevation in pulmonary vascular resistance and RV stroke work (29, 71). Although the early period of intensive care is usually characterized by respiratory alkalosis (with decreased CO_2 production during hypothermia and anesthesia), an increase in $PaCO_2$ is likely during rewarming, especially if shivering is present (another reason to inhibit shivering as previously described). Weaning from ventilatory support and extubation can be performed when the following criteria have been achieved: neurologic state adequate to protect and clear the airway, cardiovascular stability, minute ventilation less than 30% above normal, normocapnia, and adequate arterial oxygen saturation on PEEP of 5 cm H_2O and FIO_2 of 0.5 or less (30).

Renal and Metabolic Considerations

Preservation of renal function is a priority in postoperative management (Table 22.4). Notable diuresis is one characteristic of the normal recovery pattern after moderate hypothermia cardiopulmonary bypass. As a result, urine output is not a reliable indicator of adequate perfusion in the first 6–12 hours of intensive care. Early intravenous infusion of low doses of dopamine (1–2 mg/kg/min) may be beneficial by causing splanchnic vasodilation-maintained diuresis (without significant tachy-

Table 22.4
Renal Support

Postoperative changes
  Hypothermia: marked diuresis, hypomagnesemia
  Later: Hypochloremic metabolic alkalosis
    Consider low-dose dopamine infusion, correct magnesium and potassium deficiencies
    Loop diuretics for negative fluid balance
    Postoperative day 1–3:
    Potassium chloride repletion for metabolic alkalosis

cardia) (27, 28, 35). Because volume expansion is always associated with cardiopulmonary bypass, loop diuretics to augment a negative fluid balance can be given as early as the 1st day after surgery. The resulting diuresis may induce a hypochloremic metabolic alkalosis, which can best be corrected by aggressive replacement of potassium chloride. Hypochloremic metabolic alkalosis generally is not threatening to patient well-being unless compensatory hypoventilation (with CO_2 retention) becomes significant, in which case, promoting a bicarbonate diuresis with intravenous acetazolamide may accelerate correction (5).

Hypomagnesemia is commonly associated with chronic administration of digoxin or diuretics, as in patients with congestive heart failure. Perioperative administration of osmotic diuretics (e.g., mannitol) may exaggerate this deficiency. Hypomagnesemia alone or in combination with hypokalemia may induce tachyarrhythmias, coronary arterial spasm, or renal or myocardial dysfunction (31, 73). Electrocardiographic abnormalities mimicking potassium deficiency are readily reversed with intravenous administration of magnesium sulfate. Slow infusion is recommended to avoid vasodilation and hypotension.

Control of Bleeding and Coagulation

Excessive postoperative bleeding may result in life-threatening consequences, including tamponade (Table 22.5). Although

Table 22.5
Coagulation Support

Postoperative changes
  Hypothermia: impaired coagulation and
    platelet function
  Rewarming/shivering: residual heparin
    effect
    Evaluate coagulation studies and throm-
      boelastogram (TEG)
    Correct thrombocytopenia, heparin effect
      (protamine), and coagulopathies if
      bleeding present
    Surgical reexploration for bleeding in the
      absence of coagulopathy

the need for reexploration to control hemorrhage reportedly is rare (around 4% (13)), moderate drainage (more than 200 ml of blood per hour) is more common. Numerous factors can promote bleeding during the early postoperative period. Bleeding can result from a wide variety of coagulopathies, including fibrinolysis, dilution or consumption of clotting factors, thrombocytopenia, and thrombocytopathy. Through mechanisms that remain elusive, extracorporeal circulation appears to be the major source of thrombocytopathy, which in turn is a frequent cause of hemorrhage. Anticoagulation produced with heparin during cardiopulmonary bypass can be reversed with protamine sulfate, which normalizes the activated clotting time (sometimes determined by individual dose-response curves (11)). Rare but severe adverse reactions have occurred with protamine, and may be mediated through elaboration of the complement fraction C5a and the prostanoid thromboxane (49) through direct myocardial depression (34). These reactions include profound hypotension with vasodilation and heart failure, noncardiogenic pulmonary edema, pulmonary vasoconstriction, and bronchospasm (61). Caution during protamine administration (especially in patients previously exposed to protamine in preparations of NPH insulin) is appropriate. The transfusion of blood products to correct coagulopathy is best guided by standard tests such as platelet count, prothrombin, and partial thromboplastin times as well as by assessments of overall clot formation and reaction using thromboelastography (70). Should bleeding persist despite all corrective efforts, at more than approximately 200 ml/hour (with a hematocrit in the chest-tube blood greater than half that of the circulating blood), surgical reexploration is necessary.

UNIQUE SUBGROUPS OF CARDIAC SURGICAL PATIENTS

Cardiac Transplant Recipients

It has only been recent that transplantation of the human heart has become a routine life-saving procedure with low postoperative mortality and high-quality, long-term survival. Implantation of the donor heart into the recipient requires a redundant remnant of the recipient's native atria for anastomosis (43). As a result, two autonomous atrial depolarizations may appear on the ECG after surgery, which confuses the interpretation. Maneuvers that increase vagal tone will not alter the denervated heart's ventricular rate, because the donor heart is completely excluded from all normal sympathetic and parasympathetic innervation. This is most likely a permanent condition (47, 48, 66).

Arrhythmias are particularly common after cardiac transplantation (32), with supraventricular and transient ventricular tachycardia occurring in as many as 60% of these patients. Bradyarrhythmias are also common, but necessitate permanent cardiac pacing in fewer than 20% of such cases (37). Antiarrhythmic pharmacotherapy must be independent of direct autonomic activities to be effective. Thus, atropine is ineffective for bradycardia, which must be treated instead with β-receptor agonists or epicardial pacing. Digoxin is much less useful for acute control of atrial fibrillation because its vagotonic actions are ineffectual. Instead, procainamide is used to control many supraventricular and ventricular tachyarrhythmias (65).

In general, cardiopulmonary support is provided as previously described, but with a few words of caution. First, the donor heart is particularly sluggish after profound hypothermia induced during preservation and before transplantation. In addition, the heart rate tends to be quite slow with cardiac output depending on the heart rate during this early period of denervation unless appropriately supported. Therefore, all cardiac transplant recipients are treated with chronotropic and inotropic support for several days after surgery. Second, RV dysfunction is a particular concern, especially in the presence of the pulmonary hypertension that often results from congestive heart failure and cardiomyopathy. Patients with severe pulmonary hypertension (generally, a transpulmonary pressure gradient greater than 15 mm Hg that is unresponsive to vasodilators such as prostaglandin E_1 during pretransplant evaluation) are excluded from orthotopic transplantation because of the associated increase in morbidity and mortality levels (24, 50). Nonetheless, mild pulmonary hypertension is common in transplant recipients, and the newly transplanted right ventricle, unaccustomed to an environment of increased afterload, must be supported. Dobutamine and isoproterenol are preferred agents in these circumstances. The pulmonary vasodilating eicosanoid prostaglandin E_1 is also of value, as it may effectively reduce RV afterload and improve pump function (2) without significantly impairing hypoxic pulmonary vasoconstriction or exacerbating shunt (33). The implantation of moderately oversized donor hearts in patients with increased levels of pulmonary vascular resistance before transplantation is also effective in minimizing postoperative RV failure.

The consequences of immunosuppressive therapy that are relevant to the early postoperative period include increased susceptibility to infection and renal function impairment (with cyclosporine (4) and, perhaps to a lesser extent, FK506). Pulmonary function may thus be compromised by fluid retention or by pneumonia, and aggressive diagnostic and therapeutic maneuvers should be performed for all abnormalities that appear on the radiograph (58). With pneumonia, diagnosis of specific pathogens is often difficult, and bronchoalveolar lavage (63, 67) may be necessary.

Delayed deterioration in pulmonary function with hypoxemia may herald cardiac dysfunction with cardiogenic pulmonary edema. Endomyocardial biopsy is then used to evaluate the possibility of rejection and the need for adjustment in immunotherapy (6). Rejection is most common during the first 6 months after transplantation and is suggested by any evidence of decreased ventricular compliance, new pericardial effusion, new tachyarrhythmias, or systolic dysfunction (57). Echocardiography that reveals a reduction in isovolumetric relaxation time and pressure half-times also may support this diagnosis (18).

Patients with Valvular Heart Disease

Aortic Stenosis

The consequences of aortic stenosis include notable LV hypertrophy as a compensatory response to chronic pressure overload. Ventricular compliance is decreased and LV cavity size is generally reduced. As a result, small changes in volume loading may markedly change pressures and stroke volume. Maintenance of adequate preload and sustenance of normal sinus rhythm are critical to pump function. Myocardial protection during cardiopulmonary bypass is complicated by the tremendous increase in LV mass, and postoperative LV dysfunction may occur. If the left ventricle is well preserved, a hyperdynamic state with marked hypertension may predominate the early postoperative period as a result of the unloading of the left ventricle following relief of the aortic stenosis. Intravenous infusion of the ultrashort-acting β-blocker esmolol is particularly useful to control this hyperdynamic state. On the other hand, if significant preoperative LV dysfunction exists before surgery, the LV ejection fraction and systolic function may not always normalize (56), and aggressive pharmacologic support may be needed.

Aortic Regurgitation

In contrast, the chronically volume-overloaded left ventricle of the patient with long-standing aortic regurgitation (frequently as a result of myxomatous degeneration or a rheumatic or bicuspid aortic valve) is usually highly compliant and dilated, although LV hypertrophy does occur. Over time, the left ventricle will continue to dilate and eventually develop irreversible dysfunction. Only at this point will LV end-diastolic pressure increase and congestive heart failure become evident. Valve replacement is best done early, before ventricular decompensation. If the ventricle has reached end-stage dilation, surgery is poorly tolerated. Support with counterpulsation via intraaortic balloon pump is contraindicated under these dire circumstances as the diastolic cycling is likely to increase the regurgitant fraction and cause further volume overload of the left ventricle. Postoperative persistence of the reduced peripheral resistance (usually accompanying the increased stroke volumes seen with aortic regurgitation) may require the temporary use of α-adrenergic agents to support diastolic blood pressure and coronary perfusion. Similarly, the intraortic balloon pump can be used to support diastolic coronary perfusion. Hypotension and hypoperfusion after valve surgery indicate a particularly poor prognosis, despite these aggressive maneuvers, with a 1-month survival rate of only 50% (23), although the overall rate of survival after aortic valve surgery is above 96% in some institutions (44).

Mitral Valve Disease

Mitral stenosis generally preserves LV function, as both pressure and volume overload are absent. However, significant pulmonary hypertension and RV compromise with tricuspid regurgitation may be present. These problems are even more common in patients with mitral regurgitation, who are generally older and more debilitated than others with valvular heart disease. Atrial fibrillation, increased levels of total body water, and left atrial thrombi all may accompany mitral valve disease. The right ventricle is particularly susceptible to injury in the perioperative period (7, 12, 69), and life-threatening RV dysfunction may occur, particularly in the presence of persistent pulmonary hyper-

tension. Infusion of prostaglandin, as previously mentioned for patients with a cardiac transplant, may improve RV function through pulmonary vasodilation in patients with mitral valve disease (16), as well as with patients with coronary bypass (19) and severe pulmonary hypertension or congestive heart failure. Even pulmonary artery balloon counterpulsation (68) or a mechanical right ventricle assist device has occasionally been applied to save patients with severe RV dysfunction leading to biventricular failure and hypoperfusion.

CONCLUSION

Cardiothoracic surgery has evolved remarkably in the last several decades. Improvements in preoperative stabilization, intraoperative myocardial protection and preservation, and postoperative critical care have resulted in improved survival rates for patients with debilitating cardiovascular diseases. As our understanding of the pathophysiology of these disease states and the physiologic consequences of our interventions improves, so will the quality of our care of these patients.

References

1. Ardehali A, Ports TA. Myocardial oxygen supply and demand. Chest 1990;98:699–705.
2. Armitage JM, Hardesty RL, Griffith BP. Prostaglandin E_1: an effective treatment for right heart failure after orthotopic heart transplantation. J Heart Transplant 1987;6:348–351.
3. Beerthuizen GI, Goris RJ, Bredee JJ, et al. Muscle oxygen tension, hemodynamics, and oxygen transport after extracorporeal circulation. Crit Care Med 1988;16:748–750.
4. Bennet WM, Pulliam JP. Cyclosporine nephrotoxicity. Ann Intern Med 1983;99:851–854.
5. Berthelson P. Cardiovascular performance and oxyhemoglobin dissociation after acetazolamide in metabolic alkalosis. Intensive Care Med 1982;8:269–274.
6. Billingham ME. Diagnosis of cardiac rejection by endomyocardial biopsy. J Heart Transplant 1980;1:25–30.
7. Boldt J, Kling D. Moosdorf R, Hempelmann G. Influence of acute volume loading on right ventricular function after cardiopulmonary bypass. Crit Care Med 1989;17:518–522.
8. Boldt J, Kling D, Thiel A, et al. Revascularization of the right coronary artery: influence on thermodilution right ventricular ejection fraction. J Cardiothorac Anesth 1988;2:140–146.
9. Breisblatt WM, Stein KL, Wolfe C, et al. Acute

myocardial dysfunction and recovery: a common occurrence after coronary bypass surgery. J Am Coll Cardiol 1990;15:1261–1269.

10. Brister NW, Barnette RE, Schartel SA, McClurken JB, Alpern J. Isradipine for treatment of acute hypertension after myocardial revascularization. Crit Care Med 1991;19:334–338.

11. Bull BS, Huse W, Brauer F, et al. Heparin therapy during extracorporeal circulation. II. The use of a dose-response curve to individualize heparin and protamine dosage. J Thorac Cardiovasc Surg 1975;69:685–689.

12. Christakis GT, Fremes SE, Weisel RD, et al. Right ventricular dysfunction following cold potassium cardioplegia. J Thorac Cardiovasc Surg 1985;90:243–250.

13. Cosgrove DM, Loop FD, Lytle BW, et al. Determinants of blood utilization during myocardial revascularization. Ann Thorac Surg 1985;40:380–384.

14. Cruise CJ, Skrobik Y, Webster RE, Marquet-Julio A, David TE. Intravenous labetalol versus sodium nitroprusside for treatment of hypertension post coronary bypass surgery. Anesthesiology 1989;71:835–839.

15. Czer LSC, Shoemaker WC. Optimal hematocrit value in critically ill postoperative patients. Surg Gynecol Obstet 1978;147:363–368.

16. D'Ambra MN, LaRaia PJ, Philbin DM, Watkins WD, Hilgenberg AD, Buckley MJ. Prostaglandin E_1. A new therapy for refractory right heart failure and pulmonary hypertension after mitral valve replacement. J Thorac Cardiovasc Surg 1985;89:567–572.

17. Davis SV, Olichwier KK, Chakko SC. Reversible depression of myocardial performance in hypophosphatemia. Am J Med Sci 1988;295:183–187.

18. Desruennes M, Corcos T, Cabrol A, et al. Doppler echocardiography for the diagnosis of acute cardiac allograft rejection. J Am Coll Cardiol 1988;12:63–70.

19. Dewhirst WE. Prostaglandin E_1 for refractory right heart failure after coronary artery bypass grafting. J Cardiothorac Anesth 1988;2:56–59.

20. Dhainaut JF, Brunet F, Monsallier JF, et al. Bedside evaluation of right ventricular performance using a rapid computerized thermodilution method. Crit Care Med 1987;15:148–152.

21. Dhainaut JF, Schremmer B, Lanore JJ. The coronary circulation and the myocardial oxygen supply/uptake relationship: a short review. J Crit Care 1991;6:52–60.

22. Donovan KD, Dobb GJ, Lee KY. Hemodynamic benefit of maintaining atrioventricular synchrony during cardiac pacing in critically ill patients. Crit Care Med 1991;19:320–326.

23. Downing TP, Miller DC, Stofer R, Shumway ME. Use of the intra-aortic balloon pump after valve replacement. J Thorac Cardiovasc Surg 1986;92:210–217.

24. Erickson KW, Costanzo-Nordin MR, O'Sullivan EJ, et al. Influence of preoperative transpulmonary gradient on late mortality after orthotopic heart transplantation. J Heart Transplant 1990;9:526–537.

25. Estefanous FG, Tarazi RC. Systemic arterial hypertension associated with cardiac surgery. Am J Cardiol 1980;46:685–694.

26. Galleazzi RL, Benet LZ, Sheiner LB. Relationship between pharmacokinetics and pharmacodynamics of procainamide. Clin Pharmacol Ther 1976;20:278–289.

27. Goldberg LI. Cardiovascular and renal actions of dopamine: potential clinical implications. Pharmacol Rev 1972;24:1–29.

28. Goldberg LI. Dopamine-clinical uses of an endogenous catecholamine. N Engl J Med 1974;291:707–710.

29. Guyton RA, Chiaverelli M, Padgett CA, et al. The influence of positive end-expiratory pressure on intrapericardial pressure and cardiac function after coronary artery bypass surgery. J Cardiothorac Anesth 1987;1:98–107.

30. Hall JB, Wood LD. Liberation of the patient from mechanical ventilation. JAMA 1987;257:1621–1628.

31. Harris MN, Crowther A, Jupp RA, Aps C. Magnesium and coronary revascularization. Br J Anaesth 1988;60:779–783.

32. Harrison DC, Mason JW, Schroeder JS, et al. Effects of cardiac denervation on cardiac arrhythmias and electrophysiology. Br Heart J 1978;40:17–23.

33. Heerdt PM, Yee LL. Differential effect of prostaglandin E_1 and sodium nitroprusside on intrapulmonary shunt fraction in a cardiac transplantation patient. Anesth Analg 1989;69:665–667.

34. Hendry PJ, Taichman GC, Keon WJ. The myocardial contractile responses to protamine sulfate and heparin. Ann Thorac Surg 1987;44:263–268.

35. Hilberman M, Maseda J, Stinson EB, et al. The diuretic properties of dopamine in patients after open-heart operations. Anesthesiology 1984;61:489–494.

36. Ivanov J, Weisel RD, Mickleborough LL, Hilton JD, McLaughlin PR. Rewarming hypovolemia after aortocoronary bypass surgery. Crit Care Med 1984;12:1049–1054.

37. Jacquet L, Ziady G, Stein K, et al. Cardiac rhythm disturbances early after orthotopic heart transplantation: prevalence and clinical importance of the observed abnormalities. J Am Coll Cardiol 1990;16:832–837.

38. Jalonen J, Heikkila H, Arola M, et al. Myocardial oxygen balance and cardiopulmonary bypass in patients undergoing coronary artery bypass grafting. J Cardiothorac Anesth 1989;3:311–320.

39. Karanko MS, Laaksonen VO, Meretoja OA. Effects of concentrated albumin treatment after aortocoronary bypass surgery. Crit Care Med 1987;15:737–742.

40. Komatsu T, Shibutani K, Okamoto K, et al. Critical level of oxygen delivery after cardiopulmonary bypass. Crit Care Med 1987;15:194–197.

41. Knudsen F, Pedersen JO, Juhl O, et al. Complement and leukocytes during cardiopulmonary bypass: effects on plasma C3d and C5a, leukocyte count, release of granulocyte elastase and granulocyte chemotaxis. J Cardiothorac Anesth 1988;2:164–170.

42. Lang RM, Borow KM, Neumann A, Janzin D. Systemic vascular resistance: an unreliable index of left ventricular afterload. Circulation 1986;74:1114–1123.

43. Lower RR, Shumway NE. Studies on orthotopic transplantation of the canine heart. Surg Forum 1960;2:18–19.

44. Lytle BW, Cosgrove DM, Taylor PC, et al. Primary isolated aortic valve replacement. Early and late results. J Thorac Cardiovasc Surg 1989;97:675–694.

45. Maggart M, Stewart S. The mechanisms and management of noncardiogenic pulmonary edema following cardiopulmonary bypass. Ann Thorac Surg 1987;43:231–236.

46. Mangano DT, Van Dyke DC, Ellis RJ. The effect of increasing preload on ventricular output and ejection in man. Circulation 1980;62:535–541.

47. Mason JW, Stinson EB, Harrison DC. Autonomic nervous system and arrhythmias: studies in the transplanted denervated human heart. Cardiology 1976;61:75–87.

48. McLaughlin PR, Kleiman JH, Martin RP, et al. The effects of exercise and atrial pacing on left ventricular volume and contractility in patients with innervated and denervated hearts. Circulation 1978;58:476–483.

49. Morel DR, Zapol WM, Thomas SJ, et al. C5a and thromboxane generation associated with pulmonary vaso- and broncho-constriction during protamine reversal of heparin. Anesthesiology 1987;66:597–604.

50. Murali S, Kormos RL, Uretsky B, et al. Preoperative pulmonary hypertension and mortality after orthotopic cardiac transplantation [Abstract]. J Heart Transplant 1990;9:56.

51. Newman JH, Neff TA, Ziporin P. Acute respiratory failure associated with hypophosphatemia. N Engl J Med 1977;296:1101–1103.

52. O'Connor LR, Wheeler WS, Bethune JE. Effect of hypophosphatemia on myocardial performance in man. N Engl J Med 1977;297:901–903.

53. Phillips BA, McConnel JW, Smith MD. The effects of hypoxemia on cardiac output. A dose-response curve. Chest 1988;93:471–475.

54. Pinsky MR, Guimond JG. The effects of positive end-expiratory pressure on heart-lung interactions. J Crit Care 1991;6:1–11.

55. Ralley FE, Wynands JE, Ramsay JG, Carli F, MacSullivan R. The effects of shivering on oxygen consumption and carbon dioxide production in patients rewarming from hypothermic cardiopulmonary bypass. Can J Anaesth 1988;35:332–337.

56. Rediker DE, Boucher CA, Block PC, Akins CW, Buckley MJ, Fifer MA. Degree of reversibility of left ventricular systolic dysfunction after aortic valve replacement for isolated aortic valve stenosis. Am J Cardiol 1987;60:112–118.

57. Renlund DG, Bristow MR, Lee HR, et al. Medical aspects of cardiac transplantation. J Cardiothorac Anesth 1988;2:500–512.

58. Schulman LL, Smith CR, Drusin R, Rose EA, Enson Y, Reemtsma K. Respiratory complications of cardiac transplantation. Am J Med Sci 1988;296:1–10.

59. Schwenzer KJ, Kopel RF. Hemodynamic and metabolic effects of dobutamine in 18 patients after open heart surgery. Crit Care Med 1990;18:1107–1110.

60. Seward JB, Khandheria BK, Oh JK, et al. Transesophageal echocardiography: technique, anatomic correlations, implementation, and clinical applications. Mayo Clin Pro 1988;63:649–680.

61. Shapira N, Scheff HV, Piebler JM, et al. Cardiovascular effects of protamine sulfate in man. J Thorac Cardiovasc Surg 1982;84:505–514.

62. Shepherd RF, Zachariah PK, Shub C. Hypertension and left ventricular diastolic function. Mayo Clin Proc 1989;64:1521–1532.

63. Singer C, Armstrong D, Rosen PP, et al. Diffusion pulmonary infiltrate in immunosuppressed patients: a prospective study of 80 cases. Am J Med 1979;66:110–120.

64. Stein KL, Breisblatt W, Wolfe C, Gasior T, Hardesty R. Depression and recovery of right ventricular function after cardiopulmonary bypass. Crit Care Med 1990;18:1197–1200.

65. Stein KL, Darby JD, Grenvik A. Intensive care of the cardiac transplant recipient. J Cardiothorac Anesth 1988;2:543–553.

66. Stinson EB, Griepp RB, Schroeder JS, et al. Hemodynamic observations one and two years after cardiac transplantation in man. Circulation 1972;45:1183–1194.

67. Stover DE, Zaman MB, Hadju SI, et al. Bronchoalveolar lavage in the diagnosis of diffuse pulmonary infiltrates in the immunosuppressed host. Ann Intern Med 1985;101:1–7.

68. Symbas PN, McKeown PP, Santora AH, Vlasis SE. Pulmonary artery balloon counterpulsation for treatment of intraoperative right ventricular failure. Ann Thorac Surg 1985;39:437–440.

69. Thomson IR, Rosenbloom M, Cannon JE, Morris A. Electrocardiographic ST-segment elevation after myocardial reperfusion during coronary artery surgery. Anesth Analg 1987;66:1183–1186.

70. Tuman KJ, Spiess BD, McCarthy RJ, Ivankovich AD. Effects of progressive blood loss on coagulation as measured by thromboelastography. Anesth Analg 1987;66:856–863.

71. Viitanen A, Salmenpera M, Heinonen J. Right ventricular response to hypercarbia after cardiac surgery. Anesthesiology 1990;73:393–400.

72. Deleted in proof.

73. Whang R. Magnesium deficiency: pathogenesis, prevalence, and clinical implications. Am J Med 1987;82:24–29.

23

Infective Endocarditis

Michel Wolff
Serge Witchitz

During the past decade, significant progess has been made in both the diagnosis and treatment of infective endocarditis. Recent advances in echocardiography and Doppler technology have led to a substantial increase in diagnostic accuracy. The current improvement in outcome is the consequence of earlier and better surgical management of cardiac complications, combined with a more rational use of antibiotics.

PREDISPOSING FACTORS AND ETIOLOGY

Predisposing Factors

Almost any type of structural heart disease can predispose to infective endocarditis. Rheumatic heart disease was the most common underlying cardiac lesion in the preantibiotic era (53). Some recent studies have emphasized the changing spectrum of recognized abnormalities underlying endocarditis. Many factors, such as antibiotic treatment of streptococcal diseases, the steadily increasing age of the population, and improved diagnostic techniques (particularly echocardiography), may explain this phenomenon. Indeed, among 330 cases of native valve endocarditis observed between 1973 and 1988 at the Claude Bernard Hospital in Paris, France, rheumatic heart disease was present in only 13%. Similar (47) or even lower (62) percentages have recently been reported in the U.S. and in the United Kingdom.

Degenerative calcific lesions are now the most commonly identified cardiac abnormalities in patients over the age of 60 (53, 62). Congenital heart disease is the predisposing factor in 6–24% of cases with a high prevalence of bicuspid aortic valve. Mitral valve prolapse, which affects as many as 5–10% of the population, was the main underlying lesion in a recent study of 63 patients with endocarditis (53). Several authors have compared the frequency of mitral valve prolapse in patients with endocarditis and in matched controls and have suggested a greater risk of endocarditis when mitral valve prolapse is present (16, 54). Recently, the frequency of this lesion was assessed by Danchin et al. (24) in patients with mitral valve endocarditis and in matched controls. Patients with prolapse were nearly 6 times more likely to have endocarditis than were the controls. In addition, the risk was 14.5 times higher in subjects with prolapse and a previously identified systolic murmur.

Other lesions, such as Marfan's syndrome with aortic insufficiency and hypertrophic obstructive cardiomyopathy, have also been associated with endocarditis. Finally, it should be emphasized that there is an increasing number of cases of endocarditis involving otherwise normal valves, especially when virulent pathogens such as *Staphylococcus aureus*, *Streptococcus pneumoniae*, and Gram-negative rods are involved. Indeed, 70% of 118 patients with *S. aureus* endocarditis seen in our institution had no preexisting disease, versus 32% when streptococci or enterococci were the causative organisms.

Etiology According to Risk Factors

Native Valve Endocarditis in Nonaddicts

Dental Procedures and Diseases

The incidence of transient bacteremia associated with tooth extraction has been reported to range from 18–85%; other procedures may also cause bacteremia. However, in a recent large retrospective study conducted by Bayliss et al. (7), only 14% of 544 cases of endocarditis had undergone any dental procedure within 3 months of the onset of the illness. Since *Streptococcus viridans*, which abounds in the mouth and nasopharynx, were responsible for half of the cases of endocarditis, other factors such as poor dental hygiene and minor or unrecognized periodontal disease might have been present. Other pathogens may be involved in valve infections of dental or buccal origins and include *Streptococcus bovis*, enterococci, staphylococci, and occasionally anaerobic bacteria.

Gastrointestinal and Urogenital Tract Lesions or Procedures

Enterococci and *S. bovis* are the most commonly isolated pathogens in these settings. A large variety of gastrointestinal procedures result in transient bacteremia, but rarely lead to endocarditis: barium enema, colonoscopy, fiberoptic gastroscopy with biopsy, and injection sclerosis of esophageal varices. Various urologic procedures also engender bacteremia, and the incidence is higher when the urine is infected. Urethral dilation and transurethral prostatic resection are the most dangerous manipulations since they cause bacteremia in 15–40% of the cases. The association of endocarditis due to *S. bovis* with carcinoma and other lesions of the colon is well known. Gastrointestinal or urogenital lesions account for 25–50% and 20–30%, respectively, of documented portals of entry in patients with enterococcal endocarditis (42, 71). This disease affects older patients more frequently. Factors that suggest endocarditis in patients with enterococcal bacteremia have been studied by Makki and Agger (56) and include preexisting heart disease, community-acquired infection, no identifiable extracardiac focus of infection, and the absence of polymicrobial bacteremia. Enterococci and group B streptococcal valve infections have been also reported in women with postpartum and postabortion urogenital infections.

Despite an increasing incidence of enteric bacillary septicemia, endocarditis due to these pathogens is uncommon. This may be due to the fact that Gram-negative bacilli adhere less avidly to the endothelium than other bacteria such as streptococci and staphylococci (38). In the same way, nonstreptococcal anaerobic bacteria are rarely involved in this disease.

Hospital-Acquired Endocarditis

Nosocomial bacteremia is a serious complication of hospitalization that occurs mainly in patients with intravascular catheters. However, in most retrospective (37, 51, 61) and prospective (64) studies concerning nosocomial *S. aureus* bacteremia, the incidence of endocarditis is surprisingly very low. Indeed, Tsao and Katz (84) have extensively reviewed 32 studies involving 1950 patients with central venous catheters. There were only three valve infections among these patients, although the rate of catheter-associated bacteremia ranged from 3 to 44%.

By contrast, other authors have found a higher incidence of nosocomial endocarditis. In a prospective study of 55 consecutive patients who underwent autopsy and who had undergone flow-directed pulmonary artery catheterization, 53% had one or more right-sided endocardial lesions. Moreover, four patients (7%) had valve infections with positive antemortem blood cultures with the catheter in place (74). In a recent study, nosocomial episodes represented 14% of all endocarditis cases seen. Intravascular devices and urogenital tract surgery instrumentation were the source of infection in 45% and 27% of the 22 cases, respectively (82). In 199 cases of *S. aureus* endocarditis observed in a Danish study between 1976 and 1981, 38% were hospital-acquired (36). Staphylococci (both *S. aureus* and coagulase-negative) are the predominant pathogens in nosocomial cardiac infections, being far more frequent than streptococci and Gram-negative rods. Prolonged placement of an intravenous catheter is also a predisposing factor for fungal endocarditis.

Risk Factors for S. aureus Endocarditis

Staphylococcus aureus causes 20–30% of all cases of native valve endocarditis and is the etiologic agent in most acute infections. Approximately half of all patients have no clinically detectable underlying cardiac disease. In 50–60% of these cases, no obvious portal of entry is detected, although the skin is probably the source in many cases. In addition to valvular vegetations detected by echocardiography, three parameters are significantly predictive of endocarditis in staphylococcemic patients: community acquisition, absence of a primary site of infection, and metastatic complications (5).

Predisposing factors for *S. aureus* endocarditis (other than drug addiction and prostheses) are less well defined. The relationship between nasal carriage of *S. aureus* and infections has been established in specific subsets of patients such as those on hemodialysis. In one study (18), diabetic patients with *S. aureus* bacteremia were more likely than those without diabetes to have valve infections in the presence of primary foci. Finally, the typical *S. aureus* left-sided native valve endocarditis occurs in subjects with or without previous disease and often with no obvious predisposing factor.

Other Risk Factors

Immunosuppressed Patients. Various pathogens, including fungi, have been implicated in a limited number of valve infections in immunosuppressed patients because of major underlying disease or treatment with steroids or radiation. Despite frequent bacteremic episodes, endocarditis appears to be uncommon in hematologic patients. However, in a recent prospective study reported by Martino et al. (58), 5% of 141 bone marrow transplant recipients developed catheter-related right-sided endocarditis predominantly due to *Staphylococcus epidermidis*. The incidence of valve infection among AIDS patients is not higher than in the population without AIDS, except for drug addicts

Infective Endocarditis Caused by Ani-mal Exposure. *Brucella* sp. continue to be important etiologic agents in some countries, e.g., Saudi Arabia, where the organisms are responsible for nearly 10% of endocarditis cases. In addition, animal exposure is a major risk factor for the following agents: *Coxiella burnetii*, *Chlamydia psittaci*, *Erysipelothrix rhusiopathiae*, and *Haemophilus aphrophilus*.

Endocarditis in Parenteral Drug Abusers

Addiction to intravenous drugs has become an increasingly important predisposing factor in the development of endocarditis. In the U.S., the incidence of this disease among drug abusers is about 1.5–2% per year (50). Two types of maladies are most commonly seen: tricuspid valve infection, accounting for 60–80% of episodes in this population, and left-sided endocarditis, the aortic and mitral valve each being infected in 10–20% of cases. Pulmonic valve involvement is present in less than 1% of cases and is either isolated (50%) or associated with tricuspid valve infection (22). *Staphylococcus aureus* is the most frequently identified pathogen, especially in right-sided infection where it is isolated in approximately 80% of cases. Tuazon and Sheagren (85) have shown that drug abusers themselves are generally the source of the infecting organism. In a recent study, 61% of drug abusers were carriers of *S. aureus* in the throat, nose, or on the skin (8). Almost all cases of *S. aureus* right-sided endocarditis in the setting of drug addiction are caused by methicillin-sensitive strains. However, Levine et al. (50) have reported that community-acquired methicillin-resistant *S. aureus* accounts for half of the cases of bacteremia due to this species in heroin abusers in the Detroit area. There is a correlation between self-treatment with antistaphylococcal antibiotics such as cefazolin and the isolation of resistant strains from drug addicts. Streptococci, enterococci, and *S. epidermidis* are far less frequently involved (2% each). Groups A and G streptococcal endocarditis have recently been observed in patients using the femoral veins for heroin injection (20).

In drug addicts, aerobic Gram-negative endocarditis occurs sporadically with clusters of cases in particular areas. There is also a definite geographic predominance. In Detroit, 13.5% of cases between 1982 and 1983 were due to *Pseudomonas aeruginosa*. In Chicago, the percentage of cases of endocarditis caused by this pathogen among drug abusers increased from 23% in 1978 to 68% in 1980. Most cases occurred in persons who took pentazocine and tripelennamine and were due to contaminated needles and syringes (76).

Drug addiction is also a predisposing factor for fungal infections. The pathogens isolated most often are generally other than *Candida albicans* (*C. parapsilosis*, *C. tropicalis*, *C. guillermondi* and *C. kruzei*) (77). Unusual organisms include diphtheroids, *Lactobacillus*, *Pseudomonas* sp., various *Neisseiria* species, and anaerobic bacteria. Reports of polymicrobial endocarditis are rare and most are related to heroin abuse; the tricuspid and mitral valves are most commonly affected. Occult polymicrobial right-sided endocarditis has recently been reported in intravenous drug abusers. The patients had unsuspected polymicrobial valve infection due to *Haemophilus parainfluenzae*, which was identified between several days and weeks after the isolation of another microorganism from the blood (in most cases *S. viridans*). The practice of cleaning needles with saliva was probably the main mechanism (69). Finally, culture-negative endocarditis is rarely encountered in drug abusers, probably because virulent pathogens are usually involved.

Prosthetic Valve Endocarditis

Infection of the intracardiac prosthesis is a serious, often life-threatening complication of valve replacement surgery. Although the prognosis has improved during the past decade, prosthetic valve endocarditis is still a significant cause of morbidity and mortality.

Incidence and Risk Factors

The current incidence of prosthethic valve endocarditis is about 3%. In recent reports, the actuarial risk is approximately 6% at 5 years after surgery (11). Risk factors that play a role in the development of this infection have been evaluated by several investigators (11, 43). The incidence is higher in recipients of mechanical valves during the first 3 postoperative months; in patients who receive biological valves, it is higher after 12 months. However, there is no difference after 5 years according to the type of prosthesis. Replacement of more than one valve, advanced age, longer cardiopulmonary bypass time, and preoperative native valve endocarditis are additional risk factors. The site most commonly involved is an aortic prosthesis, but the infection rate is identical when adjusted for the number of valves implanted.

Source and Microbiology

By convention, prosthetic valve endocarditis is termed "early" when it appears within 60 days of valve replacement, and "late" when it occurs after this period. The two categories show significant difference in clinical features, microbial etiology, and mortality. However, Calderwood et al. (11) have shown that the microbiological pattern is similar in infections occurring within 2 months of valve insertion (early endocarditis) and those occurring up to 12 months after valve insertion (semilate endocarditis). In both groups, methicillin-resistant coagulase-negative staphylococci were the major pathogens. By contrast, after the 1st year (late endocarditis) there is a predominance of streptococci. Early and semilate prosthetic valve infections are usually acquired during the perioperative period. Several studies have shown the potential role of intraoperative contamination from sources such as the patient's skin, the operating room personnel, or contaminated blood in the bypass pump. Predisposing conditions in the postoperative period include bacteremia from infected intravascular catheters, postoperative pneumonia, chest wound infections, or infections from other sites. By contrast, the pathogenesis of late infections appears similar to that of native valve endocarditis. Conditions predisposing to late infections are dental diseases or procedures and intestinal or urogenital tract infections. The microorganisms responsible for prosthetic

Table 23.1
Distribution of Pathogens in Patients with Prosthetic Valve Endocarditis by Time of Onset after Surgery [a]

Pathogen	Time of Onset After Valve Replacement (Months)							
	<2		2–12		>12		Total	
	B	P	B	P	B	P	B	P
Coagulase-negative staphylococci	22	3	19	3	10	6	51	9
S. aureus	2	14	3	1	5	16	10	31
Streptococci	0	1	1	2	12	18	13	21
Enterococci	0	0	2	2	4	8	6	10
Gram-negative bacilli	2	4	1	1	1	5	4	10
Diphtheroids	4	0	0	0	1	4	5	4
Fastidious gram-negative coccobacilli	0	0	1	0	7	0	8	0
Fungi	2	1	2	1	1	1	5	3
Miscellaneous	3	2	2	0	1	2	6	4
Culture-negative	3	3	3	0	2	2	8	5
Total	38	28	34	10	44	62	116	97

[a] Boston group, 1975–1982 (11); P, Paris group, 1978–1988 (Claude Bernard Hospital).

valve endocarditis in two institutions are shown in Table 23.1. Staphylococci are the major cause of early and semilate infections, *S. epidermidis* being predominant in the Boston study (11), while *S. aureus* accounts for the majority of cases in the Paris study. In the latter study, *S. aureus* was isolated as frequently as streptococci in late infections. In both groups, staphylococci, streptococci, and enterococci accounted for 70% of the pathogens.

DIAGNOSIS AND MANAGEMENT

Definition

Infective endocarditis is usually categorized as definite, probable, or possible according to the criteria of von Reyn et al. (87). Briefly, definite endocarditis is defined as positive blood cultures with fresh valvular vegetations and/or destruction at autopsy or surgery. Probable endocarditis is defined as positive blood cultures and new or changing heart murmur along with at least one of the following: vegetation seen on echocardiography, emboli, and vascular phenomena. Possible endocarditis is defined as positive blood culture or changing heart murmur, but no other clinical manifestations and no vegetations seen on echocardiography.

The most precise and useful definition of prosthesis infection has been proposed by Calderwood et al. (11). The diagnosis is accepted if there are at least two of the following: (a) a compatible clinical syndrome with at least two of these criteria: fever, new murmur, skin manifestations, peripheral embolus, splenomegaly; (b) two or more positive blood cultures with the same pathogen; and (c) histologic or microbiologic evidence of infective endocarditis in a surgical or autopsy specimen. If there is a possible noncardiac source of bacteremia, valvular involvement has to be confirmed by a new or changing murmur, vegetations at echocardiography, or pathologic evidence of infective endocarditis.

Clinical Features and Blood Cultures

The symptoms and signs of endocarditis are multiple and the clinical presentation is variable. The mean duration of symptoms prior to diagnosis is usually shorter in prosthetic than in native valve infections (71). This probably reflects a heightened awareness of the risk of infection among patients with prosthetic valves. Fever is common, but may be absent in 5–10% of the cases. It must be emphasized that there is an increasing number of patients with endocarditis who have no initially detectable murmur. This is partly due to the higher frequency of acute disease caused by virulent pathogens. In subacute valve infection, a change in the character of the murmur or the appearance of a new murmur are observed in only 5–10% and 3–5% of the cases, respectively (77). By contrast, these features are common in both acute and prosthetic valve infections (50–90%) (19). The cause of the change is usually the destruction of the valve and its supporting structure. Indeed, the great majority of patients who have a new or changing regurgitant murmur develop heart failure. Skin manifestations are found in 20–50% of cases. "Classic" lesions such as Osler nodes (<20%), Janeway lesions (<10%), and Roth's spots have become less common. The most frequent skin abnormalities are petechiae (30%) caused by either vasculitis or emboli, particularly when *S. aureus* is the etiologic agent. Splenomegaly is found in one-third of all cases. Embolic complications, which occur in 30–50% of the patients, may be the first clinical manifestation, concomitant with fever, especially in patients with *S. aureus* infection. Finally, septic shock may occur with either native or early prosthetic valve infection.

The cornerstone of the diagnosis of infective endocarditis is isolation of the etiologic organism from the blood. The bacteremia is continuous, and blood cultures are positive on multiple samplings in more than 92% of patients. In approximately two-thirds of cases, all the blood cultures drawn are positive. One of the major causes of a negative result is treatment with antimicrobial agents before the diagnosis is established. In a retrospective study, 100% of blood cultures were positive in patients without antibiotic exposure versus 64% in those who had received antibiotics before hospitalization (67). The addition of antibiotic inhibitors to the media could be useful, but this technique has yet to be assessed. Fastidious bacteria, Q fever, Chlamydiae, and fungi are the main etiologic agents in negative blood culture endocarditis.

Echocardiography

Echocardiography is the method of choice in the investigation of patients with infective endocarditis. A series of major technical advances has significantly improved the value of this procedure, with transthoracic two-dimensional echocardiography, transesophageal imaging, and color-flow Doppler scanning for the detection of vegetations and perivalvular extension of the infection. Moreover, these procedures are used to assess valve dysfunction and hemodynamic status, therefore aiding in decisions on the indication and timing of cardiac surgery. The combined use of M-mode and transthoracic two-dimensional echocardiography can detect the valvular vegetations in about 75% of cases (evaluation of 14 studies involving 755 patients) (cited in 63). In patients with right-sided endocarditis, the rate of detection is approximately 85%. By contrast, these latter techniques are not as helpful in patients with prosthetic infections since echoes generated by a mechanical prosthesis are usually too intense for small vegetations to be visualized. Although it is not possible to rule out infective endocarditis on the basis of negative echocardiographic findings alone, the introduction of transesophageal echocardiography has led to a substantial improvement in the rate of detection of vegetations. This is related to the use of high-frequency transducers and scanning in the near field without interposition of the chest wall.

Convincing data have recently been reported by a team in Hanover, Germany, who provided a detailed comparison between anatomic and echocardiographic findings in 80 patients undergoing surgery or necropsy. The overall detection rate was 90% in transesophageal compared to only 58% for transthoracic echocardiography. The most striking results were obtained in patients with prosthetic valve endocarditis in whom the detection rate was increased from 27% to 77%. Finally, in this series the transesophageal procedure identified a vegetation and/or valve destruction in 90% of the patients (63). Similar results have been reported by Erbel et al. (35) in 96 patients with native valve endocarditis. Although the specificity was 98% for both approaches, the sensitivity of transesophageal echocardiography was 100% compared to 63% for the transthoracic approach. The authors emphasized the superiority of transesophageal echocardiography when vegetations were small, since only 25% of those <5 mm in diameter and detected by this technique were also observed in the transthoracic procedure.

Echocardiography has been used extensively to detect perivalvular abscesses and, more generally, perivalvular extension of infection. In a study of 14 retrospective series involving 380 patients and analyzed by Carpentier (13), the sensitivity of two-dimensional transthoracic echocardiography was near 70%. However, it must be emphasized that sensitivity values ranged from 0 to 100%, with a rate of only 18% in one prospective study (27). The specificity of transesophageal echocardiography in the identification of abscess is higher than 90%. The best investigation documenting the usefulness of this technique for the detection of abscess was the Hanover prospective study (26). During surgery or at autopsy, 44 of 118 consecutive patients (37%) had 46 definite regions of abscess associated with endocarditis. The sensitivity and specificity were 28% and 98.5%, respectively, for transthoracic echocardiography and 87% and 94.5% for transesophageal echocardiography. The latter had a significant improvement in the diagnosis of abscess in both native and prosthetic valve endocarditis. These findings have clear practical implications because patients with perivalvular infection are usually candidates for early cardiac surgery (Fig. 23.1).

There are conflicting conclusions in the literature with respect to the relation between the presence of vegetations identified by echocardiography and the incidence of complications such as embolic events, congestive heart failure (30, 52), and death (3, 77, 78). Some studies suggest an association for systemic emboli (66, 80), while others do not (53, 57). There are also discrepancies among the various studies concerning the prognostic implications of vegetation size. In a recent report, Mügge et al. (63) have suggested that vegetations >10 mm in diameter and located in native mitral valve are associated with a higher incidence of embolic episodes. The role of the offending pathogen is also debated. Although some agents such as fungi are responsible for large vegetations, the latter vary greatly in size, irrespective of the etiology. In a recent study done at the Mayo clinic of 207 patients with native valve endocarditis, the relative risk for embolic events associated with vegetation identified by echocardiography was microorganism-dependent. A significantly increased risk was observed in patients with *S. viridans* infection (79).

Other echocardiographic techniques such as Doppler imaging are most useful in the setting of infective endocarditis. Continuous wave Doppler echocardiography is important in the diagnosis of prosthetic obstruction. When color flow Doppler is used, blood flow is visually superimposed on the anatomic information. This procedure is very useful for the diagnosis of regurgitation in native valves and bioprostheses. Contrast echocardiography is able to detect fixed anatomic complications of infection such as Valsalva aneurysms.

Other Procedures

There are only limited data on the utility of computed tomography and magnetic resonance imaging in the evaluation of endocarditis. Several cases of perivalvular infections have been identified by these techniques, especially aortic root aneurysms and abscess (44, 88). These procedures could be useful in patients with suspected perivalvular extension of infection when echocardiography is negative or inconclusive.

There are few data on the use of gallium

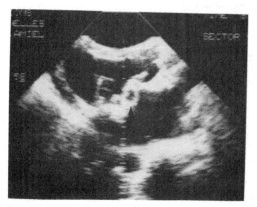

Figure 23.1. Prosthetic endocarditis on the mitral valve: annulus abscess *(arrow)*.

and indium scans for the detection of vegetations on valves or perivalvular abscess (13). The role of this technique remains to be defined in prospective studies. Progress in echocardiography technology has limited the current role of cardiac catheterization to specific situations. Angiography may provide additional information of use to the surgeon in cases of perivalvular extension of infection. When hemodynamic status is compromised, right cardiac catheterization is necessary to optimize medical treatment before valve replacement surgery.

Finally, transthoracic two-dimensional echocardiography is the standard procedure for patients with definite or suspected endocarditis. Doppler technology should also be used since it is much more sensitive in the diagnosis of regurgitation, prosthetic dysfunction, and intracardiac shunts. By contrast, transesophageal echocardiography should not be used as a screening technique (68) because it is not a truly noninvasive procedure; although rare, serious or minor complications have been reported (25). The best indications may be summarized as follows: (a) when transthoracic examination is not technically adequate or when negative results are obtained, especially when mitral valve involvement is suspected; (b) in prosthetic valve endocarditis; and (c) in the detection of perivalvular abscess, particularly in patients with heart block or those who do not respond to antibiotic treatment.

COMPLICATIONS AND MANAGEMENT

Cardiac Complications and Management

Heart failure occurs in about 50% of patients with endocarditis and is the consequence of various anatomic lesions. In native valve infections, aortic regurgitation because of valve destruction is the most frequent and life-threatening cause of heart failure. Chordal ruptures and/or perforation of mitral valve can also lead to pulmonary edema. Hemodynamically important valvular stenosis is a consequence of large vegetations (e.g., fungal infections). In prosthetic valve endocarditis, stenosis

occurs most commonly with bioprostheses in the mitral position (2). In bioprosthetic infections, the predominant lesions are leaflet tears and perforation.

One of the most serious intracardiac complications of endocarditis is the development of perivascular abscess, the exact incidence of which is difficult to assess. The rates differ according to the type of endocarditis (native versus prosthesis), the involved site, and the type of series (surgical, autopsy, or echocardiographic). Autopsy series of patients with native valve endocarditis show a 30% incidence of perivalvular abscess with left-sided valves, especially the aortic valve. By contrast, surgical series have shown a lower incidence (<10%), except in a recent study in which 34 of 103 patients had intracardiac abscesses. The aortic valve was involved in 70% of the cases (26). Approximately 30% of abscesses extend to the ventricular septum, sinus of valsalva, or, less often, the pericardium. Perivalvular abscess and annular destruction is reported to occur most frequently with highly virulent organisms such as *S. aureus*.

The pathologic hallmark of mechanical prosthetic valve endocarditis is valve ring abscess. This complication is found in 50–100% of cases (1, 2, 73). Paravalvular leak caused by a valve ring abscess may lead to heart failure subsequent to progressive valvular regurgitation. These lesions are more frequent at the aortic than the mitral position. Myocardial abscess occurs in 30–40% of mechanical valve infections, again more often in the aortic position. Valve ring abscess is less frequent in bioprosthetic infections, with an incidence <20%; myocardial abscess is rare.

The development of varying degrees of heart block, especially complete block, in association with persistent fever should alert the physician to the possibility of a perivalvular abscess. Surgical intervention is usually required in the management of intracardiac complications of endocarditis. Heart valve operations are now frequently performed in patients with active disease. Increased experience, better surgical techniques in patients with extensive destruction of the left ventricular inflow and outflow tracts, and the progress in the management of patients undergoing intensive care explain the improvement in the surgical results. Patients with infection limited to the leaflet of native or bioprosthetic valves are usually treated by standard valve replacement.

In selected subsets of patients, mitral (and less often tricuspid) valve reconstruction is possible with highly satisfactory results. For the mitral valve, the surgical techniques include leaflet resection, leaflet patching, direct suture, chordal shortening, or transposition and annular remodeling, with or without insertion of a prosthetic ring (33). If the infection extends to the annulus, aggressive debridement of infected tissue is necessary. If the mitral ring annulus is not excessively damaged, the valve is replaced in the original position. When there is extensive destruction of the mitral annulus, circumferential reconstruction is undertaken with a strip of pericardium. The mitral prosthesis is secured in the pericardial patch (23, 28). The new mitral valve with a Dacron flange may be implanted in the left atrium 1.5–2 cm above the mitral ring and sutured to the atrial wall (39). Simultaneous reconstruction of the aortic and mitral annuli may be done with a single patch sutured to the base of the left ventricle (29).

Occasionally, aortic native valve or prosthetic valve endocarditis results in destruction of the annular and aortic roots so that a prosthesis cannot be implanted in standard fashion. Very sophisticated operations have been performed successfully in these situations and include translocation of the aortic valve to the ascending aorta (70), combined with oversewing of the coronary ostia and bypass of coronary arteries, insertion of a valved conduit into the ascending aorta with coronary bypass grafts, and replacement of the aortic root with a Dacron tube graft, and reimplantation of the coronary ostia. The prosthetic valve is located either in the aorta itself by transfixing stitches or directly in the Dacron tube (10).

Extracardiac Complications and Management

Almost any organ may be involved in infective endocarditis. Extracardiac lesions are the consequence of either metastatic localizations or immunologic phenomonena. The description of all these manifestations is beyond the scope of this review. This chapter will be focused on neurologic events and splenic emboli.

Neurologic Events

Central nervous system complications occur in 20–40% of patients who develop endocarditis. The overall mortality rate may be as high as 60% in patients with cerebral hemorrhage. In a recent series of 175 patients reported by Salgado et al. (75), the types and frequencies of neurologic events were the same in both native and prosthetic valve endocarditis. Emboli from vegetations result in various manifestations including occlusion of large cerebral arteries, hematoma, brain abscess, meningitis, and encephalopathy. In most series, *S. aureus* is correlated with the development of neurologic complications and death. The majority of neurologic events occur before the start of antibiotic treatment and may be among the earliest symptoms of endocarditis. The time between the diagnosis of endocarditis and the first neurologic signs is sometimes longer in patients developing intracranial mycotic aneurysm, particularly those with streptococcal infection.

A computerized tomography scan is the procedure of choice for patients with neurologic symptoms. In two recent studies involving 79 patients, the results were as follows: bland or hemorrhagic infarct ($n = 28$), intracerebral hematoma ($n = 19$), and abscess ($n = 7$). In the remaining patients, no lesion was identified (75, 89). Cerebrospinal fluid (CSF) is usually analyzed only in patients with meningism or those with impaired consciousness but no focal neurological signs. Pleocytosis is commonly observed, but the CSF may be normal. There is a good correlation between CSF findings and the nature of the infecting organism. Virulent pathogens such as *S. aureus* and *S. pneumoniae* are frequently associated with purulent CSF. Indeed, *S. aureus* was isolated form 37% of 25 CSF specimens from patients with *S. aureus* infective endocarditis and neurologic complications at our institution (89).

By contrast, streptococci are usually associated with a normal or aseptic CSF.

There is still controversy concerning the management of neurologic complications of endocarditis. However, patients with ruptured aneurysms, deepening coma, and extensive mass lesion should undergo surgery. Large cerebral abscesses are drained if the cardiac condition is stable. Aneurysms without significant mass lesions or rupture must be monitored with serial angiography. If they appear to enlarge, surgery should be performed (86). Small abscesses and meningitis invariably resolve under antibiotic therapy. If there is cardiac failure, valve replacement will be undertaken regardless of the neurologic picture. However, for patients with hemorrhagic intracerebral lesions, cardiac surgery may be delayed or even precluded by neurologic status. Because neurologic complications occur early in the course of infective endocarditis, their prevention is difficult. Cerebrovascular accidents are more frequent among anticoagulated patients (31), so an anticoagulant should not be administered in native valve or bioprosthetic endocarditis. Heparin sodium instead of warfarin is advisable in mechanical valve infections (49).

Splenic Septic Emboli

Septic emboli to the spleen lead to foci of ischemic infection that may progress to abscess formation. In the preantibiotic era, 10% of patients who died of endocarditis had purulent lesions in the spleen. At present, the incidence of splenic infarcts or abscess is unknown. Since diagnostic techniques have improved, it is probable that the true incidence of splenic lesions was previously underestimated. In a recent series of 108 patients with left-sided endocarditis requiring valve replacement, the incidence of confirmed splenic infection and/or abscess was 19% (20 of 108). However, during the earlier period of the study, abdominal CT scan screening was not routinely performed in asymptomatic patients. During the later period, occult splenic infarcts were found in 38% of 29 asymptomatic patients (83). The distinction between infarct and abscess is not just academic; splenic infarcts do not warrant specific therapy unless they are large and peripheral, while splenectomy is often necessary in cases of splenic abscess. In this setting, CT scan findings are not always specific and have to be compared with the history and clinical signs and symptoms.

The proper management of the patient with infective endocarditis and suspected splenic abscess is not standardized, especially for patients who require valve replacement therapy. Magilligan (55) has proposed the following approach: immediately after valve replacement, the sternotomy incision is extended to the umbilicus and needle aspiration of the spleen is performed. If the spleen contains pus, white blood cells, or bacteria (Gram stain), splenectomy is undertaken; if the aspiration is negative, splenectomy is not performed. This approach was successfully used in 10 of 15 patients with active infective endocarditis who underwent splenectomy and valve replacement. In the remaining five patients, splenectomy was performed either before ($n = 1$) or after ($n = 4$) cardiac surgery (55). In the study by Ting et al. (83), all 10 splenectomies were staged and performed after valve replacement, with a mean time interval of 11 days. The indications were persistent sepsis ($n = 6$), large or peripheral lesions ($n = 3$), and spontaneous splenic rupture ($n = 1$). One patient died of uncontrolled bleeding from the splenic bed. There was no apparent seeding of the prosthetic valve with microorganisms originating from the spleen in the other nine patients, although two died from cardiac causes.

Table 23.2 summarizes the frequency of the main complications observed among the 446 patients with endocarditis seen between 1973 and 1988 at our institution.

Indications for Cardiac Surgery

Although many patients suffering from infective endocarditis are cured by medical therapy alone, urgent surgical intervention may be required. An increasing number of retrospective studies show that the presence of active infection is not a contraindication to cardiac surgery. Moreover, there are now sufficient data to suggest an aggressive approach to the management

Table 23.2
Cardiac and Extracardiac Complications in 456 Patients with Infective Endocarditis: Claude Bernard Hospital, 1973–1988[a]

	NVE (n = 330)		PVE Early (n = 39)		PVE Late (n = 87)	
Complications	n	%	n	%	n	%
Cardiac lesions[b]	162	49	19	49	49	56
Neurologic events	96	29	11	28	28	32
Renal lesions[c]	90	27	14	36	23	26.5
Emboli	45	14	10	25.5	10	11.5
Mycotic aneurysms	28	8.5	1	2.5	8	9

[a]NVE, native valve endocarditis; PVE, prosthetic valve endocarditis.
[b]Renal failure and/or renal abscesses and/or glomerulonephritis.
[c]Valve destruction and/or perivalvular extension of infection.

Table 23.3
Outcome of Surgical Therapy for Active Prosthetic Valve Endocarditis

Study	Period of Study	No. of Patients Treated Surgically	In-hospital Mortality (%)[a]
Richardson et al. (72)	1967–1977	35	43 (Early, 67; late, 18)
Present	1978–1988	59	25 (Early, 33; late, 23)
Suryapranata et al. (81)	1973–1983	9	22
Baumgartner et al. (4)	1966–1981	63	25 (Early, 57; late, 21)
Karchmer (45)	1976–1981	29[b]	34 (Early, 36; late, 33)
Rocchiccioli et al. (73)	1979–1983	24	26 (Early, 43; late, 19)
Hanania et al. (41)	1982–1986	91	23 (Early, 30; late, 24)
Leport et al. (49)	1981–1985	11[c]	18
David et al. (28)	1978–1989	24	12.5

[a]Early, early prosthetic valve endocarditis; late, late prosthetic valve endocarditis.
[b]All mechanical prostheses.
[c]All late prosthetic valve endocarditis.

of severely injured valves. This attitude is supported by the high mortality rate in subsets of medically treated patients such as those with heart failure or prosthetic valve infection. By contrast, a recent study reported the actuarial 5-year survival rate of 38 patients with native valve infections who underwent valve operation during active disease was 86% (28). In prosthetic valve endocarditis the overall mortality among patients managed with antibiotics alone is 60% compared to 38% for those who undergo valve replacement. More recently, in four studies involving 171 patients with prosthetic valve endocarditis who were operated on early in the course of the disease, the perioperative mortality was 27% (4, 28, 41, 73) (Table 23.3). Although there is an increased risk of death when surgery is performed during active infection, this should not be used as an argument for prolonging medical therapy in the case of uncontrolled infection or worsening congestive heart failure. Persistence of infection on the prosthetic valve due to the original microorganism is surprisingly uncommon (0–15%). In addition, even if hemodynamically significant paravalvular leak is more frequent when surgery is performed during the active phase, this complication has an incidence of <10% in most series.

The indications for cardiac surgery in patients with endocarditis may be summarized as follows:

Congestive heart failure that is moderate to severe in prosthetic infections or that does not respond to intensive medical management in native valve endocarditis. In the latter, heart failure from mitral regurgitation is usually easier to manage with medical treatment than failure from aortic insufficiency.

Refractory sepsis (positive blood cultures) despite appropriate bactericidal therapy after about a week.

Presence of a septal abscess and, more often, perivalvular extension of infection.

Prosthetic valve endocarditis with either valve obstruction or instability revealed by fluoroscopy or echocardiography, or new-onset heart block.

Repeated embolic episodes; however, there are no data indicating after precisely how many episodes the decision should be made.

Fungal endocarditis; the poor prognosis is because of large bulky vegetations, the frequency of embolic complications, and the poor penetration of antifungal agents into the vegetations.

In addition, valve replacement should be considered in prosthetic valve infections in the presence of one of the following criteria: mild congestive heart failure due to valve dysfunction, organisms other than a "susceptible" streptococcus or fastidious Gram-negative rods (60), embolism, vegetations revealed by echocardiography, relapse following completion of therapy, early-onset prosthesis infection, of perivalvular leak. Medical therapy is most likely to succeed in natural (65) rather than in mechanical prosthesis and when penicillin-sensitive streptococci are involved. Thus, there are a large number of situations in which early surgical intervention is warranted in prosthetic valve infections, especially when staphylococci are the etiologic agents. Conversely, there is general agreement that indications for surgery are now very limited in the setting of right-sided endocarditis since the prognosis for cure by medical therapy alone is very good (32).

ANTIMICROBIAL THERAPY: PHYSIOPATHOLOGY AND DATA FROM EXPERIMENTAL MODELS

The experimental model of infective endocarditis provides a highly useful test of antibiotic efficacy. It gives considerable information about the activity of different drugs and about their diffusion into the vegetations. Moreover, this model has been used to study the impact of antibiotic dosages and the effect of various antibiotic regimens on efficacy (12).

Antibiotic Combinations

Numerous studies have shown that, with streptococci, enterococci, and staphylococci, the combination of a β-lactam plus an aminoglycoside, synergystic in vitro, is faster and more efficient in sterilizing vegetations than the β-lactam alone. Therefore, a combined regimen, usually with an aminoglycoside for the first 2 weeks, is recommended in the following situations: penicillin-susceptible streptococcal endocarditis in patients who have been ill for more than 3 months prior to therapy or with complications such as extracardiac foci of infection, enterococcal infections, and prosthetic valve endocarditis caused by *S. aureus*. By contrast, penicillin alone for 4 weeks is an adequate regimen in uncomplicated forms caused by penicillin-susceptible streptococci. The benefit of an additional aminoglycoside has not been clinically established in *S. aureus* native valve endocarditis, except for a 2-week regimen for right-sided infections in drug addicts (15). However, the synergistic bactericidal effect of a β-lactam plus an aminoglycoside may help clear bacteremia more rapidly. This combination should thus be used for at least 5–7 days, especially in left-sided *S. aureus* valve infection.

Activity and Diffusion of Drugs into Vegetations

A plethora of drugs has been studied with respect to their activity in models of endocarditis. Among the recent compounds, the newer quinolones are highly active against both methicillin-susceptible and resistant staphylococci and Gram-negative rods. A recent preliminary trial of ciprofloxacin in combination with rifampin in the treatment of right-sided endocarditis in drug addicts has shown promising results (34). Quinolones, together with β-lactams and aminoglycosides, have been shown to penetrate into fibrin vegetations. However, there are substantial differences from one compound to another and diffusion may differ according to the valve involved. Indeed, Bayer et al. (6) found higher peak levels of ceftazidime and amikacin in right-sided vegetations than in left-sided ones. They suggested that more favorable pharmacokinetics within tricuspid rather than aortic vegetations may partly explain the better outcome in endocarditis involving the right side of the heart.

It should be emphasized that the determination of the antibiotic content in homogenates of vegetations may not reflect the potential heterogenicity of the diffusion. Indeed, autoradiographic studies have shown different patterns of antibiotic distribution in vegetations. Aminoglycosides and, to a lesser extent, β-lactam are homogenously distributed, while teicoplanin, a new glycopeptide, is concentrated at the periphery (21).

Impact of Various Regimens on the Efficacy of Antibiotics

Various studies with β-lactams in infective endocarditis models have shown that the therapeutic effect of these drugs is not

Table 23.4
Suggested Therapeutic Regimens for Endocarditis due to Gram-Positive Cocci

Pathogens	Drugs Standard	Drugs Penicillin-allergic Patients[a]	Duration of Therapy (weeks) NVE[b]	Duration of Therapy (weeks) PVE[c]
Penicillin-susceptible streptococci (minimal inhibitory concentration ≤0.1 μg/ml)	Penicillin G	Cefazolin or ceftriaxone or vancomycin or teicoplanin	4	NR[d]
	Penicillin G + gentamicin[e]		2	NR
	Penicillin G + Gentamicin		4 / 2	4 / 2
Enterococci (or streptococci with a minimal inhibitory concentration ≥0.5 μg/ml)	Ampicillin + gentamicin[e]	Vancomycin or teicoplanin	4–6	6
Enterococci with high-level resistance to gentamicin	Ampicillin or vancomycin or teicoplanin	Vancomycin or teicoplanin	8–12	8–12
Methicillin-susceptible S. aureus	Oxacillin or nafcillin[f] + Gentamicin[e]	Vancomycin or teicoplanin	4–6[g] / ≥1	≥6 / ≥2
Methicillin-resistant S. aureus	Vancomycin (or teicoplanin) + Rifampin[h]		4–6 / 4–6	≥6 / ≥6
Methicillin-resistant coagulase-negative staphylococci	Vancomycin (or teicoplanin[i]) + Rifampin + Gentamicin[j]		4–6 / 4–6 / 2	≥6 / ≥6 / ≥2

[a] Penicillin replaced by the agents listed.
[b] NVE, native valve endocarditis.
[c] PVE, prosthetic valve endocarditis.
[d] Not recommended.
[e] Gentamicin may be replaced by netilmicin.
[f] Fluoroquinolones are potentially effective (see text).
[g] A 2-week regimen has been found effective in noncomplicated right-sided endocarditis in drug abusers.
[h] The use of rifampin in S. aureus endocarditis is controversial. Fosfomycin and fusidic acid have been successfully used in combination with vancomycin.
[i] The minimal inhibitory concentration should be determined since some strains are found resistant to teicoplanin.
[j] There is an increasing number of gentamicin-resistant strains.

strongly peak level-dependent, but depends mainly on the time that an appropriate level is maintained. In other words, serum levels have to exceed the minimum bactericidal concentration of the etiologic agent during the entire dose interval. Therefore, intervals must be planned on the basis on the serum elimination half-life and the dose administered (12). This is also true for glycopeptides. Like vancomycin, teicoplanin has a relatively low bactericidal rate. In addition, because of a high degree of protein binding, low free-drug concentrations result in less activity in vivo than in vitro, as shown recently in a rabbit model of *Streptococcus sanguis* infective endocarditis (14). Sustained concentrations in serum that are several times greater than the minimum bactericidal concentration may therefore be important for efficacy in vivo. Suboptimal dosages (<400 mg, once daily) might explain treatment failures in a series of severe staphylococcal infections (40). However, two recent studies involving 43 patients with endocarditis caused by a variety of Gram-positive cocci have shown satisfactory results with higher dosages (48, 59)

Finally, both experimental and clinical studies support the use of a triple combination of vancomycin, rifampin, and an aminoglycoside in the treatment of prosthetic valve endocarditis caused by methicillin-resistant coagulase-negative staphylococci (46).

Detailed recommendations for antibiotic treatment of infective endocarditis have been published elsewhere (9) and are summarized in Table 23.4.

References

1. Anderson D, Buckley B, Hutchins G. A clinico-pathologic study of prosthetic valve endocarditis in 22 patients: morphologic basis for diagnosis and therapy. Am Heart J 1977;94:325–332.
2. Arnett EN, Roberts WC. Prosthetic valve endocarditis: clinicopathology analysis of 22 necropsy patients with comparison of observations in 74 necropsy patients with active infective endocarditis involving natural left-sided cardiac valves. Am J Cardiol 1976;38:281–292.
3. Bardy GH, Talano JV, Reisberg B, Lesch M. Sensitivity and specificity of echocardiography in a high-risk population of patients for infective endocarditis. Significance of vegetation size. J Cardiovasc Ultrasonogr 1983;2:23–27.
4. Baumgartner, WA, Craig Miller D, Reitz BA, et al. Surgical treatment of prosthetic valve endocarditis. Ann Thorac Surg 1983;35:87–104.
5. Bayer A, Lam K, Ginzton L, Norman DC, Chiu CY, Ward JI. *Staphylococcus aureus* bacteremia. Clinical, serologic, and echocardiographic findings in patients with and without endocarditis. Arch Intern Med 1987;147:457–462.
6. Bayer AS, Crowell DJ, Yih J, Bradley DW, Norman DC. Comparative pharmacokinetics and pharmacodynamics of amikacin and ceftazidime in tricuspid and aortic vegetations in experimental Pseudomonas endocarditis. J Infect Dis 1988;158:355–359.
7. Bayliss R, Clarke C, Oakley C, Somerville W, Whitfield AGW. The teeth and infective endocarditis. Br Heart J 1983;50:506–512.
8. Berman DS, Schaefler S, Simberkoff MS, Rahal JJ. S. aureus colonization in intravenous drug abusers, dialysis patients and diabetics. J Infect Dis 1987;115:829–831.
9. Bisno AL, Dismukes WE, Durack DT. Antimicrobial treatment of infective endocarditis to viridans streptococci, enterococci, and staphylococci. JAMA 1989;261:1471–1477.
10. Brown JW, Salles CA, Kirsh MM. Extra-anatomical bypass of the aortic root: an experimental technique. Ann Thorac Surg 1977;24:433–438.
11. Calderwood SB, Swinski LA, Waternaux CM, Karchmer AW, Buckley MJ. Risk factors for the development of prosthetic valve endocarditis. Circulation 1985;72:31–37.
12. Carbon C. Impact of the antibiotic dosage schedule on efficacy in experimental endocarditis. Scand J Infect Dis 1991;74 (suppl):163–172.
13. Carpentier JL. Perivalvular extension of infection in patients with infectious endocarditis. Rev Infect Dis 1991, 13:127–138.
14. Chambers HF, Kenedy S. Effects of dosage, peak and trough concentrations in serum, protein bindings and bactericidal rate on efficacy of teicoplanin in a rabbit model of endocarditis. Antimicrob Agents Chemother 1990;34:510–514.
15. Chambers HF, Miller T, Newman MD. Right-sided *Staphylococcus aureus* endocarditis in intravenous drug abusers: two week combination therapy. Ann Intern Med 1988;109:619–624.
16. Clemens JD, Horwitz RI, Jaffe CC, Feinstein AR, Stanton BF. A controlled evaluation of the risk of bacterial endocarditis in persons with mitral-valve prolapse. N Engl J Med 1982;307:776–781.
17. Come PC, Isaacs RE, Rilley MF. Diagnostic accuracy of M-mode echocardiography in active infective endocarditis and prognostic implications of ultrasound detectable vegetations. Am Heart J 1982;103:839–847.
18. Cooper G, Platt R. *Staphylococcus aureus* bacteremia in diabetic patients: endocarditis and mortality. Am J Med 1982;73:658–662.
19. Cowgill LD, Addonizio VP, Hopeman AR, Harken AH. A practical approach to prosthetic valve endocarditis. Ann Thorac Surg 1987;43:450–457.
20. Craven DE, Rixinguer A, Bisno AL, Goularte TA, Mac Cabe WR. Bacteremia caused by group G streptococci in parenteral drug abusers: epide-

miological and clinical agents. J Infect Dis 1986;153:98–99.

21. Cremieux AC, Maziere B, Vallois JM, et al. Evaluation of antibiotic diffusion into cardiac vegetations by quantitative autoradiography. J Infect Dis 1989;159:938–944.

22. Cremieux AC, Witchitz S, Malergue MC. Clinical and echocardiography observation in pulmonary valve endocarditis. Am J Cardiol 1985;56:610–613.

23. D'Agostino RS, Miller DC, Stinson EB, et al. Valve replacement in patients with native valve endocarditis: what really determines operative outcome? Ann Thorac Surg 1985;40:429–438.

24. Danchin N, Voiriot P, Briancon S, et al. Mitral valve prolapse as a risk factor for infective endocarditis. Lancet 1989;i:743–745.

25. Daniel WG, Erbel R, Kasper W, et al. Safety of transesophageal echocardiography: a multicenter survey of 10,419 examinations. Circulation 1991;83:817–821.

26. Daniel WG, Mügge A, Martin RP, Lindert O, Hausmann D, Nonnast-Daniel B, Laas J, Lichtlen PR. Improvement in the diagnosis of abscesses associated with endocarditis by transesophageal echocardiography. N Engl J Med 1991;324:795–800.

27. Daniel WG, Schroder E, Nonnast-Daniel B, Lichtlen PR. Conventional and transesophageal echocardiography in the diagnosis of infective endocarditis. Eur Heart J 1987;8 (suppl J):287–292.

28. David TE, Bos J, Christakis GT, Brofman PR, Wong D, Feindel CM. Heart valve operations in patients with active infective endocarditis. Ann Thorac Surg 1990;49:701–705.

29. David TE, Komeda M. Surgical treatment of aortic root abscess. Circulation 1989;80 (suppl 1):269–274.

30. Davis RS, Strom JA, Frishman W, Becker R, Matsumoto M, Lejemtel TH, Sonnenblick EH, Frater RWM. The demonstration of vegetations by echocardiography in bacterial endocarditis. An indication for early surgical intervention. Am J Med 1980;69:57–63.

31. Delahaye JP, Poncet PH, Malquarti V, Beaune J, Gare JP, Mann JM. Cerebrovascular accidents in infective endocarditis: role of anticoagulation. Eur Heart J 1990;11:1074–1078.

32. Dinubile M. Surgery for addiction-related tricuspid valve endocarditis; caveat emptor. Am J Med 1987;82:811–813.

33. Dreyfuss G, Serraf A, Jebara VA, Deloche A, Chauvaud S, Couetil JP, Carpentier A. Valve repair in acute endocarditis. Ann Thorac Surg 1990;49:706–711.

34. Dworkin RJ, Lee BL, Sande MA, Chambers HF. Treatment of right-sided endocarditis in intravenous drug users with ciprofloxacin and rifampicin. Lancet 1989;ii:1071–1073.

35. Erbel R, Rohmann S, Drexler M, et al. Improved diagnostic value of echocardiography in patients with infective endocarditis by transoesophageal approach. A prospective study. Eur Heart J 1988;9:43–53.

36. Espersen F, Frimodt-Moller N. Staphylococcus au-

reus endocarditis. A review of 119 cases. Arch Intern Med 1986;146:1118–1121.

37. Finckelstein R, Sobel JD, Nagler A, Merzbach D. Staphylococcus aureus bacteremia and endocarditis: comparison of nosocomial and community-acquired infection. J Med 1984;15:193–211.

38. Freedman LR, Valone JR. Experimental infective endocarditis. Prog Cardiovasc Dis 1979;22:169–180.

39. Gandjbackch I, Laskar M, Pavie A, Mesnildrey P, Cabrol C. Implantation intra-atriale de la valve mitrale. Presse Med 1982;12:1723–1724.

40. Gilbert DN, Wood CA, Kimbrough RC, and the Infectious Diseases Consortium of Oregon. Failure of treatment with teicoplanin at 6 milligrams/kilogram/day in patients with Staphylococcus aureus intravascular infection. Antimicrob Agents Chemother 1991;35:79–87.

41. Hanania G, Thoma D, Montely JM et al. Endocardite infectieuse sur prothèse valvulaire. Etude multicentrique (179 cas). Arch Mal Coeur 1989;82:509–515.

42. Herstein J, Ryan JL, Mangi RJ, Greco TP, Andriole VT. Optimal therapy for enterococcal endocarditis. Am J Med 1984;76:186–191.

43. Ivert TSA, Dismukes WE, Cobbs CG, Blackstone EH, Kirklin JW, Bergdahl LA. Prosthetic valve endocarditis. Circulation 1984;69:223–232.

44. Jeang MK, Fuentes F, Gately A, Byrnes J, Lewis M. Aortic root abscess: initial experience using magnetic resonance imaging. Chest 1986;89:613–615.

45. Karchmer AW. Prosthetic valve endocarditis. Mechanical valve. In: Magilligan DJ, Quinn EL, eds. Endocarditis: medical and surgical treatment. New York: Marcel Dekker, 1986:241–252.

46. Karchmer AW, Archer GL, Dismukes WE. Staphylococcus epidermidis causing prosthetic valve endocarditis: microbiologic and clinical observations as guides to therapy. Ann Intern Med 1983;98:447–455.

47. Kaye D. Changing pattern of infective endocarditis. Am J Med 1985; 78 (suppl 6B):157–162.

48. Leport C, Perronne C, Massip P, et al. Evaluation of teicoplanin for treatment of endocarditis caused by Gram positive cocci in 20 patients. Antimicrob Agents Chemother 1989;33:871–876.

49. Leport C, Vildé JL, Bricaire F, et al. Fifty cases of late prosthetic valve endocarditis: improvement in prognosis over a 15 year period. Br Heart J 1987;58:66–71.

50. Levine DP, Crane LR, Zervos MJ. Bacteremia in narcotic addict at the Detroit Medical Center. II. Infectious endocarditis: a prospective comparative study. Rev Infect Dis 1986;8:374–396.

51. Libman H, Arbeit RD. Complications associated with Staphylococcus aureus bacteremia. Arch Intern Med 1984;144:541–545.

52. Lutas EM, Roberts RB, Devereux RB, Prieto LM. Relation between the presence of echocardiographic vegetations and the complication rate in infective endocarditis. Am Heart J 1986;112:107–113.

53. Mac Kinsey DS, Ratts TE, Bisno AL. Underlying cardiac lesions in adults with infective endocar-

ditis. The changing spectrum. Am J Med 1987;82:681–688.

54. Mac Mahon SW, Hickey AJ, Wilcken DEL, Wittes JT, Feneley MP, Hickie JB. Risk of infective endocarditis in mitral valve prolapse with and without precordial systolic murmurs. Am J Cardiol 1986;58:105–108.

55. Magilligan DJ. Splenic abscess. In: Magilligan DJ, Quinn EL, eds. Endocarditis: medical and surgical management. New York: Marcel Dekker, 1986:197–204.

56. Makki DG, Agger WA. Enterococcal bacteremia: clinical features, the risk of endocarditis and management. Medicine 1988;67:248–269.

57. Mannolis AS, Melitta H. Echocardiographic and clinical correlates in drug addicts with infective endocarditis. Implications of vegetation size. Arch Intern Med 1988;148:2461–2465.

58. Martino P, Micozzi A, Venditti M, et al. Catheter-related right-sided endocarditis in bone marrow transplant recipients. Rev Infect Dis 1990;12:250–257.

59. Martino P, Venditti M, Micozzi A, et al. Teicoplanin in the treatment of gram positive bacterial endocarditis. Antimicrob Agents Chemother 1989;33:1329–1334.

60. Meyer DJ, Gerdine DN. Favorable prognosis of patients with prosthetic valve endocarditis caused by Gram-negative bacilli of the HACEK group. Am J Med 1988;85:104–107.

61. Mirimanoff RO, Glauser MP. Endocarditis during Staphylococcus aureus septicemia in a population of non-drug addicts. Arch Intern Med 1982;142:1311–1313.

62. Moulsdale MT, Eykyn SJ, Phillips I. Infective endocarditis, 1970–1979. A study of culture positive cases in St Thomas Hospital. Q J Med 1980;49:315–328.

63. Mügge A, Daniel WG, Frank G, Lichtlen PR. Echocardiography in infective endocarditis: reassessment of prognostic implications of vegetation size determined by the transthoracic and the transesophageal approach. J Am Coll Cardiol 1989;14:631–638.

64. Mylotte JM, Mac Dermott C, Spooner JA. Prospective study of 114 consecutive episodes of Staphylococcus aureus bacteremia. Rev Infect Dis 1987;9:891–907.

65. Nunez L, de la Lana R, Aguado MG, Iglesias A, Larrea JL, Calemin D. Bioprosthetic valve endocarditis: indicators for surgical intervention. Ann Thorac Surg 1983;35:262–270.

66. O'Brien JT, Geiser EA. Infective endocarditis and echocardiography. Am Heart J 1984;108:386–394.

67. Pazin GJ, Saul S, Thompson ME. Blood culture positivity. Suppression by outpatient antibiotic therapy in patient with bacterial endocarditis. Arch Intern Med 1982;142:263–268.

68. Pearlman AS. Transeosophageal echocardiography. Sound diagnostic technique or two-edged sword? N Engl J Med 1991, 324:841–843.

69. Raucher B, Dobkin J, Mandel L, Edberg S, Levi M, Miller M. Occult polymicrobial endocarditis with Haemophilus parainfluenzae in intravenous drug abusers. Am J Med 1989;186:169–172.

70. Reitz BA, Stinson EB, Watson D, Baumgartner WA, Jamieson JW. Translocation of the aortic valve for prosthetic endocarditis. J Thorac Cardiovasc Surg 1981;81:212–218.

71. Rice LB, Calderwood SB, Eliopoulos GM, Farber BF, Karchmer AW. Enterococcal endocarditis: a comparison of prosthetic and native valve disease. Rev Infect Dis 1991;13:1–7.

72. Richardson JV, Karp RB, Kirklin JW, Dismukes WE. Treatment of infective endocarditis: a 10-year comparative analysis. Circulation 1978;58:589–597.

73. Rocchiccioli C, Chastre J, Lecomte Y, Gandjbakch I, Gibert C. Prosthethic valve endocarditis. The case for prompt surgical management. J Thorac Cardiovasc Surg 1986;92:784–789.

74. Rowley KM, Clubb KS, Walker-Smith GJ, Cabin HS. Right-sided infective endocarditis as a consequence of flow-directed pulmonary-artery catheterization: a clinical-pathological study of 55 autopsied patients. N Engl J Med 1984;311:1152–1156.

75. Salgado AV, Furlan AJ, Keys TF, Nichols MS, Beck GJ. Neurologic complications of endocarditis: a 12-year experience. Neurology 1989;39:173–178.

76. Schekar P, Rice TW, Zierdt CH, Kallick CA. Outbreak of endocarditis caused by Pseudomonas aeruginosa serotype 011 among pentazocine and tripelennamine abusers in Chicago. J Infect Dis 1985;151:203–208.

77. Scheld WM, Sande MA. Endocarditis and intravascular infections. In: Mandell GL, Douglas RE, Benett JE, eds. Principles and practice of infectious disease. New York: Churchill Livingstone, 1990:670–706.

78. Staffort WJ, Petch J, Radford DJ. Vegetation in infective endocarditis: clinical relevance and diagnosis by cross sectional echocardiography. Br Heart J 1985;53:310–313.

79. Steckelberg JM, Murphy JG, Ballard D, et al. Emboli in infective endocarditis: the prognosis value of echocardiography. Ann Intern Med 1991;114:635–640.

80. Stewart JA, Silimperi D, Harris P, Wise NK, Fraker TD Jr, Kisslo JA. Echocardiographic documentation of vegetation lesions in infective endocarditis: clinical implications. Circulation, 1980;61:374–380.

81. Suryaprana H, Roeland T, Haalebos M, Degener J, Bos E, Hugenholz PG. Early cardiac valve replacement in infective endocarditis: a 10-year experience. Eur Heart J 1987;8:464–470.

82. Terpenning MS, Buggy BP, Kauffman CA. Hospital-acquired infective endocarditis. Arch Intern Med 1988;148:1601–1603.

83. Ting W, Silverman NA, Arzouman DA, Levitsky S. Splenic septic emboli in endocarditis. Circulation 1990; 82 (suppl IV):105–109.

84. Tsao MPP, Katz D. Central venous catheter-induced endocarditis: human correlate of the animal experimental model of endocarditis. Rev Infect Dis 1984;6:783–790.

85. Tuazon CU, Sheagren JN. Staphylococcal endocarditis in parenteral drug abusers: source of the organism. Ann Intern Med 1975;82:788–790.

86. Vittecoq D, Monsuez JJ, Rozenbaum A, et al.

Prognosis of ruptured intracranial myotic aneurysms: a review of 12 cases. Eur Heart J 1989;10:821–825.

87. von Reyn CF, Levy BS, Arbeit R, Friedland G, Crumpackers CS. Infective endocarditis: an analysis based on strict case definitions. Ann Intern Med 1981;94:505–518.

88. Winkler ML, Higgins CB. MRI of perivalvular infectious pseudo-aneurysms. AJR 1986;147:235–256.

89. Wolff M, Witchitz S, Regnier B, Pichon F, Clair B, Vachon F. Neurologic complications of *S. aureus* endocarditis (abstract). Program and abstracts of the 27th Interscience Conference on Antimicrobial Agents and Chemotherapy. New York, 1987:119.

24

Ventilation-Perfusion Relationships

Robert Rodriguez-Roisin

PHYSIOLOGIC PERSPECTIVE

The prime function of the lung is to exchange the respiratory gases, oxygen (O_2) and carbon dioxide (CO_2). When the lung fails as a gas exchanger, major abnormalities appear in arterial blood respiratory gases. As a result, arterial blood is not adequately oxygenated or there is CO_2 retention. The levels of Pao_2 and $Paco_2$, which are said to determine respiratory failure, are somewhat arbitrary, since normal values are always influenced by age, climate, geographic location (altitude), and metabolic conditions. From a clinical viewpoint, however, and as a general consensus, a Pao_2 of less than 60 mm Hg or a $Paco_2$ of greater than 50 mm Hg while breathing air, are values that indicate a serious respiratory compromise consistent with the concept of respiratory failure. The first part of this chapter deals with some aspects of the basic physiology of pulmonary gas exchange, with special emphasis on the behavior of ventilation-perfusion ($\dot{V}_A/\dot{Q}$) relationships, the most influential determinant of abnormal respiratory gases. The second part focuses extensively on the most important findings concerning pulmonary gas exchange in the adult respiratory distress syndrome and other common acute respiratory failure conditions in light of the results of clinical studies using the inert gas elimination approach, a technique that gives a detailed picture of $\dot{V}_A/\dot{Q}$ ratio distributions.

Factors Governing Blood Respiratory Gases

If we exclude a reduced inspired Po_2, only observed under very special circumstances (i.e., extreme altitude), the four major causes or mechanisms of arterial hypoxemia are: $\dot{V}_A/\dot{Q}$ mismatch, intrapulmonary shunt, alveolar hypoventilation, and al-

Table 24.1
Principal Mechanisms of Abnormal Arterial Blood Respiratory Gases in the Most Common Acute Respiratory Failure Conditions[a]

Mechanism	ARDS	Pneumonia	COPD	Asthma
$\dot{V}_A/\dot{Q}$ mismatch	+	+ +	+ + +	+ + +
Intrapulmonary shunt	+ + +	+ + +	+	0
Hypoventilation	0	0	0/ + *	0/ + *
Diffusion Limitation	0	0	0	0

[a] +, mild; + +, moderate; + + +, severe; 0, absent; *, may also be moderate or severe.

veolar end-capillary diffusion limitation to O_2 (Table 24.1). Alternatively, there are two principal causes of CO_2 retention: alveolar hypoventilation and $\dot{V}_A/\dot{Q}$ inequalities (98). However, while $\dot{V}_A/\dot{Q}$ mismatching may or may not be associated with hypercapnia according to the underlying individual ventilatory conditions, alveolar hypoventilation is always accompanied by hypercapnia. From a clinical standpoint, $\dot{V}_A/\dot{Q}$ abnormalities, intrapulmonary shunt, and alveolar hypoventilation are the three principal causes of abnormal respiratory gases. In contrast, diffusion disequilibrium to O_2 becomes a negligible component of pulmonary gas exchange such that it appears to play an additional role as a cause of hypoxemia only under conditions of severe hypoxia (83) or in patients with idiopathic pulmonary fibrosis, either at rest or during exercise (2).

At present, the most common mechanism contributing to hypoxemia in pulmonary medicine is $\dot{V}_A/\dot{Q}$ mismatch, including intrapulmonary shunt (zero $\dot{V}_A/\dot{Q}$ ratio). It should be pointed out, however, that while intrapulmonary shunt becomes the most conspicuous mechanism of hypoxemia in acute lung disease, especially in those disorders characterized by collapsed alveoli, $\dot{V}_A/\dot{Q}$ inequality is of utmost importance in chronic lung disease, where the role of collateral ventilation in preventing alveolar collapse beyond the obstructed airways is thought to be very efficient (91) (Table 24.1).

Thus, the adult respiratory distress syndrome or severe bacterial pneumonia are the two best examples of acute pulmonary disorders in which severe intrapulmonary shunt plays a crucial role in determining arterial hypoxemia. In contrast, patients with acute respiratory failure secondary to chronic obstructive pulmonary disease or due to acute severe asthma *(status asthmaticus)* are the two most representative examples of acute exacerbations of chronic lung conditions in which severe $\dot{V}_A/\dot{Q}$ mismatch but little shunt is the most outstanding factor contributing to gas exchange. Furthermore, both respiratory muscle fatigue (77) and weakness (68) may emerge as an additional cause of hypercapnia by inducing alveolar hypoventilation or an inefficient breathing pattern in patients with chronic airway obstruction during exacerbations.

Ideally, it would be of great clinical interest to physicians to be able to manage respiratory blood gas measurements only, including their most common derived (calculated) variables (alveolar-arterial P_{O_2} difference [$A_{a}P_{O_2}$], venous admixture ($\dot{Q}_s/\dot{Q}_T$), and physiologic dead space [V_D/V_T]), as a general index of the status of the lungs, at least as a gas exchanger. Thus, impaired or improved results of all these variables, whose principal merits are their simplicity and relative ease of access to measurement (or calculation), could correspond to impaired or improved pulmonary gas exchange, respectively. Unfortunately, all these variables reflect not only the state of the lung, and thereby its intrapulmonary factors (namely, $\dot{V}_A/\dot{Q}$ inequality, shunt, and diffusion limitation for O_2 transfer), but also the conditions under which the lung is operating. These conditions, which uniquely determine the P_{O_2} and P_{CO_2} in any single gas exchange unit of the lung, include three principal factors, namely the $\dot{V}_A/\dot{Q}$ ratio, the composition of the inspired gas, and the composition of the mixed venous blood (99).

Note that all these simple (respiratory blood gases) or relatively simple (derived indices) measurements of the degree of abnormal gas exchange may change in either direction even though the levels of both alveolar ventilation and pulmonary blood flow matching remain unaltered. By using multicompartmental lung modeling, West (96) has shown that venous admixture (poorly oxygenated mixed venous blood going across the lung) rises or that physiologic dead space (dead space that alone would explain the differences between arterial and mixed expired P_{O_2}) falls when total blood flow (cardiac output) increases or overall ventilation decreases provided that the $\dot{V}_A/\dot{Q}$ ratio distribution remains constant (Fig. 24.1). Conversely, venous admixture decreases and physiologic dead space increases if overall ventilation going to alveolar units is raised. Accordingly, calculated physiologic dead space rises following the increase in inspired P_{O_2}, regardless of whether or not

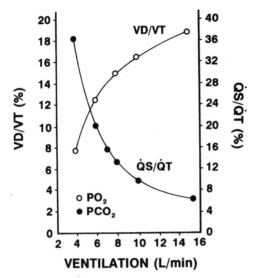

Figure 24.1. Example of the dependence of two common respiratory-derived indices (physiologic dead space [V_D/V_T] versus venous admixture [$\dot{Q}_S/\dot{Q}_T$]) of $\dot{V}_A/\dot{Q}$ mismatching *(y axis)* to overall ventilation *(x axis)* in a lung model with mild to moderate $\dot{V}_A/\dot{Q}$ inequality. Note that as ventilation is increased, physiologic dead space rises and venous admixture falls; as a result, Pao_2 increases and $Paco_2$ decreases. An increase in overall blood flow would have the opposite effect. (From West JB. Ventilation-perfusion inequality and overall gas exchange in computer lung models of the lung. Respir Physiol 1969;7:88–110.)

$\dot{V}_A/\dot{Q}$ mismatching changes or remains constant. Moreover, when true shunt (venous admixture) is measured using the oxygen method, the administration of 100% O_2 may inflict by itself considerable perturbation on pulmonary circulation or bronchomotor tone (6).

It has been shown that breathing 100% O_2 may either relieve hypoxic pulmonary vasocontriction (15) or induce reabsorption atelectasis (29), or both, thereby leading to substantial changes in the underlying degree of $\dot{V}_A/\dot{Q}$ abnormalities with further deterioration of $\dot{V}_A/\dot{Q}$ mismatch. Accordingly, the use of the respiratory gases and their related indices to assess $\dot{V}_A/\dot{Q}$ relationships may easily lead to unsatisfactory results and, hence, to common misinterpretations in the clinical setting. This is why these three classic indices based on the physiologic gases (alveolar-arterial Po_2

difference, venous admixture, and physiologic dead space) all behave as if they were indicators of the degree of ventilation-perfusion heterogeneity. Indeed, they are "lumped parameter" estimates that rely on simple two-compartment models of the lung (29). Further, these variables are highly sensitive to the composition of the inflowing mixed venous blood. Consequently, the variables calculated may be substantially in error, particularly when serial measurements are made, unless a pulmonary catheter is in place. In summary, neither venous admixture can separate $\dot{V}_A/\dot{Q}$ mismatch from true intrapulmonary shunt, nor can physiologic dead space differentiate $\dot{V}_A/\dot{Q}$ inequality from changes in the airway dead space.

It is important to understand the major contribution of the three factors governing the respiratory gases ($\dot{V}_A/\dot{Q}$ relationships, the composition of the inspired gas and that of mixed venous blood) in any single gas exchange unit. Figure 24.2 illustrates the behavior of gas exchange (more specifically, the end-capillary Po_2 and Pco_2 and the arterial O_2 content) in a single functional unit of the lung as the $\dot{V}_A/\dot{Q}$ ratio is increased. Note that as the $\dot{V}_A/\dot{Q}$ ratio rises above 0.1, Pao_2 increases steadily, whereas there is still little change in $Paco_2$ until a $\dot{V}_A/\dot{Q}$ ratio of 1.0 is reached. Also note that while the latter two variables still progress in their respective changes from a $\dot{V}_A/\dot{Q}$ ratio of 1.0, the arterial O_2 content rises little from a $\dot{V}_A/\dot{Q}$ ratio of 2.0.

The influence of O_2 on Pao_2 depends on the degree of underlying $\dot{V}_A/\dot{Q}$ mismatch. Figure 24.3 shows that the end-capillary O_2 content rises as inspired O_2 is increased for conditions in which the levels of $\dot{V}_A/\dot{Q}$ inequality are mild to moderate (up to 0.1). In contrast, as the $\dot{V}_A/\dot{Q}$ mismatch becomes more severe (below 0.1), the rise in the end-capillary O_2 content is much slower, reaching similar values to those obtained in moderate conditions but using much higher inspired Po_2 (400–500 mm Hg). The inspired Po_2 thus needs to be increased considerably, at least to the range of 600–700 mm Hg.

Figure 24.4 shows the relationship with Pao_2 of the influence of mixed venous Po_2

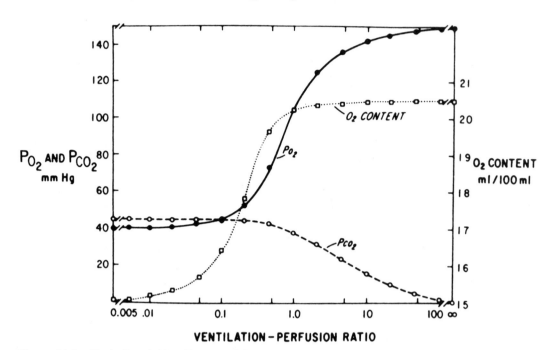

Figure 24.2. Variations in Po_2, Pco_2, and O_2 content in a gas exchange lung unit as its ventilation-perfusion ratio is progressively increased. This lung unit is assumed to be breathing air and the mixed venous blood Po_2 and Pco_2 are 40 and 45 mm Hg, respectively. See text for details. (From West JB. Ventilation-perfusion relationships. Am Rev Respir Dis 1977;116:919–943.)

$P\bar{v}O_2$ on gas exchange under three different gas exchange settings. In all three conditions there is a substantial fall in $P\bar{v}O_2$ as Pao_2 is reduced, the decrease being greatest with more abnormal respiratory gases. It is of the utmost importance to emphasize the crucial influence of the $P\bar{v}O_2$ on Pao_2, a well-known concept that is too often overlooked in the clinical arena. According to the Fick principle,

$$\dot{Q}_T = \frac{\dot{V}o_2}{Cao_2 - C\bar{v}o_2} \quad (1)$$

$$C\bar{v}o_2 = Cao_2 - \frac{\dot{V}o_2}{\dot{Q}_T} \quad (2)$$

where $\dot{V}o_2$ and $\dot{Q}_T$ represent O_2 uptake (consumption) and cardiac output, respectively. Accordingly, mixed venous hypoxemia may result from decreased arterial O_2 content, increased O_2 uptake, or from depressed cardiac output. The first variable may be influenced by changes in the factors that modulate the oxyhemoglobin dissociation curve, namely altered hemoglobin concentration or changes in temperature, P_{50} or pH, among others. However, these factors are considered to be of minor influence.

By using a lung model essentially representing intrapulmonary shunt, Wagner (85) showed that Pao_2 may be fairly sensitive to O_2 consumption changes, such that an increase from 300 to 600 ml/min, acting alone, would decrease Pao_2 by 10 mm Hg. In contrast, in a model characterized by pure $\dot{V}_A/\dot{Q}$ mismatch, a 10% change in O_2 uptake can vary the Pao_2 by 10 mm Hg in either direction. The different behavior of each model (lower sensitivity of Pao_2 in the shunt model) is related to the different levels of Pao_2 in the two situations. When Pao_2 is located in the lower, steeper, linear part of the oxyhemoglobin dissociation curve, as happens in the shunt model, changes in O_2 utilization induce smaller changes in Pao_2.

In practice, there are three possible ways in which cardiac output may modulate $P\bar{v}O_2$ (23). The most influential is through the effect on mixed venous O_2 content. A second way is by varying the transit time of the red cell through the pulmonary cap-

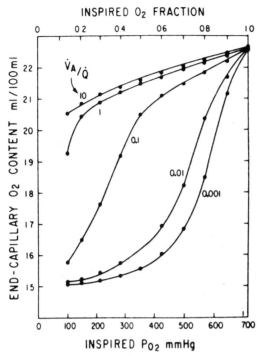

Figure 24.3. Changes in the end-capillary O_2 content *(y axis)* as inspired o_2 fraction *(top)* (or Po_2 *[bottom]*) *(x axis)* is increased. Each line represents a particular ventilation-perfusion ($\dot{V}_A/\dot{Q}$) ratio. The modeling conditions are the same as in Figure 24.2. See text for details. (From West JB. Ventilation-perfusion relationships. Am Rev Respir Dis 1977;116:919–943.)

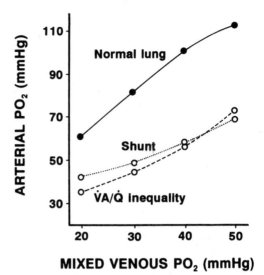

MIXED VENOUS PO₂ (mmHg)

Figure 24.4. Plots of arterial Po_2 *(y axis)* against mixed venous Po_2 *(x axis)* for different ventilation-perfusion distributions. Oxygen uptake has been allowed to decrease while both minute ventilation and cardiac output remain unaltered. *Solid line,* normal lung; *dotted line,* 30% shunt; *dashed line,* severe ventilation-perfusion. (From Dantzker DR. The influence of cardiovascular function on gas exchange. Clin Chest Med 1984;4:149–159.)

illary, which is only possible, however, when there is also a diffusion disequilibrium for the transfer of O_2. The third way is by redistributing pulmonary perfusion within the lung by releasing hypoxic pulmonary vasoconstriction, through the strong "cardiac-output shunt" relationship, or by increasing pulmonary venous pressure.

In summary, there are several determinants governing Po_2 and Pco_2 in pulmonary medicine (Fig. 24.5) (74). The most conspicuous intrapulmonary factors are $\dot{V}_A/\dot{Q}$ mismatching and intrapulmonary shunt;

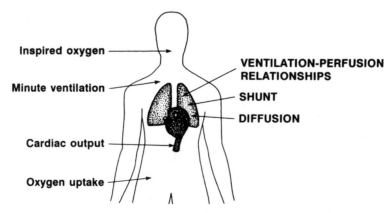

Figure 24.5. Principal intrapulmonary *(right)* and extrapulmonary *(left)* factors governing arterial blood respiratory gases.

in contrast, diffusion limitation to O_2 plays a minor role. Among the extrapulmonary factors, inspired Po_2, overall ventilation, cardiac output, and O_2 uptake are considered to be the most influential. Notice that Pao_2 may fall if inspired Po_2, overall ventilation, or cardiac output decrease, or O_2 utilization increases, even though the intrapulmonary factors remain unaltered. Conversely, if inspired Po_2, ventilation, cardiac output increase, or O_2 uptake decreases, Pao_2 may increase regardless of the changes that may operate at the level of the intrapulmonary determinants. Notice also that the three intrapulmonary factors along with overall ventilation constitute the four classic mechanisms of hypoxemia and hypercapnia. It is of interest to point out that changes in the minor factors modulating the oxyhemoglobin dissociation curve may also determine Pao_2, although less influentially, just as changes in acid-base status or in CO_2 production, in addition to overall ventilation, may regulate the levels of $Paco_2$ (95).

The development of the multiple inert gas elimination technique (MIGET) by Wagner and associates (31, 90, 92) 2 decades ago, introduced a new era in our understanding of the pathophysiology of pulmonary gas exchange in respiratory medicine. The MIGET allows investigation of the distributions (quantities) of $\dot{V}_A/\dot{Q}$ ratios and their profiles, and also the exploration and unraveling of other mechanisms of abnormal arterial blood gases. Further, the information provided by this technique permits a more complete analysis of the changes induced by O_2 on the distribution of $\dot{V}_A/\dot{Q}$ ratios because the tracer nature of the method does not alter, by itself, pulmonary gas exchange. The principles governing the inert gas technique are based on classic mass/balance equations under steady-state conditions for gas exchange in the lungs and the peripheral tissues (44). Accordingly, the uptake (referred to as retention, $Pc' / P\bar{v}$) or elimination (known as excretion, $PA / P\bar{v}$) of an inert gas in any homogenous area of the lung is given by the following equation:

$$Pc'/P\bar{v} = PA/P\bar{v} = \lambda \ / \ (\lambda + \dot{V}_A/\dot{Q}) \qquad (3)$$

where Pc', $P\bar{v}$, and PA correspond to end-capillary, mixed venous, and alveolar partial pressures, respectively, and λ to solubility (or the blood:gas partition coefficient).

If a 5% dextrose solution of a mixture of six gases (sulfur hexafluoride, ethane, cyclopropane, enflurane or halothane, ether, and acetone) is infused into a peripheral vein, thereafter samples of heparinized arterial and mixed venous blood and mixed expired gas can be collected simultaneously. Alternatively, mixed venous inert gas concentrations can be calculated by mass balance equation from arterial and mixed expired samples using the cardiac output measured by other methods. For each infused gas, the ratio of arterial to mixed venous concentration (retention) or mixed expired to mixed venous concentration (excretion) is calculated and retention-solubility and excretion-solubility curves are drawn, yielding a sort of "fingerprint" of a particular distribution of pulmonary blood flow and of alveolar ventilation, respectively.

The use of these six inert gases has two major advantages (44). First, the limitations due to a nonlinear dissociation curve on gas exchange, present for the respiratory gases, are avoided. Second, a large range of solubilities, approximately 10^5 between that of sulfur hexafluoride (the most insoluble) and acetone (the most soluble), is used. West (97) has shown that the gas exchange behavior of any gas in the event of $\dot{V}_A/\dot{Q}$ mismatching is a function of its dissociation curve in blood, namely its solubility. Figure 24.6 includes representative examples of a multicompartment $\dot{V}_A/\dot{Q}$ distribution corresponding to a young healthy individual, breathing air, at rest, and also to the most common chronic respiratory disorders.

At present, the multiple inert gas elimination approach is visualized as a powerful research tool that is able to:

1. estimate qualitatively and quantitatively the patterns of alveolar ventilation and pulmonary blood flow;
2. calculate numerical variables that describe quantitative abnormalities;
3. infer the coexistence of diffusion disequilibrium to O_2 transfer;
4. partition the alveolar end-capillary Po_a dif-

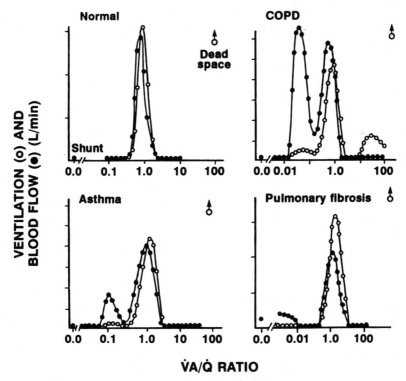

Figure 24.6. Representative examples of ventilation *(open symbols)* and blood flow *(closed symbols)* distributions *(y axis)* plotted against ventilation-perfusion ($\dot{V}_A/\dot{Q}$) ratio on a log scale *(x axis)*. *Top left*, healthy individual (symmetrical distributions, well-positioned on a $\dot{V}_A/\dot{Q}$ ratio of 1.0, with little dispersion (narrowness). Note the absence of shunt (zero $\dot{V}_A/\dot{Q}$ ratio). *Top right*, advanced COPD (bimodal distributions of blood flow and ventilation). *Bottom left*, acute severe asthma (marked bimodal blood flow pattern). *Bottom right*, idiopathic pulmonary fibrosis (modest bimodal perfusion profile). Note the practical absence of shunt in the three pulmonary diseases. *Closed circle, left*, shunt; *open circle, right*, dead space. See text for details.

ference into components due to shunt, $\dot{V}_A/\dot{Q}$ inequality, or diffusion limitation for O_2; and,

5. apportion arterial oxygenation changes into intrapulmonary and extrapulmonary determinants of respiratory blood gases.

ADULT RESPIRATORY DISTRESS SYNDROME (ARDS)

Gas Exchange and Structure

ARDS was originally described in 1967 (5). It is a common entity that is presently believed to be not a specific disease, but rather a constellation of multiple diseases with a unique category of respiratory failure distinguished from several others. This elusive syndrome, a poorly understood but often fatal prototype of increased perme-

ability pulmonary edema, is considered to be one of the most life-threatening manifestations of acute respiratory failure. Irrespective of the most appropriate definition severe refractory hypoxemia is a mainstay among the diagnostic criteria of ARDS (57). Since the introduction of the MIGET, 10 clinical studies (26, 36, 54–56, 61–64, 66) of ARDS encompassing approximately a hundred patients, have been reported (Table 24.2). Severe bacterial pneumonia, aspiration of gastric content, and sepsis accounted for more than half the cases. All the studies were performed while the patients were mechanically ventilated, using routine ventilatory strategies, and were breathing high-inspired fractions of O_2 (FIO_2) (range, 0.41–1.0). Most were performed applying an external positive end-

Table 24.2
Mean Values of Respiratory and Inert Gas Indices in Patients with ARDS[a]

Study	Pao₂ (mm Hg)	$\dot{Q}_S/\dot{Q}_T$ (%)	Shunt (%)	Low $\dot{V}_A/\dot{Q}$ Mode (%)	Dead Space (%)
Dantzker et al. (26)	77	NR	48*	NR	29**
Gerdeaux et al. (36)	80	35	31	5	NR
Matamis et al. (54)	74	38	30	7	44
Ralph et al. (64)	80	NR	39	17	40
Mélot et al. (56)	87	25	23	NR	52
Radermacher et al. (61)	103	42	34	9	46
Reyes et al. (66)	78	29	29	7	39
Mélot et al. (55)	99	20	21	0	41
Radermacher et al. (62)	113	25	18	6	NR
Radermacher et al. (63)	92	29	29	4	26

[a]$\dot{Q}_S/\dot{Q}_T$, venous admixture; shunt, % of $\dot{Q}_T$ to $\dot{V}_A/\dot{Q}$ <0.005; low $\dot{V}_A/\dot{Q}$ mode, % of $\dot{Q}_T$ to $\dot{V}_A/\dot{Q}$ <0.1 (excluding shunt); dead space, % of $\dot{V}_A$ to $\dot{V}_A/\dot{Q}$ >100; *, includes % of $\dot{Q}_T$ to $\dot{V}_A/\dot{Q}$ <0.01; **, dead space was minimized; NR, not reported.

expiratory pressure (PEEP) (range, 5–20 cm H₂O). Measurements were done during the first days of mechanical ventilation. While one of the studies (36) was essentially descriptive, three others (26, 54, 64) assessed the effects of PEEP on pulmonary gas exchange, and the remaining six evaluated the transient effects of vasoactive agents of $\dot{V}_A/\dot{Q}$ distributions.

Two common profiles of $\dot{V}_A/\dot{Q}$ ratio distributions were observed in most of the studies. On the one hand, half of the patients exhibited a considerable intrapulmonary shunt together with a modest bi-modal pulmonary perfusion pattern (Fig. 24.7). In addition to shunt, a substantial amount of blood flow was diverted to both areas of normal alveolar units ($\dot{V}_A/\dot{Q}$ ratios between 0.1 and 10) and low $\dot{V}_A/\dot{Q}$ units ($\dot{V}_A/\dot{Q}$ ratios between 0.005 and 0.1). It is of note, however, that in all studies except that of Ralph et al. (64), the amount of pulmonary blood flow to low $\dot{V}_A/\dot{Q}$ areas was moderate, averaging less than 10% of cardiac output. On the other hand, approximately 40% of the patients presented a pure shunt alone. Regardless of the $\dot{V}_A/\dot{Q}$ ratio profiles, the amounts of shunt were

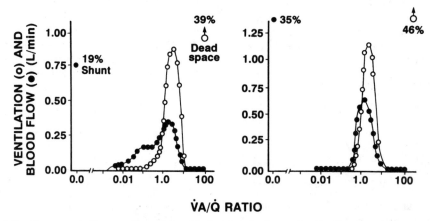

Figure 24.7. Representative profiles of ventilation-perfusion ratio distributions corresponding to two different ARDS patients. *Left,* shunt plus a modest low $\dot{V}_A/\dot{Q}$ mode (left shoulder). *Right,* pure shunt together with both unimodal blood flow and ventilation distributions. Note that shunt *(closed circle, left)* is considerably increased, whereas dead space *(open circle, right)* is slightly increased. No areas of high $\dot{V}_A/\dot{Q}$ peaks are shown. (From, in part, Reyes A, Roca J, Rodrigue.'-Roisin R, Torres A, Ussetti P, Wagner PD. Effect of almitrine on ventilation-perfusion distribution in adult respiratory distress syndrome. Am Rev Respir Dis 1988;137:1062–1067.)

for the most part, linearly related to the severity of the underlying acute lung injury, but there was no correlation between the etiologic causes of ARDS and the presence of a specific $\dot{V}_A/\dot{Q}$ distribution pattern. A small group of patients (less than 10%) disclosed a bimodal ventilation pattern in which a moderate percentage of alveolar ventilation was distributed to areas of high $\dot{V}_A/\dot{Q}$ units ($\dot{V}_A/\dot{Q}$ ratios between 10 and 100), along with the presence of pure shunt. Finally, three patients exhibited a bimodal profile of pulmonary perfusion and ventilation with pure shunt only.

In most of these studies, inert dead space was increased. The dispersion of pulmonary blood flow and ventilation distributions, two common descriptors of the degree of $\dot{V}_A/\dot{Q}$ mismatching, ranged between mild to moderate (55, 56) and moderate to severe (61) values in the studies. Also of interest was the fact that in three studies (26, 36, 56) there was close agreement between predicted Pao_2 and measured Pao_2. If alveolar end-capillary diffusion limitation for o_2 had contributed to hypoxemia, a significant discrepancy between the last two parameters, resulting in a higher predicted Pao_2, would have been detected (Fig. 24.8). In contrast, the two values were very close, with significant correlation coefficients (above 0.90). Further, no significant differences between the lines of identity and of regression were shown. This finding initially rules out the coexistence of an additional mechanism of abnormal arterial blood gases other than shunt or $\dot{V}_A/\dot{Q}$ mismatching. Moreover, these findings are consistent with the results of an experimental study on a canine model of oleic acid pulmonary edema (13) designed to test whether the apparent increase in venous admixture caused by an increase in cardiac output could be a manifestation of incomplete diffusion equilibration for O_2.

Overall, these inert gas data are largely in agreement with the original description of $\dot{V}_A/\dot{Q}$ inequalities in ARDS by Dantzker et al. (26), who essentially concluded that pulmonary blood flow is distributed mainly to two types of lung units, those normally ventilated and those completely unventi-

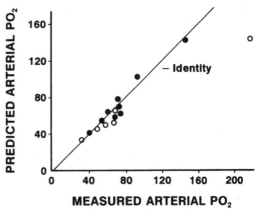

Figure 24.8. Predicted Pao_2 (mm Hg) *(y axis)* versus measured Pao_2 (mm Hg) *(x axis)* from the recovered $\dot{V}_A/\dot{Q}$ ratio distributions in ARDS patients. Note that both variables are in close agreement, ruling out the presence of diffusion limitation for o_2 as an additional cause of arterial hypoxemia. Had o_2 transfer been diffusion-limited, most of the points would have to lie above the line of identity. See text for details. (From Dantzker DR, Brook CJ, Dehart P, Lynch JP, Weg JG. Ventilation-perfusion distributions in the adult respiratory distress syndrome. Am Rev Respir Dis 1979;120:1039–1052.)

lated. According to these authors, this "all or none" or "open and closed" phenomenon is consistent with previous experimental pathologic findings (80) that showed that alveolar flooding was either complete or absent in a model of pulmonary edema in the dog.

Despite the heterogeneity of the constellation of disorders that induce diffuse alveolar damage in ARDS, it is widely accepted that during the early acute phase of the disease, human lungs show a uniform pattern of tissue injury with little specificity. Consequently, both fluid and protein flow into the lungs at a rate that exceeds that at which it can be removed. The predominant finding is, therefore, interstitial and alveolar edema, a "leaky blood-gas barrier," as termed by Bachofen and Weibel (7). The consequences of increased permeability edema on gas exchange depend on the amount of edema accumulated and also on the severity of the causative disorder. Surfactant is both quantitatively and qualitatively altered. Alveoli are heterogeneously filled with proteinaceous fluid, blood cells, macrophages, cell debris, and remnants of surfactant; hyaline membranes are always present.

Along with the consequences of edema accumulation, other effects of acute lung injury probably depend on the etiology and extent of the pulmonary insult (33). Thus, bronchoconstriction and airway inflammation due to direct airway injury or mediator release may be present under some clinical circumstances such as aspiration pneumonia or inhalation of toxic fumes and noxious gases (100). Likewise, the hypoxic vascular response of the pulmonary circulation may be altered and the pulmonary vascular resistance may be increased. Vascular abnormalities may be provoked by increased interstitial pressure, cellular edema and proliferation, or deformities (39). Briefly, the earliest changes are characterized by widespread alveolar and interstitial edema and hemorrhage. Later, after 7–10 days, during the subacute phase, the hallmarks of the lesion are inflammatory and proliferative tissue reactions to diffuse pulmonary microvascular injury. Accordingly, there are progressive and heterogeneous alterations in the septal tissue and the alveolar architecture. There are also important changes at the interstitial level, with cellular immigration, proliferation of connective tissue, persistent interstitial edema, and organized alveolar damage. Microvasculature is dramatically reduced in number and volume; the pulmonary vascular bed may be either partially or completely obliterated with marked alterations in its surface area (101).

It has been shown experimentally that pulmonary gas exchange abnormalities and lung structure correlate poorly (14). In a canine model of ARDS in which the MIGET was used, it was shown that the lung injury can be so devastating that pathophysiologic correlations may be impossible (79). However, in such a model it was observed that intrapulmonary shunt at day 1 was the principal gas exchange abnormality inducing hypoxemia; likewise, either a widening of the blood flow dispersion (as a common descriptor of $\dot{V}_A/\dot{Q}$ deterioration) or the appearance of a moderately low $\dot{V}_A/\dot{Q}$ mode were shown. Thereafter,

serial measurements denoted a progressive improvement in gas exchange abnormalities most evident at day 4, disappearing almost completely 7 days later. Thus, in animal models this all-or-none profile appears to remain to progress to resolution such that shunt gradually diminishes without conversion to areas of low $\dot{V}_A/\dot{Q}$ units.

Despite these poor structure-function correlations, the most common pathologic findings described herein may be compatible to some extent with the gas exchange findings mentioned above. Thus, the presence of a considerable intrapulmonary shunt, either alone or accompanied by alveolar units with low $\dot{V}_A/\dot{Q}$ ratios, is consistent with the underlying major morphologic changes. Lung regions with low $\dot{V}_A/\dot{Q}$ units (poorly but still ventilated) may not only represent alveolar spaces with partial filling but also suggest the coexistence of airway narrowing with increased airway resistance (100) or parenchymal areas with lung fibrosis (2). Alternatively, both the increased dead space shown in most of the patients and the high $\dot{V}_A/\dot{Q}$ mode observed in a small number of patients may denote not only the effects of external PEEP over the lung parenchyma, by developing areas completely unperfused or poorly perfused (59), but also the consequences and the effects of intrinsic PEEP (16, 70, 76), which has been demonstrated to be actively present in more than 50% of the series of ARDS patients who need mechanical ventilation (73).

Lamy et al. (47) correlated respiratory gas exchange variables (specifically, Pa_{O_2} and venous admixture at different $F_{I_{O_2}}$ and levels of external PEEP) with pathologic findings from open lung biopsies and autopsies in one of the largest series of ARDS patients. They defined three distinct profiles. Group 1, which included a third of the patients, had the most severe hypoxemia, a minimal Pa_{O_2} response to increased levels of PEEP, and an unaltered venous admixture of all $F_{I_{O_2}}$ levels. These patients exhibited essentially pathologic acute changes of ARDS, but few proliferative changes. Group 2 included another third of the individuals with less severe hypoxemia and a moderate Pa_{O_2} response to PEEP. In contrast to group 1 patients, the major pathologic findings observed were fibrotic changes. Finally, group 3, which has the least hypoxemia and the best Pao_2 response to 10 cm H_2O of PEEP, showed similar pathologic findings to group 1, but they were less severe. In the latter population, an important physiologic finding was that venous admixture increased while Fio_2 decreased. Consequently, these authors hypothesized that, while pure shunt was the principal intrapulmonary determinant of hypoxemia in group 1, both $\dot{V}_A/\dot{Q}$ mismatching and diffusion disequilibrium to O_2 constituted the principal intrapulmonary mechanisms of abnormal blood gases in the other two-thirds of the patients.

Two years earlier, King et al. (45) had already reached a similar conclusion in a smaller series of ARDS patients and also invoked diffusion limitation for o_2, in addition to shunt and $\dot{V}_A/\dot{Q}$ inequality, as another mechanism of hypoxemia to explain the profile of the change in Pao_2 while increasing Fio_2. Interestingly, Bachofen and Weibel (8) investigated the morphologic findings most relevant to pulmonary gas exchange corresponding to subacute phases of ARDS and showed that the gas exchange surface was substantially decreased while the blood-gas barrier was greatly thickened. More importantly, there was a marked reduction in capillary volume and a very low capillary hematocrit, indicating that the remaining capillaries were inadequately perfused. One consequence of these abnormalities was a decreased diffusing capacity (D_L) to less than 10% of normal. Since D_L estimated morphometrically reflects the maximum o_2 transfer capacity of the lung, the observed limitation suggests that additional impairment of hypoxemia, caused by intrapulmonary shunt or $\dot{V}_A/\dot{Q}$ mismatch, may induce a level of hypoxemia incompatible with life. However, as alluded to above, diffusion limitation for O_2 has not been proved using the principles of the MIGET.

Breen et al. (13) concluded that diffusion disequilibrium for O_2 does not contribute to the increase in venous admixture when total blood flow increases in an experimental setting. Rather, from the re-

sults of the inert gas elimination studies, the finding of an increased venous admixture as a response to decreasing values of Fio_2 by Lamy et al. (47) in two-thirds of their patients, or those of King et al. (45), can be exclusively explained on the grounds of the presence of a low $\dot{V}_A/\dot{Q}$ mode.

Influence of External PEEP

When ventilatory support is used, external PEEP is one of the hallmarks of the therapeutic strategy of ARDS. Three studies have addressed the influence of external PEEP on pulmonary gas exchange in ARDS patients. In the first, Dantzker et al. (26) took measurements at increasing levels of PEEP. Two distinct patterns emerged (Fig. 24.9). In five patients, the pattern of $\dot{V}_A/\dot{Q}$ ratio distributions remained essentially unaltered despite progressive increases of PEEP to more than 20 cm H_2O. Yet, the amount of intrapulmonary shunt progressively decreased, while that of ventilation to areas with infinity $\dot{V}_A/\dot{Q}$ ratios (dead space) increased. In the other seven patients, in addition to less intrapulmonary shunt, the shape of $\dot{V}_A/\dot{Q}$ ratio distributions changed in response to increased levels of PEEP. Thus, there was a broadening of the dispersion of ventilation distribution (because of the increase in high $\dot{V}_A/\dot{Q}$ areas) and a redistribution of ventilation from the high $\dot{V}_A/\dot{Q}$ mode (with finite $\dot{V}_A/\dot{Q}$ ratios) to dead space (infinity $\dot{V}_A/\dot{Q}$ ratios). In each patient, PEEP ultimately led to both a substantial reduction in the percentage of cardiac output distributed to unventilated or poorly ventilated $\dot{V}_A/\dot{Q}$ units and also to a marked increase in dead space, the final result being an increased Pao_2. No results were shown on $P\bar{v}o_2$. However, because lung volumes were not measured, it is not possible to determine from these data whether the increase in poorly or completely unperfused lung areas was representative of the expected increment of the increased functional residual capacity resulting from the effects of PEEP.

In the second study, Matamis et al. (54) investigated the $\dot{V}_A/\dot{Q}$ ratio distributions response to external PEEP in ARDS patients while cardiac output was main-

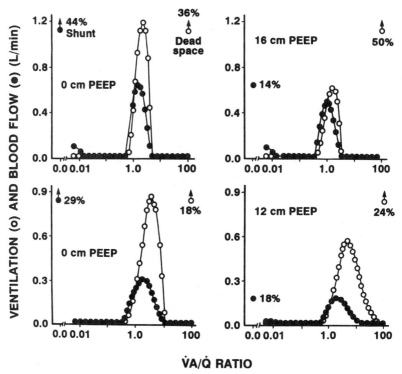

Figure 24.9. Effects of PEEP on $\dot{V}_A/\dot{Q}$ ratio distributions in patients with ARDS. *Top (from right to left),* PEEP (16 cm H$_2$O) induces a reduction in shunt *(closed symbol)* along with an increase in dead space *(open symbol)* without any marked change in the pattern of distributions. *Bottom (from right to left),* PEEP (12 cm H$_2$O) decreases shunt and increases dead space while the distribution of ventilation widens. The presence of high or infinity $\dot{V}_A/\dot{Q}$ ratios suggests the development of areas with poorly perfused or unperfused alveoli, respectively, due to the simultaneous depression of cardiac output. (From, in part, Dantzker DR, Brook CJ, Dehart P, Lynch JP, Weg JG. Ventilation-perfusion distributions in the adult respiratory distress syndrome. Am Rev Respir Dis 1979;120:1039–1052.)

tained at control values with a continuous infusion of dopamine, a drug with inotropic effects that considerably facilitates venous return. During the application of PEEP, Pao$_2$, P$\bar{v}$o$_2$ and O$_2$ delivery increased significantly, whereas venous admixture decreased markedly. Similarly, intrapulmonary shunt susbtantially dereased, in that pulmonary blood flow was redistributed from nonventilated alveolar units with zero $\dot{V}_A/\dot{Q}$ ratios to areas with normally ventilated $\dot{V}_A/\dot{Q}$ units. In other words, there was reperfusion at lung sites with normal $\dot{V}_A/\dot{Q}$ ratios. Dead space increased slightly but significantly; in contrast, the shape of the alveolar ventilation distribution remained unchanged and no additional areas of high $\dot{V}_A/\dot{Q}$ units emerged.

Because PEEP does not reduce extravascular lung water (it causes redistribution from alveoli to peribronchial and perivascular spaces (42) and may even increase it (17), these results suggest that the amelioration in both pulmonary and peripheral gas exchange may be explained by the hypothesis that external PEEP facilitates the reopening of collapsed airways and alveoli, a mechanism previously postulated by others (81). While these data are somewhat at variance with those of Dantzker et al. (26), conceivably because of the application of lower levels of PEEP, they are consistent with former data (81) that documented that progressive increments of PEEP did not increase alveolar dead space as long as cardiac output was not depressed. From a clinical standpoint, the most important conclusion of the study by Matamis et al. (54) though is that when the reduction of cardiac output may be prevented pharmacologically, i.e., by an inotropic agent such as dopamine, the beneficial effects of external PEEP in ARDS patients are maintained by means of improving both pulmonary and peripheral gas exchange. However, these results need to be tempered because the gas exchange response to PEEP alone was not assessed before restoring the cardiac output. Thus, it is unknown whether the reduction in shunt following the application of PEEP would have been mitigated or would even have been greater without the effects of dopamine.

Because of systematic investigation of the effects on $\dot{V}_A/\dot{Q}$ ratio distributions when external PEEP is serially increased in a controlled manner in ARDS patients was lacking, Ralph et al. (64) studied the gas exchange response to incremental increases in PEEP. In most of the patients, Pao_2 improved substantially either because of a decrease in intrapulmonary shunt only, in the low $\dot{V}_A/\dot{Q}$ mode alone, or a derecruitment of blood flow from shunt to areas with low or normal $\dot{V}_A/\dot{Q}$ units. Reductions in the amount of blood flow to low $\dot{V}_A/\dot{Q}$ areas were more unpredictable and, in some cases, a moderate percentage of cardiac output to low $\dot{V}_A/\dot{Q}$ units emerged following the PEEP trial. When Pao_2 remained unaltered in response to PEEP increases, there were no changes in the profiles of the $\dot{V}_A/\dot{Q}$ ratio distributions. Occasionally, an increase either in poorly perfused $\dot{V}_A/\dot{Q}$ units or in dead space was shown in some patients. In no way could the beneficial effect of PEEP on Pao_2 following the increments in PEEP be predicted by the etiology of ARDS or the severity of abnormal gas exchange on entry of the study before PEEP was applied. Cardiac output decreased progressively as PEEP was increased, a reduction not associated with a decrease in $P\bar{v}o_2$. Moreover, this hemodynamic change took place in the presence of adequate filling pressures before the application of PEEP. The mean change in cardiac output was essentially similar between PEEP trials regardless of whether or not there was improvement in Pao_2. Under the conditions of this study, therefore, the beneficial effects of PEEP on Pao_2 were attributed essentially to the opening of closed airways and alveoli due to an increase in functional residual capacity, a hypothesis similar to that postulated by Matamis and co-workers (54).

From a clinical viewpoint, these three studies are important for two reasons. First, overall the data indicate that the beneficial influence on pulmonary gas exchange in ARDS following the application of external PEEP is essentially related to the decrease of intrapulmonary shunt with redistribution of blood flow to either poorly or normally ventilated alveolar units. Besides, this mechanism seems to be strongly mediated through the reopening of collapsed alveoli and airways instead of the decrease of cardiac output per se. The depression of output by itself may lead, in turn, to a reduction in shunt or in poorly ventilated $\dot{V}_A/\dot{Q}$ units (22). This is of interest because of the well known, but poorly understood, positive association documented between shunt and cardiac output (22, 28, 50, 53). It has been shown in both the clinical (50) and experimental (22, 28) setting of ARDS, either pharmacologically using different vasoactive drugs or mechanically, that changes in cardiac output lead to directionally similar changes in intrapulmonary shunt (as assessed either by the MIGET or the oxygen method). Likewise, in many instances the shunt fraction also changes in a similar direction to changes in the $P\bar{v}o_2$ and inversely with pulmonary vascular resistance (50).

Second, of paramount importance is that in two of the three studies in which the values of $P\bar{v}o_2$ were reported, this variable either increased (54) or remained stable (64) when cardiac output was reduced. These findings represent, to some extent, an elegant example of the difficult but fascinating interplay between intrapulmonary and extrapulmonary factors governing arterial blood gases in pulmonary medicine. Overall, Pao_2 increased following the application of external PEEP because the beneficial effects on Pao_2 caused essentially by the the reduction in shunt (intrapulmonary factor) were not offset by the simultaneous expected deleterious effect on Pao_2 due to depression of cardiac output (extrapulmonary factor), which had allowed $P\bar{v}o_2$ to decrease, other things being equal. However, had the reduction of cardiac output been more severe, Pao_2 would have remained unchanged or would even have decreased despite the improvement in intrapulmonary shunt. Similarly, the finding that $P\bar{v}o_2$ did not change in the same direction as cardiac output in one of the studies (64) makes note of the observation of the pathologic supply dependence between oxygen delivery and oxygen uptake (27). Accordingly, such patients respond to the depression of cardiac output mediated by external PEEP by reducing oxygen uptake (21).

Finally, it should be noted that high $\dot{V}_A/\dot{Q}$ peaks appear, along with moderate to severe increases in dead space, following the application of PEEP. Although these responses to PEEP were not identical in all subjects and may differ from those shown experimentally in different models of ARDS (21), individual patients showed the appearance of such areas with high $\dot{V}_A/\dot{Q}$ ratios and increasing PEEP, a change also reported in a canine model of oleic acid lung injury (30). This is essentially consistent with the data obtained by Hedenstierna et al. (40), who found that the reduction of cardiac output and the depression of perfusion in the uppermost regions of the lung determined a bimodal ventilation pattern with PEEP.

Effects of Breathing 100% O_2

According to a theoretical analysis of the gas exchange factors involved in the development of shunt while breathing 100% O_2 (29), it was shown that low inspired $\dot{V}_A/\dot{Q}$ ratios (named "critical") could result in a condition of absent expired ventilation, hence inducing reabsorption atelectasis in the alveoli. By increasing the inspired O_2, such a critical unit will no longer eliminate gas but may continue gas uptake. Moreover, this unit becomes unstable and may ultimately collapse, thereby leading to the development of reabsorption atelectasis, a classic observation in critical care medicine (82). The critical $\dot{V}_A/\dot{Q}$ units depend on the Fio_2 such that they rise considerably as the latter reaches 100%.

Alternatively, these critical units may remain open and not collapse by increasing their inspired ventilation from other units. Gas uptake would be reduced in these open critical units since some of their inspired gas will have come from units in which gas exchange has already taken place. It is of note that for each level of inspired Po_2, the amount of shunt was lower when release of hypoxic pulmonary vasoconstriction accompanied the change in Fio_2. Alveolar units with moderately low $\dot{V}_A/\dot{Q}$ ratios would be able to redistribute ("steal") blood flow from those lung areas with very low or zero $\dot{V}_A/\dot{Q}$ units as their vascular resistance falls.

However, there are no reliable data so far concerning the effects of breathing 100% O_2 on gas exchange using the MIGET in patients with ARDS, except for a few anecdotal cases (87; Wagner PD, unpublished data). In a series of patients with acute respiratory failure, not clearly defined as ARDS (48), the amount of intrapulmonary shunt measured with the inert gas method remained completely unaltered during breathing 100% O_2. Similarly, the apparent stability of the very low $\dot{V}_A/\dot{Q}$ units (below 0.01) while patients were breathing 100% O_2 in the first ARDS description of $\dot{V}_A/\dot{Q}$ ratio distributions (26), led to the hypothesis that these critical alveolar units may remain partly open to facilitate some O_2 transfer. This would account for the increase in Pao_2 shown in previous studies while breathing 100% O_2 (45, 47). Efficiency of collateral ventilation, interdependence of the surrounding lung parenchyma, or the interaction of mechanical forces exerted during mechanical ventilation might contribute to this paradoxical situation (29).

Very recent data in five patients with ARDS demonstrate, however, an increase in shunt and in the dispersion of blood flow while breathing 100% O_2 for 1 hour (Santos C, Roca J, Torres A, and Rodriguez-Roisin R, unpublished data). This would indicate that breathing 100% O_2 does induce reabsorption atelectasis and abolishes hypoxic pulmonary vasoconstriction in the ARDS condition. This differs partly from former observations from the same group that were made of patients with severe bacterial pneumonia (35) or with acute respiratory failure due to chronic obstructive pulmonary disease (84). In these patients, hypoxic pulmonary vasoconstriction is always reduced while intrapulmonary shunt remains unaltered. The latter findings may be explained, however, by the influencing role of an efficient collateral ventilation. In contrast, patients with status asthmaticus who need mechanical ventilation (69) show a considerable hypoxic vascular response together with the development of moderate amounts of shunt while breathing 100% O_2, thereby suggesting the development of reabsorption atelectasis or a vascular recruitment in areas of small preexisting shunts.

An additional point of interest was the close correlation between the measurements of venous admixture ($\dot{Q}_S/\dot{Q}_T$) and of inert gas shunt at maintenance FIO_2 in most studies. This may suggest that the delayed increment in Pao_2 due to a slow washout of nitrogen in lung areas with low $\dot{V}_A/\dot{Q}$ units plays a minor role in ARDS patients (35).

Response to Vasoactive Agents

During the administration of vasodilating drugs, pulmonary artery pressure and vascular resistance values decreased in all but two studies (during the infusion of ketanserin [61], a potent inhibitor of serotonin, and of nitroglycerin [62], a well-known vasodilator) (55, 56, 61–63). Cardiac output increased after the administration of prostaglandin E_1 (PGE_1) (55, 62) a vasodilator formerly shown to improve survival in ARDS (Fig. 24.10), and prostacyclin I_2 (PGI_2) (63), a natural vasodilator and platelet aggregation inhibitor with cytoprotective properties, only. Shunt increased substantially and areas of low $\dot{V}_A/\dot{Q}$ units remained unchanged during the perfusion of all vasodilators except ketanserin (61); dead space increased after the administration of ketanserin and sodium nitroprusside, a traditional vasodilator, only. Accordingly, Pao_2 decreased in all studies except those involving ketanserin and PGI_2; $Paco_2$ increased slightly but significantly during the administration of sodium nitroprusside (61) alone. Interestingly, $P\bar{v}o_2$ remained unaltered after the infusion of all vasodilators except PGI_2 which increased O_2 delivery and decreased O_2 uptake markedly. In contrast, with almitrine (66), a peripheral chemoreceptor agonist with potential pulmonary vasoconstricting effects, both pulmonary artery pressure and vascular resistance values increased slightly but significantly, whereas shunt dramatically fell. As a result, both Pao_2 and $P\bar{v}o_2$ improved substantially, but O_2 delivery did not change.

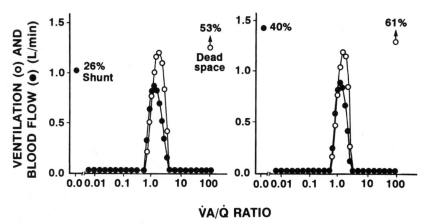

Figure 24.10. A substantial increase in shunt *(closed symbol)* is the principal deleterious effect of infusing PGE_1 *(right)* on $\dot{V}_A/\dot{Q}$ ratio distributions in an ARDS patient *(left*, baseline conditions). As a result, pulmonary gas exchange further deteriorates and Pao_2 falls substantially. (From Mélot C, Lejeune P, Leeman M, Moraine JJ, Naeije R. Prostaglandin E_1 in the adult respiratory distress syndrome. Am Rev Respir Dis 1989;139:106–110.)

These results show by and large a remarkable consistency. Notice that as pulmonary vascular pressure or resistance are depressed following vasodilators, gas exchange worsens (55, 56, 61–63). As overall pulmonary vascular pressure or resistance are increased during almitrine administration, gas exchange improves (66). Conceivably, pulmonary blood flow is diverted to damaged, hypoxic, nonventilated lung areas, thereby increasing (worsening) intrapulmonary shunt. The increase in $Paco_2$ after sodium nitroprusside may be due to the increased dead space, possibly reflecting the derecruitment of the pulmonary vasculature caused partly by the vasodilating effect of the drug by itself (61). After ketanserin, the effects of increased dead space on arterial respiratory blood gases were negligible as lone as shunt remained constant (61).

At first glance, the simplest interpretation is that all these vasoactive drugs exert their principal influence on pulmonary vascular tone in the abnormally injured, hypoxic regions of the lung. Whenever there is a high pulmonary vascular tone in disease states, as happens in primary pulmonary hypertension (25) or idiopathic pulmonary fibrosis (2), $\dot{V}_A/\dot{Q}$ matching may be enhanced. In contrast, an abnormally low pulmonary vascular reactivity, as shown in patients with liver cirrhosis (71), may worsen pulmonary gas exchange. In a canine model of lung edema (20), it was shown that sodium nitroprusside further worsened both shunt and $\dot{V}_A/\dot{Q}$ distributions and reduced pulmonary vascular resistance when the animals were ventilated with air, but not while they were breathing 100% O_2. This suggests the release of hypoxic pulmonary vasoconstriction, hence leading to further $\dot{V}_A/\dot{Q}$ mismatch. Other experimental studies using vasodilators have reported similar results either because hypoxic vasoconstriction is ablated (20, 94), or pulmonary blood flow is increased (11, 101), or both (11, 12, 101).

Several potential mechanisms have been postulated to explain the well-known but still poorly understood relationship between cardiac output and shunt fraction in acute respiratory failure, regardless of the method of inducing the increase in cardiac output (either mechanically or pharmacologically) (13, 91). Thus, an increased diffusion disequilibrium to O_2 transfer due to a reduced transit time in the pulmonary capillary network has not been demonstrated. Another hypothesis, an increased pulmonary blood flow causing more pulmonary edema, has been also refuted since extravascular lung water remained stable as both blood flow and shunt increased. Interestingly, if fractional blood flow does not increase at the lobar level while increasing total lung perfusion, it might be that, as cardiac output is increased at the intralobar level, there is preferential increase in perfusion in completely flooded alveoli but not at dry lung sites. Alternatively, the possibility that hematocrit distribution changes while cardiac output is altered has not been ruled out.

The increase (worsening) in shunt following the rise in cardiac output caused by an increased $P\bar{v}o_2$, hence releasing hypoxic pulmonary vasoconstriction, may be an alternative appealing hypothesis. There is evidence that if $P\bar{v}o_2$ increases while blood flow is kept constant, shunt is impaired; conversely, if $P\bar{v}o_2$ remains unchanged as flow increases, shunt is unaltered. Payen et al. (58) very elegantly showed in patients with ARDS that changes in $P\bar{v}o_2$ appeared to be a major determinant of venous admixture changes when the increase in cardiac output by application of lower body positive pressure was compared to that induced by dopamine infusion. Venous admixture remained unchanged as the cardiac index was increased mechanically; in contrast, when dopamine was infused, the shunt fraction deteriorated (increased) dramatically.

From a clinical viewpoint, this cardiac output-shunt strong relationship highlights the complexity of the interplay between intrapulmonary and extrapulmonary factors contributing to gas exchange. It may be that the deterioration in shunt tending to reduce Pao_2 is balanced by the increase in arterial oxygenation (due to the increase in $P\bar{v}o_2$, while other things remain unchanged), with the final Pao_2 being unaltered or just slightly decreased. Further, the increased cardiac output that may follow the administration of some vasodilators (55, 62, 63) may facilitate a better O_2 delivery. Thus, it appears that sacrificing pulmonary gas exchange (the increased shunt does not seem by itself to induce more lung injury) to reduce cardiac afterload might represent the desirable therapeutic strategy, at least theoretically, if a vasodilator is given (91).

Recent preliminary evidence suggests that gaseous nitric oxide (NO) may itself have a vasodilator therapeutic role when administered by inhalation. In two patients with ARDS who breathed an O_2/NO (36 ppm) mixture for 30 minutes (32), while mean pulmonary artery pressure decreased selectively and right ventricular ejection fraction ameliorated, gas exchange improved without any deleterious toxicologic effects; cardiac output remained unchanged. By inducing a preferential vasodilatation of alveolar units with well-matched ventilated $\dot{V}_A/\dot{Q}$ ratios, Pao_2 increased and intrapulmonary shunt fell substantially. It is noteworthy that subsequent formation of nitric and nitrous acids, which cause parenchymal damage, may therefore not be a relevant problem clinically, even with lengthy exposure.

Alternatively, the administration of almitrine at a low dosage was associated with a significant improvement in arterial oxygenation without associated changes in cardiac output (Fig. 24.11) (66). The only deleterious effect, though, was a mild but significant increase in the levels of the basal pulmonary hypertension. Almitrine, considered to be a drug that can enhance hypoxic pulmonary vasoconstriction (75), may prove to be of therapeutic usefulness to replace or complement other strategies (PEEP or high Fio_2) in ARDS provided that a low dosage (to avoid undesirable effects), to achieve a sustained beneficial effect on Pao_2, is found. Recently, it has been demonstrated that a low dose of almitrine ameliorates venous admixture in patients with ARDS to the same extent as an external PEEP of 10 cm H_2O (60). However, this benefit needs to be balanced against the unwanted increase in heart afterload that may ensue, hence exacerbating by itself the poor outcome of ARDS. There is recent hopeful evidence that almitrine may induce a sustained improvement in Pao_2 over a period of 48 hours without inflicting impediment on the right ventricular function (65).

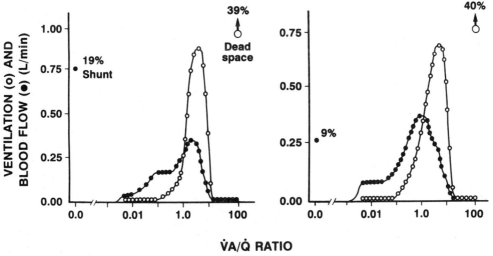

Figure 24.11. A marked reduction in shunt *(closed symbol)* is the major beneficial effect of intravenous almitrine *(right)* on $\dot{V}_A/\dot{Q}$ ratio distributions in patients with ARDS (*left*, baseline conditions). Accordingly, overall gas exchange improves and Pao_2 increases dramatically. (From Reyes A, Roca J, Rodriguez-Roisin R, Torres A, Ussetti P, Wagner PD. Effect of almitrine on ventilation-perfusion distribution in adult respiratory distress syndrome. Am Rev Respir Dis 1988;137:1062–1067.)

In summary, the profile of pulmonary gas exchange abnormalities in ARDS characteristically includes a considerable increase in intrapulmonary shunt; in almost one-half of the patients, this is accompanied by mild to moderate amounts of blood flow distributed to areas of poorly ventilated alveoli, with low $\dot{V}_A/\dot{Q}$ units. These are the principal intrapulmonary determinants of the severe refractory hypoxemia seen in patients with ARDS. Likewise, occasional areas of high $\dot{V}_A/\dot{Q}$ units together with a constantly increased dead space are shown, particularly when external PEEP is applied. Alternatively, diffusion disequilibrium for O_2, as an additional cause of hypoxemia, has been ruled out using the MIGET. There is growing evidence that the improvement (reduction) in intrapulmonary shunt following the application of external PEEP is related more to the increased lung volume (functional residual capacity), due to the recruitment of closed airways and alveoli, than to the fall in cardiac output.

The effects on gas exchange of vasoactive drugs seem to be consistently similar. Overall, vasodilating drugs worsen pulmonary gas exchange (they increase shunt and reduce Pa_{O_2}), whereas vasoconstrictors improve it (they decrease shunt and increase Pa_{O_2}). From a clinical standpoint, the titration of cardiac output using conventional therapeutic strategies, either mechanically (by applying PEEP) or pharmacologically (by infusing vasodilators), induces a well-known, but poorly explained, linear association between cardiac output and shunt. In brief, the analysis of the interplay between intrapulmonary factors (i.e., shunt) and extrapulmonary factors (i.e., cardiac output), which ultimately modulate arterial blood gases, appears to be the most complete approach to appropriately interpret gas exchange abnormalities in ARDS patients, thereby optimizing their clinical management.

SEVERE BACTERIAL PNEUMONIA

In patients with severe bacterial pneumonia and acute respiratory failure who need mechanical support, arterial hypoxemia is determined by the presence of a substantial shunt together with moderate to severe amounts of blood flow diverted to low $\dot{V}_A/\dot{Q}$ units (35, 65). Accordingly, the pattern of the $\dot{V}_A/\dot{Q}$ ratio distributions displays a bimodal profile in the blood flow distribution (Fig. 24.12). Dead space is slightly augmented (35, 46) and, in a few patients, there are mild high $\dot{V}_A/\dot{Q}$ peaks (35). These gas exchange abnormalities essentially concur with those reported experimentally (38, 87), in which intrapul-

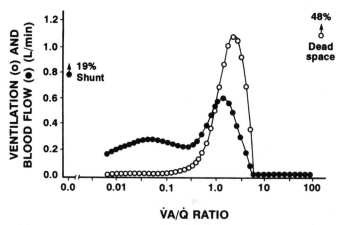

Figure 24.12. Typical bimodal blood flow distribution with a considerable amount of shunt *(closed symbol)* corresponding to a patient with severe bacterial pneumonia requiring artificial ventilation. Dead space is slightly increased *(open symbol)*, probably because of the application of PEEP. (From Gea J, Roca J, Torres A, Agusti AGN, Wagner PD, Rodriguez-Roisin R. Mechanisms of gas exchange in patients with pneumonia. Anesthesiology 1991;75:782–789.)

monary shunt is the principal determinant of hypoxemia in the early phase of the disease; thereafter, during recovery, shunt diminishes and areas with low $\dot{V}_A/\dot{Q}$ units become more marked. Likewise, they are in keeping with the underlying major pathologic findings, namely areas of consolidation with alveoli completely or partially filled with edema, leukocytes and other cells, causative bacteria, and fibrin. The discrete high $\dot{V}_A/\dot{Q}$ mode and the increased dead space may be due to the application of PEEP. The close correlation between predicted Pao_2 and measured Pao_2 is a further point of interest, in that it suggests that additional intrapulmonary factors (diffusion disequilibrium to O_2, increased intrapulmonary O_2 uptake, and postpulmonary shunt) other than intrapulmonary shunt and $\dot{V}_A/\dot{Q}$ mismatch governing hypoxemia can be ruled out (35). Both increased intrapulmonary O_2 consumption in an experimental setting (52) and postpulmonary shunt (i.e., increased bronchial circulation) in humans (3) had been suggested previously as an additional mechanism contributing to hypoxemia.

Interestingly, breathing 100% O_2 demonstrates no changes in inert gas shunt or in venous admixture (35), as might be expected in patients whose lungs include abundant critical alveolar units that are at risk of collapse, thereby developing reabsorption atelectasis. This is consistent with the findings shown in patients with acute respiratory failure (not ARDS) who need mechanical ventilation (48), but at variance with the study that is currently being investigated in patients with ARDS who do increase shunt. Besides, there is further $\dot{V}_A/\dot{Q}$ deterioration, as assessed by the simultaneous marked increase in the blood flow dispersion, strongly suggesting that hypoxic pulmonary vasoconstriction is ablated. This finding indicates a considerable hypoxic vascular response of the lung, which may likely play a protective role against further worsening in pulmonary gas exchange.

In contrast to patients with ARDS, another characteristic finding in one of the studies was that, regardless of the Fio_2, inert gas shunt was always less than venous admixture (35). Likewise, no differences were found between venous admixture and the sum of the inert gas shunt and the areas with low $\dot{V}_A/\dot{Q}$ ratio alveolar units. At maintenance Fio_2, this is explained because both the inert gas shunt and the low $\dot{V}_A/\dot{Q}$ areas are included in the conventional measurement of venous admixture $(\dot{Q}_S/\dot{Q}_T)$. During 100% O_2 breathing, however, this is an unexpected finding since it is traditionally accepted that nitrogen washout abolishes all those alveolar units with poorly ventilated $\dot{V}_A/\dot{Q}$ ratios. Although the precise mechanism for these differences still needs to be elucidated, the release of hypoxic vasoconstriction while breathing 100% O_2 both in the pulmonary and in the bronchial circulations, resulting in an increased perfusion to areas with low $\dot{V}_A/\dot{Q}$ units, could be an alternative explanation.

The intravenous administration of acetylsalicylic acid (ASA) in a preliminary study made of patients with severe pneumonia improved overall $\dot{V}_A/\dot{Q}$ mismatching (34), probably derecruiting blood flow from unventilated and poorly ventilated areas to regions with normal $\dot{V}_A/\dot{Q}$ units. These findings are in keeping with a former experimental study of pneumonia following the administration of ASA (51), which supports the hypothesis that a vasodilator prostaglandin is likely involved in maintaining blood flow to consolidated areas of the lung.

CHRONIC OBSTRUCTIVE PULMONARY DISEASE (COPD)

The profiles of the distributions of $\dot{V}_A/\dot{Q}$ relationships in COPD with acute respiratory failure are qualitatively similar to those found in advanced disease under stable clinical conditions, but quantitatively worse than in patients with less severe disease (24, 84). Figure 24.13 is a representation of $\dot{V}_A/\dot{Q}$ ratio distributions in a patient with COPD requiring mechanical ventilation. As shown, the patterns of blood flow and of ventilation distributions are bimodal. In other patients, however, there is a bimodal profile of each distribution alone. Intrapulmonary shunt is discrete and dead space is, for the most part,

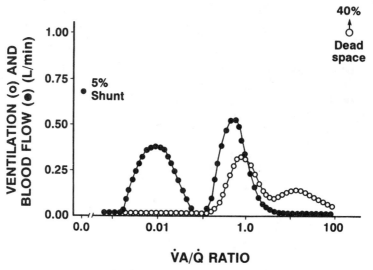

Figure 24.13. "Low" and "high" $\dot{V}_A/\dot{Q}$ ratio patterns in a patient with advanced COPD and acute respiratory failure needing mechanical support. Note that both shunt *(closed symbol)* and dead space *(open symbol)* are modestly increased.

slightly increased. Thus, gas exchange behavior in acute respiratory failure due to COPD may mimic the full spectrum of patterns of $\dot{V}_A/\dot{Q}$ inequality originally described by Wagner et al. (86). The "low" $\dot{V}_A/\dot{Q}$ profile corresponds to lung areas with a considerable proportion of blood flow diverted to low $\dot{V}_A/\dot{Q}$ alveolar units, most likely representing regions in which airways are narrowed by secretions, bronchial wall hypertrophy, bronchoconstriction, or distortion. Alternatively, the "high" $\dot{V}_A/\dot{Q}$ pattern, which indicates that a percentage of the alveolar ventilation is distributed to lung areas with poorly perfused $\dot{V}_A/\dot{Q}$ units, most likely reflects emphysematous lung areas in which alveolar destruction with loss of the pulmonary vasculature is the predominant morphologic finding.

In patients with mild COPD, however, it has been shown that, while both small airway abnormalities and pulmonary emphysema contribute to the degree of $\dot{V}_A/\dot{Q}$ mismatching, pulmonary emphysema emerges as the major morphologic correlate of abnormal arterial blood respiratory gases (9). Further, a significant correlation between a low hypoxic vascular response and the severity of wall thickening in pulmonary arteries and, also, the degree of

small airway inflammation has been found in early COPD (10). Despite the fact that COPD patients have frequently retained secretions and abundant mucus plugging, particularly during acute exacerbations, the amount of intrapulmonary shunt is usually modest (overall, below 10% of the blood flow) (37). It may be that collateral ventilation plays an important role in preventing collapse of alveoli beyond the occluded peripheral airways. Although a small component of diffusion limitation to O_2 has been assessed in stable COPD patients without accompanying respiratory failure (1), its influence, as an additional cause of hypoxemia seems to be almost negligible. Likewise, patients with COPD show a substantial hypoxic vascular response as assessed by a further worsening in $\dot{V}_A/\dot{Q}$ mismatch while breathing 100% O_2: blood flow distribution increases (deteriorates), suggesting release of hypoxic pulmonary vasoconstriction (84). In contrast, shunt remains unaltered.

It is noteworthy that the combined influence of changes in breathing pattern and in cardiac output on $\dot{V}_A/\dot{Q}$ relationships, during routine successful weaning, further deteriorates pulmonary gas exchange (84). After cessation of mechanical support, COPD patients develop rapid and shallow breathing while cardiac output increases dramatically (venous return rises abruptly). As a result, $Paco_2$ increases and pH decreases, yet Pao_2 remains constant. The interaction between intrapulmonary ($\dot{V}_A/\dot{Q}$ mismatch) and extrapulmonary (ventilation and cardiac output) determinants of gas exchange results in an unaltered Pao_2. Under these circumstances, an increased O_2 uptake, usually seen during weaning in COPD (4, 43), may further aggravate pulmonary oxygenation. Perhaps the expected rise in $P\bar{v}o_2$ following the inordinately high cardiac output may be sufficient to offset the simultaneous fall in Pao_2 due to further $\dot{V}_A/\dot{Q}$ worsening. If, however, patients fail to be successfully weaned from the ventilator, O_2 consumption dramatically increases and Pao_2 may ultimately fall, as shown in patients with a critical myocardial function (49).

The oral administration of almitrine during weaning (18) considerably improves the matching of pulmonary blood flow and alveolar ventilation, thereby ameliorating arterial blood gas abnormalities. It is hypothesized, thus, that almitrine causes a redistribution of blood flow from alveoli with poorly ventilated $\dot{V}_A/\dot{Q}$ units to those with normal $\dot{V}_A/\dot{Q}$ ratios. It would be of interest, however, to investigate the effects on $\dot{V}_A/\dot{Q}$ relationships and overall pulmonary gas exchange following the administration of the most common β_2-agonist bronchodilators in COPD patients with acute respiratory failure, just as it has been assessed in patients with stable clinical conditions (72). It is hoped that these clinical advances will help clinicians to maximize the efficiency of therapeutic strategy during acute exacerbations in these patients and have an impact on future treatment.

ACUTE SEVERE ASTHMA (STATUS ASTHMATICUS)

Patients with acute severe asthma who require mechanical ventilation develop the most abnormal gas exchange abnormalities of the $\dot{V}_A/\dot{Q}$ spectrum of bronchial asthma, but have essentially the same profile as patients with less severe disease (Fig. 24.14) (69). At maintenance F_{IO_2}, the baseline pattern of mismatch of blood flow and ventilation is characterized by a con-

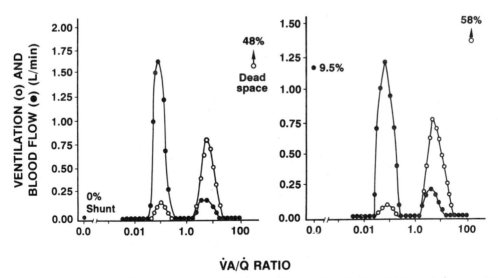

Figure 24.14. Patient with acute severe asthma requiring mechanical ventilation. *Left*, at maintenance F_{IO_2}, there is marked bimodal blood flow $\dot{V}_A/\dot{Q}$ ratio distribution with a slightly increased dead space *(open symbols)*, but no shunt *(closed symbol)*. *Right*, while breathing 100% O_2, there is moderate shunt and broadening of the blood flow distribution, suggesting further $\dot{V}_A/\dot{Q}$ worsening. See text for details. (From, in part, Rodriguez-Roisin R, Ballester E, Roca J, Torres A, Wagner PD. Mechanisms of hypoxemia in patients with status asthmaticus requiring mechanical ventilation. Am Rev Respir Dis 1989;139:732–739.)

siderable bimodal blood flow distribution without intrapulmonary shunt. In contrast, the distribution of alveolar ventilation is never bimodal and dead space is within normal range (or slightly increased due to the application of mechanical ventilation). Arterial Po_2 and the amount of $\dot{V}_A/\dot{Q}$ inequality are not closely related, probably because of the influence of some extrapulmonary factors, such as inspired Po_2, minute ventilation, and cardiac output, in addition to $\dot{V}_A/\dot{Q}$ mismatching. However, the coexistence of diffusion limitation to O_2, as a complementary mechanism of hypoxemia, has been ruled out because of the lack of systematic differences between predicted Pao_2 and measured Pao_2 (69).

Although these gas exchange findings are consistent with the most common $\dot{V}_A/\dot{Q}$ abnormalities seen in patients with less severe asthma (67, 88), they are partly at variance with postmortem studies (41), which invariably show diffuse mucosal wall edema and abundant gross, tenacious, mucus plugging in the airway together with considerable airway narrowing. One could hypothesize, therefore, that patients who suffer from the most life-threatening clinical form of asthma may show marked intrapulmonary shunt due to massive mucus impaction. Likewise, it could be reasoned that these patients may have considerable air trapping and hyperinflation, causing high intraalveolar pressures by check-valve mechanisms. Accordingly, this would partly or completely reduce perfusion in such lung areas, hence developing regions of high $\dot{V}_A/\dot{Q}$ units or increased dead space, respectively. Nevertheless, both shunt and high $\dot{V}_A/\dot{Q}$ peaks were conspicuously negligible and dead space was essentially within normal limits. Widespread airway obstruction with peripheral airway narrowing, along with an efficient collateral ventilation thus precluding alveolar occlusion beyond the obstructed airways, appears to be the most likely explanation for the presence of a marked bimodal blood flow profile without shunt in patients with status asthmaticus. Alternatively, the very little shunt may also suggest that hypoxic vasoconstriction is highly efficient, or that massive

mucus plugging is functionally incomplete, or both.

Interestingly, breathing 100% O_2 induces in these patients moderate amounts of shunt (mean, 0–9% of cardiac output), which suggests either the presence of critical alveolar units that lead to reabsorption atelectasis (29) or redistribution of pulmonary perfusion of preexisting small shunts (Fig. 24.14). Besides, $\dot{V}_A/\dot{Q}$ mismatch is substantially deteriorated (as assessed by the increase in the dispersion of pulmonary blood flow), suggesting release of hypoxic pulmonary vasoconstriction. Both findings are, nevertheless, consistent with a recent morphologic postmortem study in sudden fatal asthma (78), in which the muscular pulmonary arteries adjacent to occluded peripheral bronchioles showed a marked inflammatory wall involvement not consistent with features of chronic hypoxia. It may be that these structural abnormalities reflect microvascular leakage (increased permeability) within the airway induced by the release of potent inflammatory mediators.

Acknowledgment. This work was supported by Grant 91/0290 from the Fondo de Investigación Sanitaria (FIS), Madrid Spain.

References

1. Agustí AGN, Barberà JA, Roca J, Wagner PD, Guitart R, Rodriguez-Roisin R. Hypoxic pulmonary vasoconstriction and gas exchange in chronic obstructive pulmonary disease. Chest 1990;97:268–275.
2. Augustí AGN, Roca J, Gea J, Wagner PD, Xaubet A, Rodriguez-Roisin R. Mechanisms of gas-exchange impairment in idiopathic pulmonary fibrosis. Am Rev Respir Dis 1990;143:219–225.
3. Alexander JK, Takewaza H, Abu-Nassar HJ, York EM. Studies on pulmonary blood flow in pneumococcal pneumonia. Cardiovasc Res Cent Bull 1963;1:86–92.
4. Annat G, Viale JP, Dereymez CP, Bouffard YM, Delafosse BX, Motin JP. Oxygen cost of breathing and diaphragmatic pressure-time index. Measurement in patients with COPD during weaning with pressure support ventilation. Chest 1990;98:411–414.
5. Ashbaugh DG, Bigelow DB, Petty TL, et al. Acute respiratory distress in adults. Lancet 1967;2:319–323.
6. Astin TW. The relationships between arterial blood oxygen saturation, carbon dioxide tension, and pH and airway resistance during 30 percent oxygen breathing in patients with chronic obstruc-

tive pulmonary disease. Am Rev Respir Dis 1970;102:382–387.

7. Bachofen M, Weibel ER. Alterations of the gas exchange apparatus in adult respiratory distress syndrome. Am Rev Respir Dis 1977;116:267–284.

8. Bachofen M, Weibel ER. Sequential morphologic changes in the adult respiratory syndrome. In: Fishman AP, ed. Pulmonary diseases and disorders. New York: McGraw Hill Book Co, 1988:2215–2222.

9. Barberà JA, Ramirez J, Roca J, Wagner PD, Sánchez-Lloret J, Rodriguez-Roisin R. Lung structure and gas exchange in mild chronic obstructive pulmonary disease. Am Rev Respir Dis 1990;141:895–901.

10. Barberà JA, Riverola A, Ramirez J, et al. Pulmonary vascular structure and ventilation-perfusion relationships in patients with mild COPD (abstract). Eur Respir J 1991;3(suppl 10):184S.

11. Bishop MJ, Cheney FW. Vasodilators worsen gas exchange in dog oleic-acid lung injury. Anesthesiology 1986;64:435–439.

12. Bishop MJ, Huang T, Cheney FW. Effect of vasodilator treatment on the resolution of oleic acid pulmonary edema. Am Rev Respir Dis 1985;131:421–425.

13. Breen PH, Schumacker PT, Hedenstierna G, Ali J, Wagner PD, Wood LDH. How does increased cardiac output increase shunt in pulmonary edema? J Appl Physiol 1982;53:1273–1280.

14. Brigham KL, Kariman K, Harris T, Snapper JR, Bernard GR, Young SL. Correlation of oxygenation with vascular permeability surface area but not with lung water in humans with acute respiratory failure and pulmonary edema. J Clin Invest 1983;72:339–348.

15. Briscoe WA, Cree EM, Filler J, Houssay HEJ, Cournand A. Lung volume, alveolar ventilation and perfusion interrelationships in chronic pulmonary emphysema. J Appl Physiol 1960;15:785–795.

16. Broseghini C, Brandolese R, Poggi R, Bernasconi M, Manzin E, Rossi A. Respiratory resistance and intrinsic positive end-expiratory pressure (PEEP) in patients with the adult respiratory distress syndrome (ARDS). Eur Respir J 1988;1:726–731.

17. Caldini P, Leith D, Brennen M. Effects of continuous positive pressure ventilation on edema formation in dog lung. J Appl Physiol 1975;40:568–574.

18. Castaing Y, Manier G, Guénard H. Improvement in ventilation-perfusion relationships by almitrine in patients with chronic obstructive pulmonary disease during mechanical ventilation. Am Rev Respir Dis 1986;134:910–916.

19. Coffey RL, Albert RK, Robertson HT. Mechanism of physiological dead space response to PEEP after acute oleic acid lung injury. J Appl Physiol: Respirat Environ Exercise Physiol 1983;55:1550–1557.

20. Colley PS, Cheney FW, Hlastala MP. Ventilation-perfusion and gas exchange effects of sodium nitroprusside in dogs with normal and edematous lungs. Anesthesiology 1979;50:489–495.

21. Danek SJ, Lynch JP, Weg JG, Dantzker DR. The dependence of oxygen uptake on oxygen delivery in the adult respiratory distress syndrome. Am Rev Respir Dis 1980;122:387–398.

22. Dantzker DR. Gas exchange in the adult respiratory distress syndrome. Clin Chest Med. 1982;3:57–67.

23. Dantzker DR. The influence of cardiovascular function on gas exchange. Clin Chest Med 1983;4:149–159.

24. Dantzker DR. Gas exchange. In: Montenegro HD, ed. Chronic obstructive pulmonary disease. Edinburgh: Churchill Livingstone, 1984:141–160.

25. Dantzker DR, Bower JS. Pulmonary vascular tone improves $\dot{V}_A/\dot{Q}$ matching in obliterative pulmonary hypertension. J Appl Physiol 1981;51:607–613.

26. Dantzker DR, Brook CJ, Dehart P, Lynch JP, Weg JG. Ventilation-perfusion distributions in the adult respiratory distress syndrome. Am Rev Respir Dis 1979;120:1039–1052.

27. Dantzker DR, Foresman B, Gutierrez G. Oxygen supply and utilization relationships. A reevaluation. Am Rev Respir Dis 1991;143:675–679.

28. Dantzker DR, Lynch JP, Weg JG. Depression of cardiac output is a mechanism of shunt reduction in the therapy of acute respiratory failure. Chest 1980;77:636–642.

29. Dantzker DR, Wagner PD, West JB. Instability of lung units with low $\dot{V}_A/\dot{Q}$ ratios during O_2 breathing. J Appl Physiol 1975;38:886–895.

30. Dueck R, Wagner PD, West JB. Effects of PEEP on gas exchange in dogs with normal and edematous lungs. Anesthesiology 1977;47:359–366.

31. Evans JW, Wagner PD. Limits on $\dot{V}_A/\dot{Q}$ distributions from analysis of experimental inert gas elimination. J Appl Physiol 1977;42:889–898.

32. Falke K. Rossaint R, Pison U, et al. Inhaled nitric oxide selectively reduces pulmonary hypertension in severe ARDS and improves gas exchange as well as right heart ejection fraction (abstract). Am Rev Respir Dis 1991;143(suppl):A248.

33. Flick MR. Pulmonary edema and acute lung injury. In: Murray JF, Nadel JA, eds. Textbook of respiratory medicine. Philadelphia: WB Saunders Co, 1988:1359–1409.

34. Gea J, Agustí AGN, Rodriguez-Roisin R, Roca J, Wagner PD, Agustí-Vidal A. Effects of aspirin on gas exchange in human pneumonia (abstract). Eur Respir J 1988;1:282.

35. Gea J, Roca J, Torres A, Agustí AGN, Wagner PD, Rodriguez-Roisin R. Mechanisms of gas exchange in patients with pneumonia. Anesthesiology 1991;75:782–789.

36. Gerdeaux M, Lemaire F, Matamis D, Lampron N, Teisseire B, Becker J, Harf A. Syndrome de détresse respiratoire aiguë de l'adulte. Distribution des rapports ventilation/perfusion. Presse Méd 1984;13:1315–1318.

37. Glauser FL, Pollaty RC, Sessler CN. Worsening oxygenation in the mechanically ventilated patient. Causes, mechanisms, and early detection. Am Rev Respir Dis 1988;138:458–465.

38. Goldzimer EL, Wagner PD, Moser KM. Sequence of ventilation/perfusion alterations during experimental pneumococcal pneumonia in the dog. Chest 1973;64:394–395.

39. Greene R, Zapol W, Snider MT, et al. Early bedside detection of pulmonary vascular occlusion during acute respiratory failure. Am Rev Respir Dis 1981;124:593–601.

40. Hedenstierna G, White FC, Mazzone RB, Wagner PD. Redistribution of pulmonary blood flow in the dog with PEEP ventilation. J Appl Physiol 1979;46:278–287.

41. Hogg JC. Varieties of airway narrowing in severe fatal asthma. J Allergy Clin Immunol 1987;80(suppl part 2):417–419.

42. Hopewell PC, Murray JF. Effects of continuous positive-pressure ventilation in experimental pulmonary edema. J Appl Physiol 1975;39:672–679.

43. Hubmayr RD, Loosbrock LM, Gillespie DJ, Rodarte JR. Oxygen uptake during weaning from mechanical ventilation. Chest 1988;94:1148–1155.

44. Ketty S. The theory and applications of the exchange of inert gas at the lungs and tissues. Pharmacol Rev 1951;3:1–41.

45. King TKC, Weber B, Okinaka A, Friedman SA, Smith JP, Briscoe WA. Oxygen transfer in catastrophic respiratory failure. Chest 1974;65:405–425.

46. Lampron N, Lemaire F, Teisseire B, et al. Mechanical ventilation with 100% oxygen does not increase intrapulmonary shunt in patients with severe bacterial pneumomia. Am Rev Respir Dis 1985;131:409–413.

47. Lamy M, Fallat RJ, Koeniger E, et al. Pathologic features and mechanisms of hypoxemia in ARDS. Am Rev Respir Dis 1976;114:267–284.

48. Lemaire F, Matamis D, Lampron N, Teisseire B, Harf A. Intrapulmonary shunt is not increased by 100% oxygen ventilation in acute respiratory failure. Bull Eur Physiopathol Respir 1985;21:251–256.

49. Lemaire F, Teboul JL, Cinotti L, et al. Acute left ventricular dysfunction during unsuccessful weaning from mechanical ventilation. Anesthesiology 1988;69:171–179.

50. Lemaire F, Teisseire B, Harf A. Oxygen exchange across the acutely injured lung. In: Zapol WM, Falke KJ, eds. Acute respiratory failure. Vol 24. New York: Marcel Dekker, 1985:521–553.

51. Light RB. Indomethacin and acetylsalicylic acid reduce intrapulmonary shunt in experimental pneumococcal pneumonia. Am Rev Respir Dis 1986;134:520–525.

52. Light RB. Intrapulmonary oxygen consumption in experimental pneumococcal pneumonia. J Appl Physiol 1988;64:2490–2495.

53. Lynch JP, Mhyre JG, Dantzker DR. Influence of cardiac output on intrapulmonary shunt. J Appl Physiol 1979;46:315–321.

54. Matamis D, Lemaire F, Harf A, Teisseire B, Brun-Buisson C. Redistribution of pulmonary blood flow induced by positive end-expiratory pressure and dopamine infusion in acute respiratory failure. Am Rev Respir Dis 1984;129:39–44.

55. Mélot C, Naeije R, Mols P, Hallemans R, Lejeune P, Jaspar N. Pulmonary vascular tone improves pulmonary gas exchange in the adult respiratory distress syndrome. Am Rev Respir Dis 1987;136:1232–1236.

55. Mélot C, Lejeune P, Leeman M, Moraine JJ, Naeije R. Prostaglandin E_1 in the adult respiratory distress syndrome. Am Rev Respir Dis 1989;139:106–110.

57. Murray JF, Matthay MA, Luce JM, Flick MR. An expanded definition of the adult respiratory distress syndrome. Am Rev Respir Dis 1988;138:720–723.

58. Payen DM, Carli PA, Brun-Buisson CJL, et al. Lower body positive pressure vs. dopamine during PEEP in humans. J Appl Physiol 1985;58:77–82.

59. Pepe PP, Marini JJ. Occult positive end-expiratory pressure in mechanically ventilated patients with airflow obstruction. Am Rev Respir Dis 1982;126:166–170.

60. Prost JF, Desché P, Jardin F, Margairaz A. Comparison of the effects of intravenous almitrine and positive end-expiratory pressure on pulmonary gas exchange in adult respiratory distress syndrome. Eur Respir J 1991;4:683–687.

61. Radermacher P, Huet Y, Pluskwa F, et al. Comparison of ketanserin and sodium nitroprusside in patients with severe ARDS. Anesthesiology 1988;68:152–157.

62. Radermacher P, Santak B, Becker H, Falke KJ. Prostaglandin E_1 and nitroglycerin reduce pulmonary capillary pressure but worsen ventilation-perfusion distributions in patients with adult respiratory distress syndrome. Anesthesiology 1989;70:601–606.

63. Radermacher P, Santak B, Wüst HJ, Tarnow J, Falke KJ. Prostacyclin for the treatment of pulmonary hypertension in the adult respiratory distress syndrome: effects on pulmonary capillary pressure and ventilation-perfusion distributions. Anesthesiology 1990;72:238–244.

64. Ralph DD, Robertson HT, Weaver LJ, Hlastala MP, Carrico CJ, Hudson LD. Distribution of ventilation and perfusion during positive end-expiratory pressure in the adult respiratory distress syndrome. Am Rev Respir Dis 1985;131:54–60.

65. Rekik N, Plaisance P, Brun-Buisson C, Lemaire F. Almitrine infusion improves PaO_2 without deleterious effects on RV function in ARDS patients (abstract). Am Rev Respir Dis 1990;141:A487.

66. Reyes A, Roca J, Rodriguez-Roisin R, Torres A, Ussetti P, Wagner PD. Effect of almitrine on ventilation-perfusion distribution in adult respiratory distress syndrome. Am Rev Respir Dis 1988;137:1062–1067.

67. Roca J, Ramis LI, Rodriguez-Roisin R, Ballester E, Montserrat JM, Wagner PD. Serial relationships between $\dot{V}_A/\dot{Q}$ inequality and spirometry in acute severe asthma requiring hospitalization. Am Rev Respir Dis 1988;137:605–612.

68. Rochester DF. Respiratory muscle weakness, pattern of breathing, and CO_2 retention in chronic obstructive pulmonary disease. Am Rev Respir Dis 1991;143:901–903.

69. Rodriguez-Roisin R, Ballester E, Roca J, Torres A, Wagner PD. Mechanisms of hypoxemia in patients with status asthmaticus requiring mechanical ventilation. Am Rev Respir Dis 1989:139;732–739.

70. Rodriguez-Roisin R, Roca J. Advances in pulmonary gas exchange: update on inert gas studies in adult respiratory distress syndrome (ARDS). Appl Cardiopulm Pathophysiol 1991;3:295–305.
71. Rodriguez-Roisin R, Roca J, Agustí AGN, Mastai R, Wagner PD, Bosch J. Pulmonary vascular reactivity in patients with liver cirrhosis. Am Rev Respir Dis 1987;135:1085–1092.
72. Rodriguez-Roisin R, Roca J, Barberà JA. Intrapulmonary and extrapulmonary determinants of pulmonary gas exchange. In: Marini JJ, Roussos C, eds. Ventilatory failure. Berlin: Springer-Verlag, 1991:18–36
73. Rodriguez-Roisin R, Rossi A. Assessment of lung function in the critically ill patient. Clin Intensive Care 1991;2:97–103.
74. Rodriguez-Roisin R, Wagner PD. Clinical relevance of ventilation-perfusion inequality determined by inert gas elimination. Eur Respir J 1989;3:469–482.
75. Romaldini H, Rodriguez-Roisin R, Wagner PD, West JB. Enhancement of hypoxic pulmonary vasoconstriction by almitrine in the dog. Am Rev Respir Dis 1983;128:288–293.
76. Rossi A, Gottfried SB, Higgs BD, et al. Respiratory mechanics in mechanically ventilated patients. J Appl Physiol 1985;59:1849–1858.
77. Roussos C, Macklem PT. The respiratory muscles. N Engl J Med 1982;307:785–797.
78. Saetta M, Di Stefano A, Rosina C, Thiene G, Fabbri LM. Quantitative structural analysis of peripheral airways and arteries in sudden fatal asthma. Am Rev Respir Dis 1991;143:138–143.
79. Schoene RB, Robertson HT, Thorning DR, Springmeyer SC, Hlastala MP, Cheney FW. Pathophysiological patterns of resolution from acute oleic acid lung injury in the dog. J Appl Physiol: Respirat Environ Exercise Physiol 1984;56:472–481.
80. Staub NC, Nagano H, Pearce ML. Pulmonary edema in dogs, especially the sequence of fluid accumulation in lungs. J Appl Physiol 1967;38:886–895.
81. Suter PM, Fairley HB, Isenberg MA. Optimum end-expiratory airway pressure in patients with acute pulmonary failure. N Engl J Med 1975;292:284–289.
82. Suter PM, Fairley HB, Schlobohm RM. Shunt, lung volume and perfusion during short periods of ventilation with oxygen. Anesthesiology 1975;43:617–627.
83. Torre-Bueno J, Wagner PD, Saltzman GR, Gale GE, Moon RE. Diffusion limitation in normal humans during exercise at sea level and simulated altitude. J Appl Physiol 1985;58:989–995.
84. Torres A, Reyes A, Roca J, Wagner PD, Rodriguez-Roisin R. Ventilation-perfusion mismatching in chronic obstructive pulmonary disease during ventilator weaning. Am Rev Respir Dis 1989;14;1246–1250.
85. Wagner PD. Ventilation-perfusion inequality in catastrophic lung disease. In: Prakash O, ed. Applied physiology in clinical respiratory care. The Hague: Martinus Nijhoff, 1982:363–379.
86. Wagner PD, Dantzker DR, Dueck R, Clausen JL, West JB. Ventilation-perfusion inequality in chronic obstructive pulmonary disease. J Clin Invest 1977;59:203–216.
87. Wagner, PD, Dantzker DR, Dueck R, Uhl RR, Virgilio R, West JB. Continuous distributions of ventilation-perfusion ratios in acute and chronic lung disease (abstract). Clin Res 1974;22:134A.
88. Wagner PD, Dantzker DR, Iacovoni VE, Tomlin WC, West JB. Ventilation-perfusion inequality in asymptomatic asthma. Am Rev Respir Dis 1978;118:511–524.
89. Wagner PD, Laravuso RB, Goldzimer EL, Naumann PF, West JB. Distribution of ventilation-perfusion ratios in dogs with normal and abnormal lungs. J Appl Physiol 1975;38:1099–1109.
90. Wagner PD, Naumann PF, Laravuso RB. Simultaneous measurement of eight foreign gases in blood by gas chromatography. J Appl Physiol 1974;36:600–605.
91. Wagner PD, Rodriguez-Roisin R. Clinical advances in pulmonary gas exchange. Am Rev Respir Dis 1991;143:883–888.
92. Wagner PD, Saltzman HA, West JB. Measurements of continuous distributions of ventilation-perfusion ratios: theory. J Appl Physiol 1974;36:588–589.
93. Wagner PD, West JB. Ventilation-perfusion relationships. In West JB, ed. Pulmonary gas exchange. Ventilation, blood flow and diffusion. Volume I. New York: Academic Press, 1980:219–262.
94. Weigelt JA, Gewetz BL, Aurbaken CM, Snyder WH. Pharmacologic alterations in pulmonary artery pressure in the adult respiratory syndrome. J Surg Res 1982;32:243–248.
95. Weimberger SE, Schwartzstein RM, Weiss JW. Hypercapnia. N Engl J Med 1989;321:1223–1231.
96. West JB. Ventilation-perfusion inequality and overall gas exchange in computer lung models of the lung. Respir Physiol 1969;7:88–110.
97. West JB. Effect of slope and shape of dissociation of dissociation curve on pulmonary gas exchange. Respir Physiol 1969–70;8:66–85.
98. West JB. Causes of carbon dioxide retention in lung disease. N Engl J Med 1971;284;1232–1236.
99. West JB. Ventilation-perfusion relationships. Am Rev Respir Dis 1977;116:919–943.
100. Wright PE, Bernard GR. The role of airflow resistance in patients with the adult respiratory distress syndrome. Am Rev Respir Dis 1989;139:1169–1174.
101. Zapol WM, Snider MT, Rie MA, Frikker M, Quinn DA. Pulmonary circulation during adult respiratory distress syndrome. In: Zapol WM, Falke KJ, eds. Acute respiratory failure. Vol 24. New York: Marcel Dekker, 1985:241–273.

25

Acute Hypoxemic Respiratory Failure

Deborah J. Cook
Thomas A. Raffin

Acute hypoxemic respiratory failure may be caused by a variety of underlying conditions, such as pneumonia, congestive heart failure, pulmonary embolus, or the adult respiratory distress syndrome (ARDS). The remainder of this chapter will focus on the etiology, pathophysiology, and clinical characteristics of ARDS. This will serve as the conceptual framework for the management of acute hypoxemic respiratory failure.

Adult respiratory distress syndrome is a condition characterized by severe hypoxemia and acute, diffuse lung infiltrates of diverse etiology. Adult respiratory distress syndrome affects an estimated 150,000–200,000 Americans each year, most often those with no prior lung disease. Acute hypoxemic respiratory failure has an associated mortality rate of 65% (40). Despite the diverse causes of ARDS, the clinical characteristics, respiratory pathophysiology, and management of these conditions are remarkably similar.

Adult respiratory distress syndrome is caused by a diffuse lung injury that leads to a capillary leak syndrome and an increase in extravascular lung water. This syndrome has also been labeled shock lung, respirator lung, postcardiopulmonary bypass syndrome, capillary leak syndrome, and normal pressure pulmonary edema. Although there are several clinical and pathologic similarities between the adult and the infant respiratory distress syndrome, there are important differences. In the neonate, the hallmarks of the respiratory distress syndrome are immature alveolar surfactant production and a highly compliant chest wall. However, in adults, the surfactant changes represent the final common pathway of a number of sources of pulmonary injury, and the chest wall is not compliant.

ETIOLOGY

A number of conditions are associated with the development of acute hypoxemic respiratory failure (Table 25.1). Aspiration of gastric contents is one of the most common predisposing factors, with ARDS occurring in up to 35% of patients with witnessed pulmonary aspiration (11), particularly when the aspirate has a pH of less than 2.5 (55). Pulmonary and systemic infections (whether bacterial, viral, fungal, or protozoal) are all associated with the development of ARDS. Gram-negative septic shock appears to be an important risk factor, and has an associated mortality rate of 90%.

Although all forms of circulatory shock have been associated with ARDS, there have been no studies evaluating the independent contribution to risk of any one factor. Patients with hemorrhagic shock, for example, may have also sustained trauma and received multiple transfusions; it is therefore difficult to isolate hemorrhagic shock as an independent major risk factor for ARDS.

Inhalation of smoke and toxic gases can also cause ARDS. High concentrations of oxygen are toxic to the alveolar capillary membrane. Oxygen-free radicals (O_2^-, OH) and H_2O_2 are thought to be responsible.

Table 25.1
Conditions Associated with ARDS

Infection
    Bacterial/viral/fungal pneumonia
    Septic shock
Trauma
    Lung contusion
    Head injury
    Fractures/fat emboli
    Burns
    Near drowning
Shock
    Septic
    Cardiogenic
    Anaphylactic
    Hemorrhagic
Drugs/toxins
    Gastric acid aspiration
    Salicylates
    Thiazides
    Propoxyphene
    Chlordiazepoxides
    Heroin
    Methadone
    Irritant gas inhalation (oxygen, smoke, NO_2, NH_3, Cl_2, paraquat)
Hematologic disorders
    Disseminated intravascular coagulation
    Multiple transfusions
    Leukoagglutination reaction
    Postcardiopulmonary bypass
Miscellaneous
    Air emboli
    Increased intracranial pressure
    Pancreatitis
    Uremia
    Eclampsia
    High altitude
    Radiation

The adult respiratory distress syndrome has been associated with a variety of drug ingestions, most often in cases of overdose. Multiple blood transfusions have also been implicated. Rarely, leukoagglutinins may precipitate ARDS during blood transfusion (52). Disseminated intravascular coagulation has been described by Bone et al. (2) as occurring in 7 of 30 patients with ARDS. Near drowning is also a risk factor for the development of acute hypoxemic respiratory failure. Approximately 90% of near drownings in salt or fresh water involve alveolar flooding and destroy surfac-

tant; in addition, a direct osmotic alveolar injury can occur (32). Age does not seem to be an important predisposing factor to ARDS.

Often, several risk factors are involved, which appear to be additive (11). Pepe and colleagues (36) reported that the incidence of ARDS with one risk factor was 25%, with two risk factors was 42%, and with three risk factors was 85%. Multiple risk factors for ARDS exist in trauma victims, for example. These risk factors may include long bone fractures, fat embolism, pulmonary contusion, head injury, multiple transfusions, and infection.

PATHOPHYSIOLOGY: AN OVERVIEW

The adult respiratory distress syndrome is a form of noncardiogenic pulmonary edema resulting from functional disruption of the capillary-alveolar-epithelial barrier. It is characterized by increased lung water, yet is distinct from cardiogenic pulmonary edema in that pulmonary capillary hydrostatic pressures are not elevated.

The onset of ARDS follows a diffuse injury to the pulmonary capillary bed, either to the alveolar epithelium (as may occur after aspiration of gastric contents), or to the vascular endothelium (as arises from trauma or sepsis). Such injury alters the Starling forces regulating fluid transfer between the capillaries and pulmonary interstitium to favor exudation of protein-rich fluid into the interstitial spaces. In the normal lung, surfactant helps to balance surface forces and prevents alveolar collapse as fluid accumulates in the alveoli. However, in patients with ARDS, surfactant has been shown to be aggregated, oxidized, and nonfunctional. Therefore, the lungs of patients with ARDS show evidence of widespread atelectasis due to flooded and collapsed alveoli.

The early phase progresses to involve type I alveolar cells, which are replaced with proliferating type II cells, thereby creating a cuboidal microvillous metabolically active epithelium. As a result, the alveolar septum becomes thickened and the interstitium becomes infiltrated with mesenchymal and inflammatory cells. Pulmonary fibrosis subsequently develops and progressively obliterates alveoli, alveolar ducts, and capillaries.

MECHANISMS OF ARDS

Currently, the pathogenesis of ARDS is a subject of lively debate, as there are many putative mediators of pulmonary vascular injury. The four main mechanisms of pulmonary capillary endothelial damage are (1) direct lung injury (i.e., aspiration of gastric contents, toxin inhalation), (2) neutrophil injury, (3) arachidonic acid metabolite injury, and (4) coagulation product injury.

That neutrophil aggregation plays a key role in the genesis of acute lung injury has been repeatedly confirmed, both experimentally and clinically (20, 49). Neutrophils and their products have been found in increased numbers in the bronchoalveolar lavage fluid of ARDS patients when compared with controls (26, 30). Histologic studies have identified neutrophils in alveoli in models of acute lung injury (53). However, neutrophils are not the sole mediators of inflammation in ARDS; it can develop in neutropenic patients (35). Therefore, both cellular (neutrophil) and humoral factors are important.

Activation of the complement cascade is common to many diseases leading to ARDS. Hammerschmidt et al. (17) found a strong association between complement activation with ARDS, particularly an elevated plasma C5a. Craddock and colleagues (7) have shown that C5a can attract and aggregate neutrophils and provoke pulmonary dysfunction in animals. Stimulated neutrophils then release a number of toxic products, including oxygen-free radicals, proteases, arachidonic acid metabolites, and platelet-activating factor. Oxygen-free radicals and their intermediates (superoxide anions, hydrogen peroxide, singlet oxygen, and hydroxyl radicals) are thought to increase pulmonary vascular permeability and pulmonary vasoconstriction. In addition, proteases can activate a number of inflammatory pathways, including the Hageman factor and its associated intrinsic coagulation pathway, as well as the kinin system.

A number of arachidonic acid metabolites, notably thromboxane A_2 and prostaglandins E_2, F_2, and H_2, promote pulmonary vasoconstriction. Thromboxanes and leukotrienes have also been implicated in the bronchoconstriction that reduces lung compliance in ARDS. Leukotrienes C_4, D_4, and E_4 induce pulmonary vascular permeability directly, while leukotriene B_4 achieves the same effect indirectly by stimulating enzyme release and superoxide generation in neutrophils (39).

Platelet-activating factor encourages clumping of platelets and neutrophils at the site of injury in ARDS (10). Although platelet aggregation is not necessarily required for the development of ARDS, pulmonary sequestration of platelets can aggravate existing pulmonary hypertension through serotonin release. Other pathways exist for the development of ARDS, including the alveolar macrophage and the direct effects of endotoxin liberated in Gram-negative sepsis (31). The coagulation cascade may also be activated by endotoxemia, Hageman factor, exposure of collagen due to damaged endothelium, or release of proteases. Fibrinogen may interfere with surfactant production in the damaged lung.

Therefore, on the basis of existing data, we can now construct a model outlining the pathogenesis of ARDS (Fig. 25.1).

CLINICAL CHARACTERISTICS
Diagnosis

In the absence of a specific diagnostic test for ARDS, identification rests on a clinical description of the syndrome. Criteria include:

1. History of a pulmonary or nonpulmonary catastrophic event
2. Significant hypoxemia refractory to increased concentrations of inspired oxygen
3. New diffuse pulmonary infiltrates on chest x-ray
4. Pulmonary artery wedge pressure less than 18 mm Hg

The early clinical signs include tachypnea and dyspnea. Arterial blood gas mea-

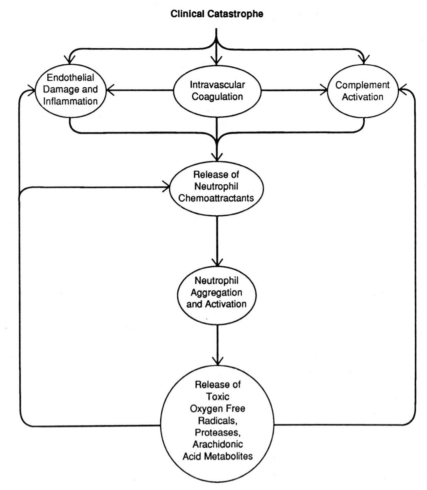

Figure 25.1. Pathophysiologic events in the development of ARDS.

surement may reveal a decreased Pao_2 despite a decreased $Paco_2$, indicating an increased alveolar-arterial oxygen gradient. At this stage, administration of supplemental oxygen can usually significantly increase the Pao_2, indicating that ventilation-perfusion mismatching, and possibly diffusion impairment, accounts for the widened gradient.

With the progression of ARDS, there is a dramatic increase in the work of breathing, with recruitment of the accessory muscles of respiration. Crackles may be heard throughout the lung fields. Agitation, lethargy, and obtundation may occur. The result of alveolar flooding is surfactant dysfunction and widespread atelectasis. The resulting reduced functional residual capacity and decreased lung compliance are the hallmarks of ARDS. Reduced lung compliance is primarily the result of interstitial and alveolar edema and fibrosis. Dynamic lung compliance is further decreased by severe bronchoconstriction induced by arachidonic acid metabolites. These changes are clinically manifested as the need for high-peak pressures to deliver an adequate tidal volume to the patient.

The profound hypoxemia refractory to administration of oxygen that characterizes the late progressive phase of ARDS is a product of the ventilation-perfusion (V/Q) mismatch and pulmonary shunting of blood past fluid-filled or collapsed alveoli. At this point in the natural history of ARDS, endotracheal intubation and mechanical ventilation are necessary.

The Chest Radiograph

The radiographic changes of ARDS are not specific for the syndrome. The chest x-ray may initially reveal bilateral interstitial markings. These may progress to diffuse, fluffy alveolar infiltrates. Although it may be difficult to distinguish between ARDS and cardiogenic pulmonary edema, in ARDS, pulmonary vascular redistribution, pleural effusions, and cardiomegaly are often absent. Over time, the alveolar infiltrates in ARDS may consolidate and take on a patchy or nodular pattern. If the disorder progresses, a pattern of diffuse interstitial fibrosis may ensue. However,

if the patient improves, the radiograph may revert to normal.

MANAGEMENT: OVERVIEW

The first priority in managing a patient with ARDS is reversal of life-threatening hypoxemia. Further management includes supportive therapy, diagnosis, and treatment of the underlying cause. Unfortunately, no therapeutic modalities are available that halt or reverse either the capillary leak syndrome or the sequela of pulmonary fibrosis. The conceptual approach to the current management of ARDS is displayed in Figure 25.2.

The critical care physician faces three major challenges in dealing with ARDS. The first is the short-term goal of establishing adequate pulmonary gas exchange. The second is successfully withdrawing

Stabilization Phase

1. Reverse Hypoxemia
   - oxygen
   - mechanical ventilation
   - positive end-expiratory pressure

2. Diagnosis and Treatment of Underlying Cause

3. Supportive Therapy
   - judicious fluid administration
   - pulmonary artery catheterization
   - vasoactive medication

Weaning From Mechanical Ventilation

1. Respiratory Muscle Exercise

2. Nutrition

3. Optimal Fluid Management

4. Emotional Support

5. Avoidance of Complications

Figure 25.2. Conceptual approach to the management of patients with ARDS.

mechanical ventilation. This is best achieved by means of a comprehensive management plan that involves attention to nutrition and the underlying cause of lung injury, as well as treatment of secondary infections and other complications. The third challenge in caring for a patient with ARDS is a realistic assessment of prognosis—recognizing that for many patients with ARDS, there comes a time when life support is no longer appropriate and the only appropriate interventions are those designed to permit a peaceful and pain-free death.

Oxygenation

Oxygen is the cornerstone of management for acute hypoxemic respiratory failure. Nasal prongs and high-flow oxygen masks provide immediate bedside management. The lowest inspired concentration of oxygen to achieve an oxygen saturation of 90% should be used. Monitoring blood gases and following pulse oximetry, using the oxyhemoglobin dissociation curve, can guide therapy (Figure 25.3). At a Po_2 of 60, hemoglobin is approximately 90% saturated. Therefore, a reasonable objective is to achieve a Pao_2 of 60, since high levels of oxygen may be toxic to the lung.

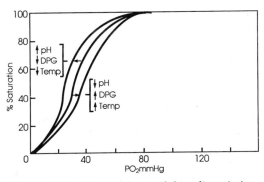

Figure 25.3. The oxyhemoglobin dissociation curve of normal blood. An increase in plasma pH or a decrease in temperature and 2,3-diphosphoglyceric acid (2,3-DPG) causes an increase in the oxygen affinity of hemoglobin (shift to the left) and a relative decrease in oxygen unloading. Conversely, a decrease in pH or an increase in temperature and 2,3-diphosphoglyceric acid (2,3-DPG) causes a decrease in oxygen affinity (shift to the right) and a relative increase in oxygen unloading.

High concentrations of oxygen may increase existing lung injury in several ways. It can cause the release of chemotaxins that recruit neutrophils (12), and can promote superinfection by causing mucociliary depression (42) by impairing migration of alveolar macrophages (51) and by increasing adherence of Gram-negative organisms to the lower respiratory tract epithelium (19).

If supplemental oxygenation is inadequate, and the patient is alert and able to protect his airway, face mask continuous positive airway pressure (CPAP) in 2.5 cm water increments can be used. The administration of CPAP by face mask may avoid endotracheal intubation, an important factor that increases the risk of nosocomial pneumonia. However, the potential complications include gastric dilation, aspiration, patient discomfort, and necrosis from facial pressure. Several studies have reported successful use of CPAP by face mask (6, 15, 47). In the only study that has compared spontaneous ventilation with CPAP to mechanical ventilation with positive end-expiratory pressure (PEEP), the former was more efficacious than the latter in improving oxygenation, and had no effect on cardiac output (43). Therefore, CPAP may be a temporizing maneuver in the alert, cooperative, spontaneously breathing patient. However, in most patients, when mask oxygen is inadequate, prompt endotracheal intubation and mechanical ventilation is performed.

Mechanical Ventilation

In one series by Fowler and colleagues (11), 90% of patients with ARDS had been intubated within 72 hours of diagnosis. When ARDS patients require assisted ventilation, an endotracheal tube with an internal diameter of 8 mm is the desired minimal size. Smaller tubes disproportionately increase airway resistance, hinder suctioning, and may preclude bronchoscopy, should it become indicated, later in the course of illness.

One common approach to mechanical ventilation in these patients is to employ large tidal volumes (15 ml/kg) and slower rates than the spontaneous rate of respiration in order to reduce the likelihood of atelectasis in the supine, relatively immobile patient. However, often the respiratory system is sufficiently stiff so that high inflation pressures are required. If the patient makes inspiratory efforts during the inflation cycle, peak inspiratory pressures may increase to dangerous levels, increasing the possibility of barotrauma. Barotrauma may lead to a pneumothorax or subcutaneous, mediastinal, retroperitoneal, or intraperitoneal emphysema. Therefore, downward adjustment of the tidal volume or rate is advisable if the peak inspiratory pressure exceeds 50 cm H_2O. Sedation with benzodiazepines or paralytic agents is often instituted, and paralysis can offer the additional advantage of reducing oxygen consumption.

Positive end-expiratory pressure was the first therapeutic modality shown to reduce mortality in ARDS (1); it is usually applied in increments of 2.5–5.0 cm H_2O (14, 54). Positive end-expiratory pressure improves functional residual capacity by increasing the gas volume of partially flooded alveoli and reversing atelectasis, thereby reducing $\dot{V}/\dot{Q}$ mismatch and shunting. However, there is no evidence of a beneficial effect of PEEP on extravascular lung water, nor is there evidence of a prophylactic role for PEEP in patients with incipient ARDS. Nevertheless, PEEP is conventionally used in mechanical ventilation and is adjusted to achieve adequate oxygenation (i.e., arterial saturation of 90% or more) using a nontoxic F_{IO_2} of less than 0.6. The major cardiovascular effect of PEEP is a decrease in cardiac output due to two mechanisms. First, increased intrapleural pressures may impede venous return directly, an effect that is, to a variable extent, offset by peripheral venoconstriction. Second, increases in lung volume may increase pulmonary vascular resistance, leading to increased pulmonary pressure and dilation of the right ventricle, which in turn displaces the intraventricular septum toward the left. This displacement decreases left ventricular filling and results in a decreased cardiac output. Therefore, although the "optimal" level of PEEP has been variably defined as that which maximizes respiratory system compliance and that which decreases shunt fraction to less

than 15%, we favor the definition of the level of PEEP that permits reduction of inspired oxygen to minimal levels without decreasing cardiac output (54). Other side effects of PEEP include impediment of thoracic venous return and increased cerebral venous and intracranial pressure. These effects could produce critical reductions in cerebral perfusion pressure since

cerebral perfusion pressure = mean arterial pressure − intracranial pressure

The reported effects of PEEP on glomerular filtration rate, total renal blood flow, and the renin-angiotensin system are not established with certainty (14), although it has been postulated that decreased urinary output in patients with PEEP is secondary to increased secretion of antidiuretic hormone.

Occasionally, at very high levels of PEEP, there may be a paradoxic decrease in Pao₂. The reason is as follows: high levels of PEEP may overdistend some alveoli that are already open. Overdistension of these units can increase the vascular resistance in these regions and increase the degree of shunt. The solution is to adjust the PEEP level downwards again.

The possible contribution of a patient's position on decreased arterial oxygenation should always be considered before escalating therapeutic interventions. Although patients with ARDS appear to have diffuse lung disease, there may be some regional variation in the extent of disease such that one side of the lung is more severely involved than the other. Since the distribution of pulmonary blood flow is so heavily determined by gravity, having the more diseased lung, with its minimal ventilation, in the more dependent position results in a measurable increase in intrapulmonary shunting, manifesting as a dramatic fall in Pao₂. Therefore, the less involved lung should be dependent when the patient is in a lateral supine position to maximize oxygenation.

Supportive Care

Fluid Management

Fluid management in the treatment of ARDS is a challenge; the colloid/crystalloid debate is ongoing. Colloid solutions contain large molecules ranging from 4×10^4 (dextran) or 6.9×10^4 (albumin) daltons. Crystalloid solutions contain sodium chloride, often with other electrolytes or glucose. Examples include lactated Ringer's solution, 0.9% sodium chloride, and dextrose in water. Colloid enthusiasts argue that colloid solutions are better volume expanders than crystalloids, and that a large proportion of crystalloid solutions end up in the pulmonary interstitium and alveoli, worsening gas exchange. Large volumes of crystalloid infusion may also lower colloid oncotic pressure, increasing the propensity for pulmonary edema formation. However, crystalloid enthusiasts argue that colloids are expensive, and that the large molecules in colloid solutions leak through damaged capillaries, accumulate in the interstitium, increase tissue oncotic pressure, and exacerbate pulmonary edema. As may be expected when there are such polarities of opinion, there is no strong evidence to support the use of crystalloid over colloid or vice versa in ARDS (45).

Pulmonary Artery Catheterization

The cardiovascular management of ARDS is complex and still evolving. In general, the goals of therapy are to achieve the lowest intravascular hydrostatic pressure consistent with adequate tissue perfusion. In many patients, insertion of a flow-directed pulmonary artery catheter (right heart catheter) may provide useful information to help guide fluid therapy and titrate vasoactive drugs. From the right heart catheter, information can be obtained about cardiac filling pressures, including the pulmonary artery occlusion pressure, cardiac output, and systemic vascular resistance. A methodologically sound, definitive trial that sufficiently addresses the question of whether pulmonary artery catheterization impacts on ICU morbidity or mortality has yet to be performed (16).

Fluid administration is titrated to ensure adequate cardiac output and tissue perfusion. In the absence of hypotension, judicious diuresis may help to decrease lung water and improve oxygenation. Humphrey and colleagues (21) found that sur-

vival was 75% in patients whose pulmonary artery occlusion pressure was lowered to a mean of 7 mm Hg, but was only 29% in patients whose mean pulmonary artery occlusion pressure was 13 mm Hg or higher. However, this study has methodologic shortcomings; the data were retrospectively collected and factors other than a lower pulmonary artery occlusion pressure may have contributed to the observed differences in outcome. It is of concern that organ perfusion, which is commonly altered in septic shock, may be aggravated by lowering intravascular volume. Moreover, excessive diuresis, especially when coupled with positive pressure ventilation and PEEP, may markedly reduce preload, cardiac output, and oxygen delivery. Therefore, in the absence of a sound prospective trial, no firm policy recommendations can be made for aggressive lowering of the pulmonary artery occlusion pressure in ARDS (22).

Inotropic agents such as dobutamine, and vasodilators such as nitroprusside and hydralazine, have been used to lower pulmonary artery occlusion pressure while maintaining or increasing cardiac output. However, it must be recognized that many agents that increase cardiac output will also increase intrapulmonary shunting, thereby increasing oxygen requirement. Moreover, there is no ideal cardiovascular agent that lowers pulmonary artery occlusion pressure, maintains or increases cardiac output, and reduces intrapulmonary shunting.

In addition to causing real changes in cardiac output, PEEP introduces uncertainties in the measurement and interpretation of the pulmonary artery occlusion pressure. Because left ventricular compliance can be effected by PEEP and because PEEP-induced changes in intrathoracic pressure are transmitted directly to the heart, a change in pulmonary artery occlusion pressure may not reflect a change in transmural cardiac filling pressure or in left ventricular end-diastolic volume. However, if the pulmonary artery catheter is located in a nondependent area of the lung where PEEP exceeds intravascular pressure, measured pulmonary artery occlusion pressure may reflect airway pressure (PEEP), not intravascular pressure (44).

Therefore, if pleural pressures are greater than atmospheric pressure when PEEP is being used, the true effective (i.e., intravascular minus pleural) pressure will be overestimated and could lead to errors in management. To avoid these problems, PEEP is sometimes removed while pulmonary artery occlusion pressure is measured; however, the steady state is destabilized, and measurements may be of dubious value. Moreover, the transient removal of PEEP for measurement of pulmonary capillary wedge pressure has been shown to cause a marked fall in arterial oxygen tension (8). A reasonable estimate of the true wedge pressure can be obtained by examining vascular pressures just before inflation, then subtracting one half of the PEEP. However, in ARDS patients who have very low compliance, transmission of atmospheric pressure may be minimal and the foregoing adjustment may be unnecessary.

Recently, Pinsky et al. (38) have demonstrated that if the pulmonary arterial catheter is inflated to wedge position and then the patient is rapidly disconnected from the ventilator, pulmonary artery occlusion pressure will quickly fall to a nadir in about 2 seconds prior to again increasing to a new plateau. This initial decrease in pulmonary artery occlusion pressure reflects the withdrawal of PEEP-induced increased intrathoracic pressure, whereas the subsequent rise in pulmonary artery occlusion pressure represents the associated increase in venous return reaching the left ventricle. Accordingly, these workers demonstrated that in postoperative cardiac patients, this nadir pulmonary artery occlusion pressure accurately reflects on-PEEP left ventricular filling pressure, as defined by the difference between left atrial pressure and pericardial pressure. Although their study examined the effect of airway disconnection on estimates on left ventricular filling pressures in patients on up to 15 cm H_2O PEEP, all their patients were in the immediate postoperative period and had no evidence of air trapping. If air trapping occurs, then following airway disconnection, intrathoracic pressure may remain elevated. Thus, nadir pulmonary artery occlusion pressure will also overestimate on-PEEP left ventricular filling

pressure. However, to the extent that no airflow obstruction exists and the pulmonary arterial catheter is in a dependent position in the lung, measures of nadir pulmonary artery occlusion pressure should accurately reflect on-PEEP left ventricular filling pressure.

As soon as the patient with ARDS has stabilized, the focus of management shifts. The goal is to keep the patient alive for as long as it takes to repair the pulmonary damage and allow the patient to breathe without assisted ventilation. This process may take anywhere from 1–8 weeks. Unfortunately, some chronically ventilated patients never gain sufficient strength to be weaned from the ventilator and may ultimately succumb to complications or have life support systems withdrawn. Nevertheless, it behooves the intensive care physician to have an approach to dealing with the ARDS patient who is difficult to wean from mechanical ventilation.

THE DIFFICULT-TO-WEAN ARDS PATIENT

A protocol that emphasizes rehabilitation as well as acute care provides the best conceptual framework for managing difficult-to-wean ARDS patients. An effective protocol has five major components: exercise, nutrition, fluid management, emotional support, and sleep.

Exercise

Adequate rehabilitation for the chronically ventilated patient should focus on pulmonary and whole-body conditioning. The goal is to achieve a training effect and ensure that the patient and staff are aware that progress is being made. There are several commonly employed methods of weaning patient with ARDS. Two commonly used approaches are the intermittent mandatory ventilation mode and T-piece trials. The intermittent mandatory ventilation mode allows the patient to take independent breaths in between ventilator breaths. This rate is adjusted according to the degree of independent function achieved. A second approach to weaning, assist-control ventilation, involves alternating rest periods with vigorous T-piece trials. There is no evidence to suggest that one mode is more effective than the other in weaning ARDS patients. Physiotherapy and isometric exercises, if possible, are also beneficial for the bedridden ventilated patient in order to prevent contractures and bedsores and minimize muscle atrophy.

Nutrition

Patients with ARDS often require 35–45 kcal/kg/day to meet their nutritional requirements. Failure to meet nutritional requirements results in negative nitrogen balance, decreased respiratory muscle strength, and increased susceptibility to infection. Conversely, overfeeding can result in volume overload, hepatic dysfunction, and increased CO_2 production. The proportion of calories contributed to by fat versus carbohydrates is crucial to decrease the respiratory quotient (the ratio of the carbon dioxide production to the oxygen consumption). Nutritional support with a diet rich in carbohydrates will increase CO_2 production and increase minute ventilation requirements. Enteral feeding is generally preferred, as it involves fewer complications and is less costly than parenteral feeding. However, enterally fed patients must be monitored closely to avoid aspiration.

Fluid Management

Optimal fluid management is crucial in patients with ARDS. A balance must be achieved between maintenance of adequate tissue perfusion (i.e., adequate cardiac output, renal and cerebral perfusion) and elimination of excess pulmonary fluid. The patient who is optimally dry may require judicious use of vasoactive drugs or diuretics.

Emotional Support and Sleep

Any conscious patient who remains in the ICU for more than several days is at risk of depression, agitation, and feelings of hopelessness. Understandably, patients who are in pain or who receive sedatives may find it difficult to feel like participants in their own recovery. Continuity of care, communication, and encouragement are crucial throughout the rehabilitation pe-

riod. An adequate sleep-wake cycle is desirable in these patients, which requires scheduling of activities such as exercise and bathing during daylight hours and darkness, silence, or short-acting benzodiazepines at night.

COMPLICATIONS AND PROGNOSIS

The patient with ARDS is predisposed to a number of complications during the ICU course. These include pulmonary barotrauma, pulmonary emboli, hypotension, arrhythmias, sepsis, gastrointestinal hemorrhage, and renal failure (37).

Respiratory insufficiency appeared to be a major cause of death in 75% of patients who died in the retrospective study by Fowler et al. (11). However, in a prospective study of 47 patients with ARDS, only 5 of 32 deaths (16%) were from irreversible pulmonary failure. Most deaths in the first 3 days could be attributed to underlying illness or injury; 16 of 22 late deaths (75%) were due to sepsis. The final common pathway for most patients who succumb is sepsis and multisystem organ failure.

Given the diverse etiologies of ARDS and the comorbid conditions associated with this condition, it is difficult to give accurate prognostic figures. Mortality for the general ARDS population is approximately 65% (11, 33). Mortality approaches 90% for patients who develop ARDS secondary to sepsis or whose respiratory failure occurs in the setting of leukemia or lymphoma.

In those patients who survive, however, structural derangements of the lung appear to be partly reversible; only one-third of survivors have a permanent reduction in vital capacity or obstruction of air flow (25, 41). A widened alveolar arterial oxygen difference persisted in all patients in whom it was measured in another study, suggesting residual interstitial or vascular abnormalities in survivors. (9).

NEW APPROACHES TO THERAPY

In the early to mid 1980s, it was hypothesized that high-dose steroids would be efficacious in acute hypoxemic respiratory failure. In 1981, a study of methylprednisolone and dexamethasone on alveolar capillary permeability in septic patients with ARDS was performed (46). In 19 patients, the clearance of [131]iodine human serum albumin was reduced by corticosteroid, while in 5, it was unaffected. The latter group of patients was more severely ill than the former, however. The authors concluded that high-dose corticosteroid therapy may reduce alveolar capillary permeability in septic ARDS if used early in the course of illness.

This finding, combined with the biologic rationale that high-dose steroids may favorably alter the oxyhemoglobin dissociation curve (29), improve cardiac output (28), reduce pulmonary venospasm (24), and reduce complement activation (18), has led to further investigation. In an open prospective study executed in 1985, severely ill trauma patients were selected to receive or not receive prophylactic methylprednisolone (50). The 47 patients receiving steroids had a significantly lower rate of ARDS development than the 45 patients who did not receive steroids. However, the methodologic limitations of such a study design limit the inferences that can be made from these data.

In the late 1980s, several large placebo-controlled trials were performed to evaluate steroids in the sepsis syndrome (3, 48, 51); these did not show a significant reduction in mortality in the treatment groups. These studies bear indirectly on the potential role for steroids in ARDS in that sepsis is a major risk factor for ARDS. However, based on the results of the foregoing, steroids cannot be recommended for prophylaxis or treatment of ARDS.

Prostaglandin E$_1$ has also been compared to placebo in a randomized double-blind multicenter study to determine whether prostaglandin therapy enhances survival of patients with ARDS (4). An improvement in oxygen availability and consumption was observed; however, there was a trend toward increased mortality in the prostaglandin group.

The involvement of the complement cascade, neutrophil aggregation, the coagulation system, and prostaglandins in acute endothelial injury provide a basis for new pharmacologic approaches to ARDS. For example, pentoxifylline may provide a protective effect on tumor necrosis factor-induced lung injury (27), and may attenuate the side effects of interleukin-2-induced acute lung injury (23). However, at present, there are no specific therapies proven to speed healing of the damaged lung or reverse the disease process.

In 1979, in a randomized controlled study of extracorporeal membrane oxygenation, 48 patients were treated with conventional mechanical ventilation and 42 were treated with mechanical ventilation and partial venoarterial bypass (56). The mortality rate between the groups was not significantly different (9.8% and 8.3%, respectively). This study effectively halted further use of extracorporeal membrane oxygenation for ARDS in adults, although research in the pediatric population has continued.

However, new therapy for ARDS developed using different modes of ventilation. The hypothesis is that the inhomogeneously injured lung in ARDS may become overexpanded with the usual modes of ventilation, sustaining damage to the remaining small fraction of compliant lung still capable of gas exchange, thereby superimposing iatrogenic lung injury on ARDS. One uncontrolled study using low-frequency positive pressure ventilation with extracorporeal carbon dioxide removal to treat severe respiratory failure was published in 1986 (13). Patients were treated with three to five positive pressure breaths per minute at low peak inspiratory pressures of 35–40 cm H$_2$O. Lung function improved in 73% of patients, and 49% of patients survived. A controlled clinical trial of low-frequency positive pressure ventilation with extracorporeal carbon dioxide removal using three-step therapy versus traditional therapy is now underway (34).

Recently, a promising new development in septic shock research has been published (57). There is a human monoclonal IgM antibody that binds specifically to the lipid A domain of endotoxin called HA-1A. A randomized double-blind trial was performed in patients with sepsis and a presumed diagnosis of Gram-negative infection. The 1-month mortality rate was significantly lower in the treated group with Gram-negative sepsis (49% versus 30%). Moreover, analyses that stratified according to the severity of illness at entry showed improved survival with HA-1A treatment in both severely ill and less severely ill patients. These findings illustrate the potential of human monoclonal immunotherapy in clinical medicine. Further trials of immunotherapy in ARDS will likely be forthcoming.

References

1. Ashbaugh DG, Bigelow DB, Petty TL, et al. Acute respiratory distress in adults. Lancet 1967;2:319–323.
2. Bone RC, Francis PB, Pierce AK. Intravascular coagulation associated with the adult respiratory distress syndrome. Am J Med 1976;61:585–589.
3. Bone RC, Fisher CJ, Clemmer TP, et al. A controlled clinical trial of high dose methylprednisolone in the treatment of severe sepsis and septic shock. N Engl J Med 1987;317:653–658.
4. Bone RC, Slotman G, Maunder R, et al. Randomized double-blind multicenter study of Prostaglandin E1 in patients with the Adult Respiratory Distress Syndrome. Chest 1989;96:114–119.
5. Bowles AL, Dauber, JH, Daniele RP. The effect of hyperoxia on migration of alveolar macrophages in vitro. Am Rev Respir Dis 1979;120:541–545.
6. Covelli HD, Weled BJ, Beekman JF. Efficacy of continuous positive airway pressure administered by face mask. Chest 1982;81:147–150.
7. Craddock PR, Hammerschmidt D, White JG, et al. Complement (C5a)-induced granulocyte aggregation in vitro: a possible mechanism of complement-mediated leukostasis and leukopenia. J Clin Invest 1977;60:260–264.
8. De Campo T, Civetta JM. The effect of short-term discontinuation of high level PEEP in patients with adult respiratory failure. Crit Care Med 1979;7:47–49.
9. Elliott CG, Morris AH, Cengiz M. Pulmonary function and exercise gas exchange in survivors of adult respiratory distress syndrome. Am Rev Respir Dis 1981;123:492–495.
10. Fink A, Geva D, Zung A, et al. Adult respiratory distress syndrome: roles of leukotriene C_4 and platelet activating factor. Crit Care Med 1990;18:905–909.
11. Fowler AA, Hamman RF, Good JT, et al. Adult respiratory distress syndrome: risk with common predispositions. Ann Intern Med 1983;98:593–597.
12. Fox RB, Shasby DM, Harada RN, et al. A novel mechanism for pulmonary oxygen toxicity: phagocyte mediated lung injury. Chest 1981;80 (suppl):3S–4S.
13. Gattinoni L, Pasenti A, Mascheroni D, et al. Low-frequency positive pressure ventilation with extracorporeal CO_2 removal in acute respiratory failure. JAMA 1986;256:881–886.
14. Gong H. Positive pressure ventilation in the adult respiratory distress syndrome. Clin Chest Med 1982;3:69–88.
15. Greenbaum DM, Millen JE, Eross B, et al. Continuous positive airway pressure without tracheal intubation in spontaneously breathing patients. Chest 1976;69:615–620.
16. Guyatt GH, Tugwell P, Feeny DH, et al. The role of before-after studies of therapeutic impact in the evaluation of diagnostic technologies. J Chron Dis 1986;39:295–304.
17. Hammerschmidt DE, Weaver LJ, Hudson LD, et al. Association of complement activation and elevated plasma C5a with adult respiratory distress syndrome. Lancet 1980;1:947–949.
18. Hammerschmidt DE, Whyte JG, Craddock PR, et al. Corticosteroids inhibit complement-induced granulocyte aggregation. J Clin Invest 1979;63:798–803.
19. Higuchi JH, Coalson JJ, Johanson WG. Effect of hyperoxia on tracheal mucosal adherence, lower respiratory tract colonization and infection [abstract]. Am Rev Respir Dis 1980;121 (suppl):353.
20. Hogg JC. Neutrophil kinetics and lung injury. Physiol Rev 1987;67:1249–1295.
21. Humphrey H, Hall J, Sznajder I, et al. Improved survival in ARDS patients associated with a reduction in pulmonary capillary wedge pressure. Chest 1990;97:1176–1180.
22. Hyers TM. ARDS: The therapeutic dilemma [Editorial]. Chest 1990;97:1025.
23. Ishizaka A, Hatherill JR, Harada H, et al. Prevention of interleukin 2-induced acute lung injury in guinea pigs by pentoxifylline. J Appl Physiol 1989;67:2432–2437.
24. Kusajima K, Wax SD, Webb WR. Effects of methylprednisolone on pulmonary microcirculation. Surg Gynecol Obstet 1974;139:1–5.
25. Lakshminarayan S, Stanford RE, Petty TL. Prognosis after recovery from adult respiratory distress syndrome. Am Rev Respir Dis 1976;113:7–16.
26. Lee CT, Fein AM, Lippman M, et al. Elastolytic activity in pulmonary lavage fluid from patients with adult respiratory distress syndrome. N Engl J Med 1981;304:192–196.
27. Lilly CM, Sandhu JS, Ishizaka A, et al. Pentoxifylline prevents tumor necrosis factor-induced lung injury. Am Rev Respir Dis 1989;139:1361–1368.
28. Lozman J, Dutton RE, English M, et al. Cardiopulmonary adjustments following single high dose administration of methylprednisolone in traumatized man. Ann Surg 1975;181:317–324.
29. McConn R, Del Guercio LRM. Respiratory function of blood in the acutely ill patient and the effect of steroids. Ann Surg 1971;174:436–450.
30. McGuire WW, Spragg RG, Cohen AB, et al. Studies on the pathogenesis of the adult respiratory distress syndrome. J Clin Invest 1982;69:543–553.
31. Meyrick BO, Ryan US, Brigham KL. Direct effects of E. Coli endotoxin on structure and permeability of pulmonary and endothelial monolayers and the endothelial layer of intimal implants. Am J Pathol 1986;122:140–151.

32. Modell JH. Biology of drowning. Ann Rev Med 1978;29:1–8.

33. Montgomery AB, Stager MA, Carrico CJ, et al. Causes of mortality in patients with the adult respiratory distress syndrome. Am Rev Resp Dis 1985;132:485–489.

34. Morris AH, Menlove RL, Rollins RJ, et al. A controlled clinical trial of a new 3-step therapy that includes extracorporeal CO_2 removal for ARDS. Trans Am Soc Artif Intern Organs 1988;11:48–53.

35. Ognibene FP, Martin SE, Parker MM, et al. Adult respiratory distress syndrome in patients with severe neutropenia. N Engl J Med 1986;315:547–551.

36. Pepe PE, Potkin RT, Reus DH, et al. Clinical predictors of the adult respiratory distress syndrome. Am J Surg 1982;144:124–130.

37. Pingleton SK. Complications associated with the adult respiratory distress syndrome. Clin Chest Med 1982;3:143–155.

38. Pinsky MR, Vincent JL, DeSmet JM. Estimating left ventricular filling pressure during positive end-expiratory pressure in humans. Am Rev Resp Dis 1991;143:25–31.

39. Raffin TA. ARDS: mechanisms and management. Hosp Prac 1987;22:65–80.

40. Rinaldo JE, Rogers RM. Adult respiratory distress syndrome: changing concepts of lung injury and repair. N Engl J Med 1982;306:900–909.

41. Rotman HH, Lavelle TF, Dimcheff DG, et al. Long term physiologic consequences of the adult respiratory distress syndrome. Chest 1977;72:190–192.

42. Sackner MA, Landa J, Hirsch J, et al. Pulmonary effects of oxygen breathing: a 6 hour study in normal men. Ann Intern Med 1976;82:40–43.

43. Shah DM, Newell JC, Dutton RE. Continuous positive airway pressure verus positive end-expiratory pressure in respiratory distress syndrome. J Thorac Cardiovasc Surg 1977;74:557–562.

44. Shasby DM, Dauber IM, Pfister S, et al. Swan-Ganz catheter location and left atrial pressure determine the accuracy of the wedge pressure when positive end-expiratory pressure is used. Chest 1981;80:666–670.

45. Shoemaker WC, Hauser CJ. Critique of crystalloid versus colloid therapy in shock and shock lung. Crit Care Med 1979;7:117–124.

46. Sibbald WJ, Anderson RR, Reid B, et al. Alveolocapillary permeability in human septic ARDS. Chest 1981;79:133–142.

47. Smith RA, Kirby RR, Gooding JM, et al. Continuous positive airway pressure (CPAP) by face mask. Crit Care Med 1980;8:483–485.

48. Sprung CL, Caralis PC, Marcial EH, et al. The effects of high dose corticosteroids in patients with septic shock: a prospective controlled study. N Engl J Med 1984;311:1137–1143.

49. Tate RM, Repine JE. Neutrophils and the adult respiratory distress syndrome. Am Rev Respir Dis 1983;128:552–559.

50. Van Der Merwe CJ, Louw AF, Welthagen D, et al. Adult respiratory distress syndrome in cases of severe trauma—the prophylactic value of methylprednisolone sodium succinate. S Afr Med J 1985;67:279–284.

51. The Veterans Administration Systemic Sepsis Cooperative Study Group. Effect of high dose glucocorticoid therapy on mortality in patients with clinical signs of systemic sepsis. N Engl J Med 1987;317:659–665.

52. Ward HN. Pulmonary infiltrates associated with leukoagglutinin transfusion reactions. Ann Intern Med 1970;73:689–694.

53. Weiland JE, Davis WB, Holter JF, et al. Lung neutrophils in the adult respiratory distress syndrome. Am Rev Respir Dis 1986;133:218–225.

54. Weisman IM, Rinaldo JE, Rogers RM. Positive end-expiratory pressure in adult respiratory failure. N Engl J Med 1982;307:1381–1384.

55. Wynne JW, Modell JH. Respiratory aspiration of stomach contents. Ann Intern Med 1977;87:466–474.

56. Zapol WM, Snider MT, Hill JD, et al. Extracorporeal membrane oxygenation in severe acute respiratory failure. A randomized prospective study. JAMA 1979;242:2193–2196.

57. Ziegler EJ, Fisher CJ, Sprung CL, et al. Treatment of gram negative bacteremia and septic shock with HA-1A human monoclonal antibody against endotoxin. N Engl J Med 1991;324:429–436.

26

Acute Exacerbation of Chronic Airflow Obstruction

Michel Aubier
Marie-Christine Dombret

The respiratory system functions in an integrated fashion, in health and disease. Thus, one must understand the syndromes of acute and chronic respiratory failure in terms of the interactions among the different parts of the respiratory system, with particular emphasis on respiratory control, the muscles used in breathing, and the efficiency of gas exchange.

Most of the conditions that predispose to the development of hypercapnic respiratory failure are characterized either by increasing the work of breathing or by respiratory muscle weakness. There are three types of disorders that increase the work of breathing: those that reduce pulmonary compliance, those that impede the motion of the chest wall, and those that increase the resistance to airflow.

By far the commonest cause of respiratory failure is severe obstruction of the intrapulmonary or lower airway. It is well recognized that respiratory failure is an occasional complication of asthma attack, but hypercapnia occurs much more frequently in chronic obstructive pulmonary disease (COPD). Therefore, most of the published data concerning the pathophysiology of respiratory failure has been obtained from patients with COPD. This chapter will deal mainly with the acute respiratory failure of COPD patients and particularly with the modifications of central respiratory drive and respiratory muscle function secondary to the increased load of breathing observed in these patients.

PATHOLOGIC STUDIES AND STRUCTURE-FUNCTION CORRELATIONS

Several pathologic changes are responsible for the marked airway obstruction observed in COPD patients. Before we discuss the mechanical aspect of airway obstruction, we will give a brief overview of the structural changes that have been observed in these patients.

COPD

Structure-function study correlations in severe COPD are difficult to obtain because patients with documented chronic airway obstruction (CAO) who come to autopsy often have a long interval between death and measurement of pulmonary function. Lungs or lobes removed by surgery supply only partial data because they are affected with mild CAO. However, autopsy performed during functional studies provide relevant data about severe CAO, as in the Intermittent Positive Pressure Breathing Trial (85) and NIH Nocturnal Oxygen Therapy Trial (59).

Chronic airflow obstruction is a syndrome that is produced by a variety of lesions that may occur in bronchi, bronchioles, and lung parenchyma. These lesions occur together in various combinations because of a common etiologic agent, tobacco smoke (113). In large airways, intraluminal inflammation can be easily documented during fiberoptic bronchoscopy. It can be assessed by visual inspection of

427

the airway and bronchial lavage, and is significantly more evident in chronic bronchitis than in either asymptomatic smokers or normal subjects (111). Visual evidence of airway inflammation is quantified by a bronchitis index. In a bronchial lavage specimen, inflammation is characterized by a higher number of cells and a higher percentage of neutrophils. Several studies have shown that patients with a higher percentage of neutrophils had significantly lower FEV_1, FEV_1/FVC and $FEF_{25\%-75\%}$ than did the subjects with lower percentage of neutrophils. Nevertheless in patients with moderate to severe CAO, there was no demonstrated relationship between bronchial inflammation and expiratory flow (85, 107, 113).

Others lesions of the large airways include mucous gland enlargement, smooth muscle hyperplasia, cartilage atrophy, and bronchial wall thickening; these yield uncertain functional consequences. Bronchiolar lesions are frequently found in CAO, but their relative importance may differ in patients with mild CAO and with severe CAO. In mild CAO, inflammation is a major factor, and narrowing fibrosis and goblet cell metaplasia are important contributory causes.

The relation between airflow limitation and bronchiolitis is more difficult to show because the more severe state of emphysema is causing airflow obstruction. Significant correlations were found between flow rates and residual volume and the proportion of airway under 400 μm in diameter (85). However, in goblet cell metaplasia, the proportion of bronchioles less than 400 μm in diameter were higher in patients with the most severe emphysema and slower flow rates. It is possible that bronchial deformity may be a consequence of emphysema and loss of radial alveolar traction. Goblet cell metaplasia has been shown to be related to expiratory flow obstruction. Nagai et al. (85) conclude that goblet cell metaplasia is a significant cause of airway obstruction, particularly because it is the only lesion associated with airway resistance.

Goblet cell metaplasia can cause obstruction by intraluminal mucus or by displacement of the surface active layer of bronchiole. Emphysema is the prominent lesion in persons with severe airflow obstruction due to COPD. Hale and associates (52) compared the interaction of bronchial gland enlargement, bronchiolar pathology, and emphysema in a group of nonsmokers, a group of smokers who died without known pulmonary disease, and a group of smokers who died with severe airflow obstruction. They examined the relationship between FEV_1 and morphologic indices. In a study of multiple regression analysis, only emphysema entered at a significant level. Most persons dying with COPD have severe emphysema. However, it is not definitely known which lesions are responsible for acute respiratory failure.

Asthma

Knowledge of the pathologic features of status asthmaticus is derived from autopsy examination in fatal cases (112). At autopsy, lungs are markedly hyperinflated and do not collapse when removed from the thorax. Airways are occluded by thick mucous plugs from the upper airways to respiratory bronchioles. These plugs are composed of a mixture of mucus and proteinaceous exudate containing a large number of eosinophils, Charcot-Leyden crystals, and shed epithelial cells. In some patients there are areas of atelectasis, subpleural fibrosis, and bronchiectasia. Emphysema is seldom seen. The bronchial mucosa shows extensive goblet cell metaplasia; the mucous glands are enlarged; the bronchial smooth muscle is thickened by muscle cell hyperplasia. There is a marked inflammation in the airway with infiltration of inflammatory cells, particularly eosinophils, and disruption of airway epithelium (33).

Similar but less severe pathologic changes have also been found in bronchial biopsy specimens from even mildly affected patients. Fresh biopsy specimens in mild to severe asthma may show a profound epithelial destruction of the airways (60, 64). The degree of epithelial cell loss has been correlated with the degree of hyperactivity (60). Laitinen et al. (64) observed the superficial location of nerves in the bronchial epithelium and concluded that exposure of mucosal afferent nerves by the sloughing of cells is possible and could explain hyperresponsiveness. Mucociliary clearance is obviously disturbed. The reticular lamina of the basement membrane becomes thickened; this change begins early during the course of the illness.

PATHOPHYSIOLOGY OF ACUTE RESPIRATORY FAILURE IN COPD

The Consequences of Airway Obstruction

Pattern of Breathing

Chronic obstructive pulmonary disease patients with severe airway obstruction exhibit a marked reduction in forced inspiratory and expiratory flow. The latter is secondary to the pathologic changes (see above) that occur in the airway, but also to an alteration of lung parenchyma elastic recoil due to centrolobular emphysema, which renders the airway more collapsible and closure occurs prematurely (31). To overcome this airway closure during positive pleural pressure breathing, the patients have to breathe at a high pulmonary volume, with the flow-volume curve being shifted to the left on the volume axis (Fig. 26.1).

In order to cope with the extra load imposed by the airway obstruction and to maintain a level of minute ventilation adapted to the metabolic needs of the body, COPD patients have to increase their inspiratory flow and lung volume. These increases are compensated for by a change in breathing pattern, which can be deduced from the following equations:

$$\dot{V}_E = V_T . f \qquad (1)$$

Minute ventilation ($\dot{V}_E$) is the product of total volume (V_T) and respiratory frequency (f). F is the opposite of the total breath duration (T_{TOT}). Equation 1 can be rewritten:

$$\dot{V}_E = V_T . 1/T_{TOT} \text{ when } T_{TOT} = T_I + T_E \quad (2)$$

where T_I is inspiratory time and T_E is expiratory time. Equation 2 can be rewritten as follows:

$$\dot{V}_E = V_T/T_I . T_I/T_{TOT} = V_T/T_E . T_E/T_{TOT} \quad (3)$$

where V_I/T_I is inspiratory flow, V_T/T_E is expiratory flow, and T_I/T_{TOT} is the duty cycle, i.e., the time fraction when the inspiratory muscles are on duty.

In COPD patients, V_T/T_E is decreased. To maintain $\dot{V}_E$ at the same level, T_E/T_{TOT} must be increased; and therefore, T_I/T_{TOT} must be decreased and V_T/T_I increased. Thus, in order to keep the same ventilation when there is expiratory flow limitation, these patients have to increase their mean

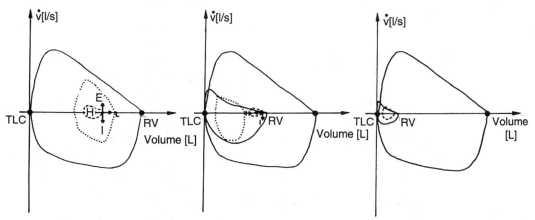

Figure 26.1. Flow-volume curves of a normal subject (*left panel*), a patient with severe COPD (*middle panel*), and a COPD patient with acute respiratory failure (*right panel*). *Solid line*, forced loop; *dashed line*, normal breathing; *dotted line*, maximal exercise. (From Derenne JP, Fleury B, Pariente R. Acute respiratory failure of chronic obstructive pulmonary disease. Am Rev Respir Dis 1988;138:1006–1033.)

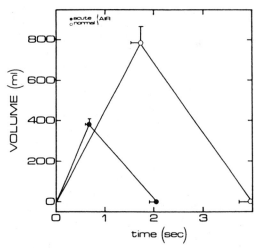

Figure 26.2. Average respiratory cycle during room air breathing in 20 COPD patients in acute respiratory failure (○) and 11 normal individuals (●). Bars indicate 1 SE. Note the rapid shallow breathing pattern in COPD patients. (From Aubier M, Murciano D, Fournier M, Milic-Emili J, Pariente R, Derenne JP. Central respiratory drive in acute respiratory failure of patients with chronic obstructive pulmonary disease. Au Rev Respir Dis 1980;122:191–199.)

inspiratory flow and decrease their duty cycle. This causes the characteristic rapid and shallow breathing that these patients exhibit, particularly during acute respiratory failure (19, 90) (Fig. 26.2).

Central Respiratory Drive

It has long been believed that the central respiratory drive of patients with severe COPD was depressed, leading to hypercapnia. Recent studies using more specific and sensitive techniques to study the activity of the respiratory centers have shown that, in fact, the respiratory centers in these patients were very active (9). These results were obtained by using the mouth (or tracheal) occlusion pressure technique (9, 108). The latter, which is not invasive and can be easily repeated in a given patient, is the pressure generated 100 msec after the onset of an inspiratory effort performed at functional residual capacity against closed airways ($P_{0.1}$).

This $P_{0.1}$ is an index of the respiratory neuromuscular drive, which depends on the respiratory center activity and the ability of the systems to transform this activity into pressure by the respiratory muscles. This index is not influenced by the mechanical alteration that may occur in the respiratory system because, during its measurement, these zero flow and almost no change in lung volume due to the occlusion. Therefore, $P_{0.1}$ is independent of airway resistance and lung compliance, contrary to minute ventilation ($\dot{V}_E$). This index has been found to be elevated in COPD patients, whether they are normocapnic or hypercapnic (108), suggesting that the increased Pa_{CO2} observed in these patients is not secondary to a decreased respiratory center output. This is further supported by the fact that $P_{0.1}$ has been found to be even much higher (4 times that of normal subjects) in COPD patients with acute respiratory failure as compared to the same COPD patients in a stable state (8 cm H_2O versus 4 cm H_2 on the average, respectively) (9). Such a level of $P_{0.1}$ will correspond to the inspiratory neuromuscular output of normal subjects who ventilate at 70/80 liter/min (30, 126). Such a high load cannot be sustained by the respiratory muscles for a long time without the occurrence of fatigue.

Respiratory Muscle Fatigue

As seen above in subjects with COPD in acute respiratory failure, some factors predispose to the occurrence of respiratory muscle fatigue. The respiratory centers are hyperstimulated, which increases the work load of the respiratory muscles (108). This work load is likewise increased by the high airway resistances. The efficiency of the respiratory muscles is impaired by hyperinflation (69, 114) and by airway resistances. In the extreme case, the diaphragm contracts isometrically, i.e., with energy demand without production of work. Furthermore, the acute respiratory acidosis itself decreases the contractility and endurance time of the diaphragm in humans, which could lead to respiratory muscle fatigue (62).

The oxygen cost of breathing is increased in COPD patients (45), but it is unclear whether muscle blood flow is maintained at an adequate level in relation to muscle work load. It is known that muscle blood flow increases when contractile activity increases. However, beyond a critical level (16), mechanical compression of diaphragmatic vessels decreases blood flow. When one adds the effect of cor pulmonale and right heart failure, which may impair cardiac output, respiratory blood flow may decrease below levels required to adequately supply substrates and oxygen.

Diaphragmatic fatigue can be detected in various ways (34). The assessment of diaphragmatic fatigue is more difficult than for other skeletal muscles because one cannot measure the generated tension directly; only the mechanical transformation of that tension into pressure can be measured. The transdiaphragmatic pressure, defined as the difference between the gastric pressure and esophageal pressure, closely reflects the tension produced by the contracting muscle. The clinical manifestations of inspiratory muscle fatigue, which is a paradoxic inward abdominal motion during inspiration (abdominal paradox) and an alteration between abdominal and rib cage breathing (respiratory alternans), have been described by Cohen *et al.*, (25). These investigators studied 12 patients intubated and ventilated for acute respiratory failure who exhibited difficulties during discontinuation of artificial ventilation. When respiratory support was discontinued, the investigators searched for clinical signs of respiratory muscle fatigue that could be correlated to electromyographic (EMG) signs of fatigue (low high/low ratio of the diaphragm and intercostal EMGs).

The EMG evidence of inspiratory muscle fatigue was described in six patients with a sequence of events leading to respiratory acidemia; EMG fatigue followed or accompanied by an increased respiratory rate was, in turn, followed by abnormalities of the thoracoabdominal mechanics (respiratory alternans, abdominal paradox) (100). These clinical manifestations were followed by an increase in $Paco_2$. It was concluded that these abnormal respiratory movements may be a reliable index of inspiratory muscle fatigue. Apart from diaphragmatic fatigue, abdominal paradox has been described only in diaphragmatic paralysis (86). Tobin *et al.* (115) recently studied normal subjects breathing against severe resistive loads and concluded that rib cage-abdominal paradox is predominantly due to an increase in respiratory load rather than to respiratory muscle fatigue because the paradox observed in this study was at a level of exercise that can be sustained indefinitely.

Diaphragmatic function can be assessed by recording transdiaphragmatic pressure and analyzing two parameters, the peak transdiaphragmatic pressure and the rate of relaxation of the transdiaphragmatic pressure. Impairment in diaphragmatic contractility reduces peak transdiaphragmatic pressure during maximum static inspiration effort (Pdi max) or during maximum sniff (Pdi sniff). However, the values of peak transdiaphragmatic pressure depend not only on diaphragmatic contractility, but also on the subject's ability and motivation to cooperate. Furthermore, the comparison of peak transdiaphragmatic pressure obtained at two different times is possible only if the abdominal compliance and also the muscle length and geometry (lung volumes) remained unchanged.

Changes in diaphragmatic contractility are also accompanied by changes in muscle relaxation time (fatigued muscles relaxing more slowly than fresh muscle) (36). This change in diaphragmatic relaxation time, which appears before the decrease in muscular tension, can be quantified by measuring the maximum transdiaphragmatic pressure relaxation rate or the time constant (τ) of the latter monoexponential phase of relaxation (38, 71). The latter index is interesting because it is not influenced by the amplitude of the peak transdiaphragmatic pressure but only by lung volume (τ decreases when lung volume increases). When τ is greater than 75 msec, diaphragmatic dysfunction may be suspected.

Changes in the frequency content of the diaphragmatic EMG during spontaneous breathing also provide information concerning diaphragmatic fatigue. Diaphragmatic muscle fatigue is associated with EMG redistribution from high to low frequencies. The technique is to ascertain the ratio of power in a high-frequency band to that of a low-frequency band (high to low ratio) of the diaphragmatic EMG. The high to low ratio of the diaphragm decreases with fatigue (51), with a time course and extent that closely match the prolongation of relaxation (38). As τ, the modification of the high to low ratio precedes overt fatigue. It is then possible to detect diaphragmatic mechanical impairment before the muscle fails as a pressure generator.

The other ways of assessing diaphragmatic function, i.e., the force frequency curve (8) or bilateral phrenic stimulation with single pulses (11), are difficult to use routinely in the intensive care unit.

The work of breathing can be increased if there is an occult PEEP or auto PEEP or intrinsic PEEP. In this case, there is a failure to reach the relaxation volume of the respiratory system. This will necessarily result in positive expiratory pressure because of lung elastic recoil at the end of expiratory time (91). This implies that the inspiratory muscles must develop sufficient force to overcome the opposing positive recoil pressure before inspiratory airflow can be initiated. Thus, a significant additional burden is placed on the inspiratory muscles, which are already disadvantaged. Intrinsic PEEP is positively correlated with mean expiratory resistance, indicating that the higher the resistance, the more inflated is the patient at the end-expiration (47).

Intrinsic PEEP is related to dynamic pulmonary hyperinflation, which is defined by an increase in functional residual capacity above relaxation volume due to dynamic factors. Three mechanisms can determine dynamic hyperinflation:

Discrepancy between the time needed to breathe out to relaxation volume and the time really available,
An increase in the postinspiratory inspiratory muscle activity,
Glottic constriction during inspiration.

Pepe and Marini (91) documented the presence of a positive end expiratory alveolar pressure during a brief occlusion of the expiratory part of the ventilator at the end of the total expiration in ventilated patients. This positive pressure, due to end-expiratory elastic recoil pressure, is related to an incomplete lung emptying.

In mechanically ventilated patients with acute exacerbation of COPD, there is an increased airway resistance and expiratory flow limitation, and a long time (i.e., more than 20 sec) is necessary to breathe out to residual volume. Such an expiration time cannot be used in any respiratory setting, and the expiration is suddenly cut off by the onset of mechanical inflation. In the early days of mechanical ventilation, functional residual capacity can be more than 1 liter above relaxation volume in COPD patients and intrinsic PEEP can be as high as 20 cm H_2O or more (21).

This intrinsic PEEP can have deleterious effects on cardiac output and oxygen transport. It is well known that intrinsic PEEP has adverse effects during the weaning phase of respiratory support. In respiratory modes requiring the patient's effort, intrinsic PEEP is added to the triggering pressure and the total pressure needed by inspiratory muscles to initiate inspiratory flow is increased. A slight degree of dynamic hyperinflation is present in COPD patients in stable condition. The difference between relaxation volume and FRC has not been measured directly, but the presence of intrinsic PEEP has been measured on the esophageal (pleural) pressure. PEEP is assumed by the difference between the onset of the negative deflection and the point corresponding to the beginning of the inspiratory flow (28). PEEP averaged 2.5 ± 1.5 cm H_2O in stable COPD patients (28) and 8.8 ± 2.3 cm H_2O in acutely ill but spontaneous breathing patients with COPD (47).

Ventilation-Perfusion Mismatching

Gas Exchange Abnormalities

It has long been postulated that ventilation is decreased and central drive impaired in COPD during acute failure. However, it is now well known that total ventilation is the same in normal subjects and stable COPD patients, while central drive assessed by $P_{O.1}$ is increased. It is still unclear why Pao_2 is decreased and $Paco_2$ increased in COPD patients. In fact, hypoxemia results mainly from the mismatching of ventilation to perfusion, which is one of the first disturbances to appear in COPD (118). This mismatching has been assessed by the multiple inert gas method (72).

The determinants of $Paco_2$ are metabolic and respiratory (121, 123). In COPD, $Paco_2$ is mainly related to respiratory variables. The relationship between $Paco_2$ and ventilation is given by the following equation:

$$Paco_2 = K.\dot{V}co_2/V(1-V_D/V_T) \qquad (4)$$

Where $\dot{V}co_2$ is the metabolic production of CO_2, $\dot{V}_E$ is minute ventilation, V_D is the dead space, and V_T is the tidal volume (23). In most cases, $\dot{V}co_2$ is normal in acute respiratory failure (12, 124), except in patients who are given food with very high carbohydrate contents during the weaning process from respiratory support. A high carbohydrate supply increases the respiratory requirements by increasing CO_2 production (29).

Minute ventilation is about the same during acute respiratory failure as in the stable state. It follows that the main reason for hypercapnia is the increased V_D/V_T ratio. This ratio, which amounts to 0.35 in a normal subject, can amount to 0.6 in stable COPD and even more (0.75–0.80) in cases of acute respiratory failure for the same $\dot{V}_E$ and $\dot{V}co_2$ values. Thus, a very different change in $Paco_2$ follows the same variation of V_D/V_T, if the starting V_D/V_T is low or high. For a 5% increase in ratio, the increment of $Paco_2$ is 25.9 mm Hg if starting $V_D/V_T = 0.75$, but only 2.56 mm Hg if starting $V_D/V_T = 0.3$ (31). If minute ventilation is not impaired, the pattern of breathing in a patient with COPD is different than that of a normal patient. They exhibit a significant lower tidal volume and higher respiratory frequency (Fig. 26.2). Therefore, there is a drop in alveolar ventilation, and a high v_D ventilation.

This abnormal breathing pattern can be improved by airway anesthesia. Murciano and associates (84) alleviated a depressant effect on airway receptors, particularly irritant receptors, by fiberoptic xylocaine administration from the larynx to the subsegmental bronchi in intubated or tracheotomized patients. They observed a small decrease in minute ventilation along with a significant increase in V_T. This new breathing pattern resulted in a 6 mm Hg fall of $Paco_2$ and an 8 mm Hg increase of $Paco_2$; these changes were associated with increased inspiratory efforts as reflected by $P_{0.1}$, which rose to very high values that would be expected to rapidly lead to fatigue of inspiratory muscles. In this connection it should be noted that in their study, all the patients required respiratory assistance after airway anesthesia (83). It can therefore be hypothesized that the breathing pattern in COPD patients is an economical one for inspiratory muscles and that their rapid shallow breathing is a compensatory mechanism to cope with the load imposed on the respiratory system.

Effects on O_2 Administration

Administration of O_2-enriched Air. It has often been postulated in the past that O_2 administration to COPD patients in acute respiratory failure may be dangerous because it removes the "hypoxic drive," leading to decreased minute ventilation and increased $Paco_2$. This theory was based entirely on indirect evidence (increased $Paco_2$) as $\dot{V}_E$ has not been measured in the past. As shown in Table 26.1, after 30 minutes of administration of O_2-enriched air ($Fio_2 = 0.4$) there was only a small decrease in $\dot{V}_E$ (from 11.4 ± 0.9 to 9.8 ± 0.7 liter min), averaging about 14% of the room air, value (9). This was due to the small reduction in V_T and respiratory function (Fig. 26.3). On the whole, however, the

Table 26.1
Mean Values ($\pm$ SE) in 20 COPD Patients in Acute Respiratory Failure Breathing Room Air and O_2-Enriched Air for 30 Minutes ($Fio_2 \simeq 0.4$)[a]

	Room Air	O_2-Enriched Air
$Paco_2$ (mm Hg)	61 ± 2	68 ± 3
Pao_2 (mm Hg)	38 ± 2	120 ± 13
$\dot{V}_E$ (liter/min)	11.4 ± 0.9	9.8 ± 0.7
P_{O1} (cm H_2O)	8.3 ± 0.8	4.9 ± 0.9

[a]From Aubier M, Murciano D, Fournier M, Milic-Emili J, Pariente R, Derenne JP. Central respiratory drive in acute respiratory failure of patients with chronic obstructive pulmonary disease. Am Rev Respir Dis 1980;122:191–199.

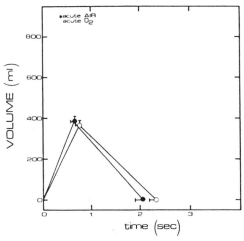

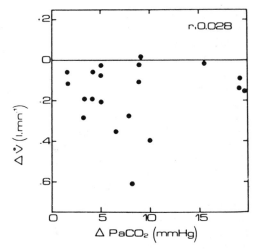

Figure 26.3. The average respiratory cycle in 20 COPD patients in acute respiratory failure during room air breathing (○) and after 30 minutes of administration of O_2-enriched air (0). Bars indicate 1 SE. (From Aubier M, Murciano D, Fournier M, Milic-Emili J, Pariente R, Derenne JP. Central respiratory drive in acute respiratory failure of patients with chronic obstructive pulmonary disease. Am Rev Respir Dis 1980;122:191–199.

Figure 26.4. The relationship between change in ventilation ($\Delta\dot{V}$) and in arterial $Paco_2$ ($\Delta Paco_2$) following 30 minutes of inhalation of O_2-enriched air in COPD patients in acute respiratory failure. No significant correlation is found ($r = 0.028$). (From Aubier M, Murciano D, Fournier M, Milic-Emili J, Pariente R, Derenne JP. Central respiratory drive in acute respiratory failure of patients with chronic obstructive pulmonary disease. Am Rev Respir Dis 1980;122:191–199.

breathing pattern was not very affected. The Pao_2, on the other hand, rose to 120 ± 13 mm Hg (Table 26.1), a value at which most of the peripheral hypoxic stimulus is removed.

Thus, in acutely ill COPD patients, removal of the hypoxic stimulus does not necessarily result in a substantial drop in $\dot{V}_E$. The $Paco_2$ rose during inhalation of O_2-enriched air by an average of 7 mm Hg; however, no significant correlation was found between the increase in $Paco_2$ and the drop of $\dot{V}_E$ resulting from the administration of O_2-enriched air (Fig. 26.4). Interestingly enough, after inhalation of O_2-enriched air for 30 minutes, $P_{0.1}$ decreased to an average of 4.9 ± 0.9 cm H_2O, the drop amounting to 40% of the corresponding room air value.

The $P_{0.1}$ values of this magnitude (4.9 cm H_2O) are found in COPD patients in the stable state (9, 108) and hence can probably be sustained in the absence of respiratory muscle fatigue. In this context it should be stressed that in these 20 patients administration of O_2-enriched air resulted in a much smaller drop of $\dot{V}_E$ and

V_T/T_I (both averaging 14%) than of $P_{0.1}$ (40%) (9). This implies a decrease in the "effective inspiratory impedance" because following the administration of O_2-enriched air, both V_T/T_I and $\dot{V}_E$ relative to $P_{0.1}$ were proportionately much greater than during room air breathing. This phenomenon has been found in stable COPD patients previously subjected to O_2-enriched air (9, 108) and is consistent with the decrease in airway resistance found by Astin (6) in stable COPD patients following inhalation of 30% O_2 in nitrogen.

Thus, in most COPD patients in acute respiratory failure, administration of O_2-enriched air appears to result in a drop of $P_{0.1}$ values that can probably be sustained without the development of muscle fatigue. This is associated with little change in $\dot{V}_E$, substantially increased Pao_2, and only moderately increased $Paco_2$.

Administration of 100% O_2. Table 26.2 shows the effect of 100% O_2 administration in a group of 22 COPD patients in acute respiratory failure. (12). During room air breathing, their values of $\dot{V}_E$ and Pao_2 and

Paco$_2$ were similar to those of the patients in Table 26.1. The administration of o$_2$ for 15 minutes resulted in a very small drop of minute ventilation, averaging about 7% of the room air value. Inasmuch as the values of Paco$_2$ and $\dot{V}_E$ during room air breathing were similar in these patients and in the 20 patients in Table 26.1, these results suggest that 100% o$_2$ administration causes, if anything, a smaller drop in $\dot{V}_E$ than administration of o$_2$-enriched air. Thus, the tenet that pure o$_2$ administration by removing the hypoxic stimulus causes a drop in $\dot{V}_E$, which in turn results in increased Paco$_2$, cannot be sustained. In this connection it should be noted that neither V_T nor respiratory function was significantly changed after 15 minutes of 100% o$_2$ administration to the patients listed in Table 26.2.

Administration of pure o$_2$ resulted in a much greater increase of Paco$_2$ (Table 26.2) than observed following the administration of o$_2$-enriched air (Table 26.1), namely 23 versus 7 mm Hg. As only a small fraction (about 5 mm Hg) of the total Paco$_2$ observed following 100% O$_2$ breathing could be attributed to the concomitant drop in $\dot{V}_E$, the data in Table 26.2 imply that most of the increase in Paco$_2$ resulting of administration of pure o$_2$ must have been due to other factors. Since Vco$_2$ was not significantly affected by o$_2$ inhalation in these patients, it follows from equation 4 that V$_D$ must have increased substantially. Indeed, the percent V$_D$/V$_T$ ratio was 77 ± 2 (SE) during room breathing, and rose to 82 ± 2 after 15 minutes of 100% o$_2$ inhalation, a significant difference (p < 0.01). The

increase in V$_D$ (reflecting increased arterial to alveolar Pco$_2$ difference) could be attributed both to the "Haldane effect" (67) and to changes in $\dot{V}_A/\dot{Q}$ distribution secondary to a shift of blood flow from poorly ventilated areas in the lung resulting from release of hypoxic vasoconstriction (66, 122). In addition, lung units with a low $\dot{V}/\dot{Q}$ ratio may become unstable and collapse when 100% o$_2$ is inhaled, thus increasing the shunt (122).

The results obtained with 100% o$_2$ administration confirm previous observations, namely that in COPD patients in acute respiratory failure the increase in Paco$_2$ is more marked with pure o$_2$ administration than with inhalation of o$_2$-enriched air. Contrary to previous belief, however, these results show that the more pronounced increase of Paco$_2$ during 100% o$_2$ breathing is not due to a depression in $\dot{V}_E$, it rather reflects an impairment of gas exchange within the lung.

PATHOPHYSIOLOGY OF ACUTE RESPIRATORY FAILURE IN PATIENTS WITH ASTHMA

Airway Dynamics and Lung Volumes

During acute asthma attacks the increase in bronchial smooth muscle tone tends to induce closure of small airways at higher than normal volumes. Airway resistances are increased 5 to 15 times the normal amount (98). The closure of subsegmental airways results in a large increase in residual volume and functional residual capacity, a shift of maximal expiratory flow volume curve without a change in its slope, and a severe reduction of FVC and FEV$_1$ without an important decrease in the FEV$_1$/FVC ratio. The only way to keep the airway open is to increase lung volume and transpulmonary pressure, resulting in an increased outward radial traction on the airway. The higher the bronchial tone closing the distal airway, the higher the lung volume must be to keep them open (41). Functional residual capacity could be 100% or more of predicted total lung capacity (92). Martin and De Troyer (73) have shown that, during histamine-induced broncho-

Table 26.2
Mean Values (± SE) in 22 COPD Patients in Acute Respiratory Failure Breathing Room Air and 100% o$_2$ for 15 Minutes [a]

	Room Air	100% o$_2$
Paco$_2$ (mm Hg)	65 ± 3	88 ± 5
Pao$_2$ (mm Hg)	38 ± 2	225 ± 23
$\dot{V}_E$ (liter/min)	10.2 ± 0.5	9.5 ± 0.7

[a] From Aubier M, Murciano D, Milic-Emili J, et al. Effects of administration of O$_2$ on ventilation and blood gases in patients with chronic obstructive pulmonary disease during acute respiratory failure. Am Rev Respir Dis 1980;122:747–754.

constriction, there was a significant postinspiratory muscle activity. Inspiratory intercostal and accessory muscle activity account for displacement of the rib cage compartment of chest wall. The diaphragm may also be actively involved during expiration. (82). This increased lung volume, which is seen radiologically, can be underestimated by the helium dilution method because of impaired ventilation in obstructed areas.

The Work of Breathing

Many factors increase the work of breathing:

hyperinflation through its effects on the Laplace's relationship,
airway obstruction and need for active expiratory muscle work,
postinspiratory muscle activity,
decreased dynamic lung compliance caused by overinflation in nonobstructed units, and
reduced pressure volume relationship of the thorax at high lung volumes.

Permutt (93) has calculated that an increase in functional residual capacity of 2.5 liters with a tidal volume of 500 ml lead, to an 11-fold increase in the work of breathing. Oxygen consumption by the respiratory muscle increases and may lead to respiratory muscle fatigue and hypercapnic ventilatory failure.

Gas Exchange

The uneven distribution of inspired gas leads to marked variations in time constants of different lung units and ventilation-perfusion ratio mismatching. These disturbances are reflected in arterial blood gas change.

There is a strong correlation between hypoxemia and severe airway obstruction (70) Fig. 26.5). A complete airway obstruction caused by plugging secretions can lead to a right and left anatomic shunting. Hypoxic vasoconstriction may reduce this shunt by diverting blood flow from nonventilated areas. Dead volume may be increased in some instances, but diffusion limitation does not contribute to arterial hypoxemia.

Arterial hypoxemia may be worsened by the administration of certain drugs such isoproterenol that increase $\dot{V}/\dot{Q}$ inequality by increasing blood flow in poorly ventilated areas (44). Finally, if airway obstruction worsens or if respiratory muscle fatigue appears, alveolar ventilation may fall and hypoxemia occurs with concomitant hypercarbia. There is no linear relationship between FEV_1 and $Paco_2$, but hypercapnia is more often observed with very low FEV_1 values (below 25% of predicted values) (70) (Fig. 26.5).

Lactic acidosis may be seen with severe asthma (3). It is believed to result from a combination of lactate overproduction by the respiratory muscles and lactate underutilization resulting from hypoperfusion of the liver and skeletal muscle. This metabolic disturbance reflects severe airway obstruction and life-threatening respiratory failure.

TREATMENT

There is no single approach to treatment of acute respiratory failure in patients with COPD. Endotracheal intubation and mechanical ventilation are not indicated for all the patients. Assisted or controlled ventilation allows rapid improvement of gas exchange and easy suction of secretions. It exposes the patient to a variety of complications, including a decrease in cardiac output, complete dependence of the patient on the machine and on the people who control him or her, and to secondary problems, particularly those linked to complications of intubation and tracheostomy of the vocal cords and the trachea.

The treatment of acute respiratory failure is conservative if the patient is managed without intubation or tracheostomy and mechanical ventilation. A majority of cases of acute respiratory failure in COPD can be treated in this manner. However, it is still difficult to predict which patients will require mechanical ventilation and when it should be instituted. Furthermore, there is no general agreement about which kind of ventilatory support is preferable. In any case, the patients should be treated in an intensive care unit if at all possible.

Conservative treatment is preferable if the correction of life-threatening hypox-

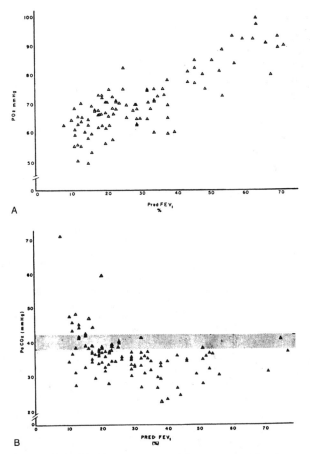

Figure 26.5. **A,** percent predicted FEV_1 versus arterial oxygen tension in acute asthma. **B,** percent predicted FEV_1 versus arterial carbon dioxide tension in acute asthma. The normal range of $Paco_2$ is shown by the shaded area. (From McFadden ER Jr, Lyons HA. Arterial-blood gas tension in asthma. N Engl J Med 1968;278:1027–1030.)

emia is possible, i.e., that the administration of oxygen increases oxygen saturation of the arterial blood above 90% and that the oxygen-induced acidemia does not reach dangerous values. The aims of conservative treatment are improvement of oxygen saturation, removal of secretions, decrease of mechanical load, improvement of respiratory muscle force and endurance, correction of electrolyte abnormalities, and treatment of primary or secondary infection and thrombosis, while at the same time avoiding complications.

Metabolic Disorders

Although an important goal of treating air pump failure is to improve the contractility endurance of the respiratory muscle by pharmacologic agents, another one is also to recognize and treat electrolyte disturbance that by itself, can compromise muscle function.

Acidosis

Metabolic Acidosis

Metabolic acidosis has been shown to be an important determinant in the contractile process of skeletal muscle. Indeed, *in vitro*, an excellent correlation has been found between the degree of acidosis and the decrease in contractile force (46). The same phenomenon has also been recently demonstrated in the dog *in vivo* (102).

Respiratory Acidosis

Juan et al. (62) have recently studied the effect of acute changes in $Paco_2$ on diaphragmatic contractility in normal subjects. This was achieved by measuring the ability of the diaphragm to generate pressure at a given level of excitation by determining the relation between the electrical activity of the diaphragm and transdiaphragmatic pressure during a voluntary quasi-isometric inspiratory effort carried out at different levels of end-tidal carbon dioxide. They found that acute respiratory acidosis equivalent to an $Paco_2$ of about 54 mm HG decreases the contractility and endurance time of the diaphragm in humans.

Electrolyte Disorders

The influence of various electrolyte disorders on the contractility of the respiratory muscles is still not well known. We recently studied the effect of hypophosphatemia, a frequent laboratory finding in patients with respiratory illness, in eight patients with acute respiratory failure who were artificially ventilated (10). Diaphragmatic function was evaluated in each patient before and after correction of hypophosphatemia; the contractile properties of the diaphragm were assessed by measuring the transdiaphragmatic pressure generated at functional residual capacity during bilateral supramaximal electrical stimulation of the phrenic nerves. In all the patients, the increase in serum phosphorous was accompanied by a marked increase in transdiaphragmatic pressure after phrenic stimulation; the mean increase in transdiaphragmatic pressure for the eight patients averaged 70% (Fig. 26.6). These results clearly demonstrate that diaphragmatic function is impaired by hypophosphatemia, which may lead to weaning difficulties and thus may prolong artificial ventilation. This illustrates, therefore, the importance of the treatment of metabolic disorders in critically ill patients.

Oxygen Therapy

Oxygen therapy is the first priority in acute failure COPD because of the potentially

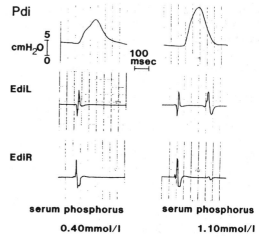

Figure 26.6. Typical tracings of transdiaphragmatic pressure (Pdi) and electrical activity of the left hemidiaphragm (EdiL) and the right hemidiaphragm (EdiR) generated during phrenic stimulations in one patient before *(left panel)* and after *(right panel)* correction of hypophosphatemia. (From Aubier M, Murciano D, Lecocguic Y, et al. effect of hypophosphatemia on diaphragmatic contractility in patients with acute respiratory failure. N Engl J Med 1985;313:420–424.)

lethal effects of severe hypoxemia. Methods of administration of oxygen were carefully set forth by Campbell (22) 20 years ago, and whatever method is chosen—Venturi mask (103) or low flow by nasal prongs—the same clinical risks linked to hypercapnia should be watched. Although the reasons for the increase in $Paco_2$ when oxygen is administered may be different from what was generally accepted some years ago, it remains an unquestionable fact that uncontrolled oxygen administration can cause dangerous respiratory acidosis. On the other hand, the risks of respiratory acidosis should not be overestimated and oxygen should be administered in order to obtain oxygen saturation <90% (22).

Antibiotics

The role that respiratory tract infection plays in the onset of exacerbation in patients with chronic bronchitis is unclear. There are conflicting data on the role of tracheobronchial microflora and the usefulness of antibiotics in this disease. Many studies demonstrated a limited benefit for anti-microbial treatment in acute exacerbations of chronic bronchitis.

Nicotra and associates (88) did not find any subjective or objective improvement in any parameters in patients who received tetracycline. However, Anthonisen and associates (2) studied the effects of doxycycline or trimethoprim versus placebo in 173 patients with acute exacerbation of COPD and found a 63% success rate with antibiotics and 55% with placebo (p<0.01). To assess the role of respiratory tract infection, Fagon and associates (43) studied 54 patients with acute exacerbation of COPD who had been receiving mechanical ventilation. To overcome the major problem of contamination by upper respiratory tract secretions and to rule out a simple colonization, the authors used a protected specimen brush that is passed through a fiberscope. The use of a double-lumen catheter with a protected brush has been documented to have reasonable precision in identifying the causative organisms in pneumonia (24) and should lead to a more accurate description of the pathogens responsible for distal bronchial infection in acute exacerbation of COPD. A threshold $>10^3$ colony-forming units per milliliter was usually used for distinguishing colonization from infection in patients with pneumonia. Twenty-four patients had quantitative cultures $>10^3$ colony-forming units per milliliter, which probably reflected a heavy small airway infection. Twenty-seven patients had a sterile protective specimen brush culture. *Haemophilus parinfluenzae* were the bacteria most frequently isolated, followed by *Streptococcus pneumoniae* and *H. influenzae*. Nine patients with sterile culture did not receive antibiotics. Their short-term outcome did not differ from that of other patients without infection treated by empiric antibiotherapy. Distal bronchial infection is probably not the sole cause of acute exacerbation of COPD. The role of non-bacterial infection needs to be investigated. The use of antibiotics seems appropriate when infection is proved, but the clinical practice of systematically giving antimicrobial treatment for exacerbations of COPD should probably be reassessed.

Heparin

Pulmonary emboli are a frequent cause of acute respiratory failure. Furthermore, they often complicate the course of acute respiratory failure (54) and must be treated with heparin. Although some investigators disagree (81), there is a general consensus for the preventive use of a low-dose heparin treatment in COPD patients with acute respiratory failure without contraindications such as bleeding, severe liver disease, or malignant hypertension (54).

Bronchodilators

Acute respiratory failure is characterized primarily by an increased resistive load on the respiratory muscles. With the threat of respiratory muscle fatigue, alleviation of the load is one of the major goals of therapy. Because smooth muscle contraction as well as inflammation are generally considered prominent mechanisms of the increased airway obstruction (26, 95), bronchodilators are generally indicated. However, in COPD patients the role of smooth muscle tone in causing airway obstruction has not been proven. In an extensive study based on the examination of the lungs of 48 patients who died during the NIH clinical trial of Intermittent Positive Pressure Breathing, Nagai and colleagues (85) reported that they could not find any relationship between central airway muscle and air flow reversibility. Furthermore, they found that emphysema and two of its closely related lesions (pigmentations and proportion of airway less than 0.4 mm in diameter) were negatively related to bronchodilator response.

There are six classes of agents (methylxanthines, calcium channel blockers, β_2-adrenergic agonists, anticholinergics, inflammatory mediator release blockers, and glucocorticoids) that are known to have bronchodilator effects, but only two (methylxanthines and β_2-stimulants) are commonly used in acute respiratory failure of COPD. Both act directly on the smooth muscle cells through an increase of intracellular phosphorylase activity (77, 89). Methylxanthines inhibit the degradation of 3'5'-cyclic adenosine monophosphate (cyclic AMP) by phosphodiesterase, whereas β-adrenergic agonists increase the conversion of adenosine triphosphate cyclic into AMP. Thus, both types of drugs tend to raise intracellular cyclic AMP by different mechanisms, allowing a possible combined use of these drugs (32). However, other mechanisms responsible for the bronchodilator effect of theophylline have also been reported: calcium antagonist effect, inhibition of histamine and leukotriene release from mast cells, and inhibition of the effects of prostaglandins on smooth muscle (77).

Both methylxanthines and β_2-stimulants have been used in the treatment of acute respiratory failure for many years. However, in the last decade, other pharmacologic properties of these drugs have been emphasized. It has been shown that the force of contraction of the diaphragm is increased by aminophylline in the dog (13, 104), in normal human subjects (7), and in COPD patients (83).

The force of contraction of the fatigued diaphragm can be improved in various animals by aminophylline (14, 58, 117), isoproterenol (58), terbutaline (14, 15) or milrinone (99), but not by salbutamol (58). Caffeine, another methylxanthine, has been shown to potentiate the maximal twitch force and to increase the force at low frequency of stimulation in strips of diaphragm from albino mice and in strips of human sternomastoids (61). In humans, improvement in pressure frequently curves of the fatigued diaphragm was observed after aminophylline (7). In stable hypoxemic and hypercapnic COPD patients, theophylline increases diaphragmatic contractility and resistance to fatigue (83). Caffeine increases diaphragmatic contractility in humans (110).

The mechanisms of action of methylxanthines on diaphragmatic contractility are not fully understood (14). Caffeine increases the release and inhibits the uptake of calcium in isolated sarcoplasmic reticulum (37) and increases the sensitivity of the myofilaments to calcium (42). At low dose, it increases myoplasmic-free calcium and initiates contraction by calcium release from storage sites (48); at high dose, it inhibits relaxation by preventing released calcium reaccumulation (55). Theophylline

affects contractility by a different mechanism. There are experimental results supporting the hypothesis that theophylline may influence transmembrane calcium movements (106, 116) by a mechanism that is not fully understood. The main effects of theophylline on respiration are as follows: (a) it improves forced expiratory flow rates in variable manner (39, 57, 120); (b) it stimulates the central nervous system and respiratory center (57, 77); (c) it stimulates ciliary beat frequency, increases the water flux toward the lumen, augments net ion secretion, promotes the secretion of mucus, at least in the lower airways (119), and enhances mucociliary clearance (75, 119); and (d) it increases diaphragmatic contractility (14) but does not seem to affect other muscles, in particular, it does not prevent or reverse sternomastoid fatigue in humans (68). It follows that the analysis of the net effects of theophylline on minute ventilation, arterial blood gases, and respiratory response to stimulants such as Pa_{CO_2} and Pa_{O_2} will depend on the relative importance of each of these effects in individual subjects.

On the other hand, it has been shown that aminophylline improves and may even normalize right ventricular ejection fraction in COPD patients, with concomitant increments in left ventricular ejection fraction. Whether this is a direct effect on myocardial muscle of the drug or whether it is secondary to changes in airway resistance and pleural pressure needs further evaluation (74).

It is still debatable whether or not theophylline and caffeine are major therapeutic agents in acute respiratory failure of COPD. Although respiratory muscle fatigue is likely to be a major clinical problem, the clinical efficacy of methylxanthines in acute respiratory failure of patients with COPD has not been undoubtedly proven up to now. Rice and associates (97) were unable to show that the administration of aminophylline provided significant additional benefit to an otherwise standard treatment, which is in agreement with the findings of Eaton and colleagues (35) in the stable chronic state. The regimen recommended by Mitenko and Ogilvie (80) may not be appropriate in the case of severe airway obstruction; the clearance of the drug is increased and interindividual variability of clearance is higher, making the plasma theophylline concentration resulting from any dosage relatively uncertain (96). Therapy caused a 26% reduction of cerebral blood flow in patients with severe COPD studied by Bowton and co-workers (20). Furthermore, theophylline has many toxic side effects, with a therapeutic dosage situated in a range close to serum levels that are susceptible to cause "major" or "minor" deleterious effects (19, 56, 105). In addition, theophylline disposition has been found abnormal in patients with severe COPD (27) and in acutely ill patients (96). Loading and maintenance dosage of the drug should be carefully controlled by repeated serum level measurements. In general, a mean serum level of about 10–15 $\mu g/ml$ should be obtained.

β-Adrenergic stimulants are potent bronchodilators (77). Terbutaline improves mucociliary clearance (101). Furthermore, terbutaline improves systolic ventricular function mainly by decreasing pulmonary and systemic vascular resistances, i.e. biventricular afterload in patients with severe COPD (17). Terbutaline has a positive inotropic effect on the fatigued diaphragm in the dog (14), but the clinical implications of this finding are unknown.

β-Adrenergic stimulants may be administered by different routes. Aerosols may be administered with compressor-powered nebulizers or by mechanical assistance. Whether or not metered-dose inhalers are as effective as powered nebulizer therapy remains to be proven (94, 127). Tablets or parenteral preparations may be prescribed, depending on the clinical status of the patient and the physician's habits (77). The most common side effect of β_2-adrenergic agonists is tremor. When theophylline is given in association with β_2-agonists, the possibility of myocardial toxicity has been hypothetized (87).

The efficacy of anticholinergic drugs has been reported as superior to sympathomimetics in stable COPD patients (76, 105). Whether anticholinergic drugs are indicated in acute respiratory failure of COPD patients is still unknown.

Corticosteroids

Long-term studies have reported some benefit from corticosteroids in some but not all patients with stable COPD (53, 65, 76, 94). Yet other studies have shown negative results (40, 109). In stable COPD patients, randomized placebo-controlled crossover trials of corticosteroids have recently shown beneficial results (18, 78) that cannot be explained by significant psychological test ratings (79).

In COPD patients with acute respiratory failure, the prescription of corticosteroids remains controversial. Albert and associates (1) have reported in a double-blind study that methylprednisolone improved spirometric parameters in a group of patients undergoing acute respiratory failure. However, corticosteroids have adverse reactions, including hypokalemia (which may impair respiratory muscle function), sodium retention, psychiatric disorders, and, particularly, gastric ulcer and bleeding. Furthermore, there is no evidence that steroids improve the prognosis of acute failure. It follows that until sufficient evidence is provided, the prescription of corticosteroids should not be generalized, but may be indicated when severe bronchospasm or excessive inflammation is present, *i.e.*, when past history and behavior suggest some component of asthma. Because of the potential severity of their complications, the prescription of steroids should require careful control.

Nutritional Support

The institution of nutritional support should be preceded by nutritional assessment, i.e., history-taking, clinical examination, and laboratory measures including serum albumin and transferin, prealbumin and retinol-binding protein, 24-hr output of creatinine and creatinine height index, and determination of 24-hr nitrogen balance (124). Ideally, nutritional support should provide substrates qualitatively and quantitatively adapted to meet the body's demand. Unfortunately, the changes in metabolism and energy expenditure in acute respiratory failure are not accurately known. Patients with stable COPD have a higher metabolic rate (50). Metabolic requirements may be increased in acute respiratory failure.

However, there are insufficient data to make definitive recommendations regarding the optimal pattern of nutritional support in acute respiratory failure (124). In the early 1970s, it was not unusual for patients to receive 4000–5000 kcal per day (63). Excessive nutritional support may cause hypercapnia (29). High carbohydrate loading is generally well tolerated in COPD patients (49), although fat emulsions produce smaller CO_2 production than glucose (4). Protein and amino acids can modify the respiratory response to hypoxia (128) and CO_2 (5, 128). In stable emphysematous patients, nutritional repletion increases body weight and respiratory muscle strength (125). In acute respiratory failure, significant gains in lean body mass are unlikely, and all that can be expected is to prevent the "step" decline in the nutritional status (124). The optimal proportion of protein, lipid, and carbohydrate is still not universally accepted (124); the optimal amount of kilocalories is probably around 2500 to 3000 (63), although that is still a matter of debate.

References

1. Albert RK, Martin TR, Lewis SW. Controlled clinical trial of methylprednisolone in patients with chronic bronchitis and acute respiratory insufficiency. Ann Intern Med 1980;92:753–758.
2. Anthonisen NR, Manfred J, Warren CPW, Hershfield ES, Harging GKM, Nelson NA. Antibiotic therapy in exacerbations of chronic obstructive pulmonary disease. Ann Intern Med 1987;106:196–204.
3. Appel D. Lactic acidosis in severe asthma. Am J Med 1983;75:580–585.
4. Askanazi J, Nordenstrom J, Rosenbaum SH, et al. Nutrition for the patient with respiratory failure: glucose vs. fat. Anesthesiology 1981;54:373–377.
5. Askanazi J, Weissman C, Lasala PA, Milic-Emili J, Kinney JM. Effect of protein intake on ventilatory drive. Anesthesiology 1984;60:106–110.
6. Astin T. The relationship between arterial blood oxygen saturation carbon dioxide tension, and pH and airway resistance during 30% oxygen breathing in patients with chronic bronchitis with airway obstruction. Am Rev Respir Dis 1970;102:382–387.
7. Aubier M, De Troyer A, Sampson M, Macklem PT, Roussos C. Aminophylline improves diaphragmatic contractility. N Engl J Med 1981;305:249–252.
8. Aubier M, Farkas G, De Troyer A, Mozes R, Roussos C. Detection of diaphragmatic fatigue in man by phrenic stimulation. J Appl Physiol 1981;51:499–508.
9. Aubier M, Murciano D, Fournier M, Milic-Emili J, Pariente R, Derenne JP. Central respiratory drive in acute respiratory failure of patients with chronic obstructive pulmonary disease. Am Rev Respir Dis 1980;122:191–199.
10. Aubier M, Murciano D, Lecocguic Y, et al. Effect of hypophosphatemia on diaphragmatic contractility in patients with acute respiratory failure. N Engl J Med 1985;313:420–424.
11. Aubier M, Murciano D, Lecocguic Y, Viires N, Pariente R. Bilateral phrenic stimulation: a simple technique to assess diaphragmatic fatigue in humans. J Appl Physiol 1985;58:58–64.
12. Aubier M, Murciano D, Milic-Emili J, et al. Effects of administration of O_2 on ventilation and blood gases in patients with chronic obstructive pulmonary disease during acute respiratory failure. Am Rev Respir Dis 1980;122:747–754.
13. Aubier M, Murciano D, Viires N, Lecocguic Y, Palacios S, Pariente R. Increased ventilation due to improved diaphragmatic efficiency during aminophylline infusion. Am Rev Respir Dis 1983;148:54–59.
14. Aubier M, Murciano D, Viires N, Lecocguic Y, Pariente R. Respiratory muscle pharmacotherapy. Bull Eur Physiopathol Respir 1984;20:459–466.
15. Aubier M, Viires N, Murciano D, Medrano G, Lecocguic Y, Pariente R. Effects and mechanism of action of terbutaline on diaphragmatic contractility and fatigue. J Appl Physiol 1984;56:922–929.
16. Bellemare F, Wight C, Lavigne M, Grassino A. Effect of tension and timing of contraction in the blood flow of the canine diaphragm. J Appl Physiol, 1983;54:1597–1606.
17. Berger HJ, Matthay RA, Loke J, Marshall RC, Gottschalk A, Zaret BL. Assessment of cardiac performance with quantitative radionucleide angiocardiography: right ventricular ejection fraction with reference to findings in chronic obstructive pulmonary disease. Am J Cardiol 1978;41:897–905.
18. Blair GP, Light RW. Treatment of chronic obstructive pulmonary disease with corticosteroids. Comparison of daily vs. alternate-day therapy. Chest 1984;86:524–528.
19. Bone RC. Treatment of respiratory failure due to advanced chronic obstructive lung disease. Arch Intern Med, 1980; 37:49–50.
20. Bowton DL, Alford PT, McLees BD, Prough DS, Stump DA. The effect of aminophylline on cerebral blood flow in patients with chronic obstructive pulmonary disease. Chest 1987;91:874–877.
21. Broseghini C, Brandolese R, Poggi R, et al. Respiratory mechanics during the first day of mechanical ventilation in patients with pulmonary oedema and chronic airway obstruction. Am Rev Respir Dis 1988;138:355–361.

22. Campbell EJM. The Burns Amberson Lecture. The management of acute respiratory failure in chronic bronchitis and emphysema. Am Rev Respir Dis 1967;96:626–639.

23. Campbell EJM. Respiratory failure: definition, mechanisms and recent developments. Bull Eur Physiopathol Respir 1979;15:1–12.

24. Chastre T, Viau F, Brun P, et al. Prospective evaluation of protected specimen brush for the diagnosis of pulmonary infections in ventilated patients. Am Rev Respir Dis 1984;13:924–929.

25. Cohen CA, Zagelbaum G, Cross D, Roussos C, Macklem PT. Clinical manifestations of inspiratory muscle fatigue. Am J Med 1982;73:308–316.

26. Cosio MG, Guezzo M, Hogg JC, et al. The relations between structural changes in small airways and pulmonary function tests. N Engl J Med 1977;298:1277–1281.

27. Cusack BJ, Crowley JJ, Mercer GD, Charn NB, Vestal RE. Theophylline clearance in patients with severe chronic obstructive pulmonary disease receiving supplemental oxygen and the effect of acute hypoxemia. Am Rev Respir Dis 1986;133:1110–1140.

28. Dal-Vecchio L, Polese G, Poggi R, Rossi A. "Intrinsic" positive end expiratory pressure in stable patients with chronic obstructive pulmonary disease. Eur Resp J 1990;3:74–80.

29. Dark DS, Pingleton K, Kerby GR. Hypercapnia during weaning, a complication of nutritional support. Chest 1985;88:141–143.

30. Derenne JP, Couture J, Iscoe S, Whitelaw WA, Milic Emili J. Occlusion pressures in man rebreathing CO_2 under methoxyflurane anesthesia. J Appl Physiol 1976;40:805–814.

31. Derenne JP, Fleury B, Pariente R. Acute respiratory failure of chronic obstructive pulmonary disease. Am Rev Respir Dis 1988;138:1006–1033.

32. Dull WL, Alexander MR, Sadoul P, Woolson RF. The efficacy of isoproterenol inhalation for predicting the response to orally administered theophylline in chronic obstructive pulmonary disease. Am Rev Respir Dis 1982;126:656–659.

33. Dunnil MS. The pathology of asthma with special reference to changes in the bronchial mucosa. J Clin Pathol 1960;13:27–33.

34. Dureuil B, Aubier M. Assessment of diaphragmatic function in the intensive care unit. Intensive Care Med 1988;14:83–85.

35. Eaton ML, Green BA, Church TR, McGowan T, Niewoehner DF. Efficacy of theophylline in "irreversible" airflow obstruction. Ann Intern Med 1980;92:758–761.

36. Edwards RHT. Physiological analysis of skeletal muscle weakness and fatigue. Clin Sci Mol Med 1978;54:463–470.

37. Endo M. Mechanism of action of caffeine on the sarcoplasmic reticulum of skeletal muscle. Proc Jpn Acad 1975;51:479–484.

38. Esau SA, Bellemare F, Grassino A, Permutt S, Roussos C, Pardy RL. Changes in relaxation rate with diaphragmatic fatigue in humans. J Appl Physiol 1983;54:1353–1360.

39. Estenne M, Yernault JC, De Troyer A. Effect of parenteral aminophylline on lung mechanics in normal humans. Am Rev Respir Dis 1980;121:967–971.

40. Evans JA, Morrison IM, Saunders KB. A controlled trial of prednisolone in low dosage, in patients with chronic airways obstruction. Thorax 1974;29:401–406.

41. Even P, Sors H, Safran D. Interaction between ventilation and circulation in bronchial asthma and pulmonary emphysema. In: Cumming G, Bensignore G, eds. Pulmonary circulation in health and disease. New York: Plenum Press, 1980.

42. Fabiato A. Effects of cyclic AMP and phophodiesterase inhibitors on the contractile activation and the Ca^{2+} transient detected with segonin in skinned cardiac cells from rat and rabbit ventricules. J Gen Phyiol 1981;78:15a–16a.

43. Fagon JY, Chastre J, Trouillet JL, et al. Characterization of distal bronchial microflora during acute exacerbation of chronic bronchitis. Am Rev Respir Dis 1990;142:1004–1008.

44. Field GB. The effects of posture, oxygen, isoproterenol and atropine on ventilation-perfusion relationships in the lung in asthma. Clin Sci 1967;32:279–285.

45. Field S, Kelly S, Macklem PT. The oxygen cost of breathing in patients with cardiorespiratory disease. Am Rev Respir Dis 1982;126:9–13.

46. Fitts RH, Holloszy O. Lactate and contractile force in frog muscle during development of fatigue and recovery. Am J Physiol 1976;231:430–433.

47. Fleury B, Murciano D, Talamo C, Aubier M, Pareinte R, Milic Emili J. Work of breathing in patients with chronic obstructive pulmonary disease in acute respiratory failure. Am Rev Respir Dis 1985;131:816–821.

48. Ford LE, Podolsky RJ. Intracellular calcium movements in skinned muscle fibres. J Physiol (Lond) 1972;223:21–33.

49. Giseke T, Gurushanthaiah G, Glauser FL. Effects of carbohydrates on carbon dioxide excretion in patients with airway disease. Chest 1977;71:55–58.

50. Golstein S, Askanazi J, Weissman C, Thomashow B, Kinney JM. Energy expenditure in patients with chronic obstructive pulmonary disease. Chest 1987;91:222–224.

51. Gross D., Gassino A, Ross WDR, Macklem PT. Electromyogram pattern of diaphragmatic fatigue. J Appl Physiol 1979;46:1–7.

52. Hale KA, Ewing SL, Gosnell BA, Niewoehner DE. Lung disease in long-term cigarette smokers with and without chronic airflow obstruction. Am Rev Respir Dis 1984;130:716–721.

53. Harding SM, Freedman SA. A comparison of oral and inhaled steroids in patients with chronic airways obstruction: features determining response. Thorax 1978;33:214–218.

54. Harris SK, Bone RC, Ruth WE. The efficacy of low dose heparin for prevention of pulmonary embolism in a respiratory intensive care unit. Am Rev Respir Dis 1977;114:115–118.

55. Hellam DC, Podolsky RJ. Forced measurements in skinned muscle fibres. J Phiol (Lond) 1969;200:807–819.

56. Hendeles L, Weinberger M. Poisoning patients

with intravenous theophylline. Am J Hosp Pharm 1980;37:49–50.

57. Hendeles L, Weinberger M. Slow release theophylline. Rationale and basis for product selection. N Engl J Med 1983;308:760–764.

58. Howell S, Fitzgerald RS, Roussos CS. Effects of aminophylline, isopreterenol, and neostigmine on hypercapnic depression of diaphragmatic contractility. Am Rev Respir Dis 1985;132:241–247.

59. Jamal K, Cooney TP, Fleetman JA, Thurlbeck WM. Chronic bronchitis. Correlation of morphologic findings to sputum production and flow rates. Am Rev Respir Dis 1984;129–719–722.

60. Jeffery PK, Wardlow AJ, Nelson FC, Collins JV, Kay AB. Bronchial biopsies in asthma. Am Rev Respir Dis 1989;140:1745–1753.

61. Jones DA, Howell S, Roussos C, Edwards RHT. Low frequency fatigue in isolated skeletal muscles and the effects of methylxanthines. Clin Sci 1982;63:161–167.

62. Juan G, Calverey P, Talamo C, Schnader J, Roussos C. Effect of carbon dioxide on diaphragmatic function in human beings. N Engl J Med 1985;310:874–879.

63. Koretz RL. Nutritional support: whether or not some is good, more is not better. Chest 1985;88:2–3.

64. Laitinen LA, Heino M, Laitinen A, Kava T, Haahtela T. Damage of the airway epithelium and bronchial reactivity in patients with asthma. Am Rev Respir Dis 1985;131:599–606.

65. Lam UK, So SY, Yu DYC. Response to oral corticosteroids in chronic airway obstruction. Br J Dis Chest 1983;77:189–197.

66. Lee J, Read J. Effects of oxygen breathing on distribution of pulmonary blood flow in chronic obstructive lung disease. Am Rev Respir Dis 1967;96:1173–1180.

67. Lenfant C. Arterial-alveolar difference in PaCO$_2$ during air and oxygen breathing. J Appl Physiol 1966;21:1356–1362.

68. Lewis MI, Belham MJ, Sieck GC. Aminophylline and fatigue of the sternomastoid muscle. Am Rev Respir Dis 1986;133:672–675.

69. Macklem PT. Hyperinflation. Am Rev Respir Dis 1984;129:1–2.

70. McFadden ER Jr, Lyons HA. Arterial-blood gas tension in asthma. N Engl J Med 1968;278:1027–1030.

71. Mal H, Aubier M, Pamela F, Murciano D, Pariente R. Evaluation of the transdiaphragmatic pressure (Pdi) relaxation rate in COPD patients during respiratory failure. Bull Eur Physiopathol Respir 1987;23(suppl 12):359S.

72. Marthan R, Castaing Y, Manier G, Guenard H. Gas exchange alteration in patients with chronic obstructive lung disease. Chest 1985;87:470–475.

73. Martin JG, De Troyer A. The thorax and control of functional residual capacity. In: Roussos C, Macklem PT, eds. The thorax, Part B. New York: Marcel Dekker, 1985;899–921.

74. Matthay RA, Berger HJ, Loke J, Gottschalk A, Zaret BL. Effects of aminophylline upon right and left ventricular performance in chronic obstructive pulmonary disease. Am J Med 1978;65:903–910.

75. Matthys H. Effect of theophylline on mucociliary clearance. Eur J Respir Dis 1980;61(suppl):98–110.

76. Mendella LA, Manfreda J, Warren CPW, Anthonisen NR. Steroid response in stable obstructive pulmonary disease. Ann Intern Med 1982;96:17–21.

77. Miller WF, Geumei AM. Respiratory and pharmacological therapy in COLD. In: Petty TL, ed. Chronic obstructive pulmonary disease. 2nd ed. New York: Marcel Dekker, 1985:205–338.

78. Mitchell DM, Gildeh P, Rehahn M, Dimond AH, Collins JV. Effects of prednisolone in chronic airlow limitation. Lancet 1984;2:193–195.

79. Mitchell DM, Gildeh P, Rehahn M, Dimond AH, Collins JV. Psychological changes and improvement in chronic airflow limitation after corticosteroid treatment. Thorax 1984;39:924–927.

80. Mitenko PA, Ogilvie RI. Rational intravenous doses of theophylline. N Engl J Med 1973;289:600–603.

81. Moser KM, Lemoine JR, Nachtwey FJ, Spragg RG. Deep venous thrombosis and pulmonary embolism. JAMA 1981;246:1422–1424.

82. Muller N, Bryan AC, Zamel N. Tonic inspiratory muscle activity as a cause of hyperinflation in histamine induced asthma. J Appl Physiol 1980;49:869–875.

83. Murciano D. Aubier M, Lecocguic Y, Pariente R. Effects of theophylline on diaphragmatic strength and fatigue in patients with chronic obstructive pulmonary disease. N Engl J Med 1984;311:349–353.

84. Murciano D, Aubier M, Viau F, et al. Effects of airway anesthesia on patterns of breathing and blood gases in patients with COPD during acute respiratory failure. Am Rev Respir Dis 1982;126:113–117.

85. Nagai A, West WW, Thurlbeck WM. The National Institutes of Health Intermittent Positive Pressure Breathing Trial: pathology studies II: Correlation between morphologic findings, clinical findings, and evidence of expiratory air-flow obstruction. Am Rev Respir Dis 1989;32:946–953.

86. Newson Davis J, Goldman M, Casson M. Diaphragm function and alveolar hypoventilation. Q J Med 1976;45:89–100.

87. Nickles RA, Whitehusrt VE, Dohonoe RF. Combined use of beta adrenergic agonists and methylxanthines. N Engl J Med 1982;307:55–58.

88. Nicotra MB, Rivera M, Awe RJ. Antibiotic therapy of acute exacerbations of chronic bronchitis. A controlled study using tetracycline. Ann Intern Med 1982;97:18–21.

89. Olgivie RI. Clinical pharmacokinetics of theophylline. Clin Pharmacokinet 1978;3:267–293.

90. Parot S, Miara B, Milic Emili J, Gauthier H. Hypoxemia, hypercapnia and breathing pattern in patients with chronic obstructive pulmonary disease. Am Rev Respir Dis 1982;126:882–886.

91. Pepe PE, Marini JJ. Occult positive end expiratory pressure in mechanically ventilated patients with airflow obstruction. The auto PEEP effect. Am Rev Respir Dis 1982;126:166–70.

92. Peress L, Sybrecht G, Mackiem PT. The mechanisms of increase in total lung capacity during acute asthma. Am J Med 1976;61:165–169.

93. Permutt S. Some physiological aspects of asthma: bronchomuscular contraction and airways calibre. In: Porter R, Birch J, eds. Identification of asthma. CIBA Foundation Study Group no. 38. Londen: Churchill Livingston, 1971:63.

94. Petty TL. Rational respiratory therapy. N Engl J Med 1986;315:317–319.

95. Petty TL, Silvers EW, Stanford RE, Baird MD. Small airways pathology is related to increased closing capacity and abnormal slope of phase III in excised human lungs. Am Rev Respir Dis 1980;121:449–456.

96. Powell JR, Vozeh S, Hopewell P, Costello J, Sheiner LB, Rigelman S. Theophylline disposition in acutely ill hospitalized patients. The effect of smoking, heart failure, severe airway obstruction, and pneumonia. Am Rev Respir Dis 1978;118:229–238.

97. Rice KL, Leatherman JW, Duane PG, et al. Aminophylline for acute exacerbations of chronic obstructive pulmonary disease. A controlled trial. Ann Intern Med 1987;107:305–309.

98. Rochester DF, Arona NS. The respiratory muscles in asthma. In: Lavietes MH, Reichman L, eds. Symposium on bronchial asthma. Diagnostic aspects and management of asthma. New York: Purdue Frederick Co, 1982:27–38.

99. Rossing TH, Shannon K, Miller MJ. Effects of milrinone on contractility of rat diaphragm *in vitro*. Am Rev Respir Dis 1987;136:841–844.

100. Roussos Ch, Fixley M, Gross D, Macklem PT. Fatigue of respiratory muscles and their synergic behaviour. J Appl Physiol 1979;46:867–904.

101. Santa Cruz R, Landa J, Hirsch J, Sackner MA. Tracheal mucous velocity in normal men and patients with obstructive lung disease. Effects of terbutatline. Am Rev Respir Dis 1974;109:458–463.

102. Schader JY, Juan G, Howell S, Fitzgerald R, Roussos C. Arterial CO$_2$ partial pressure effects on diaphragmatic function. J Appl Physiol 1985;58:823–829.

103. Schiff MM, Massaro D. Effect of oxygen administration by a venturi apparatus on arterial blood gas values in patients with respiratory failure. N Engl J Med 1967;277:950–953.

104. Sigrist S, Thomas D, Howelle S, Roussos C. The effect of aminophylline on inspiratory muscle contractility. Am Rev Respir Dis 1982;126:46–50.

105. Skorodin MS. Pharmacologic management of obstructive lung disease. Am J Med 1986;81(suppl 5A):8–15.

106. Smith PA, Wight FF, Lehne RA. Potentiation of Ca^{2+} dependent K$^+$ activation by theophylline is independent of cyclic nucleotide elevation. Nature (Lond) 1979;280:400–402.

107. Snider GL. Chronic obstructive pulmonary disease: a definition and implications of structural determinants of airflow obstruction for epidemiology. Am Rev Respir Dis 1989;140:53–58.

108. Sorli J, Grassino A, Lorange G, Milic Emili J. Control of breathing in patients with chronic obstructive lung disease and acute respiratory failure. Clin Sci Mol Med 1977;52:395–403.

109. Stokes TC, Shaylor JM, O'reilly JF, Harrison BDW. Assessment of responsiveness in patients with chronic airflow obstruction. Lancet 1982;2:345–348.

110. Supinski GS, Kelsen SG. Comparison of the effects of aminophylline and caffeine on diaphragmatic contractility in man. Am Rev Respir Dis 1983;127(suppl):231.

111. Thompson AB, Daughton D, Robbins RA, Ghafouri MA, Oehlerking M, Rennard SI. Intraluminal airway inflammation in chronic bronchitis characterization and correlation with clinical parameters. Am Rev Respir Dis 1989;140:1527–1537.

112. Thurlbeck WM. Pathology of status asthmaticus. In: Weiss EB, ed. Status asthmaticus. Baltimore, University Park Press, 1978.

113. Thurlbeck WM. Pathophysiology of chronic obstructive pulmonary disease. Clin Chest Med 1990;11:389–403.

114. Tobin MJ. Respiratory muscles in disease. Clin Chest Med 1988;9:263–286.

115. Tobin MJ, Perez W, Guenther SM, Lodato RF, Dantzer DR. Does rib cage abdominal paradox signify respiratory muscle fatigue? J Appl Physiol 1987;63:851–860.

116. Varagic VM, Prostran M, Kentera D. Temperature dependence of the effects of isoprenaline, aminophylline and calcium ionophores on the isometric contractions of the isolated hemidiaphragm of the rat. Eur J Pharmacol 1979;55:1–9.

117. Viires N, Aubier M, Murciano D, Fleury B, Talamo C, Pariente R. Effect of aminophylline on diaphragmatic fatigue during acute respiratory failure. Am Rev Respir Dis 1984;129:396–402.

118. Wagner PD, Dautzker DR, Dueck R, Clausen JL, West JB. Ventilation-perfusion inequality in chronic obstructive pulmonary disease. J Clin Invest 1977;59:203–216.

119. Wanner A. Effects of methylxanthines on airway mucociliary function. Am J Med 1985;79(suppl 6A):16–21).

120. Weinberger M, Riegelman S. Rational use of theophylline for bronchodilatation. N Engl J Med 1974;291:151–153.

121. Weinberger SE, Schwartzstern RM, Woodrow JW. Hypercapnia. N Engl J Med 1989;321:1223–1231.

122. West JB. Pulmonary pathophysiology. The essentials. Baltimore: Williams & Wilkins, 1977.

123. West JB. Causes of carbon dioxide retention in lung disease. N Engl J Med 1987;284:1232–1236.

124. Wilson DD, Rogers RM, Hoffman RM, Nutrition and chronic lung disease. Am Rev Respir Dis 1985;132:1347–1365.

125. Wilson DO, Rogers RM, Sanders MH, Pennock BE, Reilly JJ. Nutritional intervention in malnourished patients with emphysema. Am Rev Respir Dis 1986;134:672–677.

126. Withelaw WA, Derenne JP, Milic Emili J. Occlusion pressure as a measure of respiratory center output in conscious man. Respir Physiol 1975;23:181–199.

127. Zibrak JD, Rosetti P. Wood E. Effect of reduction in respiratory therapy on patient outcome. Am Rev Respir Dis 1986;315:292–295.

128. Zwillich CW, Sahn SA, Weil JV. Effects of hypermetabolism on ventilation and chemosensitivity. J Clin Invest 1977;60:900-960

27

Weaning from Respiratory Support in Hypoxemic Pulmonary Parenchymal Failure

Peter M. Suter

Numerous critically ill patients develop pulmonary dysfunction and some degree of hypoxemia during their illness. (Conditions associated primarily with hypoventilation and elevated Paco$_2$ levels are discussed in the next chapter.) Although patients with severe gas exchange and parenchymal abnormalities can usually be maintained adequately by artificial respiratory means (see Chapter 25, "Acute Hypoxemic Respiratory Failure"), it is often not clear when disease resolution has progressed far enough to permit weaning from respiratory support. Furthermore, general principles governing initiation weaning are influenced by risk-benefit considerations. Prolonged intubation is associated with nocosomial pneumonia and tracheal mucosal damage. Prolonged positive-pressure ventilation can induce further parenchymal injury due to regional overdistension. However, premature weaning from respiratory support can severely worsen gas exchange and induce hemodynamic instability (10), cardiac arrhythmias, and death. Thus, decisions about weaning from respiratory support can be difficult.

Since extubation is the goal of weaning from mechanical respiratory support, patients should be evaluated as to how they may function if this support were removed either in part or in toto. Guidelines to define when weaning from artificial ventilation should be started in patients with hypoxemic respiratory failure cannot be uniform; the clinical course and the evolution of pulmonary failure are the most important considerations. The time to start withdrawing ventilatory support for these patients should clearly be during an interval of hemodynamic and metabolic stability. It is difficult to assess the patient's tolerance of the weaning process, and weaning may be unsuccessful in the unstable patient despite otherwise adequate intrinsic respiratory status. Furthermore, although patients can be weaned from positive-pressure ventilation while still receiving positive end-expiratory pressure (PEEP), requirements for a high F$_I$O$_2$ (>0.5) and high levels of PEEP (>15 cm H$_2$O) suggest severe gas exchange abnormalities that may result in worsening hypoxemia during weaning due to exercise-induced (spontaneous ventilation) decreases in mixed venous oxygen saturation.

The ideal conditions for weaning are situations in whom the acute process appears to have resolved, in whom cardiovascular and metabolic status are normal, and who require an F$_I$O$_2$ <0.5 and a PEEP of <10 cm H$_2$O to maintain gas exchange. Few critically ill patients with these characteristics present difficulties in weaning. When previously healthy patients resolve their acute illness without residual respiratory impairment, weaning from mechanical ventilation is rarely a problem. The problems usually arise when patients have coexistent cardiorespiratory dysfunction. It is the management of these patients that is discussed in this chapter.

PATHOPHYSIOLOGY

Patients requiring mechanical ventilation support for the treatment of acute pul-

447

monary parenchymal failure have two typical pathologic changes: (1) respiratory mechanics of an acute severe restrictive type due to interstitial alveolar edema, cellular infiltrates, or consolidation of lung parenchyma (8, 9); and (2) gas exchange abnormalities due to gross ventilation-perfusion mismatching. The acute restrictive changes in respiratory mechanics are very important to the choice of the weaning technique and the evaluation of clinical progress during this period. All lung volumes are markedly decreased. This is particularly important for functional residual capacity because this volume determines the alveolar surface available for pulmonary gas exchange.

Tidal volume and vital capacity are decreased by the same amount or more, i.e., to about one-third or less of the normal values. This reduction in tidal volume prevents significant alveolar recruitment, which is necessary to maintain adequate gas exchange space during spontaneous inspiration. Lung compliance is considerably lower than normal due to edema or consolidation of pulmonary parenchyma. This stiffening of the lung is the major reason for the low tidal volume observed in these patients. Because the lungs are stiffer, the work performed by the respiratory muscle (work cost of breathing) is increased.

The relation between ventilation to perfusion throughout the lung is altered. Under normal circumstances, dependent parts of the lung receive a greater proportion of both perfusion and spontaneous ventilation. This is very different in hypoxemic pulmonary parenchymal failure where a marked proportion of the dependent lung is consolidated by massive interstitial edema, cellular infiltration, and compression by overlying altered lung tissue (8, 9). As a consequence, most of the ventilation, whether mechanical or spontaneous, is distributed preferentially to nondependent parts of the lung. This pathologic situation results in a marked ventilation to perfusion maldistribution. An increased dead space ventilation is observed in nondependent regions where perfusion is more impaired than ventilation, and an increased venous admixture in dependent lung zones, where ventilation is more impaired than perfusion.

Pathophysiologic Considerations for Weaning

The reduced lung volume and gas exchange surface area can be offset, at least in part, by distending pulmonary parenchyma as a direct physiologic consequence of increased airway pressure. Positive airway pressure applied during mechanical ventilation or as continuous positive airway pressure (CPAP) during spontaneous breathing increases the functional residual capacity and arterial oxygenation.

The low compliance increases the work-cost of breathing considerably, making some degree of respiratory support necessary to achieve a sufficient alveolar ventilation in most patients with acute hypoxemic respiratory failure. This respiratory support should maintain adequate CO_2 elimination. Techniques such as intermittent mandatory ventilation or inspiratory pressure support can be used for this purpose. Their levels of support adjusted upward or downward as necessary are defined by $Paco_2$ levels and arterial pH.

Newer methods of respiratory support such as airway pressure release ventilation and biphasic positive airway pressure ventilation can theoretically combine a certain amount of pressure support to offset the work-cost of breathing and a continuous positive airway pressure to maintain appropriate gas exchange.

TECHNIQUES APPLIED TO IMPROVE PULMONARY GAS EXCHANGE DURING WEANING AND TO FACILITATE TRANSITION TO SPONTANEOUS BREATHING

There are essentially two types of methods allowing improved gas exchange for oxygen and co_2 in acute parenchymal lung failure: (*a*) increasing transpulmonary pressure and (*b*) partial support of respiratory work.

During both respiratory support and weaning in acute hypoxemic pulmonary parenchymal failure, PEEP and CPAP improve functional residual capacity, alveolar-capillary surface area and gas exchange for oxygen by increasing transpulmonary pressure. The level of positive airway pressure required to give a good result will depend on the initial reduction of lung volume, the previous lung condition, and the amount of recruitable gas exchange units. For instance, patients with underlying chronic obstructive lung disease (COPD) will require lower levels of positive airway pressure than those with previously healthy lung and severe acute parenchymal failure to derive similar benefits of oxygenation.

During weaning, PEEP and CPAP is usually set at 5–15 cm H_2O. The most appropriate level of end-expiratory airway pressure should be chosen by close monitoring of clinical signs of respiratory distress, spontaneous tidal volumes and frequency, arterial blood gases, and pulse oximetry. Either too little or too much PEEP or CPAP will impair gas exchange. PEEP and CPAP can alter cardiac function as well.

The goal of CPAP therapy should be to maximize pulmonary oxygen uptake in order to maintain an appropriate oxygen transport to all vital organs and tissues, and also maintain an adequate CO_2 elimination by the lung. The optimal level of CPAP to achieve these goals must be determined by titration for each individual patient. In addition to its effects on gas exchange, CPAP can also influence respiratory work. When functional residual capacity and total intrathoracic volume are severely decreased, the application of a positive airway pressure can decrease respiratory work by opening collapsed alveolar units, improving respiratory compliance and breathing pattern. This can be seen clinically by a higher tidal volume and a lower respiratory frequency (19). In patients with normal or increased functional residual capacity however, PEEP and CPAP can increase respiratory work by placing the inspiratory muscles on an unfavorable part of the pressure-volume relationship and potentially producing overdistension of lung tissue.

In severe airflow obstruction, Smith and Marini (17) noted a decrease in inspiratory work by 20–53% with the addition of 5 or 10 cm H_2O positive pressure. Similarly, Petrof et al. (13) observed a progressive reduction in inspiratory work and the inspiratory muscle and diaphragm pressure-time product with increasing levels of CPAP, as well as an improvement in dyspnea during weaning of patients presenting with an acute exacerbation of COPD. From these data it can be concluded that CPAP can also be used in a patient with COPD if the clinical status, the respiratory pattern, and the pulmonary gas exchange is monitored carefully.

Airway pressure release ventilation has been shown to provide both an increased mean transpulmonary pressure, thereby improving gas exchange, and a partial support of respiratory work (16). By allowing a slowly progressive reduction of both parts of this support, airway pressure release ventilation could potentially be beneficial for those patients who are particularly difficult to wean from mechanical aids. The clinical experience reported to date is, however, insufficient to confirm this idea.

Biphasic positive airway pressure ventilation has similar characteristics and potential indications for weaning patients with hypoxemic pulmonary parenchymal failure (2). Again, more clinical application and controlled studies will hopefully help determine the value and indications for this technique.

Position changes of the patient in the bed can help to improve regional and global ventilation-perfusion relationship. By placing relatively normal parts of the lung in a dependent situation, perfusion will be increased in these regions, promoting improved gas exchange. This is a simple and efficient way to improve systemic oxygenation in patients with marked unilateral lung disease pneumonia (6, 14). In contrast to adults, children with predominantly unilateral lung disease should be placed with the good lung up, i.e., in the nondependent position, to see a similar positive effect on gas exchange.

Partial Support of Respiratory Work During Weaning

Intermittent mandatory ventilation (IMV) was proposed 20 years ago to facilitate weaning in patients with increased respiratory work or decreased respiratory muscle strength (5). In hypoxemic pulmonary parenchymal failure, these conditions can apply secondary to a stiff lung and a compliance that is so low that it does not allow an appropriate spontaneous tidal volume. For many years, this technique has been used very frequently in this indication, although no controlled clinical trial has shown an advantage or a benefit compared to other methods of weaning.

The primary disadvantage of IMV in patients with pulmonary parenchymal consolidation is the high-peak airway pressures produced by the intermittent mechanical breath if the tidal volume is delivered too large or the patient fights the respirator. In addition, recent evidence suggests that IMV, even at relatively high rates, does not substantially decrease respiratory work (12). In clinical practice, IMV is being replaced more and more by the inspiratory pressure support mode, which seems to allow a better patient-respirator collaboration. Again, no prospective clinical trials have documented the superiority of either form of partial respiratory support in patients with respiratory failure.

Inspiratory pressure support has been shown to allow a substantial improvement of respiratory pattern (4). This includes an increase in spontaneous tidal volume, a decrease in electromyographic and mechanical activity of the diaphragm, a lower oxygen cost of breathing, less diaphragmatic fatigue, and a decrease in respiratory frequency (3). Furthermore, the patient regulates the inspiratory and expiratory times as well as the respiratory rate. It seems that the patient's comfort is improved during inspiratory pressure support ventilation, and less sedation is required (11). This technique is also a simple means to compensate for the additional resistance induced by the endotracheal tube, and the tubing and valves of the respiratory circuit.

Inspiratory pressure support ventilation is applied routinely today during weaning in hypoxemic pulmonary parenchymal failure. Substantial technological improvements in the delivery of inspiratory gas during pressure support ventilation have occurred. These improvements have resulted in a decrease in the delay and resistance of the trigger mechanisms, and the inspiratory resistance in general of this form of respiratory support. However, since pressure support ventilation only augments spontaneous respiratory efforts and does not initiate positive pressure breaths of its own, it has to be stressed that the use of pressure support ventilation requires an intact respiratory drive. It can be used in sedated patients, but an appropriate monitoring of cardiovascular and respiratory function is mandatory. A reasonable safety feature is to give pressure support ventilation with a backup assisted-ventilation rate slow enough as to not deliver positive pressure breaths unless apnea occurs.

Newer forms of pressure support techniques include biphasic positive airway pressure (2), airway pressure release ventilation (7, 18), intermittent mandatory pressure release ventilation (16), and proportional assist ventilation (21, 22). With these methods airway pressure is changed regularly by the respirator to provide adequate alveolar ventilation with the aim of reducing total respiratory load, lowering peak airway pressure, and enhancing patient comfort. These forms of pressure support ventilation are presently being evaluated.

NONRESPIRATORY ASPECTS OF WEANING

Fluid Retention

Positive pressure ventilation for acute hypoxemic pulmonary parenchymal failure frequently leads to water retention, a positive fluid balance, and diffuse edema. This phenomenon is due to a number of factors, including: (a) an increase in central venous pressure; (b) change in hormonal status (elevated secretion of antidiuretic hormone and a decrease in atrial natriuretic peptide have been reported); (c) a depression of excretory function of the kidney; (d) concurrent diffuse disturbances in capillary permeability due to the underlying disease; and *(e)* septicemia or mediators altering capillary endothelial cell function.

When weaning is started, intrathoracic pressure decreases in most patients due to the more negative pleural pressure produced by spontaneous breathing movements. In this situation, the venous return to the heart may increase and the relative central hypervolemia can require a diuretic treatment to maintain a good or optimal cardiovascular function and prevent the development or worsening of pulmonary edema.

Superinfection

Respiratory infection such as tracheobronchitis and pneumonia can render weaning difficult by adding an additional burden to respiratory work, airway resistance, and clearing of bronchial secretions. Special attention has been given to appropriate respiratory physiotherapy to remove airway secretions, to recognize early and treat appropriately any clinically important respiratory infection.

Associated vital organ dysfunction such as renal failure, liver or cardiac insufficiency (10), and metabolic imbalances make weaning more difficult. These problems require adequate treatment and stabilization before extubation is considered. However, complete correction of all other organ dysfunctions need not be achieved before respiratory support is discontinued. A good global clinical management and close surveillance are mandatory in these situations. Clearly, a stable patient has more ability to adapt to the stress of weaning than does an unstable one.

THE RIGHT TIME FOR EXTUBATION

The endotracheal tube should be removed as early as possible to decrease the risk for respiratory superinfection and for other side effects such as sinusitis, laryngeal ulcers, and tracheal stenosis. The usual clinical, respiratory, and gas exchange criteria are helpful for this important decision (15, 20). Most important, however, remains the clinical cause of respiratory failure and the level of respiratory support needed. The maximal level of CPAP that allows extubation is between 5 and 10 cm H_2O; a T-piece trial of patients is seldom necessary to make the decision to extubate. Furthermore, lung volume is lower on T-piece than with 5 cm H_2O CPAP or after extubation in this type of patient (1).

Similarly, an inspiratory pressure support ventilation level of 5–10 cm H_2O corresponds, in general, to the 5–10 cm H_2O resistance of endotracheal tube and breathing circuit. Accordingly, extubation can be performed safely at these levels in most cases. When there is doubt as to the patient's ability to breathe spontaneously, a "stress test" using a T-piece can facilitate the decision of extubation. Following extubation, supplemental oxygen by mask with good humidification and a regular chest physiotherapy should be provided because tracheal mucosal injury may preclude normal tracheal mucociliary clearance function for some time following extubation.

References

1. Annest SJ, Gottlieb M, Paloski W, Stratton H, Newell JC, Dutton R, Powers SR. Detrimental effects of removing end-expiratory pressure prior to endotracheal extubation. Ann Surg 1980; 191:539–545.
2. Baum M, Benzer H, Putensen CH, Koller W, Putz G. Biphasic positive airway pressure (BIPAP)—Eine neue Form der augmentierenden Beatmung. Anaesthesist 1989;38:452–458.
3. Brochard L, Harf A, Lorino H, Lemaire F. Inspiratory pressure support prevents diaphragmatic fatigue during weaning from mechanical ventilation. Am Rev Respir Dis 1989;139:513–521.
4. Brochard L, Pluskwa F, Lemaire F. Improved efficacy of spontaneous breathing with inspiratory pressure support. Am Rev Respir Dis 1987;136:411–415.
5. Downs JB, Klein EF Jr, Desautels D, Modell JH, Kirby RR. Intermittent mandatory ventilation: a new approach to weaning patients from mechanical ventilators. Chest 1973;64:331–335.
6. Fishman AP. Down with the good lung. N Engl J Med 1981;304:537–538.
7. Garner W, Downs JB, Stock MC, Räsänen J. Airway pressure release ventilation (APRV). A human trial. Chest 1988;94:779–781.
8. Gattinoni L, Pelosi P, Vitale G, Pesenti A, D'Andrea L, Mascheroni D. Body position changes redistribute lung computed-tomographic density

in patients with acute respiratory failure. Anesthesiology 1991;74:15–23.

9. Gattinoni L, Pesenti A, Bombino M, Baglioni S, Rivolta M, Rossi F, Rossi GP, Fumagalli R, Marcolin R, Mascheroni D, Torresin A. Relationship between lung computed tomographic density, gas exchange and PEEP in acute respiratory failure. Anesthesiology 1988;69:824–832.

10. Lemaire F, Teboul JL, Cinotti L, Giotto G, Abrouk F, Steg G, Macquin-Mavier I, Zapol WM. Acute left ventricular dysfunction during unsuccessful weaning from mechanical ventilation. Anesthesiology 1988;69:171–179.

11. MacIntyre NR. Respiratory function during pressure support ventilation. Chest 1986;89:677–683.

12. Marini JJ, Rodriguez RM, Lamb V. The inspiratory workload of patient-initiated mechanical ventilation. Am Rev Respir Dis 1986;134:902–909.

13. Petrof BJ, Legare M, Goldberg P, Milic-Emili J, Gottfried SB. Continuous positive airway pressure reduces work of breathing and dyspnea during weaning from mechanical ventilation in severe chronic obstructive pulmonary disease. Am Rev Respir Dis 1990;141:281–289.

14. Remolina C, Khan AU, Santiago TV, Edelman NH. Positional hypoxemia in unilateral lung disease. N Engl J Med 1981;304:523–525.

15. Romand JA, Suter PM. Weaning from mechanical ventilation in the elderly postoperative cardiac surgery patient. Eur Heart J 1989;10 (suppl H):13–16.

16. Rouby JJ, Ben Ameur M, Jawish D, Cherif A, Andreev A, Dreux S, Viars P. Continuous positive airway pressure (CPAP) vs. intermittent mandatory pressure release ventilation (IMPRV) in patients with acute respiratory failure. Intensive Care Med 1992;18:69–75.

17. Smith TC, Marini JJ. Impact of PEEP on lung mechanics and work of breathing in severe airflow obstruction. J Appl Physiol 1988;65:1488–1499.

18. Stock MC, Downs JB, Froelicher DA. Airway pressure release ventilation. Crit Care Med 1987;15:462–466.

19. Venus B, Jacobs HK, Lim L. Treatment of the adult respiratory distress syndrome with continuous positive airway pressure. Chest 1979;76:257–261.

20. Yang KL, Tobin MJ. A prospective study of indexes predicting the outcome of trials of weaning from mechanical ventilation. N Engl J Med 1991;324:1445–1450.

21. Younes M. Proportional assist ventilation, a new approach to ventilatory support. Theory. Am Rev Respir Dis 1992;145:114–120.

22. Younes M, Puddy A, Roberts D, Light RB, Quesada A, Taylor K, Oppenheimer L, Cramp H. Proportional assist ventilation. Results of an initial clinical trial. Am Rev Respir Dis 1992;145:121–129.

28

Ventilatory Management of Severe Airflow Obstruction

John J. Marini

PATHOPHYSIOLOGY OF AIRFLOW OBSTRUCTION

Complex physiology renders patients with decompensated airflow obstruction difficult to manage during the acute phase of illness, and similarly problematic in the process of withdrawal from ventilatory support (6). Nevertheless, once a few key physiologic principles are clearly understood, safe and effective treatment decisions can be approached with confidence. Because the phase of weaning from ventilator support is an extension of management strategy implemented from the initial stages of therapy, some material presented in other chapters of this volume deserve reemphasis here.

As detailed elsewhere, many diverse factors contribute to the difficulties of the acutely decompensated patient with airflow obstruction. Hypoxemia, pulmonary hypertension, and heart failure predominate in some cases and contribute in many others. However, the primary difficulty that leads to ventilator dependence is most often a simple disparity between ventilatory capability and demand.

To accomplish adequate ventilation, the ventilatory pump must repeatedly expand the chest against the flow-resistive and elastic impedance of the ventilatory system. The number of breathing cycles required per minute is a function of the metabolic load of CO_2 and ventilatory efficiency, as expressed indirectly by the deadspace fraction. Tidal ventilation can be partitioned into that part of the tidal volume (V_t) which participates in gas exchange in the respiratory zone of the lung,

referred to as alveolar ventilation ($\dot{V}_{alv}$), and that which does not, referred to as deadspace ventilation ($\dot{V}_D$). Since O_2 uptake and CO_2 elimination occur only through alveolar ventilation, one can define ventilatory efficiency indirectly by the deadspace fraction of the breath (V_D/V_T). When these interactions are considered over a minute, rather than per breath, alveolar minute ventilation ($\dot{V}_{alv}$) can be expressed as a function of both total minute ventilation ($\dot{V}_E$) and V_D/V_T:

$$\dot{V}_{alv} = \dot{V}_E \left(1 - V_D/V_T\right)$$

Exhalation usually occurs passively, driven by the recoil energy (in the form of elastic pressure) stored in the tissues of the lungs and chest wall during the inspiratory half cycle. The simplified equation of motion for the ventilatory system can be considered as the sum of its flow-resistive and elastic pressure components:

$$P_{Itot} = P_{res} + P_{el}$$

where P_{Itot}, P_{el}, and P_{Pres} are the total, elastic and nonelastic ("resistive") inspiratory pressures applied across the respiratory system. The elastic pressure can be viewed as comprised of the tidal pressure needed to inflate the respiratory system by the tidal volume (P_{elt}) and any residual elastic pressure (P_{ex}) remaining at end-exhalation that must be overcome before gas begins to flow into the chest, as explained below. Therefore this equation can be rewritten:

$$P_{Itot} = P_{res} + P_{elt} + P_{ex}$$

The individual components of this equation can be expressed in terms of the vari-

453

ables that influence them. Thus, P_{res} is influenced by inspiratory resistance (R_i) and average inspiratory flow rate [$\dot{V}_E/(t_i/t_{tot})$]; P_{elt} by tidal volume $V_t = V_E/f$) and compliance (C); and P_{ex} by pressures intentionally applied (positive and expiratory pressure [PEEP] and spontaneously generated in the process of dynamic hyperinflation (auto-PEEP [AP]):

$$P_I tot = [\dot{V}_E/(t_i/t_{tot})]\ Ri + \dot{V}_E/(fc) + (PEEP) + AP)$$

The flow-resistive, tidal elastic, and residual elastic components of this equation are each elevated in the setting of a chronic obstructive pulmonary disease (COPD) exacerbation (Fig 28.1). The flow-resistive element is increased by numerous factors, which include airway secretions, bronchospasm, mucosal edema, as well as a reduced number of functional conducting pathways.

Once the bronchi are seriously narrowed, further reductions in airway caliber cause marked increases in the pressure required to drive airflow. Although maximal flow rates may be similar, the nature of the flow resistance undoubtedly varies with the specific disease process. For example, the severity of flow resistance can be markedly different in inspiration and expiration if tissue recoil pressure is diminished by emphysema. Here the problem is not so much with the innate caliber of the native airway itself, but rather with its collapsible nature during exhalation. Such expiratory flow-resistive problems are accentuated by vigorous breathing efforts and increases of minute ventilation. Other types of airflow obstruction (e.g., asthma) may be associated with a smaller discrepancy between inspiratory resistance (R_i) and expiratory respiratory resistance (R_x) and less sensitivity of the R_x/R_i ratio to vigorous breathing. As the equation of motion indicates, a reduction in the inspiratory time fraction, without modification of the V_E requirement, will increase the flow resistive pressure loss.

DYNAMIC HYPERINFLATION
Definitions

Dynamic hyperinflation describes the process that occurs whenever insufficient exhalation time between adjacent tidal cycles prevents the respiratory system from decompressing to its resting end-expiratory equilibrium volume (15). Auto-PEEP ("intrinsic" PEEP) is defined as the positive difference between alveolar pressure and the end-expiratory alveolar pressure selected by the clinician (PEEP or continuous positive airway pressure (CPAP)) (Fig. 28.2). This positive pressure difference ensures that flow continues throughout exhalation, until deflation is actively interrupted by the subsequent inspiratory cycle. Auto-PEEP is therefore the residual flow-driving *expiratory* pressure that remains at the outset of *inspiratory* effort. It should be noted that dynamic hyperinflation and auto-PEEP are not necessarily a linked phenomena. When hyperinflation occurs gradually, there may be sufficient remodeling of thoracic and pulmonary structure to attenuate or eliminate auto-PEEP. Even in the acute setting, auto-PEEP does not necessarily imply hyperinflation, as discussed below.

Determinants of Auto-PEEP

If no PEEP is applied, P_{ex} is composed solely of auto-PEEP, a dynamic pressure that may vary greatly from breath to breath.

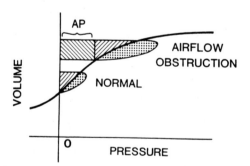

Figure 28.1. Influence of dynamic hyperinflation on the work of breathing. The heavy *solid line* indicates the volume-pressure relationship for the respiratory system. *Cross-hatched* and *stippled areas* represent elastic and nonelastic (flow resistive) work, respectively. Auto-PEEP (AP) adds significantly to the pressure cost of inspiring each tidal volume. (From Marini JJ. Ventilatory management of COPD. In: Cherniack NS, ed. Chronic obstructive pulmonary disease. Philadelphia: WB Saunders, 1991.)

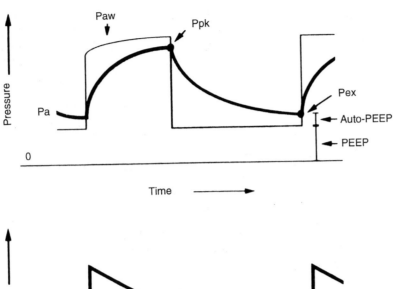

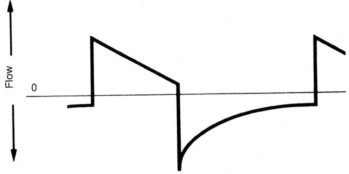

Figure 28.2. Schematic diagram of airway pressure (Paw), alveolar pressure (P_A), and flow in a patient experiencing dynamic hyperinflation during controlled volume cycled ventilation with decelerating flow. P_{PK} denotes maximum alveolar pressure achieved at end-inspiration. Note that end-expiratory alveolar pressure (P_{ex}) is the sum of PEEP and auto-PEEP. This positive pressure drives flow at the very end of exhalation, until counterbalanced by pressure developed in the central airway by the next machine-delivered cycle (volume control, decelerating flow). From Ravenscraft SA, Burke WE, Marini JJ. Volume cycled decelerating flow: an alternative form of mechanical ventilation. Chest 1992;101:1342–1351.

Since auto-PEEP impacts directly on ventilatory efficiency, an understanding of its determinants proves useful in managing patients with airflow obstruction. Assuming passive deflation with no PEEP externally applied, the progressive reduction in alveolar pressure can be characterized to a first approximation by the following uniexponential function of the time elapsed since deflation onset (t), the end-inspiratory alveolar pressure (P_S), and the deflation tendency of the respiratory system, as expressed in the exhalation time constant ($R \times C = 1/k$):

$$P_{alv} = P_S \, e^{\infty tt} = P_S \, [e^{-/R \times C}]$$

Here and in the subsequent equations, e is the numerical base of the natural logarithm system (2.7183). At end-exhalation, t = te, and therefore:

$$P_{ex} = P_S [e^{-te/R \times C}]$$

This last equation can be placed in clinical perspective by considering that at end-inspiration, P_S is the sum of end-tidal elastic pressure and residual elastic pressure. Accordingly, this expression can be rewritten:

$$P_{ex} = (P_{ex} + V_t/C) \, e^{-te/R \times C}$$
$$P_{ex} = V_t/[C(e^{te/R \times C} - 1)]$$
$$P_{ex} = V_E/[fC(e^{(1-z)60/(fR \times C)} - 1)]$$

Here, f, V_t, C, te, Rx, V_E and z represent frequency, tidal volume, compliance, expiratory time, expiratory resistance, minute ventilation, and the inspiratory time

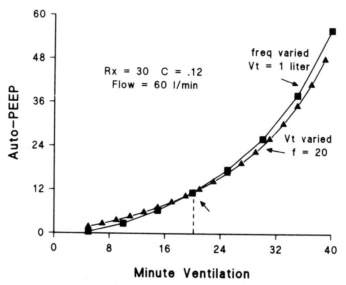

Figure 28.3. Computer-simulated comparison of different breathing patterns on auto-PEEP during constant flow, volume-cycled ventilation. The curvilinear nature of these auto-PEEP/V_E relationships is due to the increase T_i/t_{TOT} that develops as minute ventilation rises at a fixed inspiratory flow rate. Note that for a given minute ventilation, the magnitude of auto-PEEP does not depend strongly on the precise values of tidal volume or frequency.

fraction (t_i/t_{tot}), respectively. These equations indicate that the longer the inspiratory time fraction, the longer the expiratory time constant (R_xC), or the greater the minute ventilation, the higher auto-PEEP and P_{ex} will be. Interestingly, if $\dot{V}_E$, z, and all other variables input to this equation remain unchanged, auto-PEEP is not strongly influenced by the pattern of breathing; i.e., the f/Vt ratio makes little difference to its measured value (Fig. 28.3). Similarly, P_{ex} does not appear to be greatly altered by changes in compliance. The same is not true of the volume "trapped" at end-exhalation, which for the same P_{ex} is directly proportional to C. Although these mathematical formulae appear somewhat impractical to implement and detached from clinical medicine, they succinctly describe interrelationships useful in the daily management of patients with severe airflow obstruction, as the following discussion emphasizes.

Types of Auto-PEEP

Given the multiple determinants of auto-PEEP, as well as the marked variations among different individuals with regard to

airway collapsibility, perhaps it is not surprising that there are several variants of this phenomenon worthy of clinical consideration (21). Such variablility has implications for the response of patients to therapeutic interventions.

Auto-PEEP without Proportionate Hyperinflation

Because auto-PEEP reflects only alveolar pressure (P_{alv}) and not *transalveolar* pressure (the *difference* between alveolar and pleural pressures), it is possible to have auto-PEEP without hyperinflation. This happens when expiratory muscle effort displaces the respiratory system from the relaxed equilibrium position appropriate to that alveolar pressure (Fig. 28.4). Indeed, during exertion or when breathing with moderately high PEEP, most normal subjects strive to prevent or limit PEEP-induced chest distension. Forcing the system below its equilibrium position occurs routinely in healthy persons during upright exercise and may be a method of work sharing between the inspiratory and expiratory phases of respiration.

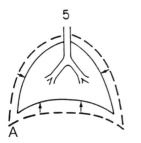 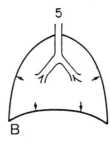

Figure 28.4. Mechanism of inspiratory "work sharing" during active exhalation against applied PEEP. As the expiratory muscles force the respiratory system below the equilibrium position appropriate to 5 cm H_2O PEEP placed at the airway opening, end-expiratory lung distension is prevented or minimized **(A)**. At the onset of inspiration, however, recoil energy stored during exhalation is released to aid inflation **(B)**. (From Marini JJ. Ventilatory management of COPD. In: Cherniack NS, ed. Chronic obstructive pulmonary disease. Philadelphia: WB Saunders, 1991:496.)

Auto-PEEP with Hyperinflation

Without active muscular activity, the persistence of alveolar pressure at end-exhalation implies distension of the respiratory system to an extent determined by lung and chest wall compliance. Expiratory narrowing of the airway may be structural, functional, or any combination of the two. When primarily structural (e.g., mild asthma), there may be little tendency for expiratory airway collapse. Dissipated or frictional pressure losses (characterized as the pressure drop across "resistance") depend on flow rate, which itself is a variable function of minute ventilation, inspiratory time fraction, and the pressure-flow relationship of the exhalation pathway: $P_R = k\dot{V}^\epsilon$. During purely laminar flow $\epsilon \sim 1$, and during fully developed turbulent flow, $\epsilon \sim 2$. The P_R for exhalation is the driving pressure for expiratory flow, i.e., the difference between alveolar and atmospheric pressures. As $\dot{V}_E$ rises, the inspiratory time fraction has an increasingly important influence on overall expiratory flow rate, airway resistance, and the average pressure drop across the airway. Auto-PEEP detected in "nonobstructive" clinical settings often originates primarily at the level of the expiratory valve, the resistance of

which rises in proportion to the average flow across it: $[\dot{V}_E/(1 - (t_i/t_{tot}))]$. Expiratory valve resistance, in conjunction with a reduced number of patent airways and expiratory muscle action, helps to account for the extraordinary incidence of auto-PEEP reported in the setting of adult respiratory distress syndrome (ARDS)—inherently a *restrictive* disease (4).

When the expiratory airway collapses during tidal exhalation, flow limitation similar to that which occurs during voluntary forced spirometry may occur, even in the course of passive deflation. Expiratory efforts by the subject intensify the obstruction, tending to accentuate air trapping, rather than speed deflation. It is highly likely that flow limited and nonflow limited exhalation pathways exist in parallel within the same obstructed patient, along with marked interregional differences in air trapping. The presence or absence of dynamic tidal airway compression has significant implications for the therapeutic management of such patients, as will be discussed later.

Physiologic Consequences of Dynamic Hyperinflation

Dynamic hyperinflation holds physiologic implications which often contribute to protracted ventilator dependence of patients with airflow obstruction. Failure to address auto-PEEP may lead to significant management errors, increased breathing effort, and/or hemodynamic compromise.

Breathing Effort

Work of Breathing

The process of dynamic hyperinflation moves the average lung volume to a higher position on the pressure volume curve of the respiratory system (Fig. 28.1). This distension tends to increase airway caliber but reduce compliance. The total elastic pressure required to inspire a given tidal volume rises for two reasons: first, the system has increased stiffness; and second, auto-PEEP represents an expiratory bias or threshold that must be overcome to produce the subatmospheric airway pressures necessary to initiate inspiration

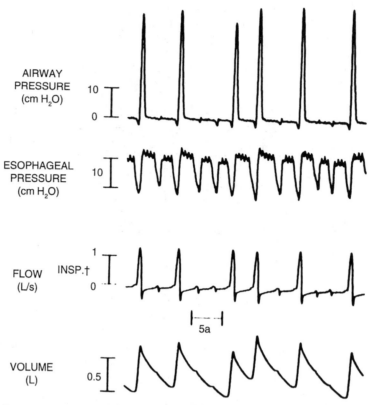

Figure 28.5. Experimental record demonstrating triggering inhibition during assist-controlled ventilation in a patient with severe chronic airflow obstruction and dynamic hyperinflation. Note the cycle-to-cycle variation in lung volume. (From Gottfried SB. The role of PEEP in the mechanically ventilated COPD patient. In: Berlin: Springer-Verlag, Marini JJ, Roussos, C, eds. Ventilatory Failure. Berlin: Springer-Verlag, 1991:399.

(41). This expiratory bias pressure may be sufficiently high so as to impede or prevent triggering of the ventilator during assisted mechanical ventilation, or synchronized intermittent mandatory ventilation (SIMV) (Fig. 28.5). Auto-PEEP also interferes with the ventilatory efficiency of pressure preset (pressure control or pressure support) forms of ventilation, at times drastically increasing the work of breathing.

Respiratory Muscle Function

Not only is the respiratory workload increased during dynamic hyperinflation, but the pumping action of the acutely distended ventilatory system is also compromised (20). Acute hyperinflation shortens the resting length of the inspiratory muscle fibers (reducing preload) and alters the configuration of the muscle groups which must interact effectively to power inspiration (Fig. 28.6). As the diaphragm flattens, it loses its zone of apposition with the lowermost rib cage, so that positive intraabdominal pressures do not have the same inspiratory action as before. Furthermore, the horizontal orientation of the diaphragmatic muscle fibers tends to convert their tension into an *expiratory* rather than inspiratory force vector. Conversely, the extradiaphragmatic respiratory muscles become increasingly important in accomplishing inspiration because they lose relatively little of their precontractile length and inherent strength at high volumes. The compliance of the distended chest wall

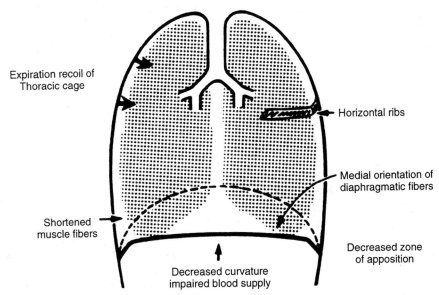

Expiration recoil of
Thoracic cage

Horizontal ribs

Medial orientation of
diaphragmatic fibers

Shortened
muscle fibers

Decreased zone
of apposition

Decreased curvature
impaired blood supply

Figure 28.6. Schematic diagram of the detrimental effects of hyperinflation on respiratory muscle function. (Adapted from Tobin MJ. Respiratory muscles in diseases. Clin Chest Med 1988;9:264)

declines at high lung volumes (greater than ~ 60% of vital capacity), as inwardly directed recoil of the chest cage supplants the outwardly directed recoil that normally assists inspiration at lower lung volumes. How important these latter changes are during *chronic* hyperventilation is an unsettled question at present. Almost certainly, the process of chronic hyperinflation is better tolerated than the acute variant (35).

The relative importance of the nondiaphragmatic ventilatory musculature in breathing during hyperinflation helps to account for two commonly observed phenomena. First, the key role of the skeletal (postural) muscles of the thoracic cage in stabilizing the thorax for optimal breathing efficiency may account for the dyspnea experienced by many such patients when arm activity diverts contractile power to other uses (5). Patients with extreme hyperinflation may become seriously dyspneic with only moderate activities of daily living that involve arm extension. Second, the diaphragm normally is pivotal during sleep, especially in the rapid eye movement (REM) stage. During REM, the activity of extradiaphragmatic muscles is significantly inhibited, and the diaphragm

tends to bear the breathing workload. If the diaphragm is ineffective, as it is often in severe COPD, relative hypoventilation occurs during these periods, with resulting hypoxemia and possible sleep disruption (10). Such disturbances may be instrumental to the evolution of decompensation or the failure of attempted ventilator withdrawal.

Hemodynamic Importance of Dynamic Hyperinflation

Raising mean right atrial pressure relative to that present elsewhere in the systemic vasculature impedes venous return (14). As dynamic hyperinflation develops under passive conditions, mean alveolar pressure must rise because distension of the lung and passive chest wall requires positive distending force. This rise, in turn, causes mean pleural and right atrial pressures to increase. Quite different dynamic prevail during spontaneous breathing, however. Here, *net* intrathoracic pressure actually *falls* as the vigor of inspiratory effort increases (42). Simultaneously, *end-expiratory* pressure may remain stable, decline slightly, or, more commonly, rise to a higher level. Although these relationships were first described in studies of spontaneously breathing asthmatic children (42), similar observations have been made anecdotally in adult patients with COPD being weaned from ventilatory support (18). Abrupt cardiovascular stress often tends to occur during sudden transitions from mechanical ventilation to spontaneous breathing. It would appear, therefore, that spontaneously breathing patients with auto-PEEP are more at risk for right heart decompensation (due to the increased right ventricular afterload that accompanies hyperinflation), to flooding (due to increased venous return and higher cardiac output), or to left heart compromise (due to ischemia, diastolic dysfunction, or increased afterload) than to falling venous return and insufficient cardiac output.

An overt crisis of low cardiac output is frequently precipitated when mechanical ventilation is first initiated in patients with severe airflow obstruction (32). As sedatives and paralytics are given to establish passive conditions, mean intrathoracic pressure rises, tending to impede venous return. At the same time, vascular compensatory mechanisms that normally tend to preserve the pressure-driving gradient are blunted by pharmacologic vasodilation in conjunction with elimination of skeletal muscle tone and phasic pumping activity. It is not uncommon, therefore, to find the recently intubated patient with COPD or asthma arrive hypotensive to the intensive care unit after intubation has been accomplished elsewhere. In the presence of auto-PEEP, measured central venous and pulmonary artery occlusion (wedge) pressures may be misleading high (32).

The "Panic" Cycle

Knowing the problems inherent in dynamic hyperinflation with regard to increased work of breathing, functionally diminished muscle power, and tendency for cardiovascular dysfunction, it comes as little surprise that seriously obstructed patients often enter a "panic" cycle whenever increasing minute ventilation elicits forceful breathing (Fig. 28.7). Increased muscular effort increases the $\dot{V}o_2$ and $\dot{V}co_2$. As a rising $\dot{V}_E$ accentuates dynamic hyperinflation and auto-PEEP, both the work per liter of ventilation as well as the number of liters required per minute increase simultaneously, even as acute hyperinflation progressively impairs the action of the thoracic pump. Central vascular congestion and ventricular ischemia may further compromise muscular efficiency, boost the breathing workload, increase anxiety, and contribute to discoordinate breathing. Fortunately, this self-reinforcing cycle can often be broken by verbal coaching, enhanced ventilatory support, or by timely reduction of anxiety, airway resistance, or the raised $\dot{V}_E$ requirement itself. Sudden transitions between levels of ventilatory support are particularly likely to precipitate problems, a fact that argues against the use of intermittent T-piece, or "blow-by" periods as a

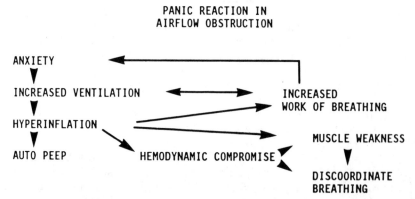

Figure 28.7. Positive feedback panic cycle often observed in patients with severe airflow obstruction and accentuated minute ventilation requirements.

weaning method. For some patients, appropriate cardiovascular therapy may be a crucial adjunct.

Monitoring Cardiac and Ventilatory Function During Dynamic Hyperinflation

The pulmonary artery occlusion pressure (P_{pao}) is characteristically assessed at end-exhalation, where the intrathoracic pressure is relatively free from fluctuations induced by the ventilatory cycle. Auto-PEEP, however, increases the measured P_{pao} by an amount determined by the relative compliances of the lung and chest wall, as well as by any active contribution of the respiratory muscles to the end-expiratory alveolar pressure. Under passive conditions, the fraction of alveolar pressure transmitted to the pleural space is: δ Pp1 = δ Pap [C1/Cl + Cw)]. (Here, δ represents the change in pleural or alveolar pressure.) During forceful activation of the expiratory muscles without dynamic hyperinflation, auto-PEEP may be generated entirely by pressures originating in the pleural space. Vigorous muscular activity predictably produces striking elevations P_{pao} that can be quantified by reestablishing passive conditions or approximated using a published nomogram (40). When a serious question exists regarding the significance of a measured P_{pao}, true transmural pressures are perhaps best assessed by simultaneous measurement of intraesophageal as well as P_{pao}.

Unaccounted for auto-PEEP can also influence computations of chest compliance (Cw) (36). Characteristically, compliance is estimated as the quotient of tidal volume and the difference between static end-inspiratory and end-expiratory airway pressures, which reflect their alveolar counterparts under these conditions. If flow does not cease at end-exhalation, the divisor of this ratio will be inappropriately high, so that the compliance will be underestimated. The error will be greatest at low tidal volumes (Fig. 28.8).

PRACTICAL MANAGEMENT OF AIRFLOW OBSTRUCTION

The foregoing discussion provides the pathophysiologic background for developing an appropriate strategy for the ventilatory management of patients with severe airflow obstruction. As noted elsewhere in this volume, nutrition, infection management, secretion clearance, bronchodilation, appropriate humidification, and skillful fluid-electrolyte management are key elements in the therapeutic scheme. With specific reference to the patient requiring weaning from protracted mechanical ventilation, several areas require special consideration.

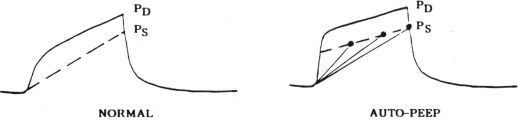

NORMAL   **AUTO–PEEP**

Figure 28.8. Influence of auto-PEEP and changing tidal volume on measurements of respiratory system compliance. These schematic diagrams depict the airway pressure waveforms observed during the constant flow, volume-cycle mechanical ventilation in a passive normal subject *(left)* and a passive subject with severe airflow obstruction. Normally tidal volume (which under these constant inspiratory flow conditions is proportionate to the length of the horizontal axis) requires an alveolar pressure change approximated by the peak static pressure (P_S). The slope of the *dashed line* reflects elastance (the inverse of compliance). In a patient with dynamic hyperinflation, auto-PEEP must be subtracted from (P_S) to derive the appropriate slope, indicated by the *dashed line*. When auto-PEEP is ignored, computed compliance is artifactually lower (and elastance higher) than actual, as indicated by the steeper slopes of the *solid lines*. The magnitude of the error for a given level of auto-PEEP increases as tidal volume is reduced.

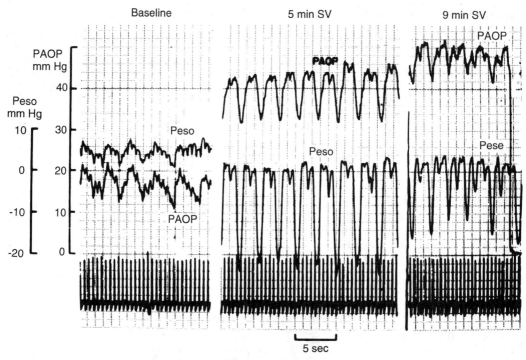

Figure 28.9. Changes in esophageal (P_{eso}) and in wedge pressure (PAOP) during a brief trial of spontaneous breathing in a patient with COPD and cardiac dysfunction. As the transition is made from full ventilator support (*baseline*) to spontaneous ventilation (*SV*), wedge pressure rises dramatically and mean esophageal pressure falls. Note that end-expiratory esophageal pressure falls modestly at first, and then begins to rise as the patient fatigues. (From LeMaire F, Teboul JL, Cinotti L, et al. Acute left ventricular dysfunction during unsuccessful weaning from mechanical ventilation. Anesthesiology 1988;69:171–179.)

Cardiovascular Function and Mechanical Ventilation

Relief by effective mechanical support of the very high breathing workload associated with severe airflow obstruction can allow marked and parallel reductions of the $\dot{V}O_2$ and the associated requirement for cardiac output (7). Such energy savings can make a crucial difference to the patient with stressed or inadequate cardiovascular reserve. Conversely, sudden resumption of a very high breathing workload can precipitate coronary ischemia, diastolic dysfunction, and pulmonary vascular congestion (Fig. 28.9) (18). In some patients, right heart strain produced by alveolar hypoxemia and lung overdistension result in right heart dilation, left ventricular crowding (via cardiac interdependence), and consequent pulmonary vascular congestion.

Although providing adequate ventilatory support aids ventricular function, it is important to proceed cautiously, not giving more than is needed to ensure comfort and acceptable blood gases. To provide more ventilatory support than needed may accentuate the tendency for dynamic hyperinflation.

Sedation and Paralysis

Sedation, complemented by paralysis when necessary, may be required in the early stages of ventilatory support to allow well-coordinated mechanical ventilation and effective muscle rest. As a general rule, 12–72 hr of deep sedation or paralysis are appropriate to facilitate adequate resting of the ventilatory muscles, assure sleep quality, and provide sufficient time for initial therapy to reverse the underlying or precipitating problem. Yet, after 24–48 hr of complete rest, deconditioning and protein catabolism are well underway. Furthermore, silencing of muscular effort eliminates coughing and encourages widespread pooling of airway secretions, especially in dependent areas. Very recently it has been shown that certain neuromuscular blocking agents may result in prolonged weakness (13) or overt myopathy, particularly when used in conjunction with corticosteroids (8). When sepsis complicates the picture, patients are also at risk for critical illness polyneuropathy, a selective motor deficit that may require months for full recovery (46).

Circuit Considerations

During acute exacerbations of airflow obstruction, the primary site of expiratory flow resistance usually resides in the small airways (<2 mm diameter). Nonetheless, care should be taken to insert with a tube of appropriate width, to facilitate the extraction of central airway secretions by suctioning. Sufficient pressure support should be provided to overcome endotracheal tube resistance during all spontaneous cycles. The pressure level must be carefully monitored and frequently readjusted, however, to provide adequate support without impeding exhalation (see below). Although the efficiency of the circuit (valves, resistance) in providing spontaneous breaths is important to maintain (38), these considerations may be somewhat less important for the patient with severe airflow obstruction than for patients with higher flow demands (e.g., those with ARDS).

PARTIAL VENTILATORY SUPPORT

In the present clinical setting, the primary options for partial ventilatory support include assist/control, pressure control (time-cycled) ventilation, synchronized intermittent mandatory ventilation with volume-limited, flow-controlled cycles (SIMV), pressure support (PSV), continuous positive airway pressure (CPAP), and others. Certain options (e.g., CPAP or biphasic CPAP) are particularly well adapted to noninvasive support.

Assist Control

Volume-controlled, flow-limited assisted mechanical ventilation (AMV) is the primary full support mode applied by most clinicians in the initial phase of acute support. Here, a relatively rapid inspiratory flow setting is selected (~5–6 times the minute ventilation requirement) in order to minimize end-expiratory gas trapping. Early on, moderate sedation is usually appropriate and often required to avoid overt dysynchrony between patient and machine. Should inspiratory flow prove inadequate or the patient experience dyspnea for other reasons (e.g., depressed *effective* triggering sensitivity due to auto-PEEP), considerable inspiratory work may be done during machine cycles (24, 41). Sedation or paralysis may be also required to employ the strategy of permissive hypercapnia (discussed below). A very brief end-inspiratory pause (0.2–0.3 sec) (11) or the use of the decelerating flow waveform (34) should be employed to enhance gas distribution at end-inspiration among many heterogeneously affected lung units. Care must be taken, however, always to keep the total t_i/t_{tot} <0.4. Using PEEP in patients with expiratory flow limitation may reduce dyspnea secondary to dynamic collapse of central airways (31), as well as improve the threshold for initiating inspiration (33, 41). In my practice, I apply at least 3 cm H_2O PEEP in all intubated patients who make active breathing efforts. The PEEP is titrated to the level at which end-inspiratory pressure begins to rise with further PEEP increments. Usually, this is somewhat less than the original level of auto-PEEP observed at ambient end-expiratory pressure. (I have never used more than 8 cm H_2O of added PEEP for this purpose, but others have reported benefit in well-selected patients with considerably more.)

Pressure Control

Pressure-controlled, time-cycled ventilation (PCV) would appear at present to have a rather limited place in the clinical management of patients with serious airflow obstruction. The ventilatory efficiency of PCV is dramatically influenced by the frequent changes in airflow imped-

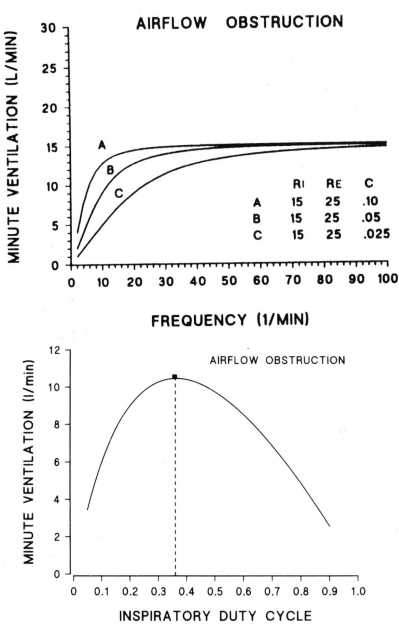

Figure 28.10. Influence on minute ventilation of frequency *(top)* and inspiratory duty cycle *(bottom)* during pressure-controlled ventilation of a patient with severe airflow obstruction. *Top,* note that for a given level of applied pressure there is a distinct upper bounding limit for minute ventilation as frequencies increases. Compliance affects the minute ventilation observed at any given frequency, but does not influence the bounding limit itself. Optimal ventilatory efficiency is normally achieved at slow frequencies. *Bottom,* in a typical flow-obstructed patient, there is a well-defined optimum duty cycle needed to achieve a given minute ventilation for the same applied pressure.

ance, chest wall compliance, impedance, and auto-PEEP that characterize such patients. Moreover, the ventilation of patients with severe airflow obstruction is markedly affected by the clinician's choice of frequency and t_i/t_{tot} (Fig. 28.10) (23). For these reasons, minute ventilation and blood gases should be monitored especially closely when PCV is employed. Carefully controlled clinical data comparing pressure and flow controlled ventilation in these patients are badly needed.

Pressure Support

Pressure support (PSV) aids greatly in overcoming endotracheal tube resistance and should be routinely employed for this purpose in patients taking spontaneous breaths (Fig. 28.11). Yet, PSV used as a "stand alone" power source and mode for weaning presents many potential problems for the patient with severe COPD. Like PCV and other forms of pressure-limited ventilation, its ventilatory efficacy

is susceptible to the vagaries of lung or chest wall compliance (23). When auto-PEEP develops or increases (e.g., as part of a panic cycle or due to increased airway resistance), it effectively negates a proportion of the applied PSV, forcing the patient to inspire with greater effort. Furthermore, most PSV circuits cannot keep pace with the timing or vigor of forceful inspiratory efforts, especially if no CPAP is used to offset auto-PEEP and thereby help improve effective triggering sensitivity (33, 41). Although such limitations can be partially overcome by increasing the PSV level, overdistension and discomfort may arise when the patient calms sufficiently to reduce $\dot{V}_E$.

Relatively few clinicians realize that the patient with severe COPD receiving PSV is often obligated to *actively* turn off machine pressure, as inspiratory flow cannot passively decay quickly enough to the requisite off-trigger value within a time frame consistent with length of the inspiratory duty cycle set by the patient's own respi-

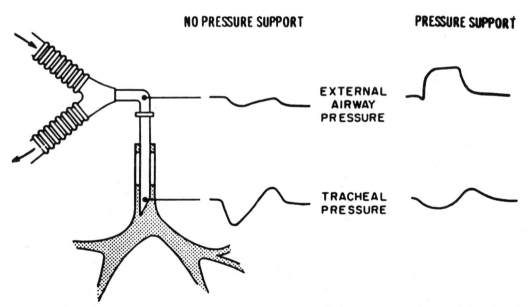

NO PRESSURE SUPPORT   PRESSURE SUPPORT

EXTERNAL AIRWAY PRESSURE

TRACHEAL PRESSURE

Figure 28.11. Influence of endotracheal tube resistance on spontaneous work of breathing, with and without the benefit of pressure support. No matter how efficient an external CPAP circuit may be in keeping airway pressure constant, marked fluctuations of tracheal and esophageal pressure must occur to inspire through the resistance of the endotracheal tube. Pressure support helps to overcome endotracheal tube resistance, minimizing tracheal pressure fluctuations. (From Marini JJ. Minimizing breathing effort during mechanical ventilation. Crit Care Clin 1990;6:653.)

ratory drive center. In fact, the level of auto-PEEP can actually *increase* as pressure support is augmented, both because the $\dot{V}_E$ may rise and because delayed "off-switching" effectively lengthens t_i/t_{tot} and shortens t_e/t_{tot} (17). It should also be understood that during PSV withdrawal, the rate at which the ventilatory muscles are reloaded accelerates with the final few decrements of supporting pressure (19). Finally, PSV used alone does not provide a guaranteed backup ventilation. Despite these major shortcomings, PSV does have a defined place as a primary power source for the patient with COPD who has relatively few secretions, stable ventilatory drive, a modest $\dot{V}_E$, and only moderate severity of illness. In well selected patients, properly adjusted PSV often proves more comfortable than SIMV for this purpose (19).

Synchronized Intermittent Mandatory Ventilation

Despite its relative age, SIMV remains an attractive mode of ventilation that combines some characteristics of AMV and CPAP. Properly adjusted, SIMV can be a comfortable mode that does not present the same problems of overt, pressure-limiting dysynchrony between patient and ventilator so prevalent during AMV. SIMV should virtually always be combined with "low-level" CPAP and "low-level" PSV to optimize the triggering characteristics of the spontaneous and machine-assisted cycles, as well as to offset endotracheal tube resistance. Some cycle-to-cycle variation of patient effort is expected during quiet and moderately vigorous breathing during SIMV. However, it is noteworthy that in the dyspneic patient, effort (assessed by the inspiratory pressure-time product) may not vary greatly cycle-to-cycle at any given level of machine support (26). In this limited sense and in this confined but common clinical setting, SIMV is similar to pressure support, a mode in which there is great similarity among the effort profiles of contiguous breaths. Levels of dyspnea and anxiety also may not vary greatly between these modes at similar levels of machine-delivered power (16).

Proportional Assist Ventilation

In the near future, many of the drawbacks of PSV just mentioned may be addressable with a newly described technique of partial ventilatory assistance, termed proportional assist ventilation (PAV) (44, 45). The basic idea behind PAV is that the ventilator should act as an auxiliary set of muscles whose output varies in direct proportion to patient effort (Fig. 28.12). Although the clinician selects the strength and character of these "auxiliary muscles," all timing and depth components of the breathing cycle are under direct patient control, a feature that should help assure comfort and safety. PAV derives its exquisite instantaneous sensitivity from information gathered by monitoring the flow and volume entering the lung. By adjusting independent gains for flow and volume, the

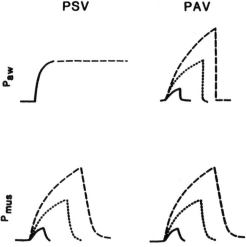

Figure 28.12. Conceptual difference between pressure support ventilation (*PSV*) and proportional assist ventilation (*PAV*). As muscular pressures generated by the patient vary, note that pressure support and proportional assist respond differently. During PSV, P_{aw} remains constant, so that the delivered flow and volume may be quite different—greater or less—than those needed by or acceptable to the patient. With PAV, airway pressure remains proportional to muscular effort at all points in the inspiratory cycle. (From Younes M. Proportional assist ventilation and pressure support ventilation: similarities and differences. In: Marini JJ, Roussos C, eds. Ventilatory failure. Berlin: Springer-Verlag, 1991:361–380.)

clinician is able to adjust the overall proportionality constant or amplification factor (power assist), as well as how the machine's assistance is partitioned across the elastic and nonelastic impedance elements defined by the equation of motion. Although PAV is an exciting new concept that has features especially attractive to the management of patients with severe airflow obstruction, it is currently unproven and undergoing clinical evaluation. Nonetheless, such delicate flow control and power assist may eventually prove crucial to the ease with which machine support may be withdrawn.

Noninvasive Ventilation

The potential for noninvasive ventilatory support (NIV), applied continuously for brief periods, or intermittently on an indefinite basis, is only now being explored. The concept of noninvasive ventilatory assistance with positive pressure was originally developed to facilitate the application of CPAP for treatment of obstructive sleep apnea. As a broad extension of that successful experience, numerous pressure- and volume-based modes of ventilatory assistance can now be applied using a tightly fitting facial mask or occlusive nasal appliance (Fig. 28.13) to deliver modest airway pressures (generally less than 25 cm H_2O). Benefits in terms of improved blood gases or reduced effort are expected and are clearly demonstrable during the period of pressure application. Recent studies have strongly suggested the value of NIV as a temporizing measure to avert intubation or facilitate extubation (2). Furthermore, a growing number of studies now indicate that benefits persist well after each ventilation period (1, 12). Using intermittent ventilation, reduced dyspnea and improved activity levels, in association with better strength, blood gases (unsupported), and sleep quality have been reported in various investigations of patients with neuromuscular weakness or COPD.

The use of nocturnal nasal ventilation is especially intriguing. Because patients with severe airflow obstruction depend heavily on the intact function of the extradiaphragmatic musculature, provision of

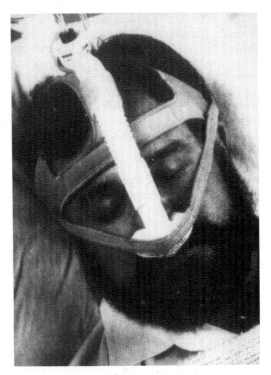

Figure 28.13. Application of noninvasive, positive pressure ventilation using a nasal occlusion appliance (Adam circuit, courtesy of Puritan-Bennett, Carlsbad, CA.)

adequate ventilatory assistance during the REM period may greatly improve sleep quality and preserve adequate blood gases. These benefits may help explain recent enthusiastic reports of this technique as an adjunct for both inpatient and outpatient use (1, 2, 12, 27). Such reports also lend rationality to the practice of providing increased ventilatory support during sleep periods in all intubated, hospitalized, ventilator-dependent patients.

Pressure-limited modes of ventilatory support, such as biphasic CPAP and airway pressure release ventilation (APRV, a mode with similar characteristics) (9) tend to compensate well for moderate leaks that develop between appliance and patient, but are inherently limited in their ability to ventilate the patient with serious airflow obstruction. To give adequate support, pressures are sometimes required beyond those that can be comfortably applied, and circuit leaks commonly develop. In addition, the efficacy of ventilation relies on the exponential buildup and decay of alveolar pressure and volume, a process retarded by airflow obstruction (23). Despite the great potential value of NIV, much remains to be proven before these techniques can be considered to have a confirmed place in patient care. Nonetheless, reports now emerging strongly suggest the benefit of these adjuncts for well-selected patients.

WEANING FROM VENTILATORY SUPPORT

Whereas it is rather easy to predict the success or failure of a weaning attempt in obvious cases, the prediction of outcome is much more difficult in others (22). Clearly, the development of cardiac failure, coronary ischemia, severe arterial hypoxemia, psychogenic decompensation, and other "nonventilatory" problems can perpetuate machine dependence. These are somewhat difficult, however, to quantify or incorporate into a meaningful predictive index. In recent years it has become clear that even for the most common cause of machine dependence, ventilatory insufficiency, isolated measures of workload (e.g., V_E) or muscle strength (e.g., maximal inspiratory pressure (MIP)) have only limited value. This may be because the ventilatory pump and the neural center that controls it interact closely in an attempt to avoid both CO_2 retention and catastrophic muscle fatigue (37). The most successful weaning indexes, therefore, seem to take the ratio between power requirement and power output reserve into account, either indirectly through observations of involuntary patient response, or by direct measurement (e.g., the ratio between the pressure required per breath and the MIP, the ratio of tidal volume to vital capacity, or the ratio of V_E to maximum voluntary ventilation). In my view, such involuntary measures as the $P_{0.1}$ (30, 39) and the CO_2-stimulated $P_{0.1}$ (28) hold promise, but are technically difficult for routine use. Similarly, complex scoring systems seem to work well in a research setting (29), but are difficult to implement in routine practice. As recently emphasized by Yang and Tobin (43), qualitative and quantitative as-

sessment of the breathing rhythm, pattern of muscle activation, and muscular coordination in response to monitored stress may be an effective clinical compromise.

In recent years, a great deal has been written regarding the serious problem of protracted ventilator dependence in patients with airflow obstruction. Certain modes have been suggested as markedly preferable to others, often with little substantive scientific information to underpin these assertions. Patients with severe airflow obstruction must be weaned gradually and with considerable skill in order to avoid panic reactions, intolerable fluid shifts, or cardiovascular dysfunction as well as to allow a period of readaptation to the ongoing stress of tidal breathing (22). Although a recent European multicenter trial of weaning modes (3) strongly indicated that stand alone pressure support was clearly preferable to SIMV in difficult cases, this conclusion runs counter to the clinical experience of others, including myself. Because of the difficulty in designing a truly fair comparative trial, and because several fundamental principles of weaning were not adhered to in the protocol (e.g., providing adequate nocturnal support, allowing sufficient pressure assistance for each spontaneous breath of SIMV to overcome tube resistance), these rather startling findings require confirmation and may not apply directly to routine clinical practice.

A Personal Approach to Weaning from Ventilatory Support

Taking into consideration the advantages and shortcomings of the techniques described above, the complex underlying physiology of severe airflow obstruction, and influenced by my own clinical experience, I have settled on a strategy that seems to facilitate machine withdrawal in the difficult patient with airflow obstruction. The key elements are as follows:

1. Reverse the underlying process that led to the acute worsening. Several days of nearly complete ventilatory rest may be required initially. As outlined elsewhere in this volume, attention to cardiovascular, fluid, electrolyte, nutritional, comfort, and mental status are crucial. Positional effects, air

swallowing, gastric distension, cough fractures, muscular strain, and constipation are frequently overlooked reasons for discomfort and agitation.

2. Do not stress the patient beyond the point of incipient fatigue or obvious dyspnea. Chaotic breathing rhythms, vigorous use of the accessory muscles of breathing, diaphoresis, an elevated frequency to tidal volume ratio, and irregular or discoordinate breathing (paradox, alternans) must be avoided.

3. Assure adequate sleep. This often requires an increased level of ventilatory support with AMV, high-level SIMV, or increased PSV at night. A mild sedative may be helpful.

4. Maintain effective bronchodilation, secretion clearance, and infection control throughout the weaning period, both before and *after* extubation has been accomplished.

5. Minimize the use of corticosteroids (and paralytic agents) in the "full-support" phase that precedes the weaning period. Personally, I do not advocate using more than the daily equivalent of 40 mg prednisone in the acute period (first 2–3 days), and I taper the steroid dose quickly after obvious progress has been made.

6. For all intubated patients drawing spontaneous breaths during CPAP or SIMV, endotracheal tube resistance must be offset with a level of pressure support, commensurate with tube diameter and minute ventilation ($\sim$ 4–7 cm H_2O).

7. In general, patients with severe airflow obstruction, neuromuscular weakness, or cardiac dysfunction do not easily tolerate abrupt transitions from full support to spontaneous breathing. Therefore, machine power should be withdrawn gradually, with the rate of withdrawal an empirical function of patient tolerance. The ability of the patient to resume responsibility for breathing should be frequently retested, as this can change with surprising suddenness, even after a rather lengthy period of ventilatory support.

8. The precise method of gradually reducing machine power (SIMV or PSV) may not be terribly crucial, provided that with any technique used, attention is paid to overcoming tube and circuit resistance, maintaining adequate end-expiratory lung volume, and periodically giving one more "sigh" breaths to help prevent atelectasis during monotonous shallow breathing (Fig. 28.14). When SIMV is used as the power source, CPAP and PSV are also employed in low levels: when PSV is used as the power source, a few large ($\sim$10–12 ml/kg), volume-controlled breaths are provided each minute to help maintain recruitment. Decrements in machine support are made with due respect for the relative weakness of the patient in relation to the workload. An empirical 3–5 minute minitrial at the bedside often proves invaluable, especially when there is demonstrated minute-to-minute stability or trend-like deterioration of the monitored parameters (Fig. 28.15). During this brief assessment period, the f/Vt ratio may provide guidance, quickly demonstrating the likely tolerance or intolerance of an intended setting adjustment (22, 43). Heart rate and clinical signs of comfort or distress help to define the appropriate level of support.

9. The patient must be continually reassessed with respect to the suitability for a weaning attempt. Marked changes may occur quickly

PRESSURE SUPPORT	SIMV
• PSV$_{max}$ ---> PSV$_5$	• AMV ---> SIMV$_2$
• SIMV 0.5 - 2/min	• PSV 3 - 7 cmH$_2$O
• CPAP 3 - 5 cmH$_2$O	• CPAP 3 - 5 cmH$_2$O

Figure 28.14. Two alternatives for weaning from mechanical ventilation. In both instances, a similar strategy is followed. Priority is given to: *(a)* overcoming endotracheal tube resistance with pressure support during each spontaneous breathing cycle; *(b)* ensuring periodic large breaths (with *SIMV*) for volume recruitment; *(c)* maintaining a sufficient end-expiratory lung volume with low-level CPAP; and *(d)* providing ventilatory support adequate for high-quality sleep. When pressure support is used as the primary source of machine power, it is varied from PSV$_{max}$ (providing a large tidal volume of approximately 7–10 ml/kg) to a value of 5 cm H_2O. When *SIMV* is used for this purpose, the frequency of machine cycles is tapered from every breath (assist control, *AMV*) to two breaths per minute.

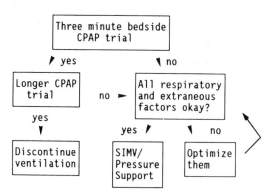

Figure 28.15. Making decisions for weaning based on empirical observation of the patient's response to brief and extended trials of spontaneous or partially supported breathing. During the trial, the patient is observed continuously at the bedside over a 3-minute period after the change in ventilatory support is made, during which trends in the ECG, breathing frequency, tidal volume, breathing rhythm, and pattern of muscular activation provide valuable clues as to tolerance of the intervention. Because most such changes occur quickly, these brief periods of observation should be repeated whenever there is a significant change in the level of ventilatory support prescribed.

in these patients, especially if a good night's sleep or a noticeable reduction in the V_E has occurred between points of evaluation. Muscular coordination, for example, frequently improves over very brief intervals. For some patients, maintaining a specific posture may be essential to optimize muscle strength and efficiency.

10. In most patients, extubation should occur from 5–7 cm H_2O of pressure support and 3–5 cm H_2O CPAP. Postextubation, there should be special care directed toward maintaining secretion clearance, effective oxygenation, appropriate cardiovascular support, and adequate sleep. Although it is important to provide an adequate number of calories, oral feedings are hazardous in the first few hours to days postextubation; impaired swallowing must be recognized and respected in order to avoid aspiration.

11. Noninvasive ventilation may help to provide a temporary bridge across the unstable postextubation period in certain tenuous patients.

References

1. Branthwaite, MA, Elliott MW, Simonds AK. Ventilatory failure: innovative support techniques. In: Marini JJ, Roussos C, eds. *Ventilatory failure.* Berlin: Springer-Verlag, 1991:430–443.
2. Brochard L, Isabey D, Piquet J, Piedode A, Mancebo J, Messadi A, Brun-Buisson C, Rauss A, Lemaire F, Harf A. Reversal of acute exacerbations of chronic obstructive pulmonary disease by inspiratory assistance with a face mask. N Engl J Med 1990;323:1523–1530.
3. Brochard L, Rauss A, Benito S, Conti G, Mancebo J, Rekik N, Lemaire F. Comparison of three techniques of weaning from mechanical ventilation. Results of an European multicenter trial. Am Rev Respir Dis 1991;143:A602.
4. Broseghini C, Brandolese R, Poggi R. Respiratory mechanics during the first day of mechanical ventilation in patients with pulmonary edema and chronic airway obstruction. Am Rev Respir Dis 1988;138:355–361.
5. Celli BR, Rassulo J, Make B. Dyssynchronous breathing during arm but not leg exercise in patients with chronic airflow obstruction. N Engl J Med 1986;314:1485–1490.
6. Cherniack NS, ed. Chronic obstructive pulmonary disease. Philadelphia: WB Saunders, 1991.
7. Cherniack RM. The oxygen consumption and efficiency of the respiratory muscles in health and emphysema. J Clin Invest 1959;38:494–499.
8. Douglass JA, Tuxen DV, Horne M, et al. Acute myopathy following treatment of severe life-threatening asthma (SLTA). Am Rev Respir Dis 1990;141 (suppl):A97.
9. Downs JB, Stock MC. Airway pressure release ventilation: a new concept in ventilatory support. Crit Care Med 1987;15:459–461.
10. Elliott MW, Carroll M, Simonds AK, Wedzicha JA, Branthwaite MA. Domiciliary nasal ventilation improves sleep and daytime blood gas tensions in patients with COPD. Am Rev Respir Dis 1991 (in press).
11. Fuleihan SF, Wilson RS, Pontoppidan H. Effect of mechanical ventilation with end-inspiratory pause on blood-gas exchange. Anesth Analg 1976;55:122–130.
12. Gay PC, Patel AM, Viggiano RW, Hubmayr RD. Nocturnal nasal ventilation for treatment of patients with hypercapnic respiratory failure. Mayo Clin Proc 1991;66:695–703.
13. Gooch J, Suchyta MR, Balbierz JM, Petajan JH, Clemmer TP: Prolonged paralysis after treatment with neuromuscular junction blocking agents. Crit Care Med 1991;19:1125–1131.
14. Guyton AC, Lindsey AW, Abernathy JB, Richardson T. Venous return at various right atrial pressures and the normal venous return curve. Am J Physiol 1957;189:609–618.
15. Kimball WR, Leith DE, Robins AG. Dynamic hyperinflation and ventilator dependence in chronic obstructive pulmonary disease. Am Rev Respir Dis 1982;126:991–995.
16. Knebel A, Marini J, Janson-Bjerklie S. Dyspnea, anxiety, and inspiratory effort during weaning with intermittent mandatory ventilation (IMV) and pressure support ventilation (PSV) [Abstract]. Am Rev Respir Dis 1991;4:A603.
17. Kuwayama N, Takezawa J, Hotta T, Shitaokoshi A, Takahashi T, Shimado Y. Application of pressure control ventilation (PCV) in overcoming auto-

peep created by pressure support ventilation (PSV) [Abstract]. Chest 1991;100:3S.

18. LeMaire F, Teboul JL, Cinotti L, et al. Acute left ventricular dysfunction during unsuccessful weaning from mechanical ventilation. Anesthesiology 1988;69:171–179.

19. MacIntyre NR. Respiratory function during pressure support ventilation. Chest 1986;89:677–683.

20. Macklem PT. Hyperinflation. Am Rev Respir Dis 1984;129:1–2.

21. Marini JJ. Should PEEP be used in airflow obstruction?. Am Rev Respir Dis 1989;140:1–3.

22. Marini JJ. Weaning from mechanical ventilation. N Engl J Med 1991;324:1496–1498.

23. Marini JJ, Crooke PS, Truwit JD. Determinants and limits of pressure preset ventilation: a mathematical model of pressure control. J Appl Physiol 1989;67:1081–1092.

24. Marini JJ, Rodriguez RM, Lamb VJ. The inspiratory workload of patient-initiated mechanical ventilation. Am Rev Respir Dis 1986;134:902–909.

25. Martin J, Shores S. Engel LA. Effect of continuous positive airway pressure on respiratory mechanics and pattern of breathing in induced asthma. Am Rev Respir Dis 1982;126:812–817.

26. Marini JJ, Smith TC, Lamb VJ. External work output and force generation during synchronized intermittent mechanical ventilation. Effect of machine assistance on breathing effort. Am Rev Respir Dis 1988;138:1169–1179.

27. Meduri GU, Conoscenti CC, Menashe P, Nair S. Noninvasive face mask ventilation in patients with acute respiratory failure. Chest 1989;95:865–870.

28. Montgomery AB, Holle RHO, Neagley SR, et al. Prediction of successful ventilatory weaning using airway occlusion pressure and hypercapnic challenge. Chest 1987;4:496–499.

29. Morganroth ML, Morganroth JL, Nett LM, et al. Criteria for weaning from prolonged mechanical ventilation. Arch Intern Med 1984;144:1012–1016.

30. Murciano D, Boczkowski J, Lecocguic Y, et al. Tracheal occlusion pressure: a simple index to monitor respiratory muscle fatigue during acute respiratory failure in patients with chronic obstructive pulmonary disease. Ann Intern Med 1988;108:800–805.

31. O'Donnell DE, Sanii R, Anthonisen NR, Younes M. Effect of dynamic airway compression on breathing pattern and respiratory sensation in severe chronic obstructive pulmonary disease. Am Rev Respir Dis 1987;135:912–918.

32. Pepe PE, Marini JJ. Occult positive end-expiratory pressure in mechanically ventilated patients with airflow obstruction. Am Rev Respir Dis 1982;126:166–170.

33. Petrof BJ, Legare M, Goldberg P, Milic-Emili J, Gottfried SB. Continuous positive airway pressure reduces work of breathing and dyspnea during weaning from mechanical ventilation in severe chronic obstructive pulmonary disease. Am Rev Respir Dis 1990;141:281–289.

34. Ravenscraft SA, Burke WC, Marini JJ. Volume cycled decelerating flow: an alternative form of mechanical ventilation. Chest 1992;101:1342–1351.

35. Rochester DF. The diaphragm in COPD. Better than expected but not good enough. N Engl J Med 1991;325:961–962.

36. Rossi A, Gottfried SB, Zocchi L, et al. Measurement of static compliance of the total respiratory system in patients with acute respiratory failure during mechanical ventilation: the effect of intrinsic positive end-expiratory pressure. Am Rev Respir Dis 1985;131:672–677.

37. Roussos, C. and Moxham, J. Respiratory muscle fatigue. In: Roussos C, Macklem PT, eds. The Thorax. New York: Marcel Dekker, 1985:829–870.

38. Samodelov LF, Falke KJ. Total inspiratory work with modern demand valve devices compared to continuous flow CPAP. Intensive Care Med 1988;14:632–639.

39. Sassoon CSH, TE TT, Mahutte CK, Light RW. Airway occlusion pressure: an important indicator for successful weaning in patients with chronic obstructive pulmonary disease. Am Rev Respir Dis 1987;135:107–114.

40. Schuster DP, Seeman MD. Temporary muscle paralysis for accurate measurement of pulmonary artery occlusion pressure. Chest 1983;84:593–597.

41. Smith TC, Marini JJ. Impact of PEEP on lung mechanics and work of breathing in severe airflow obstruction. The effect of PEEP on Auto-PEEP. J Appl Physiol 1988;65:1488–1499.

42. Stalcup SA, Mellins RB. Mechanical forces producing pulmonary edema in acute asthma. N Engl J Med 1977;297:592–596.

43. Yang KL, Tobin MJ. A prospective study of indexes predicting the outcome of trials of weaning from mechanical ventilation. N Engl J Med 1991;324:1445–1450.

44. Younes M. Proportional assist ventilation and pressure support ventilation: similarities and differences. In: Marini JJ, Roussos C, eds. Ventilatory Failure. Berlin: Springer-Verlag, 1991:361–380.

45. Younes M. Proportional assist ventilation. A new approach to ventilatory support. Am Rev Respir Dis 1991 (in press).

46. Zochodne DW, Bolton CF, Wells GA, et al. Critical illness polyneuropathy: a complication of sepsis and multiple organ failure. Brain 1987;110:819–841.

29

Heart-Lung Interactions

Michael R. Pinsky

The primary goal of the cardiovascular and respiratory systems is to supply adequate amounts of oxygen to the tissues to meet their metabolic demand and to excrete the carbon dioxide produced by this process. Furthermore, the primary role of critical care resuscitative efforts is to ensure the adequacy of these systems. It is clear, therefore, that an understanding of cardiopulmonary physiology and the effects of disease and therapeutic interventions on cardiopulmonary status is central to the management of the critically ill patient. Within this broad framework lies the effects of ventilation on the circulation and the effects of the circulation on ventilation. Other factors remote to central hemodynamic considerations such as oxygen extraction in the periphery and hemoglobin affinity for oxygen are also clinically important but beyond the scope of this discussion. In this chapter we will define the primary determinants of heart-lung interactions during health and disease. Numerous review articles, chapters, and books have been written on this subject (7, 28, 29, 32, 38–44, 46, 52). The reader is referred to these references if greater detail is desired.

AN APPROACH TO THE ASSESSMENT OF CARDIOPULMONARY INTERACTIONS

Cardiopulmonary interactions include numerous aspects of cardiopulmonary function that span the entire spectrum of cardiopulmonary physiology. They can be studied by an analysis of venous return, right ventricular (RV) function, pulmonary blood flow, intrapulmonary gas exchange, ventricular interdependence, left ventricular (LV) systolic function, cardiac output, work-cost of breathing, and the effect of ventilation on systemic blood flow distribution. The specific clinical focus and analysis used is more dependent on the perceived condition at hand than on the global interactions of the various factors listed above. Thus, if one is primarily interested in how ventilation is altering right ventricular function in a patient with acute cor pulmonale, the analysis would be considerably different from that which would ensue if the same patient had recovered from acute right heart failure, but with severe obstructive lung disease, was now being actively weaned from mechanical ventilatory support.

How then does one focus on the specific physiologic factors operative in a given patient that determine steady-state cardiac output and cardiopulmonary stability? The answer is often not easy to come by, because confounding processes often coexist. At any given moment, it may be impossible to determine exactly how all these factors interact. However, if the clinical problem is first defined relative to specific interactions and then put within the context of the present pathophysiologic state, then it is possible to reasonably predict what will happen during specific interventions and what the significance of these responses will mean relative to the outcome of the patient. What follows then is an approach that utilizes this physiologic construct to understand and manage the critically ill patient in whom cardiopulmonary instability is or may become a significant aspect of his or her problem.

We will first define the isolated cardiopulmonary interactions that occur during ventilation, then describe the series and parallel interactions that occur between and among these forces, ending with specific clinical scenarios which may be relevant to the practicing intensivist.

EFFECTS OF VENTILATION ON THE CIRCULATION

The vast majority of clinically relevant problems associated with heart-lung interactions revolve around the effects of ventilation on the circulation. Ventilation can be spontaneous, partially assisted, or totally supported by mechanical means. Spontaneous inspiration decreases intrathoracic pressure (ITP), whereas positive-pressure inspiration increases ITP. Assisted ventilation has a variable effect on ITP, sometimes decreasing ITP (especially during early inspiration of patient-triggered breaths) and sometimes increasing ITP (especially at end-inspiration). All forms of ventilation clinically available, however, maintain gas exchange by cyclically varying lung volume so as to induce tidal air movement into and out of the lungs. Thus, changes in ITP and lung volume can occur in the same or opposite directions during ventilation. Since changes in lung volume reflect a common aspect of all forms of ventilation, the heart-lung interactions of changes in lung volume will be considered first. However, except with marked overdistension or profound alveolar collapse, most heart-lung interactions are attributable to changes in ITP, not changes in lung volume.

Hemodynamic Effects of Changes in Lung Volume

The primary hemodynamic effects of changes in lung volume revolve around changes in autonomic tone, pulmonary vascular resistance, and mechanical heart-lung interactions. Most of these effects are of minor clinical importance except at the extremes of lung volume.

Reflex Cardiovascular Changes

Increases in lung volume within the normal range (≤ 10 ml/kg) increase heart rate

due to withdrawal of sympathetic tone. This is referred to as respiratory sinus arrhythmia (1). Except in children and in patients with abnormal sinus node function, this heart rate varying effect of inspiration is of minimal clinical relevance in the ICU. Larger tidal volumes (>10 ml/kg), however, can induce a vasodilation cardiodepressive effect that is directly proportional to tidal volume. This inflation cardiodepressor effect may be due to many factors, including withdrawal of sympathetic tone (20) and release of vasodilating arachodonic acid metabolites from the lung (5). This negative inotropic effect appears to be related more to changing lung volume than to static levels of lung inflation.

Pulmonary Vascular Resistance

Changes in lung volume also alter pulmonary vascular resistance (Fig. 29.1). Normal pulmonary vascular resistance is low and only decreases further as blood flow increases, due to recruitment and distension of the pulmonary capillary net-

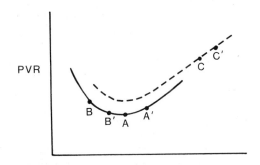

Figure 29.1. Schematic relation between lung volume and pulmonary vascular resistance. *Dotted line* reflects this relation for a patient with severe chronic airflow obstruction. Minimal resistance resides around volumes seen at end-expiration in normal subjects (*point A*). Acute hypoxemic respiratory failure decreases end-expiratory lung volume (*point B*), whereas hyperinflation seen in acute exacerbation of obstructive lung disease increases end-expiratory lung volume (*point C*). Positive end-expiratory pressure increases end-expiratory lung volume and may either decrease (point B') or increase (points A' and C') resistance.

work (18). However, if lung volume decreases below normal end-expiratory levels, usually referred to as functional residual capacity (FRC), as may occur in patients with acute lung injury (ARDS) or neuromuscular weakness and paralysis, then pulmonary vascular resistance will increase. This increase in pulmonary vasomotor tone is primarily due to increased extraalveolar vessel vasomotor tone (24). The cause of this increase in pulmonary vasomotor tone is twofold. As lung volume decreases, the lung interstitial radial forces also decrease. They become unable to maintain terminal airway patency. Thus, the terminal airways collapse, allowing alveolar hypoxia to rapidly develop. Reactive hypoxic pulmonary vasoconstriction occurs in those hypoxic lung units. Although hypoxic pulmonary vasoconstriction is a useful local reflex mechanism in maintaining ventilation-perfusion matching in the setting of regional alveolar collapse, if global collapse occurs, then pulmonary vascular resistance will rise and may impair RV ejection. Increasing lung volume back toward normal FRC by recruitment of collapsed alveoli (sighs, bag-sigh-suctioning, positive end-expiratory pressure, body positioning) will decrease pulmonary vasomotor tone, and thus pulmonary arterial pressure.

Increases in lung volume above FRC also increase pulmonary vascular resistance. However, this increase in resistance is not due to an increase in pulmonary vasomotor tone, but rather to an increase in extravascular pressure relative to alveolar capillary pressure (10). The greater the increase in lung volume, the greater the increase in pulmonary vascular resistance (62). Furthermore, in patients with both a reduced number of alveolar capillaries and preexistent hyperinflation (emphysema and chronic bronchitis), similar increases in lung volume above an already hyperinflated level can markedly increase pulmonary vascular resistance, precipitating acute pulmonary hypertension, RV failure, and circulatory shock (acute cor pulmonale). Ventilatory therapies that minimize or reverse hyperinflation will decrease the pressure load for RV ejection.

Mechanical Heart-Lung Interactions

Increasing lung volume also compresses the heart within the cardiac fossa. The expanding lungs push the chest wall out laterally and depress the diaphragm downward, but the heart within the cardiac fossa is, in essence, trapped, unable to be displaced by the expanding lung. Although the heart cannot be displaced laterally, it does tend to move anteriorly toward the sternum with hyperinflation. Increases in lung volume increase juxtacardiac pleural pressure more than lateral chest wall or diaphragmatic pressures (8). This translates into a bilateral compressive force on the heart that decreases biventricular end-diastolic volumes. Both right and left ventricular free walls collapse into the septum. This mechanical heart-lung interaction manifests itself as a type of tamponade in which pulmonary artery occlusion pressure relative to atmosphere is increased for the same LV end-diastolic volume, stroke volume and cardiac output, whereas the relation between pulmonary artery occlusion pressure relative to pericardial pressure and LV end-diastolic volume is unaltered (30). Furthermore, the clinician may misinterpret this interaction as impairment in LV contractility. This interaction is most commonly seen when hyperinflation occurs, either due to excessive amounts of PEEP (13, 48) or airtrapping (35).

Clinical Correlates

Increasing lung volume above FRC (hyperinflation) both increases pulmonary arterial pressure (increasing RV afterload) and compresses the right ventricle (decreasing RV end-diastolic volume); thus, cardiac output may fall. This is the proposed mechanism for hypotension and syncope in cough-syncope (60). Intravascular fluid replacement may mitigate this process by increasing RV end-diastolic volume. However, the definitive therapy for this process would be to reverse the hyperinflation that originally caused the deterioration.

Hyperinflation can occur because the

terminal airways collapse prematurely, preventing further expiration, or because expiratory time is sufficient to allow for complete exhalation. The former process is often called air-trapping, whereas the latter process is called either dynamic hyperinflation or auto-PEEP.

Air-trapping occurs in patients with emphysema due to loss of tissue elastic recoil pressure. To a large extent, air-trapping is irreversible. Air-trapping also occurs due to reversible airways obstruction owing to bronchospasm, excess mucus secretion into the airways, or airway mucosal edema. Bronchodilator therapy by reducing bronchomotor tone, antibiotic therapy by reducing mucus secretion, decreasing mucus viscosity, mucosal inflammation (edema), and pulmonary toilet by removing airways secretions will all reduce hyperinflation and may improve cardiac output independent of their specific effects on gas exchange.

Dynamic hyperinflation occurs when expiratory time is insufficient to allow for complete exhalation to FRC. Expiration is normally passive. The time required for complete exhalation is a function of the elastic recoil of the lungs, airway resistance, and the amount of gas in the lungs at end-inspiration (6). If either airway resistance or lung compliance increases, it will take longer for the inspired breath to be exhaled. Thus, in patients with either increased airway resistance or increased lung compliance, what would otherwise be normal tidal breaths may result in significant hyperinflation. Furthermore, if respiratory rate should increase, all else being constant, less time will be available for exhalation, and hyperinflation will also ensue. Patients with acute exacerbations of chronic airway obstruction are often tachypneic and have an increase in airways resistance caused by active expiratory dynamic compression of the airways and bronchospasm. Furthermore, otherwise stable ventilatory-dependent patients with chronic airflow obstruction who are being weaned from mechanical ventilatory support may become tachypneic, hyperinflate, and thus become hypotensive, independent of the effects of hyperinflation

on the mechanical efficiency of the respiratory muscles.

Maintenance of or return to a normal FRC should be a primary cardiopulmonary goal of ventilatory therapy. In patients at risk for alveolar collapse, this goal may be realized by the use of periodic sighs (large tidal breaths ≥ 15 ml/kg), positive end-expiratory pressure (PEEP or CPAP), and proper positioning of the patient in the bed to minimize diaphragmatic compression of the basilar lobes. In patients at risk for hyperinflation, this goal may be realized by therapies that reduce bronchomotor tone, airway secretions, and premature terminal airways collapse, and by modifying ventilation patterns so as to maximize the time necessary for adequate exhalation. Examples of such modifications of the ventilatory pattern include increased inspiratory flow rates, use of smaller tidal volumes, PEEP or CPAP therapy, and intentional hypoventilation.

Hemodynamic Effects of Changes in Intrathoracic Pressure

The heart within the thorax is, in essence, a pressure chamber within a pressure chamber. Thus, changes in ITP will passively effect the pressure gradients for systemic venous return to the right ventricle and LV ejection into the aorta independent of the heart itself.

Venous Return

Since venous return determines steady-state cardiac output in most patients, the primary hemodynamic effects of ventilation in most patients are directly due to the effects that changes in ITP have on venous return (23). The pressure gradient for venus return is equal to the upstream pressure in the venous reservoirs (often called mean systemic pressure) and right atrial pressure (or CVP) (Fig. 29.2). Since the right atrium is a highly compliant structure, changes in ITP are directly transferred to the atrium. Decreases in ITP, as occur during spontaneous inspiratory efforts, will increase venous return by decreasing right atrial pressure. This spontaneous inspiration-induced increase in

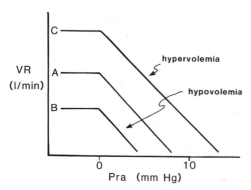

Figure 29.2. Schematic relation between right atrial pressure *(Pra)* and steady-state venous return *(VR)* under normal *(curve A)*, hypovolemic *(curve B)*, and hypervolemic *(curve C)* conditions. Note that for an identical Pra, venous return can vary, depending on blood volume. Similar curve shifts could be drawn for decreased or increased peripheral vasomotor tone *(curves B* and *C, respectively)*. Thus, changes in venous return can be induced by changes in either Pra, blood volume, or peripheral vasomotor tone.

venous return has been referred to as the thoracic pump. If ITP decreases much below atmospheric pressure, however, venous return reaches a maximal rate and further decreases in ITP will not increase venous return further (Fig. 29.2). This flow-limitation of venous return occurs because the large venous conduits collapse as they enter the thoracic cage in a fashion analogous to a wet paper straw collapsing when sucked on too hard. However, to the extent that the venous reservoirs can increase their drainage and right atrial pressure falls, decreases in ITP will almost always increase RV end-diastolic volume and subsequently RV output (22, 37). In patients with intravascular volume overload or increased pulmonary capillary permeability, spontaneous inspiratory efforts (by increasing venous return) will increase intrathoracic blood volume (7, 63) and may precipitate or exacerbate pulmonary edema formation.

Likewise, steady-state increases in ITP, as occur during hyperinflation or positive-pressure inspiration, increase right atrial pressure impeding venous return (37); whereas, phasic increases in ITP, as occur during a cough or positive-pressure inspi-

ration, only phasicly decrease venous return (Fig. 29.2). Any ventilatory process that increases ITP will impede venous return, decreasing cardiac output. Prolonged inspiratory flow rates during positive-pressure ventilation, large tidal volume ventilation, decreased expiratory time, positive end-expiratory pressure, and hyperinflation will all decrease cardiac output (14). Therapeutic strategies that aim to minimize hyperinflation (as described above) and that keep ITP at the lowest level compatible with normal gas exchange will be associated with the least degree of impairment in venous return.

Left Ventricular Ejection

Left ventricular ejection reflects the balance between several interrelated forces that can be grouped into the categories of heart rate, preload, contractility, and afterload. Assuming that heart rate and intrinsic contractility are relatively constant, then LV ejection is primarily altered by changes in LV preload and afterload.

Left Ventricular Preload

Series Interactions. Left ventricular preload is proportional to end-diastolic volume. If venous return is reduced, then LV filling must eventually decrease as well. This is what commonly occurs in shock states associated with acute cor pulmonale. However, LV preload can also be decreased by either extrinsic compression of the heart by hyperinflated lungs or by parallel increases in RV end-diastolic volume decreasing LV diastolic compliance (ventricular interdependence) (58). The former occurs with acute exacerbations of chronic airflow obstruction and asthma (50) and was described above under changes in lung volume, while the latter occurs with exaggerated negative inspiratory swings in ITP (57).

Parallel Interactions. Venous return to the RV increases as ITP decreases increasing RV end-diastolic volume. Right ventricular distension decreases LV diastolic compliance by mechanical interaction between the dilating RV and either ventricular septal shift or common free wall myofibral interactions (58). This ventricular interdependence is the primary process thought responsible for pulsus paradoxus in acute asthma (49, 50). It follows that pulsus paradoxus may increase if inspiratory efforts increase, airflow obstruction increases, or venous return increases (because of fluid resuscitation). Furthermore, pulsus paradoxus may decrease in patients with acute asthma either because the bronchospasm resolves, allowing inspiration to occur without great negative swings in ITP, or because respiratory muscle fatigue limits inspiratory efforts. Thus, decreasing pulsus in a patient with acute exacerbations of airflow obstruction may be either a good or a bad event, but it is rarely of no consequence.

Left Ventricular Afterload

Changes in ITP also alter LV afterload. The left ventricle ejects its stroke volume into a thoracic aortic with relatively free extrathoracic drainage. Thus, changes in ITP, although affecting the pressure surrounding the left ventricle, will have no direct effect on the pressure surrounding the systemic arterial circuit. Left ventricular ejection pressure can be defined as the pressure gradient between the inside of the left ventricle (intralumenal pressure) and outside the heart (pericardial pressure). Assuming no pericardial restraint or aortic outflow obstruction, then LV transmural ejection pressure can be estimated as aortic pressure minus ITP. It follows that for a constant aortic pressure (mean arterial pressure), increasing ITP will decrease the pressure gradient for LV ejection, whereas decreasing ITP will increase the pressure gradient for LV ejection (11). In patients with normal cardiac function, changes in LV ejection pressure minimally affect cardiac output because under these conditions the LV is relatively insensitive to changes in ejection pressure (6). However, in patients with LV failure, changes in LV ejection pressure may be the primary determinant of steady-state cardiac output (7, 47). Thus, changes in ITP will alter LV performance to the extent that LV ejection depends on ejection pressure.

Clinical Correlates

The hemodynamic effects of changes in ITP will depend on the degree to which cardiac output and left ventricle performance depend on loading conditions.

When ventricular function is normal, steady-state cardiac output primarily depends on venous return, and small changes in LV ejection pressure have little hemodynamic effects (7). At the present time, this clinical scenario represents the majority of patients and heart-lung interactions encountered in intensive care settings. In such patients, decreases in ITP will maximize venous return and thus cardiac output. Increases in ITP, on the other hand, will decrease cardiac output to the extent that venous return is decreased. Ventilatory strategies that attempt to use spontaneous inspiratory efforts will be associated with less impairment in venous return than other strategies that use only positive-pressure ventilation.

When ventricular function is impaired and intravascular volume expanded, as in congestive heart failure, small decreases in the pressure gradient for venous return do not alter cardiac output (12). Indeed, a major therapy of patients in congestive heart failure is often to decrease intravascular blood volume and venous return. In such patients, decreasing ITP will both increase venous return and further impair LV ejection, increasing intrathoracic blood volume and possibly precipitating acute pulmonary edema formation. Either removing the negative spontaneous inspiratory swings in ITP by adding positive pressure to the airway or applying positive-pressure ventilation will decrease the pressure gradients for both venous return and LV ejection, decreasing intrathoracic blood volume and increasing LV ejection. Thus, in the volume-resuscitated patient in heart failure, positive-pressure ventilation does not decrease cardiac output and may actually increase steady-state cardiac output (21). Furthermore, it may be hemodynamnically superior to intubate and ventilate hemodynamically unstable patients with acute LV failure than to allow them to continue to breathe spontaneously (27).

Work-Cost of Breathing

Ventilation, like all muscular activities, requires energy for its action. The diaphragm is the primary muscle of inspiration. Unlike all other skeletal muscles, it has an extremely well-developed blood supply network relative to its mass, such that even at maximal levels of activities blood flow is usually adequate to prevent anaerobic metabolism (53). Normally the oxygen cost of ventilation is small and adds little to the overall oxygen consumption of the patient. However, in acute respiratory failure states or when profound tachypnea is present, the work-cost of breathing can approach 30–40% of the total systemic oxygen consumption (18). Under these conditions, which include all forms of acute respiratory failure, mixed venous oxygen tension will be low, reflecting the increased extraction of oxygen by the working respiratory muscles. Examples of conditions associated with increased work-cost of breathing are listed in Table 29.1

Markedly increased levels of oxygen consumption due to spontaneous ventilatory efforts can have significant effects on arterial oxygen tension (Pao_2) and systematic oxygen delivery in certain disease states. These effects are due to the resultant decrease in mixed venous oxygen saturation ($S\bar{v}o_2$) and to the selective increase in blood flow to the diaphragm. For example, in patients with increased intrapulmonary shunt fraction, increased oxygen extraction, by decreasing $S\bar{v}o_2$ will also result in a lower Pao_2. Placing such patients on mechanical ventilatory support, by reducing the work-cost of breathing, may improve arterial oxygenation by increasing $S\bar{v}o_2$ without altering intrapulmonary gas exchange (18, 41, 53, 61). Furthermore, if cardiac output is limited, then the increased work-cost of breathing seen in acute respiratory failure may stress the compensatory blood delivery system, resulting in a fall in blood flow to other organs. This could induce anaerobic metabolism, as manifest by increased arterial blood lactate levels (2). Again, placing such a patient on mechanical ventilatory support, by reducing the work-cost of

Table 29.1
Clinical Examples of Increased Work-Cost of Breathing

Increased airway resistance
  Intrinsic
    Asthma
    Chronic airflow obstruction (bronchitis and emphysema)
    Tracheal stenosis
    Vocal chord paralysis
  Extrinsic
    Small artificial airway
    Ventilator apparatus flow resistance
Decreased lung compliance
  Intrinsic
    Pulmonary fibrosis
    Pulmonary edema (including ARDS)
    Bilateral pleural effusions (massive)
  Extrinsic
    Thoracic eschar
    Tense ascites or abdominal binding
    Respiratory circuit demand valve delay in opening
Altered ventilatory patterns
  Normal ventilation
    Tachypnea (increased frequency)
    Hyperpnea (increased tidal volume)
  Abnormal ventilation
    Hyperinflation (decrease diaphragmatic muscle efficiency)
    Paradoxic respiration (asynchronous movement of chest wall and diaphragm)

breathing, may improve tissue oxygenation and lower arterial lactate levels without altering cardiac output or Pao_2 (18, 51, 53).

Effects of Ventilation on Blood Flow Distribution

Ventilation by altering steady-state cardiac output, right atrial pressure, and diaphragmatic position will alter blood flow distribution. First, if cardiac output should decrease, then sympathetic tone should reflexly increase. This will induce an immediate decrease in renal cortical blood flow (56) and, via right atrial volume receptor-mediated release of antidiuretic hormone, a delayed decrease in cortical blood flow increasing renal sodium resorption. Most ventilator-dependent patients tend to retain sodium due to the above two processes. Thus, most of the patients may need less maintenance fluids than similar patients who are not intubated. To the extent that sodium retention is mild, however, this can be usually ignored. Furthermore, fluid replacement that restores cardiac output back to its original pre-positive-pressure ventilation level will result in a return of normal baseline renal function (34). Ventilation also alters both intrahepatic blood flow distribution and the handling of substances cleared by the liver (33). The implications of these interactions are still unknown, but may explain some of the altered pharmacokinetics and clearance capabilities seen in the intubated and ventilated patient.

Hemodynamic Effects of Ventilation: A Mixed Expression of Effects

Ventilation alters numerous aspects of the balance between venous return, ventricular function, and cardiac output. If examined during steady-state, sustained increases or decreases in lung volume, or ITP appear to be definable. However, most patients breathe, and breathing is not a steady state but a dynamic and recycling state of balance that can not be defined by the hemodynamic characteristics of only one part of the ventilatory cycle. Variables, such as ventricular filling pressures and cardiac output measured at end-expiration, for example, will not reflect steady-state values during the ventilatory cycle in the same patients (41, 43, 44). Furthermore, lung disease (restrictive or obstructive) is rarely uniform, but displays marked inhomogeneity over lung units (17). Thus, alveolar collapse and overdistension can coexist. This inhomogeneity may make predictions about the effect of airway pressure on lung volume and ITP invalid. How then does one assess either steady-state cardiovascular status during ventilation or the hemodynamic effects of ventilation? These can be formidable questions. One method of addressing these complicated issues is to simplify the cardiopulmonary interactions, so as to isolate the specific process described above that is of concern.

Defining the Question

The three most common clinical situations that are encountered regarding the effects of ventilation on the circulation are (1) the initiation of mechanical ventilatory support, (2) continued maintenance or modification of mechanical ventilatory support, and (3) the withdrawal of ventilatory support. In all these conditions it is important to predict beforehand what the hemodynamic effects will be, and if potentially detrimental, to take precautionary steps to prevent their subsequent occurrence. For example, in the spontaneously breathing patient with combined cardiopulmonary dysfunction (i.e., some degree of respiratory failure and cardiovascular instability), one is often interested in predicting the immediate hemodynamic effect of applying supplemental mechanical ventilatory support. Will the patient's blood pressure and cardiac output be maintained, impaired, or improved? The answers to these questions depend, to a great deal, on the existing cardiovascular and respiratory status. Identical ventilatory maneuvers can have opposite effects in patients with differing baseline cardiopulmonary function. Thus, it is important to determine what cardiopulmonary variables may modify with the above cardiopulmonary interactions to derive the final cardiovascular response.

Determining the Variables

As described above, both cardiovascular and respiratory variables modify the hemodynamic effects of ventilation (Table 29.2). The cardiovascular variables operative in these interactions, in rough order of their importance, are effective circulating blood volume, peripheral vasomotor tone, intrinsic cardiac contractility and mechanical ejection efficiency, and pulmonary vascular conductivity.

The above hierarchy of interactions may be somewhat different for specific clinical conditions. However, it easily describes the cardiovascular interactions potentially seen in a trauma patient. If the patient has lost significant amounts of blood, the effective circulating blood volume will be

Table 29.2
Cardiovascular and Respiratory Variables
that Modify Cardiopulmonary Interactions[a]

Cardiovascular variables
  Effective circulating blood volume
  Peripheral vasomotor tone
  Intrinsic cardiac contractility and mechanical
    ejection efficiency
  Pulmonary vascular conductivity
Respiratory variables
  Global pulmonary compliance
  Airway resistance
  Degree of homogeneity of lung unit function
  Respiratory drive

[a]By order of their relative influence on the cardiovascular response.

reduced. Clearly, any increase in ITP in such a hypovolemic patient will reduce cardiac output and may induce a hypotensive response by impeding venous return. Furthermore, if the patient is unable to increase peripheral vasomotor tone further following the increase in ITP, as would normally occur to compensate for the increase in Pra (increasing mean systemic pressure), then the hypotensive state may persist. This may be the case because the patient is already maximally stressed or because peripheral sympathetic tone is impaired (spinal shock). Similarly, if the patient has either baseline-impaired cardiac contractility or in the presence of valvulopathy or asymmetric septal hypertrophy (reduced ejection efficiency) or trauma-induced ventricular dysfunction (e.g., RV dysfunction with anterior chest trauma), the increased-ITP-induced reduction in LV preload may induce a greater degree of cardiovascular impairment, if the LV end-diastolic volume is reduced below a level necessary to maintain LV ejection. Finally, if pulmonary vascular resistance is increased (status-postpulmonary emboli, lung contusion), the increased lung volume associated with positive-pressure ventilation may increase pulmonary artery pressure, impeding RV ejection.

The respiratory variables operative in these interactions, in rough order of their importance, are global pulmonary compliance, airway resistance, degree of homogeneity of lung unit function, and level of central respiratory drive. In patients with normal or increased pulmonary compliance, increases in airway pressure will distend the lung more than in patients with reduced lung compliance. Increased airway resistance may reduce the degree to which peak airway pressure is transmitted to the alveoli, but it also predisposes to hyperinflation because of incomplete exhalation. Thus, mean alveolar pressure may increase to a greater amount in patients with increased airways resistance (asthma and chronic airflow obstruction) than in patients with normal or stiff lungs. Accordingly, ITP and end-expiratory lung volume may increase more for the same ventilatory settings in patients with obstructive lung disease than either patients with normal or stiff lungs. Similarly, in patients with stiff lungs, increases in mean airway pressure may not be reflected by either increased lung volume or ITP. However, if the lung disease is nonhomogeneous, the increased airway pressure will inflate the more compliant parts of the lung and may induce identical changes in ITP, despite smaller increases in absolute lung volume. This latter consideration complicates the analysis of all heart-lung interactions, making even the best predictions of these interactions rough approximations. Finally, if combined increased respiratory drive and increased work-cost of breathing coexist, mechanical ventilatory assistance may profoundly alter global oxygen supply-demand relations.

Defining a Steady State

During ventilation there is a constantly varying venous return and LV output. Therefore, a true steady state that can be defined by one aspect of the ventilatory cycle does not exist. Ventilation, by cyclically varying lung volume and ITP will cyclically vary venous return and cardiac output (23, 63). During spontaneous inspiration, venous return increases as ITP falls. This increases RV volumes and output and may decrease LV volumes and output. The opposite directional changes then occur on expiration. Similarly, positive-pressure inspiration increases ITP. This decreases RV volumes and output and may

Table 29.3
Cardiovascular Variables Altered by the Ventilatory Cycle[a]

Marked variations with the ventilatory cycle
  Right atrial pressure (central venous pressure)
  Pulmonary arterial pressure
  Pulmonary artery occlusion pressure
  Cardiac output (by thermodilution)[b]
Variations with the ventilatory cycle
  Aortic pulse pressure
  Mean arterial pressure
Minimal variations with the ventilatory cycle
  Mixed venous oxygen saturation
  Pulse oximetry
  Arterial blood gas tensions[b]

[a]By order of their degree of variability throughout the ventilatory cycle, with most variability first.
[b]Not a continuous trend recording.

increase LV volumes and outputs. The causes for these interactions represent both series (phase relation of blood flow) and parallel (interdependence and ITP) factors.

Measures of cardiovascular function that do not vary over the ventilatory cycle may be more useful monitoring tools than those variables that show significant variation of the ventilatory cycle. Table 29.3 lists several measured variables that show differing degrees of ventilatory cycle sensitivity in their measurement. The most variable measures include intrathoracic vascular pressures and cardiac output as measured by thermodilution (35). The least variable measures include mixed venous oxygen saturation and arterial blood gas tensions, with mean arterial pressure lying somewhere in between.

Since measures of LV filling pressure, cardiac output, and mean arterial pressure are thought to be important in the management of critically ill patients, how can the measurement of these variables be made more accurate? Clearly, if the patient's ventilatory efforts can be minimized and the swings in lung volume and ITP kept small, the degree of variability of the measures will diminish. Furthermore, if the measures could be averaged over the entire ventilatory cycle and, at least for vascular pressures, measured relative to ITP, a more useful measure of these variables could be made. Since most of the change

in pulmonary artery occlusion pressure measurements during ventilation reflects changes in ITP (48), it appears to be reasonable to measure of pulmonary artery occlusion pressure immediately prior to any forceful respiratory effort, such as inspiration. Examination of mean arterial pressure from a central catheter using an oscillograph usually allows for the accurate estimate of arterial perfusion pressure. Finally, distributing the timing of the thermal injections randomly throughout the ventilatory cycle (25), or at specific intervals evenly distributed in a controlled ventilation ventilatory cycle may decrease the ventilation-induced error in thermodilution estimates of cardiac output. If these measures are taken, then accuracy of thermodilution cardiac output measurements can approach a $\pm 10\%$ level, which is usually adequate for clinical analysis.

Using Ventilation as a Test of Cardiovascular Status

Since ventilation and ventilatory maneuvers alter several variables concurrently, they are occasionally used as methods of stressing the overall cardiovascular system to ascertain relative preload-dependency and cardiac responsiveness. Traditionally, aortic pulse pressure and aortic diastolic pressure are examined to ascertain preload or afterload dependency in these maneuvers. The assumption is that increasing ITP decreases both venous return and LV ejection pressure.

Sustained increases in ITP (Valsalva maneuver) induce differing aortic pulse pressure responses depending on whether the patient is normal (preload-dependent, e.g., hypotension immediately following release from the strain), has moderately impaired LV function (absence of pressure overshoot during recovery from release hypotensive response), or is in congestive heart failure (square-wave response during strain without either hypotension or recovery response) (55). Initially, clinicians used only sustained increased ITP without a change in lung volume (Valsalva maneuver) to assess cardiovascular responsiveness (64). This aortic pressure response to a voluntary Valsalva maneuver is useful in determining cardiac responsiveness in the cooperative nondyspneic patient, but is of limited value in most critically ill patients.

Recently it has been proposed that the hemodynamic changes seen during phasic increases in ITP during ventilation can also be examined (36). If increases in ITP decrease aortic pulse pressure and aortic diastolic pressure, then cardiac output is primarily preload-dependent and may respond favorably to volume expansion. If, however, increasing ITP also increases aortic pulse pressure and aortic diastolic pressure (reverse pulsus paradoxus) (31), the patient is most likely in heart failure with adequate intravascular volume. Such a patient may benefit from further afterload reduction or additional inotropic agents. Clinical and animal studies support the use of this analysis in the interpretation of aortic pressure responses to positive-pressure ventilation.

An important caveat to this dynamic pressure analysis needs to be remembered. Series interactions between the right and left ventricles often complicate this analysis. Cyclical changes in ITP first alter venous return to the RV. If venous return changes, LV preload will subsequently change in the same direction, but on later beats (usually two to three beats later). For example, increasing ITP decreases venous return, decreasing RV output. This subsequently decreases LV filling and LV output. When LV output, and thus aortic pulse pressure, falls relative to the ventilatory cycle depends on the heart rate, ventilatory frequency, and tidal volume delivered (54). One may incorrectly interpret a falling arterial pulse pressure during expiration as representing impaired LV contractility (incorrectly seen as an increasing aortic pulse pressure during inspiration) when it actually means a phasic reduction in LV filling. One need only observe arterial pressure during the subsequent beats during a prolonged expiration, noting that aortic pulse pressure increases again despite an increase in ITP, to correctly show that fluctuations in venous return and not in LV ejection pressure were responsible for the aortic pulse pressure changes.

EFFECTS OF THE CIRCULATION ON VENTILATION

Circulatory disturbances can alter blood flow within the lungs (lesser circulation) as well as within the systemic circulation. Furthermore, profound systemic hypotension associated with increased pulmonary vascular resistance can induce RV ischemic dysfunction, further compromising pulmonary blood flow, intrapulmonary gas exchange, and cardiac output (9, 19). It is not clear, however, to what extent these ventilatory effects occur. Clearly, the hemodynamic effects are easier to demonstrate in most critically ill patients. However, this lack of a clinically apparent effect of circulation on ventilation may be more a function of our inability to continuously monitor shunt and dead space ventilation changes induced by cardiovascular status, rather than of dearth of interaction. Still, the ventilatory effects of circulatory changes appear to be less common, although clearly as important in the extreme.

Effects of Blood Flow on Intrapulmonary Gas Exchange

Changes in cardiac output can alter arterial blood gas content in several ways, as described below and itemized in Table 29.4. Specifically, changes in cardiac output can alter Pao_2 by varying either $S\bar{v}o_2$ or shunt fraction. Furthermore, changes in cardiac output and pulmonary arterial perfusion pressure can alter $Paco_2$ by varying either dead space ventilation or the co_2 load placed on the lungs (because of changing metabolic demands and supplemental anaerobic metabolism). Finally, both Pao_2 and $Paco_2$ may vary by changes in ventilation-perfusion ratios, which are not due to changes in shunt blood flow or dead space ventilation. The latter processes are described in greater detail in Chapter 24, "Ventilation-Perfusion Relationships."

Arterial Oxygenation

Arterial oxygenation is the final balance of alveolar gas exchange and intrapulmonary,

Table 29.4
Effect of Circulation on Intrapulmonary Gas Exchange

Worsened By	Improved By
Arterial oxygenation (Pao_2)	
Increased shunt fraction (Qs/Qt)	Decreased Qs/Qt
Overdistension of aerated lung units	Reverse hyperinflation
Overcome hypoxic pulmonary vasoconstriction	Increased $S\bar{v}o_2$
Decreased $S\bar{v}o_2$, increased systemic oxygen uptake ($\dot{V}o_2$) (work-cost of breathing)	Decreased $\dot{V}o_2$ (Mechanically assisted ventilation)
Decreased systemic oxygen delivery ($\dot{D}o_2$) (decreased cardiac output)	Increased $\dot{D}o_2$ (Reduction of LV afterload by abolishing negative swings in ITP)
Carbon dioxide excretion and $Paco_2$	
Increased dead space ventilation (Vd/Vt)	Decreased Vd/Vt
Increased West zones 1 and 2	Reverse hyperinflation
Increased co_2 production ($\dot{V}co_2$) (because of increased work-cost of breathing and anaerobic metabolism and bicarbonate buffering of lactic acid)	Decreased $\dot{V}co_2$ (Mechanically assisted ventilation)
Both Pao_2 and $Paco_2$	
Ventilation-perfusion ratios (V/Q) imbalance	
Overdistension in nonhomogenous lung disease	

shunt blood flow. If shunt fraction increases or $S\bar{v}o_2$ decreases, Pao_2 also decreases.

As described above, if hyperinflation overdistends aerated alveoli, their local vascular resistance will increase, tending to promote more blood flow through nondistended lung units whose vascular resistance has not changed. This differential effect on regional pulmonary vascular beds may increase blood flow to nonaerated lung units that, because of hypoxic pulmonary vasoconstriction, were normally not perfused (3, 15, 16, 26). The clinical observation associated with this phenomena would be for Pao_2 to fall as mean airway pressure increased (e.g., increasing level of PEEP), without a change in $S\bar{v}o_2$ or cardiac output. This scenario is most graphically represented in patients with unilateral lung disease (57), but potentially could also occur in all ventilated patients with nonhomogenous lung disease.

Arterial oxygenation can also be altered without a change in shunt blood flow. If $S\bar{v}o_2$ should fall for a constant shunt blood flow, then Pao_2 would also fall. Similarly, increasing $S\bar{v}o_2$ would increase Pao_2 without altering gas exchange. This effect of $S\bar{v}o_2$ on Pao_2 is often employed in patients with acute hypoxemic respiratory failure in which shunt fraction is large and relatively nonresponsive to other interventions. The strategy here is to reduce global oxygen consumption by use of paralytic agents and hypothermia. In patients with markedly increased work-cost of breathing, institution of ventilatory assist will reduce global oxygen uptake (2, 51) and should also result in an increase in Pao_2. Theoretically, similar beneficial effects of increasing $S\bar{v}o_2$ on Pao_2 should also occur if cardiac output were to increase while global oxygen uptake remained constant. Thus, measures that primarily improve cardiac output, such as fluid resuscitation, inotropic support, mechanical ventricular assist, or LV afterload reduction (removing large negative swings in ITP by institution of positive-pressure ventilation) should also improve Pao_2 without altering intrapulmonary gas exchange. In this instance, progressive circulatory shock should be associated with a worsening arterial oxygenation.

Carbon Dioxide Excretion and $Paco_2$

If cardiac output decreases enough, pulmonary arterial pressure will also decrease. During hyperinflation, since venous return often falls because of an increase in Pra, RV output will also fall. Thus, under conditions of increased alveolar pressure, as may occur during hyperinflation and the application of PEEP, alveolar pressure may exceed pulmonary arterial pressure within a large region of the pulmonary vascular bed (West zones 1 and 2) (16). Areas of the lung that are ventilated but not perfused are dead space. Excessive levels of PEEP in hypotensive shock can induce an increase in dead space ventilation and a rise in $Paco_2$. If the level of PEEP cannot be reduced, measures aimed at increasing cardiac output and pulmonary arterial pressure usually result in a decrease in $Paco_2$ levels because dead space ventilation decreases. The increased alveolar pressures may also shift intrapulmonary blood flow from ventilated lung units that sense alveolar pressure to less well-ventilated lung units increasing shunt fraction. Under these conditions, increasing cardiac output and pulmonary arterial pressure may also reduce shunt fraction, but this effect is less well described in man (16).

Effects of Blood Flow on Ventilation

Since spontaneous ventilation is an active muscular process, if blood flow to the respiratory muscles were to decrease, as may occur during circulatory shock, respiratory muscle failure may occur, leading to a respiratory death (51, 72). It is not clear, however, how often this scenario develops in the normal progression to death in patients with circulatory shock. However, in animals with acute tamponade shock, a respiratory death ensues within 2 hours of induction of circulatory shock. This respiratory failure appears to be a primary muscle fatigue type of failure since it is char-

acterized by failure of the diaphragm to generate an effective transdiaphragmatic pressure in response to increasing phrenic nerve activity. Furthermore, if these animals are artifically ventilated at the moment of respiratory arrest, they do not die but remain viable for several hours more (2), suggesting that death, when it occurred in the nonventilated animals, was due entirely to respiratory muscle failure.

Right Ventricular Function During Shock

Right ventricular myocardium is at risk of becoming ischemic in patients with combined cardiopulmonary disease despite adequate arterial oxygenation and normal coronary artery anatomy. The right ventricle receives its blood flow primarily during systole (58). Furthermore, the right ventricle is larger than the left ventricle and has a thinner free wall. Thus, the potential exists for the right ventricle to dilate and to experience a greater wall stress than the left ventricle. These points, coupled with the systolic timing of myocardial blood flow, make the right ventricle susceptible to ischemic dysfunction if the perfusion pressure for myocardial blood flow were to decrease at the same time that the right ventricle dilated. Examples of this scenario include acute cor pulmonale induced by either a massive pulmonary embolism, profound hyperinflation, or anaphylaxis-associated pulmonary hypertension. In all these cases, systemic hypotension and pulmonary hypertension coexist. When the pressure gradient from arterial to pulmonary arterial pressure narrows, the pressure gradient for right coronary blood flow decreases (9). Besides attempting to maintain contractility at acceptable levels by the use of inotropic agents, treatment is directed at reducing pulmonary arterial pressure and increasing systemic arterial pressure (19). Both measures are more easily said than done. Prostaglandin E, prostacyclin, hydralazine, or nitrates may reverse pulmonary vasomotor tone. Such pharmacotherapy often induces systemic hypotension and is thus coupled with left atrial infusion of a vasopressor. Usually these are only temporizing measures performed until definitive therapies such as embolectomy or cardiopulmonary bypass can be employed to treat the underlying problem.

THE PATIENT-VENTILATOR INTERFACE

Based on the above physiologic framework and the complicated interactions described, it is clear that in complicated patients it may never be possible to understand all the contributory cardiopulmonary interractions. However, most patients have disease processes that conveniently separate them into one of several groups. Those who are primarily preload-dependent, which comprise most critically ill patients, need measures that minimize detrimental heart-lung interactions. Whereas those who have some degree of impaired cardiac contractility or reduced LV ejection efficiency, although still sensitive to detrimental heart-lung interactions, may benefit from specific modes of ventilation that reduce the afterload to either the right or the left ventricle. Furthermore, these forces are all modified by the characteristics of the ventilatory system, including pulmonary compliance, airway resistance, homogeneity of lung function, and respiratory drive. Cardiopulmonary therapeutic strategies can then be separated into those that minimize detrimental hemodynamic effects and those that maximize beneficial hemodynamic effects. These measures are described below and summarized in Table 29.5.

Guidelines to *Minimize* Detrimental Hemodynamic Effects of Ventilation

Prevent Hyperinflation

In the general sense of the term, hyperinflation represents an increase in end-expiratory lung volume above FRC. However, FRC may be constant and larger than normal tidal volumes can result in similar detrimental effects (14). The clinician is often stuck between two opposing needs. The first is a desire to prevent alveolar collapse and maintain alveolar ventilation. The second is a concern about dynamic hyperinflation.

Table 29.5
Ventilatory Strategies to Optimize the Cardiovascular Status

Minimize detrimental hemodynamic effects of ventilation
Prevent hyperinflation
   "Least" PEEP
   Prolonged expiratory time
   Increased inspiratory flow rate[a]
Keep peak and mean airway pressure low
   Promote spontaneous inspiratory efforts
   Decrease inspiratory flow rate[a]
Keep the swings in ITP to a minimum (but mainly negative during inspiration)
Decrease the work-cost of breathing (in spontaneously breathing patient)
   Match machine ventilatory pattern to patient's ventilatory pattern
   Decrease inspiratory trigger threshold for assisted breath
   Offset Auto-PEEP with extrinsic PEEP

Maximize beneficial hemodynamic effects of ventilation
Maintain end-expiratory lung volume near FRC
   Prevent hyperinflation in obstructive lung disease
   Give minimal level of PEEP in hypoxemic respiratory failure
Prevent large negative swings in ITP
   Decrease inspiratory pressure threshold
   Increase CPAP or PEEP to offset inspiratory effort
   Decrease extrinsic airway resistance
Add increased ITP only when venous return is adequate
   Fluid resuscitation and inotropic support as necessary
   Allow for spontaneous respiratory efforts with assisted breaths

[a]These two goals are often in conflict with each other.

Since alveolar collapse has significant detrimental effects on its own, efforts directed at preventing alveolar collapse are warranted. These may include frequent turning of the patient in bed, sitting the patient up, use of periodic sighs, and bronchopulmonary suctioning. Furthermore, use of the least level of PEEP or CPAP associated with adequate gas exchange and fluid restriction to prevent alveolar flooding are all reasonable guidelines.

Efforts that allow for adequate time for exhalation to normal FRC are also useful. This can be accomplished by increasing expiratory time, usually by increasing inspiratory flow rate, or by using the lowest tidal volume to frequency ratio compatible with adequate carbon dioxide excretion.

Keep Peak and Mean Airway Pressure Low

Efforts that reduce bronchomotor tone, increase airway caliber, and decrease inspiratory flow rate will all decrease peak inspiratory pressure. Furthermore, promotion of spontaneous inspiratory efforts will offset the increase in alveolar pressure for the same tidal volume. In patients with increased airway resistance, some degree of hyperinflation and gas exchange abnormalities may be necessary to prevent markedly elevated alveolar pressures and the resultant barotrauma and cardiovascular sequelae.

Keep the Swings in ITP to a Minimum, but Mainly Negative During Inspiration

Large swings in ITP will result in large swings in the pressure gradients for venous return and LV ejection, and will require increased energy requirements for maintenance. To the extent that the swings in ITP can be minimized, these changes and energy requirements will be reduced. Some slight negative swing in ITP during inspiration is useful both for maintaining optimal venous return and for matching the inspiration-induced increase in pulmonary blood flow with inspiration-induced alveolar ventilation. Thus, gas exchange is always slightly better in healthy subjects during spontaneous ventilation than during positive-pressure ventilation (15, 16).

Decrease the Work-Cost of Breathing

Clearly, a primary goal of ventilatory support is to reduce the work-cost of breathing. Since respiratory muscle oxygen requirements can be great in the dyspneic patient with lung disease, efforts that min-imize the work-cost of breathing will reduce the metabolic load on the cardiovascular system (41, 42). If this is true, why are all intubated patients not paralyzed and sedated? Besides the obvious reasons of patient safety, comfort, and autonomy, global paralysis will require maximal mechanical ventilatory support to ensure adequate alveolar ventilation. Such a situation will be associated with a lower cardiac output and worse gas exchange efficiency than occurs during spontaneous ventilation. It is not clear if newer modes of ventilatory support such as pressure-support ventilation uniformly decrease the work-cost of breathing, especially in the dyspneic patient with severe obstructive lung disease. However, any mode of ventilatory assistance that decreases patient effort while not violating any of the above constraints should have beneficial cardiovascular consequences. These concepts are discussed in greater detail in Chapter 28.

At least three potential strategies can be used that should reduce the work-cost of breathing. The first one is to match the ventilator inspiratory flow pattern and tidal volume to the patient's intrinsic ventilatory pattern. Assuming that the patient's respiratory drive is not excessive for the required gas exchange requirements, both adequate gas exchange and improved matching of the patient to the ventilator should be achieved. A significant problem exists with this strategy. Patients with stiff lungs (restrictive lung disease, neuromuscular weakness), metabolic acidosis, or inflammation of the serosal lining of the gut, thorax, or brain (peritonitis, pleuritus, and meningitis, respectively), or those patients who are in pain or are agitated may have an inappropriately elevated respiratory drive. In these patients, matching the ventilator to the patient's own ventilator pattern will result in hyperventilation. This problem can be addressed by giving supplemental sedation as necessary and by employing methods that decrease the intrinsic respiratory drive, such as imposing a brief end-inspiratory pause, increasing mean inspiratory flow rate, or using a nondecelerating inspiratory flow pattern.

The second method is to decrease the inspiratory trigger threshold for assisted breaths so that the patient need not strain prior to receiving a mechanically delivered breath. This approach can often be accomplished by the use of a continuous flow-by CPAP system placed in parallel to the ventilatory circuit.

Finally, as described by Marini et al., (29), if the ventilatory end-expiratory pressure can be increased until it equals that amount of auto-PEEP coexistent in the patient, itself a product of air-trapping and hyperinflation, then the degree of inspiratory effort necessary to trigger a mechanical breath will be reduced. Clearly, extrinsic PEEP will have no beneficial effects on the work of breathing in a patient who passively receives mechanical breaths.

Guidelines to *Maximize* Beneficial Hemodynamic Effects of Ventilation

Ventilation benefits the circulation in several ways. First, by augmenting systemic venous return during spontaneous inspiration ("thoracic pump"), it maintains the maximal steady-state cardiac output possible for the specific conditions of blood volume, vasomotor tone, and cardiac pump function. Second, by refreshing alveolar gas through its actions to open collapsed lung units and maintain alveolar ventilation to poorly ventilated lung units, it reduces alveolar hypoxia, thereby decreasing hypoxic pulmonary vasoconstriction. Thus, RV ejection is less impeded. Furthermore, positive pressure ventilation by abolishing large negative swings in ITP during spontaneous inspiration in the setting of stiff lungs (hypoxic respiratory failure, pulmonary edema, interstitial lung disease) or increased inspiratory resistance (vocal cord paralysis, extrathoracic airway obstruction, bronchospasm), LV afterload is reduced, increasing LV ejection efficiency.

Maintain End-Expiratory Lung Volume Near FRC

It is not clear what level of end-expiratory lung volume should be sought in the management of the patient in acute respiratory failure. However, if the aim is to minimize over- or underdistension of lung units and to maintain alveolar aeration, one should aim to restore end-expiratory lung volume back toward that value thought to have been present prior to the acute insult (FRC). In patients with chronic airflow obstruction, that almost uniformly means to prevent further hyperinflation and, if possible, to reverse it. Measures that allow sufficient time for exhalation (as described above) will be beneficial. Potentially useful therapies that await further investigation before they can be used clinically include the use of CPAP in the spontaneously ventilated patient to decrease the work of breathing by preventing premature airway closure (16) and the addition of phosphodiesterase inhibitors to increase diaphragmatic contractility (53).

In patients with acute hypoxemic respiratory failure (ARDS), the addition of PEEP in amounts necessary to return end-expiratory lung volume to FRC will improve lung compliance and gas exchange without overdistending the lungs (4). It is not clear what level of PEEP this should be in a given patient, but it seems prudent to suggest that the minimal level of PEEP that improves Pao_2 without decreasing $S\bar{v}o_2$ would be the least harmful and may therefore be the most beneficial. These points are described further in Chapter 27.

Prevent Large Negative Swings in ITP

Since large negative swings in ITP increase LV afterload and can induce LV failure even in patients without overt signs of LV dysfunction (27), appropriate measures should be taken to minimize these large negative swings in ITP during spontaneous inspiration.

Three strategies can be used to accomplish this goal. First, the inspiratory pressure threshold for activation of the machine-derived mechanical breath can be reduced (45). Second, one can increase CPAP or PEEP to offset the spontaneous inspiratory effort so that ITP does not decrease during inspiration (59). Finally, and perhaps most importantly, the physician can decrease extrinsic airway resistance of the respiratory circuit. Small-bore endotracheal tubes and increased resistance of threshold respiratory valves can increase both the work of breathing and the negative swings in ITP during spontaneous inspiration. In this regard, pressure-support ventilation appears to be uniquely suited to automatically minimize the negative swings in ITP during inspiration because it automatically varies the inspiratory flow pattern to match patient effort. Newer "negative impedance" ventilators that apply this concept more fully are under investigation. (29).

Add Increased ITP Only When Venous Return Is Adequate

Finally, by increasing ITP in patients who are adequately fluid resuscitated, cardiac output will not fall, and may actually increase, if these patients have coexistent LV failure (44). However, it is important to emphasize that adequate fluid resuscitation and inotropic support may be necessary for the beneficial effect of increasing ITP to be seen. As an added measure to ensure adequate venous return during positive-pressure ventilation, it is useful to allow for spontaneous inspiratory efforts during assisted breaths, independent of the level of PEEP employed. This strategy is used in the recently described form of ventilation referred to as pressure-release ventilation (29).

References

1. Anrep GV, W Pascual, R Rossler. Respiratory variations of the heart II. The central mechanism of the respiratory arrhythmia and the inter-relations between the central and the reflex mechanisms. Proc R Soc Lond Ser B 1936;119:218–230.
2. Aubier M, Viires, N, Syllie G, Mozes R, Roussos Ch. Respiratory muscle contribution to lactic acidosis in low cardiac output. Am Rev Respir Dis 1982;126:648–652.
3. Ballester E, Reyes A, Roca J, Guitart R, Wanger PD, Rodriguez-Roisin R. Ventilation-perfusion mismatching in acute severe asthma: effects of salbutamol and 100% oxygen. Thorax 1989;44:258–267.
4. Benito S. Lemaire F. Pulmonary pressure-volume relationship in acute respiratory distress syndrome in adults: role of positive end-expiratory pressure. J Crit Care 1990;5:27–34.
5. Berend N, Christopher KL, Voelkel NF: Effect of positive end-expiratory pressure on functional residual capacity: role of prostaglandin production. Am Rev Respir Dis 1982;126:641–647.
6. Bergam NA. Intrapulmonary gas trapping during mechanical ventilation at rapid frequencies. Anesthesiology 1969;30:378–387.
7. Bromberger-Barnea B: Mechanical effects of inspiration on heart functions: a review. Fed Proc 1981;40:2171–2177.
8. Brookhart JM, Boyd TE. Local cardiac filling pressure. AM J Physiol 194;148:434–444.
9. Brooks H, Kirk ES, Vokonas PS, et al. Performance of right ventricle under stress: relation to right coronary flow. J Clin Invest 1971;50:2176–2183.
10. Brower RG, Gottlieb J, Wise RA, Permutt W, Sylvester JT: Locus of hypoxic vasoconstriction in isolated ferret lungs. J Appl Physiol 1987;63:59–65.
11. Buda AJ, Pinsky MR, Ingles NB, Daughters GT, Stenson E, Alderman EL. Effect of intrathoracic pressure on left ventricular performance. N Engl J Med 1979;301:453–459.
12. Calvin JE, Driedger AA, Sibbald WJ. Positive end-expiratory pressure (PEEP) does not depress left ventricular function in patients with pulmonary edema. Am Rev Respir Dis 1981;124:121–128.
13. Cassidy SS, Robertson CH, Pierce AK, et al. Cardiovascular effects of positive end-expiratory pressure in dogs. J Appl Physiol 1978;44:743–748.
14. Cournand A. Motley HL, Werko L, et al. Physiologic studies of the effect of intermittent positive pressure breathing on cardiac output in man. Am J Physiol 1948;152:162–174.
15. Dantzker DR. The influence of cardiovascular function on gas exchange. In: Matthay RA, Matthay MA, Dantzker DR, eds. Cardiovascular-pulmonary interaction in normal and diseased lungs. Vol 4. Philadelphia: WB Saunders, 1983:149–160.
16. Dantzker DR, D'Alonzo GE. The effect of exercise on pulmonary gas exchange in patients with severe chronic obstructive pulmonary disease. Am Rev Respir Dis 1986;134:1135–1139.
17. Gattinoni L, Perenti A, Avalli L, Rossi F, Bombino M. Pressure-volume curve of total respiratory system in acute respiratory failure. Computed tomographic scan study. Am Rev Respir Dis 1987;136:730–736.
18. Gherini S, Peters RM, Virgilio RW: Mechanical work of the lungs and the work of breathing with positive end-expiratory pressure and continuous positive airway pressure. Chest 1979;76:251–256.
19. Ghignone M, Girley L, Prewitt RM. Volume expansion versus norepinepherine in treatment of a low cardiac output complicating on acute increase in right ventricular afterload in dogs. Anesthesiology 1984;60:132–135.
20. Glick G. Wechsler AS, Epstein DE: Reflex cardiovascular depression produced by stimulation of pulmonary stretch receptors in the dog. J Clin Invest 1969;48:467–472.
21. Grace MP, Greenbaum DM. Cardiac performance in response to PEEP in patients with cardiac dysfunction. Crit Care Med 1982;20:358–360.
22. Guntheroth WC, Gould R, Butler J, et al. Pulsatile flow in pulmonary artery, capillary and vein in the dog. Cardiovasc Res 1974;8:330–337.
23. Guyton AC, Lindsey AW, Abernathy B, et al.

Venous return at various right atrial pressures and the normal venous return curve. Am J Physiol 1957;189:609–615.

24. Hakim TS, Michel RP, Minami H, Chang HK: Site of pulmonary hypoxic vasoconstriction studied with arterial and venous occlusion. J Appl Physiol 1983;54:1298–1302.

25. Jansen JRC, Schreuder JJ, Settels JJ, Kloek J, Vesprille A. An adequate strategy for the thermodilution technique in patients during mechanical ventilation. Intensive Care Med 1990;16:422–425.

26. Kanarek DJ, Shannon DR. Adverse effects of positive end-expiratory pressure in pulmonary perfusion and arterial oxygenation. Am Rev Respir Dis 1975;112:457–460.

27. Lemaire F, Teboul JL, Cinotti L, et al. Acute left ventricular dysfunction during unsuccessful weaning from mechanical ventilation. Anesthesiology 1988;69:171–179.

28. Lister G and Pitt BR. Cardiopulmonary interactions in the infant with congenital heart disease. In: Matthay RA, Matthay MA, Dantzker DR, eds. Cardiovascular-pulmonary interaction in normal and diseased lungs. Vol 4. Philadelphia: B Saunders, 1983:219–232.

29. Marini JJ. Strategies to minimize breathing effort during mechanical ventilation. In: MJ Tobin, ed, Mechanical ventilation, critical care clinics Philadelphia: WB Saunders, 1990:635–662.

30. Marini JJ, Culver BN, Butler J. Mechanical effect of lung distension with positive pressure on cardiac function. Am Rev Respir Dis 1980;124:382–386.

31. Massumi RA, Mason DT, Vera Z, et al. Reversed pulsus paradoxus. N Engl J Med 1973;289:1272–1275.

32. Matthay RA, Harvey JB. Cardiovascular function in cor pulmonale. In: Matthay RA, Matthay MA, Dantzker DR, eds. Cardiovascular-pulmonary interaction in normal and diseased lungs. Vol 4. Philadelphia: WB Saunders, 1983:269–296.

33. Matuschak GM, Pinsky MR, Rogers RM. Effects of positive end-expiratory pressure on hepatic blood flow and hepatic performance. J Appl Physiol 1987;62:1377–1383.

34. Meeham JP. Cardiovascular receptors and fluid volume control. Aviat Space Environ Med 1986;57:267–275.

35. O'Quinn R, Marini JJ. Pulmonary artery occlusion pressure; clinical physiology, measurement, and interpretation. Am Rev Respir Dis 1983;128:318–326.

36. Perel A, Pizov R, Cotev S. Systolic blood pressure variation in a sensitive indicator of hypovolemia in ventilated dogs subjected to graded hemorrhage. Anesthesiology 1987;67:498–502.

37. Pinsky MR. Determinants of pulmonary artery flow variation during respiration. J Appl Physiol 1984;56:1237–1245.

38. Pinsky MR. The influence of positive pressure ventilation on cardiovascular function in the critically ill. In: Sibbald W, ed. Cardiovascular crises in the critically ill. Vol. 3. Chicago: Year Book, 1985:699–717.

39. Pinsky MR. Cardiopulmonary interactions: the effects of negative and positive pleural pressure changes on cardiac output. In: Dantzker D, ed. Cardiopulmonary medicine and critical care, Orlando, Fl: Grune & Stratton, 1986:89–122.

40. Pinsky MR. Hemodynamic effects of artificial ventilation. In: Snyder JV, ed. Oxygen transport in the critically ill. Chicago: Year Book, 1986:319–332.

41. Pinsky MR. Hemodynamic effects of mechanical ventilation in the critically ill. In: Shoemaker WC, Thompson WL, Holbrook PR, eds. Textbook of critical care. 2nd ed. Philadelphia: WB Saunders, 1988:676–685.

42. Pinsky MR. The effect of changing intrathoracic pressure on the normal and failing heart. In: Cassidy S, Scharf SM, eds. Heart-lung interactions in health and disease. New York: Marcel Dekker, 1989:839–876.

43. Pinsky MR. Effects of mechanical ventilation on the cardiovascular system. In: Tobin MJ, ed. Critical care clinics: Mechanical ventilation. Vol. 6. Orlando, Fl: WB Saunders, 1990:663–678.

44. Pinsky MR. Cardiopulmonary interactions: the effects of negative and positive pleural pressure changes on cardiac output. In: Dantzker D, ed. Cardiopulmonary medicine and critical care. 2nd ed. Philadelphia: WB Saunders, 1991:87–120.

45. Pinsky MR, Hrehocik D, Culpepper JA, Snyder JV. Flow resistance of expiratory positive-pressure systems. Chest 1988;94:788–791.

46. Pinsky MR, Kramer D. The effects of intrathoracic pressure in cardiovascular performance. In: Tinker J, Zapol W, eds. Care of the critically ill. London: Springer-Verlag, 1991:41–58.

47. Pinsky MR, Summer WR. Cardiac augmentation by phasic high intrathoracic support (PHIPS) in man. Chest 1983;84:370–375.

48. Pinsky MR, Vincent JL, DeSmet JM. Estimating left ventricular filling pressure during positive end-expiratory pressure in humans. Am Rev Respir Dis 1991:143:25–31.

49. Rankin JS, Olsen CO, Arentzen CE, et al. The effects of airway pressure on cardiac function in intact dogs and man. Circulation 1982;66:108–120.

50. Rebuck AS, Read J. Assessment and management of severe asthma Am J Med 1971;51:788–798.

51. Robertson JC, Foster G, Johnson R. Relationship of respiratory failure to the oxygen consumption of, lactate production by, and distribution of blood flow among respiratory muscles during increasing inspiratory resistance. J Clin Invest 1977;59:31–42.

52. Robotham JL, Scharf SM. Effects of positive and negative pressure ventilation on cardiac performance. In: Matthay RA, Matthay MA, Dantzker DR, eds. Cardiovascular-pulmonary interaction in normal and diseased lungs. Vol. 4. Philadelphia: WB Saunders, 161–188.

53. Roussos C, Macklem PT. The respiratory muscles. N Engl J Med 1982;307:786–797.

54. Scharf SM, Brown R, Saunders N, et al. Hemodynamic effects of positive pressure inflation. J Appl Physiol 1980;49:124–131.

55. Sharpey-Schaffer EP. Effects of Valsalva maneu-

ver on the normal and failing circulation. Br Med J 1955;1:693–699.

56. Shepherd JT: The lungs as receptor sites for cardiovascular regulation. Circulation 1981;63:1–10.

57. Stalcup SA, Mellins RB: Mechanical forces producing pulmonary edema in acute asthma. N Engl J Med 1977;297:592–596.

58. Taylor RR, Corell JW, Sonnenblick EH, Ross J Jr. Dependence of ventricular distensibility on filling the opposite ventricle. Am J Physiol 1967;213:711–718.

59. Venous B, Jacobs HK, and Lim L. Treatment of the adult respiratory distress syndrome with continuous positive airway pressure. Chest 1979;76:257–261.

60. Vincent JL, Pinsky MR. Cough-induced syncope [Clinico-Pathological Conference]. Intensive Care Med 1988;14:591–594.

61. Vires N, Sillye G, Rassidakis A, et al. Effect of mechanical ventilation on respiratory muscle blood flow during shock. Physiologist 1980;23:1–8.

62. Whittenberger JL, McGregor M, Berglund E, et al: Influence of state of inflation of the lung on pulmonary vascular resistance. J Appl Physiol 1960;15:878–882.

63. Wise RA, Robotham JL, Summer WR: Effects of spontaneous ventilation on the circulation. Lung 1981;159:175–1921.

64. Zema MJ, Caccavano M, Klingfield P. Detection of left ventricular dysfunction in ambulatory subjects with the bedside Valsalva maneuver. Am J Med 1983;75:241–248.

30

Acute Asthma

François Jardin
Jean-Pierre Bourdarias

Asthma is characterized by the occurrence over short periods of time of wide variations in bronchial resistance to flow that result in episodic and paroxysmal attacks of breathlessness. In some asthmatic patients, life-threatening bronchoconstriction can occur in few minutes, while in others persistent symptoms over hours or recurrent symptoms over days (status asthmaticus) may result in progressive respiratory muscles weakness.

EPIDEMIOLOGY

Bronchial asthma occurs at all ages, but predominantly in early life. Precise epidemiologic studies concerning asthma are difficult because they must depend completely on what physicians or patients call asthma. However, it appears that asthma affects more than 5% of the population in industrialized countries. In fact, diagnosis is more reliable below age 45 because chronic bronchitis occurs with such frequency above this age that it may interfere with the diagnosis of asthma.

Pathophysiology of the disease is difficult. Preferred treatments and therapeutic approaches are quite different, depending on whether allergy specialists, chest physicians, or psychoanalysts are involved. The demonstration of allergic sensitivity in asthmatic patients is highly variable. A suspected or proven allergic cause seems to be found more often in young patients (under 16 years old) at the onset of their disease (26). An allergic cause is probably frequent in occupational asthma. Genetic factors have been implicated as possibly connected with the bronchial hyperresponsiveness that is characteristic of asthma, but never demonstrated. The role of infec-tion in the etiology and natural history of asthma is not completely proven, but viral infection as a precipitating factor has been suggested for asthma in children (19). The role of anxiety, stress, and psychosomatic factors is probably underestimated in the etiology of asthma. When discussing their cases with asthmatic patients recovering from their attacks, we often observe that an emotional stress (such as death of a parent, divorce, emigration, loss of job) has preceded the onset of their illness.

As recently emphasized (2), there is much evidence that the severity of asthma is rising (2). For a long time, it was believed that death from asthma did not occur except under extremely unusual conditions. It is now well known that approximately 4000 adults per year die from bronchial asthma in the U.S. Moreover, the mortality rate from asthma seems to be rising despite recent developments in treatment. This alarming increase in the mortality rate raises the question of the efficacy of long-term therapy.

ACUTE AIRWAYS NARROWING: PATHOPHYSIOLOGY

Acute airways narrowing in asthma results from increased airways smooth muscle tone, mucous hypersecretion, and regional inflammation of airways. The relative contribution of each of these factors is variable from one patient to another and from time to time in the same patient.

Bronchomotor tone is regulated by cholinergic parasympathetic activity. Bronchoconstriction represents a normal defense mechanism (against harmful inhalation, for example). An exaggerated bronchocon-

491

strictor response, bronchial hyperresponsiveness, is characteristic of asthma. The suddenness and severity of this response can cause instantaneous and life-threatening bronchoconstriction in asthmatics. Numerous stimuli are considered capable of triggering this "bronchospasm": viral infection (19), allergens (29), environmental (15) or occupational (20) factors, exercise (18), and so on. The role of psychologic events on bronchomotor tone in humans has also been documented, and anxiety is a potent factor that is able to acutely increase bronchomotor tone and respiratory drive, thus leading to a "vicious circle."

A second factor responsible for the acute increase in bronchial resistance to flow is mucous hypersecretion. In this state, the amount of mucous is increased and mucous tends to be more viscous. Because patients cannot cough up secretions, mucous plugs coat airway lumen and play a great part in mechanical impairment. Histologic studies performed in patients who have died from severe attacks have demonstrated that almost the entire bronchial lumen was occluded by a thick, tenacious, mucoid plug that is difficult to detach (6). In patients who die under mechanical ventilation, tidal volume delivery may remain impossible even postmortem. This finding suggests a limited role for bronchospasm and a more important role for mucous abnormality.

A third factor is represented by the regional inflammation of airways. Fatal asthma is associated with marked inflammatory changes of the mucosa and the submucosa of airways; mucosal edema, congestion, and varying degrees of cellular infiltration are present (6). Bronchoalveolar lavage has also revealed an increased proportion of eosinophils in asthmatic patients.

RESPIRATORY CONSEQUENCES

Respiratory Mechanics

During quiet breathing, only inspiration is active. The most important inspiratory muscle is the diaphragm. Contraction of the diaphragm increases the vertical dimension and transverse diameter of the thorax. Conversely, expiration is passive. Because they are elastic, the lungs and chest wall tend to return to their equilibrium position after being actively expanded during inspiration. This elastic recoil pressure supplies a sufficient force to promote expiration of the tidal volume when airways have a normal diameter.

When acute airflow obstruction is present, as in acute asthma, this obstruction predominates at expiration. As a general rule, the bronchi are supported by the radial traction of the surrounding lung tissue, and their diameter increase during inspiration and decrease during expiration. In asthma, the elastic recoil pressure supplied by inspiration of a tidal volume above a normal-ranged FRC becomes insufficient to promote expiration. An additional force should be useful. This additional force is usually obtained by increasing FRC above the normal range (17). Hyperinflation increases elastic recoil pressure and, furthermore, increased lung volume is associated with an increase in airways caliber. A second mechanism is also used by asthmatic patients to increase the expiratory force: active exhalation is facilitated by contraction of the abdominal muscles, which creates a positive pleural pressure. By compressing the lungs, this positive pleural pressure tends to promote expiration but also squeezes the small airways, which are more readily collapsible because of their reduced diameter. Thus, in asthmatic patients, active use of expiratory muscles to increase expiratory flow actually decreases the flow because of airways closure occurring with positive pleural pressure.

Ventilation-Perfusion Mismatch

Bronchial obstruction is not homogeneous, but predominates in some areas and spares other ones so that a heterogeneous distribution of airflow is created. Whereas a relatively reduced part of the tidal volume is distributed to the areas with the highest resistance, resulting in local hypoventilation, a relatively increased part is distribution to the areas with the lowest bronchial resistance, resulting in local hyperventilation. On the other hand, changes in blood flow distribution are more limited. Finally, in areas with reduced ventilation, ventilation/perfusion (V/Q) is decreased, while in areas with an increased ventilation, V/Q is increased. Consequently, blood leaving the low V/Q areas has a reduced oxygen content and an increased carbon dioxide content. In contrast, blood leaving the increased V/Q areas has a reduced carbon dioxide content and a near-normal oxygen content because of the full saturation of hemoglobin. As a result, ventilation-perfusion mismatch alters oxygen content proportionately more than carbon dioxide content and, as a general rule, produces hypoxemia without hypercapnia. If anxiety increases respiratory drive, a very common situation (hypocapnia) may occur. However, hyperventilation cannot correct hypoxemia since blood oxygen content cannot be substantially increased when full saturation of hemoglobin is reached.

When bronchial obstructions are more diffuse and pronounced, they result in global hypoventilation with hypercapnia (respiratory acidosis). In this situation, tidal volume is essentially distributed to proximal airways and do not reach alveoli (dead space ventilation).

Additional Work of Breathing

Acute asthma markedly increases the work of breathing. This work can be computed as the transthoracic pressure (pleural pressure minus atmospheric pressure) necessary to move a given volume of air. During inspiration, although the airways still dilate, they cannot reach the same dimensions as those achieved in the unobstructed state. A more negative pleural pressure is thus needed to inspire the same tidal volume, particularly in an hyperinflated lung. Inspiratory transthoracic pressure is markedly increased (27). During expiration, there occurs a further reduction of the already small-sized airways. Therefore, an increase in the expiratory driving pressure becomes necessary for expiration. This increase is partially brought about by active contraction of the expiratory muscles, creating a positive pleural pressure (10) and, in turn, an increased transthoracic pressure.

During acute asthma, the acute increase in the FRC represents an efficient compensating mechanism for offsetting elevated bronchial resistance because it is associated with a greater elastic recoil, which facilitates expiration. However, such an increase in elastic recoil cannot be achieved without additional cost. Hyperinflated lungs have a reduced compliance and thus are stiffer to inflate and thereby require an additional work of breathing (17).

Persistent increase in the mechanical work of breathing causes fatigue. As it does in skeletal muscle, respiratory muscle fatigue occurs when the rate of energy consumption of these muscles is higher than the rate of energy supplied by blood flow (16). Lactic acidosis, indicating oxygen debt, is often observed in acute asthma (1, 7). Unfavorable hemodynamic conditions may precipitate muscle failure (10). Hypovolemia is also present during acute asthma, a finding still unexplained (28).

HEMODYNAMIC CONSEQUENCES
Pulmonary Artery Hypertension

The presence of hypoventilated lung areas, resulting in alveolar hypoxia, causes local vasoconstriction. Reducing blood flow through the low V/Q areas and increasing it through higher V/Q areas improves gas exchange. However, it also increases pulmonary vascular resistance because increased blood flow should pass through a reduced vascular bed.

Pulmonary hypertension in asthma also results from the negative level of pleural pressure reached at inspiration. This important mechanism was first emphasized by Permutt (14), who reported that alveolar distending pressure (i.e., alveolar pressure at atmospheric level minus pleural pressure at a markedly negative level) is sharply increased. In a more recent study, using measured transmural pulmonary artery diastolic pressure, we could confirm this concept by demonstrating an inspiratory increase in pulmonary vascular resistance (10). Compared to expiration, pulmonary artery diastolic pressure was elevated, whereas right ventricular stroke output was markedly reduced (9, 10).

Right Ventricular Failure

A very specific pattern of right ventricular failure occurs in asthma, inspiratory right ventricular failure. At expiration, examination of the right ventricle by two-dimensional echocardiography does not reveal any sign of right ventricular failure (9). At this respiratory time, only right ventricular filling is impaired, producing a progressive reduction in right ventricular outflow as expiration develops (Fig. 30.1). In fact, the positive level of pleural pressure generated by active expiration acts on the right ventricle as a Valsalva maneuver, and reduces right ventricular inflow from venous return. Turgor of jugular vein observed at expiration results from mechanical impairment of venous return and not from actual right ventricular systolic dysfunction. It should also be noted that venous return impairment is usually associated with a trend toward hypovolemia (28).

At inspiration, the very low level of pleural pressure efficiently promotes venous return to the right heart cavities. As evidenced by two-dimensional echocardiography, right ventricular preload is markedly increased at inspiration, even if vena caval collapse tends to limit right ventricular distension (9, 10). Despite this increase in right ventricular preload, right ventricular stroke output is markedly reduced, a finding highly suggestive of inspiratory right ventricular systolic failure. As we have proposed, this right ventricular systolic failure may be interpreted as resulting from the external application of a very negative pleural pressure on the right ventricular free wall, whereas the external pressure exerted on the intraalveolar part of the pulmonary circulation is the alveolar distending pressure (i.e., the transpulmonary pressure) that is highly positive in this situation. The external negative pressure applied to the right ventricle appears strong enough to hold the right ventricular free wall and impede its systolic inward motion (9). During systole, contraction of the normal right ventricle

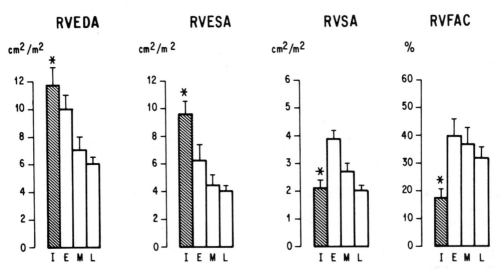

Figure 30.1 Average values for two-dimensional echocardiographic measurements of right ventricular *(RV)* end-diastolic *(ED)* and end-systolic *(ES)* areas *(A)* in a group of 20 patients during acute asthmatic attacks. Four successive cardiac beats occurred on a whole respiratory cycle, one during inspiration *(I, hatched bars)* and three during expiration *(E, early expiration; M, midexpiration; L, late expiration; open bars)*. A progressive reduction in RV dimensions, stroke area *(RVSA)*, and RV fractional area contraction *(RVFAC)* was observed along with expiration, acting as a Valsalva maneuver. During inspiration, RVSA and RVFAC were markedly reduced despite RV enlargement*, P < 0.05.

can only develop a positive pressure of about 30 mm Hg, and at inspiration during an asthmatic attack, a negative pressure of approximately the same level is generated by the diaphragm. Admittedly, one should bear in mind that thoracic and cardiac pumps compete with one another.

Paradoxical Pulse

Inspiratory reduction in peripheral arterial pulse is a common finding in acute asthma, but it does not involve any clinical significance about the severity of dyspneic attacks. Reduction in pulse pressure implies that the decrease in systolic pressure is greater than that in diastolic pressure. Thus, transmission of pleural pressure to the arterial tree cannot account for the appearance of paradoxical pulse. Furthermore, if aortic compliance is assumed to be constant, this phenomenon should imply a reduction in left ventricular stroke output. In fact, negative pleural swings at inspiration impair both diastolic and systolic left ventricular functions.

In a study using two-dimensional echocardiography, we could demonstrate that left ventricular preload is reduced at inspiration (10). Two main mechanisms are thought to contribute to the reduction in the left ventricular preload: (1) decreased right ventricular output reduces pulmonary venous return; and (2) acute right ventricular distension in a stiff pericardial space reduces left ventricular compliance. In addition, an inspiratory increase in left ventricular afterload may interfere since negative pleural pressure increases the pressure gradient against which the left ventricle must eject a given stroke volume into the extrathoracic compartment (25). In other words, at inspiration, the left ventricle should increase its hydraulic power to eject the same stroke volume (23). In clinical studies performed in asthmatic patients having a normal baseline left ventricular function, the inspiratory left ventricular afterloading is usually cancelled by a prominent reduction in left ventricular preload (10).

Regarding the paradoxic pulse mechanism, the "Windkessel" concept as applied to thoracic aorta deserves considera-

tion. As previously stated, the widely accepted assumption that an inspiratory reduction in pulse pressure reflects a decrease in left ventricular stroke output implies that compliance of thoracic aorta remains unaltered despite wide changes in pleural pressure. As a matter of fact, an inspiratory increase and an expiratory decrease in aortic compliance are likely to occur, and these changes can modify the Windkessel function of thoracic aorta. When a negative external pressure is exerted at inspiration, systolic expansion of the thoracic aorta is facilitated. Thus, the damping effect of this vessel on phasic left ventricular stroke is more pronounced. Conversely, when a positive pleural pressure is applied to the aortic wall, systolic expansion of the thoracic aorta is reduced and pulse pressure increases.

CLINICAL PRESENTATION

Asthma characteristically occurs in attacks of variable duration; some are brief, but others may last several days. Between attacks, patients are free of symptoms because their pulmonary function is normal or nearly normal.

The onset of an asthmatic attack is more frequent at night. Asthmatic attack is characterized by expiratory dyspnea, wheezing, cough, and ronchi. Because the bronchial lumens enlarge upon inspiration and narrow upon expiration, dyspnea is more pronounced and wheezing and ronchi are audible during expiration. A characteristic alteration in breathing pattern thus occurs, including a rapid inspiration followed by a prolonged expiration. During inspiration, the negative intrathoracic pressure is accompanied by retraction of the soft tissues of the intercostal, suprasternal, and supraclavicular spaces. Violent use of accessory respiratory muscles (scalenes muscles, sternomastoids) may be visible. Expiratory dyspnea requires the use of abdominal wall muscles.

Asthmatic patients are usually anxious, particularly when they are hospitalized in a respiratory intensive care unit. Dyspnea limits speech, which is interrupted by frequent pauses for breath. The patients are fatigued, sweating, and often agitated.

Regular tachycardia is present. Blood pressure may be slightly elevated due to catecholamine release, and an inspiratory depression in pulse is present. External jugular veins are prominent at expiration and they collapse at inspiration. When present, cyanosis is the feature of advanced hemoglobin desaturation.

A pulse rate greater than 130 beats/min, occurrence of obtundation, reduced thoracic excursion with pardoxic disappearance of wheezing, are symptoms indicating severity. When they are associated, they may indicate an immediate need for mechanical ventilation.

Routine chest x-ray is of limited value in a typical asthmatic attack; it confirms lung distension and usually does not provide additional information that will influence therapy. Because of the duration of the expiration, an x-ray is usually taken at this time; the cardiac silhouette appears reduced in relation to lung distension (Fig. 30.2).

Results of blood gas analysis also do not influence therapeutic options. Hypoxemia is present in all patients hospitalized in a respiratory intensive care unit, and can be easily corrected by oxygen administration. In many patients, some degree of hyperventilation is present that produces hypocapnia. On the other hand, hypercapnia indicates a severe attack associated with more diffuse or pronounced obstructions or complicated by respiratory weakness. However, acute hypercapnia can resolve rapidly and the level of $Paco_2$ per se is not a guideline for deciding whether mechanical ventilation should be instituted. Some degree of metabolic acidosis is also present in the majority of asthmatic patients hospitalized in a respiratory intensive care unit (1, 7). When associated with respiratory acidosis, metabolic acidosis may produce a substantial shift in arterial pH, but this finding does not require special management; plasma alkalinization, for example, would be meaningless in this situation. We also noticed that hemoconcentration was present in about 90% of

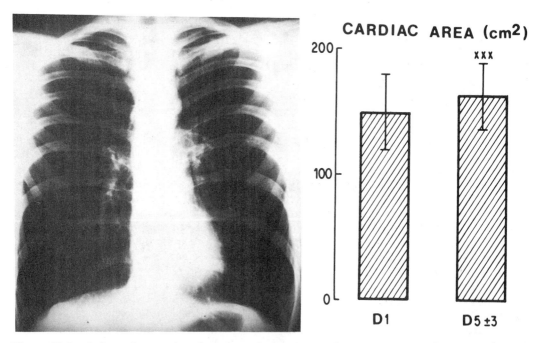

Figure 30.2. *Left panel,* a routine chest x-ray in a young asthmatic patient is shown, illustrating the acute pulmonary distension. *Right panel,* the average value of heart area, mapped from chest x-ray in 50 asthmatic patients, is significantly reduced from admission (day 1) to recovery (day 5 +/−3). XXX, P < 0.05.

our patients. The exact mechanism of this hemoconcentration, associated with hypovolemia, remains unclear, but an isolated increase in hemoglobin and plasma proteins concentration, without any change in electrolytes or BUN concentration, suggests an acute leak of fluid from the circulatory compartment to the extracellular compartment. An elevated pressure at the venous side of capillaries during prolonged expiration, modifying Starling's equilibrium, is consistent with this mechanism.

TREATMENT

Therapeutic Goals

Long-term treatment for asthma appears to be a recurring challenge for chest physicians. For respiratory intensive care specialists, however, management of the disease is easier: the therapeutic goals are primarily the resolution of the acute attack, and the avoidance of an early relapse after discharge.

An asthmatic patient that is admitted to an emergency department or intensive care unit should be managed with calm, avoiding unnecessary agitation and invasive procedures.

Oxygen

The first therapeutic measure in a severe attack of asthma is oxygen administration. Hypoxemia can usually be corrected by a flow of 4 to 6 liters/min given by a nasal tube (or by a face mask, and used as a vector for nebulization). Acute hypercapnia observed in asthma does not limit oxygen use, and the potential risk of increasing $Paco_2$ by decreasing respiratory drive or reducing hypoxic vasoconstriction appears trivial in asthma; dilation of peripheral airways by oxygen administration overrides its slight depressive effect. However, this risk actually exists in chronic hypercapnic patients who often exhibit "asthmatic" exacerbation of their dyspnea. Chronic hypercapnia is easily recognized on blood gas analysis when some degree of metabolic alkalosis is present, an unusual finding in pure asthma.

Bronchodilators

The most effective bronchodilators in current use are β-adrenergic agonists (21, 22). Inhaled β-adrenergic agonists are the treatment of choice for acute asthma. This mode of administration appears most efficient and preferable to intravenous infusion. In our current practice, we use salbutamol administered by an oxygen face mask. β-adrenergic agonists increase the heart rate. Thus, tachycardia caused by excessive β-adrenergic agonist administration can be misleading in the appreciation of asthma severity.

Theophylline or aminophylline are less effective bronchodilators than β-agonist agents. In an acute attack they are only effective when given intravenously. Theophylline has a relatively high incidence of unwanted side effects, such as nausea, headache, and cardiac arrhythmias. The therapeutic theophylline plasma level ranges from 10–20 μg/ml (13), but monitoring of plasma concentration does not totally protect against side effects because they can be present in patients in whom plasma concentration remains within the therapeutic range.

Steroids

Steroids, given by inhalation in the majority of patients, or orally in a minority, are effective to control asthma on a long-term basis. Since they do not have a rapid bronchodilator effect and do not provide immediate relief of symptoms, they do not represent a first-choice therapy during an acute asthma attack. Steroids are usually given intravenously when the initial treatment does not sufficiently improve the patient's status (5). Some authors recommend using steroids systematically in acute asthma (3, 14). It is argued that steroids have a beneficial effect in the prevention of early relapses after intensive care treatment (3).

Treatment of Anxiety

Asthmatic patients are markedly anxious during an acute attack, and hospitalization in an emergency room or in an intensive care unit may aggravate their anxiety. We do not agree with the general reluctance against sedation in these patients who do not exhibit chronic hypercapnia but only an acute episode of hypoventilation. Mild sedation using, for instance, benzodiazepine compounds, is very useful; adverse side effects in a continuously monitored patient are usually not likely unless chronic obstructive pulmonary disease and chronic hypercapnia are present.

Mechanical Ventilation

In severe asthmatic attacks, mechanical ventilation may be required. Association of the above-mentioned symptoms of severity usually leads to this decision. Measurement of peak flow with a disposable flowmeter may confirm a clinical impression of severity. The controlled mode is necessary in these exhausted patients. A complete adaptation to the respirator should be obtained to suppress useless and energy-consuming muscular activity. For this purpose, we use intravenous sedation with benzodiazepines combined with morphinic drugs, despite their theoretical bronchoconstrictor effect, which is trivial in this setting. In some patients, curarization may be required when intravenous sedation alone does not induce complete muscular inactivity. Institution of mechanical ventilation in an asthmatic patient indicates definite failure of bronchondilator agents, which can thus be withdrawn.

Airflow obstruction often rends mechanical ventilation difficult. It may even be impossible in few cases, as illustrated in Figure 30.3. To avoid mechanical complications such as subcutaneous or mediastinal emphysema or tense pneumothorax, airway pressure should be limited (peak airway pressure less than or equal to 40 cm H_2O is our current upper limit). With this limitation in airway pressure, tidal delivery remains usually low in severely obstructed patients. With the use of an increased FiO_2 (up to 0.4 or 0.5), hypoxemia can be corrected and arterial oxy-

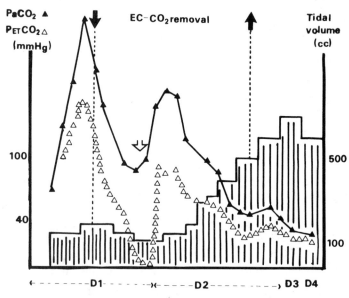

Figure 30.3 In a 22-year-old asthmatic woman, a substantial tidal delivery could not be obtained despite profound sedation and curarization, even with a high peak airway pressure (50 cm H_2O). When the $Paco_2$ level reached 200 mm Hg and higher, circulatory failure developed along with a rapid increase in lactate blood level. Extracorporeal co_2 (EC-co_2) removal was decided and performed during 36 hours (12). After 12 hours, some improvement was observed, allowing progressive increase in tidal delivery. The patient was extubated after 5 days of mechanical ventilation. *Open arrow* denotes a reduction in extra-corporeal blood flow (from 3 to 1.5 liters/min). ▲, $Paco_2$; △, $Petco_2$ (end-tidal Pco_2).

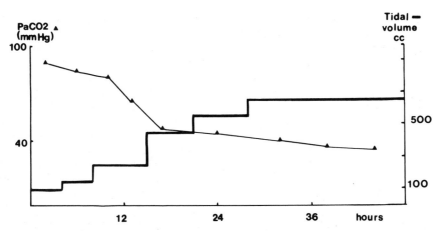

Figure 30.4. Time course of Paco$_2$ and tidal delivery in a 30-year-old male asthmatic patient requiring mechanical ventilation. Complete adaptation to the respirator was obtained by profound sedation and curarization. Mechanical ventilation was run on the controlled mode with low frequency (8 to 12 cycles per minute) and limited peak airway pressure (40 cm H$_2$O initially and 30 cm H$_2$O after the 28th hour). ▲, Paco$_2$

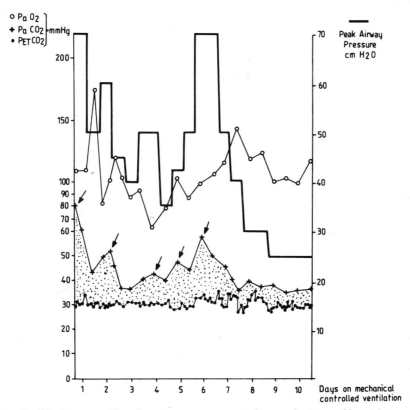

Figure 30.5. In this 35-year-old asthmatic woman, several exacerbations of bronchospasm *(arrows)* were observed under mechanically controlled ventilation, despite profound sedation, which produced large discrepancies (materialized by *dotted area*) between arterial *(a)* and end-tidal *(ET)* Pco$_2$. Note the excessive airway pressure that resulted in major subcutaneous emphysema in this case. Despite this serious complication, the patient ultimately recovered, but 10 days of respiratory support were necessary. ○, Pao$_2$; +, Paco$_2$; ●, Petco$_2$;

gen saturation sufficiently improved despite a relatively small tidal volume. However, if hypercapnia persists under controlled ventilation, its rapid correction should not be attempted (4). Intrinsic PEEP is present at the onset of mechanical ventilation. A sufficient time for expiration should be allowed to avoid excessive gas trapping (at least two times the insufflation length). When bronchial obstruction progressively resolves, peak airway pressure decreases; at this time, tidal delivery should be progressively increased if the patient remains hypercapnic (Fig. 30.4). When normocapnia is obtained with moderate airway pressure, sedation can be progressively reduced. Some relapse is often observed when the patient is being awakened. Weaning from mechanical ventilation is usually obtained within several days in pure asthma (1–10 days, in our experience).

When mechanical ventilation is difficult, invasive arterial pressure monitoring is indicated since a drop in arterial pressure may require hemodynamic support by blood volume expansion. It also facilitates blood sampling for repeated blood gas analysis. Conversely, end-tidal P_{CO_2} (PETCO$_2$) monitoring is not very useful (11). This is particularly true in asthma because large discrepancies between end-tidal and arterial P_{CO_2} have been noted, as illustrated by Figures 30.3 and 30.5.

Hemodynamic Support

During acute asthma, the cardiac index has been reported to be elevated (10). This is not an unexpected finding because when muscular work is increased, a high level of cardiac output is required. However, mechanical conditions of breathing in asthma are associated with an alteration of the pulmonary circulation, which tends to limit the spontaneous increase in cardiac output (8). These mechanical conditions prevent an increase in stroke output so that asthmatic patients can only adapt cardiac output by increasing heart rate. We readily use blood volume expansion which can markedly improve the hemodynamic pattern of these patients. The risk of iatrogenic pulmonary edema advocated by some

authors (27) is low in asthma insofar as the blood volume present in the pulmonary capillary bed is markedly reduced.

References

1. Appel D, Rubenstein R, Schrager K, Williams H. Lactic acidosis in severe asthma. Am J Med 1983; 75:580–584.
2. Benatar S. Fatal asthma. N Engl J Med 1986;314:423–429.
3. Chapman K, Verbeek R, White J, Rebuck A. Effect of a short course of prednisone in the prevention of early relapse after the emergency room treatment of acute asthma. N Engl J Med 1991;324:788–794.
4. Darioli R, Perret C. Mechanical controlled hypoventilation in status asthmaticus. Am Rev Respir Dis 1984;129:385–387.
5. Franklin W. Asthma in the emergency room. N Engl J Med 1981;305:826–827.
6. Hayes J. The pathology of bronchial asthma. In: Weiss E, Segal M, eds. Bronchial asthma. Boston: Little, Brown and Company, 1976:347–382.
7. Jardin F. Fréquence de l'acidose métabolique au cours de l'état de mal asthmatique de l'adulte. Press Med 1977;6:329–332.
8. Jardin F, Bourdarias JP. Influence of abnormal breathing conditions on right ventricular function. Intensive Care Med 1991;17:129–135.
9. Jardin F, Dubourg O, Margairaz A, Bourdarias JP. Inspiratory impairment in right ventricular performance during acute asthma. Chest 1987; 92:789–795.
10. Jardin F, Farcot JC, Boisante L, Prost JF, Gueret P, Bourdarias JP. Mechanism of paradoxical pulse in bronchial asthma. Circulation 1982; 66:887–894.
11. Jardin F, Genevray B, Bazin M, Margairaz A. Inability to titrate PEEP in patients with acute respiratory failure using end-tidal carbon dioxide measurements. Anesthesiology 1985;62:530–533.
12. Jardin F, Genevray B, Steg G, Margairaz A. Epuration extra-corporelle du gaz carbonique au cours d'une crise d'asthme sévère. Presse Med 1986;15:9.
13. Koch-Weser J. Bronchodilator therapy. N Engl J Med 1977;297:476–482, 758–764.
14. Littenberg B, Gluck E. A controlled trial of methylprednisolone in the emergency treatment of acute asthma. N Engl J Med 1986;314:150–152.
15. Lopez M, Wessels F, Salvaggio J. Environmental influences in asthma. In: Weiss E, Segal M, eds. Bronchial asthma. Boston: Little, Brown and Company, 1976:503–516.
16. Macklem P. Respiratory muscle: the vital pump. Chest 1980;78:753–758.
17. McFadden E. Respiratory mechanics in asthma. In: Weiss E, Segal M, eds. Bronchial asthma. Boston: Little, Brown and Company, 1986:259–278.
18. McFadden E. Exercise and asthma. N Engl J Med 1987;317:502–504.
19. Minor T, Elliot D, DeMeo A, Ouellette J, Cohen M, Reed C. Viruses as precipitants of asthmatics attacks in children. JAMA 1974;227:292–298.

20. Murphy R. Industrial disease with asthma. In: Weiss E, Segal M, eds. Bronchial asthma. Boston: Little, Brown and Company, 1976:517–536.
21. Newhouse M, Dolovitch M. Control of asthma by aerosols. N Engl J Med 1986;315:870–874.
22. Oates J, Wood A. A new approach to the treatment of asthma. N Eng J Med, 1989;321:1517–1527.
23. Olsen C, Tyson G, Maier G, Davis J, Rankin S. Diminished stroke volume during inspiration: a reverse thoracic pump. Circulation 1985;72:668–679.
24. Permutt S. Relation between pulmonary arterial pressure and pleural pressure during the acute asthmatic attack. Chest 1973;63 (suppl) 25S–26S.
25. Robotham J, Lixfeld W, Holland L, McGregor M, Bryan C, Rabson J. Effects of respiration on cardiac performance. J Appl Physiol 1978;44:703–709.
26. Speizer F. Epidemiology, prevalence and mortality in asthma. In: Weiss E, Segal M, eds. Bronchial asthma. Boston: Little, Brown and Company, 1976:43–52.
27. Stalcup A, Mellins R. Mechanical forces producing pulmonary edema in acute asthma. N Engl J Med 1977;297:592–596.
28. Straub P, Bühlman A, Rossier P. Hypovolemia in status asthmaticus. Lancet 1969;2:923–925.
29. Van Arsdel P. Etiological factors in asthma: allergens and others provoking factors. In: Weiss E, and Segal M, eds. Bronchial asthma. Boston: Little, Brown and Company, 1976:473–480.

31

Cardiopulmonary Resuscitation

Sheldon Magder

A 62 year-old-man developed diffuse ST segment elevations and suffered a cardiac arrest due to dissection of the left main coronary artery during cardiac catheterization. Cardiopulmonary resuscitation was commenced but he failed to respond to defibrillation; arrangements were made for an immediate aortocoronary bypass procedure. For the next 40 minutes and until the operating room was ready, he received closed chest cardiac massage; in the operating room, open chest massage was continued for another 10 minutes until he was put on bypass. During this period, the heart was perforated. He underwent a three-vessel aortocoronary bypass procedure and repair of his ventricle and was successfully weaned from the pump. Postoperatively, he was hemodynamically stable but remained comatose. Over the next few months he had a slow neurologic recovery. By 4 months following the event he was able to communicate but appeared withdrawn and not completely appropriate in his responses. He also had numerous contractures and significant muscle atrophy.

This case illustrates a number of important points about cardiopulmonary resuscitation (CPR). It shows how CPR can successfully maintain the circulation (16), for this man survived ventricular fibrillation that lasted for more than 45 minutes. However, it also shows the limitations of CPR, for although he survived, he was left with significant neurologic dysfunction due to inadequate perfusion. Finally, it illustrates an important complication of open chest massage, cardiac perforation.

BRIEF HISTORY

The history of CPR has been covered in a number of recent reviews (35, 71, 127, 128) and only a few major landmarks will be considered. Although the Academy of Science of Paris certified mouth-to-mouth breathing in 1740 as the treatment of choice for drowning, this approach was abandoned in favor of techniques that employed chest compression and passive recoil of the chest for ventilation. This was allegedly because of the mistaken belief that expired gas concentrations were inadequate for oxygenation, although I suspect that aesthetic concerns may also have been operative. In the 1950s, Safar and colleagues (104) clearly established the superiority of mouth-to-mouth ventilation over arm-lift techniques, and it is now no longer debated that ventilation should be provided by positive pressure ventilation, whether from the mouth of a resuscitator or by a bag mask ventilator. The normal expired O_2 is 17–18% and therefore more than adequate for oxygenation.

Artificial circulatory support lagged behind the development of ventilatory support. There had been early animal experiments that showed that chest compressions could produce blood flow (35, 128), but these did not receive much attention, possibly because the heart could not be defibrillated. The major advance occurred with the report by Zoll and co-workers (131) on the reversal of ventricular fibrillation with an external countershock. This made it possible to defibrillate the heart, and it became necessary to develop temporary means of artificially sustaining the circulation until the heart could be defibrillated. Until the 1960s this was done by open chest direct compression of the heart. The present approach of closed chest CPR began with a fortuitous event. Kouwenhaven noted a rise in arterial pressure of dogs every time the defibrillator paddles were applied with a great force. In association with Knickerbocker and Jude, he developed the present-day approach of external chest compression (71). The combination of mouth-to-mouth breathing and external chest compression was standardized for basic life support in 1966.

DEFIBRILLATION

The success of CPR ultimately depends on the ability to defibrillate the heart, and the faster this is accomplished, the better the results (48, 67).

Hypoxia and acidosis decrease the efficacy of debrillation; therefore, delay is an important factor (67). For this reason, the AHA recommends that chest compressions be performed for 2–3 minutes before defibrillation in an unwitnessed arrest (14). This will potentially increase myocardial oxygenation and decrease acidosis because tissue PCO_2 is an important part of the tissue acidosis and it will decrease as flow is increased (54, 116).

Defibrillation was originally performed with AC current, but this was superseded by DC current. The first reason is practical since DC current can be obtained from a portable unit, whereas AC current requires a constant source from the wall. The DC current also allows a better quantitation of the energy and is of less risk to bystanders.

An important factor in defibrillation is the energy delivered, which is the product of the voltage and current (amperage). The amount of energy that gets to the chest is determined by the resistance between the energy source and the heart (3, 65, 103, 114). This can be decreased by increasing the paddle size, but, if they are too large, the density of charge is decreased. Gelled or soaked pads will also help decrease the resistance. Pressing hard on the chest wall decreases thoracic impedance by decreasing the thoracic volume. Finally, the paddles must be sufficiently far apart to make sure that the heart is exposed to the current and that the current does not simply travel from paddle to paddle.

A point that is often debated is whether body size is of importance in determining the energy needed (3, 65, 67, 114). In animal studies, the energy requirements vary considerably and do not seem to depend on the animal size. Thus, most do not believe that the amount of energy has to

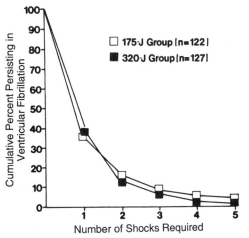

Figure 31.1. Electrocardiogram and aortic pressure in patient 3. Ventricular fibrillation followed right coronary injection. Patient remained conscious for 39 seconds with the application of external pressures followed by cough-induced cardiopulmonary resuscitation and conversion to sinus rhythm was achieved with 400 w/sec shock. (From Weaver WD, Fahrenbruch CE, Johnson DD, Hallstrom AP. Effect of epinephrine and lidocaine therapy on outcome after cardiac arrest due to ventricular fibrillation. Circulation 1990;82:2027–2034.)

be increased for large individuals (3, 49), although others feel that this is important (114). An important study by Weaver et al. (120) showed that two shocks with low energy (175 J) followed by a third with high energy (320 J), if necessary, produced the same results as three high-energy shocks (Fig. 31.1). A critical variable in the delivery of the energy to the heart is the impedance of the chest wall; defibrillators have been designed that can measure this and then allow better quantitation of the energy needs (66). By and large, however, the risks of myocardial damage with 175 J appears low, and the approach suggested by Weaver et al. is very practical. Of interest, there has recently been a report of defibrillation with an esophageal electrode that requires less energy (2).

GENERATION OF BLOOD FLOW

Kouwenhaven et al. (71) thought that the mechanism of blood flow during closed chest CPR was direct compression of the heart between the sternum and spine. Indeed, they called the technique closed-chest cardiac massage. This requires that the force be preferentially transmitted to the ventricle so that ventricular pressures increase more than atrial pressure and close the atrioventricular valves. This is called the cardiac pump theory. If this is the correct explanation for blood in the CPR, then where compressions are applied on the chest is important.

In 1980, Rudivoff and associates (102) noted that it was difficult to generate a pulse pressure during CPR in patients with flail chests, despite the fact that it was easier to directly compress their hearts. They proposed that the mechanism of blood flow in CPR is therefore the generation of intrathoracic pressure, and that the failure of CPR in patients with flail chests is because intrathoracic pressure cannot be increased in someone with a flail chest. According to this theory, compression of the chest increases the pressure throughout the chest and all the intrathoracic blood volume is compressed and ejected. Backward flow is prevented by valves in the superior vena cava (47) and a greater potential for the veins to collapse than the arteries with the rise in intrathoracic pressure. This is called the thoracic pump model. If this theory is correct, blood flow in CPR will be improved by increasing intrathoracic pressure. Which of these two theories, i.e., cardiac pump or thoracic pump, is correct, continues to be debated (6, 13, 20, 57, 83, 100, 123, 125).

Before discussing the mechanisms of the generation of blood flow in CPR, it is useful to review the generation of blood flow by the beating heart. The beating heart ejects blood essentially by a rapid decrease in ventricular compliance during systole. Sagawa (105) called this a "time-varying elastance." Increasing stiffness of the ventricle results in a progressive rise in intraventricular pressure, which eventually ejects blood from the ventricle when the ventricular pressure exceeds the aortic pressure and the aortic valve opens. Backward flow is prevented by the atrioventricular valves. The aortic pressure remains elevated in diastole because of the discharge of the compliant volume of the

aorta, reflected waves, and the time taken for blood to drain through the arterial resistance. The pressure generated by the ventricles and the volume ejected depend on the degree of filling of the ventricles (i.e., Frank-Starling mechanism), the afterload which is a function of aortic pressure, and cardiac contractility. Furthermore, a large part of the return of blood to the heart takes place during the ventricular ejection phase because the atrial pressures normally remain low, at least until the end of systole. (See Chapter 8 for a discussion of the factors that determine the return of blood to the heart.) The determinants of venous return to the heart include the stressed volume of the vasculature, venous compliance, resistance to venous return, the distribution of blood flow, and right atrial pressure (assuming that the right atrial pressure is greater than zero and greater than pleural pressure).

No matter which model of CPR is correct (i.e., thoracic pump or cardiac pump), some common basic principles apply to the generation of flow. Flow occurs when a pressure gradient develops between two loci, whether this pressure difference is created by direct cardiac compression or compression of intrathoracic blood volume by an increase in intrathoracic pressure. There must also be a volume of blood that can be transferred by this pressure difference; this is the left ventricular volume in the direct cardiac compression model, and intrapulmonary and cardiac volumes in the thoracic pump model. There must be a mechanism that only allows unidirectional flow. This is the atrioventricular valves in the cardiac compression model and the venous valves and venous collapse in the thoracic pump model. There must be a mechanism for venous return that results in a gradient in pressure from the periphery to the right atrium. In the direct cardiac compression model, this occurs with the release of the compression of the ventricles and in the thoracic pump model by the decrease in intrathoracic pressure.

Theoretic Considerations

Wise and co-workers (94, 127, 128) developed a theoretical model to analyze blood

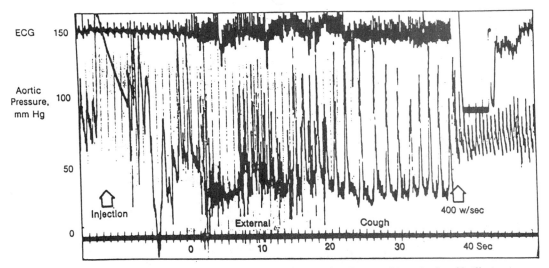

Figure 31.2. Effectiveness of 175 and 320 J shocks in defibrillation. Ventricular fibrillation was converted at least transiently in over 60% of patients after one shock and in more than 8% after two shocks. Defibrillation rates were virtually the same in the two treatment groups. Defibrillation occurred in all patients. Shocks of 320 J were delivered to both treatment groups when three or more shocks were required. The tracings show that the aortic pressure was actually higher during cough than with the application of external pressures. With a cough, peak aortic pressures were >100 mmHg. (From Criley JM, Blaufuss AH, Kissel GL. Cough-induced cardiac compression. JAMA 1976;236:1246–1250.)

flow in CPR and tested many of the predictions of their analysis (Fig. 31.2). These workers support the thoracic pump model, but their analysis still applies to any closed chest CPR model. There are different implications for open chest massage that will be discussed later. In their model, the circulation has two compliant regions; one contains the thoracic blood volume and the other contains the peripheral volume. These two compartments are connected by two lumped variable conduits with characteristics of resistance and collapsibility. These represent venous and arterial circuits. The direction of flow is determined by one-way valves in each conduit. When flow is stopped, the pressure is the same throughout the system and determined by the sum of the two compliances and stressed volume. An increase in pressure around the thoracic compartment, whether this is the left ventricle in the cardiac pump model or pleural pressure around the pulmonary blood volume in the thoracic pump model, produces a gradient from the thorax to the periphery that generates flow and transfers volume from the thoracic compartment to the peripheral region. The pressure thus rises in the peripheral region. Relaxation of the thoracic pressure, whether it is the ventricular pressure in the direct compression model or pleural pressure with the thoracic pump model, allows flow to occur from the peripheral compartment back to the thoracic compartment. These workers developed an equation to describe the model mathematically, which is based on the following: (*a*) the total volume change that can occur in the thoracic compartment if it is first allowed to fill to equilibrium during the filling condition, and then empty to equilibrium during the emptying phase by compression (V_m); (*b*) the time constant of emptying, τe, which is the product of the resistance and compliance of the arterial circuit; (*c*) the time constant of filling, τf, which is the product of venous resistance and compliance; (*e*) the fraction of the total cycle, α, spent in the emptying phase, which is also called the duty cycle; and (*f*) the fraction of the cycle spent in the filling phase, $1-\alpha$. Since time is required for filling and emptying, as is given by the time constant τe and τf, and these events must occur independently, not all Vm will be available for flow if the filling and emptying phase are not long enough. The actual equation is:

$$Q = \frac{Vm}{\tau e/\alpha + \tau f/(1-\alpha)} \quad (1)$$

where Q is flow in liters per minute. The final Q will thus be reduced if α is insufficient to allow adequate emptying. This is especially important if τe is long.

The volume that can be displaced, Vm, is determined by the difference in pressure in the thoracic compartment during the emptying and filling phases, whether this is the heart in the cardiac pump model or the thoracic volume in the thoracic pump model. It is also determined by the compliances of the peripheral and thoracic compartments, for these values determine how much volume is stored in each region at a given pressure. The formal equation for this is:

$$Vm = (Pple - Pplf) (CtCp / (Ct + CP)) \quad (2)$$

where Ct is the thoracic compliance, Cp is the peripheral compliance, and Pple and Pplf are the cardiac or thoracic pressures during emptying and filling, respectively.

The time constants of emptying and filling depend on the arterial (Ra) and venous (Rv) resistances and compliances. The formal equations for these are:

$$\tau e = Ra (CtCp / (Ct + Cp)) \quad (3)$$

$$\tau f = Rv (CtCp / (Ct + Cp)) \quad (4)$$

Thus, the higher the resistance or the greater the compliance, the longer it takes to empty or fill the thoracic compartment.

The above analysis assumed that the conduits were rigid tubes and not collapsible. However, both the arteries and veins are collapsible if the surrounding pressures are sufficiently high (94). This occurs when the pressures across the wall, i.e., the transmural pressure, is close to zero in the veins and at a negative value for the more rigid arteries (130). It should be emphasized that when collapse occurs it does not stop flow, but limits any further increase in flow when the downstream pressure is decreased. When flow limita-tion occurs due to collapse, the total volume of the system becomes an important determinant of Vm, along with the transmural pressures at which collapse occurs. The formal equation for this is:

$$Vm = V - (Ptm'a\ Ct) - (Ptm'v\ Cp) \quad (5)$$

where Ptm'a and Ptm'v are the collapse pressures of the arterial and venous conduits. The Ptm'v is close to zero, whereas Ptm'a is a negative number. Under these circumstances, the time constants of emptying and filling are determined solely by the compliances of the thoracic and peripheral compartments and the resistances up to the point of collapse, Ra' and Rv', respectively. This can be formally written as:

$$\tau e = Ra'\ Ct \quad (6)$$

$$\tau f = Rv'\ Cp \quad (7)$$

Implications of Theoretic Modeling of CPR

We can now compare some of the factors in the generation of blood flow with CPR to blood flow with normal cardiac function. A major difference occurs in the way blood returns to the heart. Closed chest compressions elevate pleural pressure during the ejection of blood and thus blood can only return to the heart during the relaxation phase. This is why both τe and τf occur in the denominator of equation 1. In contrast, blood returns to the beating heart during both systole and diastole (127, 128).

The arrested heart also cannot respond to changes in preload. The displaced volume, Vm, is directly proportional to the difference between the pleural pressure during emptying and filling, and the pleural pressure during emptying depends totally on the operator. There is no feedback that can alter Pple and Pplf to the volume returning to the heart. In contrast, in the beating heart, the volume that returns to the heart determines the end-diastolic pressure, which directly affects the pressure generated by the heart and the volume ejected.

The "contractility" of the arrested heart is also fixed in CPR, except for some variation in the force applied by the operator. In contrast, in the beating heart, neuro-humeral mechanisms adjust cardiac contractility to the needs of the body.

Except with open chest direct cardiac massage, the intrathoracic pressure must rise during CPR, whether the mechanism of blood flow is an increase in pleural pressure or direct cardiac compression. This can lead to collapse of the arteries and produce the condition of flow limitation (130). This never occurs with the normal contracting heart except perhaps during rapid ejection in hypertrophic cardiomyopathies. The absence or presence of flow limitation also determines the response to volume loading. When flow limitation is not present, increasing the blood volume in the heart or thorax does not increase the volume ejected, for this is simply a function of the pressures applied to the heart or chest and the compliances of the compartments (equation 2). However, when the pressures in the chest are high enough to produce flow limitation, then increasing blood volume can increase the maximal flow (equation 5).

THORACIC PUMP VERSUS DIRECT COMPRESSION MODELS

The original terminology indicated the bias of the investigators for the technique was called closed-chest cardiac massage (71). However, there is little doubt that blood flow can be generated without cardiac compressions. This was first dramatically demonstrated by Criley and co-workers (34, 85), who showed that coughing could sustain sufficient cardiac output to maintain the circulation and keep patients alive for close to a minute (Fig. 31.3). This still remains a very useful technique in the cardiac catheterization laboratory where the cardiac arrest is immediately witnessed, and continued coughing can provide sufficient time to prepare for defibrillation.

The ability of increases in intrathoracic pressure to produce blood flow with direct cardiac compressions was also confirmed by Wise and co-workers (60, 127, 128), who showed that blood flow could be generated in an isolated heart-lung prepara-

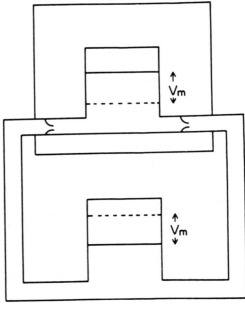

$$\dot{Q} = \frac{V_m}{\dfrac{\tau_E}{\alpha} + \dfrac{\tau_f}{1-\alpha}}$$

Figure 31.3. The lumped parameter hydraulic model of CPR is discussed in the text. The upper reservoir represents the thoracic blood volume surrounded by a pressurized chamber. The lower reservoir represents the peripheral vascular compliance. Each of the conduits is a collapsible tube with resistance partioned between segments inside and outside the thorax. One-way valves represent the cardiac and venous valves and ensure unidirectional flow. V_m is the total volume that would leave one reservoir and enter the other reservoir when the pressure is changed from conditions of filling to conditions of emptying, and the system is allowed to equilibrate. The maximum steady-state blood flow during rapid oscillation of the pressure in the thorax is given in the equation in which τ_E is the time constant of emptying, τ_f is the time constant of filling, and α is the duty cycle. (From Wise RA, Summer WR. Cardiopulmonary resuscitation. In: Dantzker DR, ed. Cardiopulmonary critical care. Philadelphia: WB Saunders Co, 1988:385–405.)

tion in a sealed Plexiglas box by changing the pressures in the box. Passerini et al. (92) were also able to document carotid blood flow in a dog model in which a plaster cast was placed around the thorax and abdomen and the lungs were inflated with a specially designed ventilator that produced a square wave of intrathoracic pressure.

Just because these studies demonstrate that blood flow can be generated without cardiac compression does not mean that cardiac compressions do not play a role in the generation of blood flow in CPR. Much of the evidence that is raised in support of the cardiac compression model comes from studies on the pattern of movement of cardiac valves. The thoracic pump model predicts that the pulmonary blood volume is mobilized during chest compression, which means that blood should flow from the pulmonary vessels through the cardiac chambers to the aorta and to the rest of the body. Thus, this model predicts that the mitral and aortic valves would be open during chest compression. In contrast, the cardiac pump mechanism requires that the mitral valve is closed during cardiac compression, otherwise there would be retrograde flow. The advocates of the thoracic pump model were indeed able to show angiographic and echocardiographic data to support the contention that the mitral valve is open during chest compression (33, 124). However, proponents of the cardiac pump model have also shown evidence that the mitral valve is closed during chest compression (39, 46). These studies thus also fail to definitively distinguish between the two theories. This can possibly be explained by realizing that echocardiographic visualization of valves cannot determine that flow is stopped through the valve, and although the atrioventricular valves may look closed, there still could be a small opening that allows flow. It is also possible that the ventricular volume empties faster than the pulmonary volume because it is compressed first, which gives the appearance that the heart is collapsed and the valves closed, especially if the compressions are directed over the heart. Angiographic studies are also contradictory. Some have shown that cardiac chambers are not compressed during CPR (33, 47, 84, 87), whereas others have shown that they are (7, 46). Once again, the site of the compression could alter the observation and, just as in the echocardi-

ographic studies, the observation of cardiac compression does not necessarily prove that this is the mechanism of blood flow in CPR. A further piece of evidence to indicate that the atrioventricular valves are not closed during CPR is that the peak right atrial pressure equals the peak aortic pressure in CPR (42); therefore, there is no pressure gradient to close the atrioventricular valve.

Another issue of concern with the thoracic pump model is control of the direction of blood flow. In the cardiac pump model, retrograde flow is prevented by closure of the atrioventricular valves, but these are believed to be open in the thoracic pump model. The absence of retrograde flow in the thoracic pump model can be explained by two mechanisms. There is angiographic evidence of a valve at the junction of the superior vena cava and right atrium, which prevents backward flow (47, 87). However, even without a true valve, backward flow would be limited by the collapse of the veins. This occurs because the intrathoracic pressure, which is the force generating flow, is greater than the pressure inside the veins exiting the thorax because of the loss of pressures from the upstream vessels due to the normal resistance through the system. Since the pressure starts the same everywhere in the thorax, even a small gradient from the pulmonary veins to the superior and inferior vena cava will allow the surrounding pressure to be higher than the pressure in the veins and prevent flow just as it does in West's zone 1 of the lungs (52).

PERIPHERAL VERSUS THORACIC LIMITATIONS

Is the primary limitation to blood flow in CPR emptying of the thoracic volume or filling of the thoracic volume? If the peripheral capacitance decreases during CPR, because of a loss of tone or leaky capillaries, one would predict that the venous return would decrease as more blood would be pumped out than enters. If, however, the problem is emptying of the thoracic volume, then the venous blood volume would increase as less blood would leave the veins than was pumped out from the thorax. Most animal and clinical observations demonstrated that the limiting factor in maintaining blood flow is getting blood out of the chest and not into it. This primary excess venous return may not be obvious in man because right atrial pressure rises with the failure to eject blood from the chest and decreases the gradient for venous return.

How then can the ejection of blood be increased from the heart? Based on the equations developed by Wise and coworkers (127, 128), we can consider the following possibilities: changes in vascular compliance, duty cycle, rate, applied force, blood volume, vascular resistance, and abdominal pressure.

Compliance

As can be seen in equations 2 through 7, the vascular compliances affect Vm, τe, and τf. A decrease in either the thoracic or pulmonary compliance will decrease the transferable volume, Vm, but will also decrease τe and τf, which can increase flow. The net effect would most likely be no change because the compliance terms affect all the other variables. It should also be emphasized that what is important in these equations is the compliance, not the capacitance. The compliance is the slope of the pressure-volume curve; the capacitance is the actual volume at a given pressure and therefore takes into account the unstressed volume as well. If a drug just changes the position of the pressure-volume relationship but does not change the slope of the pressure-volume relationship, this is the equivalent of increasing volume and does not represent a change in compliance.

Duty Cycle

One of the most important terms in equation 1 is α, the duty cycle, which is the fraction of the cycle spent during contraction. Notice that increasing α decreases the magnitude of the denominator and therefore results in a bigger flow. Of course, increasing α, also decreases 1-α, the factor modifying τf or the time for venous drainage. Therefore, there will be an optimal α that depends on the relative magnitudes

of τe and τf. The predicted responses are shown in Figure 31.4. The optimal value in an isolated heart-lung model was 0.7. In a study on humans, the optimal compression time was 60% of the cycle, but this was difficult to sustain (Fig. 31.5) (115). Furthermore, the optimal value will vary among patients. Since the optimal duty cycle depends on the relative time constants of emptying and filling, in conditions in which peripheral resistance is high, such as with catecholamines, the time constant of emptying is increased and therefore the duty cycle should be longer. Under conditions in which the time constant of emptying may be shorter, such as with low peripheral resistance as seen in sepsis, the duty cycle should be shorter. However, the time constant of emptying cannot be assessed in an individual patient. Therefore the present AHA recommendation is to use a duty cycle of 0.5, which should be close to the maximum in most patients and easier to sustain for a more prolonged time than a longer duration (14).

Rate

It may initially seem intuitive that changing the rate of compression should be important. However, rate does not come into any of the equations presented above. This is because changing the rate changes the amount of blood ejected per beat, but not the total amount of blood ejected per minute, which depends on the interaction between the inflow and outflow time constants (equation 1). This assumes that the stroke volume is small relative to the total stressed volume, which is not true at very slow rates of compression but is valid above 20–30 beats/min. Therefore, the rate should probably be at least 30–40 beats/min, but rates above this do not make much difference. This is supported by data from studies on the isolated heart-lung preparation (60), dogs (92), and humans (115). In the latter study, changes in rates between 40 and 80 compressions per minute at a duty cycle of 0.6 had no effect on blood pressure (Fig. 31.5). However, as previously noted, it is difficult to sustain prolonged duty cycles.

Pulmonary Mechanics and CPR

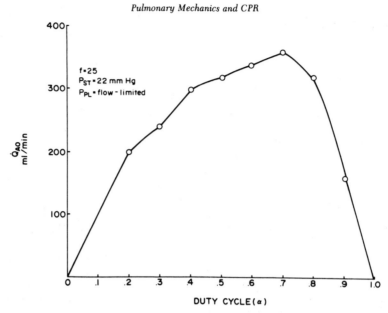

Figure 31.4. The effect of duty cycle on steady-state blood flow in an isolated model of cardiopulmonary resuscitation. A canine heart and lungs were placed within an artificial thorax and connected to a mechanical analog of the systemic circulation. Pleural pressure was cycled at a level approximately twice that at which flow limitation occurred, at various duty cycles. With a static blood pressure of 22 mm Hg, the maximum blood flow was achieved at $\alpha = 0.7$, corresponding to the fact that the time constant of emptying took considerably longer than that of filling. (From Wise RA, Summer WR. Pulmonary mechanics and artificial support of the arrested circulation. Clin Chest Med 1983;4:189–198.)

Changes in rate, though, have some indirect consequences. In the studies quoted above, the rates were changed with a constant duty cycle, but what usually happens in practice is that the compression phase occupies a constant time and takes up a greater proportion of the total cycle time when the rate is increased. Increases in rate thus usually result in an increase in duty cycle. This could explain the benefit of high-impulse rapid compressions seen by Maier et al. (78). The rapid impulses used by these investigators had a short compression time so that only at very high rates would the fraction of the cycle spent during compression be long, for the compression time did not change in their study, which means that the relaxation phase must have decreased. Therefore, the rate effect that they observed could very well have been a consequence of the change in duty cycle.

Applied Force

A major variable affecting the volume ejected, Vm, is the difference in applied pressure during emptying or the ejecting phase and the filling phase (equation 2). Thus, as should be obvious, the greater the applied force, the greater the Vm. The applied pressure depends on the operator and how the pressure is dissipated. This is especially important in the thoracic pump model. If the airway is open, the applied pressure will be dissipated as air is forced out of the chest instead of blood. However, it has been shown that even with an open airway, some air is trapped in the lungs, which still results in some increase in intrathoracic pressure even with an open airway (19). To maximize the effects of chest compressions, it has been recommended to compress the chest with either an occluded airway or simultaneously with

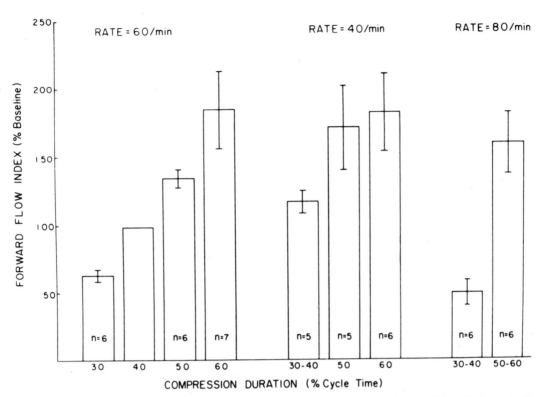

Figure 31.5. Prolonging compression duration resulting in greater forward-flow index at all compression rates studied. (Bars denote ± SEM.) Flow index is expressed as a percentage of flow at compression rate of 60 per minute and compression duration of 40% for the eight patients studied. Thus, the flow at a compression rate of 60 per minute and compression duration of 40% is indicated as 100%. The maximum flow index occurred at a compression duration of 60% whether the compression rate was 40, 60 or 80/min. (From Taylor GJ, Tucker WM, Greene HL, Rudikoff MT, Weisfeldt ML. Importance of prolonged compression during cardiopulmonary resuscitation in man. N Engl J Med 1977;296:1515–1517.)

ventilation (12, 31, 102). This was actually proposed in the early 1960s (126). The changes in lung volume produced by ventilation can, however, complicate matters. At high lung volumes, the actual blood volume ejected from the chest may decrease because the increase in transpulmonary pressure can impede the movement of fluid from the pulmonary arteries and right heart (60). Therefore, large tidal volumes should not be used. This is especially important if the vascular volume is low.

A large part of the dissipation of the force applied to the chest is through the abdomen (41). Therefore, measures that decrease the compliance of the abdomen can be very helpful for increasing intra-

thoracic pressure and augmenting blood flow. This has been tested in numerous studies in which the abdomen has been bound or compressed with the thoracic compressions (9, 61, 72). Since the abdomen is the most compliant part of the thoracoabdominal complex, it can be shown that compressing the abdomen itself can actually generate an increase in intrathoracic pressure and generate flow, for the noncompliant chest wall actually resists expansion from the rise in thoracoabdominal pressure much better than occurs when the chest is compressed and the pressure expands the lax abdominal wall. A potential problem with the application of high abdominal pressure is damage to abdominal organs (61), but most studies have shown that this can be minimized by careful technique (20, 30, 102). The subject of abdominal counterpulsation will be discussed in detail below.

A major concern with the use of high intrathoracic pressures to generate flow was that the rise in intrathoracic pressure could be transferred to the intracerebral fluid and increase intracranial pressure. This occurs both through the veins, as well as directly through the intravertebral spaces adjacent to the pleural space and can lead to an increase in the back pressure to flow in the brain, which would potentially decrease carotid blood flow (56). However, studies have shown that there is no damage to the brain with techniques that involve abdominal binding (112), and brain blood flow is improved by these techniques (71).

Although equation 2 predicts that increasing intrathoracic pressure differences will increase blood flow, there are limits to the effectiveness of these maneuvers because eventually the high intrathoracic pressure produces vascular collapse and results in flow limitation. When this occurs, further increases in intrathoracic pressure will not result in any further increase in flow as shown by equation 5. This has also been found experimentally (60, 92).

Volume

In the beating heart, the initial volume, or preload, is a major determinant of the systolic pressure and volume ejected. Below the point of flow limitation, as mathematically shown in equations 1 and 2, the total blood volume does not influence the flow, which is mainly dependent on the pressure difference between emptying and filling, $Pple - Pplf$. However, when flow limitation occurs, as is shown in equation 5, the total volume, V, becomes a factor and an increase in total volume increases Vm. This probably explains the variable results in the literature of volume infusions during CPR. In studies in which flow limitation occurs, as would be expected when high pressures are applied, increasing blood volume is important (92, 102). However, in studies in which flow limitation has not occurred, increasing the volume will not make a difference (42). In standard CPR the intrathoracic pressures are probably not high enough to produce flow limitation, and increasing the blood volume will not be of great help; however, these interactions have not been examined.

Resistance

The time constants of filling and emptying of the thoracic volume are affected by the resistances of the conduits that enter and drain this region, and therefore decreases in these resistances should decrease the time constants and increase flow. It is not easy to increase the venous time constant, although possibly a drug such as epinephrine could result in the redistribution of blood flow to areas with fast time constants of venous drainage that would decrease τf (28, 95). Decreasing the arterial resistance will result in a lower arterial pressure, and if the brain and heart already start with low resistances, decreasing the resistance of the rest of the body could actually decrease the fractional flows to the brain and heart, and increase flow to nonessential areas such as muscle. Indeed, the fractional flows to the brain and heart are higher than other regions of the body at the start of CPR (77, 113). For this reason, the usual and best approach is to give drugs such as norepinephrine, epinephrine, or methoxamine, which increase peripheral resistance. These drugs do not seem to affect the cerebral and coronary circulations as much as other regions, and the rise in diastolic pressure therefore augments flow (82, 111). They also stiffen the arteries and decrease the tendency of the arteries to collapse by allowing a more negative transmural pressure (i.e., the value $Ptm'a$ in equation 5) before the vessel collapses (123). Therefore, flow limitation occurs at a higher pressure (130) and higher pleural pressures can be used. This factor is probably one of the more important variables in determining blood flow during CPR whether closed or open chest techniques are used (123) and will be discussed further in the section on catecholamines.

Abdominal Binding

There has long been an interest in the role of abdominal binding in CPR, including a report by Criley and Dolley in 1906 (34). Redding (98) conducted a large study in dogs and found that abdominal binding greatly increased survival, particularly when performed in conjunction with the injection of an α-agonist. Abdominal compression has a number of theoretical advantages in CPR. As discussed above, abdominal compression during chest compression prevents the dissipation of the forces applied to the chest through the abdominal wall by effectively splinting the abdominal wall and reducing its compliance (41). The abdominal binding also effectively decreases the peripheral capacitance and thereby increases the stressed volume. This will be beneficial if there is no flow limitation as discussed above. High abdominal pressures could also keep abdominal vascular pressures high and thereby decrease flow through the lower part of the body. This would effectively redirect flow in a cephalad direction and help maintain aortic diastolic pressure, which is so important for coronary flow (85, 86, 108). In support of this, Redding (98) found an increase in the pressure gradient from the aorta to the central venous pressure with abdominal binding. Studies from the group at Johns Hopkins in animals and humans have also shown that abdominal binding increases blood pressure and carotid flows (30, 31, 58), although other studies in humans have been less successful (53). A number of studies have also shown an increase in brain blood flow with abdominal binding (70, 77). This is important because concerns were raised about the transmission of abdominal pressures to the central spinal fluid (56). However, despite the increase in the cerebral spinal fluid pressure, there still is an increase in flow (6).

In one of the earlier studies with abdominal binding (61), concern was raised about liver laceration from the application of abdominal pressure. The proposed mechanism was that the high abdominal pressures results in a fixation of the liver so that it is more vulnerable to injury from

the chest compressions. Later studies do not support this (22, 30, 31, 98, 102). However, because of it, investigators began using abdominal compressions interposed between chest compressions. This technique has provoked many studies that will be discussed in the next section.

Interposed Abdominal Compressions

In the interposed abdominal compression technique, the abdomen is compressed with from 100–200 mm Hg during the "diastolic" or relaxation phase of the chest compressions. Interest in this approach began with the canine studies by Ralston et al. working with Babbs (96) and showed an increase in aortic pressure, cardiac output, and the pressure gradient from the aorta to the central venous pressure with this technique. Three mechanisms were proposed to explain the benefit of interposed abdominal compression. (a) The abdominal compressions could produce aortic counterpulsations much like those that occur with an intraaortic balloon pump (8, 10, 13). (b) It could act by splinting the aorta and thereby redirecting blood in a cephalad direction by preventing the flow of blood to the legs (61, 98). (c) It could act by compressing the abdominal vascular compliant region, thereby increasing venous return and "prime" the pump (8, 10, 13).

The arterial pressure and carotid flow increase on the first beat of interposed abdominal compressions, indicating a direct aortic effect (42, 117). In the model presented previously (equation 1), the increase in abdominal pressure, if applied on release or just before the onset of chest compressions, would act by increasing α, the duty cycle, of the emptying phase. The problem is that the central venous pressure may also increase, either from a transfer of venous blood from the abdomen to the right atrium (117), or direct transmission of pressures to the chest (18) so that there is no improvement in the pressure gradient from the aorta to the right atrium, which is such an important prognostic factor (85, 86, 108). It appears that the size of the animal makes a difference, for central venous pressures do not rise as much in small animals. It is believed by some that this is because the primary mechanism of blood flow in small animals is direct compression of the heart, for the chests of small animals are easier to compress (11, 62). However, this could be explained equally by better emptying of the thoracic volume during compression in small animals or perhaps venous collapse at the level of the diaphragm, which prevents a cephalad transfer of abdominal volume through the veins even in the thoracic pump model. It is of interest that use of an intraaortic balloon pump has been shown to improve hemodynamic parameters in experimental studies of CPR (43).

The second proposed mechanism is a redirection of blood flow in a cephalad direction by effectively cross-clamping the aorta. However, Kimmel et al. (69) and Hoekstra et al. (62) found no redistribution, and Bertrand et al. (18) found that femoral flow also increased with abdominal compressions, indicating emptying of the abdominal compartment in both directions with interposed abdominal compression. Thus, this does not appear to be the primary mechanism.

Another consequence of cross-clamping the aorta, which is not intuitively obvious, is a redistribution of blood flow away from the splanchnic region, which has a slow time constant of venous drainage, to the upper extremity, which has a faster time constant of venous drainage (32, 95). This would effectively decrease the τf in equation 1 and increase flow. This, however, should not produce an increase in aortic pressure on the first beat which, as noted above, occurs.

The third mechanism proposed for the benefit of interposed abdominal compressions is an increase in the venous return by a "priming" of the pump. This mechanism can be seen as a direct effect of a transient increase in abdominal pressure that effectively decreases the abdominal compliance and acts as a second applied force. Neither of these were included in the original model of Wise and co-workers (127, 128). However, Voorhees et al (117) and Einagel et al (42) found that carotid flow and pressures increase on the very

first application of abdominal pressure, and therefore a transfer of volume from the abdomen to the chest cannot explain this initial increase in flow and pressure. Nor was there an increment with subsequent beats, although others have found a progressive increase in pressure (12).

The potential of abdominal compressions to transfer volume seems tempting at first, but it assures a model in which the thorax and abdomen are two separate compartments (8, 10, 13, 19). However, the flaccid diaphragm readily transmits abdominal pressures into the thorax so that there may not be an increase in pressure gradient for flow from the abdomen to the thorax (41). Indeed, Einagel et al. (42) found that abdominal compressions in dogs actually produced a greater increase in intrathoracic pressures than chest compressions, and in their study, carotid flows and pressures were higher during the abdominal compression phase than during the chest compression phase so that the chest compressions became the effective diastole. The exact timing of the increase in flow and pressures with interposed abdominal compressions has not always been examined so that the importance of this in other studies is difficult to ascertain, but it is probably model-dependent (11). It is clear that in human applications of interposed abdominal compressions, the pressures generated during the chest phase are higher than the abdominal phase (53, 63). In any case, Einagel et al. went so far as to suggest that chest compressions during interposed abdominal compressions may actually make matters worse, for it would decrease the gradient for venous return and decrease the gradient for coronary perfusion.

What actually has been found with interposed abdominal compressions? Ralston et al. (96) and Voorhees (117), working with Babbs, found that interposed abdominal compressions increase brain blood flow and cardiac output in canine models. Voorhees et al. found an increase in oxygen delivery and a decrease in lactate levels with interposed abdominal compressions. Brain blood flow has been found to increase as much as fourfold (118), although myocardial blood flow does not increase and the pressure gradient from aorta to central venous pressure (CVP) also does not increase (106), as may have been expected by the potential for right atrial pressure to increase with abdominal compressions (42).

In human studies, the pressure gradient from the aorta to central venous pressure has been shown to increase, which would favor coronary blood flow (17, 63), but no advantage in terms of survival was found in an extensive field study in Milwaukee (81). Improvement in hemodynamic measurements and survival was found in another randomized trial of interposed abdominal compressions and standard CPR (119). In one animal study that compared interposed abdominal compressions with standard CPR, survival was worse with interposed abdominal compressions (107). Of importance, there is now a large experience with this technique in humans and animals, and liver laceration does not appear to be a problem.

In most of the studies in which abdominal compressions have been used, they were applied during the relaxation phase. One of the earliest investigations of intermittent abdominal compressions was by Ohomoto et al. (88), who used prolonged abdominal compressions and superimposed chest compressions and found increased survival in dogs. They used simultaneous abdominal and chest compression. Neimann et al. (85) combined abdominal compressions with chest inflation and also effectively used a simultaneous abdominal and chest compression technique. Bertrand et al. (18) predicted that simultaneous chest compressions might be better than interposed abdominal compressions, and in a preliminary study found better carotid flows and aortic pressures with simultaneous interposed abdominal compressions in a canine model, although the difference was small. Indeed, in that study, abdominal compression alone was equal to interposed abdominal compressions and both were much better than chest compressions. If abdominal compressions act by increasing intrathoracic pressure, then the benefit would occur if there is not already flow limitation. Otherwise, the increase in force will not increase flow unless it prolongs the duty cycle.

In summary, the exact role of abdominal compressions in CPR is still controversial and conclusions vary with the model of CPR used for the study as well as the theoretical model used to predict results. Furthermore, the clinical results to date remain inconclusive.

OPEN CHEST VERSUS CLOSED CHEST TECHNIQUES

Prior to the report by Kouwenhoven et al. (71) of closed chest cardiac resuscitation, open chest cardiac massage was the only available technique. Today, this is largely reserved for patients with flail chests, deep hypothermia, massive pulmonary emboli, patients with their chests already open, and patients with no pulse with standard CPR (21). However, there have been calls for greater application of this approach (36) and some have recommended using it after 10 minutes of failed closed chest resuscitation (21).

There are some important theoretical advantages to open chest massage. With closed chest techniques, the cardiac output depends on the time constants of filling and emptying (equation 1) because unlike normal cardiac function, the chest and heart can only fill during the relaxation phase. However, in open chest CPR, as in normal cardiac contractions, blood can return to the atria and thorax during cardiac compressions if only the ventricles are compressed and not the atria. Under this condition, equation 1 does not hold, and flow is limited by the stressed volume divided by the time constant of venous return, as in the normal heart. Furthermore, there is no flow limitation with the open chest technique because the force is applied to the heart and not the whole thorax, and there is no high intrathoracic pressure to produce collapse of the aorta. Thus, flows can be greater than the 50% of normal predicted for standard CPR, which is unlikely with closed chest techniques (95, 127, 128). This framework allows us to consider the factors that determine flow in open chest massage.

A crucial factor is that both the right

and left ventricles must be compressed. Since the ventricles are enclosed by a common space, the pericardial sac, failure to empty the right ventricle could result in less filling of the left ventricle and therefore less left ventricular ejection, which is obviously crucial for the systemic circulation. Opening the pericardium would actually allow greater ventricular filling and potentially greater cardiac output. This has been done in only one animal study and the results were not compared with open and closed pericardial compressions (15).

The stressed volume is also an important factor. If there is a large volume loss from the thoracotomy, this will severely limit the ability of chest compressions to produce flow, for stressed volume is a major determinant of the venous return to the heart. Remember that with closed chest techniques, the volume is only a factor when there is sufficient intrathoracic pressure to produce flow limitation.

As with closed chest techniques, rate should not be a major factor, for outflow depends on the return of blood to the heart, as with the normal circulation. Most studies have found that optimal flows can be obtained with rates of 50–60 beats/min. The length of time of ejection is again important, but this is more easily monitored with direct cardiac compressions because the operator can feel when the ventricle is emptied with each compression.

As with any artificial technique, the force applied is a crucial variable. It should be noted that, unlike the normal beating heart, this force is independent of the diastolic volume. Therefore, if the rate of return of blood is increased by a volume infusion or a decrease in the time constant of venous return, and the same force is applied to the heart, there will be no increase in output for the arrested heart does not have a Frank-Starling mechanism nor does it have an intrinsic means of changing contractility. An advantage of the open chest technique is that the operator can easily observe an increase in volume and respond with an increase in force. As noted above, an increase in the force with open chest massage will not produce flow limitation as it does with closed chest techniques.

Since the output in open chest massage depends very much on the return of blood, measures that increase this should be of help. These could include the use of α-adrenergic drugs to decrease venous capacitance and even interposed abdominal compressions to increase venous return. This could potentially be much more effective than in closed chest techniques.

Based on this theoretical discussion, it would seem that the technique used during open chest massage should be very important. Both ventricles need to be compressed and the force needs to be applied adequately and long enough to eject all the blood and yet not lacerate the heart. One needs to be careful not to twist the heart, which will decrease venous return. The operator must be careful not to compress the atrium, for this will decrease the return of blood to the heart during the systolic phase and decrease the advantage of this technique. In one study, three different techniques were used (15). A two-handed approach that allowed better compression of the ventricles and a technique that compressed the heart against the sternum were superior to a one-handed approach in which a thumb was placed over the anterior left ventricle, the apex was placed in the palm, and the rest of the heart was gripped by the fingers.

How well does open chest massage actually work? There have been a number of animal studies that have addressed this question. They have generally shown a higher cardiac output (122) and higher carotid blood flow (15, 20), although aortic pressures were not much higher (20, 109, 122), and one study found no difference between open and closed chest techniques (99). This has been attributed to the small size of the dog they used, which probably optimized the closed chest technique (106). This factor needs to be considered in all CPR studies, although it is not known if humans are more similar to small or large dogs!

One study showed improved survival in dogs that were switched to open chest massage (109). In a study that optimized the pressure generation during closed chest compressions (20), the carotid blood flow was equally improved with open and closed techniques, but the carotid blood flow fell after approximately 10 minutes with an optimal closed chest technique. This could be related to a progressive decrease in the threshold for collapse in the aorta as discussed above and might have been alleviated with α-adrenergic drugs.

Open and closed chest CPR in humans was assessed by Del Guerico et al. (37, 38), who obtained cardiac output and hemodynamic measurements during cardiac arrest in 11 patients. They were able to compare open and closed techniques in three patients and found that the open technique produced higher cardiac outputs (38). This paper is often cited as evidence of the advantage of open versus closed resuscitation. A number of features are worth noting in this rather heroic study. Cardiac output and aortic pressure were higher in some of the patients with closed chest compressions than in other patients with the open chest technique. In fact, one patient had a higher cardiac index during ventricular fibrillation and chest compressions than with spontaneous contractions! No details are given about the administration of catecholamines during the resuscitations, which is crucial for the prevention of aortic collapse. This could explain why cardiac outputs were higher in the closed techniques that had shorter resuscitation times. Furthermore, although flow was higher, the pressure gradient from the aorta to central veins did not change much. This is believed to be the most important prognostic factor in CPR, and the failure to increase it indicates that the heart may not have been adequately perfused (85, 86, 108). Finally, all the patients died, no matter which technique was used.

As a final point, one has to consider the complications of open chest massage. The infection rate is cited as 10% of survivors (21). Of greater importance, a post mortem study found gross lacerations in 10% of cases (1), although others have found less complications (14).

In summary, open chest massage offers some important theoretical advantages, including the potential for higher flow and lower central venous pressures; however, the technique used is crucial and it should only be applied by well-trained operators.

CATECHOLAMINES

The administration of catecholamines with primarily α activity has been shown to be effective for increasing blood flow, arterial diastolic pressures, and survival in both animal and human studies. When CPR is prolonged, survival is rare without exogenous catecholamines.

The mechanism of action of catecholamines, however, is not clear. First, catecholamines obviously do not act by increasing cardiac contractility, and therefore must act by affecting the vasculature. One way they could act is by decreasing the time constant of filling (equation 1), either by decreasing vascular compliance or by decreasing the resistance to venous return. If anything, they tend to increase the resistance to venous return and usually decrease the capacitance with little change in compliance (5), and thus essentially produce an increase in stressed volume. As noted previously, this could be important when flow limitation is present. Also, τf could be decreased by redistributing blood flow to beds with fast time constants of drainage, i.e., muscle, but there is no evidence of this occurring during CPR. In fact, in one study, blood flow to the liver and small intestine increased with epinephrine, which would effectively increase the resistance to venous return (28).

On the arterial side, catecholamines could increase blood pressure by increasing the systemic vascular resistance, but based on equation 1, this could actually decrease flow by increasing the time constant of emptying unless countered by an increase in the duty cycle α. Furthermore, if catecholamines cause a general increase in systemic vascular resistance, then the resistance to the cerebral vascular bed, which has a lower resistance than the other beds during CPR (77), may proportionately increase more, which would actually decrease cerebral blood flow. However, we know this does not occur (82), but why?

An important mechanism of catecholamines in CPR is that they perhaps make the collapse pressure of the arteries more negative, and therefore the arteries are more resistant to collapse, as was well demonstrated by Yin et al. (130). With a more negative collapse pressure, a greater force can be applied to the chest and therefore a greater volume displaced (equation 5). A loss of tone over time and rise in the collapse pressure in the arteries probably explains the failure of closed chest techniques over time (129) and the importance of catecholamines during prolonged resuscitation.

Catecholamines have been shown to increase the pressure gradient from the aorta to CVP which, as noted previously, is an important determinant of coronary flow (27, 73–76). This could be due to an increase in total blood flow, which would produce more aortic volume to be dissipated during diastole. It could also be due to an increase in systemic vascular resistance, which is greater than the brain and heart, or else there would be no accompanying increase in flow to the heart.

There has been much debate as to the ideal catecholamine for CPR. Clearly β-agonists alone, such as isoproterenol (93) and dobutamine (91), are of no help for they do not appear to increase systemic vascular resistance or increase the collapse threshold, whereas drugs with α activity have been shown to be beneficial. It has also been debated whether α-1 or α-2 activity is more important. This debate has arisen because investigators have tried to avoid the potentially detrimental β effects of norepinephrine and epinephrine by substituting methoxamine or phenylephrine (25). However, these latter two drugs only have α-1 activity, whereas norepinephrine and epinephrine also have α-2 activity. The α_1-receptor appears to be down-regulated in hypoxia, whereas the α_2-receptor retains its activity and can still produce vasoconstriction. Therefore, the effectiveness of a pure α-agonist may decrease with time. Some studies, indeed, have found that methoxamine is less effective than norepinephrine (26, 89). Others found that it is equal to epinephrine (24), and still others have found methoxamine to be much better than epinephrine (93, 101), and phenylephrine was equal to or slightly better than epinephrine (73). Roberts et al. (101) compared high doses of methoxamine (20 mg) and epinephrine

(0.2 mg/kg) and found much better organ flows and survival in animals treated with methoxamine. However, in a recent randomized field trial, Olson et al. (89) found that 0.5 mg of epinephrine was more effective during resuscitation than methoxamine. Because of the down-regulation of the α_1-receptor with hypoxia, oxygenation could be an important variable in these studies. The doses of drugs used and the techniques of CPR is probably also important.

The effectiveness of norepinephrine and epinephrine have also been compared. Epinephrine has more β activity, particularly β_2 activity than norepinephrine. This has been shown to increase myocardial oxygen consumption (75) and, although the blood flow is higher than with norepinephrine, the extraction remains the same because of the higher oxygen need in a fibrillating heart (40, 75). This could explain why fibrillating hearts are defibrillated more easily when the animals are treated with norepinephrine and dopamine than epinephrine (74). However, in asphyxial models of cardiac arrest, better results were achieved with epinephrine than norepinephrine (74), presumably because there is less stimulation of myocardial oxygen consumption in this model and the β activity provides better maintenance of coronary flow.

The animal studies suggest that the dose of epinephrine may be larger than the currently recommended dose of 0.14 mg/kg; some have suggested that doses as high as 0.45 mg/kg are required (27, 51, 75). A recent randomized trial in adults with cardiac arrest showed a significantly higher success rate of resuscitation with high-dose epinephrine versus the standard dose, but there was no difference in the hospital discharge rate (73). The higher doses are especially important when the endotracheal route is used for the administration of the drug because of the lower absorption rate by this route (97). In summary, catecholamine administration is an important part of CPR. Current data suggest that norepinephrine is the best choice for ventricular fibrillation, and epinephrine and norepinephrine are probably equally effective in asphyxial arrest, although both may need to be given in larger doses than are currently recommended.

MONITORING DURING CPR

It would be helpful to have a simple method for monitoring patients during CPR. The current recommendation of the AHA is to monitor the carotid pulse. Unfortunately, the systolic pressure generated does not correlate with the outcome. This is probably because in animal studies it is the pressure gradient from the aorta to CVP during diastole that best predicts survival (85, 86, 108) and an increase in aortic pressure does not always mean an increase in aortic pressure. Neither do arterial gases predict outcome (150). Recently, much attention has been given to the usefulness of end-tidal Pco_2 measurements after Sanders et al. (110) found a good correlation between the end-tidal Pco_2 and outcome. In their study, all patients with an end-tidal Pco_2 of greater than 10 mm Hg survived. The end-tidal Pco_2 has also been shown to correlate with cardiac output (45, 121) and success (29). This has been attributed to a decreased ability of the lungs to clear Pco_2 (110). To better understand the role of end-tidal Pco_2 measurements, it is necessary to review the physiologic mechanisms controlling the arterial and venous Pco_2 and the end-tidal Pco_2.

Arterial Pco_2 is determined by the CO_2 production ($\dot{V}co_2$) and alveolar ventilation. Reported values of $Paco_2$ (120) during CPR indicate that the $Paco_2$ was in fact less than the reference value of 40 mm Hg during CPR. This indicates that there is actually hyperventilation and no problem clearing CO_2 by the lungs. For example, Weil et al. (121) found a $Paco_2$ of 35 mm Hg.

The mixed venous or pulmonary arterial CO_2 depends on $\dot{V}co_2$, blood flow, and the arterial CO_2 content as given by the Fick equation, which is a statement of the conservation of mass. Thus, $\dot{Q} = \dot{V}co_2/(\text{venous} - \text{arterial } CO_2 \text{ content})$. If $\dot{V}co_2$ and arterial Pco_2 do not change, and the cardiac output drops by more than 50%, the pulmonary arterial Pco_2 must rise considerably. This is strictly a function of the decrease in flow and has nothing to do

with the lungs. It is difficult to predict whether Pco_2 increases or decreases in the tissues. The decrease in metabolism would decrease $\dot{V}o_2$ and thereby decrease $\dot{V}co_2$ for CO_2 is produced only through aerobic metabolism; however, the acidosis would contribute to an increase in CO_2 production by shifting the dissociation curve of bicarbonate to carbonic acid and then H_2O and CO_2. An increase in $\dot{V}co_2$ will also increase pulmonary arterial CO_2, which is why pulmonary arterial CO_2 levels are very high during exercise.

The end-tidal Pco_2 normally is close to the $Paco_2$. This assumes minimal dead space ventilation. If dead space ventilation increases, then the end-tidal CO_2 is a mixture of alveolar air that comes in contact with the blood and air from areas that do not. A classic example of a sudden increase in dead space is a pulmonary embolism. This has allowed a decrease in the gradient between $Paco_2$ and end-tidal Pco_2 to be used to diagnose pulmonary embolism (44). The low end-tidal Pco_2 with normal $Paco_2$ in patients with failed resuscitations would then seem to suggest an increase in dead space ventilation. More than likely, the decreased pulmonary perfusion results in decreased perfusion of well-ventilated regions and an increase in dead space. This could potentially be made worse by conditions that increase airway pressures and thus increase West zone I condition of the lung. Thus, increasing the respiratory rate or increasing lung volume, could make patients appear worse off than they really are with this technique. An interesting recent failure of the use of end-tidal Pco_2 measurements was observed in a study by Martin et al. (80). They used end-tidal Pco_2 to monitor the effects of epinephrine infusions during CPR. Although coronary perfusion pressure increase, the end-tidal Pco_2 decreased. This could be explained by an increase in dead space due to redistribution of pulmonary blood flow by the norepinephrine away from ventilated areas and may not represent decreased cardiac output.

In conclusion, end-tidal Pco_2 measurements can be useful for monitoring patients during CPR, but one must be cognizant of the physiology involved in this measurement, for a decrease in this measurement may not always be a bad prognostic sign.

SODIUM BICARBONATE THERAPY

Sodium bicarbonate has long been advocated to buffer the acidosis that develops during cardiac arrest. This is believed to be important because acidosis makes it harder to defibrillate the heart and could contribute to decreased responsiveness to catecholamines. Indeed, low pH is correlated with failure of resuscitation (67). However, it should be appreciated that delay in resuscitation is probably the most important variable in these studies.

Bishop and Weisfeldt (23) showed that arterial pH can be maintained at greater than 7.25 μg when ventilation and compressions are adequate. A number of animal studies have also found no advantage of bicarbonate therapy compared to placebo (55, 68); in one study, animals were defibrillated after 30 minutes of resuscitation without any bicarbonate therapy (82).

The failure of sodium bicarbonate to improve the outcome with CPR can be understood from recent analyses of arterial and venous blood gases in the whole body (45, 121) and regional circulations (54, 116). The large part of the acid load comes from the accumulation of CO_2. As discussed in the section on end-tidal P_{CO_2} measurements, the Fick principle predicts that a decrease in flow will result in a marked increase in venous CO_2 and therefore a decrease in venous pH. The CO_2 load is excreted by ventilation, and the fact that the P_{CO_2} is normal or below normal during CPR, indicates that a steady state is established and that the clearance of CO_2 by the lungs is adequate. Little benefit will be achieved by adding a buffer. The problem is inadequate tissue perfusion and the clearance of tissue CO_2. The CO_2 is a normal byproduct of metabolism, and it is dissolved P_{CO_2} that forms carbonic acid and produces the acid load. Bicarbonate administration has the potential of paradoxically increasing the regional CO_2 level, which will diffuse into cells and increase

cellular acidosis (62, 90). The only thing that sodium bicarbonate can do is counter the acid load from lactic acid, but this does not appear to be a major factor. (54)

Sodium bicarbonate has some important negative aspects that need to be considered (55). An increase in arterial pH will shift the oxyhemoglobin saturation curve to the left and decrease the release of oxygen. Alkalosis can contribute to cardiac arrhythmias. The sodium bicarbonate adds an important osmotic load and can produce hypernatremia (79). Sodium bicarbonate is thought to inactive catecholamines and can depress cardiac function. As noted above, it can produce a paradoxic increase in intracellular pH. Finally, sodium bicarbonate can result in a marked alkalosis following the arrest when the P_{CO_2} is regulated and lactate is cleared by normal metabolism. In conclusion, the bulk of evidence indicates that sodium bicarbonate therapy should be used judiciously.

CONCLUSION

In conclusion, much work has been done on the mechanisms of the generation of flow during CPR and on how to maximize the cardiac output. Our understanding of these factors has greatly improved in the last decade, but unfortunately the ability to apply these in a practical way is still limited. The most important factors still remain rapid onset of CPR and early defibrillation.

References

1. Adelson L. A clinicopathologic study of the anatomic changes in the heart resulting from cardiac massage. Surg Gynecol Obstet 1957;104:513–523.
2. Adgey AAJ, McKeown PP, McAnderson J. Cardioversion and defibrillation: the esophageal approach. In Vincent JL, ed. Update in intensive care and emergency medicine. New York: Springer-Verlag, 1991:34–43.
3. Adgey AAJ, Patton JN, Campbell NPS, Webb SW. Ventricular defibrillation: appropriate energy levels. Circulation 1979;60:219–222.
4. American Heart Association Part IV. Advanced cardiac life support. JAMA 1980;244:479–493.
5. Appleton C, Olajos M, Morkin E, Goldman S. Alpha-1 adrenergic control of the venous circulation in intact dogs. J Pharmacol Exp Ther 1985;233:729–734.

6. Babbs CF. New versus old theories of blood flow during CPR. Crit Care Med 1980;8:191–195.
7. Babbs CF. Cardiac angiography during CPR. Crit Care Med 1980;8:189–190.
8. Babbs CF. Abdominal counterpulsation in cardiopulmonary resuscitation: animal models and theoretical considerations. Am J Emerg Med 1985;3:165–170.
9. Babbs CF, Blevins WE. Abdominal bindings and counterpulsation in cardiopulmonary resuscitation. Crit Care Clin 1986;2:319–332.
10. Babbs CF, Ralston SH, Geddes LA. Theoretical advantages of abdominal counterpulsation in CPR as demonstrated in a simple electrical model of the circulation. Ann Emerg Med 1984;13:660–671.
11. Babbs CF, Tacker WA, Paris RL, Murphy RJ, David RW. CPR with simultaneous compression and ventilation at high airway pressure in 4 animal models. Crit Care Med 1982;10:501–504.
12. Babbs CF, Voorhees WD, Fitzgerald KR, Holmes HR, Geddes LA. Influence of interposed ventilation pressure upon artificial cardiac output during cardiopulmonary resuscitation in dogs. Crit Care Med 1980;8:127–130.
13. Babbs CF, Weaver JC, Ralson SH, Geddes LA. Cardiac, thoracic and abdominal pump. Mechanisms in cardiopulmonary resuscitation: studies in an electrical model of the circulation. Am J Emerg Med 1984;2:229–308.
14. Baker CC, Thomas AN, Trunkey DD. The role of emergency room thoracotomy in trauma. J Trauma 1980;20:848–855.
15. Barnett WM, Alifimoff JK, Paris PM, Stewart RD, Safar P. Comparison of open-chest cardiac massage techniques in dogs. Ann Emerg Med 1986;15:408–411.
16. Bedell SE, Delbanco TL, Cook EF, Epstein FH. Survival after cardiopulmonary resuscitation in the hospital. N Engl J Med 1983;309:569–576.
17. Berryman CR, Phillips GM. Interposed abdominal compression-CPR in human subjects. Ann Emerg Med 1984;13:226–229.
18. Bertrand F, Einagel V, Roussos Ch, Magder SA. Effects of abdominal compression on three modes of CPR [Abstract]. Clin Invest Med 1986;9(suppl, A):A32.
19. Beyar R, Kishon Y, Kimmel E, Neufeld H, Dinnar U. Intrathoracic and abdominal pressure variations as an efficient method for cardiopulmonary resuscitation: studies in dogs compared with computer model results. Cardiovasc Res 1985;19:335–342.
20. Bircher N, Safar P. Comparison of standard and "new" closed-chest CPR and open-chest CPR in dogs. Crit Care Med 1981;9:384–385.
21. Bircher N, Safar P. Open-chest CPR: an old method whose time has returned. Am J Emerg Med 1984;2:568–571.
22. Bircher N, Safar P, Stewart R. A comparison of standard, MAST-augmentation, and open-chest CPR in dogs. Crit Care Med 1980;8:147–152.
23. Bishop RC, Weisfeldt M. Sodium bicarbonate administration during cardiac arrest. JAMA 1976;235:506–509.
24. Bleske BE, Chow MSS, Zhao H, Kluger J. Epinephrine versus methoxamine in survival post-

25. Brillman J, Sanders A, Otto CW, Fahmy H, Bragg S, Ewy GA. Comparison of epinephrine and phenylephrine for resuscitation and neurologic outcome of cardiac arrest in dogs. Ann Emerg Med 1987;16:11–17.
26. Brown CG, Davis EA, Werman HA, Ham Lin RL. Methoxamine versus epinephrine on regional cerebral blood flow during cardiopulmonary resuscitation. Crit Care Med 1987;15:682.
27. Brown CG, Werman HA, Davis EA, Hobson J, Hamlin RL. The effects of graded doses of epinephrine on regional myocardial blood flow during cardiopulmonary resuscitation in swine. Circulation 1987;75:491–497.
28. Caldini P, Permutt S, Waddell JA, Riley RL. Effect of epinephrine on pressure, flow, and volume relationships in the systemic circulation of dogs. Circ Res 1974;34:606–623.
29. Callaham M, Barton C. Prediction of outcome of cardiopulmonary resuscitation from end-tidal carbon dioxide concentrations. Crit Care Med 1990;18:358–362.
30. Chandra N, Snyder LD, Weisfeldt ML. Abdominal binding during cardiopulmonary resuscitation in man. JAMA 1981;246:351–353.
31. Chandra N, Weisfeldt ML, Tsitlik J, et al. Augmentation of carotid flow during cardiopulmonary resuscitation by ventilation at high airway pressure simultaneous with chest compression. Am J Cardiol 1981;48:1053–1063.
32. Chesnie BM, Adelman AG, Douglas BD, Magder SA, Huckell VF, Goldman BS. Results of aortocoronary bypass surgery in patients with unstable angina. Can J Surg 1979;22:137–140.
33. Cohen JM, Chandra N, Alderson PO, Van Aswegan A, Tsitlik JE, Weisfeldt ML. Timing of pulmonary and systemic blood flow during intermittent high intrathoracic pressure cardiopulmonary resuscitation in the dog. Am J Cardiol 1982;49:1883–1889.
34. Criley JM, Blaufuss AH, Kissel GL. Cough-induced cardiac compression. JAMA 1976;236:1246–1250.
35. DeBard ML. The history of cardiopulmonary resuscitation. Ann Emerg Med 1980;9:273–275.
36. Del Guerico LRM. A plea for open-chest CPR. Am J Emerg Med 1984;2:565–566.
37. Del Guerico LRM, Coomaraswamy RP, State D. Cardiac output and other hemodynamic variables during external cardiac massage in man. N Engl J Med 1963;269:1398–1404.
38. Del Guercio LRM, Feins NR, Cohn JD, Coomaraswamy RP, Wollman SB, State D. Comparison of blood flow during external and internal cardiac massage in man. Circulation 1965;31–31(suppl):I-171–I-180.
39. Deshmukh HG, Weil MH, Gudipati CV, Trevino RP, Bisera J, Rackow EC. Mechanism of blood flow generated by precordial compression during CPR. I. Studies on closed chest precordial compression. Chest 1989;95:1092–1099.
40. Ditchey RV, Lindenfeld J. Failure of epinephrine to improve the balance between myocardial oxy-

gen supply and demand during closed-chest resuscitation in dogs. Circulation 1988;78:382–389.

41. Ducas J, Roussos Ch, Karsardis C, Magder S. Thoracoabdominal mechanics during resuscitation maneuvers. Chest 1983;84:446–451.

42. Einagel V, Bertrand F, Wise RA, Roussos Ch, Magder SA. Interposed abdominal compressions and carotid blood flow during CPR. Chest 1988;93:1206–1212.

43. Emerman CL, Pinchak AC, Hagen JF, Hancock D. Hemodynamic effects of the intra-aortic balloon pump during experimental cardiac arrest. Am J Emerg Med 1989;7:378–383.

44. Eriksson MB, Wollmer P, Olsson CG, et al. Diagnosis of pulmonary embolism based upon alveolar dead space analysis. Chest 1989;96:357–362.

45. Falk JL, Rackow EC, Weil MH. End-tidal carbon dioxide concentration during cardiopulmonary resuscitation. N Engl J Med 1988;318:607–611.

46. Feneley MP, Maier GW, Gaynor JW, et al. Sequence of mitral valve motion and transmitral blood flow during manual cardiopulmonary resuscitation in dogs. Circulation 1987;76:363–375.

47. Fisher J, Vaghaiwalla F, Tsitlik J, et al. Determinants and clinical significance of jugular venous valve competence. Circulation 1982;65:188–196.

48. Gadzinski DS, White BC, Hoehner PJ, Hoehner T, Krome C, White JD. Canine cerebral cortical blood flow and vascular resistance post cardiac arrest. Ann Emerg Med 1982;11:58–63.

49. Gascho JA, Crampton RS, Cherwek ML, Sipes JN, Hunter FP, O'Brien WM. Determinants of ventricular defibrillation in adults. Circulation 1979;60:231–240.

50. Gazmuri RJ, Von Planta M, Weil MH, Rackow EC. Arterial PCO2 as an indicator of systemic perfusion during cardiopulmonary resuscitation. Crit Care Med 1989;17:237–240.

51. Gonzalez ER, Ornato JP, Garnett AR, Levine RL. Dose-dependent vasopressor response to epinephrine during CPR in human beings. Ann Emerg Med 1991;20:440–441.

52. Green, JF. Fundamental cardiovascular and pulmonary physiology. 2nd ed. Philadelphia: Lea and Febiger, 1987.

53. Groeneveld ABJ, Bronsveld W, Thijs LG. Intermittent abdominal compression during cardiopulmonary resuscitation. Lancet 1984;1076–1077.

54. Gudipati CV, Weil MH, Gazmuri RJ, Deshmukh HG. Increases in coronary vein CO2 during cardiac resuscitation. J Appl Physiol 1990;68:1405–1408.

55. Guerci AD, Chandra N, Johnson E, et al. Failure of sodium bicarbonate to improve resuscitation from ventricular fibrillation in dogs. Circulation 1986;74:75–79.

56. Guerci AD, Shi AY, Levin H, Tsitlik J, Weisfeldt ML, Chandra N. Transmission of intrathoracic pressure to the intracranial space during cardiopulmonary resuscitation in dogs. Circ Res 1985;56:20–30.

57. Guerci AD, Weisfeldt ML. Mechanical-ventilatory cardiac support. Crit Care Clin 1986;2:209–221.

58. Guyton AC, Armstrong GG, Chipley PL. Pressure volume curves of the arterial and venous system in live dogs. Am J Physiol 1956;184:253–258.

59. Halperin HR, Brower R, Weisfeldt ML, et al. Air trapping in the lungs during cardiopulmonary resuscitation in dogs: a mechanism for generating changes in intrathoracic pressure. Circ Res 1989;65:946–954.

60. Hausknecht MJ, Wise RA, Brower RG, et al. Effects of lung inflation on blood flow during cardiopulmonary resuscitation in the canine isolated heart-lung preparation. Circ Res 1986;59:676–683.

61. Harris LC, Kirimli B, Safar P. Augmentation of artificial circulation during cardiopulmonary resuscitation. Anesthesiology 1967;28:730–734.

62. Hoekstra OS, Van Lambalgen AA, Thijs LG. Abdominal interposed between thoracic compressions during cardiopulmonary resuscitation. In: Vincent JL, ed. Update in Intensive Care and Emergency Medicine. New York: Springer-Verlag 1991:3–10.

63. Howard M, Carrubba C, Foss F, Janiak B, Hogan B, Guinness M. Interposed abdominal compression-CPR: its effects on parameters of coronary perfusion in human subjects. Ann Emerg Med 1987;16:3:253–259.

64. Imai T, Kon N, Kunimoto F, Tanaka M. Exacerbation of hypercapnia and acidosis of central venous blood and tissue following administration of sodium bicarbonate during cardiopulmonary resuscitation. Jpn Circ J 1989;53:298–306.

65. Kerber RE, Grayzel J, Hoyt R, Marcus M, Kennedy J. Transthoracic resistance in human defibrillation: influence of body weight, chest size, serial shocks, paddle size and paddle contact pressure. Circulation 1981;63:676–682.

66. Kerber RE, Kouba C, Martins J, et al. Advance prediction of transthoracic impedance in human defibrillation and cardioversion: importance of impedance in determining the success of low-energy shock. Circulation 1984;70:303–308.

67. Kerber RE, Sarnat W. Factors influencing the success of ventricular defibrillation in man. Circulation 1979;60:226–230.

68. Kette F, Weil MH, Von Planta M, Gazmuri RJ, Rackow EC. Buffer agents do not reverse intramyocardial acidosis during cardiac resuscitation. Circulation 1990;81:1660–1666.

69. Kimmel E, Beyar R, Dinnar U, Sideman S, Kishon Y. Augmentation of cardiac output and carotid blood flow by chest and abdomen phased compression cardiopulmonary resuscitation. Cardiol Res 1986;20:574–580.

70. Koehler RC, Chandra N, Guerci AD, et al. Augmentation of cerebral perfusion by simultaneous chest compression and lung inflation with abdominal binding after cardiac arrest in dogs. Circulation 1983;67:266–275.

71. Kouwenhoven WB, Jude JR, Knickerbocker CG. Closed-chest cardiac massage. JAMA 1960;173:1064–1067.

72. Lee HR, Wilder RJ, Downs P, Massion W, Blank WF. MAST augmentation of external cardiac compression: role of changing intrapleural pressure. Ann Emerg Med 1981;10:560–565.

73. Lindner, KH. Vasopressor therapy in cardiopulmonary resuscitation. In: Vincent JL, ed. Update in intensive care and emergency medicine. New York: Springer-Verlag, 1991:18–24.

74. Lindner KH, Ahnefeld FW. Comparison of epinephrine and norepinephrine in the treatment of asphyxial or fibrillatory cardiac arrest in a porcine model. Crit Care Med 1989;17:437–441.

75. Lindner KH, Ahnefeld FW, Bowdler IM. Comparison of different doses of epinephrine on myocardial perfusion and resuscitation success during cardiopulmonary resuscitation. Am J Emerg Med 1991;9:27–31.

76. Lindner KH, Ahnefeld FW, Schuermann W, Bowdler IM. Epinephrine and norepinephrine in cardiopulmonary resuscitation. Effects on myocardial oxygen delivery and consumption. Chest 1990;97:1458–1462.

77. Luce JM, Ross BK, O'Quin J, et al. Regional blood flow during cardipulmonary resuscitation in dogs using simultaneous and nonsimultaneous compression and ventilation. Circulation 1983; 67:258–264.

78. Maier GW, Tyson GS, Graig QO, et al. The physiology of external massage: high-impulse cardiopulmonary resuscitation. Circulation 1984;70:86–101.

79. Maltar JA, Weil MH, Shubin H, Stein L. Cardiac arrest in the critically ill. Hyperosmolar states following cardiac arrest. Am J Med 1974;56:162–168.

80. Martin GB, Gentile NT, Paradis NA, Moeggenberg J. Effect of epinephrine on end-tidal carbon dioxide monitoring during CPR. Ann Emerg Med 1990;19:396–398.

81. Mateer JR, Stueven HA, Thompson BM, Aprahamian C, Darin JC. Prehospital IAC-LPR verdus standard CPR. Ann Emerg Med 1985;3:143–146.

82. Michael JR, Guerci AD, Koehler RC, et al. Mechanisms by which epinephrine augments cerebral and myocardial perfusion during cardiopulmonary resuscitation in dogs. Circulation 1984;69:822–835.

83. Newton JR, Glower DD, Wolfe JA, et al. A physiologic comparison of external cardiac massage techniques. J Thorac Cardiovasc Surg 1988;95:892–901.

84. Niemann JT, Rosborough JP, Hansknecht M, Gardiner D, Brilley JM. Pressure-synchronized cineangiography during experimental cardiopulmonary resuscitation. Circulation 1981;64:985–991.

85. Niemann JT, Rosborough JP, Niskanen RA, Alferness C, Criley JM. Mechanical "cough" cardiopulmonary resuscitation during cardiac arrest in dogs. Am J Cardiol 1985;55:199–204.

86. Niemann JT, Rosborough JP, Ung S, Criley JM. Coronary perfusion pressure during experimental cardiopulmonary resuscitation. Ann Emerg Med 1982;11:127–131.

87. Niemann JT, Rosborough JP, Ung S, Criley JM. Hemodynamic effects of continuous abdominal binding during cardiac arrest and resuscitation. Am J Cardiol 1984;53:269–274.

88. Ohomoto T, Miura I, Konno S. A new method of external cardiac massage to improve diastolic augmentation and prolong survival time. Ann Thorac Surg 1976;21:284–290.

89. Olson DW, Thakur R, Stueven HA, Thompson B. Randomized study of epinephrine versus methoxamine in prehospital ventricular fibrillation. Ann Emerg Med 1989;18:1258–1259.

90. Ornato JP, Levine RL, Young DS, Racht EM. The effect of applied chest compression force on systemic arterial pressure and end-tidal carbon dioxide concentration during CPR in human beings. Ann Emerg Med 1989;18:732–737.

91. Otto CW, Yakaitis RW, Redding JS, Blitt CD. Comparison of dopamine, dobutamine, and epinephrine in CPR. Crit Care Med 1981;9:640–643.

92. Passerini L, Wise RA, Roussos Ch, Magder SA. Maintenance of circulation without chest compression during CPR. Crit Care Med 1988;3:62–106.

93. Pearson JW, Redding JS. Influence of peripheral vascular tone on cardiac resuscitation. Anesth Analg 1965;44:746–752.

94. Permutt S, Riley S. Hemodynamics of collapsible vessels with tone: the vascular waterfall. J Appl Physiol 1963;18:924–932.

95. Permutt S, Wise RA, Sylvester JT. Interaction between the circulation and ventilatory pumps. In: Lenfant C, Roussos, Ch, eds. The Thorax. New York: Marcel Dekker, 1985.

96. Ralston SH, Babbs CF, Niebauer MS. Cardiopulmonary resuscitation with interposed abdominal compression in dogs. Anesth Analg 1982;61:645–651.

97. Ralston SH, Tacker WA, Showen L, Carter A, Babbs CF, Lafayette W. Endotracheal versus intravenous epinephrine during electromechanical dissociation with CPR in dogs. Ann Emerg Med 1985;14:1044–1048.

98. Redding JS. Abdominal compression in cardiopulmonary resuscitation. Anesth Analg 1971; 50:668–675.

99. Redding JJ, Cozino RA. A comparison of open chest and closed chest cardiac massage in dogs. Anesthesiology 1961;22:280–285.

100. Redding JS, Haynes RR, Thomas JD. "Old" and "new" CPR manually performed in dogs. Crit Care Med 1981;9:386–387.

101. Roberts D, Landolfo K, Dobson K, Light RB. The effects of methoxamine and epinephrine on survival and regional distribution of cardiac output in dogs with prolonged ventricular fibrillation. Chest 1990;98:999–1005.

102. Rudikoff MT, Maughan WL, Effron M, Freund P, Weisfeldt ML. Mechanisms of blood flow during cardiopulmonary resuscitation. Circulation 1980;61:345–352.

103. Safar P, Bircher NG. Cardiopulmonary cerebral resuscitation. 3rd ed. London: WB Saunders, 1988.

104. Safar P, Escarraga LA, Elam JO. A comparison of the mouth-to-mouth and mouth-to-airway artificial respiration with the chest-pressure, arm-life method. N Engl J Med 1958;258:675.

105. Sagawa K. The ventricular pressure-volume diagram revisited. Circ Res 1978;43:677–687.

106. Sanders AB, Ewy GA. Open-chest CPR: not yet. Am J Emerg Med 1984;2:566–567.

107. Sanders AB, Ewy A, Alferness A, Taft T, Zimmerman M. Failure of one method of simultaneous chest compression, ventilation, and abdominal binding during CPR. Crit Care Med 1982;10:509–513.

108. Sanders AB, Ewy GA, Taft TB. The importance of aortic diastolic blood pressure during cardiopulmonary resuscitation. Crit Care Med 1984;12:871–873.

109. Sanders AB, Kern KB, Ewy GA, Atlas M, Bailey L. Improved resuscitation from cardiac arrest with open-chest massage. Ann Emerg Med 1984;13:672–675.

110. Sanders AB, Kern KB, Otto CW, Milander MM, Ewy GA. End-tidal carbon dioxide monitoring during cardiopulmonary resuscitation. JAMA 1989;262:1347–1351.

111. Schleien CL, Dean JM, Koehler RC, et al. Effect of epinephrine on cerebral and myocardinal perfusion in an infant preparation of cardiopulmonary resuscitation. Circulation 1986;73:809–817.

112. Schleien CL, Koehler RC, Shaffner DH, Traystman RJ. Blood-brain barrier integrity during cardiopulmonary resuscitation in dogs. Stroke 1990;21:1185–1191.

113. Sharff JA, Pantley G, Noel E. Effect of time on regional organ perfusion during two methods of cardiopulmonary resuscitation. Ann Emerg Med 1984;13:649–665.

114. Tacker WA, Ewy GA. Emergency defibrillation dose: recommendations and rationale. Circulation 1979;60:223–225.

115. Taylor GJ, Tucker WM, Greene HL, Rudikoff MT, Weisfeldt ML. Importance of prolonged compression during cardiopulmonary resuscitation in man. N Engl J Med 1977;296:1515–1517.

116. Von Planta M, Weil MH, Gazmuri RJ, Bisera J, Rackow EC. Myocardial acidosis associated with CO2 production during cardiac arrest and resuscitation. Circulation 1989;80:684–692.

117. Voorhees WD, Niebauer MJ, Babbs CF. Improved oxygen delivery during cardiopulmonary resuscitation with interposed abdominal compressions. Ann Emerg Med 1983;12:128–135.

118. Walker JW, Bruestle JC, White BC, Evans AT, Indreri R, Bialek H. Perfusion of the cerebral cortex by use of abdominal counter pulsation during cardiopulmonary resuscitation. Am J Emerg Med 1984;2:391–393.

119. Ward KR, Sullivan RJ, Zelenak RR, Summer WR. A comparison of interposed abdominal compression CPR and standard CPR by monitoring end-tidal PCO2. Ann Emerg Med 1990;19:1201–1202.

120. Weaver WD, Fahrenbruch CE, Johnson DD, Hallstrom AP. Effect of epinephrine and lidocaine therapy on outcome after cardiac arrest due to ventricular fibrillation. Circulation 1990;82:2027–2034.

121. Weil MH, Rackow EC, Tevino R, Grundler W, Falk JL, Griffel MI. Difference in acid-base state between venous and arterial blood during cardiopulmonary resuscitation. N Engl J Med 1986;315:153–156.

122. Weiser FM, Adler LN, Kuhn L. Hemodynamic effects of closed and open cardiac resuscitation in normal dogs and those with acute myocardinal infarction. Am J Cardiol 1962;10:555–561.

123. Weisfeldt ML, Halperin HR. Cardiopulmonary resuscitation: beyond cardiac massage. Circulation 1986;74:443–448.

124. Werner JA, Greene HL, Janko CL, Cobb LA. Visualization of cardiac valve motion in man during external chest compression using two-dimensional echocardiography. Circulation 1981;63:1417–1421.

125. Wexler HR, Gelb AW. Controversies in cardiopulmonary resuscitation. Crit Care Clin 1986;2:335–345.

126. Wilder RJ, Weir D, Rush BF, Ravitch MM. Methods of coordinating ventilation and closed chest cardiac massage in the dog. Surgery 1963;53:186–194.

127. Wise RA, Summer WR. Pulmonary mechanics and artificial support of the arrested circulation. Clin Chest Med 1983;4:189–198.

128. Wise RA, Summer WR. Cardiopulmonary resuscitation. In: Dantzker DR, ed. Cardiopulmonary Critical Care. Philadelphia: WB Saunders, Co., 1988:385–405.

129. Yakaitis RW, Ewy GA, Otto CW, Taren DL, Moon TE. Influence of time and therapy on ventricular defibrillation in dogs. Crit Care Med 1980;8:157–163.

130. Yin FCP, Cohen JM, Tsitlik J, Zola B, Weisfeldt ML. Role of carotid artery resistance to collapse during high-intrathoracic-pressure CPR. Am J Physiol 1982;243:H259–H267.

131. Zoll PM, Linenthal AS, Gibson W., Paul MH, Norman LR. Termination of ventricular fibrillation in man by externally applied electrical countershock. N Engl J Med 1956;254:727.

32

Community-Acquired Acute Pneumonia and Respiratory Failure

Jean Chastre
Jean-Yves Fagon

Acute infectious pneumonia is defined as the recent onset of inflammation of the normally sterile lung parenchyma due to a microbe that is distinguished from infections of the larger airways alone, e.g., tracheobronchitis, even though many organisms can cause both conditions. Pneumonia that develops outside the hospital, without iatrogenic procedures, is considered to be community-acquired. This infection remains an important cause of morbidity and mortality in adults. In one study of 858 infections in individuals of all ages seen in an emergency department, 65% were of respiratory origin (64). Pneumonia is the sixth most common cause of death in the United States and the most common cause of infection-related mortality, accounting for an estimated 55,000 deaths annually (1). Despite progress in diagnostic techniques and treatments, management of respiratory tract infections remains challenging because the precise etiology remains uncertain in as many as nearly 50% of the cases (26). Moreover, new agents have been implicated as causes of community-acquired pneumonia. Given the broad spectrum of diagnostic possibilities, management has become more complex, as empiric therapy is usually required at the outset and precise etiologic diagnosis requires results of laboratory tests, which may not be available immediately.

Our goal in this review is to provide current information on these different issues so that an updated approach to diagnosis and management can be rationally formulated.

PATHOGENESIS

Pneumonia results from microbial invasion of the normally sterile lung parenchyma caused by either a defect in host defenses or challenge by a particularly virulent microorganism or an overwhelming inoculum. Organisms can enter the lung and cause infection in several ways: *(a)* by direct inhalation of infectious particles from ambient air, *(b)* by aspiration of secretions from the mouth and nasopharynx, *(c)* by deposition in the lung vasculature following hematogenous spread from another site, and rarely, *(d)* by penetration of lung tissue or spread from a contiguous site across the chest wall or diaphragm. Aspiration of microbes colonizing the naso-oropharynx provides the most frequent entry to the lung. Both the upper and lower respiratory tracts have an elaborate array of defenses against the source of contamination of pulmonary parenchyma. These defenses include anatomic barriers such as nasopharyngeal filtration and the epiglottis, cough reflexes, tracheobronchial secretions, cell-mediated and humoral immunity, and polymorphonuclear neutrophils (37). When these components are functioning properly, invading microbes are eliminated and clinical disease is avoided, but if these defenses are impaired or if they are overcome by virtue of

525

a high inoculum of organisms or organisms of unusual virulence, pneumonitis results.

A number of factors are known to interfere with normal host defenses and thus to predispose to infection. Alterations in the level of consciousness due to any cause (stroke, seizures, drug intoxication, alcohol abuse, and even normal sleep) can compromise epiglottic closure and lead to aspiration of microorganisms present in the oropharynx into the lower respiratory tract. Other factors that impair pulmonary clearance of pathogens include cigarette smoking, hypoxemia, chronic obstructive lung disease, pulmonary edema, malnutrition, immunosuppressive agents, viral infection, and mechanical obstruction (22).

When microbes adhere to alveolar macrophages, chemotactic substances relatively specific for neutrophils are released (41). Proteases released by these neutrophils can, in turn, activate the complement cascade, the kinin system, and fibrinolysis. These products induce a capillary leak, resulting in accumulation of exuded fluid in the interstitium and alveoli (42). Consequently, gas exchange in those areas is severely compromised. Although blood flow to the affected areas decreases, a ventilation-perfusion mismatch may result that, if severe, can lead to the development of arterial hypoxemia. Finally, the proteases released by the neutrophils may activate various mediators of inflammation that have been implicated in the pathogenesis of the intense inflammatory response in the lung that results in the clinical adult respiratory distress syndrome (ARDS).

ETIOLOGIC AGENTS

The etiologies of community-acquired pneumonia appear to have changed over the last decade (22, 26) (Table 32.1). Additional pathogens have been implicated, old pathogens have assumed new significance, and new pathogens, such as *Legionella* species or *Chlamydia pneumoniae*, have emerged. All of this makes it more difficult to predict the microbial etiology of pneumonia solely on the basis of clinical evaluation alone or the presence of an underlying disease. With the diagnostic tests presently available, a microbiologic diagnosis can be made in approximately 45–70% of pneumonia cases, depending on the percentage of patients who had received antibiotics before admission (26).

Even if its relative importance has decreased, *Streptococcus pneumoniae* remains the predominant organism in most recent studies, causing 15–60% of the cases of acute community-acquired pneumonia (22, 26) (Table 32.2). Advanced age, cigarette smoking, dementia, seizures, and the presence of chronic illnesses, such as chronic obstructive pulmonary disease, congestive heart failure, splenectomy, and cerebrovascular disease, have been identified as significant risk factors for the development of pneumococcal pneumonia (52). Despite antibiotic therapy, mortality continues to be as high as 25–30% in patients 50 years of age and older, those with multilobar disease, leukopenia, or severe concomitant diseases, in patients with bacteremic pneumonia, and in those infected with type 1 and type 3 pneumococcus (5, 22, 79).

Overwhelming pneumococcal sepsis with disseminated intravascular coagulation has been described in asplenic patients and in patients with functional asplenia, such as those with sickle cell anemia (56, 99). Recently, Hook et al. (40) were unable to decrease mortality, despite intensive care unit support of patients with bacteremic pneumococcal pneumonia. Intensive care support only shifted mortality from the first 24 hours to late in the hospitalization. In recent years, antibiotic-resistant *S. pneumoniae* have increasingly been identified (2). Although most of these pneumococci are only moderately resistant to penicillin, with minimal inhibitory concentrations (MICs) of 0.1–1.0 μg/ml, emergence of pneumococci highly resistant to penicillin alone and pneumococci multiresistant to various antibiotics have been found throughout the world (2). These data underscore the need to test pneumococcal isolates on a routine basis for penicillin susceptibility.

Haemophilus influenzae is now more frequently recognized as an important cause of community-acquired pneumonia, responsible for an estimated 4–15% of the

Table 32.1
Etiologic Agents of Community-Acquired Pneumonia

Agent	Common	Uncommon
Bacterial	*Streptococcus pneumoniae* *Staphylococcus aureus* *Haemophilus influenzae* *Legionella* spp. Mixed anaerobes Enterobacteriaceae *Escherichia coli* *Klebsiella pneumoniae* *Enterobacter* spp. *Serratia* spp. *Pseudomonas aeruginosa*	*Acinetobacter* spp. *Actinomyces* spp. *Aeromonas hydrophilia* *Branhamella catarrhalis* *Campylobacter fetus* *Francisella tularensis* *Neisseria meningitidis* *Nocardia* spp. *Pasteurella multocida* *Pseudomonas pseudomallei* *Salmonella* spp. *Enterococcus faecalis* *Streptococcus pyogenes* *Yersinia pestis*
Viral	Influenza A and B viruses Adenovirus Respiratory syncytial virus	Parainfluenza virus Varicella-zoster virus Herpes simplex virus Cytomegalovirus Measles virus Rhinovirus Enteroviruses
Bacteria-like organisms	*Mycoplasma pneumoniae* *Chlamydia pneumoniae*	*Chlamydia psittaci* *Chlamydia trachomatis* *Coxiella burnetii* *Rickettsia rickettsii*
Mycobacterial	*Mycobacterium tuberculosis*	
Fungal	*Histoplasma capsulatum* *Coccidioides immitis* *Blastomyces dermatitidis*	*Candida* spp. *Aspergillus* spp. *Cryptococcus neoformans* *Mucor* spp.
Parasitic	*Pneumocystis carinii*	*Toxoplasma gondii* *Strongyloides stercoralis* *Ascaris lumbricoides*

cases (26). In most studies, *Hemophilus* species are ranked among the top five etiologies (Table 32.2). The true incidence of this organism is, however, obscured by the difficulty encountered in isolating it from sputum and identifying it in Gram-stained sputum smears, and because of the inability to distinguish true infection from colonization in earlier studies. Claims of a pathogenic relationship in individual cases are usually based on the finding of heavy or pure cultures from material obtained by transtracheal aspiration or from the Gram staining of such specimens, or by identification of the organism in blood or pleural fluid cultures. The use of coun-terimmunoelectrophoresis to identify the antigen(s) in sputum and blood is of uncertain efficacy because of the high incidence of colonization and the high frequency of uncategorized organisms causing disease. In adults, *H. influenzae* infection occurs most often in compromised hosts with chronic bronchopulmonary disease, alcoholism, diabetes, or an immunoglobin defect (90). However, a few patients appear to be free of underlying disease (3, 96). The mortality rate from bacteremic *H. influenzae* pneumonia has been estimated to be 34%, a reflection of the severity of patients' underlying illness (26, 90, 92). Treatment is complicated by the increasing

Table 32.2
Literature Review of Studies on Community-Acquired Pneumonias including more than 100 Patients[a,b]

Site	Year	No. of Cases	Organism Rank (%)					Unknown (%)	Ref. No.
			First	Second	Third	Fourth	Fifth		
Edinburgh	1960–62	141	S. pneumo (44 ?)	H. influ (22)	Virus ? (?)	S. aureus (9)	Mycoplasma (?)	38	12
Baltimore	1965–66	100	S. pneumo (62)	Virus (12)	Mycoplasma (3)	K. pneumo (2)	S. aureus (1)	34	27
Atlanta	1967–68	292	S. pneumo (62)	Gram-neg. (20)	Virus (11)	S. aureus (10)	H. influ (8)	43	85
Milwaukee	1969–70	148	S. pneumo (53)	S. aureus (7)	Klebsiella (6)	Influ A. (5)	Mycoplasma (4)	17	23
Baltimore	1970–71	144	S. pneumo (47)	H. influ (46)	S. aureus (14)	Klebsiella (14)	Proteus (8)	13	65
Nottingham, UK	1980–81	127	S. pneumo (76)	Legionella (15)	C. psittaci (6)	Virus (6)	H. influ (3)	3	54
Hartford	1981	204	S. pneumo (36)	H. influ (15)	Legionella (14)	S. aureus (8)	K. pneumo (7)	0	47
Göteborg, Sweden	?	127	S. pneumo (54)	Mycoplasma (14)	Influ A (12)	H. influ (4)	C. psittaci (2)	21	14
Nova Scotia	1981–82	138	Aspiration (15)	S. pneumo (15)	H. influ (9)	CMV (6)	Chlamydia (4)	44	57
Oreboro, Sweden	1982	147	S. pneumo (39)	H. influ (5)	Mycoplasma (5)	Influ A (5)	B. catarrhalis (2)	29	39
Britain	1982–83	453	S. pneumo (42)	Mycoplasma (10)	Influ A (7)	H. influ (6)	C. psittaci (3)	33	75
France	1982–83	274	S. pneumo (12)	Legionella (11)	Mycoplasma (9)	H. influ (6)	Klebsiella (3)	49	4
Nova Scotia	1981–84	301	Aspiration (11)	S. pneumo (9)	H. influ (9)	TWAR (6)	Influ A (5)	37	58
Paris, France	1983–84	116	S. pneumo (26)	H. influ (12)	M. tb (10)	Gram-neg. (7)	Legionella (4)	35	50
Nottingham, UK	1984–85	236	S. pneumo (36)	Influ A (6 ?)	Other viruses (12)	H. influ (10)	S. aureus (1)	45	97
Pittsburgh	1986–87	359	S. pneumo (15)	H. influ (11)	Legionella (7)	TWAR (6)	Gram-neg. (6)	33	26

[a]Abbreviations: S. pneumo, Streptococcus pneumoniae; H. influ, Haemophilus influenzae; Mycoplasma, Mycoplasma pneumoniae; K. pneumo, Klebsiella pneumoniae; Gram-neg., aerobic Gram-negative rod; Influ A, influenzae A; C. psittaci, Chlamydia psittaci; CMV, cytomegalovirus; B. catarrhalis, Branhamella catarrhalis; TWAR, Chlamydia pneumoniae; M. tb, Mycobacterium tuberculosis.
[b]From Fang GD, Fine M, Orlott J, et al. New and emerging etiologies for community-acquired pneumonia with implications for therapy. A prospective multicenter study of 359 cases. Medicine (Baltimore) 1990;69:307–316.

incidence of ampicillin resistance, which appears to be due to the production of a β-lactamase. The degree of resistance is now estimated to be about 20% in children and 10% in adults (67). In addition, penicillin-resistant organisms are now showing resistance to chloramphenicol, the previously recognized back-up antibiotic for ampicillin. Fortunately, the recently released second- and third-generation cephalosporins are very β-lactamase stable and most *Hemophilus* species are exquisitely sensitive (67).

Staphylococcus aureus accounts for 1–10% of the cases of acute community-acquired pneumonia (22). The incidence of staphylococcal pneumonia has been reported to be particularly high in elderly patients institutionalized in nursing homes or during outbreaks of viral influenza (78). In this latter situation, *S. aureus* may be responsible for up to 20% of the encountered pneumonias, even if pneumococcus remains the most frequent pathogen, accounting for about 46% of the cases in two studies (59, 78). A small percentage of staphylococcal pneumonia may result from hematogenous embolization to the lungs from primary extrapulmonary infections, usually in the setting of right-sided endocarditis or venous septic thrombophlebitis in IV drug abusers, in patients undergoing hemodialysis, or on home IV therapy (91). There are no clinical or radiologic features typical of *S. aureus* pneumonia except possibly rapid cavitation of a bronchopneumonia and the development of a pleural empyema. The diagnosis is based on identification of the organism in pleural fluid or blood, or by Gram staining. Sputum culture is unreliable because up to 40% of adults are asymptomatic carriers (27).

Aerobic Gram-negative rods of Enterobacteriaeceae and nonfermentative organisms are a relatively uncommon cause of community-acquired pneumonia (Table 32.2). *Klebsiella pneumoniae* is most often considered, but *Escherichia coli*, *Pseudomonas aeruginosa*, *Enterobacter cloacae*, *Acinetobacter* and *Serratia* spp., *Proteus*, and many other aerobic Gram-negative bacilli may also cause disease (Table 32.1). Although these organisms can infect previously healthy patients, they are more likely to cause disease in older patients and patients with chronic underlying disease (26, 47, 50, 84). For example, in the study of Fang et al., (26), 88% of the patients with Gram-negative rod pneumonia had an underlying illness, while only 50% of the patients with chlamydial pneumonia had a comorbid illness. Surprisingly, however, chronic obstructive pulmonary disease was the most common underlying disease in these patients with Gram-negative pneumonias. Immunosuppression, defined as hematologic malignancy, solid tumor, neutropenia, and taking corticosteroids, was unexpectedly low (38%), but all deaths in patients with Gram-negative pneumonias occurred in immunosuppressed patients. Although prior antibiotic therapy has been suggested as a predisposing factor for Gram-negative pneumonia, this was corroborated for only 28% of the patients with Gram-negative pneumonia, a frequency of usage that is not significantly different from that observed in other etiologies of pneumonia in one study (26).

The importance of *Legionella* spp. in causing community-acquired pneumonia varies greatly according to the geographic area. While incidences as high as 17–22% have been reported, many localities report significantly lower rates (54, 84, 98). Routine testing using selective medium for culture, direct fluorescent antibody labeling, serology (both acute and convalescent), and urinary antigen detection are crucial in uncovering the diagnosis. Community-acquired legionnaires' disease seem to be more frequent among males, persons 50 years of age and older, persons requiring renal dialysis or transplantation, smokers, immunosuppressed patients, and persons with a comorbid disease, such as chronic bronchitis or diabetes mellitus (25).

Recently, *Moraxella (Branhamella) catarrhalis* has been identified as a cause of pneumonia. The overall incidence of disease due to this bacterium is low, but it is an important pathogen in elderly patients with underlying lung disease or carcinoma (80).

The true incidence of anaerobic etiologies of community-acquired pneumonias is uncertain. In some studies using invasive diagnostic methods, anaerobes have been cultured from lower respiratory tract specimens in 20–30% of the cases (9). However, other reports suggest that anaerobic pneumonias account for only 3–4% of the cases of community-acquired pneumonia (22, 26). Anaerobic pulmonary infections are usually recognizable by the characteristic clinical and radiographic findings. Commonly, the patient's oral hygiene is poor and he or she may have some underlying disease in which there is prior evidence of altered consciousness, a diminished gag reflex, or an abnormal swallowing mechanism (e.g., epilepsy, alcoholism, esophageal carcinoma, or drug overdose). An insidious low-grade fever is typical, and the chest radiography demonstrates segmental involvement of dependent areas of the lung, often with cavitation (8).

Mycoplasma pneumoniae is a common cause of community-acquired pneumonia, accounting for 10–40% of the infections in some studies (28, 30, 93). Although nearly all infections with this organism are mild, *M. pneumoniae* can also mimic bacterial pneumonia and some unusual pulmonary manifestations, such as lung abscess, lobar consolidation, or ARDS, have been reported (48, 72). Most laboratories do not culture *M. pneumoniae* and the diagnosis is usually made on serologic evidence.

Chlamydia pneumoniae (TWAR) is a newly discovered pulmonary pathogen. Grayston et al. (35) reported that *C. pneumoniae* was the etiology for 12% of the community-acquired pneumonia in Seattle University students. *Chlamydia pneumoniae* has been associated with pneumonia epidemics in teenagers, young adults, and military conscript populations (35, 36). In the study of Fang et al. (26) (Table 32.2) this microorganism constituted 6.1% of the pneumonias and was a common etiology for pneumonia in older adults (mean age, 65 years) and patients with chronic underlying illness.

Although much more frequent in children, viral pneumonia remains a significant problem in adults. Viral pneumonia typically presents subacutely as an upper respiratory tract infection, but may have an acute onset, with severe pulmonary damage and ARDS (51). Of the viral agents associated with pneumonia in adults, influenza A and B virus and adenovirus are the most common (Table 32.1), but respiratory syncytial virus, the predominant respiratory pathogen in infants and children, is now recognized as an etiology of pneumonia in adults. While the number of cases is small, groups at particularly high risk appear to be the elderly and patients who are immunosuppressed. The definitive diagnosis of viral pneumonia requires detection of the virus from sputum or nasopharyngeal swabs. Information based on serology is often not clinically relevant at the time of the acute illness.

Fungal infections are being recognized with increasing frequency. Fungi can cause human pulmonary disease by several mechanisms. Some organisms (such as *Histoplasma capsulatum, Coccidioides immitis, and Blastomyces dermatitidis*) are primary pathogens that most frequently infect health individuals. They are found in specific geographic areas and usually cause asymptomatic or mild infection, evidenced only by the development of positive skin tests. However, fulminant primary infection or chronic pulmonary disease with or without systemic dissemination can cause significant morbidity and can occasionally be fatal (33). A second group of organisms (particularly *Aspergillus* and *Candida* species) are essentially opportunistic organisms that chiefly affect immunocompromised hosts or grow in association with underlying systemic or pulmonary disease. In addition, some fungi (particularly *Aspergillus* spp.) can cause disease through an exaggerated hypersensitivity reaction without actually invading tissue. Finally, the inhalation of massive amounts of fungi can itself provoke a toxic nonallergic pulmonary reaction.

Patients with acute tuberculosis (TB) may present with a syndrome indistinguishable from acute community-acquired pneumonia, with infiltrates involving primarily the middle and lower lung fields without apical disease (46). On occasion, patients with miliary TB present with a syndrome reminiscent of ARDS. Therefore, TB must be considered in patients with acute respiratory failure and fever who do not respond to the usual antibacterial therapy. This was highlighted by Bobrowitz (15), who retrospectively identified 20 patients in whom TB was the primary cause of death but was not diagnosed until autopsy.

Although *Nocardia* was originally described as a primary disease in normal patients, it is essentially observed in patients with various underlying conditions, such as organ transplant patients, patients with lymphoreticular neoplasms, hepatic cirrhosis, chronic pulmonary disorders, and almost any situation requiring prolonged corticosteroid therapy (13). Pulmonary nocardiosis can produce a variety of chest radiography abnormalities, including lobar infiltrate, abscess, nodules, and patchy bronchopneumonia or interstitial infiltrates mimicking ARDS (31). The diagnosis of pulmonary nocardiosis requires a high index of suspicion in the patient at risk because this organism grows slowly. Although cases of *Nocardia* colonization have been described, the finding of branching Gram-positive, partially acid-fast filaments in the sputum virtually establishes the diagnosis (31).

With the emergence of AIDS, *Pneumocystis carinii* is now appearing as a major pathogen in a selected population with community-acquired pneumonia. Given the striking variation in the prevalence of AIDS in different communities, AIDS patients who develop pneumonia should be viewed as a distinct entity and not part of the general rubric of community-acquired pneumonia. In addition to the more common bacterial agents usually observed in patients with acute pneumonia, cytomegalovirus, *Mycobacterium tuberculosis*, and *Cryptococcus neoformans* also play important roles as etiologic agents in patients with AIDS.

In summary, recent studies have demonstrated a change in reported etiologies for community-acquired pneumonia. Several factors may be contributory. First, new microbial agents have been recognized and are now identifiable with readily available tests. Secondly, a population of patients increasingly susceptible to opportunistic infections has emerged, such as patients with AIDS or an organ transplant. Finally, it must be stressed that in virtually every clinical series recording etiologic agents for community-acquired pneumonia, there is a sizable number of cases for which no specific etiology could be determined. This fact is probably explained for the most part by the increasing use of broad-spectrum antibiotic therapy in the community. Antibiotics given before admission decrease the ability to isolate a specific pathogen and, in particular, prevent the detection of pneumococcus (26).

CLINICAL EVALUATION

History-taking should attempt to determine the clinical setting in which the pneumonia is occurring. Special attention should be given to pneumonia developing in unusual settings. For example, outbreaks of *M. pneumoniae* or *C. pneumoniae* pneumonia have frequently been reported in relatively closed populations of young adults, i.e., at military bases or colleges (30, 35). Specific etiologic agents of pneumonia have been associated with certain underlying diseases. As previously discussed, an increased incidence of staphylococcal pneumonia has been noted during epidemics of influenza (51, 59). Cystic fibrosis is associated with pseudomonas and staphylococcal pulmonary infections. Recent dental work, sedative overdose, seizure, or loss of consciousness for any reason should raise the suspicion of anaerobic infection due to aspiration of oropharyngeal bacteria (8). Needless to say, exposure resulting from an unusual occupation or from travel must be considered (e.g., travel to a Q-fever zone or frequent handling of psittacine birds).

Patients with community-acquired pneumonia typically present with chills, cough, sputum production, fever, and pleuritic chest pain. Mental status changes, confusion, or disorientation are also frequently observed and occur significantly more frequently in elderly patients. Although the above clinical manifestations are useful in diagnosing pneumonia, individual symptoms or signs are not specific for defining the etiologic agent. Fang et al. (26) compared the clinical manifestations of the five most common etiologies (pneumococcus, *H. influenzae*, *Legionella* spp., *C. pneumoniae*, and Gram-negative bacilli) of community-acquired pneumonia found in their study. In contrast to previous studies (25, 63), they demonstrated that abdominal pain, vomiting, relative bradycardia, neurologic changes, hyponatremia, and abnormal liver function tests did not occur significantly more frequently in pneumonia caused by *Legionella* spp. than in those caused by other microorganisms. However, *Legionella* cases had much more frequently a temperature $\geq 40°C$ and a slightly higher incidence of diarrhea than in pneumonias of other origins (Table 32.3). Patients with *Legionella* spp. pneumonias were also more frequently admitted to intensive care units (26).

The atypical pneumonia syndrome includes viral, mycoplasmal, and chlamydial infections and is thought to be distinguishable from bacterial pneumonias by the presence of gradual onset, viral prodrome, absence of rigors, nonproductive cough, lower degree of fever, absence of pleurisy, absence of consolidation, low leukocyte count, and an ill-defined infiltrate on chest

Table 32.3
Comparison of Underlying Conditions, Symptoms, Physical Signs, Laboratory Data, Prognostic Factors, and Mortality Associated with Major Etiologies in Community-Acquired Pneumonia[a]

	S. pneumoniae	*H. influenzae*	*Legionella* spp.	*C. pneumoniae*	Gram-negative
Underlying conditions					
Mean age, years (range)	65 (27–92)	62 (30–97)	63 (23–92)	63.3 (32–84)	67 (21–89)
Sex (M:F)	56:44	48:52	54:46	80:20	87:13
Smoking history (%)	59	60	70	62	50
Chronic obstructive pulmonary disease (%)	50	41	38	30	56
Alcohol (%)	36	42	44	29	47
Immunosuppression (%)[b]	28	39	44	36	38
No underlying disease (%)	26	26	33	50	12
Symptomatology					
Shortness of breath (%)	67	66	50	60	83
Chest pain (%)	46	33	14	32	18
Sputum production (%)	74	87	75	62	80
Hemoptysis (%)	17	8	13	20	11
Chills (%)	58	35	42	53	50
Diarrhea (%)	4	5	21	20	5
Abdominal pain (%)	4	16	17	0	11
Viral prodrome (%)	27	39	29	37	35
Physical signs					
Temperature $\geq 40°C$ (%)	6	5	21	5	0
Mental changes (%)	15	13	22	38	23.8
Hypotension (%)	11	18	17	18	14.3
Consolidation (%)	35	21	33	32	15.0
Laboratory data					
Na <131 mEq/liter (%)	13	10	17	18	14
SGOT mean, Units/liter	35.8	24.8	31.8	37.7	24.94
SGPT mean, Units/liter	27.1	37.0	20.4	27.4	18.47
WBC mean x $1000/mm^3$	15.6	13.2	13.6	15.6	12.4
Creatinine mean, mg/dl	1.2	1.6	1.4	1.3	1.7
BUN mean, mg/dl	19.9	21.0	21.3	22.4	24.0
Po_2 mean, mm Hg	55.7	64.3	63.0	59.6	61.5
Prognostic factors and mortality					
Respiratory support (%)	11	8	17	5	10
ICU admission (%)	16	15	25	14	10
Mortality (%)	9	5	17	5	14

[a] Adapted from Fang GD, Fine M, Orlott J, et al. New and emerging etiologies for community-acquired pneumonia with implications fo therapy. A prospective multicenter study of 359 cases. Medicine (Baltimore) 1990; 69:307–316.
[b] Immunosuppression defined as solid tumor, hematologic malignancy, neutropenia or steroid treatment.

radiographies. Atypical pneumonia is said to be less serious and these patients have a better prognosis than those with bacterial pneumonias. In fact, when these findings, which are considered classical for atypical pneumonias, were compared to observations made in patients with proven viral, *M. pneumoniae*, and *C. pneumoniae* infections and in patients with known bacterial pneumonia, they were essentially nonspecific (Table 32.3) (26). Therefore, it is probably unlikely that this classification will offer sufficient specificity on which to base the selection of treatment.

RADIOLOGIC EXAMINATION

The chest film may show different radiographic characteristics that can be useful in management decisions. However, it is unusual that the pattern of infiltrate will indicate an etiology. Although a long list of pattern-etiology associations has been developed, there are as many exceptions as there are examples of conformity to the rules. It must be also recognized that chest films are only helpful in conjunction with the clinical history and physical examination.

Three principal radiographic patterns are usually delineated. The first one, air space or alveolar ("lobar") pneumonia, is characteristic of pneumococcal infection but can also occur with other organisms, such as *K. pneumoniae* (Fig. 32.1). It appears as a homogeneous consolidation that is relatively sharply demarcated from adjacent uninvolved parenchyma. The lack of respect for segmental boundaries is of major importance in differentiating between acute air space pneumonia and bronchopneumonia. Contrary to the implication of the

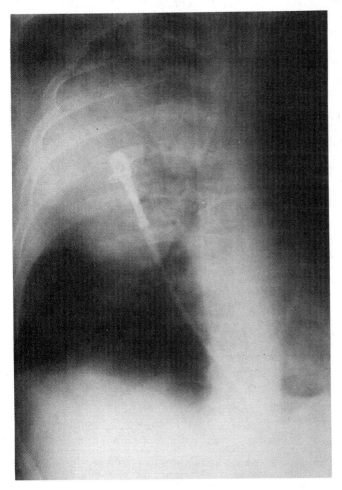

Figure 32.1. Acute air space pneumonia due to *S. pneumoniae*. A detailed view of the right lung from a posteroanterior chest radiography discloses massive air space consolidation in the axillary portion of the right upper lobe. The irregular margin of the lesion superomedially and air bronchograms define the more typical signs of an air space lesion.

common term lobar pneumonia, only rarely is a complete lobe consolidated. The larger bronchi usually remain patent and air-containing, thus creating an air bronchogram. Most frequently, the disease is confined to one lobe, but the infection may develop simultaneously in two or more lobes.

The second pattern corresponds to bronchopneumonia (lobular pneumonia) as exemplified by *S. aureus* infection (Fig. 32.2). Since the pathogenesis of this type of infection is related to the bronchial tree, resultant parenchymal consolidation is typically segmental in distribution. Depending on the severity of involvement, the process may be patchy or more homogeneous. The disease is frequently bilateral. Abscess formation with subsequent communication with the bronchial tree and the appearance of fluid-containing cavities occurs in 25–75% of the patients with *S. aureus* pneumonia (91). As in children, the cavity may become enlarged, resulting in the development of thin-walled pneumatoceles. Although pneumatoceles are characteristic of staph-

ylococcal infection, they may be seen in pneumonias of other etiologies, including *K. pneumoniae, H. influenzae, S. pneumoniae,* and more rarely, *P. carinii* (21, 53). Pulmonary infections due to Pseudomonas and aspiration pneumonia also have a marked tendency toward cavitation and empyema (77).

Interstitial pneumonia (Figure 32.3) usually caused by viruses, and *M. pneumoniae* are anatomically characterized by edema and an inflammatory cellular infiltrate situated predominantly within interstitial lung tissue. Subsequent involvement may include terminal bronchioles and adjacent alveoli. Therefore, the radiographic patterns are varied; diffuse and localized involvement with both interstitial and alveolar patterns have been noted (19).

Studies have been done to discover whether radiographic patterns can distinguish between the various causes of pneumonia (55, 86). A panel of six radiologists who had no prior knowledge of the clinical data were only 67% accurate in the identification of 16 bacterial pneumonias and

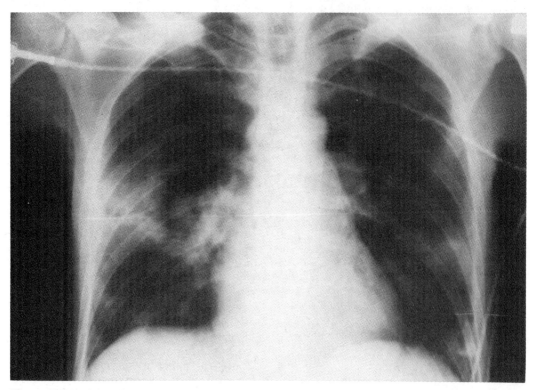

Figure 32.2. Acute bronchopneumonia due to *S. aureus*. The chest radiography discloses several areas of inhomogeneous consolidation in both lungs; some are excavated with thin walls.

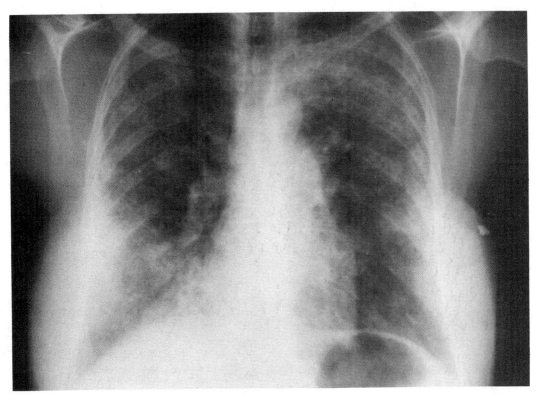

Figure 32.3. Acute interstitial and air space pneumonia due to *M. pneumoniae*. The chest radiography discloses bilateral interstitial and alveolar infiltrates.

65% correct in 9 cases of viral etiology; moreover, no consistent pattern was identified in any specific group of pneumonia (86). In a comparative study of the radiographic features of community-acquired legionnaires' disease, pneumococcal pneumonia, mycoplasmal pneumonia, and acute psittacosis, investigators found that homogeneous opacities (air-space disease) were more frequent in legionnaires' disease and pneumococcal infection than in mycoplasmal pneumonia (55). In both of these studies, the pattern of mycoplasmal pneumonia could be confused with air-space bacterial pneumonia in at least 50% of the cases (55, 86).

NONINVASIVE BACTERIOLOGIC DIAGNOSTIC TECHNIQUES

Sputum Examination

Microscopic examination and culture of expectorated sputum remain the mainstays of the laboratory evaluation of patients with community-acquired pneumonia, despite ongoing controversy concerning their sensitivity and specificity. These procedures are noninvasive and, while sputum culture requires 24–48 hrs, Gram staining can give valuable information in a matter of minutes, provided certain guidelines and precautions are followed. The first and most important of these guidelines is to obtain a proper specimen. Therefore, the patient should be carefully instructed and supervised by a physician or a respiratory therapist to obtain secretions resulting from a deep cough. The patient should be told specifically that nasopharyngeal secretions and saliva are not adequate. Seriously ill and debilitated patients are often unable to follow instructions and should be particularly helped. Although most patients with pneumonia have a productive cough, some may require aerosol induction of sputum with hypertonic saline, as described for AIDS patients with *P. carinii* infection. One alternative for some patients unable to expectorate anything other than oropharyngeal secretions is to blindly pass a small catheter through the upper respiratory tract into the trachea to directly sample distal secretions. As a general rule, sputum specimens should be transported promptly to the laboratory for processing. Transportation delays for 2–5 hr at room temperature result in reduced isolation rates of pneumococci, staphylococci, and Gram-negative bacilli, and increased number of microorganisms that are indigenous to the upper respiratory tract (43).

In all cases of acute pneumonia and, when possible, prior to the initiation of antibiotics, a Gram stain of sputum should be prepared. In order to maximize the diagnostic yield of the sputum examination, only samples free of oropharyngeal contamination should be reviewed. Various criteria based on cytologic characteristics have been suggested for scoring the quality of sputum specimens (7, 68). In a study in which parallel cytologic and microbiologic analyses of sputa and transtracheal aspirates from patients with pneumonia were performed, Geckler et al. (32) found that the results of sputum culture containing >25 squamous epithelial cells per low-power field (magnification ×100) showed poor agreement with those of transtracheal aspiration, regardless of the number of leukocytes that were present. Such samples are therefore nondiagnostic and should be discarded. On the other hand, the presence of <10 epithelial cells and >25 leukocytes per field suggests that the specimen actually represents lower respiratory tract secretions (68). Unfortunately, in a study conducted at the Mayo Clinic, only 25% of the sputum specimens submitted to the clinical microbiology laboratory fit these criteria, underlining the difficulty encountered in obtaining a good-quality sputum specimen (68).

Gram-stained smears of acceptable specimens should then be examined under oil immersion (magnification ×1000) to determine whether bacteria of a specific or characteristic morphologic type are present. Neither the fields being examined nor any of the immediately adjacent fields should contain any squamous epithelial cells, but at least several neutrophils or alveolar macrophages should be present. The morphologic and staining characteristics of any bacteria should be recorded and a semiquantitative estimate of their number should be made. This method has proved useful for the identification of *S. pneumoniae* in the sputum. Rein et al. (74) have suggested that when strict criteria for Gram-stain positivity are used (predominant flora or >10 Gram-positive, lancet-shaped diplococci per oil immersion field), the specificity of the technique is 85% with a sensitivity of 62%. Whether this approach is equally useful for the identification of other bacterial causes of pneumonia remains unclear. However, Tillotson and Lerner (88) noted that Gram-negative bacilli were seen in smears of all sputum specimens taken from 20 cases of *E. coli* pneumonia. Small Gram-negative coccobacillary organisms are characteristic of *H. influenzae*. Staphylococci appear as Gram-positive cocci in tetrads and small clusters. Gram-stained smears may also support a diagnosis of atypical pneumonia or legionnaires' disease when sputum examinations repeatedly show no bacteria in a patient who has received no antimicrobial treatment prior to admission.

A variety of diagnostic techniques have recently been developed that provide the potential for more accurate and rapid identification of the etiologic agents of pneumonia by sputum analysis. The most frequent application of direct immunofluorescence to the examination of sputum is in the detection of *Legionella* species. Using positive cultures or antibody titers to define legionnaires' disease, Edelstein et al. (24) found that the sensitivity of direct immunofluorescence of respiratory tract secretions was 50% with a specificity of 94%. Direct immunofluorescence and genetic probes may also be used to detect chlamydial species, *M. tuberculosis*, and some viruses. While many of these techniques are of great interest, their general applicability remains to be determined.

The utility of sputum cultures as a means of establishing the agents responsible for pneumonia has been questioned. Patients with bacteremic pneumococcal pneumonia have been reported to have negative sputum cultures in 45%–50% of the cases, even when large numbers of organisms have been noted on Gram-stained preparations (6). Similarly, 34–47% of sputum cultures are negative with proven *H. influenzae* pneumonia (49, 92). Furthermore, cultures of expectorated sputum often yield multiple organisms and it is difficult to tell whether these bacteria are causative or are merely colonizing the upper respiratory tract. For example, contamination with Gram-negative bacilli has been noted in 32% of sputum cultures (45). Semiquantitative cultures, washing of sputum samples, and the use of mucolytic agents have been proposed to improve the clinical utility of sputum cultures; however, results have been variable and the practicality of these techniques for routine use is questionable. In fact, the main role of sputum cultures in clinical practice is to permit definitive identification of the organisms that are present in predominance in the Gram-stained smear and to determine their susceptibility to antibiotics. In other words, results of sputum cultures should always be used as a function of the results of the Gram-staining.

Other Noninvasive Diagnostic Techniques

Approximately 20–30% of the patients with bacterial pneumonia are bacteremic and therefore blood cultures should not be overlooked as a means of identifying the bacterial etiology of pneumonia (22). Pleural fluid cultures, when positive, are also specific for the etiology of the underlying pneumonia.

Counterimmunoelectrophoresis and latex agglutination techniques have been used to detect *S. pneumoniae*, *H. influenzae*, and *Pseudomonas* antigens in urine, serum, and pleural fluid, but results have been variable and frequently disappointing. For example, detection of the pneumococcal capsular antigen by counterimmunoelectrophoresis has been reported to have a sensitivity varying from 20–90% with 8–20% of false-positive results (59, 70).

Serologic tests are used to diagnose a variety of pulmonary pathogens including *Legionella* species, *M. pneumoniae*, *Chlamydia* spp., and many viruses. Since these tests usually require two blood specimens drawn at a minimum of a 2-week interval, they are of help only in confirming a clinical diagnosis, not for initiating treatment.

INVASIVE DIAGNOSTIC TECHNIQUES

Transtracheal Aspiration

Transtracheal aspiration was originally discribed by Pecora and Yeagin (69) in 1959 as a means to obtain specimens from the lower respiratory tract that are free of contamination by the normal flora present in the upper airways. When done correctly and in the proper clinical setting, transtracheal aspiration has been shown to be safe and more reliable than expectorated sputum cultures. The theoretical basis for transtracheal aspiration is that the oropharyngeal flora stops abruptly at the level of the larynx and, therefore, that samples obtained from the subglottic trachea reflect the bacteria present in the pulmonary parenchyma. The most extensive study of the diagnostic accuracy of transtracheal aspiration for diagnosing bacterial pneumonia involved 488 patients, including 383 who satisfied clinical criteria for bacterial pneumonia (Table 32.4) (8). Likely pulmonary pathogens were recovered from 335 of the 383 patients with pneumonia (sensitivity 87%), but 44 of the 48 false-negative cultures were from patients who had received antimicrobial treatment prior to the procedure. Restricting analysis to untreated patients, the incidence of false-negative cultures was only 1%. The diagnostic accuracy of the procedure in that study was further documented by showing that the same organism recovered from blood cultures in 23 pneumonia patients with bacteremia was also present in the companion transtracheal aspiration specimen. A false-positive rate of approximately 21% was, however, noted due to oropharyngeal contamination of the specimen or presence of subglottic colonization, especially in patients with chronic obstructive lung disease or lung carcinoma. Analogous results have been reported by numerous other investigators (38, 45, 76).

Table 32.4
Correlation Between 488 Cultures of Transtracheal Aspirates and Clinical Diagnoses[a]

Culture Findings	No.
Pulmonary pathogen	369
Bacterial pneumonia[b]	335
Exacerbation of chronic bronchitis	16
No clinical evidence of bacterial infection	18
No pulmonary pathogen	119
No bacterial pneumonia	71
Bacterial pneumonia	48
Antimicrobial drugs given prior to transtracheal aspiration	44
No prior antimicrobial treatment	4

[a]Adapted from Bartlett JG. Diagnostic accuracy for transtracheal aspiration bacteriologic studies. Am Rev Respir Dis 1977;115:777–782.
[b]As defined by the three following criteria: *(a)* fever, *(b)* pulmonary infiltrate on chest radiograph, and *(c)* clinical response with radiographic clearing after treatment with antimicrobial drugs or an autopsy diagnosis of bacterial pneumonia.

Transtracheal aspiration should not be performed in patients with significant hemostatic abnormalities, especially thrombocythemia, in patients with severe hypoxemia or uncontrolled hemodynamic status, and when the anatomic landmarks are not easily located. Caution should also be taken in patients with uncontrollable cough and in patients who cannot or will not cooperate (45, 73). The transtracheal aspiration method is not without risk, even if the overall incidence of serious complications in several large series of patients appears to be low and a review of the reports of fatal complications shows that most of these patients had factors contraindicating the procedure (73). Complications at the needle puncture site include bleeding, puncture of the posterior tracheal wall, cutaneous or paratracheal abscess, and subcutaneous emphysema that may spread to the face, mediastinum, or cause a pneumothorax. Catheter placement in the lower airways may produce severe cough paroxysm, precipitate severe hypoxemia with acute respiratory failure, or cause severe cardiac arrhythmias, hypotension, or myocardial ischemia. A few cardiorespiratory arrests have been also reported (73, 81).

It is difficult to describe specific indications for transtracheal aspiration in patients with community-acquired pneumonia. A general guideline is that this technique is best justified in clinical situations where: *(a)* bacterial pathogens are suspected, *(b)* alternative specimens using less invasive techniques are inconclusive or not available, *(c)* the severity of the illness justifies the risk incurred, *(d)* technical expertise is available, *(e)* patient's contraindications do not apply, *(f)* fiberoptic bronchoscopy is not justified, and *(g)* no prior antimicrobial treatment was administered to the patient (8). Settings that appear to satisfy these guidelines probably include some patients with severe underlying disease in whom multiple etiologic possibilities are often considered and some patients with severe necrotizing pneumonia.

Fiberoptic Bronchoscopy

Flexible fiberoptic bronchoscopy is a safe, common, easily performed procedure that is well tolerated by most patients. It not only enables direct visualization of the endobronchial tree but also affords an opportunity to obtain specimens for culture and histology by various techniques directly from the site of inflammation in the lung. Initial studies concerning the reliability of specimens obtained for culture directly by suction through the inner channel have been disappointing. Bartlett et al. (11) demonstrated that, in patients without lower respiratory tract infections, cultures of aspirates obtained during bronchoscopy were frequently contaminated, producing an average of five different bacterial species. Therefore, this type of specimen collection has the same potential drawbacks as those observed with expectorated sputum, thus stressing the importance of examining a Gram-stained preparation of bronchoscopic secretions before interpreting the results of such cultures (29).

The development of the protected specimen brush technique by Wimberley et al. (95) has significantly decreased, but not eliminated, this problem. This technique uses a double-catheter system with two telescoping cannulas, a distal occluding plug, and a small brush that calibrates the volume of respiratory secretions collected. Using $\geq 10^3$ colony-forming units (CFU)/ml as a "breakpoint" on quantitative cultures for the determination of the clinical significance of an isolate, the protected specimen brush has been proven experimentally and clinically to be both sensitive (70–97%) and specific (95–100%) for the diagnosis of bacterial pneumonia (8, 17, 66, 71, 94, 95). For example, in a study on 172 patients, Pollock et al. (71) found that 75 of 78 patients (96%) with a clinical diagnosis of pneumonia had a likely pulmonary pathogen in significant concentration, whereas high counts were recovered in only 2 of 35 control patients (Table 32.5). As with other techniques, however, specimens obtained from patients with pneumonia who had received prior antibiotic treatment were frequently negative, emphasizing the fact that previous treatment negates to a large extent the potential utility of this method (98).

Bronchoalveolar lavage, in which a segment of lung is "washed" with sterile saline, has proved to be an excellent means of diagnosing respiratory infections. Lavage is indeed a safe and practical method for obtaining cells and secretions from the lower respiratory tract. This technique samples a relatively large area of the lung (about 10^6 alveoli). The cells and liquid recovered can be examined microscopically immediately after the procedure and are also suitable for culture and other techniques. Bronchoalveolar lavage is therefore now the procedure of choice for diagnosing opportunistic pulmonary infections in immunosuppressed patients (16, 83). In patients with AIDS, the sensitivity of the procedure for detecting *P. carinii* and cytomegalovirus pneumonia ranges from 89–98% (16). By using immunofluorescent monoclonal antibodies to viral antigens and rapid culture technique, the diagnosis of cytomegalovirus pneumonia may be made within hours (20). Bronchoalveolar lavage may be also useful for detecting other pathogens (fungi, mycobacteria, *Toxoplasma gondii*, *Nocardia*), even if its accuracy has not been thoroughly evaluated in these infections. Generally, bronchoscopy yields better diagnostic results in immunosuppressed patients when several techniques are applied, including bronchoalveolar lavage, protected specimen brush, sampling, and transbronchial biopsies (16).

Cytologic screening and microbiologic quantitation of bronchoalveolar lavage fluid may also enable the detection of conventional bacteria (Figure 32.4). Thorpe et al.

Table 32.5
Results of Quantitative Cultures of Specimens Obtained with a Protected Specimen Brush in 78 Patients with Bacterial Infection of the Lower Airways and in 35 Control Patients[a]

Patient Category	No. of Patients with Bacterial Counts (CFU/ml) of	
	$\geq 10^3$	$< 10^3$
Lower respiratory tract infection		
Pneumonia	75	3
Acute bronchitis	11	0
Controls (no infection)	2	33

[a] Adapted from Pollock HM, Hawkins EL, Bonner JR, et al. Diagnosis of bacterial pulmonary infections with quantitative protected catheter cultures obtained during bronchoscopy. J Clin Microbiol 1983;17:255–259.

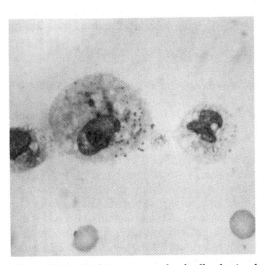

Figure 32.4 Light micrograph of cells obtained from a patient with pneumonia due to *S. pneumoniae*. Most alveolar macrophages and neutrophils contain numerous oval or lancet-shaped diplococci. (Diff Quik stain, original magnification × 1000)

(87) performed bronchoalveolar lavage with the bronchoscope introduced either transnasally or through an endotracheal tube in a heterogeneous group of 92 hospitalized patients, 15 of whom were thought to have active bacterial pneumonia. Thirteen of the 15 patients with clinically active bacterial pneumonia had a bronchoalveolar lavage culture of $>10^5$ CFU/ml of bronchoalveolar lavage fluid, whereas none of the other patients, including those with resolving pneumonia or chronic bronchitis, had counts of $>10^4$ CFU/ml. Furthermore, Gram-staining of cytocentrifuged bronchoalveolar lavage fluid was positive (one or more organisms seen per $1000 \times$ field) only in those patients with active bacterial pneumonia. In a similar study, Kahn and Jones (44) evaluated 75 patients (most of whom were immunocompromised) by fiberoptic bronchoscopy and bronchoalveolar lavage for the presence of lower respiratory tract bacterial infection. In 18 "control" patients without evidence of respiratory infection, the presence of $>1\%$ squamous epithelial cells in the bronchoalveolar lavage sample accurately predicted the presence of heavy contamination of the sample by oropharyngeal flora. In the remaining patients with possible infections, potential pathogens were recovered at concentrations of $>10^5$ CFU/ml in 16 of 18 patients with bacterial infections (none has $>1\%$ squamous epithelial cells in their bronchoalveolar lavage sample). No patient without evidence of bacterial infection and with $<1\%$ of squamous epithelial cells had $>10^5$ CFU/ml in bronchoalveolar lavage cultures, but contamination of the lavage fluid occurred in a relatively large number (26%) of patients.

Fiberoptic bronchoscopy is regarded as a relatively safe technique with few serious complications. Postbronchoscopy fever with increasing infiltrates may be observed. There is also a 10–20 mm Hg decrease in Pao_2, which could pose a problem for some patients with severe hypoxemia. The use of supplemental oxygen with a nonrebreather mask and an F_{IO_2} of 100% has been stressed in this setting. Pneumothorax may follow transbronchial biopsy or the use of a protected specimen brush (60).

Transthoracic Needle Aspiration

Percutaneous transthoracic needle aspiration enables collection of uncontaminated specimens directly from the pulmonary parenchyma for cytologic and microbiologic analyses. The use of smaller (ultrathin) gauge needle has reduced the frequency of pneumothorax as a complication (89). Problems with the procedure include a relatively high rate of false-negative cultures and potentially serious complications in patients with severe underlying disease (10). This technique may be particularly attractive in children, since respiratory secretions may be difficult to obtain and transtracheal aspiration is infrequently performed (10).

Open Lung Biopsy

Open lung biopsy remains the definitive invasive procedure for making an etiologic diagnosis of pneumonia in immunosuppressed patients. The diagnostic yield in this setting ranges from 55–91% and averages about 60% (18, 61, 62, 82). Even if the overall complication rate of open lung biopsy is probably low (11% in six combined series of patients), this procedure should probably be performed only after fiberoptic bronchoscopy combined with transbronchial biopsy and segmental bronchoalveolar lavage fails to provide a diagnosis (60). Even in this situation, some have questioned whether open lung biopsy provides meaningful information that significantly affects the patient's clinical outcome (61, 62).

TREATMENT

Initial therapy of community-acquired pneumonia is based on the clues provided by clinical, epidemiologic, and radiologic information and by evaluation of stained sputum smears. In the case of a presumed bacterial pneumonia in which an etiologic agent is identified on the Gram-stained sputum smear, selection of an appropriate therapy is relatively straightforward (Table 32.6).

When the clinician is confronted with no sputum or with a poor-quality sputum specimen, or when the patient has already

Table 32.6
Selection of Initial Antimicrobial Treatment in Adult Patients with Community-Acquired Pneumonia Based on Results of a Gram-Stained Sputum Smear[a]

Morphologic and Staining Characteristics of Predominant Bacteria	Suspected Pathogen	Presumptive Therapy
Gram-positive, oval, or lancet-shaped diplococci	*S. pneumoniae*	Penicillin G
Small pleomorphic Gram-negative coccobacilli	*H. influenzae*	Amoxycillin/clavulanic acid
Gram-negative, biscuit-shaped diplococci	*M. catarrhalis*	Amoxycillin/clavulanic acid
Large Gram-positive cocci in tetrads or clusters	*S. aureus*	Nafcillin plus aminoglycoside
Large Gram-negative encapsulated bacilli	*K. pneumoniae*	Third-generation cephalosporin plus aminoglycoside
Gram-negative rods	Enterobacteriaceae or other Gram-negative bacilli	Third-generation cephalosporin plus aminoglycoside
No bacteria[b]	*L. pneumophila* *C. pneumoniae* *M. pneumoniae*	IV Erythromycin

[a]Only Gram-stained smears containing ≤10 epithelial cells and ≥25 neutrophils under low-power magnification ($\times$100) should be considered.
[b]In patients who have not received prior antimicrobial treatment.

received prior antimicrobial treatment, the choice of antibiotics becomes more difficult. One option would be to perform an invasive diagnostic procedure, such as transtracheal aspiration or fiberoptic bronchoscopy with bronchoalveolar lavage or protected specimen brush. However, for an uncomplicated case of community-acquired pneumonia or for an uncooperative patient (e.g., an agitated hypoxemic patient or a combative alcoholic), it is unlikely that invasive techniques will be needed or feasible. In these cases, empiric therapy should be designed to treat the most likely or the most potentially lethal possibilities. Since detailed analysis of a large series of patients revealed that the clinical manifestations of community-acquired pneumonia are rarely specific for various microbial agents and that the popular classification scheme differentiating "atypical" pneumonia from "bacterial" illness does not withstand the rigor of statistical analysis, therapy in seriously ill patients should include coverage for *S. pneumoniae, H. influenzae, L. pneumophila, C. pneumoniae*, as well as *S. aureus* and Gram-negative rods in some cases. Selec-

tion of antibiotics should also take into account the possibility of ampicillin-resistant *H. influenzae*, unless it is known that no such resistant organisms have been isolated from the community. While the newer β-lactam agents, including the extended-spectrum penicillins and cephalosporins, are often applied as empiric therapy in this setting (34), these agents are ineffective against *Legionella* spp. and *C. pneumoniae*, two of the most common etiologies. Therefore, a more appropriate choice, in our opinion, would be the association of amoxycillin/clavulanic acid with erythromycin or with a new quinolone such as ciprofloxacin.

In patients with a milder illness, no history of cigarette abuse, and no severe underlying disease, empiric use of erythromycin as the sole treatment may be strongly considered. This agent will provide adequate therapy against the pneumococcus as well as against *M. pneumoniae, C. pneumoniae*, and *Legionella* spp. While experience is limited with erythromycin in the treatment of *H. influenzae*, the organism is generally sensitive in vitro. This policy will minimize overprescription of expensive broad-spectrum agents, while maximizing the use of established agents for specific pathogens.

Acknowledgments. The authors wish to thank Catherine Brun for her invaluable help in the preparation of the manuscript.

References

1. Anonymous. Statistical abstract of the US. 108th ed. Washington, DC: US Dept of Commerce, Bureau of the Census, 1988.
2. Applebaum PC. Worldwide development of antibiotic resistance in pneumococci. Eur J Clin Microbiol 1987;6:367–377.
3. Ashworth M, Ross G, Loehry C. Lobar pneumonia caused by *Haemophilus influenzae* type B. Br J Dis Chest. 1985;79:95–97.
4. Aubertin J, Dabis F, Fleurette J, et al. Prevalence of legionellosis among adults: a study of community-acquired pneumonia in France. Infection 1987;15:328–331.
5. Austrian R, Gold J. Pneumococcal bacteremia with special reference to bacteremic pneumococcal pneumonia. Ann Intern Med 1964;60:759–776.
6. Barrett-Connor E. The non-value of sputum culture in the diagnosis of pneumococcal pneumonia. Am Rev Respir Dis 1971;103:845–848.
7. Bartlett RC. Medical microbiology: quality cost and clinical relevance. New York: John Wiley Sons, 1974:27–36.
8. Bartlett JG. Diagnostic accuracy of transtracheal aspiration bacteriologic studies. Am Rev Respir Dis 1977; 115:777–782.
9. Bartlett JG. Anaerobic bacterial infections of the lung. Chest 1987;91:901–909.
10. Bartlett JG. Invasive diagnostic techniques in respiratory infections. In: Pennington JE, ed. Respiratory infections: diagnosis and management. New York: Raven Press, 1989:69–96.
11. Bartlett JG, Alexander J, Mayhew J, et al. Should fiberoptic bronchoscopic aspirates be cultured? Am Rev Respir Dis 1976;114:73–78.
12. Bath JC, JL, Boissard GPB, Calder M, Moffat M. Pneumonia in hospital practice in Edinburgh, 1960–1962. Br J Dis Chest 1964;58:1–16.
13. Beaman BL, Burnside J, Edwards B, Causey W. Nocardial infections in the United States, 1972–1974. J Infect Dis 1976;134:286–292.
14. Berntsson E, Blomberg J, Lagergard T, Trollters B. Etiology of community-acquired pneumonia in patients requiring hospitalization. Eur J Clin Microbiol 1988;4:268–272.
15. Bobrowitz ID. Active tuberculosis undiagnosed until autopsy. Am J Med 1982;72:650–686.
16. Broaddus C, Dake MD, Stalburg MS, et al. Bronchoalveolar lavage and transbronchial biopsy for the diagnosis of pulmonary infections in the acquired immune deficiency syndrome. Ann Intern Med 1986;102:747–752.
17. Chastre J, Viau F, Brun P, et al. Prospective evaluation of the protected specimen brush for the diagnosis of pulmonary infections in ventilated patients. Am Rev Respir Dis 1984;130:924–929.
18. Cockerill FR III, Wilson WR, Carpenter HA, et al. Open lung biopsy in immunocompromised patients. Arch Intern Med 1985; 145:1398–1404.
19. Conte P, Heitzman ER, Markarian B. Viral pneumonia. Roentgen pathological correlations. Radiology 1970;95:267–272.
20. Crawford SW, Bowden RA, Hackman RC, et al. Rapid detection of cytomegalovirus pulmonary infection by bronchoalveolar lavage and centrifugation culture. Ann Intern Med 1988;108:180–185.
21. Dines DE. Diagnostic significance of pneumatoceles of the lung. JAMA 1968;204:1169–1172.
22. Donowitz GR, Mandell GL. Acute pneumonia. In: Mandell GL, Douglas RG Jr, Bennett JE, eds. Principles and Practice of Infectious Diseases. 3rd ed. New York: Churchill Livingstone, 1990:540–555.
23. Dorff G, Rytel M, Farmer S, Scanlon G. Etiologies and characteristic features of pneumonias in a municipal hospital. Am J Med Sci 1973;266:349–358.
24. Edelstein PH, Meyer RD, Finegold SM. Laboratory diagnosis of Legionnaires' disease. Am Rev Respir Dis 1980;121:317–327.
25. England AC, Fraser DW, Plikaytis DB, et al. Sporatic legionellosis in the United States: the first thousand cases. Ann Intern Med 1981;84:164–168.
26. Fang GD, Fine M, Orlott J, et al. New and emerging etiologies for community-acquired pneumonia with implications for therapy. A prospective multicenter study of 359 cases. Medicine (Baltimore) 1990;69:307–316.
27. Fekety FR Jr. The epidemiology and prevention of staphylococcal infection. Medicine (Baltimore) 1964;43:593–601.
28. Fekety FR, Caldwell J, Gump D, et al. Bacteria, viruses, and mycoplasmas in acute pneumonia in adults. Am Rev Respir Dis 1971;104:499–507.
29. Flataver FE, Chabalko JJ, Wolinski E. Fiberoptic bronchoscopy in bacteriologic assessment of lower respiratory tract secretions. JAMA 1980;244:2427–2429.
30. Foy HM, Kenny GE, Cooney MK, Allan ID. Long term epidemiology of infections with *Mycoplasma pneumoniae*. J Infect Dis 1979;139:681–685.
31. Fragier AR, Rusenow EC III, Roberts GD. Nocardiosis. A review of 25 cases occurring during 24 months. Mayo Clin Proc 1975;50:657–663.
32. Geckler RW, Gremillon DH, McAllister CK, Ellenbogen C. Microscopic and bacteriological comparison of paired sputa and transtracheal aspirates. J Clin Microbiol 1977;6:396–399.
33. Goodwin RA, Lloyd JE, DesPrez RM. Histoplasmosis in normal hosts. Medicine (Baltimore) 1981;60:231–266.
34. Grasela TH, Timm E, Welage L. A nationwide survey of antibiotic utilization in bacterial pneumonia [Abstract]. Los Angeles: Twenty-eighth Intersci Conf Antimicrob Agents Chemother. 1988;761.
35. Grayston JT, Kuo CC, Wang SP, Altman J. A new *Chlamydia psittaci* strain called TWAR from acute respiratory tract infections. N Engl J Med 1986;315:161–168.

36. Grayston JT, Wang SP, Kuo CC, Campbell LA. Current knowledge of *Chlamydia pneumoniae* strain TWAR, an important cause of pneumonia. Eur J Clin Microbiol Infect Dis 1989;8:191–202.

37. Green G. In defense of the lung. Am Rev Respir Dis 1970;102:691–703.

38. Hahn HH, Beaty HN. Transtracheal aspiration in the evaluation of patients with pneumonia. Ann Intern Med 1970;72:183–187.

39. Holmberg H. Aetiology of community-acquired pneumonia in hospital patients. Scand J Infect Dis 1987;19:491–501.

40. Hook EW III, Horton CA, Schaberg DR. Failure of intensive care unit support to influence mortality from pneumococcal bacteremia. JAMA 1983;240:1055–1058.

41. Hunninghake GW, Gradek JE, Fales HM, Crystal RG. Human alveolar macrophage-derived chemotactic factor for neutrophils. J Clin Invest 1980;66:473–478.

42. Jacobs ER, Bone RC. Mediators of septic lung injury. Med Clin North Am 1983;62:701–714.

43. Jefferson H, Dalton HP, Escobar MR, Allison MJ. Transportation delay and the microbiological quality of clinical specimens. Am J Clin Pathol 1975;64:689–693.

44. Kahn FW, Jones JM. Diagnosing bacterial respiratory infection by bronchoalveolar lavage. J Infect Dis 1987;155:862–868.

45. Kalinske RW, Parker RH, Brandt D, et al. Diagnostic usefulness and safety of transtracheal aspiration. N Engl J Med 1967;276:604–608.

46. Khan MA, Kovnat DM, Bachus B, et al. Clinical and roentgenographic spectrum of pulmonary tuberculosis in the adult. Am J Med 1977;62:31–38.

47. Klimek JJ, Ajemian E, Fontecchio S, Gracewski J, Klemas B, Jiminez L. Community-acquired bacterial pneumonia requiring admission to hospital. Am J Infect Control 1983;11:79–82.

48. Koletsky RJ, Weinstein AJ. Fulminant *Mycoplasma pneumoniae* infection. Report of a fatal case, and a review of the literature. Am Rev Respir Dis 1980;122:491–493.

49. Levin D, Schwartz M, Matthay R. et al. Bacteremic *Haemophilus influenzae* pneumonia in adults. A report of 24 cases and review of the literature. Am J Med 1977;62:219–224.

50. Levy M, Dromer F, Brion N, Leturder F, Carbon C. Community-acquired pneumonia: importance of initial noninvasive bacteriologic and radiographic investigations. Chest 1988;92:43–48.

51. Lindsay MI Jr, Herrmann EC Jr, Morrow GW Jr, Brown AL Jr. Hong Kong influenza. Clinical, microbiologic, and pathologic features in 127 cases. JAMA 1970;214:1825–1829.

52. Lipsky BA, Boyko EJ, Invi TS, et al. Risk factors for acquiring pneumococcal infections. Arch Intern Med 1986;146:2179–2185.

53. Luddy RE, Champion LA, Schwartz AD. *Pneumocystis carinii* pneumonia with pneumatocele formation. Am J Dis Child. 1977;131:470.

54. MacFarlane JT, Finch RG, Ward MJ, Macrae AD. Hospital study of adult community-acquired pneumonia. Lancet 1982;2:255–258.

55. MacFarlane JT, Miller AC, Roderick-Smith WH, et al. Comparative radiographic features of community-acquired Legionnaires disease, pneumococcal pneumonia, mycoplasma pneumonia, and psittacosis. Thorax 1984;39;28–34.

56. Mafson MA, Oley G, Hughey D. Pneumococcal disease in a medium-sized community in the United States. JAMA 1982;248:1486–1489.

57. Marrie TJ, Grayston JT, Wang SP, Kwo CC. Pneumonia associated with the TWAR strain of *Chlamydia*. Ann Intern Med 1987;106:507–511.

58. Marrie TJ, Haldane EV, Faulkner R, Durant H, Kwan C. Community-acquired pneumonia requiring hospitalization. Is it different in the elderly? J Am Geriatr Soc 1985;33:671–680.

59. Martin CM, Kunin C, Gottlieb LS, et al. Asian influenza A in Boston, 1957–1958. II. Severe staphylococcal pneumonia complicating influenza. Arch Intern Med 1959;103:532–542.

60. Matthay RA, Moritz ED. Invasive procedures for diagnosing pulmonary infection. A critical review. Clin Chest Med 1981;2:3–18.

61. McCabe RE, Brooks RG, Mark JBD, et al. Open lung biopsy in patients with acute leukemia. Am J Med 1985;78:609–616.

62. McKenna RJ, Mountain CF, McMurtrey MJ. Open lung biopsy in immunocompromised patients. Chest 1984;86:671–674.

63. Meyer RD, Edelstein PH, Kirby BD, et al. Legionnaires' disease: unusual clinical and laboratory features. Ann Intern Med 1980;93:240–245.

64. Moffet HL. Common infections in ambulatory patients. Ann Intern Med. 1978;89:743–746.

65. Moore M, Merson M, Charache P, Shepard R. The characteristics and mortality of out patient-acquired pneumonia. Johns Hopkins Med J 1977;140:9–14.

66. Moser KM, Maurer J, Jassy L, et al. Sensitivity, specificity and risk of diagnostic procedures in a canine model of *Streptococcus pneumoniae* pneumonia. Am Rev Respir Dis 1982;125:436–442.

67. Moxon ER. Haemophilus influenzae. In: Mandell GL, Douglas RG Jr, Bennet JE, eds. Principles and practice of infectious diseases. 3rd ed. New York: Churchill Livingstone, 1990:1722–1729.

68. Murray PR, Washington JA II. Microscopic and bacteriologic analysis of expectorated sputum. Mayo Clin Proc 1975;50:339–344.

69. Pecora DV, Yeagin D. Bacteriology of lower respiratory tract in health and chronic disease. N Engl J Med 1958;258:71–74.

70. Perlino CA. Laboratory diagnosis and pneumonia due to *Streptococcus pneumoniae*. J Infect Dis 1985;150:139–144.

71. Pollock HM, Hawkins EL, Bonner JR, et al. Diagnosis of bacterial pulmonary infections with quantitative protected catheter cultures obtained during bronchoscopy. J Clin Microbiol 1983;17:255–259.

72. Ponka A. Clinical and laboratory manifestations in patients with serological evidence of *Mycoplasma pneumoniae* infection. Scand J Infect Dis 1978;10:271–280.

73. Pratter MR, Irwin RS. Transtracheal aspiration: guidelines for safety. Chest 1979;76:518–520.

74. Rein MF, Gwaltney JM Jr, O'Brien WM, Jennings RH, Mandell GL. Accuracy of Gram's stain in

identifying pneumococci in sputum. JAMA 1978;239:2671–2673.

75. Research Committee of the British Thoracic Society and the Public Health Laboratory Service. Community-acquired pneumonia in adults in British hospitals in 1982–1983: a survey of aetiology, mortality, prognostic factors and outcome. Q J Med 1987;239:195–220.

76. Ries K, Lewison ME, Kaye D. Transtracheal aspiration in pulmonary infection. Arch Intern Med 1974;133:453–458.

77. Scanlon GT, Unger JD. The radiology of bacterial and viral pneumonias. Radiol Clin North Am 1973;11:317–338.

78. Schwarzmann SW, Adler JL, Sullivan RJ, et al. Bacterial pneumonia during the Hong Kong influenza epidemic of 1968–1969. Experience in a city-county hospital. Arch Intern Med 1971; 127:1037–1041.

79. Shlaes DM, Mandell R, Bass S, et al. Bacteremia caused by *Streptococcus pneumoniae* of non-vaccine serotypes. Am Rev Respir Dis 1982;126:712–716.

80. Slevin NJ, Aitken J, Thornleg PE. Clinical and microbiological features of *Branhamella catarrhalis* bronchopulmonary infections. Lancet 1987;1:782–783.

81. Spencer CD, Beaty HN. Complications of transtracheal aspiration. N Engl J Med 1972;286:304–306.

82. Springmeyer SC, Silvestri RC, Sale GE, et al. The role of transbronchial biopsy for the diagnosis of diffuse pneumonias in immunocompromised marrow transplant recipients. Am Rev Respir Dis 1982;116:763–765.

83. Stover DE, Zaman MB, Hajdin SI, et al. Bronchoalveolar lavage in the diagnosis of diffuse pulmonary infiltrates in the immunosuppressed host. Ann Intern Med 1984;101:1–7.

84. Stratton CW. Bacterial pneumonia. An overview with emphasis on pathogenesis, diagnosis and treatment. Heart Lung 1986;15:226–244.

85. Sullivan R, Dowdle WR, Marine W, Hierholzer JC. Adult pneumonia in a general hospital. Arch Intern Med 1972;129:935–942.

86. Tew J, Calenoff L, Berlin BS. Bacterial or non-bacterial pneumonia: accuracy of radiographic diagnosis. Radiology 1977;124:607–612.

87. Thorpe JE, Baughman RP, Frame PT, et al. Bronchoalveolar lavage for diagnosing acute bacterial pneumonia. J Infect Dis 1987;155:855–861.

88. Tillotson JR, Lerner AM. Characteristics of pneumonias caused by *Escherichia coli*. N Engl J Med 1967;277:115–122.

89. Torres A, Jimenez P, Puig de la Bellacasa J, Celis R, Gonzales J, Gea J. Diagnostic value of non-fluoroscopic percutaneous lung needle aspiration in patients with pneumonia. Chest 1990;98:840–844.

90. Trollfors B, Claesson B, Lagergard T, et al. Incidence, predisposing factors and manifestations of invasive *Haemophilus influenzae* infections in adults. Eur J Clin Microbiol 1984;3:180.

91. Waldvogel FA. *Staphylococcus aureus* (including toxic shock syndrome). In: Mandell GL, Douglas RG Jr, Bennett JE, eds. Principles and practice of infectious diseases. 3rd Ed. New York: Churchill Livingstone, 1990:1489–1510.

92. Wallace RJ Jr. Musher DM, Martin RR. *Haemophilus influenzae* pneumonia in adults. Am J Med 1978;64:87–93.

93. White RJ, Blainey AD, Harrison KJ, Clarke SKR. Causes of pneumonia presenting to a district general hospital. Thorax 1981;36:566–568.

94. Wimberley NW, Bass JB, Boyd BW, et al. Use of a bronchoscopic protected catheter brush for the diagnosis of pulmonary infections. Chest 1982;81:556–562.

95. Wimberley NW, Faling LJ, Bartlett JG. A fiberoptic bronchoscopy technique to obtain uncontaminated lower airway secretions for bacterial cultures. Am Rev Respir Dis 1979;119:337–342.

96. Woodhead MA, MacFarlane JT. *Haemophilus influenzae* pneumonia in previously fit adults. Eur J Respir Dis 1987;70:218–221.

97. Woodhead MA, MacFarlane JT, McCracken JS, Rose DH, Finch RG. Prospective study of the aetiology and outcome of pneumonia in the community. Lancet 1987;1:671–674.

98. Yu VL, Kroboth FJ, Shonnard J, et al. Legionnaires' disease: new clinical perspective from a prospective pneumonia study. Am J Med 1982; 73:357–361.

99. Zarrabi MH, Rosner F. Serious infections in adults following splenectomy for trauma. Arch Intern Med 1984;144:1421–1424.

33

Hospital-Acquired Pneumonia

Jean-Yves Fagon
Jean Chastre

Nosocomial bacterial pneumonia is one of the three most common hospital-acquired infections, along with urinary tract infection and wound infection. Pneumonia is the leading cause of death from nosocomial infection in all countries. In the US, hospital-acquired pneumonia affects almost 250,000 patients; 17,500 deaths are directly attributed to nosocomial pneumonia each year (14, 44, 46). Moreover, the extra hospitalization time directly attributable to the pneumonia is evaluated at approximately 2.5 million days annually, a very heavy economic burden (20, 37).

Rates of pneumonia are considerably higher among patients hospitalized in the intensive care unit compared to patients on hospital wards, and the risk of pneumonia is increased several-fold for the intubated patient receiving mechanical ventilation (13, 38, 101). Despite the use of more accurate methods for diagnosing pneumonia in this setting and the development of potent broad-spectrum antibiotics, fatality rates for nosocomial pneumonia remain high in the mechanically ventilated patient, ranging from 40–80% of the cases (23, 29, 33, 44, 101).

Therefore, definition of high-risk populations, more rapid identification of infected patients, and accurate selection of antimicrobial therapy for treatment of nosocomial pneumonia represent important clinical goals, since it appears that prevention or better treatment of this infection may result in fewer deaths per year and in fewer days of hospitalization per year.

EPIDEMIOLOGY OF NOSOCOMIAL PNEUMONIA

Standardized criteria for diagnosis have not been used in most of the reported studies, despite the fact that (as indicated below) the precise diagnosis of pneumonia in critically ill, ventilated patients is often difficult. Consequently, nearly all previous epidemiologic investigations in this setting have relied solely on clinical diagnostic criteria, and therefore have probably included patients who did not have pneumonia. Furthermore, most of these studies have used the results of cultures of tracheal secretions as the major culture source for microbiological analyses, despite the fact that the upper respiratory tract of most ventilated patients is frequently colonized by multiple potential pathogens. On the other hand, studies that have restricted the diagnosis to cases involving bacteremia or empyema have probably included only a limited portion of the clinical spectrum of the disease.

Incidence

The incidence of hospital-acquired pneumonia depends on the patient setting. The National Nosocomial Infection Study (NNIS), reporting for the year 1983, recorded an annual incidence of nosocomial lower respiratory infection of approximately 0.55% (14). The incidence was much lower in nonteaching hospitals (0.41%) and small teaching hospitals (0.46%) compared to large teaching hospitals (0.75%). The incidence of nosocomial pneumonia ranged widely among various inpatient services in the NNIS report, with highs of 0.5–1.0% on medical-surgical wards, and lows of 0.03–0.3% on obstetrics, gynecology, and pediatrics wards. Many studies have noted an even higher incidence of nosocomial pneumonia in certain settings, such as adult intensive care units (ICUs), postoperative and neonatal ICUs (23, 38, 47). The incidence of nosocomial pneumonia in general ICU populations ranges from 2–51% (25); however, a majority of studies have reported rates varying between 8 and 20% (21, 23, 25, 29, 33, 47, 53, 63, 94).

In ICU patients, the risk of pneumonia seems to be considerably higher in intubated patients receiving mechanical ventilation. Cross and Roup (24) found rates of pneumonia in ventilated patients were increased 10-fold compared to patients with no respiratory therapy device. In the Study on the Efficacy of Nosocomial Infection Control (SENIC), only 1% of the patients were treated with continuous ventilatory support, but the rate of pneumonia was 21-fold higher for these patients than for patients who were not receiving mechanical ventilation. Celis et al. (13) examined 120 consecutive episodes of nosocomial pneumonia and found intubation increased the risk of nosocomial pneumonia approximately sevenfold. In ventilated patients receiving mechanical ventilation, several investigators have reported different rates, ranging from 9–67%. Table 33.1 indicates rates reported in the more recent studies. With the exception of the study conducted by Kerver and associates in 1987 (57), the incidence of pneumonia varies only from 9–24%. In the study conducted by our group on 567 ventilated patients, using quantitative culture of specimens obtained with a protected brush catheter during fiberoptic bronchoscopy for defining pneumonia, the rate of nosocomial pneumonia was 9% (33). More interestingly, using an actuarial method, the cumulative risk of pneumonia in this setting was estimated to be 6.5% at 10 days and 19% at 20 days after the onset of mechanical ventilation (Fig. 33.1). Furthermore, the incremental risk of pneumonia was

Table 33.1
Incidence and Mortality Rate of Nosocomial Pneumonia in Ventilated ICU Patients

Author (Reference)	Type of Study (No. of Patients)	Incidence (%)	Bacteriological Criteria	Mortality (%)
Salata et al. (94)	Prospective (51)	41	Tracheal aspirate + Quantitative cultures	76
Kerver et al. (57)	Prospective (39)	67	Tracheal aspirate	30
Craven et al. (23)	Prospective (233)	21	Tracheal aspirate	55
Jimenez et al. (50)	Prospective (77)	23	Protected specimen brush + Quantitative cultures	28
Fagon et al. (33)	Prospective (567)	9	Protected specimen brush + Quantitative cultures	71
Torres et al. (107)	Prospective (322)	24	Protected specimen brush and/or pleural fluid	33

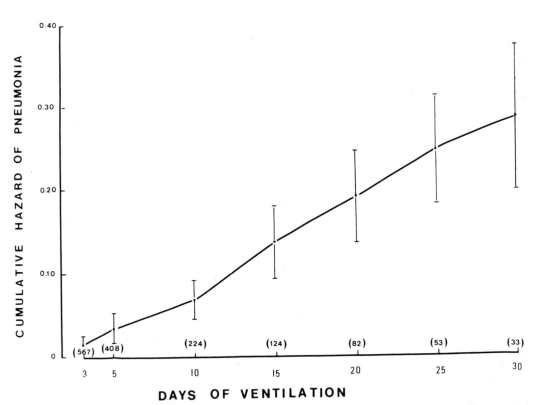

Figure 33.1. Cumulative hazard of ventilator-associated pneumonia in 567 patients. Data points are mean values (±SD). Figures in parentheses along the abscissa refer to the number of patients being followed at the start of the subsequent interval.

virtually constant through the entire ventilation period, with a mean rate of about 1% per day.

Morbidity and Mortality

It is impossible to estimate accurately the morbidity and excess costs associated with nosocomial pneumonia. However, with respect to morbidity measures, the excess stay in the hospital as a direct consequence of the pneumonia has been estimated to be 7–9 days per patient (20, 37, 66). The mortality associated with nosocomial pneumonia has been more clearly identified.

Nosocomial pneumonia contributed to 60% of the fatal infections in a study of 200 consecutive hospital deaths by Gross et al. (46). Stevens et al. (101) reported fatality rates of 50% for ICU patients with hospital-acquired pneumonia compared to 3.5% for patients without pneumonia.

Several studies have confirmed this result, reporting death rates varying between 40 and 50% (13, 20, 23). Mortality rates observed in ventilated patients are indicated in Table 33.1. Despite variations between studies, the risk of death for ventilated patients with nosocomial pneumonia seems to be higher than for nonventilated patients, exceeding 70% in two studies. For example, 71% of the patients who developed pneumonia in our series died during their hospitalization resulting in a significant twofold increase in mortality as compared to nonpneumonia patients (33).

Of particular interest is the relationship between etiologic agents and mortality from nosocomial pneumonia. It is clear that the prognosis associated with aerobic, Gram-negative bacillary pneumonias is considerably worse than that with Gram-positive agents. Graybill et al. (44) reported a 56% mortality rate in cases of Gram-negative bacilli pneumonia and 24% in cases of

Gram-positive pneumonia. Similarly, Stevens et al. (101) found a mortality rate of 50% in pneumonia due to Gram-negative and 5% in pneumonia due to Gram-positive organisms. Death rates associated with *Pseudomonas* spp. pneumonia are particularly high, with rates of 70% to more than 80% reported in several studies (11, 33, 101, 104, 105). In our series, mortality associated with *Pseudomonas* or *Acinetobacter* pneumonia was 87%, compared to only 55% in case of pneumonia due to other organisms (Fig. 33.2). It is worth noting that the majority of patients who developed pneumonia due to these multiresistant organisms had been receiving antimicrobial therapy prior to the onset of pneumonia.

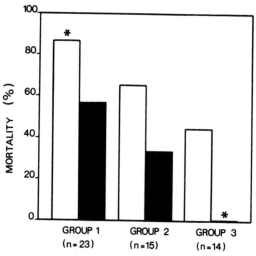

Figure 33.2. Mortality in patients with ventilator-associated pneumonia. Shown are the overall mortality *(open bars)* and the mortality specifically attributed to pulmonary infection *(closed bars)* in subgroups according to the responsible agents. Group 1, episodes of pneumonia involving *Pseudomonas* or *Acinetobacter* spp. Group 2, episodes of pneumonia involving *Staphylococcus* spp. but not *Pseudomonas* or *Acinetobacter* spp. Group 3, episodes of pneumonia involving other organisms. Asterisks indicate P<0.05 for the comparison of patients in this subgroup with other patients. (From Fagon JY, Chastre J, Domart Y, et al. Nosocomial pneumonia in patients receiving continuous mechanical ventilation. Prospective analysis of 52 episodes with use of a protected specimen brush and quantitative culture techniques. Am Rev Respir Dis 1989;139:877–884.)

Other risk factors for death in ventilated patients who developed pneumonia have been investigated systematically in only one recent study by Torres et al. (107). Using multiple logistic regression analysis, these authors demonstrated that worsening of the respiratory failure, presence of an ultimately or rapidly fatal underlying condition, presence of shock, inappropriate antibiotic therapy, and type of ICU where the pneumonia developed were factors with a negative influence on the prognosis of nosocomial pneumonia.

In summary, although the direct relationship between lung infection and mortality in ventilated patients has not been formally demonstrated, results observed in several studies indicate that nosocomial pneumonia is indeed associated with mortality in excess of that due to the underlying disease alone.

Etiologic Agents

The importance of Gram-negative bacilli as pathogens in nosocomial respiratory infections has been repeatedly documented (6, 11, 14, 33, 62, 67, 100, 104). Regardless of the bacteriologic method used for defining the precise etiology of pneumonia, several studies have reported that more than 60% of nosocomial pneumonias are caused by aerobic, Gram-negative bacilli. In the National Nosocomial Infection Study, Gram-negative accounted for six of the top seven etiologic agents identified in the last reported survey (14). In rank order, these organisms were *Pseudomonas aeruginosa* (16.9%), *Staphylococcus aureus* (12.9%), *Klebsiella* spp. (11.6%), Enterobacteriaceae (9.4%), *Escherichia coli* (6.4%), *Serratia marcescens* (5.8%), and *Proteus* spp. (4.2%). As indicated in Table 33.2, the results obtained in our study of patients with ventilator-associated pneumonia in whom bacteriologic studies were restricted to uncontaminated specimens confirm these results: 75% of all episodes of pneumonia included at least one Gram-negative bacillus (33). The predominant organisms were *P. aeruginosa*, *Acinetobacter* spp., and *Proteus* spp. A relatively high rate of Gram-positive pneumonias was also reported in this study, with *S. aureus* involved in 33%

Table 33.2
Organisms Recovered from Protected Brush Specimens in 52 Episodes of Ventilator-associated Pneumonia[a]

Organism	Total Number	% Total Episodes (n = 52)	% Mono-microbial Episodes (n = 31)	% Poly-microbial Episodes (n = 21)
Gram-negative bacteria	51	75	65	95
P. aeruginosa	16	31	29	33
Acinetobacter spp.	8	15	6	29
Proteus spp.	8	15	13	14
B. catarrhalis	5	10	3	19
Haemophilus spp.	5	10	3	19
E. coli	4	8	3	14
Klebsiella spp.	2	4	3	5
Enterobacter cloacae	1	2	0	5
Citrobacter freundii	1	2	0	5
Legionella pneumophila	1	2	3	0
Gram-positive bacteria	32	52	35	71
S. aureus	17	33	26	43
S. pneumoniae	3	6	3	10
Other streptococci	8	15	3	38
Corynebacterium spp.	4	8	3	14
Anaerobes	1	2	0	5

[a] From Fagon FY, Chastre J, Domart Y, et al. Nosocomial pneumonia in patients receiving continuous mechanical ventilation. Prospective analysis of 52 episodes with use of a protected specimen brush and quantitative culture techniques. Am Rev Respir Dis 1989; 139:877–884.

of them. Moreover, it is noteworthy that one-third of the pneumonias in this study were caused by or included organisms such as streptococci other than *Streptococcus pneumoniae*, *Corynebacterium* spp., *Haemophilus* spp., or *Branhamella catarrhalis*. Other studies have demonstrated a high incidence of pneumonia due to enterococcus spp. (9), *Haemophilus influenzae* (99), or anaerobic bacteria, especially in cases occurring after large-scale aspirations. It is now evident that *Legionella* spp. account for a certain number of cases of nosocomial pneumonia. Estimates of frequency range from 3–10% (58). In hospital settings with contamination of potable water by *Legionella* spp., this pathogen may account for up to 30% of all nosocomial pneumonias (19). However, using prospective monitoring, others have documented extremely low frequencies of *Legionella* nosocomial pneumonia (40).

A number of less frequent etiologies exist for nosocomial pneumonia. Several may be more common than is generally acknowledged. This potential for underre-porting is due to difficulties experienced with the diagnostic techniques necessary for identifying certain etiologic agents. For example, epidemic viral pneumonia has been recognized in the hospital setting (41). In one survey, it was reported that viral agents accounted for 20% of all nosocomial lower respiratory infections observed during a 17-month surveillance period in a general hospital (114). However, the majority of nosocomial viral pneumonia cases occur on pediatric wards (120). Finally, it should be emphasized that certain hospital centers, and particularly certain ICUs, may experience sporadic outbreaks of nosocomial pneumonia, associated or not with local factors such as contamination of specific respiratory equipment or fluids, or by pathogens carried on the skin of individual health-care personnel.

Recently, the high rate of polymicrobial infection in nosocomial pneumonia has been underlined by several authors. Using transtracheal aspiration to study nosocomial pneumonia occurring in nonventilated patients, Bartlett and associates (6) demonstrated that 54% of infections were polymicrobial. In a study of 172 episodes of bacteremic nosocomial pneumonia reported by Bryan and Reynolds (11), 13% of pneumonias were also caused by multiple agents. Similarly, using the protected specimen brush as described by Wimberley et al. (122) to establish the causative agent(s) in 52 consecutive cases of nosocomial pneumonia in ventilated patients, Fagon et al. (33) found a 40% incidence of polymicrobial infection.

Predisposing Factors

A number of factors that increase the risk of pneumonia in the hospital setting have been suspected or identified. However, no study has sought to examine in detail prehospitalization risk factors for hospital-acquired pneumonia. Importantly, only a few studies of potential risk factors have utilized available statistical modeling to define independent risk determinants. The study conducted by Celis et al. (13) evidenced that nasotracheal or orotracheal intubation, depressed level of consciousness, chronic lung disease, thoracic or abdominal surgery, a previous episode of a large-volume aspiration, and age over 70 years were the factors significantly predisposing to the development of pneumonia, after adjusting for confounding factors. These results confirm the major role that intubation of the respiratory tract and mechanical ventilation plays in the development of nosocomial pneumonia; the risk of pneumonia in ventilated patients was evaluated to be 4 times (24) to 21 times (in the SENIC project) higher than for nonintubated patients. Respiratory equipment itself may serve as a source of bacteria; for example, side-arm medication nebulizers may become contaminated with bacteria after a single use (31, 80).

Postsurgical patients clearly are at increased risk for pneumonia (13, 38). In one hospital's experience, 50% of all nosocomial pneumonias occurred in postoperative patients (32). In a study reported in 1981 by Garibaldi et al. (38), the incidence of pneumonia during the postoperative period was 17.5%. In that study, the authors stated that acquisition of pneumonia was closely associated with preoperative mark-

ers of the severity of the underlying disease, such as low serum albumin concentration and high American Society of Anesthesiologists preanesthesia physical status classification. A history of smoking, longer preoperative stays, longer surgical procedures, and thoracic or upper abdominal intervention sites were also significant risk factors for postoperative pneumonias.

The use of antibiotics in the hospital setting has been associated with increased risk of nosocomial pneumonia (53, 68, 104). These so-called superinfections presumably occur as a consequence of selection for more resistant bacterial pathogens during treatment of a primary infection. In one report, 149 patients treated in the hospital with penicillin or erythromycin for community-acquired pneumonia experienced a 16% incidence of pulmonary superinfection (104). In the study conducted by our group (33), patients receiving prior antimicrobial therapy were not at higher risk for developing pneumonia. However, we noted that 65% of the pneumonias among patients receiving broad-spectrum antimicrobial drugs, but only 19% of pneumonia among patients not having received prior antibiotics included *Pseudomonas* or *Acinetobacter* spp. as the responsible organisms.

In the group of ventilated patients, two studies have systematically examined risk factors for the development of pneumonia using logistic regression analysis to eliminate confounding variables. Table 33.3 summarizes results of these two studies conducted by Craven et al. (23) in 233 patients and by Torres and associates (107) in 322 patients. The data indicate specific high-risk patients (COPD) and treatment modalities (intracranial pressure monitoring, use of cimetidine, 24-hr circuit changes, reintubation); moreover, they underline the importance of gastric colonization (cimetidine, gastric aspiration) and the negative role played by the severity of respiratory disease requiring mechanical ventilation (use of PEEP, duration of mechanical ventilation). Recently, Dreyfuss et al. (28) confirmed and extended the findings of Craven et al. on the lack of reduction in the incidence of ventilator-associated pneumonia with frequent circuit changes. They found that not changing ventilator circuits

Table 33.3
Factors Selected by Logistic Regression Analysis Associated with a Higher Risk of Acquiring Nosocomial Pneumonia During Mechanical Ventilation[a]

Risk Factor	Relative Odds Ratio	95% Confidence Interval	p Value
Craven 1986 (23)			
Intracranial pressure monitoring	4.2	1.7–10.5	0.002
Cimetidine	2.5	1.2–5.0	0.01
24-hr circuit changes	2.3	1.2–4.7	0.02
Fall-winter season	2.1	1.1–4.2	0.04
Torres 1990 (107)			
Reintubation (>1)	5.0	3.5–7.0	0.00001
Gastric aspiration	5.05	3.35–7.8	0.0002
MV duration (>3 days)	1.17	1.15–1.19	0.015
COPD	1.89	1.38–2.59	0.048
Use of PEEP	1.85	1.30–2.64	0.092

[a]MV, mechanical ventilation; COPD, chronic obstructive pulmonary disease; PEEP, positive end-expiratory pressure.

had no adverse effects on the rate of nosocomial pneumonia and the colonization of patients and circuits. In the same way, results observed by Torres et al. (107) suggest that routine periodic changes of endotracheal tubes should be strongly discouraged.

In conclusion, identification of those predisposing factors amenable to intervention and definition of high-risk populations should be the first steps undertaken to implement effective monitoring and initiate therapeutic or prophylactic measures.

PATHOGENESIS

General Factors Affecting Susceptibility

The normal human respiratory tract is provided with a variety of defense mechanisms that protect the lungs from infection. The lower respiratory tract is protected by the glottis and the larynx, and material passing these barriers stimulates the expulsive cough reflex. Removal of small particles from lower airways is facilitated by their mucociliary lining. Finally, growth of bacteria reaching normal alveoli is inhibited by their relative dryness and by a dual phagocytic system that involves both granulocytes and alveolar macrophages (91, 106, 118). Any anatomic or physiologic disturbance of these coordinated defenses tends to augment the susceptibility of lungs to infection. Anesthesia, alcoholic intoxication, or convulsions depress the cough reflex. Alterations in the tracheobronchial tree leading to anatomic changes in the epithelial lining or to localized obstruction increase the vulnerability of the lungs to infection. Local or generalized pulmonary edema resulting from viral infection, inhalation of irritant gases, cardiac failure, or contusion of the chest wall provides a fluid exudate in the alveoli for the growth of bacteria. Common factors that adversely affect pulmonary macrophage function in the nosocomial setting are summarized in Table 33.4. These factors are frequently present in association in ICU patients.

Table 33.4
Factors that Adversely Influence Pulmonary Macrophage Function in the Nosocomial Setting

Community exposures
  Viruses
  Cigarette smoke
  Air pollutants
Hospital exposures
  Inhalation of anesthetic agents
  Hyperoxia
  Chemotherapeutic and immunosuppressive agents
Associated clinical condition
  Cancer
  Acidosis
  Pulmonary edema
  Uremia

Sources and Modes of Acquisition

Although hospital-acquired pneumonias may occur as metastatic infections secondary to bacteremia, the infrequent association of nosocomial pneumonia with bacteremias suggests that primary respiratory infection is by far the most common route. The majority of nosocomial pneumonias appears to result from aspiration of potential pathogens that have colonized the mucosal surfaces of the upper airways (52, 81, 88). In an important study published in 1972, Johanson and co-authors (52) demonstrated that 45% of 213 patients admitted to a medical ICU became colonized with aerobic, Gram-negative bacilli by the end of 1 week in the hospital. Of these 95 colonized patients, 22 (23%) developed subsequent nosocomial pneumonia. By comparison, only 4 of the 118 colonized patients (3.4%) developed pneumonia. In the same study, the risk of airway colonization increased as a function of time in the hospital. As determined in this study and in several others, risk factors for upper airway colonization with Gram-negative bacilli appear to be more advanced degrees of illness, longer duration in the hospital, prior or concomitant use of antibiotics, intubation, azotemia, and underlying pulmonary disease (51, 52, 68, 115).

Data are now available to describe mechanisms for bacterial colonization of the respiratory epithelium. Recent observations have indicated that the respiratory epithelium in hospitalized patients has increased affinity for the attachment of Gram-negative bacilli (51, 55, 74) and that *in vitro* bacterial adherence assays using buccal or tracheal cells from various patient groups may predict subsequent bacterial colonization of the airways (75). The mechanisms by which aerobic, Gram-negative bacilli become more adherent to the airway mucosa of hospitalized patients have also been studied. Bacterial lectins, such as the pili on cell membranes of *P. aeruginosa* have been identified as an important factor (124). Receptors on respiratory epithelial cells may also be important in mediating attachment of Gram-negative bacilli (85). Also, considerable data have been collected suggesting that the mucosal cell surface glycoprotein, fibronectin, plays an integral part in modulating oropharyngeal bacterial ecology (1, 123).

The most common interpretation of the relationship between colonization of the oropharynx and pneumonia is that when the oropharynx become colonized by enteric, Gram-negative bacteria, pneumonia is more likely to occur because any aspiration that occurs in this setting potentially involves pathogenic organisms (21). However, aspiration is a common event in many patients (49, 76) who do not develop pneumonia. Another and probably more accurate interpretation of all the data concerning colonization and pneumonia may be that colonization of the oropharynx is a marker for critically ill patients who have multiple deficiencies in the host-defense system of their respiratory tract. Thus, the patient whose oropharynx is colonized by Gram-negative bacteria is also likely to have other impairments in his or her cellular and humoral responses to bacterial invasion of the lung, and it is these defects that predispose the patient to the development of pneumonia, once Gram-negative organisms have entered the tracheobronchial tree.

The source of organisms colonizing the upper airway has been a controversial subject. Over the past decade, more evidence has emerged on the role of the gastrointestinal tract as a source of oropharyngeal colonization by Gram-negative bacilli. Studies of nosocomial infection have demonstrated an association between infection with a particular organism and the intestinal presence of the same organism (3, 96). In one study, daily cultures were monitored from rectal, hypopharyngeal, and tracheal sites in 21 patients requiring prolonged intubation (96). Enterobacteriaceae were commonly cultured from the hypopharynx and rectum before their appearance in tracheal cultures, suggesting that patients may become colonized by endogenous flora. Le Frock et al. (65) confirmed these data by demonstrating a correlation between newly appearing Gram-negative bacilli in the oropharynx and those predominating in the fecal flora; as the fecal flora changed during hospitalization, so did the oropharyngeal flora.

A direct fecal-to-oral pathway for bacterial contamination of the airways is one of the possible mechanisms suspected in bedridden patients. Others have advanced that the most important vector for transmission of environmental flora is the hands of health-care personnel (69, 102). While hand washing and other infection control methods may reduce cross-contamination with certain potential pathogens, it appears that the patient's endogenous flora will continue to provide a source for upper airway colonization.

Recent data suggest that the use of gastric alkalinization to prevent stress ulcers and bleeding in hospitalized patients is producing larger numbers of patients with extensive bacterial overgrowth in the upper gastrointestinal tract. Normally, the stomach maintains near-sterility by its acid pH. Changes in the gastric flora occur in patients of increased age, with malnutrition, achlorhydria, or other gastrointestinal diseases (27, 43). Reduced gastric acid in the intubated ICU patient may result from the intrinsic decrease of gastric acid production or from the use of antacids or histamine type 2 blockers, which neutralize or block gastric acid secretion (22, 89, 93).

Table 33.5 summarizes studies of gastric colonization and pH in relation to nosocomial pneumonia. Most of the data emphasize gastric colonization with aerobic Gram-negative bacilli, but high numbers of Gram-positive bacteria may occur as well. A clear sequence of colonization were demonstrated by Du Moulin et al. (30), Daschner et al. (25), and Goularte et al.

Table 33.5
Studies of Gastric Colonization and pH in Relation to Nosocomial Pneumonia[a]

Authors (Reference)	No. of Patients	Results/Comments
Atherton and White (3)	10	Gastric overgrowth in 90% Retrograde colonization of trachea from stomach in 33% Gastric colonization reaches 10^6 organisms/ml
Du Moulin et al. (30)	30	Gastric colonization up to 10^8 GNB/ml Retrograde colonization of trachea from stomach in 65%
Goularte et al. (42)	40	Retrograde colonization of GNB from stomach to trachea in 40% Gastric colonization: 10^7 GNB/ml
Donowitz et al. (26)	153	Gastric colonization in 59% of cases when pH ≥ 4; 14% when pH < 4
Pingleton et al. (83)	18	100% gastric colonization Retrograde colonization from stomach to trachea in 36% Pneumonia 63%
Craven et al. (23)	233	Pneumonia 38% in patients receiving AA and cimetidine 36% in patients given cimetidine 18% in patients given AA alone
Tryba et al. (113)	100	Pneumonia 34% in patients given AA 10% in patients given sucralfate
Driks et al. (29)	130	Pneumonia 23% in patients given AA 12% in patients given sucralfate Gastric colonization higher in patients receiving antacids/H_2
Daschner et al. (25)	142	Retrograde tracheal colonization from stomach with GNB in 32%

[a]GNB, Gram-negative bacteria; AA, antacids.

(42) with gastric colonization preceding colonization of the pharynx in a large subset of patients. The possible direct role of gastric colonization in the pathogenesis of pneumonia was supported by the prospective study conducted by Craven et al. (23). Although the number of patients was small, the administration of H_2 blockers with and without antacids was independently associated with the development of pneumonia.

In contrast, although sucralfate protection against stress bleeding appears to be similar to that provided by antacids and H_2 blockers (10), two recent randomized trials (29, 113) found lower rates of pneumonia in mechanically ventilated patients given sucralfate than in those given conventional agents (Fig. 33.3). Driks et al. (29) also reported that gastric colonization by Gram-negative bacilli was significantly lower in patients given sucralfate compared to patients given conventional therapy.

Increased pH due to tube feeding may increase gastrointestinal colonization by Gram-negative bacilli. Pingleton et al. (83) demonstrated gastric colonization in 100% of 18 ventilated patients receiving enteral feeding without antacid or H_2 blocker therapy, and 63% of them subsequently developed nosocomial pneumonia.

In intubated and ventilated patients, nearly all the factors and mechanisms cited above are associated with an increased risk of nosocomial pneumonia. Table 33.6 summarizes the effects of intubation on oropharyngeal colonization and the pathogenesis of pneumonia.

DIAGNOSIS

In contrast to community-acquired pneumonia, it may be difficult to determine whether or not pneumonia has developed in a hospitalized patient, and particularly in a ventilated ICU patient.

Clinical Diagnosis

The classic clinical findings for pneumonia, such as new fever, new pulmonary infiltrate, cough, sputum production and elevated leukocyte count, may not be present in the hospitalized patient with nosocomial pneumonia. Alternatively, these findings may be present, but may not be caused by pneumonia. Most critically ill patients have serious underlying disease,

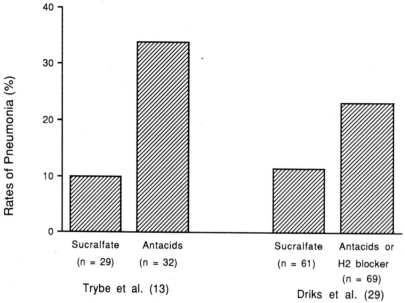

Figure 33.3. Rates of pneumonia reported by Tryba et al. (113) for patients randomized to receive prophylaxis with sucralfate or antacids, and rates of pneumonia reported by Driks et al. (29) for patients randomized to receive sucralfate versus antacids, H_2 blockers, or both.

Table 33.6
Effects of Intubation on Oropharyngeal
Colonization and Pathogenesis of Pneumonia

Patient immobility and decubitus
  Delays gastric emptying
  Increases gastric pressure
  Increases regurgitation of stomach content
Endotracheal tube
  Bypasses the nasopharynx
  Alters air temperature and humidity
  Acts as a foreign body
  Traumatizes epithelium in pharynx and
    trachea
  Impairs cilia clearance
  Alters cough
  Causes retention of secretions
  Requires suctioning
  Impairs swallowing
  Changes mouth flora
  Cuff may cause local trauma or leak
    contaminated secretions from the
    oropharynx
Nasogastric tube
  Acts as a foreign body
  Impairs swallowing
  Causes stagnation of oropharyngeal
    secretions
  Impairs lower esophageal sphincter
  Increases reflux
  Acts as a conduit for bacterial migration

increased oropharyngeal colonization with hospital flora, and numerous reasons for elevated body temperature and leukocytosis. Chest radiographic changes consistent with pneumonia may be caused by pulmonary edema, pulmonary infection, or atelectasis. Furthermore, microscopic evaluation and culture of tracheal secretions are frequently inconclusive since the upper respiratory tract of most ventilated patients is colonized with potential pulmonary pathogens, whether or not deep pulmonary infection is present (17). Therefore, results of studies evaluating the usefulness of clinical parameters or cultures of tracheal secretions in identifying ventilated patients with nosocomial pneumonia have generally been disappointing.

Andrews et al. (2), when comparing clinical criteria used for the diagnosis of pneumonia with histologic findings in the lungs of 24 acute respiratory distress syndrome patients who died during treatment, found that clinical diagnoses were in error in 29% of patients; pneumonia was correctly predicted using clinical data in 9 patients (64%), and was misdiagnosed in 5 patients (36%). The following clinical variables were present in the groups with and without pneumonia, respectively: fever, 100% versus 80%, leukocytosis or leukopenia, 100% versus 80%, pathogens in the sputum, 86% versus 70%, and asymmetric infiltrates on chest films, 57% versus 30%. Interestingly, only 2 of 14 patients subsequently proven to have pneumonia improved with the administration of antimicrobial agents. Similar improvement was noted in 3 of 10 patients who did not have pneumonia; hence, the response of the patient to antibiotic treatment was therefore also an unreliable indicator of the presence or absence of bacterial infection.

In a similar study from the same institution conducted by Bell et al. (8) in 47 adult respiratory distress syndrome patients who died, 38% of the 35 patients with pneumonia were also misdiagnosed. Pneumonia was clinically suspected in 21 patients and confirmed histologically in 19 patients (10% false-positive rate); it was not suspected clinically in 26 patients, but it was found histologically in 16 (62% false-negative rate). Likewise, in the study conducted by our group in 147 ventilated patients suspected of having lung infections, we found that, in the 24-hr interval preceding the availability of the results of protected specimen brush cultures, the attending physicians were as likely to initiate or modify antibiotic treatment in patients with pneumonia as in those without pneumonia (34). Moreover, when 16 clinical variables such as fever, leukocytosis, hypoxemia, or radiologic findings were evaluated by stepwise regression analysis, no combinations were found that were useful in distinguishing between patients with and without bacterial pneumonia.

As a consequence, unless further evaluation is undertaken, most patients with fever and pulmonary infiltrates are treated with one or more antibiotics. This policy, based only on clinical evaluation and the results of cultures of tracheal aspirates, has several potential disadvantages. First, large numbers of patients who do not have bacterial pneumonia are treated with antibiotics, thus exposing them to unnecessary toxicity, delaying the diagnosis of the true etiology of the pulmonary infiltrates and increasing hospital costs. Antibiotic therapy prior to the development of true nosocomial pneumonia influences the frequency of various types of pneumonia. Second, some patients with nosocomial pneumonia may not be recognized clinically since they may have an atypical presentation. Finally, even if the diagnosis of pneumonia is accurate, results of cultures of tracheal aspirates could be misleading in directing the choice of antibiotics. For these reasons, a number of specialized microbiologic assays and several invasive techniques for obtaining specimens have been described as being potentially useful for improving diagnostic specificity for nosocomial pneumonia.

Bronchoscopic Specimens

Bronchoscopy provides direct access to the lower airways for sampling bronchial and parenchymal tissues. To reach the bronchial tree, however, the bronchoscope must traverse the endotracheal tube and proximal airways where contamination is likely to occur. Therefore, distal secretions directly aspirated through the bronchoscope suction channel are frequently contaminated, thus limiting their clinical specificity. In a study of 16 nonventilated patients without lung infection who underwent flexible fiberoptic bronchoscopy, Bartlett et al. (5) found that all bronchoscopic aspirates were contaminated by oropharyngeal bacteria, with an average of 5 bacterial species per aspirate. By spraying a methylene blue marker in the posterior pharynx, they demonstrated that passage of the bronchoscope resulted in the introduction of oropharyngeal contaminants into the suction channel.

Recently, two techniques have been proposed as being of value in establishing a specific diagnosis of pneumonia in critically ill patients. First, the use of a double-lumen catheter with a protected specimen brush to collect uncontaminated culture specimens directly from affected areas in the lower respiratory tract and, second,

the use of bronchoalveolar lavage, since this technique is a safe and practical method for obtaining cells and secretions from the lower respiratory tract.

Protected Specimen Brush

To reduce contamination of lower airway aspirates collected by bronchoscopy, Wimberley and colleagues (122) in the late 1970s developed the protected specimen brush technique, which became commercially available in 1979. This method is in fact based on the combination of four different techniques: (1) the use of fiberoptic bronchoscopy to directly sample the site of inflammation in the lung; (2) the use of a special double-catheter brush system with a distal occluding plug to reduce contamination of lower airway aspirates by flora colonizing proximal airways; (3) the use of a brush to calibrate the volume of respiratory secretions obtained; and (4) the use of a quantitative culture technique to aid in distinguishing between airway colonization and serious underlying infection, with a cutoff point of 10^3 colony-forming units (CFU)/ml for establishing this distinction.

The usefulness of the protected specimen brush technique in evaluating patients receiving mechanical ventilation and suspected of having pneumonia has been extensively investigated in both human and animal studies (4, 7, 15–17, 34, 48, 54, 72, 73, 79, 90, 109–111, 119, 126). However, in only four studies (17, 48, 54, 73) was the relative cultural accuracy of the protected specimen brush method determined with an acceptable "gold" standard, i.e., in comparison with both histologic features and quantitative cultures from the same area of the lung. Moser et al. (73) found in a canine model of *S. pneumoniae* pneumonia that the sensitivity of the protected specimen brush technique was high, ranging between 90 and 100%. Higuchi et al. (48) found that 7 of the 10 baboons with nosocomial pneumonia had positive protected specimen brush cultures and no false-positive results were observed. In studies evaluating the appearance of pneumonia in ventilated baboons with permeability pulmonary edema,

Johanson et al. (54) also found that quantitative cultures of protected specimen brush specimens showed a good correlation with the bacterial content of lung tissue, even if the results were inferior to those obtained with bronchoalveolar lavage.

To determine the operating characteristics of the protected specimen brush technique for diagnosing lung infection in patients undergoing mechanical ventilation, 26 of our intubated patients in respiratory failure were subjected to bronchoscopy just after their deaths, while mechanical ventilation was continued (17). Cultures of the protected specimen brush yielded 15 of the 19 bacteria present in the lung cultures of the 6 patients with histologically proven pneumonia and no additional organisms. All protected specimen brush cultures from these patients had at least one microorganism growing at a concentration of $>10^3$ CFU/ml. Using the cutoff point of 10^3 CFU/ml to define a positive protected specimen brush culture, no false-negative results were observed. In the 20 patients without pneumonia, the false-positive rate was 45% (58% in patients receiving antibiotics prior to death and only 23% in patients who received no antibiotics).

More recently, the clinical utility of protected specimen brush has been investigated by Fagon et al. (34) in a large group of intubated patients, most of whom were ventilated for respiratory insufficiency after cardiac surgery. Results of quantitative culture of the protected specimen brush sample showed that only 45 patients (30%) had at least one microorganism growing above the cutoff point of 10^3 CFU/ml. The diagnosis of pneumonia was confirmed in 34 of these patients. One hundred two patients had either no growth (77 patients) or the protected specimen brush culture yielded $<10^3$ CFU/ml. None of them had bacterial pneumonia. The positive predictive value of a positive culture ($\geq 10^3$ CFU/ml) was greater than 75%.

The reliability of the protected specimen brush technique in the diagnosis of lower respiratory tract infection was also studied by Baughman et al. (7). Cultures of the protected specimen brush specimen from the affected lung in all 8 cases of bacterial

pneumonia had one or more organisms present at >100 CFU/ml, whereas only one of the 13 cases of nonpneumonia had a culture from the affected area of >100 CFU/ml.

Despite the need for caution in interpreting the results, these studies indicate that the protected specimen brush technique offers a sensitive and specific approach in critically ill patients to determine the organisms responsible for the pneumonia and to differentiate between colonization of the upper respiratory tract and distal lung infection. When the results of the 15 studies that have evaluated the protected specimen brush technique in ventilated patients (36), including more than 300 patients, are pooled together, the overall accuracy of this technique for diagnosing nosocomial pneumonia was 93%, with a sensitivity of 91% and a specificity of 95%.

Before initiating extensive clinical use of the protected specimen brush technique, some potential limits or drawbacks of this method should be considered. They are listed in Table 33.7. Three of these limits seem to be of particular importance. First, the results of protected specimen brush specimen cultures from patients given prior antimicrobial therapy can be difficult to interpret. As demonstrated by ourselves and Johanson et al. (54), the protected specimen brush technique appears to work well in cases in which pneumonia develops as a superinfection in patients who had been receiving systemic (but not topical) antibiotics for several days before the appearance of the new pulmonary infiltrates, because the bacteria responsible for

Table 33.7
Potential Limits and Drawbacks of the Protected Specimen Brush Technique

1. Patients with diffuse lung injury
2. Patients given prior antimicrobial therapy
3. Inherent risks on bronchoscopy in ICU patients
4. Hospital costs
5. False-positive results
6. False-negative results
7. Absence of information to guide initial therapy

the new infection are then resistant to the antibiotics given previously. In contrast, the protected specimen brush technique is probably of little value in patients with a recent pulmonary infiltrate who have received new antibiotics for this reason, even for less than 24 hours. In this case, a negative finding could indicate that either the patient has been successfully treated for pneumonia and the bacteria are eradicated, or there was no lung infection to begin with. These two different clinical situations should be clearly distinguished before interpreting a protected specimen brush result in a patient given antibiotics prior to recognized lung infection. In the latter situation, no conclusion concerning the presence or absence of pneumonia can be drawn if the protected specimen brush result is "negative," thereby emphasizing the need to make every effort to obtain the protected specimen brush specimens before new antibiotics are administered, as for all types of microbiological samples.

Second, fiberoptic bronchoscopy is generally regarded as safe, based on surveys of endoscopists. The inherent risk in such an examination appears slight, even in critically ill patients requiring mechanical ventilation, although the associated occurrence of cardiac arrhythmias, hypoxemia, or bronchospasm is not unusual. A recent study conducted by Trouillet et al. (112) in 107 ventilated patients has shown that fiberoptic bronchoscopy under midazolam sedation is practicable in this setting. No death or cardiac arrest occurred during or within the 2 hours immediately following the procedure. However, patients in the ICU are at risk of relative hypoxemia during fiberoptic bronchoscopy, even when high levels of oxygen are provided to the ventilator, and gas leaks around the endoscope are minimized by a special adaptor. Careful methodical attention must be paid to the anesthetic protocol with the addition of a short-acting neuromuscular blocking agent. Monitoring of patients during bronchoscopy should enable rapid correction and more frequent prevention of hypoxemia in this setting and therefore should further decrease the morbidity of this procedure.

Third, protected specimen brush samples must be cultured for 24–48 hours, and therefore no information is available to guide the initial decisions concerning the appropriateness of antimicrobial therapy and which antibiotics should be used.

Bronchoalveolar Lavage

The evaluation of bronchoalveolar lavage seems to be a logical next step since this technique has been extremely helpful in diagnosing a wide range of lung infections in immunocompromised individuals. Indeed, several considerations indicate that bronchoalveolar lavage might be useful in establishing the diagnosis of bacterial pneumonia. Lavage is a safe and practical method for obtaining cells and secretions from the lower respiratory tract. The technique is used to obtain samples from a relatively large area of the lung; the cells and liquid recovered can be examined microscopically immediately after the procedure and are also suitable for culture using quantitative techniques.

Two reports indicate that bronchoalveolar lavage in association with quantitative bacteriologic techniques can accurately diagnose bacterial pulmonary infections in nonventilated patients (56, 103). The utility of bronchoalveolar lavage in nosocomial pneumonia has also been reported in ventilated animals and humans. Quantitative bronchoalveolar lavage cultures were performed by Johanson et al. (54) in 35 mechanically ventilated baboons; 6 received no antibiotic and 29 received systemic or topical antibiotic treatment. Quantitative bronchoalveolar lavage cultures correlated well with the bacterial count in the lung, provided culture results were expressed as a "bacterial index". The bacterial index was calculated by adding the $\log_{10}$ concentrations of the individual bacterial species. Only animals given topical antibiotic therapy had negative bronchoalveolar lavage cultures and no pneumonia. In the 6 animals not given antibiotic therapy, bronchoalveolar lavage cultures were positive and pneumonia was found. Therefore, the utility of bronchoalveolar lavage cultures in a situation analogous to clinical airway colonization (without definite pneumonia) is not known.

Quantitative bronchoalveolar lavage and protected specimen brush cultures have also been compared in ventilated patients by Chastre et al. (15), who evaluated 21 ventilated patients clinically suspected of nosocomial pneumonia because of the presence of new pulmonary infiltrates and purulent tracheal aspirates. Pneumonia was diagnosed in five patients with $>10^3$ CFU/ml by protected specimen brush and verified by rapid cavitation of lung infiltrates or by lung histopathology. When quantitative bronchoalveolar lavage cultures were evaluated, no clear threshold separated these patients with from those without pneumonia, in contrast to quantitative protected specimen brush cultures.

More recently, Torres et al. (110) compared bronchoalveolar lavage and protected specimen brush in 34 mechanically ventilated patients. Pneumonia was diagnosed clinically only. Agreement was excellent (88.5%) between bronchoalveolar lavage and protected specimen brush with respect to the type of organism recovered; disagreement existed in only one case.

Several factors probably explain the apparent differences in the usefulness of lavage fluid cultures for identifying patients with pneumonia in these various studies. First, criteria used for identifying patients with pneumonia and distinguishing them from patients with only airway colonization were more or less stringent. Second, different populations of patients were included in these studies. Finally, it is important to note that even if the number of organisms recovered per milliliter of lavage fluid from patients with pneumonia was statistically higher than that recovered from patients without pneumonia, some patients with true lung infection had low bacterial indexes or no bacteria recovered in high concentrations from lavage fluid.

Recently, a modified bronchoalveolar lavage technique was described by Meduri et al. (72) and is based on a protected transbronchoscopic balloon-tipped catheter designed to avoid exposing the instilled and aspirated bronchoalveolar lavage solution to the contaminants present in the suction lumen of the bronchoscope. Using a threshold of 10^4 CFU/ml, only one false-positive result and one false-negative result were observed for a diagnostic sensitivity of 97% and a specificity of 92%.

Chastre et al. (16) recently demonstrated in a series of 61 patients suspected of having nosocomial pneumonia that microscopic examination of cytocentrifuged preparations obtained from bronchoalveolar lavage fluid enabled the very easy and rapid determination of the presence or absence of intracellular or extracellular bacteria in the cells and secretions lining the lower respiratory tract (Fig. 33.4). Fourteen patients had a definite diagnosis of pneumonia established by either autopsy, rapid cavitation of pulmonary infiltrates, or positive pleural culture. Among the 47 patients without pneumonia, the protected specimen brush culture showed no growth in 39 and insignificant growth in 8. In the group with pneumonia, 12 patients had significant growth ($>10^3$ CFU/ml) and 2 had no growth, a 14% false-negative rate. Microscopic analysis of bronchoalveolar lavage showed intracellular organisms in more than 7% of the recovered cells in 12 of 14 patients with pneumonia (86% sensitivity) and in only 2 of 47 without pneumonia (96% specificity). Furthermore, in patients with pneumonia, the morphology and Gram staining of such bacteria closely correlated with the results of protected specimen brush bacterial culture (Fig. 33.5).

Microscopic analysis of the bronchoalveolar lavage, therefore, may provide rapid identification of patients with pneumonia because results are available immediately, enabling early formulation of a specific antimicrobial therapy that can later be adapted to the results of the protected specimen brush culture and sensitivity. In addition, it is likely that the lavage procedure samples a greater area of lung tissue than the protected specimen brush. Therefore, this technique may enable the identification of some of the false-negative results observed with the protected specimen brush method. Combining the two techniques may then improve the overall diagnostic accuracy. These results suggest that microscopic examination of bronchoalveolar lavage fluid can be easily incorporated into a protocol in conjunction with the quantitative cultures of protected

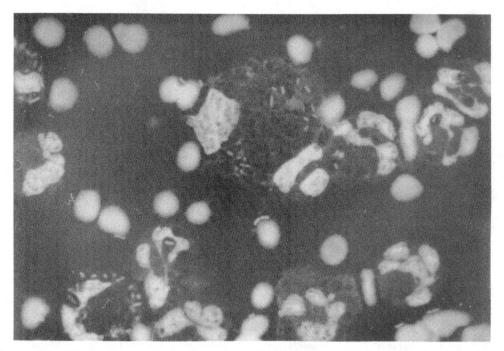

Figure 33.4. Light micrograph of cells recovered by bronchoalveolar lavage from a patient with pneumonia due to *P. aeruginosa*. Shown are one alveolar macrophage and many neutrophils containing multiple intracellular bacilli (Diff Quick stain, original magnification × 1000).

specimen brush samples. Interestingly, the usefulness of this technique was confirmed in two recent studies evaluating bronchoalveolar lavage efficacy in the diagnosis of lung infection (71, 84). In each study, either the Giemsa or the Gram stain was positive in all patients with pneumonia, enabling early and accurate diagnosis of lower respiratory tract infection before cultures results were available.

Nonbronchoscopic Procedures

Respiratory secretions obtained by nonprotected endotracheal aspiration should be examined microscopically. Unfortunately, these specimens are often contaminated with upper airway flora and do not enable a distinction to be made between colonization and true nosocomial lung infection (53).

The direct needle aspiration of a pulmonary infiltrate through the chest wall is a promising older technique that has been recently revived (108, 125). Although highly specific, this technique may show low sensitivity, probably because of the small sam-

pling area and small inoculum volume obtained for microbiological examination and the difficulty in precisely localizing the infected area. In addition, this procedure carries a considerable risk of pneumothorax among ventilated patients, which prohibits its routine use.

Isolation of a single organism from blood cultures may help to distinguish between contaminating and infecting bacterial isolates in tracheal aspirate or sputum. Blood cultures are, however, positive in fewer than 10% of patients with nosocomial pneumonias (11, 33).

In order to simplify procedures and to reduce costs, new developments in the protected specimen brush techniques and bronchoalveolar lavage were recently proposed.

A modification of the protected specimen brush technique was suggested by Torres et al. (109), who developed a nonbronchoscopic method to perform protected brushing, using a Metras catheter without fluoroscopy through an endotracheal tube. In a study of 25 ventilated patients, these authors demonstrated that

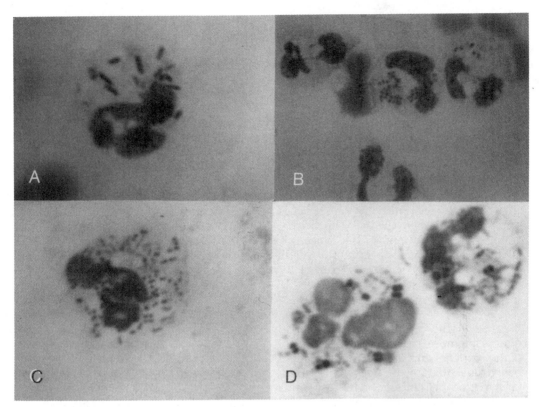

Figure 33.5. Light micrographs of neutrophils recovered by bronchoalveolar lavage from: **(A)** a patient with pneumonia due to *P. aeruginosa*, **(B)** a patient with pneumonia due to *S. aureus*, **(c)** a patient with pneumonia due to *H. influenzae*, and **(D)** a patient with pneumonia due to *Moraxella catarrhalis* and nonpneumococcal streptococci. In all patients, the morphology and Gram staining of intracellular bacteria closely correlated with the results of protected specimen brush bacterial cultures.

the sensitivities of the nonbronchoscopic and the bronchoscopic protected specimen brush were nearly the same (64% versus 71%), with a predicted value of 100% for both. A second study was based on the use of a new device composed of a plugged telescoping catheter used with or without fiberoptic bronchoscopy (79). In a study of 78 suspected episodes of nosocomial pneumonia in 55 patients, Pham et al. (79) found that this device gave results similar to those obtained with the protected specimen brush technique in 74% of the cases. A major discrepancy was observed between the two techniques in only 20 episodes, including 6 false-negatives for protected specimen brush in patients with proven pneumonia, 4 possible false-positives for protected specimen brush, and 10 possible false-positives for the plugged

catheter. Furthermore, the blinded non-bronchoscopic plugged telescoping catheter sampling was as accurate as directed sampling via bronchoscopy using plugged telescoping catheter or protected specimen brush.

A technique described by Rouby et al. (92) was recently proposed to circumvent the problem of contamination of bronchoalveolar lavage fluid by the flora present in proximal airways, and is based on the use of a plugged double catheter blindly wedged into the distal airways for performing a small lavage with 20 ml of saline. The value of this new technique was tested in a control group of 21 patients free of any pulmonary disease throughout their stay in the ICU and a pneumonia group of 30 patients who died in the ICU with histologically and bacteriologically proven nosocomial pneumonia. In that study, the sensitivity of a positive (using only a qualitative technique) protected lavage was 80%, while the specificity was 66%. Among the 43 microorganisms isolated in the lung cultures, 74% were recovered by the lavage. Although these techniques appear promising, more information is needed before it will be possible to use them routinely in clinical practice.

Finally, immunologic methods for the diagnostic evaluation of respiratory specimens have been described, including a direct fluorescent antibody for *Legionella* spp. Unfortunately, the vast majority of nosocomial pneumonias are caused by pathogens for which no immunologic diagnostic techniques currently exist.

TREATMENT

Because of the difficulty encountered in diagnosing nosocomial pneumonia in ventilated patients and in selecting antimicrobial drugs, therapy of nosocomial pneumonia is often empiric, with the initial antimicrobial regimen based on local experience and sensitivity patterns, immune competence of the patient, and severity of disease. Two factors appear to render the choice of antibiotics particularly difficult in such patients. First, nosocomial pneumonias are likely to result from highly resistant organisms (33, 105). Second, multiple organisms are frequently cultured from patients considered to have pneumonia (6, 11, 33). Moreover, the difficulty experienced in differentiating patients with colonization from those with true distal infection requiring antibiotic treatment suggests that overtreatment could occur commonly if only clinical criteria were used. The undue use of antibiotics in patients without pneumonia as well as the use of drugs ineffective against the responsible pathogens in patients with pneumonia not only represents a considerable additional cost, but increases the risk of side effects and toxicity, contributes to the development of resistant strains of bacteria, and increases the risk of serious superinfections (104). Consequently, as stressed above, it is reasonable that evaluation of ventilated patients suspected of having

nosocomial pneumonia includes the use of a reliable technique to identify patients with pneumonia and to guide the choice of antimicrobial treatment.

When no technique (or an unreliable technique) is used, empiric choices of initial antimicrobial agents must be made for suspected cases of nosocomial pneumonia. Selected therapy must be broad enough to ensure coverage for aerobic, Gram-negative bacilli, including such highly resistant organisms as *P. aeruginosa*, *S. marcescens*, and *Acinetobacter* spp.; moreover, treatment must not ignore the increasing role that Gram-positive bacteria like methicillin-resistant *Staphylococcus* spp. play in numerous cases. On the basis of these considerations, several regimens have been employed for empiric treatment of nosocomial pneumonia. Combination therapy with an aminoglycoside and a β-lactam has long been the cornerstone of therapy (78). In special situations, coverage of other organisms must also be included, e.g., oral anaerobes when obvious aspiration has occurred, *H. influenzae* in patients with chronic lung disease, and *Legionella* spp. in certain hospitals.

The development of new broad-spectrum antibiotics, such as monobactams, third-generation cephalosporins, and imipenem, has introduced the possibility of monotherapy for the treatment of nosocomial pneumonia. For example, the acylamino penicillins are very active against a wide variety of aerobic, Gram-negative rods and have the major advantage of being less toxic than aminoglycosides. In general, monotherapy has proven to be a useful alternative to combination therapy. Table 33.8 lists theoretical advantages and disadvantages of monotherapy and combination therapy and Table 33.9 summarizes results of controlled studies that have compared the therapeutic outcome of monotherapy or combination therapy (70, 71, 87, 95). Success rates were somewhat higher in the monotherapy group (88%) when compared to results obtained with combination therapy (76%). However, an important potential limiting factor for the use of monotherapy is the development of resistance during therapy. Superinfection and colonization rates observed in mon-

Table 33.8
Theoretical Advantages and Disadvantages of Monotherapy and Combination Therapy for the Treatment of Nosocomial Pneumonia

Combination Therapy	Monotherapy
Advantages	
Broad-spectrum coverge	Lower cost
Synergistic effects	Less toxicity
High bactericidal activity	
Limitation of the emergence of resistant organism(s)	
Disadvantages	
Aminoglycosides	
Toxicity	Failure to treat *P. aeruginosa*
Necessity of monitoring plasma levels	and possibly other multi-resistant organisms
	Superinfection
	Emergence of resistant flora
2 β-lactams in association:	
Relapse infection	
Emergence of multiple β-lactam-resistant organisms	
Fungal infection	
Cost	

otherapy versus combination therapy studies are shown in Table 33.9. Superinfection rates were higher among patients treated with combination therapy (18% versus 12%), while colonization rates were higher in monotherapy-treated patients (30% versus 20%).

The duration of treatment of nosocomial pneumonia is also controversial. In cases such as those due to highly resistant organisms, treatment may be necessary for longer than 1 month, although there is no clear data concerning the definition of a successful bacteriologic treatment in this setting. In some cases, it will be impossible to eradicate the original pathogen from tracheal secretions despite clinical improvement. The continued presence of a tracheal prosthesis undoubtedly contributes to this persistence of pathogens in airways. Moreover, the risk for emergence of resistant microorganisms during such therapy is considerable and has been proposed as an additional reason to use two different classes of antibiotics (39).

The role of aminoglycosides in treating nosocomial pneumonia deserves further comment because of the existence of con-

flicting data. Evidence exists that aminoglycosides are more active than β-lactams against certain resistant, Gram-negative bacilli (12). On the other hand, the therapeutic ratios for aminoglycosides in serum are narrow, and the penetration of circulating aminoglycosides into the infected lung tissues may be insufficient to treat infecting organisms (77). Consequently, several new approaches have been devised to improve delivery of aminoglycosides to infected lung tissues. One of the most important is direct instillation of aminoglycoside into the respiratory tract via an endotracheal tube or tracheostomy. In a prospective randomized study (61) comparing systemic treatment alone versus systemic treatment plus sisomicin deposition into the respiratory tract, more patients improved in the group given local aminoglycoside treatment. Further investigation of on-site aminoglycoside therapy for nosocomial pneumonia will, however, be necessary before the relative risks and benefits can be definitively explained.

In the event that a specific etiologic agent is identified, questions remain regarding proper therapy in terms of duration of

Table 33.9
Comparison of Monotherapy and Combination Therapy for the Treatment of Nosocomial Pneumonia

Monotherapy (Reference)	Success/Total	Superinfection (%)	Colonization (%)	Combination	Success/Total	Superinfection (%)	Colonization (%)
Aztreonam (95)	24/26 (92%)	37	41	Tobramycin	7/14 (50%)	36	21
Cefoperazone (71)	45/52 (87%)	3		Clindamycin or Cefazolin/gentamicin	44/61 (72%)	18	
Ceftazidime (87)	15/17 (88%)		17	Tobramycin/ticarcillin	15/18 (83%)		
Ceftazidime (70)	21/24 (88%)	4		Tobramycin/cefazolin	24/26 (92%)	8	19
Total	105/119 (88%)	12	30	Total	90/119 (76%)	18	20

treatment, monotherapy versus combination therapy, and adjunction of local treatment. Nevertheless, the initial choice of antimicrobial drugs is much easier because the optimal treatment may be selected in light of the susceptibility patterns of the causative pathogens, without resorting to broad-spectrum drugs.

In addition to antibiotics, considerable interest has been expressed in the development of immunologic methods for treating nosocomial pneumonia. Passive immune sera, hyperimmune globulins, and monoclonal antibodies are potentially valuable treatments for severe, Gram-negative infections, including Gram-negative pneumonia (18), but their usefulness remains to be determined.

PREVENTION

Recommendations for prevention of nosocomial pneumonia can be discussed from the viewpoints of unit design, staff training and motivation, asepsis and antisepsis, monitoring and reporting of infection, and therapeutic measures.

The design of the ICU will have a direct effect on the potential for infection. Unfortunately, modifications of engineering and architectural elements are probably the most costly measures and consequently are difficult to undertake. Adequate space and lighting, proper functioning of ventilation systems, and facilities for hand washing will contribute to lower rates of infection (97, 121). Personnel who treat seriously ill patients should be part of the planning and design processes in the construction and renovation of intensive care facilities.

In any ICU, the most important factor is the number, quality, and motivation of its medical, nursing, and ancillary staffs. There should be enough nurses to eliminate the need for them to move between patients and they should not be constantly working under pressure or basic, aseptic, routine practices may be neglected. The importance of personal cleanliness and attention to aseptic procedures must be pointed out at every opportunity. At the same time, unnecessarily rigid restrictions should be avoided.

It is clear that careful monitoring, decontamination, and adherence to the usage guidelines of respiratory equipment will decrease the incidence of nosocomial pneumonia (82). However, a number of recommendations published for the prevention of nosocomial pneumonia are empiric rather than based on controlled observations (98). For example, the recommendation that breathing-circuit tubing be changed every 24 hr is arbitrary. Craven et al. (23) evidenced no significant increase in bacterial contamination of tubing between 24 and 48 hr of use. Recently, Dreyfuss et al. (28) reported no modifications in bacterial contamination and the incidence of pneumonia between changes every 48 hr and no change of circuit tubing. These published guidelines contain many other recommendations, such as wearing sterile gloves for endotracheal suctioning, that have not been sufficiently studied. Nonetheless, hand washing remains uncontested as the most important infection-control practice (64).

A bacterial monitoring policy could be initiated to facilitate the early recognition of colonization and infection; it could be applied to patients in the unit and to their environment. However, the focal point for infection control activities in the unit is a system of surveillance designed to establish and maintain a database that describes endemic rates of nosocomial infection. Awareness of the endemic rates enables the recognition of the onset of an epidemic when infection rates rise above a calculated threshold.

A very important but less evaluated measure is the adoption of an antibiotic policy. It would limit the emergence of resistant bacterial strains, discourage the prescription of useless antibiotics, and probably reduce the cost of treatment. The antibiotic policy is based on: (a) laboratory identification of organisms and their clinical significance, (b) changing patterns of antibiotic sensitivity, (c) the effectiveness and toxicity of antibiotic treatment, and (d) the cost of such treatment.

Therapeutic measures include the prophylactic use of endobronchial antibiotics and "selective digestive decontamination." Several authors have used prophylactic endobronchial antibiotics in an attempt to reduce the incidence of nosocomial pneumonia (45, 60). Results of studies using gentamicin aerosol (60) or an aminoglycoside-polymyxin B combination (59), were disappointing. An extensive analysis of prophylactic polymixin B aerosol for patients in a respiratory intensive care unit has been described (35, 45). After early encouraging reports, the final phase of the study evidenced emergence of antibiotic-resistant pathogens and increased pneumonia-related mortalities (45). Based on these data, routine use of prophylactic endobronchial antibiotics could not be recommended.

Recently, several groups, particularly in Europe, have used topical prophylactic antibiotics for decontamination of the oropharynx and gastrointestinal tract in patients at high risk for nosocomial pneumonia. The rationale for this preventive method is that oropharyngeal or gastrointestinal bacterial flora appear to be an important source of airway colonization in hospitalized patients (116). At this time, more than 25 reports have been published that described the impact of selective digestive decontamination on the occurrence of nosocomial infection and on the outcome of ICU patients (86, 117). Results of these studies are, however, troublesome. Despite the clear demonstration of decreases in colonization and in gram-negative pneumonia (if we accept the criteria used for defining pneumonia), very few investigations, with the exception of those involving trauma patients, have shown a reduction in mortality. The outcome of serious illness is very heavily weighted by the occurrence of infection, particularly Gram-negative infection, and these results that fail to evidence improvement in the mortality rate are disappointing. To date, there has been no significant problem encountered with antibiotic resistance. However, careful and continuous microbiologic monitoring must remain part of the protocol in any unit adopting selective digestive decontamination. Larger, controlled studies using this approach will be needed before the impact on morbidity, mortality, and emergence of resistant bacteria can be fully evaluated.

In summary, much progress has been made in our understanding of nosocomial infections of the lower respiratory tract. However, there is little evidence that significant progress has been made either in preventing or improving the treatment of nosocomial pneumonias. With the aim to reduce mortality, it seems reasonable that future studies concerning nosocomial pneumonias should examine the determinants of infection and define "high risk" patients in whom it will be possible to show the potential benefit of prophylactic or therapeutic measures.

Acknowledgements. The authors wish to thank Catherine Brun and Christelle Largenton for their invaluable help in the preparation of the manuscript.

References

1. Abraham SN, Beachey EH, Simpson WA. Adherence of *Streptococcus pyogenes, Escherichia coli* and *Pseudomonas aeruginosa* to fibronectin-coated and uncoated epithelial cells. Infect Immun 1983;41:1261–1268.
2. Andrews CP, Coalson JJ, Smith JD, et al. Diagnosis of nosocomial bacterial pneumonia in acute diffuse lung injury. Chest 1981;80:254–258.
3. Atherton ST, White DJ. Stomach as source of bacteria colonizing respiratory tract during artificial ventilation. Lancet 1978;ii:968–969.
4. Baigelman W, Bellins S, Cupples LA, Berenberg MJ. Bacteriologic assessment of the lower respiratory tract in intubated patients. Crit Care Med 1986;14:864–868.
5. Bartlett JG, Alexander J, Mayhew J, et al. Should fiberoptic bronchoscopy aspirates be cultured? Am Rev Respir Dis 1976;114:247–251.
6. Bartlett JG, O'Keefe P, Tally FP, Louie TJ, Gorbach SL. Bacteriology of hospital-acquired pneumonia. Arch Intern Med 1986;146:868–871.
7. Baughman RP, Thorpe JE, Staneck J, Rashkin M, Frame PT. Use of the protected specimen brush in patients with endotracheal or tracheostomy tubes. Chest 1987;91:233–236.
8. Bell RC, Coalson JJ, Smith JD, et al. Multiple organ system failure and infection in adult respiratory distress syndrome. Ann Intern Med 1983;99:293–298.
9. Berck SL, Verghese A, Holtsclaw SA, Smith JK. Enterococcal pneumonia. Occurrence in patients receiving broad-spectrum antibiotic regimens and enteral feeding. Am J Med 1983;74:153–154.
10. Bresalier RA, Grendell JH, Cello JP, Meyer AA. Sucralfate suspension versus titrated antiacids for the prevention of acute stress-related gastrointestinal hemorrhage in critically ill patients. Am J Med 1987;83:110–116.
11. Bryan CS, Reynolds KL. Bacteremic nosocomial pneumonia. Am Rev Respir Dis 1984;129:668–671.

12. Bundtzen RW, Gerger AU, Cohn DL, et al. Post-antibiotic suppression of bacterial growth. Rev Infect Dis 1981;3:28–37.

13. Celis R, Torres A, Gatell JH, Almela M, Rodriguez-Roisin R, Augusti-Vidal A. Nosocomial pneumonia. A multivariate analysis of risk and prognosis. Chest 1988;93:318–324.

14. Centers for Disease Control. National Nosocomial Infections Study Report. Annual Summary: 1984. MMWR 1986;35:17 SS-29 SS.

15. Chastre J, Fagon JY, Soler P, et al. Diagnosis of nosocomial bacterial pneumonia in intubated patients undergoing ventilation: comparison of the usefulness of bronchoalveolar lavage and the protected specimen brush. Am J Med 1988;85:499–506.

16. Chastre J, Fagon JY, Soler P, et al. Quantification of BAL cells containing intracellular bacteria rapidly identifies ventilated patients with nosocomial pneumonia. Chest 1989;95:190S–192S.

17. Chastre J, Viau F, Brun P, et al. Prospective evaluation of the protected specimen brush for the diagnosis of pulmonary infections in ventilated patients. Am Rev Respir Dis 1984;130:924–929.

18. Class I, Junginger W, Kloss T. Pseudomonas immunoglobin in surgical intensive care patients on mechanical ventilation. Infection 1987;15:S67–S70.

19. Cordes LG, Wiesenthal DS, Gorman GW, et al. Isolation of *Legionella pneumophila* from hospital shower heads. Ann Intern Med 1981;94:195–197.

20. Craig CP, Connelly S. Effect of intensive care unit nosocomial pneumonia on duration of stay and mortality. Am J Infect Control 1984;12:233–238.

21. Craven DE, Daschner FD. Nosocomial pneumonia in the intubated patient: role of gastric colonization. Eur J Clin Microbiol Infect Dis 1989;8:40–50.

22. Craven DE, Driks MR. Pneumonia in the intubated patient. Semin Respir Infect 1987;2:20–33.

23. Craven DE, Kunches LM, Kilinski V, Lichtenberg DA, Make BJ, McCabe WR. Risk factors for pneumonia and fatality in patients receiving continuous mechanical ventilation. Am Rev Respir Dis 1986;133:792–796.

24. Cross AS, Roup B. Role of respiratory assistance devices in endemic nosocomial pneumonia. Am J Med 1981;70:681–685.

25. Daschner F, Kappstein L, Engels I, et al. Stress ulcer prophylaxis and ventilation pneumonia: prevention by antibacterial cytoprotective agents. Infect Control Hosp Epidemiol 1988;9:59–65.

26. Donowitz GL, Page ML, Mileur BL, Guenthner SH. Alteration of normal gastric flora in critical care patients receiving antiacid and cimetidine therapy. Infect Control 1986;7:23–26.

27. Drasar BS, Shiner M. Studies of the intestinal flora. II. Bacterial flora of the small intestine in patients with gastrointestinal disorders. Gut 1969;10:812–819.

28. Dreyfuss D, Djedaini K, Weber P, et al. Prospective study of nosocomial pneumonia and of patient and circuit colonization during mechanical ventilation with circuit changes every 48 hours versus no change. Am Rev Respir Dis 1991;143:738–743.

29. Driks MR, Craven DE, Celli BR, et al. Nosocomial pneumonia in intubated patients given sucralfate as compared with antiacids or histamine type 2 blockers. N Engl J Med 1987;317:1376–1382.

30. Du Moulin GC, Hedley-Whyte J, Paterson DG, Libson A. Aspiration of gastric bacteria in antiacid-treated patients, a frequent cause of postoperative colonization of the airway. Lancet 1982;i:242–245.

31. Edmondson EB, Reinarz JA, Pierce AK, Sanford JP. Nebulization equipment. A potential source of infection in gram-negative pneumonias. Am J Dis Child 1966;111:357–360.

32. Eickhoff JC. Pulmonary infections in surgical patients. Surg Clin North Am 1980;60:175–183.

33. Fagon JY, Chastre J, Domart Y, et al. Nosocomial pneumonia in patients receiving continuous mechanical ventilation. Prospective analysis of 52 episodes with use of a protected specimen brush and quantitative culture techniques. Am Rev Respir Dis 1989;139:877–884.

34. Fagon JY, Chastre J, Hance A, et al. Detection of nosocomial lung infection in ventilated patients. Use of a protected specimen brush and quantitative culture techniques in 147 patients. Am Rev Respir Dis 1988;138:110–116.

35. Feeley TW, Du Moulin GC, Hedley-Whyte J, Bushnell LS, Gilbert JP, Feingold DS, et al. Aerosol polymyxin and pneumonia in seriously ill patients. N Engl J Med 1975;293:471–475.

36. Fitzgerald JM, Cook KJ, Oxman A, et al. The role of the protected brush catheter and bronchoalveolar lavage in the diagnosis of pneumonia [Abstract]. Am Rev Respir Dis 1991;143; A108.

37. Freeman J, Rosner BA, McGowan JE. Adverse effect of nosocomial infections. J Infect Dis 1979;140:732–740.

38. Garibaldi RA, Britt MR, Coleman ML, et al. Risk factors for postoperative pneumonia. Am J Med 1987;70:677–680.

39. Gerber AU, Vastola AP, Brandel J, et al. Selection of aminoglycoside-resistant variants of *Pseudomonas aeruginosa* in an *in vivo* model. J Infect Dis 1982;146:691–697.

40. Girod JC, Reichman RC, Winn WC Jr, Klaucke DN, Vogt RL, Dolin R. Pneumonic and nonpneumonic forms of Legionnellosis. Arch Intern Med 1982;142:545–547.

41. Glezen WP. Viral pneumonia as a cause and result of hospitalization. J Infect Dis 1983;147:765–770.

42. Goularte TA, Lichtenberg DA, Craven DE. Gastric colonization in patients receiving antiacids and mechanical ventilation: a mechanism for pharyngeal colonization. Am J Infect Control 1986;14:88–92.

43. Gray JD, Shiner M. Influence of gastric pH on gastric and jejunal flora. Gut 1967;8:574–581.

44. Graybill JR, Marshall LW, Charache P, Wallace CR, Melvin VB. Nosocomial pneumonia. A continuing major problem. Am Rev Respir Dis 1973;108:1130–1140.

45. Greenfield S, Teres D, Bushnell CS, et al. Prevention of gram-negative bacillary pneumonia

using aerosol polymixin as prophylaxis. J Clin Invest 1973;52:2935–2940.

46. Gross PA, Neu HC, Aswapokee P, et al. Deaths from nosocomial infections: experience in a university hospital and a community hospital. Am J Med 1980;68:219–223.

47. Hemming VG, Overall JC Jr, Britt MR. Nosocomial infections in a newborn intensive care unit. N Engl J Med 1976;294:1310–1316.

48. Higuchi JH, Coalson JJ, Johanson WG Jr. Bacteriologic diagnosis of nosocomial pneumonia in primates. Usefulness of the protected specimen brush. Am Rev Respir Dis 1982;125:53–57.

49. Huxley EJ, Viroslav J, Gray WR, Pierce AK. Pharyngeal aspiration in normal adults and patients with depressed consciousness. Am J Med 1978;64:564–568.

50. Jimenez P, Torres A, Rodriguez-Roisin R et al. Incidence and etiology of pneumonia acquired during mechanical ventilation. Crit Care Med 1989;17:882–885.

51. Johanson WG Jr, Higuchi JC, Chaudhuri TR, Woods DE. Bacterial adherence to epithelial cells in bacillary colonization of the respiratory tract. Am Rev Respir Dis 1980;121:55–63.

52. Johanson WG Jr, Pierce AK, Sanford JP. Changing pharyngeal bacterial flora of hospitalized patients. N Engl J Med 1969;281:1137–1140.

53. Johanson WG Jr, Pierce AK, Sanford JP, et al. Nosocomial respiratory infections with gram-negative bacilli. Ann Intern Med 1972;77:701–706.

54. Johanson WG Jr, Seidenfeld JJ, Gomez P, De Los Santos R, Coalson JJ. Bacteriologic diagnosis of nosocomial pneumonia following prolonged mechanical ventilation. Am Rev Respir Dis 1988;137:259–264.

55. Johanson WG Jr, Woods DE, Chaudhuri TR. Association of respiratory tract colonization with adherence of gram-negative bacilli to epithelial cells. J Infect Dis 1979;139:667–673.

56. Kahn FW, Jones JM. Diagnosing bacterial respiratory infection by bronchoalveolar lavage. J Infect Dis 1987;155:862–869.

57. Kerver AJH, Rommes JH, Mevissen-Verhage EAE, Hulstaert PF, Vos A, Verhoef J. Colonization and infection in surgical intensive care patients. A prospective study. Intensive Care Med 1987;13:347–351.

58. Kirby BD, Snyder KM, Meyer RD, Finegold SM. Legionnaire's disease: report of sixty-five nosocomially acquired cases and review of the literature. Medicine (Baltimore) 1980;59:188–200.

59. Klastersky J, Hensgens C, Noterman J, Mouawad E, Meunier-Carpentier F. Endotracheal antibiotics for the prevention of tracheobronchial infections in tracheotomized unconscious patients. A comparative study of gentamicin and aminoside-polymixin B combination. Chest 1975;68:302–306.

60. Klastersky J, Huysmans E, Weerts D, et al. Endotracheally administered gentamicin for prevention of infections of the respiratory tract in patients with tracheostomy. A double-blind study. Chest 1974;65:650–654.

61. Klastersky J, Meunier-Carpentier F, Kahan-Cop-

pens L, et al. Endotracheally administered antibiotics for gram-negative bronchopneumonia. Chest 1979;75:586–591.

62. LaForce FM. Hospital-acquired gram-negative rod pneumonias: an overview. Am J Med 1981;70:664–669.

63. Langer T, Mosconi P, Cigada M, Mandelli M, and the Intensive Care Unit Group of Infection Control. Long-term respiratory support and the risk of pneumonia in critically ill patients. Am Rev Respir Dis 1987;140:302–305.

64. Larson E, McGinley KJ, Grove GL, Ceyden JJ, Talbot GH. Physiologic, microbiologic, and seasonal effects of handwashing on the skin of health care personnel. Am J Infect Control 1986;14:51–59.

65. Le Frock JL, Ellia CA, Weinstein L. The relation between aerobic fecal and oropharyngeal microflora in hospitalized patients. Am J Med Sci 1979;277:275–280.

66. Leu Hsieh-Shong, Kaiser DL, Mori M, Woolson RF, Wenzel RP. Hospital-acquired pneumonia. Attributable mortality and morbidity. Am J Epidemiol 1989;129:1258–1267.

67. Levison ME, Kaye D. Pneumonia caused by gram-negative bacilli: an overview. Rev Infect Dis 1985;7:S 656–S 665.

68. Louria DB, Kaminski T. The effects of four antimicrobial drug regimens on sputum superinfection in hospitalized patients. Am Rev Respir Dis 1962;85:649–665.

69. Maki DG, Alvarado CJ, Hassemer CA, Zilz MA. Relation of the inanimate hospital environment to endemic nosocomial infection. N Engl J Med 1982;25:1562–1566.

70. Mandel LA, Nicolle LE, Ronald AK. A multicenter prospective randomized trial comparing ceftazidime with cefazolin/tobramycin in the treatment of hospitalized patients with non-pneumococcal pneumonia. J Antimicrob Chemother 1983;12:S 9–S 20.

71. Mangi RJ, Greco T, Ryan J, Thornton G, Andriole VT. Cefoperazone versus combination antibiotic therapy of hospital-acquired pneumonia. Am J Med 1988;84:68–74.

72. Meduri GU, Beals DH, Maijub AG, Buselski V. Protected bronchoalveolar lavage. A new bronchoscopic technique to retrieve uncontaminated distal airway secretions. Am Rev Respir Dis 1991;143:855–864.

73. Moser KM, Maurer J, Jassy L, et al. Sensitivity, specificity, and risk of diagnostic procedures in a canine model of *Streptococcus pneumoniae* pneumonia. Am Rev Respir Dis 1982;25:436–442.

74. Niederman MS, Merrill WM, Ferranti RD, Pagano KM, Palmer LB, Reynolds HY. Nutritional status and bacterial binding in the lower respiratory tract in patients with chronic tracheostomy. Ann Intern Med 1984;100:795–800.

75. Niederman MS, Rafferty TS, Sasaki CT, Merrill WM, Matthay RA, Reynolds HY. Comparison of bacterial adherence to ciliated and squamous epithelial cells obtained from the human respiratory tract. Am Rev Respir Dis 1983;127:85–90.

76. Olivares L, Segovia A, Revuelta R. Tube feeding

and lethal aspiration in neurological patients: a review of 720 autopsy cases. Stroke 1974;5:654–656.

77. Pennington JE. Penetration of antibiotics into respiratory secretions. Rev Infect Dis 1981;3:67–73.

78. Pennington JE. Nosocomial respiratory infection. In: Mandell GL, Douglas RG Jr, Bennett JE, eds. Principles and practice of infectious diseases. 3rd ed. New York: Churchill Livingstone, 1990:2199–2205.

79. Pham LH, Brun Buisson C, Legrand P, et al. Diagnosis of nosocomial pneumonia in mechanically ventilated patients. Comparison of a plugged telescoping catheter with the protected specimen brush. Am Rev Respir Dis 1991;143:1055–1061.

80. Pierce AK, Sanford JP. Bacterial contamination of aerosols. Arch Intern Med 1973;131:156–159.

81. Pierce AK, Sanford JP. Aerobic gram-negative bacillary pneumonias. Am Rev Respir Dis 1974;110:647–658.

82. Pierce AK, Sanford JP, Thomas GD, et al. Long-term evaluation of decontamination of inhalation-therapy equipment and the occurrence of necrotizing pneumonia. N Engl J Med 1970;282:528–531.

83. Pingleton SK, Hinthorn DP, Liu C. Enteral nutrition in patients receiving mechanical ventilation: multiple sources of tracheal colonization include the stomach. Am J Med 1986;80:827–830.

84. Pugin J, Auckenthaler R, Mili N, et al. Diagnosis of ventilator-associated pneumonia by bacteriologic analysis of bronchoscopic and nonbronchoscopic "blind" bronchoalveolar lavage fluid. Am Rev Respir Dis 1991;143:1121–1129.

85. Ramphal R, Pyle M. Evidence for mucins and sialic acid as receptors for *Pseudomonas aeruginosa* in the lower respiratory tract. Infect Immun 1983;44:38–40.

86. Ramsay G, Reidy JJ. Selective digestive decontamination in intensive care practice: a review of clinical experience. Intensive Care Med 1990;10:S 217–S 223.

87. Rapp RP, Young B, Foster TS, Tibbs PA, O'Neal W. Ceftazidime versus tobramycin/ticarcillin in treating hospital-acquired pneumonia and bacteremia. Pharmacology 1984;4:211–215.

88. Reynolds HY. Bacterial adherence to respiratory tract mucosa. A dynamic interaction leading to colonization. Semin Respir Infect 1987;2:8–19.

89. Rigaud D, Chastre J, Accary JP, Bonfils S, Gibert C, Hance AJ. Intragastric pH profile during acute respiratory failure in patients with chronic obstructive pulmonary disease; effects of ranitidine and enteral feeding. Chest 1986;90:58–60.

90. Rodriguez de Castro F, Violan JS, Lafarga Capuz B, et al. Reliability of the bronchoscopic protected catheter brush in the diagnosis of pneumonia in mechanically ventilated patients. Crit Care Med 1991;19:171–175.

91. Rose RM. Pulmonary macrophages in nosocomial pneumonia: defense function and dysfunction, and prospects for activation. Eur J Microbiol Infect Dis 1989;8:25–28.

92. Rouby JJ, Rossignon MD, Nicolas MH, et al. A prospective study of the protected bronchoalveolar lavage in the diagnosis of nosocomial pneumonia. Anesthesiology 1989;71:679–685.

93. Ruddell WSJ, Axon ATR, Findlay JM, Bartholomew BA, Hill MJ. Effects of cimetidine on the gastric bacterial flora. Lancet 1980;i:672–674.

94. Salata RA, Lederman MM, Shlaes DM, et al. Diagnosis of nosocomial pneumonia in intubated intensive care unit patients. Am Rev Respir Dis 1987;135:426–432.

95. Scentag JJ, Vari AJ, Winslade NE, et al. Treatment with aztreonam or tobramycin in critical care patients with nosocomial gram-negative rod pneumonia. Am J Med 1985;78:34–41.

96. Schwartz SN, Dowling JN, Benkovic C, De Quittner-Buchanan M, Prostko T, Yee RB. Sources of gram-negative bacilli colonizing the tracheae of intubated patients. J Infect Dis 1978;138:227–231.

97. Shirani KZ, McManus AT, Vaughan GM, McManus WF, Pruitt BA, Mason AD. Effects of environment on infection in burn patients. Arch Surg 1986;121:31–36.

98. Simmons BP, Wong ES. Guidelines for prevention of nosocomial pneumonia. Infect Control 1982;3:327–333.

99. Simon HB, Soutwick TS, Moellering RC, Sherman E. *Haemophilus influenzae* in hospitalized adults: current perspectives. Am J Med 1980;69:219–226.

100. Stamm WE, Martin SM, Bennett JV. Epidemiology of nosocomial infections due to gram-negative bacilli. Aspects relevant to development and use of vaccines. J Infect Dis 1977;136:S151–S160.

101. Stevens RM, Teres D, Skillman JJ, et al. Pneumonia in an intensive care unit. Arch Intern Med 1974;134:106–111.

102. Tafuro P, Ristuccia P. Recognition and control of outbreaks of nosocomial infections in the intensive care setting. Heart Lung 1984;13:486–494.

103. Thorpe JE, Baughman RP, Frame PT, et al. Bronchoalveolar lavage for diagnosing acute bacterial pneumonia. J Infect Dis 1987;155:855–861.

104. Tillotson JR, Finland M. Bacterial colonization and clinical superinfection of the respiratory tract complicating antibiotic treatment of pneumonia. J Infect Dis 1969;119:597–624.

105. Tillotson JR, Lerner AM. Characteristics of nonbacteremic Pseudomonas pneumonia. Ann Intern Med 1968;118:295–307.

106. Toews GB. Role of the polymorphonuclear leukocyte: interaction with nosocomial pathogens. Eur J Clin Microbiol Infect Dis 1989;8:21–24.

107. Torres A, Aznar R, Gatell JM, et al. Incidence, risk and prognosis factors of nosocomial pneumonia in mechanically ventilated patients. Am Rev Respir Dis 1990;142:523–528.

108. Torres A, Jimenez P, Puig de la Bellacasa J, et al. Diagnostic value of nonfluoroscopic percutaneous lung needle aspiration in patients with pneumonia. Chest 1990;98:840–844.

109. Torres A, Puig de la Bellacasa J, Rodriguez-Roisin R, Jimenez DE, Anta MT, Agusti-Vidal

A. Diagnostic value of telescoping plugged catheters in mechanically ventilated patients with bacterial pneumonia using the Metras catheter. Am Rev Respir Dis 1988;138:117–120.

110. Torres A, Puig de la Bellacasa J, Xaubert A, et al. Diagnostic value of quantitative cultures of bronchoalveolar lavage and telescoping plugged catheters in mechanically ventilated patients with bacterial pneumonia. Am Rev Respir Dis 1989;140:306–310.

111. Torzillo PJ, McWilliam DB, Young IH, Woog RH, Benn R. Use of protected telescoping brush system in the management of bacterial pulmonary infection in intubated patients. Br J Dis Chest 1985;79:125–131.

112. Trouillet JL, Guiguet M, Gibert C, et al. Fiberoptic bronchoscopy in ventilated patients. Evaluation of cardiopulmonary risk under midazolam sedation. Chest 1990;97:927–933.

113. Tryba M, Zevounou F, Torok M, Zenz M. Prevention of acute stress bleeding with sucralfate, antiacids, or cimetidine. Am J Med 1985;79:S55–S61.

114. Valenti WM, Hall CB, Douglas RG Jr, Menegus MA, Pincus PH. Nosocomial viral infections 1. Epidemiology and significance. Infect Control 1979;1:33–37.

115. Valenti WM, Trudell RG, Bentley DW. Risk factors predisposing to oropharyngeal colonization with gram-negative bacilli in the aged. N Engl J Med 1978;298:1108–1111.

116. Van der Waaij D, Manson WL, Arends JP, de Vries-Hospers HG. Clinical use of selective decontamination: the concept. Intensive Care Med 1990;16:S212–S215.

117. Van Saene HKF, Stoutenbeek CP, Gilbertson AA. Review of available trials of selective decontamination of the digestive tract (SDD). Infection 1990;18:S5–S9.

118. Vial WC, Toews GB, Pierce AK. Early pulmonary granulocytes recruitment in response to *Streptococcus pneumoniae*. Am Rev Respir Dis 1984;129:87–91.

119. Villers D, Derriennic M, Raffi F, et al. Reliability of the bronchoscopy protected catheter brush in intubated and ventilated patients. Chest 1985;88:527–530.

120. Wenzel RP, Deal EA, Hendley JO. Hospital-acquired viral respiratory illness on a pediatric ward. Pediatrics 1977;60:367–371.

121. Wiklund PE. Intensive care units: design, location, staffing ancillary areas, equipment. Anesthesiology 1969; 31:122–136.

122. Wimberley N, Faling LJ, Bartlett JG. A fiberoptic bronchoscopy technique to obtain uncontaminated lower airway secretions for bacterial culture. Am Rev Respir Dis 1979;119:337–343.

123. Woods DE, Straus DC, Johanson WG Jr, Bass JA. Role of fibronectin in the prevention of adherence of *Pseudomonas aeruginosa* to buccal cells. J Infect Dis 1981;143:784–790.

124. Woods DE, Straus DC, Johanson WG Jr, Berry VK, Bass JA. Role of pili in adherence of *Pseudomonas aeruginosa* to mammalian buccal epithelial cells. Infect Immun 1980;29:1146 1151.

125. Zavala DC, Schoell JE. Ultrathin needle aspiration of the lung in infectious and malignant diseases. Am Rev Respir Dis 1981;123:125–131.

126. Zucker A, Pollack M, Kate R. Blind use of the double-lumen plugged catheter for diagnosis of respiratory tract infections in critically ill children. Crit Care Med 1984;12:867–870.

34

Etiology and Pathophysiology of Acute Renal Failure

Maria Valentina Pellanda
Aldo Fabris
Claudio Ronco

Acute renal failure is a clinical situation in which renal function decreases rapidly and produces progressive elevation of BUN and nitrogen waste products. Anuria, which was a pathognomonic aspect of acute renal failure in the past, is less common today, probably because of a more aggressive and early approach to critically ill patients or because of increased prevalence of drug-induced acute renal failure (1). Acute renal failure, defined as a sudden reversible impairment of renal function, can be generated by prerenal, renal, or postrenal pathologic events. In prerenal azotemia, the decrease of glomerular filtration rate is substantially caused by renal hypoperfusion without structural damage of the kidney. This event can generally be reversed upon restoration of renal blood flow. On the contrary, intrinsic renal failure is a syndrome caused by parenchymal damages. Virtually any renal insult may result in the acute renal failure syndrome, but some circumstances can be commonly identified: (a) forms resulting from renal hypoperfusion (evolution of prerenal azotemia); (b) forms secondary to poisons or nephrotoxins; (c) acute interstitial nephritis, in which a decrease in glomerular filtration rate results from interstitial inflam-mation, (d) acute glomerulonephritis or vasculitis; and (e) acute renovascular disease.

In postrenal azotemia (or acute obstructive uropathy), the decrease of glomerular filtration rate results from an obstruction in the urinary collecting system. This classification represents a schematization of pathologic derangements that can have a clinical overlapping. For example, prerenal azotemia and acute intrinsic renal failure represent two extremes of a spectrum of renal hypoperfusion syndromes (10); on the other hand, obstructive uropathy may sometimes cause significant changes in renal hemodynamics so as to produce remarkable organic damage. Preexisting conditions associated with reduced renal perfusion present an elevated risk of acute renal failure when patients are exposed to a potentially nephrotoxic drug or to renal ischemia (14).

The risk of renal failure is increased in the following situations: extracellular fluid volume depletion that produces reduced cardiac output, diminishes renal perfusion, and increases proximal tubular reabsorption of potentially nephrotoxic agents; severe generalized atherosclerotic disease that may reduce renal perfusion by occlusion of blood vessels; myocardial dysfunction and congestive heart failure that result in diminished cardiac output and renal hypoperfusion; and advanced age, in cases of reduced renal plasma flow and glomerular filtration rate.

ETIOLOGY OF ACUTE RENAL FAILURE

Prerenal Azotemia

In prerenal azotemia, the cause of acute azotemia is a combination of hypotension, hypovolemia, and diminished renal perfusion. Hypovolemia may result from hemorrhage (traumatic, postpartum, gastrointestinal, surgical) or fluid losses in extensive burns, vomiting, diarrhea, diuretic abuse, adrenal insufficiency, or fluid sequestration in case of pancreatitis, peritonitis, traumatized tissues, or diabetic ketoacidosis. Another important cause of prerenal azotemia is decreased cardiac output resulting from impaired cardiac function, as observed in congestive heart failure; myocardial infarction, pericardial tamponade, and acute pulmonary embolism. Peripheral vasodilation occurring in bacteremia and during antihypertensive drug excess may also cause renal hypoperfusion, as well as the increased renal vascular resistance observed in anesthesia, surgical operations, and hepatorenal syndrome. Acute pathologic events such as bilateral renal vascular obstruction occurring in dissecting aneurysma of aorta and embolism or thrombosis of renal artery or renal vein can be a less common cause of transient prerenal azotemia, resulting more frequently in severe organic parenchymal damage.

All these causes of diminished renal perfusion activate compensatory systemic and renal responses, including activation of autonomic nervous system, renin-angiotensin system, ADH release, and increased tubular reabsorption of sodium and water (Fig. 34.1). The small amount of urine formed is very poor in sodium and is highly concentrated; usually urine osmolality is greater than 500 mOsm/kg and urinary sodium is less than 20 mEq/liter. Finally, there are situations of normal glomerular filtration rate in which elevated azotemia is observed; this generally occurs in cases of increased urea production after both large protein intake and increased protein catabolism (fever, severe illness, steroids, tetracyclins, surgery). It is still controversial, however, whether prerenal azotemia may occur with completely normal kidney function or at least a small reduction of the renal functional reserve must be present.

In the case of gastrointestinal bleeding, there is enhanced protein reabsorption associated with intravascular volume depletion and this may represent a further cause of acute azotemia in the absence of renal parenchymal damage (10).

Parenchymal Diseases Causing Acute Renal Failure

Intrinsic acute renal failure can be caused by different parenchymal diseases that can be classified in groups: ischemic, toxic, and those affecting interstitium, renal blood vessels, or glomeruli. Such a division is not sharp because frequent overlapping of these groups is observed and mixed pathologic mechanisms can be present. For example, acute tubular necrosis results from renal ischemia, nephrotoxins, or a combination of both (10). Ischemic causes of intrinsic renal failure include all the causes of renal hypoperfusion observed in prerenal azotemia. Depending on the severity and duration of renal ischemia, the disease can progress from the functional derangements of prerenal azotemia to the organic lesions of acute tubular necrosis: the more severe and prolonged is renal hypoperfusion, the less is the possibility of recovery at restoration of renal blood flow. Toxic causes of acute renal failure may be divided into exogenous and endogenous. Exogenous nephrotoxins include antibiotics, anesthetics, analgesics, immunosuppressive agents, contrast media, organic solvents, heavy metals, and other substances. Endogenous toxins include calcium, uric acid, myoglobin, hemoglobin, bilirubin, oxalate crystals, products of tumor lysis, and paraproteins (Fig. 34.2).

Interstitial causes of acute renal failure include infections, tumoral infiltration, and hypersensitivity reactions to drugs (Fig 34.3).

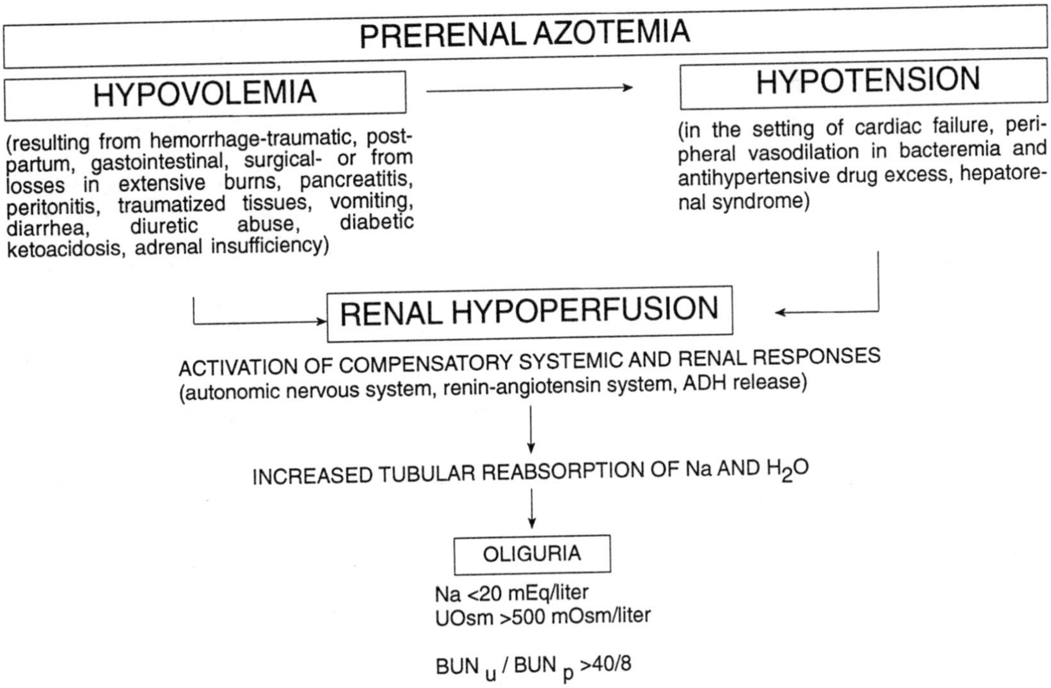

Figure 34.1. Mechanisms of prerenal azotemia.

EXOGENOUS NEPHROTOXINS

antibiotics: aminoglycosides, cephalosporins sulfonamide, tetracyclines, amphotericin B

anesthetic agents: methoxyflurane, enflurane

analgesics: aspirin, ibuprofen, naproxen, indomethacin, piroxicam, pyrazolones, phenazone, phenacetin, glaphenine

chemotherapeutic and immunosuppressive agents: *cis*-platinum, methotrexate, mitomycin, 5·azacytidine, nitrosoureas, cyclosporin A

contrast media: diatrizoate, Iothalamate, bunamiodyl, iopanoic acid

organic solvents: carbon tetrachloride, tetra- and trichloroethylene, ethylene glycol, diethylene glycol, aromatic hydrocarbons and aliphatic-aromatic hydrocarbons

heavy metals: antimony, arsenic, bismuth, barium, cadmium, copper, gold, iron, lead, lithium, mercury, silver, uranium, thallium, chrome, platinum

miscellaneous: insecticides (chlordane), herbicides (paraquat, diquat), rodenticide-containing elemental phosphorus, mushroom (i.e., *Cortinarius* genus), aniline, cresol, chlorates, potassium bromate, etc.

ENDOGENOUS NEPHROTOXINS

Calcium, (hypercalcemia)
uric acid (hyperuricemia and hyperuricosuria)
myoglobin (rhabdomyolysis)
hemoglobin (hemolysis)
bilirubin (obstructive jaundice)
oxalate crystals
paraproteins

Figure 34.2. Toxic causes of acute renal failure.

Infections: bacterial (i.e., *E. coli, Staphylococcus, Proteus*, etc.), fungal (i.e., *Candida albicans*, etc.) or viral (i.e., Hantaan virus, etc.)

Tumoral infiltration: lymphoma, leukemia, myeloma

Systemic disorders: sarcoidosis, systemic lupus erythematosus, Sjögren's syndrome

Hypersensitivity reactions to drugs: penicillin, methicillin, ampicillin, cephalotin, rifampin, sulfonamides, fenoprofen, naproxen, ibuprofen, indometacin, meclofenamate, phenylbutazone, phenazone, aspirin, diflunisal, paracetamol, glafenin, sulfinpyrazone, D-penicillamine, cimetidine, phenindione, diphenylhydantoin, phenytoin, phenobarbital, carbamazepine, interferon, thiazides, furosemide, allopurinol, azathioprine, captopril, clofibrate, amphetamine, α-methyldopa

Figure 34.3. Interstitial causes of acute renal failure.

Diseases of glomeruli and small blood vessels that may cause acute renal failure include acute postinfectious glomerulonephritis, rapidly progressive glomerulonephritis, Goodpasture's syndrome, systemic lupus erythematosus, polyarteritis nodosa and related disorders, Henoch-Schönlein purpura, hemolytic-uremic syndrome, serum sickness, malignant hypertension, and toxemia of pregnancy.

There is a prevalence of hemodynamically induced forms of acute renal failure that represent about 50% of all the cases, followed by nephrotoxin-induced cases, which may represent more than 20% of all the cases.

Postrenal Azotemia

In postrenal azotemia (or obstructive uropathy), renal failure results from obstruction of the urinary collecting system (Fig. 34.4). It occurs in 2–5% of all cases of acute renal failure. Obstruction may occur at various levels of the urinary tract. Bilateral ureteral obstructions or unilateral obstruction in a single functioning kidney are often characterized by abrupt onset of anuria. Ureteral obstruction may be secondary to intraureteral causes (stones, blood clots, edema, papillary necrosis, fungal balls, stricture) or to extraureteral causes (tumors of pelvic organs, periureteral fibrosis, retroperitoneal hemorrhage, acciden-

tal ureteral ligation during pelvic surgery). Obstruction at the level of the bladder neck may be due to organic factors, such as stones, clots, bladder carcinoma and infections, prostatic hypertrophy or malignancy, or to functional ones. Functional forms may be due to neurogenic factors or effects of ganglionic blocking agents. Obstruction may occur also at urethral level as a consequence of congenital valve, stricture, phimosis or tumors.

From a pathophysiologic point of view, acute severe obstruction has a much more rapid and severe effect on the glomerular filtration rate than slowly progressive partial obstruction does. The mechanism whereby obstruction influences glomerular filtration rate is complex. Studies in animals show that obstruction determines a rapid increase in intraureteral pressure so as to decrease the pressure gradient through the glomerular capillary wall with consequent reduction of glomerular filtra-

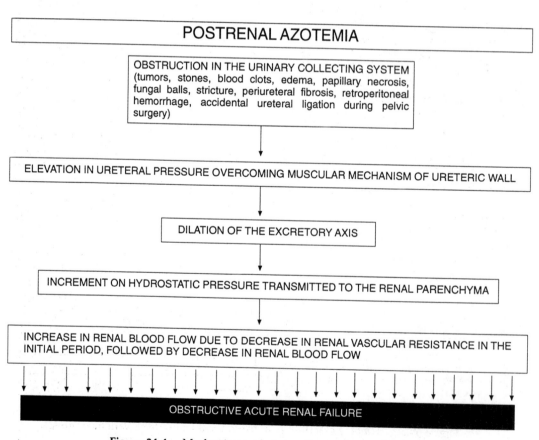

Figure 34.4. Mechanisms of obstructive acute renal failure.

tion rate. Because about 12 hours after obstruction the intraluminal pressure comes back to normal, hemodynamic modifications play an important role in the pathogenesis of obstructive uropathy (2, 32). An increase in renal blood flow has been observed experimentally in the initial period after obstruction due to a decrease in renal vascular resistance and a redistribution of blood flow to the inner cortical nephrons. This effect may be due to increased production of the potent renal vasodilator prostaglandin E_2 in the affected kidney. If obstruction persists, renal blood flow decreases. Several studies in animals emphasize the role of the renin-angiotensin system and intrarenal production of vasoconstrictory substances such as thromboxane A_2 that are responsible for glomerular filtration rate reduction in spite of a return of the intraluminal pressure to normal.

In conclusion, even though several causes have been demonstrated for this syndrome, all mechanisms involved in the pathogenesis of acute renal failure may activate a final pathologic cascade that leads to oliguria and organic damage with a similar clinical pattern (Fig. 34.5).

Diagnostic Criteria in Acute Renal Failure and Differential Diagnosis

History

To differentiate acute and chronic renal failure, and prerenal or postrenal and parenchymal forms, one has to investigate previous renal function tests and blood pressure determinations, extrarenal fluid losses, exposure to nephrotoxins, presence of heart failure, diuretic therapy, symptoms related to the genitourinary tract, or recent pelvic surgery.

Physical Examination

This type of examination must be very accurate. To determine the presence or absence of prerenal and postrenal causes of acute renal failure, one must seek signs

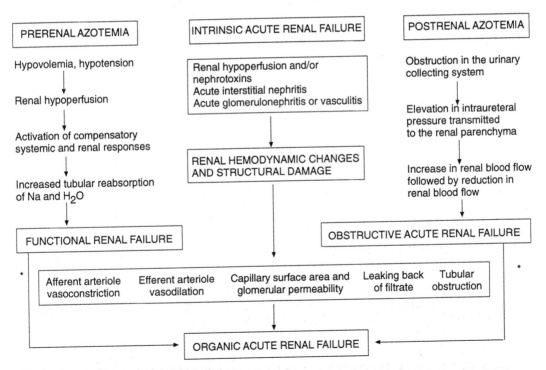

Figure 34.5. Pathologic pathways of acute renal failure from various origins.

*Depending on severity and duration of injury.

of volume depletion such as orthostatic decreases in arterial pressure, increases in pulse rate, decreased skin turgor, or signs of cardiac dysfunction, or bladder distension, flank mass due to distended renal pelvis, or signs of rectal or pelvic disorders. Physical examination must also be carried out to try to discover symptoms and signs typical of other syndromes and diseases involving the kidney such as systemic lupus, vasculitis, arthritis, infectious diseases, neoplasms, and myeloma.

Urinalysis

A normal urinalysis in the setting of acute renal failure suggests the presence of either prerenal azotemia or obstructive uropathy, whereas heavy proteinuria suggests the presence of vasculitis or glomerulonephritis. Urinary sediment containing few formed elements or hyaline casts suggests prerenal azotemia or obstructive uropathy. Red blood cells and red blood cell casts suggest the presence of glomerular or vascular inflammatory disease and are rarely seen in acute interstitial nephritis. Large numbers of polymorphonuclear leukocytes are typical of acute diffuse pyelonephritis or papillary necrosis, while eosinophils are commonly found in acute allergic interstitial nephritis.

Urinary Volume

The sudden onset of anuria or the fluctuation in urine volume are typical of obstructive uropathy. Oliguria (urinary volume less than 400 ml/day) is a pathognomonic index of renal failure even though nonoliguric forms are more common today than in the past. Many authors have investigated the cause of the increasing frequency of nonoliguric forms of acute renal failure. This has supposedly depended on an early and improved supportive management of seriously ill and traumatized patients, on the extensive use of potent diuretic agents and renal vasodilators particularly after open heart surgery, and finally on the increased incidence of acute renal failure due to nephrotoxic effects of drugs such as aminoglycosides (1).

Urine Chemistry

The kidney responds to hypoperfusion by avidly retaining salt and water with emission of urine that may reach 1030 of specific gravity. In acute intrinsic renal failure, when the kidney is unable to concentrate or dilute the urine, urinary-specific gravity is 1.010 (like that of serum). Urine osmolality is a reliable index of concentrating ability; values greater than 500 mOsm/liter suggest prerenal azotemia, while urine osmolality less than 350 mOsm/liter is found in parenchymal acute renal failure. Urinary sodium is a useful marker to distinguish prerenal azotemia from parenchymal forms: urinary sodium less than 20 mEq/liter is typical of prerenal azotemia.

Diagnostic Indices

The urine/plasma creatinine ratio is a possible diagnostic index: values greater than 40 are encountered in most prerenal acute renal failure, while low values (less than 20) are more frequent in parenchymal acute renal failure. Some patients may have intermediate values and the diagnosis cannot be made on the basis of this index. Furthermore, the sensitivity and specificity of this index are quite limited. The renal failure index (i.e., urinary sodium/([urinary creatinine/plasma creatinine]) represents a further possible diagnostic parameter: values less than 1 are found in prerenal azotemia, but not in parenchymal acute renal failure. The fractional excretion of sodium, i.e., the clearance of sodium expressed as a percentage of glomerular filtration rate, is a reliable index to distinguish prerenal azotemia (fractional excretion of sodium less than 1%) from acute tubular necrosis. Fractional excrement of sodium less than 1% also occurs in the hepatorenal syndrome, in acute renal failure due to nonsteroidal antiinflammatory agents or iodinated contrast media, in septic shock, glomerulonephritis, thrombotic thrombocytopenic purpura, and in early obstructive uropathy (Fig. 34.6) (7, 17, 42).

Diagnostic Imaging

Different forms of acute renal failure can be identified by imaging procedures. Renal

URINARY CHEMICAL INDICES IN PRERENAL AZO-
TEMIA

Urinary specific gravity 1020
Urinary osmolality >500 mOsm/liter
U_{Na} <20 mEq/liter
RFI <1
FeNa <1%

URINARY CHEMICAL INDICES IN PARENCHYMAL
ACUTE RENAL FAILURE

Urinary specific gravity 1010
Urinary osmolality <350 mOsm/liter
$U_{creatinine}/P_{creatinine}$ >40

>1% in acute tubular necrosis

FeNa   <1% in forms due to myoglobunuria,
iodinated contrast media, glomerulonephritis
thrombotic thrombocytopenic purpura

Figure 34.6. Urinary chemical indices.

ultrasonography is helpful in establishing renal size, the presence of calculi, and the presence or absence of hydronephrosis. It is not uncommon to observe obstructive uropathy without significant hydronephrosis; therefore, this finding is not necessary to make the diagnosis of obstruction. Intravenous urography should be generally avoided and, when necessary, cystoscopy and retrograde urography can be performed. Arteriography should be reserved for patients with suspected renal artery occlusion or polyarteritis, although a radionuclide scan may be just as useful and carries less morbidity. Finally, computerized tomography and nuclear magnetic resonance must be reserved for those cases in which the previous named examinations do not yield conclusive diagnoses.

Renal Biopsy

When the cause of acute renal failure is not clear and the syndrome appears to be prolonged, percutaneous biopsy is strongly indicated. This procedure must be carried out with special care to bleeding risk in patients with acute renal failure, but can be very useful to make the diagnosis of glomerulonephritis, cortical necrosis, tubular necrosis, vasculitis, or systemic disease.

PATHOPHYSIOLOGY OF ACUTE RENAL FAILURE

Renal Hypoperfusion, Vasoconstriction and Mechanisms of Decrease of Glomerular Filtration Rate Reduction

The susceptibility of the kidney to hypoperfusion is very high. This is particularly true in critically ill patients in whom hypotension, shock, or hypovolemia are often present, coupled with clinical situations requiring potentially dangerous therapies. The mortality, very high in these patients, may reach 80% in patients with respiratory failure and acute renal failure (4, 29). Other high-risk settings for the development of acute renal failure are surgical procedures on the abdominal aorta and open heart surgery (23, 37–39, 53). There is much literature dealing with experimental acute renal failure (8, 9, 11, 12, 15, 21, 30, 40, 43, 45, 46, 50, 51, 54); however, the animal models may not exactly mimic the human situation. Despite the many experimental studies that have been carried out, the pathogenetic role of different events occurring in human acute renal failure is not completely defined. Therefore, mechanisms such as afferent arteriole vasoconstriction, reduction in the capillary surface area, a decrease in glomerular permeability, efferent arteriole vasodilation, necrosis of cells lining the tubule and consequent leaking of the filtrate back into the renal interstitium, and tubular obstruction by cellular debris may act as a single factor or as a multifactorial event in the genesis of acute renal failure.

There are two major pathogenetic mechanisms of acute renal failure: vascular and tubular. Under normal circumstances, renal blood flow and glomerular filtration rate are relatively constant over a wide range of renal perfusion pressures, thanks to a phenomenon termed autoregulation. A decrease in renal perfusion pressure below the autoregulatory level can lead to a marked decrease in glomerular filtration rate. In 1947, Trueta et al. (49), studying acutely shocked animals, described striking changes in renal perfusion, suggestive of vasoconstriction. Arteriographic studies in shock patients with acute renal failure supported the original observation of intense vasoconstriction (8, 19). A decrease in the total renal blood flow can lead to a decrease in the driving force for filtration and a consequent decrease in glomerular filtration rate. Hemodynamic changes can impair glomerular filtration rate either by reducing the ultrafiltration coefficient with a parallel reduction of the filtering area, or by decreasing glomerular blood flow and glomerular capillary hydraulic pressure. Diminished glomerular capillary hydraulic pressure may result from a combination of afferent arteriolar vasoconstriction and efferent arteriolar vasodilation (10). The reduction of the ultrafiltration coefficient (Kf, i.e., glomerular permeability × surface area) is considered an important factor causing acute renal failure. In fact, several experimental and clinical conditions show a fall in glomerular filtration rate disproportionately greater than that observed in renal blood flow (10).

Therefore, it appears very difficult to evaluate the relevant role of the alterations of glomerular vascular resistances and Kf reduction in acute renal failure because both events may represent an effective response to specific hormones. These substances, such as angiotensin II, may cause mesangial contraction, a decline in Kf, afferent arteriole vasoconstriction, and efferent arteriole vasodilation (10). In experimental models and in man, a reduction in renal blood flow with a rise in renal vascular resistance has been documented during the initial phase of acute renal failure (8). During this phase a restoration of renal blood flow may restore glomerular filtration. In the established phase, however, an increase in renal blood flow toward normal values is not followed by an improvement of glomerular filtration rate (10). Many studies in experimental models and in man suggest that afferent arteriolar vasoconstriction is a major determinant of the hemodynamic modifications observed in acute renal failure. This vasoconstriction may be either neurogenically or hormonally mediated (52). The renin-angiotensin system is perhaps the best-studied hormonal mediator of renal vasoconstriction.

The observation of juxtaglomerular hypertrophy in patients with acute posttraumatic renal failure during World War II led Goormaghtigh (22) to first suggest a role for the renin-angiotensin system in the pathogenesis of this syndrome. In consideration of the important role of renin-angiotensin system in acute renal failure, some authors (33, 47) suggested that it may be related to the tubuloglomerular feedback: defective tubular sodium reabsorption at a site proximal to the macula densa induces renin release that, acting as a vasoconstrictor on the afferent arteriole, induces a decrease in glomerular filtration rate. Several evidences suggest a possible modulation of tubuloglomerular feedback by the renin-angiotensin system, but its precise role remains controversial and this hypothesis is still unproven.

Many experimental and clinical studies support the hypothesis of a pathogenetic role for renin-angiotensin system in acute renal failure (52). Some of the factors in favor of this hypothesis can be summarized as follows:

1. Plasma renin activity is high in patients with acute renal failure.
2. Dehydration that stimulates the renin-angiotensin system enhances experimental acute renal failure.
3. Sodium chloride loading that suppresses the renin-angiotensin system prevents experimentally induced renal failure.
4. Angiotensin II infusion can cause acute renal failure in animal models.
5. Inhibition of angiotensin II action by antibodies or angiotensin inhibitors can prevent acute renal failure.

Furthermore, the renal glomerulus can respond to humoral agents such as angiotensin II by reducing its overall size and possibly the surface area available for filtration. There are several data, however, against the role of the renin-angiotensin system in the pathogenesis of acute renal failure (52):

1. High circulating levels of angiotensin II, as observed in normal pregnancy and malignant hypertension, do not induce acute renal failure in itself.
2. The protective effect of volume expansion is not always proven.

3. Angiotensin-converting enzyme inhibitors do not uniformly prevent acute renal failure in animal models.

Some authors attributed the reduction of renal blood flow to other factors such as neurogenic mechanisms (8), chemical mediators such as endothelin (19, 45), cell swelling (20), and intravascular coagulation (31). Regarding neurogenic mechanisms responsible for renal vasoconstriction, in many clinical situations such as shock, surgery and anesthesia there is an association between acute renal failure and increased sympathetic activity (8). Changes in renal nerve activity may be associated with the early stages of acute renal failure, but adrenergic blockade provides only partial protection against this syndrome. On the other hand, acute renal failure also occurs in transplanted, not innervated, kidneys. Therefore, we can assume that the neural mechanisms may be present but not essential in the pathogenesis of acute renal failure. Recent studies (19, 45) support the role of endothelin as a mediator in the pathogenesis of acute renal failure. Endothelin is a 21-residual peptide produced by endothelial cells in response to hypertension and hypoxia. This substance activates transmembrane calcium flux in the muscular cells of vascular walls. It is a very potent vasoconstrictor; in the isolated perfused rat kidney, very low concentrations of this mediator cause intense long-lasting vasoconstriction. The concentration of endothelin required to reduce blood flow by 50% is 200 pmol/liter, compared with higher doses (1000 pmol/liter) required for angiotensin II to produce the same effect. Endothelin may also cause a striking reduction in the glomerular filtration rate.

Other authors (20) suggested that swelling of the endothelial cells caused by ischemic injury induces a reduction of the diameter of renal arterioles and an increased resistance to blood flow. This hypothesis, although attractive, remains unproven because experimental and morphologic studies indicate that renal blood flow does not deteriorate further after an injury, and cell swelling involves more tubular than endothelial cells. An important role of intra-vascular coagulation in reducing renal blood flow has been suggested in some clinical settings such as intravascular coagulation, but it is not fully demonstrated (31). Bilateral cortical necrosis is a typical condition in which circulatory and clotting mechanisms may mutually operate in the genesis of acute renal failure. This situation may be associated with obstetric complications such as abruptio placentae, pre- or postpartum hemorrhage, bacterial sepsis, hyperacute renal allograft rejection, pancreatitis, and severe dehydration, particularly in children. In this setting, there is severe vasospasm of renal arterioles that is followed by deposition of fibrin thrombi. Thromboplastin, released in the setting of abruptio placentae, endotoxemia, pancreatitis, and immunologic reactions, can activate clotting mechanism (18).

The important role of renal vasoconstriction is also observed in conditions characterized by systemic vasodilation. In septic shock (43) it has been experimentally demonstrated that low systemic vascular resistance is accompanied by important reductions in both effective renal plasma flow and glomerular filtration rate; the renal circulation does not contribute to the sepsis-induced systemic vasodilation. The enhanced renal excretion of PGE_2 seen in septic shock perhaps represents an attempt of the kidney to maintain renal blood flow in the setting of reduced renal perfusion pressure.

Nephrotoxic Damage and Acute Tubular Necrosis

Many experimental and clinical observations suggest that toxic insults are frequently associated with renal hypoperfusion in inducing renal tubular cell necrosis and acute renal failure (10). For this reason, it is very difficult to distinguish in every case which pathogenetic mechanism prevails. Vascular mechanisms, however, seem to have a major role in most cases because a decrease of Kf in response to hormonal agents such as angiotensin II is generally observed. Besides, a nephrotoxic drug by itself induces dose-dependent intrarenal vasoconstriction.

The susceptibility of the kidney to injury from toxins or drugs depends on effective renal blood flow, glomerular capillary surface area, glomerular ultrafiltration, tubular reabsorption, and active transport mechanisms. The precise location of damage along the length of the nephron depends on the nature of the insult. In acute renal failure due to aminoglycosides (13), lesions are typically located in the proximal tubular cells, whereas in cases of nephrotoxic effect by contrast media, renal ischemia combines with direct tubular cell damage (50). Two tubular mechanisms contribute to the decrease in glomerular filtration rate: leaking of the filtrate back through disrupted tubular epithelium into the renal interstitium, and tubular obstruction by necrotic cells or pigments (10, 36). According to the tubular leak theory, glomerular filtration is normal or slightly reduced, but filtered fluid leaks back through the damaged tubular wall into the renal interstitium and peritubular vasculature. This theory is supported by the experimental models in which destruction of tubular epithelium with relatively normal glomeruli is observed. Furthermore, micropuncture studies performed in animals with toxic and ischemic acute renal failure demonstrate that normally nonreabsorbable marker molecules are found to escape from the tubules into the interstitial space. On the other hand, other theories may also find scientific support because tubular necrosis is not a consistent finding in human acute renal failure, and many experimental models show a poor correlation between tubular necrosis and development of acute renal failure.

Tubular obstruction by necrotic cells or pigments with consequent increase in intratubular pressure has been found in many experimental models and it has been demonstrated by micropuncture in some experimental studies. In human acute renal failure this mechanism may be important in toxic or ischemic forms and in cases related to intratubular precipitation of uric acid, oxalate, and sulfonamides. However, its exact role remains uncertain (10). Acute renal failure due to antibiotic toxicity may occur particularly in seriously ill patients.

Therapy by aminoglycosides may frequently be complicated by renal failure; the precise mechanism of this nephrotoxicity is unclear. It is possible that these drugs, as they act on bacteria, bind to ribosomes in proximal tubular cell with consequent impairment of cell protein synthesis (13, 41). Amphotericin B interacts with sterols in the cell membrane, damaging it, and causing both leakage of cell content (41) and intracellular calcium deposition. In such cases, renal vasoconstriction and ultrastructural vascular alterations may also play a role as additional factors. Polymyxin B damages cell membrane because of its detergent action. The mechanism of nephrotoxicity relates to the binding of this cationic polypeptide to cell membrane (41).

The nephrotoxic effect of mercury depends on its binding with plasma-membrane sulfhydryl groups of proximal tubular membrane. This binding alters enzyme function and membrane permeability, causing intracellular mercury accumulation (41). This mechanism of injury occurs with other heavy metals and with platinum compounds like *cis*-diammino-dichloroplatinum (41). Contrast media account for 2–9% of all cases of acute renal failure; the incidence is greater in diabetic patients and in patients with preexisitng impairment of renal function. The mechanism of toxicity involves renal vasoconstriction and direct tubular damage (41, 50). The combination of direct toxic effect on tubular cells, obstruction, and circulatory effects such as hypoxia, extracellular fluid volume depletion, and shock occurs in pigment nephropathy observed in the settings of hemoglobinuria and myoglobinuria (1). Fluorinated anesthetic nephrotoxicity is related to their metabolization in the liver to oxalic acid and inorganic fluoride (41).

Acute Interstitial Nephritis

Acute interstitial nephritis is a form of acute renal failure characterized by usually nonoliguric renal failure, fever, skin rash, eosinophilia, and eosinophiluria. The histopathologic examination shows infiltration of the renal interstitium with inflammatory cells, interstitial edema, and patchy tubular lesions (24). The diagnosis of acute interstitial nephritis requires renal biopsy. The analysis of the renal cell infiltrate may explain the pathogenetic mechanisms involved because in acute bacterial infection there is a massive infiltration of polymorphonuclear neutrophils, whereas in drug-induced acute interstitial nephritis, the infiltrate is composed of lymphocytes and plasma cells or eosinophils. This form of acute renal failure has been extensively studied using animal models, based on immunization with homologous or heterologous antigens in various experimental designs (3, 6, 25, 26, 28, 34, 35). However, animal models may not exactly mimic the situation in man and the results of these studies cannot be directly transferred to human acute interstitial nephritis. Antitubular basement membrane antibodies may be found in human acute interstitial nephritis. Linear deposition of immunoglobulins (IgG) and C3 along the tubular basement membrane were reported in methicillin-related nephropathy (3, 6), suggesting that the complex hapten (methicillin) plus tubular basement membrane protein could stimulate the formation of antitubular basement membrane antibodies and could give rise to acute interstitial nephritis. Circulating immunocomplexes may also be found occasionally (28). The aspect of interstitial infiltrates, characterized by a prevalence of lymphocytes and mononuclear cells with frequently negative immunofluorescence and the presence of epithelioid and giant cell granulomas, suggest a delayed type of hypersensitivity reaction (3, 28, 35).

Pathophysiology of Acute Renal Failure at the Cellular Level

Many studies in experimental models and in cultured cells have tried to explain the mechanisms of cell injury in renal failure. Cells from the various segments of the nephron exhibit differential susceptibility to ischemic and toxic injury. The cells of the proximal tubular segments, where metabolic activity is rather high, are most

sensitive. After a period of ischemia, severe damage of the cell occurs when reperfusion takes place because of the production of toxic compounds, such as oxygen-free radicals (11). The parallel correction of acidosis permits an increase in enzymatic activity with a consequent membrane damage (44). Ischemia is followed by a rapid depletion of cellular energy stores of ATP, disturbances of electrolyte homeostasis (i.e., increased intracellular levels of calcium, sodium, and chloride, and decreased levels of potassium and phosphate), cell and organ swelling, and acidosis (11).

Functional recovery is possible if ischemia is short-lived, but when it is prolonged, progressive damage of the cell has been observed on reperfusion. During anoxia, because of the decrease of the intracellular ATP level, the activity of Na-K-ATPase, the enzyme that actively extrudes sodium from the cell, diminishes. Therefore, water enters the cell and the cell swells (11). Tissue calcium levels have been shown to correlate directly with cell damage (27); alterations of calcium homeostasis appear to be closely linked to the development of irreversible anoxic cell injury. The cytosolic calcium concentration rises due to inhibition of active calcium extrusion by the Ca-dependent ATPase because of the decreased intracellular ATP levels. Decreased ATP levels also induce reduction of calcium uptake by the endoplasmic reticulum and reduction of mitochondrial transport.

ACUTE RENAL FAILURE IN RENAL TRANSPLANT

Excluding intravascular and acute rejection episodes that can cause loss of the transplanted kidney, we term "primary graft anuria" (or "transplant acute tubular necrosis") the situation in which cadaveric renal allografts do not function immediately after transplantation. The cause of this malfunction is not clear, but in the past it has been considered analogous to acute tubular necrosis. Factors acting during "warm" and "cold" ischemia periods were considered to have an important role in the genesis of such a malfunction. Recent studies (48), however, do not support this hypothesis and this situation seems to be much more complex than acute renal failure in the native kidney. Usual factors responsible for acute tubular necrosis (such as hypovolemia, drugs, or radiographic contrast media) seem to play an important role immediately after the transplant when the kidney is very sensitive to any insult. Cyclosporin may play a role in the induction of this form, possibly acting on prostacyclin-tromboxane axis. It becomes complex sometimes to identify different clinical and pathologic patterns. Cyclosporin toxicity, acute tubular necrosis, and acute graft rejection are very similar in detail, making them nearly indistinguishable. In this case, the fine-needle aspiration biopsy may be helpful to establish an accurate diagnosis.

THE HEPATORENAL SYNDROME

The hepatorenal syndrome is a form of renal failure that occurs in patients with advanced chronic or acute liver failure due to cirrhosis, viral hepatitis, malignancy, or massive resection of the liver. At first, the term "hepatorenal syndrome" was used to designate acute renal failure complicating biliary surgery. It has a functional and potentially reversible nature and resembles prerenal azotemia. Indeed, pathologic abnormalities are minimal and xenon-133 washout examination and renal arteriography (16) show reduction in renal blood flow, particularly in cortical perfusion. Postmortem angiography shows normalization of the vascular abnormalities. The syndrome, initially based on functional derangements, can evolve to acute tubular necrosis. In early phases of liver cirrhosis there is avid sodium retention in response to a remarkable hyperaldosteronism. With a progressive decrease in liver function, hypovolemia worsens, with a consequent hypotension, fluid sequestration in the splanchnic region, and further potent stimulation of the renin-angiotension-aldosterone axis. Despite the activation of the compensatory response to effective circulating volume, renal hypoperfusion takes place and the hepatorenal syndrome becomes clinically evident.

Common precipitating causes of hepatorenal syndrome are deterioration in liver function, sepsis, exposure to nephrotoxic drugs, abuse of diuretics, diarrhea, gastrointestinal bleeding, and abdominal paracentesis. Hepatorenal syndrome is characterized by very low urinary sodium content (usually less than 10 mEq/liter) and urine osmolality two or three times higher than that of plasma. Pathogenetic mechanisms of hepatorenal syndrome include increased sympathetic tone due to systemic circulation underfilling and intrahepatic hypertension, activation of the renin-angiotensin-aldosterone axis, alteration in kallikrein-kinin system with diminished kinin formation, an increase in vasoactive intestinal peptides, endotoxins, and "false neurotransmitters." These substances are normally produced in the bowel by bacteria and cleared by the liver; in the setting of liver failure, they escape inactivation and enter systemic circulation. All these mechanisms induce renal vasoconstriction with reduction of renal blood flow and a fall in the glomerular filtration rate (5).

CONCLUSION

Recent studies on the pathogenesis of acute renal failure permitted a more profound investigation and shifted the attention from gross pathologic alterations to subtle derangements of renal circulation and electrolyte homeostasis at the cellular level. These mechanisms can explain pathophysiologic events and could permit a new diagnostic and therapeutic approach to patients affected by acute renal failure in the future.

In intensive care medicine, however, the renal involvement during systemic derangements is more and more commonly seen and the direction in which the studies will be undertaken is mostly regarding the renal damage during multiple-organ failure syndromes. Multiple-organ failure generally develops in four different steps. A physiologic shock of different origin is the first step, followed by a pulmonary dam-

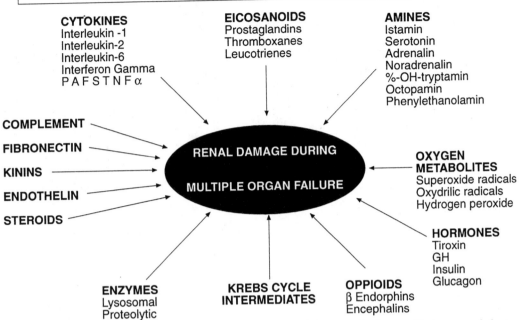

Figure 34.7. Chemical mediators involved in the renal damage during multiple organ failure.

age with gas exchange impairment and a severe condition of hypermetabolism. Then, 5–12 days later, renal and hepatic function start to deteriorate toward different degrees of organ insufficiency. There is generally a fatal progression of the multiple-organ derangement with a fatal progression of the multiple-organ derangement with an extremely high percentage of deaths. The physiology of the kidney function during multiple-organ failure recalls a condition of prerenal azotemia that may present a severe evolution toward an organic form of acute renal failure.

Several chemical mediators have been proposed to affect the evolution of the syndrome and particularly the evolution of the kidney function (Fig. 34.7). The specific action of each of these substances is still to be clarified, although vascular and metabolic mechanisms are likely to take a major part in the observed kidney function derangements. Molecular biology studies, together with ex juvantibus criteria ap-

plied to the extra corporeal renal replacement therapies carried out with different membranes and mechanisms, will certainly help to elucidate the crucial steps in the pathophysiology of this complex syndrome.

References

1. Anderson JR, Schrier RW. Acute tubular necrosis. In: Schrier RW, Gottschalk CW, eds. Diseases of the kidney. 4th ed. Boston: Little, Brown and Company, 1988:1413–1446.
2. Badr K, Ichikawa I, Brenner BM. Renal circulatory and nephron function in experimental obstruction of the urinary tract. In: Brenner BM, Lazarus JM, eds. Acute renal failure. Philadelphia: WB Saunders Co, 1983:116–135.
3. Baldwin DS, Levine BB, Mc Cluskey RT, et al. Renal failure and interstitial nephritis due to penicillin and methicillin. N Engl J Med 1968;279:1245–1254.
4. Bell RC, Coalson JJ, Smith JD, et al. Multiple organ system failure and infection in adult respiratory distress syndrome. Ann Intern Med 1983;99:293–303.
5. Better OS, Chaimovitz C. The hepatorenal syndrome. In: Schrier RW, Gottschalk CW, eds. Dis-

eases of the kidney. 4th ed. Boston: Little, Brown and Company, 1988:1489–1500.

6. Border WA, Lehman DH, Egan JD, et al. Antitubular basement membrane antibodies in methicillin nephritis. N Engl J Med 1974;291:381–394.

7. Bouffet E, Laville M, Zanettini MC, et al. Le sediment urinaire dans l'insuffisance renale aigue. La presse medicale 1984;13:2307–2310.

8. Burnier M, Schrier RW. Pathogenesis of acute renal failure. Adv Exp Med Biol 1987;212:3–13.

9. Burnier M, Schrier RW. Protection from acute renal failure. Adv Exp Med Biol 1987;212:275–283.

10. Brezis M, Rosen S, Epstein FH. Acute Renal Failure. In: Brenner BM, Rector FC, eds. The kidney. 4th ed. Philadelphia: WB Saunders Co, 1991:993–1061.

11. Canavese C, Stratta P, Vercellone A. The case for oxygen free radicals in the pathogenesis of ischemic acute renal failure. Nephron 1988;49:9–15.

12. Conger JD, Falk SA, Yuan BH, Schrier RW. Atrial natriuretic peptide and dopamine in a rat model of ischemic acute renal failure. Kidney Int 1989;35:1126–1132.

13. De Broe et al. Early effects of gentamicin, tobramycin and amikacin on the human kidney. Kidney Int 1984;25:643–652.

14. De Ritis G, Giovannini C, Pietropaoli P. Evaluation of operatory risk (R.O.) in relation to eventual presence of concomitant disease. In: Recent advances in anaesthesia, pain, intensive care and emergency. Trieste:APICE Editor 1989:481–488.

15. Epstien FH, Silva P, Spokes C, Brezis M, Rosen S. Renal medullary Na-K-ATP-ase and hypoxic injury in perfused rat kidneys. Kidney Int 1989;36:768–772.

16. Epstein M. The hepatorenal syndrome (HRS). Adv Exp Med Biol 1987;212:157–165.

17. Espinel CH. The FENa test use in the differential diagnosis of acute renal failure. JAMA 1976; 236:579–581.

18. Finn WF. Acute renal failure. In: Earley LE, Gottshalk CW, eds. Strauss and Welt's. Diseases of the kidney. 3rd ed. Boston: Little, Brown and Company, 1979:167–210.

19. Firth JD, Raine AEG, Ratcliffe PJ, Ledingham JGG. Endothelin: an important factor in acute renal failure? Lancet 1988;ii:1179–1181.

20. Flores J, Di Bona DR, Beck CH, Leaf A. The role of cell swelling in ischemic renal damage and the protective effect of hypertonic solute. J Clin Invest 1972;51:118–127.

21. Fujiwara Y, Kitamura E, Ueda N, Fukunaga M, Orita Y, Kamado T. Mechanism of action of angiotensin II on isolated rat glomeruli. Kidney Int 1989;36:985–991.

22. Goormaghtigh N. La doctrine de la cellule muscolaire, afibrillaire, endocrine en patholgie humaine. Le rein de l'eclampie puerperal. Bull Acad R Med Belg 1942;7:194–210.

23. Gornick CC Jr, Kjiellstrand CM. Acute renal failure complicating aortic aneurysm surgery. Nephron 1983;35:145–153.

24. Grunfeld JP. Kleinknecht D, Droz D. Acute Interstitial Nephritis. In: Schrier RW, Gottschalk

CW. Diseases of the kidney, 4th ed. Boston: Little, Brown and Company, 1988:1461–1488.

25. Heptinstall RH. Interstitial Nephritis. In: Pathology of the kidney. 3rd ed. Boston: Little, Brown and Company, 1983:1149–1193.

26. Hoyer JR. Tubulointerstitial immune complex nephritis in rats immunized with Tamm-Horsfall protein. Kidney Int 1988;17:284–293.

27. Humes HD. Role of calcium in pathogenesis of acute renal failure. Am J Physiol 1986–4;254(pt 2):F579–589.

28. Kleinknecht D, Vanhille P, Morel-Maroger L, et al.: Acute interstitial nephritis due to drug hypersensitivity. An up-to-date review with a report of 19 cases. Adv Nephrol 1983;12:277–308.

29. Kraman S, Khan F, Patel S, et al. Renal failure in the respiratory intensive care unit. Crit Care Med 1979;7:263–274.

30. Lugon JR, Boim MA, Ramos OL, Ajzen H, Schor N. Renal function and glomerular hemodynamics in male endotoxemic rats. Kidney Int 1989;36:570–575.

31. Mant MJ, King EG. Severe acute disseminated intravascular coagulation. Am J Med 1979;67:557–568.

32. Maschio G. Acute renal failure due to obstructive uropathy. Adv Exp Med Biol 1987;212:179–183.

33. Mason J. Tubulo-glomerular feedback in the early stages of experimental acute renal failure. Kidney Int 1976;10(suppl 6):S106–114.

34. Mc Cluskey RT. Immunologically mediated tubulointerstitial nephritis. In: Cotran RS, Brenner BM, Stein JH, eds. Tubulo-interstitial nephropaties. New York: Churchill Livingstone, 1983:121–149.

35. Mery JP, Morel-Maroger L. Acute interstitial nephritis. A hypersensitivity reaction to drugs. In: Giovannetti S, Bonomini V, D'Amico G, eds. Proceedings of the 6th International Congress of Nephrology. Basel:Karger, 1976.

36. Minetti L, Galato R, Radaelli L, Rovati G, Seveso MA. Clinical insight into the pathophysiology of drug-induced acute renal failure. Adv Exp Med biol 1987;212:115–123.

37. Myers BD, Carrie BJ, Yee RR, et al. Pathophysiology of hemodynamically mediated acute renal failure in man. Kidney Int 1980;18:495–502.

38. Myers BD, Hilbermann M, Spencer RJ, et al. Glomerular and tubular function in non-oliguric acute renal failure. Am J Med 1982;72:642–649.

39. Myers BD, Miller DC, Mehigan JT. Nature of the renal injury following total ischemia in man. J Clin Invest 1984;73:329–341.

40. Paller MS, Hoidal JR, Ferris TF. Oxygen free radicals in ischemic acute renal failure in the rat. J Clin Invest 1984;74:1156–1564.

41. Porter GA, Bennet WM. Nephrotoxin-induced acute renal failure. In: Brenner BM, Stein JH, eds. Acute renal failure. New York: Churchill Livingstone, 1980:123–162.

42. Pru C, Kjellestrand C. Urinary indices and chemistries in the differential diagnosis of prerenal failure and acute tubular necrosis. Semin Nephrol 1985;5:224–233.

43. Schaer GL, Fink MP, Chernow B, Ahmed S, Parrillo JE. Renal hemodynamics and prostaglan-

din E_2 excretion in a non human primate model of septic shock. Crit Care Med 1990;18:52–59.

44. Schrier RW, Arnold PE, van Putten VJ, Burke TJ. Pathophysiology of cell ischemia. In: Schrier RW, Gottschalk CW, eds. Diseases of the kidney. 4th ed. Boston: Little, Brown and Company, 1988: 1379–1413.

45. Shibouta Y, Suzuki N, Shino A, et al. Pathophysiological role of endothelin in acute renal failure. Life Sci 1990;46:1611–1618.

46. Stein JH, Gottschalk J, Osgood RW, Ferris TE. Pathophysiology of a nephrotoxic model of acute renal failure. Kidney Int 1975;8:27–41.

47. Thurau K, Boylan JW. Acute renal success. The unexpected logic of oliguria in acute renal failure. Am J Med 1976;61:308–315.

48. Touraine JL, Garnier JL, Mercatello A, et al.: Post-transplant acute renal failure. Adv Exp Med Biol 1987;212:205–210.

49. Trueta J, Barclay AE, Daniel PM, Franklin KJ, Prichard MML. Studies of the renal circulation. Oxford:Blackwell Scientific, 1947.

50. Vari RC, Natarajan LA, Whitescarver SA, Jackson BA, Ott CE. Induction, prevention and mechanisms of contrast media-induced acute renal failure. Kidney Int 1988;33:699–707.

51. Welch WJ, Wilcox CS. Modulating role for thromboxane in the tubulo-glomerular feedback response in the rat. J Clin Invest 1988;81:1843–1849.

52. Wilkes BM, Mailloux LU. Acute renal failure. Pathogenesis and prevention. Am J Med 1986: 1129–1136.

53. Wilkins RG, Faragher EB. Acute renal failure in an intensive care unit: incidence, prediction and outcome. Anesthesia 1983;38:628–637.

54. Zager RA. Hypoperfusion-induced acute renal failure in the rat: an evaluation of oxidant tissue injury. Circ Res 1988;62:430–435.

35

Clinical Manifestations of Acute Renal Failure and Their Pathophysiologic Bases

Frank Cosentino

The kidneys are important in regulating water excretion, acid/base and electrolyte balance, and nitrogen excretion. During acute renal failure the kidneys are unable to regulate the body's internal environment. The result is a failure of nitrogen excretion along with electrolyte, acid/base, and water imbalances.

The first part of this chapter describes the biochemical abnormalities that occur in acute renal failure. Changes in blood nitrogen products resulting from decreased renal excretion and increased catabolism will be discussed. Changes in divalent ion metabolism is also discussed. An understanding of these changes is important so that these imbalances can be treated and additional iatrogenic insult can be avoided. Specific laboratory abnormalities may also provide clues to the etiology of the acute renal failure.

The direct effect of acute renal failure on various organ systems is described. Organ system changes secondary to various disease states that may cause acute renal failure is not stressed. It is important to be aware of the effect of acute renal failure on the body systems because of enhanced morbidity and mortality associated with additional organ system dysfunction. The greater the number of complications of acute renal failure, the higher the mortality. In addition, certain types of complications such as respiratory or cardiovascular failure significantly increase the risk of dying in patients with acute renal failure. Therefore, prevention and early recognition and management of these complications is important.

BIOCHEMICAL DISTURBANCES

A variety of biochemical disturbances and associated laboratory abnormalities are known to occur in acute renal failure. However, despite these abnormalities the specific uremic toxins responsible for the signs and symptoms of the uremic syndrome continue to be elusive. This section discusses some of the biochemical abnormalities that occur in the setting of acute renal failure and that are not discussed in other chapters of this text. Topics not covered in this section include monovalent electrolyte abnormalities and acid/base disturbances.

Some of the biochemical disturbances that occur in acute renal failure are also observed in chronic renal failure. However, these changes can elicit different responses in the two settings. Patients suffering from acute renal failure have much less time to adapt to biochemical disturbances compared to those with chronic renal failure. So, at any given level of azotemia, patients experiencing acute renal dysfunction are likely to have more symptoms compared to someone who develops renal failure over a more prolonged period of time.

Blood Urea Nitrogen

Acute renal failure is defined as an acute decrease in renal function. There is a rise in blood nitrogen products, termed azotemia. The level of blood urea nitrogen in any individual depends on the amount of nitrogen ingested in the form of protein, the rate of protein metabolism, and the amount of renal nitrogen excretion. Urea is produced from hepatic metabolism of amino acids that are not used for protein synthesis. Amino acids are deaminated to produce ammonia, which is converted to urea to prevent toxic levels of ammonia from accumulating. Therefore, urea production will be influenced by protein intake and tissue catabolism.

In acute renal failure the urea nitrogen will increase because of decreased renal excretion and an increase in protein catabolism. The amount of protein intake will also have an effect. Knochel (36) has shown that a normal person taking in enough calories to prevent ketosis but taking in no protein will catabolize endogenous protein at a rate of 0.5 g/kg/day, or 35 g in a 70-kg individual. This represents 5.5 g of nitrogen. Eighty-five percent of this nitrogen is in the form of urea nitrogen, which is equivalent to 4.7 g/day. If this urea nitrogen cannot be excreted by the kidneys and this 70-kg individual has a total body water of 42 liters, then the blood urea nitrogen would increase by 11 mg/dl in 1 day (36). In contrast, a patient with major trauma may have three times the catabolism of a normal individual. This could represent the production of 17 g of nitrogen per day. If one were to go through the same calculations for a 70-kg individual, the blood urea nitrogen would increase by 40 mg/dl/day if renal excretion were not present (36).

Thus, it is apparent that one of the factors that affects the rate of increase of blood urea nitrogen is the degree of catabolism in any individual patient with acute renal failure. Hypercatabolic patients can be observed to have an increase in blood urea nitrogen levels of 20–50 mg/dl/day (4). Patients with acute renal failure who are not hypercatabolic may have an increase in urea nitrogen levels of only 10–20 mg/dl/day. A review of 462 patients with acute renal failure showed that 32% were hypercatabolic. This was defined as a daily increase of blood urea nitrogen (BUN) >30 mg/dl for 2 days. Hypercatabolic patients were more likely to have acute renal failure in the setting of trauma or surgical procedures as opposed to medical causes of acute renal failure. They were also twice as likely to die compared to those that were not hypercatabolic (10).

In a prospective study of 92 patients with acute renal failure, Anderson and coauthors (3) were able to show that the degree of renal dysfunction also influences the level of BUN. In this study patients that had nonoliguric acute renal failure seemed to suffer a less severe renal insult. For this reason they also exhibited lesser degrees of azotemia compared to oliguric patients.

The cause of increased catabolism in acute renal failure is not definitely known. It may not even be the renal failure that causes the increased catabolism, but rather the circumstances that surround the acute renal failure. For example, Long and associates (46) have shown that whole-body protein breakdown increases by 73% in trauma patients not suffering from acute renal failure compared to normal controls. Skeletal muscle protein breakdown increased by a factor of 2.7. A study of muscle protein turnover and glucose uptake in uremic rats showed that there was increased muscle protein breakdown within the initial 24 hr of acute renal failure which further increased at 48 hr (11). The authors went on to show that insulin was ineffective in decreasing the amount of muscle protein catabolism. Decreased protein synthesis was also noted at 48 hr and could not be enhanced with insulin. The authors postulated that perhaps ineffective glucose utilization secondary to decreased insulin sensitivity may contribute to the enhanced muscle protein breakdown in uremia (11). Hörl and Heidland (29) have postulated that there may be active proteases that play a role in protein wasting in hypercatabolic acute renal failure. They studied eight patients with acute renal failure and found that two of these patients exhibited hypercatabolism. They speculated that enhanced catabolism was secondary to enhanced proteolytic enzyme production or a decrease in breakdown of these enzymes.

In addition to enhanced protein catabolism from increased levels of proteolytic activity and insulin resistance, there is also evidence that increased levels of growth hormone as well as glucagon and catecholamines may contribute to the enhanced protein breakdown and catabolism in renal failure (37). Thus, it seems that the elevated urea nitrogen concentrations in acute renal failure are a result of decreased renal excretion as well as enhanced urea nitrogen generation secondary to increased catabolism. The degree of protein intake will also play a role. Likewise, patients who have experienced serious trauma, muscle damage, fever, or sepsis may also experience a hypercatabolic state secondary to these or other factors.

Serum Creatinine

The serum creatinine level is also a marker of azotemia in acute renal failure. In noncatabolic states it may increase by a factor of 1–1.5 mg/dl/day. In catabolic states the daily increase in the serum creatinine level may be much more. The serum creatinine level may also increase at accelerated rates in persons experiencing skeletal muscle injury. Breakdown of skeletal muscle will result in release of creatinine leading to a disproportionate increase in the serum creatinine relative to the level of BUN (9). Increments in plasma creatinine in the setting of skeletal muscle injury may range from 1.6–6.6 mg/dl daily (26).

Moran and Myers (53) have described the changes in serum creatinine by studying a model of creatinine kinetics during the course of acute renal failure. The authors described three separate groups of patients. The first group demonstrated an initial decrease in creatinine clearance followed by a slow increase. During the recovery phases as the creatinine clearance increased, the serum creatinine continued to rise and the urinary indices were consistent with avid sodium reabsorption. This group of patients experienced short periods of renal ischemia as a cause of their acute renal failure and carried a good prognosis. The remaining two groups of patients experienced prolonged ischemia and exhibited either a prolonged decrease in creatinine clearance or an exponential decrease in creatinine clearance with corresponding increases in serum creatinine levels. These groups experienced a worse prognosis and most often required dialysis.

CALCIUM ABNORMALITIES

Hypocalcemia

The most common abnormality of serum calcium in acute renal failure is hypocalcemia. The hypocalcemia may be associated with low, normal, or elevated serum phosphorus levels. Resistance to the action of parathyroid hormone may at least partially explain why hypocalcemia is seen in acute renal failure (67). Massry and colleagues (50) also demonstrated that a deficiency of 1,25-dihydroxyvitamin D_3 may be partially responsible for the skeletal resistance to the action of parathyroid hormone in uremia. Other reasons for depressed calcium level in acute renal failure include severe hyperphosphatemia and hypoalbuminemia.

Severe hypocalcemia that seems out of proportion to the duration and severity of acute renal failure may be seen in rhabdomyolysis (14). Lach and colleagues (41) have suggested that the hypocalcemia associated with acute renal failure in rhabdomyolysis is secondary to the severe hyperphosphatemia leading to deposition of calcium and phosphorus in tissues. Also decreased synthesis of 1,25-dihydroxyvitamin D_3 also seems to play a role. Hypocalcemia may occur with rhabdomyolysis even in the absence of acute renal failure. Akmal and colleagues (1) have demonstrated the deposition of calcium in injured tissues regardless of the presence or absence of acute renal failure.

During the course of rhabdomyolysis, hypercalcemia may actually develop in the diuretic phase of acute renal failure. It is thought that the most likely explanation for hypercalcemia in this setting is the mobilization of calcium previously deposited in injured tissues. In addition, the hypercalcemia may also be partly secondary to increased synthesis of 1,25-dihydroxyvitamin D_3 (41). This finding was substantiated in the study by Akmal et al. They suggested that extrarenal production of 1,25-dihydroxyvitamin D_3 may occur in patients in the diuretic phase of acute tubular necrosis secondary to rhabdomyolysis (1).

Hypocalcemia may also be seen in other causes of acute renal failure. For example, cisplatin can cause nephrotoxicity associated with hypocalcemia, hypomagnesemia, and hypokalemia secondary to increased urinary excretion of these cations. The incidence of cisplatin nephrotoxicity has been observed to decrease when patients are hydrated prior to receiving the drug (20). Other nephrotoxins that may be associated with hypocalcemia include mithramycin, methoxyflurane, and glycols. In addition, hypocalcemia has also been associated with renal failure in the setting of acute pancreatitis. Gordon and Calne (25) reported on six patients with pancreatitis and acute renal failure complicated by hypocalcemia.

Hypercalcemia

As indicated above hypercalcemia may be seen in the diuretic phase of acute renal failure secondary to rhabdomyolysis. Technetium pyrophosphate imaging has demonstrated the extraosseous tissue deposition of calcium in patients with rhabdomyolysis and acute renal failure (66). It is likely that this tissue deposition of calcium leads to the subsequent hypercalcemia in the diuretic phase of rhabdomyolysis-associated acute renal failure. Likewise, as noted above, during the diuretic phase there is also an increased synthesis of 1,25-dihydroxyvitamin D_3 which also likely contributes to the hypercalcemia in this setting (41). Hypercalcemia may also be more likely in this setting if patients are given supplemental calcium during the time that they exhibit hypocalcemia. Calcium supplementation should be reserved for patients with obvious clinical signs of hypocalcemia (72).

Hypercalcemia has also been noted in critically ill patients with acute renal failure not due to rhabdomyolysis (21). The mechanism may be related to enhanced parathyroid hormone secretion. Patients exhibiting hypercalcemia seem to have a higher incidence of shock, sepsis, and multiple transfusions containing citrate. The citrate may lower blood calcium levels and therefore stimulate parathyroid hormone secretion. Such a phenomenon was seen in 15% of critically ill patients in one series. Five of the 15 patients exhibiting hypercalcemia did not have acute renal failure. Hyper-

calcemia may also occur in patients with solid tumors such as breast, lung, and kidney carcinomas, as well as hematologic malignancies, including multiple myeloma and leukemias. Hypercalcemia occurring in these situations may be secondary to the malignancy itself and contribute to the development of renal failure. For example, hypercalcemia is one of several potential causes of renal failure in the setting of multiple myeloma (2).

PHOSPHORUS ABNORMALITIES

Hyperphosphatemia

Hyperphosphatemia is commonly seen in the setting of acute renal failure. Phosphorus is usually present in the range of 5–8 mg/dl (49). Decreased renal excretion of phosphorus can account for hyperphosphatemia in this setting. Phosphorus can also be released from injured tissues, contributing even more to the hyperphosphatemia. This can be seen, for example, in rhabdomyolysis where skeletal muscle injury will result in the release of intracellular phosphorus. The hyperphosphatemia may be associated with hyperuricemia and hyperkalemia from intracellular release of these substances as well. Severe hyperphosphatemia can also be associated with tumor lysis following treatment of various malignancies, especially lymphoproliferative disorders (63). Hyperphosphatemia in patients with these disorders can occur as a result of rapid cell lysis following the start of chemotherapy. There may also be an associated hyperuricemia and hyperkalemia in these situations.

Hypophosphatemia

Hypophosphatemia in the setting of acute renal failure is less common than hyperphosphatemia, but has been known to occur. Kurtin and Kouba (40) described 4 of 19 patients with acute renal failure requiring dialytic support with mean serum phosphate levels of 0.8 mg/dl. The only apparent cause was the administration of a large percentage of total calories in the form of carbohydrate for a prolonged period. It is postulated that this resulted in intracellular accumulation of phosphorus secondary to insulin-induced intracellular shifting of phosphorus. Hypophosphatemia has also been reported in acute renal failure secondary to staphylococcal toxic shock syndrome. The etiology for this is unclear (13). Proximal tubular dysfunction of Fanconi's syndrome can also lead to a renal phosphate leak and therefore hypophosphatemia in the setting of acute renal failure.

MAGNESIUM ABNORMALITIES

Hypermagnesemia

Another abnormality of divalent ion metabolism is that of hypermagnesemia in the setting of acute renal failure. Massry and colleagues (49) evaluated 10 patients with acute renal failure, 9 of whom were found to be hypermagnesemic in the oliguric phase. In this report, serum magnesium ranged from 2.2—4.6 mg/dl. It was during the oliguric phase when the magnesium reached its highest level. During the diuretic phase of acute renal failure in this study, the magnesium level decreased to a range of 1–4.0 mg/dl. It was during this phase as well as the recovery phase that several of the patients became hypomagnesemic. It has been noted that the fractional excretion of magnesium increases in the diuretic phase of acute renal failure. Even higher levels of hypermagnesemia may be encountered in acute renal failure patients if they are given magnesium-containing substances such as antacids or laxatives. For this reason, magnesium-containing products should not be administered to patients with acute renal failure, especially in the oliguric phase. It may be necessary to supplement magnesium if the patient becomes hypomagnesemic during the diuretic or recovery phase of acute renal failure.

Hypomagnesemia

Less commonly, hypomagnesemia may be seen in the setting of acute renal failure. As noted above, this may occur during the diuretic or recovery phase of acute renal failure. Hypomagnesemia can also occur in the setting of cisplatin nephrotoxicity.

Acute renal failure secondary to cisplatin can also be associated with calcium and potassium wasting as well. Pentamidine is another drug that has been associated with magnesium and calcium wasting by the kidneys. A third setting of renal failure and hypomagnesemia can be seen in bone marrow transplant recipients. Kone et al. (38) reported an 88% incidence of hypomagnesemia secondary to magnesium wasting by the kidney in bone marrow transplant recipients with hypertension and renal dysfunction. Reasons for magnesium wasting included cyclosporine and aminoglycoside antibiotics.

CARDIOVASCULAR COMPLICATIONS

Cardiovascular complications are frequently encountered in critically ill patients with acute renal failure. Bullock and colleagues (10) reported cardiovascular complications occurring 62% of the time in a series of 462 patients with acute renal failure. These complications included congestive heart failure, pulmonary edema, ventricular arrhythmias, acute myocardial infarction, and cardiac arrest. The authors went on to show that those patients who developed cardiovascular complications, 82% of them died. Multivariate analysis of risk factors showed that cardiovascular events occurring in acute renal failure increased the risk of dying by a factor of 3.4. Thus, cardiovascular complications are common in the setting of acute renal failure and imply a poor prognosis with regards to overall survival.

Volume overload is a common complication occurring in acute renal failure. Patients are prone to volume overload, especially if they are oliguric because they are frequently given large amounts of intravenous fluids for nutrition, drug administration, and fluid challenges in an effort to increase the urine output. In addition to this, there is also the endogenous production of water through metabolic pathways. Consequences of volume overload include hypertension, edema, and pulmonary vascular congestion. These can be severe enough to lead to death of the patient. In a series of 104 patients with acute renal failure, 56% of them developed congestive heart failure. Mortality for this group was 68% compared to a 42% mortality for those who did not develop congestive heart failure (52). Edema was also common in this group of patients, occurring 50% of the time.

Another potential complication in the setting of acute renal failure is that of cardiac ischemia or myocardial infarction. In a series of 276 cases of acute renal failure, McMurray and colleagues (51) demonstrated acute myocardial infarction occurring in 7% of the patients. The patients that experienced myocardial infarction had a mean age of 64 years compared to 51 years for those not developing myocardial infarction ($p < 0.001$). Myocardial infarction is more likely to occur in older populations as well as those patients who develop acute renal failure in the setting of cardiovascular or abdominal aneurysm surgery. Because of advanced age and because of underlying ischemic heart disease, these patients are at greater risk for dying.

Patients with acute renal failure are also prone to cardiac arrhythmias. In the series by McMurray and colleagues (51), 33% of the patients experienced arrhythmias in the form of atrial tachycardia, ventricular tachycardia, or complete heart block. Patients are prone to cardiac arrhythmias because of disturbances in electrolytes such as potassium, calcium, and magnesium. Also, acid-base disturbances and drug toxicities such as digoxin toxicity may contribute to cardiac arrhythmias. Cardiac ischemia leading to arrhythmias may also be induced secondary to hypotensive episodes occurring with volume depletion or dialysis-induced hypotension.

Pericarditis is another complication that may occasionally be seen in the setting of acute renal failure. However, this is more rare than other complications. Pericarditis may occur as a manifestation of the uremia itself, or may be related to some underlying disease such as a collagen vascular disease. It seems that in the older literature, pericarditis was more common when dialysis was not as common or was performed later in the course of acute renal failure compared to the way it is done today (74).

Uremic pericarditis may be present with no other symptoms or signs other than a pericardial friction rub heard during physical examination. In contrast to other causes of pericarditis, pain may not be a prominent component. Uremic pericarditis is an indication for dialysis.

Pericardial tamponade is also a potential complication in acute renal failure. A clue to the diagnosis may be a sudden onset of hypotension following fluid removal with diuresis or dialysis. Also, acute pericardial tamponade may occur during hemodialysis secondary to pericardial hemorrhage because of anticoagulation used with dialysis.

It is important to keep in mind that a systemic disease may be the cause of both cardiac disease and acute renal failure. For example, bacterial endocarditis can cause both cardiac abnormalities as well as renal failure. Other diseases that may present in this fashion include vasculitis or collagen vascular diseases such as systemic lupus erythematosus or scleroderma.

In summary, cardiovascular complications are common in the setting of acute renal failure and contribute to an increase in mortality. This is especially common in older individuals and those patients who have acute renal failure in association with cardiac surgery or major vascular surgery. For this reason it is important to correct electrolyte, acid-base, and fluid imbalances in an attempt to prevent any potential cardiovascular problems.

PULMONARY COMPLICATIONS

Pulmonary complications can be a common occurrence in the setting of acute renal failure. In a series of 462 patients with acute renal failure, 250 patients (54%) developed pulmonary complications that included aspiration pneumonia, respiratory failure, respiratory arrest, and the adult respiratory distress syndrome (10). The authors went on to show that these pulmonary complications constituted the most ominous threat to patient survival. Patients with acute renal failure and pulmonary complications had an 87.2% mortality rate. Multivariate analysis showed that patients with acute renal failure and pulmonary complications has an increased risk of dying by a factor of 8.2 (10). Similar findings were observed in a series of 686 patients with respiratory failure. Seventy-four of these patients had acute renal failure in the setting of respiratory failure. Of these 74 patients, 60 (80%) died (39).

Pulmonary edema is a common finding in patients with acute renal failure. It can be observed even in patients with normal cardiac function. Uremic pulmonary edema may be the result of alterations in the Starling forces in the pulmonary circulation as well as increases in pulmonary capillary membrane permeability (57). These changes can allow for the exudation of protein-rich fluid from the intravascular tree into the alveolar air spaces. Therefore, even though fluid overload may be absent and cardiac function may be normal, pulmonary edema may still occur. Certainly, superimposed left ventricular failure or fluid overload will also exacerbate increases in extravascular lung water.

Crosbie and Parsons (18) demonstrated the early development of respiratory compromise in the setting of acute renal failure. A series of 12 patients with acute renal failure were shown to develop arterial hypoxemia within 2–3 days despite normal or increased cardiac output. Excessive extravascular lung water was present in the lung interstitium, leading to increased shunting. The authors showed that there was a progressive deterioration in lung function if the acute renal failure failed to improve, even if cardiac function remained normal (18). Effective gas exchange was evaluated in 55 acute renal failure patients by Lee and colleagues (42). This study revealed defective gas exchange due to a reduction in diffusion capacity across the alveolar capillary membrane. The effect was related to the severity of renal dysfunction and it was present without clinical or radiologic evidence of pulmonary disease. A restrictive defect also was found to accompany the diffusion defect which was more marked in male patients. It was felt that these findings were compatible with the presence of pulmonary edema even though routine clinical studies were normal.

Patients with acute renal failure may have abnormal infiltrates on radiographs not only because of pulmonary edema but also because of pneumonia. In the series of 276 acute renal failure patients reported by McMurray et al. (51), 81 patients developed pneumonia. In this study, infectious complications showed an inverse correlation to the likelihood of survival.

Defective gas exchange and hypoxemia may be seen in association with pulmonary edema or pulmonary infection, as noted above. Also, the adult respiratory distress syndrome that is so common in critically ill patients can also be seen in association with acute renal failure. This association of acute respiratory failure and acute renal failure carries a poor prognosis, with a mortality rate of 80% (10, 39).

Defective gas exchange and hypoxemia may occur during hemodialysis (17). Blood membrane interaction can lead to the stimulation of the alternate complement pathway resulting in margination of white blood cells in the pulmonary vasculature, leading to an elevation in pulmonary arterial pressures and hypoxemia. This blood-membrane interaction depends on the type of membrane used. Complement-activating membranes like cupraphane will cause hypoxemia and pulmonary leukocyte sequestration (6). This does not occur with membranes like polymethylmethacrylate, which do not activate complement (17). Hypoventilation may also occur on dialysis secondary to a loss of CO_2 in the dialysate, further aggravating hypoxemia (6).

It is important to remember that acute renal failure in association with pulmonary disease may be secondary to the same etiology. Several disease entities including vasculitis and connective tissue diseases may present with both acute renal dysfunction and simultaneous pulmonary involvement. Some examples include Wegener's granulomatosis, Goodpasture's syndrome, systemic lupus erythematosus, polyarteritis nodosa, and idiopathic rapidly progressive glomerulonephritis. Infections may also be associated with both pulmonary disease and acute renal dysfunction. For example, right-sided bacterial endocarditis may present with pulmonary infiltrates and immune complex-mediated glomerulonephritis. Therefore, the patient presenting with an apparent pulmonary renal syndrome needs to be evaluated for vasculitis, collagen vascular diseases, and infection, along with cardiovascular disease and the possibility of pulmonary edema.

GASTROINTESTINAL COMPLICATIONS

Common gastrointestinal complications seen with acute renal failure include anorexia, nausea and vomiting, and upper gastrointestinal bleeding. In a series of 276 patients with acute renal failure, upper gastrointestinal bleeding was seen in 90 patients (51). In these 90 patients, only 25 had bleeding severe enough to require endoscopy. Four patients died because of gastrointestinal hemorrhage. Although this study showed that death secondary to gastrointestinal hemorrhage in the setting of acute renal failure is not common, other studies have shown that gastrointestinal bleeding is a common cause of death in patients with acute renal failure (69). The frequency of gastrointestinal hemorrhage contributing to death in patients with acute renal failure may depend on whether or not acute renal failure is encountered in a medical versus a surgical setting. Gastrointestinal bleeding may be more severe in surgical or trauma patients (4).

Upper gastrointestinal bleeding usually occurs because of stress ulcerations. Patients with acute renal failure have several potential reasons for why they may be predisposed to gastric mucosal abnormalities. Hypergastrinemia has been reported in patients with acute renal failure and chronic renal failure (71). In spite of the elevated gastrin levels, the pathophysiology of gastrointestinal hemorrhage in acute renal failure is not well delineated. Patients with renal failure are known to have low gastric acid output in spite of the high gastrin levels (64). The low basal acid output is accompanied by a high basal intragastric pH. These findings may be secondary to the high gastric ammonia levels that are derived from urea nitrogen. The elevated gastric ammonia content may neutralize the gastric acid.

The hypergastrinemia is seen in at least 50% of patients with acute renal failure and values may reach the ranges seen in the Zollinger-Ellison syndrome (69). Gastrointestinal inhibitory polypeptide and cholecystokinin are also elevated in renal failure.

The probability of gastrointestinal hemorrhage may actually be increased during dialysis. The use of anticoagulants probably is not the entire explanation. During the hemodialysis procedure, gastric acid secretion actually increases and this seems to be related to a fall in blood pressure (64). There is a correlation between changes in systolic blood pressure and changes in the permeability of the gastric mucosa. Hypotension increases the gastric mucosa permeability to hydrogen ions, thus increasing the likelihood of gastrointestinal hemorrhage during hemodialysis (64).

Because of the relatively high incidence of gastrointestinal hemorrhage in patients with acute renal failure and the potential for an increase in mortality secondary to bleeding, studies have been conducted to examine preventative measures in critically ill patients. In one recent study utilizing a randomized double-blind placebo-controlled design, cimetidine was shown to be superior to placebo for diminishing upper gastrointestinal bleeding and the need for transfusions (55). Eleven of the 39 patients in this study had renal failure. The dose of cimetidine must be adjusted for patients with acute renal failure. In another recent study involving 75 critically ill patients at risk for acute gastrointestinal bleeding, cimetidine was shown to be inferior to antacid therapy (56). Upper gastrointestinal bleeding occurred in seven of 38 cimetidine-treated patients but in none of 37 antacid-treated patients. A third study published in 1981 showed that both cimetidine and antacids were equally efficacious in decreasing the incidence of upper gastrointestinal bleeding in high-risk patients (8). Overall it seems that either an H_2 blocker or antacid therapy should be administered to patients with acute renal failure to prevent or decrease the incidence of upper gastrointestinal hemorrhage. It is important to remember that dosages of cimetidine and some other H_2 blockers need to be adjusted for acute renal failure. In addition, magnesium-containing antacids should not be administered to patients with acute renal failure because of the potential for the development of hypermagnesemia.

Since amylase is excreted by the kidney, hyperamylasemia is often seen in a setting of acute renal failure. For this reason, acute pancreatitis may be difficult to diagnose. The amylase-creatinine clearance ratio becomes inaccurate for the diagnosis of acute pancreatitis in patients with moderate renal insufficiency (7). Usually amylase levels rarely exceed twice the upper limit of normal in the setting of acute renal failure. Markedly elevated amylase levels may suggest the presence of acute pancreatitis. Lipase determinations can be used to assist in the diagnosis of pancreatitis in patients with acute renal failure. Acute renal failure may often be associated with acute pancreatitis. In a series of 519 cases of acute pancreatitis, 23 patients developed acute renal failure. Twenty-two of these 23 patients subsequently died (33). This study as well as others suggests that acute renal failure in the setting of acute pancreatitis carries a poor prognosis. A series reported by Imrie and colleagues included 78 patients with acute pancreatitis. Five patients developed acute renal failure and four of these patients subsequently died (32).

Another finding sometimes encountered in patients with acute renal failure is that of jaundice. In a series of 462 patients with acute renal failure reported by Bullock, 42.9% had jaundice (10). Of those 198 patients with jaundice, 84% died. Using multivariate analysis of various risk factors, jaundice was shown to increase the risk of dying in patients with acute renal failure by a factor of four. Thus, jaundice in patients with acute renal failure is an ominous sign. The jaundice may be secondary to passive hepatic congestion, septicemia, medications and toxins, hepatic ischemia, or an intraabdominal process. Hyperbilirubinemia may be nephrotoxic, but a definite mechanism has failed to be elucidated (43). In addition, hyperbilirubinemia may be aggravated by acute renal failure because of the retention of bile acids resulting in markedly elevated blood levels. Urea nitrogen retention from acute renal failure may also lead to an increase in ammonia production because of the increased availability of this substrate. This can aggravate hepatic encephalopathy.

Lastly, it is important to remember that acute renal failure may be seen in association with hepatobiliary disease of the same cause. For example, vasculitis such as polyarteritis nodosa may present with both liver and kidney involvement. Certain infections such as leptospirosis or hepatitis B may also present with kidney and liver involvement. Gram-negative infections leading to septicemia and cholangitis can also be complicated by acute renal failure.

NERVOUS SYSTEM COMPLICATIONS

Metabolic encephalopathy secondary to uremia is noted to occur both in acute and in chronic renal failure. Although standard biochemical laboratory abnormalities do not correlate with the presence or absence of uremic encephalopathy, in general uremic encephalopathy can occur when the glomerular filtration rate is less than 10% of normal (22). The signs and symptoms of uremic encephalopathy can be the same as those seen in other types of metabolic encephalopathy. Usually there is a clouding of sensorium preceding an impairment in cognitive function. Symptoms may be more severe and progression may be more rapid in acute renal failure compared to chronic renal failure (58). The earliest signs or symptoms of uremic encephalopathy may be a confusional state in which the patient exhibits inattention and alterations of alertness and awareness of the environment. Patients may then exhibit drowsiness with excessive sleepiness and fatigue. During this stage, asterixis and myoclonus may also develop. Stupor is the third stage, in which the patient may be asleep but arousable to painful stimuli. Vomiting and seizures may also be seen. The most severe stage is that of coma, in which the patient is not arousable from apparent sleep even with painful stimuli. There may be accompanying cardiovascular abnormalities and respiratory depression.

Routine biochemical laboratory values may not accurately portray the degree of renal dysfunction and therefore there exists a poor correlation between the level of blood urea nitrogen and creatinine to neurologic dysfunction in the setting of acute renal failure. This may be particularly true in patients with underlying liver disease in which the glomerular filtration rate may be less than 25 ml/min with a serum creatinine level of less than 1.5 mg/dl (54). In this series of patients, the inulin clearance was observed to decline over time without any corresponding change in the serum creatinine level. Therefore, the level of BUN and creatinine cannot be reliably used to diagnose the presence or absence of uremic encephalopathy in patients with acute renal failure and apparent central nervous system dysfunction.

The electroencephalogram (EEG) is sensitive but not specific in diagnosing neurologic dysfunction in acute renal failure. Cooper and associates demonstrated that patients with acute renal failure of less than 48-hr duration with only modest increases in plasma urea and creatinine had striking abnormalities in the EEG. Dialysis failed to affect these changes. The EEG did become normal if renal function improved (14). In general, the EEG shows slow background activity with an excess of theta and delta waves. Spike activity may be seen in patients with focal seizures. The EEG becomes slower as the uremic state worsens (58).

Psychological testing may be useful in determining that encephalopathy exists in patients but is not specific enough to diagnose uremic encephalopathy versus encephalopathy from some other cause.

Biochemical and cellular studies show that altered calcium metabolism in the central nervous system is involved in the pathophysiology of nervous system dysfunction in renal failure. The report by Cooper and colleagues showed that patients with acute renal failure had an increase in brain cellular calcium content at a level of almost twice the normal value. This was independent of plasma calcium and phosphorus products (14). In addition, there was a decrease in brain sodium content but brain water, potassium, and magnesium were normal. This increase in brain calcium content may be secondary to a direct effect of parathyroid hormone, which is elevated in acute renal failure (48). There is an alteration in cellular calcium pumps secondary to parathyroid hormone, resulting in an increase in cellular calcium content. In various models of acute renal failure the changes in intracellular calcium concentration can be prevented by parathyroidectomy. These changes can also be stimulated by the in vivo administration of parathyroid hormone (23). Calcium is an essential mediator of neurotransmitter release and also plays a critical role in many intracellular processes (48). The alteration in brain calcium content is possibly what is responsible for disrupting nervous system function.

Although patients with acute renal failure are prone to develop uremic encephalopathy, one must not forget that other causes of central nervous system dysfunction can also occur. For example, various electrolyte imbalances such as sodium imbalance, hypermagnesemia, or hypercalcemia can all lead to abnormalities in the level of consciousness. In addition, patients with acute renal dysfunction, especially if accompanied by hepatic dysfunction, are also prone to toxicities from many medications. Also other organ system dysfunction such as liver failure may contribute to the development of encephalopathy. In patients with both hepatic and renal failure, it often becomes difficult to determine which organ system is primarily responsible for alterations in central nervous system function.

Treatment of acute uremia may also contribute to central nervous system dysfunction. Dialysis disequilibrium is a syndrome that is known to occur in patients being treated with hemodialysis, whether it be for acute or chronic renal failure (22). Mild symptoms of dialysis disequilibrium include muscle cramps, anorexia, restlessness, and dizziness (62). More severe symptoms include headache, nausea and vomiting, muscle twitching, blurring of vision, tremors, and seizures. The syndrome generally occurs in patients undergoing rapid hemodialysis, usually in the setting of acute renal failure. The pathogenesis of the syndrome was initially thought to be secondary to osmolar changes that occur during the dialysis procedure. It was thought that the plasma clearance of urea exceeded urea clearance from the intracellular compartment, especially in the brain. This was thought to result in an osmotic gradient between the blood and brain causing a net movement of water into the brain (5). Subsequent reports have indicated that there are no differences in the rate of urea clearance from blood and the brain. Rather, cerebral edema may be secondary to a decrease in the intracellular pH of the cerebral cortex (22). The dialysis disequilibrium syndrome can be prevented by using less aggressive, more frequent dialysis in patients with acute renal failure, especially those presenting with markedly elevated levels of azotemia.

HEMATOLOGIC ABNORMALITIES

Bleeding diatheses are an important complication of acute renal failure and uremia in general. In a report from 1967, bleeding complications were noted to contribute to one-tenth of all deaths in acute renal failure (70). With more frequent use of dialysis, uremic bleeding has become less common but can still present problems in patients undergoing surgical or invasive procedures. The primary hemostatic defect is platelet dysfunction. Many patients with acute renal failure have an elevated bleeding time (19). The prothrombin time and partial thromboplastin time are not elevated secondary to acute renal failure itself (69). Although earlier reports of bleeding in the setting of uremia describe thrombocytopenia and/or elevated prothrombin time or partial thromboplastin time, many of these reports do not comment on the concomitant presence of vitamin K deficiency, liver disease, sepsis, disseminated intravascular coagulation, or toxicity from medications (35).

The primary hemostatic abnormality in uremia is that of a defect in platelet function. The main clinical findings consist of a prolonged bleeding time, abnormal prothrombin consumption, and decreased platelet adhesiveness. The defect in platelet adhesiveness has been shown to correlate with the level of serum urea nitrogen and creatinine, and incidence of clinical bleeding. There is also an inverse correlation between defective platelet adhesiveness and hematocrit levels (19, 44).

Platelet function abnormalities that seem to contribute to overall platelet dysfunction include defective platelet factor-III. This may be secondary to elevated levels of guanidinosuccinic acid in uremic subjects (30). Inhibition of platelet aggregation in uremic patients may also be a consequence of enhanced activity of prostacyclin from endothelial cells or altered sensitivity of platelets to prostacyclin (61). Remuzzi and colleagues showed that blood from uremic subjects exhibited an abnormality of platelet arachidonic acid metabolism with a subsequent reduction in thromboxane A_2 production. This may also contribute to defective platelet aggregation in uremia (60).

Platelet dysfunction and bleeding time abnormalities may be partially reversed in uremic individuals with hemodialysis. The amount of hemodialysis may influence the degree of correction. However, usually the bleeding time will not be corrected all the way to normal (44, 70). Platelet functional abnormalities have been corrected to normal following successful renal transplantation in previously uremic individuals.

It is important to keep in mind that the hemodialysis procedure itself may result in platelet activation with subsequent thrombocytopenia. This has been observed most commonly when cuprophane membranes are used. These membranes are known to induce complement activation, platelet activation as evidenced by an increase in thromboxane B_2 levels, and thrombocytopenia (27). The same report demonstrated that these abnormalities do not occur when a noncomplement-activating dialyzer membrane such as polymethylmethacrylate is utilized. Thus, the reactive platelet activation may be a consequence of complement activation when blood comes into contact with the artificial membrane.

Several potential treatments are available to decrease the incidence of bleeding in patients with uremia. Cryoprecipitate, which is enriched with factor VIII and von Willebrand factor, has been shown effective in correcting the bleeding time in uremic patients (68). This form of treatment is hampered because of heterogeneous preparations of cryoprecipitate, the risk of transmitting blood-borne infections, and the short duration of action. Desmopressin causes the release of autologous von Willebrand factor and also corrects the prolonged bleeding time in uremia (47). Like cryoprecipitate, vasopressin has a short duration of action. In 1986, Livio and colleagues (45) reported on the use of conjugated estrogens in the management of uremic bleeding. Five daily infusions of conjugated estrogens shortened the bleeding time in uremic patients with an effect lasting as long as 14 days. In a report published in 1990, the authors concluded that treatment with conjugated estrogens resulted in a shortening of bleeding time associated with an increase in thromboxane A_2 and β-thromboglobulin in the microvasculature. There was no effect on prostacyclin production (28). More recently, oral estrogen therapy has been shown to be effective in improving the bleeding tendency in patients with chronic renal failure (65).

As noted above, hemodialysis may also partially correct the abnormal platelet function in uremia. The degree of correction may depend on how much dialysis the patient receives (44). It has also been demonstrated that the correction of any coexisting anemia in patients with renal failure will also improve uremia-induced platelet dysfunction (69). This can be accomplished either with red cell transfusions in the setting of acute renal failure or erythropoietin therapy in patients with chronic renal failure.

INFECTIOUS COMPLICATIONS

Infectious complications account for a significant amount of morbidity and mortality in patients with acute renal failure. Acute renal failure may develop and later be complicated by infection, or conversely a patient may develop an infection or septicemia with the subsequent appearance of acute renal failure. In either case, the coexistence of infection and acute renal failure carries an ominous prognosis. In a recent study of acute renal failure in the setting of open heart surgery, sepsis was a complication in 25% of the patients (16). Other series have noted the occurrence of sepsis in the setting of acute renal failure 50–60% of the time (15). The incidence of sepsis as a cause of acute renal failure has varied from 5–58% with an overall frequency of 28% (57). However, two recent studies have shown that the presence of sepsis is not a risk factor for the subsequent development of acute renal failure. The results of multivariate analysis suggest that the way in which sepsis is associated with the development of acute renal failure may be on the basis of volume depletion of hypotension (10, 57). Even if sepsis is not a potential cause for acute renal failure, the coexistence of sepsis and acute renal failure can increase patient mortality to as high as 70–90% (15).

The frequent association of infection as a complicating factor is the subject of ongoing investigation. Patients with renal failure have several abnormalities in their host defenses that may account for a predisposition to infection. Some of the information that is present in the literature pertains to chronic renal failure patients on chronic hemodialysis, but may also be applicable to those with acute renal failure. A recent review of host defenses in patients on chronic hemodialysis delineated several immunologic alterations (24). Some of these alterations include defects in the skin barrier because of indwelling vascular catheters as well as skin changes that may be related to uremia itself. Granulocyte abnormalities include abnormal mobilization, phagocytosis, and inflammatory responses. In a rat model of acute renal failure, Clark and colleagues (12) demonstrated that uremic serum had a defective chemotactic response in vitro. Cell-mediated immunity may be depressed because of lymphopenia and shortened lymphocyte survival. Absolute lymphopenia has been described in both acute and chronic renal failure (34). However, despite the depressed level of circulating B lymphocytes, immunoglobulin levels have been reported to be normal (31). There have also been reports of depressed antibody formation in response to specific antigenic challenge in patients with acute renal failure on hemodialysis (24).

The hemodialysis procedure itself may also affect immunologic function and host defenses in patients with renal failure. Hakim and Schafer (27) demonstrated the effect of cuprophane membranes on complement activation. In a more recent report, Vanholder and coworkers (73) concluded that both uremia and the types of dialysis membrane affect the phagocytosis of leukocytes. Defective ability of leukocytes to respond to phagocytic challenge was shown to increase with advancing uremia or the use of cuprophane membranes. Dialysis using noncomplement-acting membranes did not exert the same effect on leukocyte phagocytic function.

In summary, acute renal failure and infectious complications coexist commonly. This combination carries a poor prognosis with a very high mortality. Patients with renal failure have multiple abnormalities in their immune system. In addition, the hemodialysis procedure itself can also induce defects in the immune system. Whether acute renal failure predisposes the patient to the development of infection or the clinical setting itself predisposes the patient to the development of sepsis irrespective of the presence or absence of acute renal failure is a question that cannot be answered at present.

References

1. Akmal M, Bishop JE, Telfer N, Norman AW, Massry SG. Hypocalcemia and hypercalcemia in patients with rhabdomyolysis with and without acute renal failure. J Clin Endocrinol Metab 1986;63:137–142.
2. Alexanian R, Barlogie B, Dixon D. Renal failure in multiple myeloma. Pathogenesis and prognostic implications. Arch Intern Med 1990;150:1693–1695.
3. Anderson RJ, Linas SL, Berns AS, Henrich WL, Miller TR, Gabow PA, Schrier RW. Nonoliguric acute renal failure. N Engl J Med 1977;296:1134–1138.
4. Anderson RJ, Schrier RW. Acute tubular necrosis. In: Schrier RW, Gottschalk CW, eds. Diseases of the kidney. 4th ed. Boston: Little, Brown and Company, 1988:1413–1446.
5. Arieff AI, Lazarowitz VC, Guisado R. Experimental dialysis disequilibrium syndrome: prevention with glycerol. Kidney Int 1978;14:270–278.
6. Aurigemma NM, Feldman NT, Gottleib M, et al. Arterial oxygenation during hemodialysis. N Engl J Med 1977;297:871–873.
7. Banks PA, Sidi S, Gelman ML, Lee KH, Warshaw AL. Amylase-creatinine clearance ratios in serum amylase isoenzymes in moderate renal insufficiency. J Clin Gastroenterol 1979;1:331–335.
8. Baso N, Bagarani M, Materia A, et al. Cimetidine and antacid prophylaxis of acute upper gastrointestinal bleeding in high-risk patients. Am J Surg 1981;141:339–341.
9. Better OS, Stein JH. Early management of shock and prophylaxis of acute renal failure in traumatic rhabdomyolysis. N Engl J Med 1990;322:825–829.
10. Bullock ML, Hum AJ, Finkelstein M, Keane WF. The assessment of risk factors in 462 patients with acute renal failure. Am J Kidney Dis 1985;5:96–103.
11. Clark AS, Mitch WE. Muscle protein turnover and glucose uptake in acutely uremic rats. J Clin Invest 1983;72:836–845.
12. Clark RA, Hamory BH, Ford GH, Kiball HR. Chemotaxis in acute renal failure. J Infect Dis 1972;26:460–463.
13. Chesney RW, Chesney PJ, Davis JP, Segar WE. Renal manifestations of the staphylococcal toxic-shock syndrome. Am J Med 1981;71:583–588.
14. Cooper JD, Lazarowitz VC, Arieff AI. Narrow diagnostic abnormalities in patients with acute renal failure. J Clin Invest 1978;61:1448–1455.
15. Corwin HL, Bonventre JV. Factors influencing survival in acute renal failure. Semin Dial 1989;2:220–225.
16. Corwin HL, Sprague SM, DeLaria GA, Norusis MJ. Acute renal failure associated with cardiac operations: A case controlled study. J Thorac Cardiovasc Surg 1989;98:1107–1112.
17. Craddock PR, Fehr J, Brigham KL, Kronenbery RS, Jacob HS. Complement and leukocyte-mediated pulmonary dysfunction in hemodialysis. N Engl J Med 1977;296:769–774.
18. Crosbie WA, Parsons V. Cardiopulmonary response to acute renal failure [Abstract]. Kidney Int 1976;9:380.
19. Eknoyan G, Wacksman SJ, Glueck HI, Will JJ. Platelet function and renal failure. N Engl J Med 1969;280:677–681.
20. Fillastre JP, Raguenez VG. Cisplatin nephrotoxicity. Toxicol Lett 1989;46:163–175.
21. Forster J, Querusio L, Burchard KW, Gann, DS. Hypercalcemia in critically ill surgical patients. Ann Surg 1985;202:512–518.
22. Fraser CL, Arieff AI. Nervous system complications in uremia. Ann Intern Med 1988;109:143–153.
23. Fraser CL, Sarnacki P, Budayr A. Evidence that parathyroid hormone-mediated calcium transport in rat brain synaptosomes is independent of cyclic adenosine monophosphate. J Clin Invest 1988;81:982–988.

24. Goldblum SE, Reed WP. Host defenses and immunologic alterations associated with chronic hemodialysis. Ann Intern Med 1980;93:597–613.
25. Gordon D, Calne RY. Renal failure in acute pancreatitis. Br Med J 1972;3:801–802.
26. Grossman RA, Hamilton RW, Morse BM, et al. Nontraumatic rhabdomyolysis and acute renal failure. N Engl J Med 1974;291:807–811.
27. Hakim RM, Schafer AI. Hemodialysis associated platelet activation in thrombocytopenia. Am J Med 1985;78:575–580.
28. Heistinger M, Stockenhuber F, Schneider B, et al. Effect of conjugated estrogens on platelet function and prostacyclin generation in CRF. Kidney Int 1990;38:1181–1186.
29. Hörl WH, Heidland A. Enhanced proteolytic activity—cause of protein catabolism in acute renal failure. Am J Clin Nutr 1980;33:1423–1427.
30. Horowitz HI, Stein IM, Cohen BD, White JG. Further studies on the platelet inhibitory effect of guanidinosuccinic acid and its role in uremic bleeding. Am J Med 1970;49:336–345.
31. Hosking CS, Atkins RC, Scott DF, Holdsworth SR, Fitgerald MG, Shelton MJ. Immune and phagocytic functions in patients on maintenance dialysis and post-transplantation. Clin Nephrol 1976;6:501–505.
32. Imrie CW, Whyte AS. A prospective study of acute pancreatitis. Br J Surg 1975;62:490–494.
33. Jacobs ML, Daggett WM, Civetta JM, et al. Acute pancreatitis: analysis of factors influencing survival. Ann Surg 1977;185:43–51.
34. Jensson O. Observations on the leukocyte blood picture in acute uremia. Br J Haematol 1958;4:422–427.
35. Jubelirer SJ. Hemostatic abnormalities in renal disease. Am J Kid Dis 1985;5:219–225.
36. Knochel JP. Biochemical and acid-base disturbances in acute renal failure. In: Brenner BM, Lazarus JM, eds. Acute renal failure. 2nd ed. New York: Churchill Livingstone, 1988:677–703.
37. Kokot F, Kuska J. The endocrine system in patients with acute renal insufficiency. Kidney Int 1976;10:S26–S31.
38. Kone BC, Whelton A, Santos G, Saral R, Watson AJ. Hypertension and renal dysfunction in bone marrow transplant recipients. Quart J Med 1988;69:985–995.
39. Kraman S, Kahn F, Patel S, Seriff N. Renal failure in the respiratory intensive care unit. Crit Care Med 1979;7:263–266.
40. Kurtin P, Kouba J. Profound hypophosphatemia in the course of acute renal failure. Am J Kid Dis 1987;10:346–349.
41. Lach F, Felsenfeld AJ, Haussler MR. Pathophysiology of altered calcium metabolism in rhabdomyolysis-induced acute renal failure. N Engl J Med 1981;305:117–123.
42. Lee HY, Stretton TB, Barnes AM. The lungs in renal failure. Thorax 1975;30:46.
43. Levenson DJ, Skorecki KL, Newell GC, Narins RG. Acute renal failure associated with hepatobiliary disease. In: Brenner BM, Lazarus JM, eds. Acute renal failure. 2nd ed. New York: Churchill Livingstone, 1988:535–580.
44. Lindsay RM, Moorthy AV, Koens F, Linton AL. Platelet function in dialyzed and nondialyzed patients with chronic renal failure. Clin Nephrol 1975;4:52–57.
45. Livio M, Mannucci PM, Vigano G, et al. Conjugated estrogens for the management of bleeding associated with renal failure. N Engl J Med 1986;315:731–735.
46. Long CL, Birkhahn RH, Geiger, JW, Blakemore WS. Contribution of skeletal muscle protein in elevated rates of whole body protein catabolism in trauma patients. Am J Clin Nutr 1981;34:1087–1093.
47. Mannucci PM, Remuzzi G, Pusineri F, et al. Deamino-8-d-arginine vasopressin shortens the bleeding time in uremia. N Engl J Med 1983;308:8–12.
48. Massry SG. Current status of the role of parathyroid hormone in uremic toxicity. Contrib Nephrol 1985;49:1–11.
49. Massry SG, Arieff AI, Coburn JW, et al. Divalent ion metabolism in patients with acute renal failure: studies on the mechanism of hypocalcemia. Kidney Int 1974;5:437–445.
50. Massry SG, Stein R, Garty J, et al. Skeletal resistance to the calcemic action of parathyroid hormone in uremia: Role of 1,25 $(OH)_2D_3$. Kidney Int 1976;9:467–474.
51. McMurray SD, Luft FC, Maxwell DR, et al. Prevailing patterns and predictor variables in patients with acute tubular necrosis. Arch Intern Med 1978;138:950–955.
52. Minuth AN, Terrell JB, Suki WN. Acute renal failure: a study of a course and prognosis of 104 patients and of the role of furosemide. Am J Med Sci 1976;271:317–324.
53. Moran MS, Myers BD. Course of acute renal failure studied by a model of creatinine kinetics. Kidney Int 1985;27:928–937.
54. Papadakis MA, Arieff AI. Unpredictability of clinical evaluation of renal function in cirrhosis. Am J Med 1987;82:945–952.
55. Peura DA, Johnson LF. Cimetidine for prevention and treatment of gastroduodenal mucosal lesions in patients in an intensive care unit. Ann Intern Med 1985;103:173–177.
56. Priebe HJ, Skillman JJ, Bushnell LS, Long PC, Silen W. Antacid vs cimetidine in preventing acute gastrointestinal bleeding. N Engl J Med 1980;302:426–430.
57. Rackow EC, Fein IA, Sprung C, Grodman RS. Uremic pulmonary edema. Am J Med 1978;64:1084–1088.
58. Raskin NH, Fishman RA. Neurologic disorders and renal failure. N Engl J Med 1976;294:143–148.
59. Rasmussen HH, Ibels LS. Acute renal failure. Multivariate analysis of causes and risk factors. Am J Med 1982;73:211–218.
60. Remuzzi G, Benigni A, Dodesini P, et al. Reduced platelet thromboxane formation in uremia. Evidence for a functional cyclo oxygenase defect. J Clin Invest 1983;72:762–768.
61. Remuzzi G, Mecca G, Cavenaghi AE, Donati MB, de Gaetano G. Prostacyclin-like activity and

bleeding in renal failure. Lancet 1977;2:1195–1197.

62. Rodrigo F, Shideman J, McHugh R, Buselmeir T, Kjellstrand C. Osmolality changes during hemodialysis. Natural history, clinical correlations, and influence of dialysate glucose and intravenous mannitol. Ann Intern Med 1977;86:544–561.

63. Saleh RA, Grahm-Pole J, Cumming WA. Severe hyperphosphatemia associated with tumor lysis in a patient with T-cell leukemia. Pediatr Emerg Care 1989;5:231–233.

64. Shapira N, Skillman JJ, Steinman TI, Silen W. Gastric mucosal permeability and gastric acid secretion before and after hemodialysis in patients with chronic renal failure. Surgery 1978;83:528–535.

65. Shemin D, Elnour M, Amarantes B, Abuelo G, Chazan JA. Oral estrogens decrease bleeding time and improve clinical bleeding in patients with renal failure. Am J Med 1990;89:436–440.

66. Shih WJ, Flueck J, O'Connor W, Domstad PA. Extensive extra-osseous localization of bone imaging agent in a patient with renal failure and rhabdomyolysis accompanied by combined hypercalcemia and hyperphosphatemia. Clin Nucl Med 1989;14:163–167.

67. Somerville PJ, Kaye M. Resistance to parathyroid hormone in renal failure: role of vitamin D metabolites. Kidney Int 1978;14:245–254.

68. Steiner RW, Coggins C, Carvalho ACA. Bleeding time in uremia: a useful test to assess clinical bleeding. Am J Hematol 1979;7:107–117.

69. Steinman TI, Lazarus JM. Organ system involvement in acute renal failure. In: Brenner BM, Lazarus JM, eds. Acute renal failure. 2nd ed. New York: Churchill Livingstone, 1988:705–739.

70. Stewart JH, Castaldi PA. Uremic bleeding: a reversible platelet defect corrected by dialysis. Q J Med 1967;36:409–423.

71. Taylor IL, Dockray GJ. Hypergastronemia in renal failure: the biological significance of molecular forms of gastrin. Br J Surg 1976;63:657.

72. Thyssen EP, Hou SH, Alverdy JC, Spiegel DM. Temporary loss of limb function secondary to soft tissue calcification in a patient with rhabdomyolysis-induced acute renal failure. Am J Kidney Dis 1990;16:491–494.

73. Vanholder R, Ringoir S, Dhondt A, et al. Phagocytosis in uremic and hemodialysis patients: a prospective and cross-sectional study. Kidney Int 1991;39:320–327.

74. Wacker W, Merril JP. Uremic pericarditis in acute renal failure. JAMA 1954;156:764.

36

Electrolyte Derangements in Acute Renal Failure

Aldo Fabris

PATHOPHYSIOLOGY OF SODIUM METABOLISM

Sodium is the most important cation in the extracellular fluid space; with its major anions, bicarbonate and chloride, it accounts for more than 90% of the osmotically active solutes in this compartment. By virtue of its relationship to the osmolality of body fluids, the sodium concentration indirectly influences the volume of intracellular water, and the quantity of total body sodium is the main determinant of the extracellular volume (25).

Because the control of extracellular fluid volume depends on the regulation of sodium balance, any variation of the latter will be accompanied by a modification of the former. In the case of positive sodium balance, the increased amount of the cation, predominantly located in the extracellular fluid compartment, creates an osmotic gradient between intra- and extracellular space, causing a water movement out of the cells and an expansion of extracellular fluid volume. Additionally, the increase of extracellular fluid osmolality both stimulates the thirst center with consequent increased fluid intake and leads to a release of antidiuretic hormone, which decreases water excretion by increasing tubular water permeability (3). Finally, the influence of positive sodium balance, combined with a release of antidiuretic hormone and increased thirst, leads to expansion of extracellular fluid volume.

Conversely, a negative sodium balance results in extracellular fluid volume depletion that is clinically manifested by de-creased skin turgor, dry oral mucous membranes, flat neck veins, decreased axillary sweating, tachycardia, orthostatic hypotension, and in some instances, oliguria and prerenal acute renal failure.

Decrease, increase, as well as normal total body sodium, clinically expressed by contraction of extracellular fluid volume, edema, and apparent euvolemia, respectively, can be accompanied either by hyponatremia or hypernatremia. The former is the result of an excess of total body water relative to body sodium; the latter is the expression of a relative water deficit.

Hyponatremia is often observed during extrarenal and renal losses of sodium-containing fluids that are responsible for a depletion of extracellular fluid volume. Extrarenal causes of extracellular fluid volume depletion, as observed during vomiting, diarrhea, fluid sequestration in "third space" (peritonitis, pancreatitis, rhabdomyolysis, burns) activate the various volume regulatory responses. These include stimulation of renin-angiotensin-aldosterone axis, antidiuretic hormone release, and modification of renal hemodynamics such as reduction of glomerular filtration rate and renal plasma flow, changes in filtration fraction, and in peritubular capillary hydrostatic pressure. These combined forces lead to renal sodium and water retention and reduction in urine output, thus accounting for the low urinary sodium and for the high urinary osmolality, which along with other signs are considered pathognomonic aspects of prerenal acute renal failure (Table 36.1) (10). One possible exception to the association of hypovolemia and low urinary sodium,

Table 36.1
Sodium Derangements in Acute Renal Failure [a]

Hypovolemic Hyponatremia (with low TBNa)			Hyponatremia with High TBNa			Hypovolemic Hypernatremia (with low TBNa)		
Causes	Uosm	UNa	Causes	Uosm	UNa	Causes	Uosm	UN
Vomiting (steady state)	↑	↑ or ↓	CHF	↑	↓	Excess sweating	↑	↓
Third space	↑	↓	Cirrhosis	↑	↓	Diarrhea	↑	↓
Diarrhea	↑	↓	Nephrosis	↑	↓	Nonoliguric ARF	iso	↑
Renal losses			ARF	iso	↑	Recovery phase of ARF	↓	↑
Diuretics	iso	↑				Osmotic diuresis	↓	↑
Salt-losing nephritis	iso	↑						

[a]TBNa, total body sodium; Uosm, urine osmolality; UNa, urine sodium; ↑, increased; ↓, decreased; CHF, cardiac failure; ARF, acute renal failure; iso, isotonic.

is the metabolic alkalosis often linked to vomiting, where bicarbonaturia obligates cation losses (sodium and potassium) to maintain electolyte neutrality. In this condition, low urine chloride is the best marker for extracellular fluid volume contraction (22).

When the cause of losses of sodium-containing fluids that may lead to extracellular fluid volume depletion and hyponatremia is of renal origin as occurs for example during diuretic therapy and in sodium-losing nephritis, the kidney is not able to respond appropriately to extracellular fluid volume depletion, thus eliminating an isotonic sodium-rich urine (Table 36.1) (10).

In the extrarenal and renal losses listed above, the presence of hyponatremia is ascribed to impaired water excretion. The mechanism of this impairment depends on (a) decreased delivery of filtrate to diluting segment of the nephron, secondary to reduced glomerular filtration rate and increased proximal tubular reabsorption (the capacity of generating free water will therefore be diminished), and (b) nonosmotic antidiuretic hormone release, with consequent increased urinary concentration and enhanced water retention (19).

Hyponatremia will appear when, in an individual patient who is unable to dilute urine, hypotonic infusions are administered or increased water intake, in part secondary to stimulation of thirst by angiotensin II, is present (19).

The same sequence of events described during extracellular fluid volume deple-

tion and leading to sodium and water retention can be observed in other hyponatremia conditions such as nephrotic syndrome, cirrhosis, and cardiac failure (Table 36.1), characterized by increased total body sodium, extracellular fluid volume expansion, and edema, but by reduction of effective arterial blood volume (19). In these circumstances, renal hypoperfusion can precipitate prerenal acute renal failure when factors worsening an already unstable circulatory equilibrium are superimposed.

In acute renal failure, when renal dilution is compromised by organic alterations, hyponatremia frequently occurs when water intake exceeds the losses. This situation is characterized by an increased total body sodium (19), by an isotonic urine, and by high urinary sodium (Table 36.1). To avoid this disorder, which leads to circulatory overload, and taking into account the fact that insensible water losses in uncomplicated situations are about 800 ml/day and endogenous water production are about 400 ml/day, daily water intake should be about 400 ml, plus the amount of water lost through renal and extrarenal routes. Another method to avoid hyperhydration is to watch closely the weight of the patient. Because acute renal failure is a catabolic state, a loss of 0.3–0.5 kg/day is considered to be normal; therefore, any weight gain represents an excess of fluid administration.

Extracellular fluid volume depletion, causing prerenal acute renal failure, can also be observed during hypotonic fluid losses that are not replaced by adequate water intake (11) or are partially repaired with relatively hypertonic solutions (32). In these situations, hypernatremia is the rule. If the losses are of extrarenal origin, like in profuse sweating and in gastroenteritis with profuse diarrhea, particularly in children, the kidney acts as reported above to preserve extracellular fluid volume, thus eliminating a concentrated urine low in sodium (Table 36.1) (10).

Hypotonic losses with extracellular fluid volume depletion and hypernatremia can also be noted in nonoliguric acute renal failure, in the recovery phase of acute renal failure, after relief of obstruction, or during any other variety of osmotic diuresis. In these situations, urinary sodium will be more than 20 mEq/liter and urine will be iso or hypotonic (Table 36.1).

Hypotension and other signs of hypovolemia are rarely noted in the hypernatremia that accompanies pure water losses of diabetes insipidus, either central or nephrogenic, or in the hypernatremia observed during insensible water losses through skin and lungs. Because water freely crosses cellular membranes, two-thirds of the losses will originate from the intracellular compartment and one-third from the extracellular compartment. Because intravascular water content represents $1/12$ of total body water, it will contribute only about 8% to the losses, thus accounting for the low incidence on vascular symptoms (20), unless the losses of pure water are remarkable.

Clinical Manifestations

Clinical signs of hyponatremia generally occur at serum sodium concentration below 120–125 mEq/liter and mainly involve the neuropsychiatric functions. The symptoms include lethargy, fatigue, disorientation, headache, muscle cramps, anorexia, psychosis, pseudobulbar palsy, seizures, and coma (6). The degree of symptoms depends on age (elderly persons, children, and young females in the postoperative period are more prone to manifest symptoms), sex, and rate of development of the hyponatremia (6). The serum sodium reduction that develops in

less than 24 hr frequently results in more serious symptoms than those occurring over more prolonged time (16).

The prognosis is very poor in rapidly developing severe hyponatremia, particularly in alcoholics, malnourished persons, and in patients with debilitating diseases (7). The dependency of symptoms and prognosis on the rapidity and severity of hyponatremia correlate well with alterations that occur in brain water content (16). Experimentally, it has been demonstrated that acute hyponatremia is associated with cerebral edema, while in chronic hyponatremia, brain water content and solute concentration are less than that observed in the acute form (16). This suggests that brain cells regulate their volume by extruding osmotically active solutes, such as Na^+, K^+, Cl^-, various osmolytes, and amino acids, thus causing less movement of water into brain cells (16).

Also in hypernatremia (defined as when serum sodium is greater than 150 mEq/liter), the predominant abnormalities are neurologic (15). When hypernatremia develops rapidly, initial symptoms including restlessness, irritability, ataxia, tremors, hyperreflexia, lethargy, and convulsions can progress to depression in sensorium and coma (16, 17). In the chronic form, symptoms are less marked.

Mortality, morbidity, and neurologic sequelae, particularly in children, may be very high when hypernatremia develops acutely (21).

As in hyponatremia, the symptoms of hypernatremia are linked to variations in brain water content. Experimentally, in the acute hypernatremic form, the rapid increase of plasma osmolality leads to a water movement out of the cerebral cells with shrinkage of the brain and possible hemorrhages (38). In the chronic form, the alteration in brain water content is less marked because it is attenuated by a brain increase both in known solutes, such as sodium, potassium, chloride, glucose, amino acids, and unknown substances. The latter are termed "idiogenic osmoles" (16). These substances may also have major therapeutic implications in the treatment of hypernatremia because they produce a water movement into cells during water replacement. The resultant cell swelling may account for some manifestations such as seizures, which occur in rapid correction of hypernatremia. For this reason, a slower rate of correction permits the brain to extrude the osmotic substances, thus preventing cerebral edema.

Treatment

Hyponatremia

The treatment of hyponatremia is still debated because there is no agreement about the rate of treatment. Excessively slow therapy seems to result in increased mortality, while rapid treatment appears to be associated with central pontine myelinolysis (33), a disease first described in 1959 (1). In this disease, the patient presents with hyponatremic symptoms that can be mild, such as weakness and dysarthria, or severe, such as seizures and coma. During the treatment of hyponatremia, the symptoms improve, but later on neurologic conditions worsen and new symptomats emerge. In classic cases there is a gradual onset of pseudobulbary palsy, quadriplegia, inability to speak, and impaired response to painful stimuli. The majority of patients are alcoholics, malnourished, or persons with debilitating diseases.

Knowing the problems associated with the treatment of hyponatremia, several authors have tried to indicate the best strategy to treat this disorder. Ayus et al. (7) noted that rapid treatment of severe symptomatic hyponatremia to obtain mildly hyponatremic levels at a rate of 2 mEq/liter/hr was accompanied by less mortality than that observed in patients in whom hyponatremia was treated at a rate less than 0.7 mEq/liter/hr, which is considered slow treatment. This statement was confirmed in a follow-up study in which the appearance of demyelinizating lesions in a group of patients who underwent rapid treatment of hyponatremia was attributed more to several concomitant causes—such as a delay in diagnosis and initiation of therapy and rapid increase in serum sodium to either normal or hypernatremic levels within the first 48 hr of therapy—than to rate of correction per se (8).

Cheng et al. (13) noted that the rapid

Table 36.2
Therapy for Hyponatremia [a]

Condition	Therapy
Acute symptomatic hyponatremia	Rapid restoration to mildly hyponatremic levels
Chronic severe hyponatremia	Slow treatment
Asymptomatic hyponatremia	Restriction of water intake
Hyponatremia with low total body sodium	Isotonic saline
Hyponatremia with high total body sodium	Restriction of water and sodium intake and increased excretion of both

[a]See text for details.

treatment of acute hyponatremia produced no long-term neurologic sequelae, and Arieff (24) reported permanent brain damage in those patients in whom serum sodium levels were slowly returned to mildly hyponatremic values. On the other hand, Sterns (39) stated that there was no evidence that slow treatment, defined as an increase of less than 12 mEq/liter/day, was accompanied by an increased risk of brain damage or death when compared with rapid treatment.

From the data of the literature and from our own experience, some conclusions can be drawn (Table 36.2):

1. In acute symptomatic hyponatremia (when the rate of decrease of serum sodium exceeds 0.5 mEq/liter/hr) (15), treatment to return to mildly hyponatremic levels (120–130 mEq/liter) should be rapid, at a rate of 1–2 mEq/liter/hr, with complete serum sodium restoration in several days (8, 31). In the first 48 hr sodium increase should not exceed 25 mEq/liter (8). The treatment can be accomplished with 3% (513 mEq/liter) or 5% (855 mEq/liter) saline; however, treatment with hypertonic saline can be followed by fluid overload, particularly dangerous in the elderly. On the other hand, because the sodium infused is completely excreted, plasma sodium increase is small (36). For these reasons, some authors utilize concomitant IV furosemide, which increases free water clearance (9), or ultrafiltration, when the diuretic is not effective

(37), thus augmenting the effect of hypertonic saline in correcting the hyponatremia. The excess of water that has to be excreted can be estimated as follows:

Excess water: TBW × actual plasma Na/desired plasma Na, where TBW is the body weight × 60%. For example, in a 70-kg man the water to be excreted to correct natremia from 110 to 125 mEq/liter is: $42 \times 110/125 = 37$; $42 - 37 = 5$ liters.

2. In severe chronic hyponatremia, some authors advise slow treatment, at a rate less than 0.5 mEq/liter/hr (15) or less than 12 mEq/liter/day for the 1st day and even slower for the following days (40). In the presence of severe neurologic symptoms, it has been suggested that aggressive therapy designed to increase the serum sodium by 1–2 mEq/liter/hr should be stopped after 4 hr or as soon the clinical situation improves (40).
3. In asymptomatic hyponatremia it is generally sufficient to restrict water and wait for the evaporative and urinary losses to correct the hyponatremia (31).
4. The hyponatremia with a low tidal body sodium and extracellular flow volume depletion rarely necessitates infusion of hypertonic saline. In this setting it is sufficient to administer isotonic saline until the volume deficit is repaired. The reexamination of intravascular volume, by normalizing renal blood flow, glomerular filtration rate, proximal tubular reabsorption, and by suppressing antidiuretic hormone release, will reverse the pathophysiologic factors that had caused the impaired water excretion. With this therapy, serum sodium concentration may return to normal within a few hours, but this rapid treatment does not seem dangerous (31).
5. The hyponatremia with increased total body sodium and edema is best managed by restriction of sodium and water intake and by increasing the excretion of both these elements. This can be accomplished by diuretic therapy or by ultrafiltration.

Hypernatremia

In volume-depleted hypernatremic patients, the initial step to recovery is to reverse the symptoms linked to hypovolemia, such as hypotension, tachycardia, and flat neck veins, by isotonic saline. Then 0.45% saline or 5% dextrose is administered to lower the plasma osmolality.

As above reported, fluid administration should be given at a rate that lowers plasma osmolality by about 2 mOsm/hr to avoid any cerebral edema (19). The water deficit can be calculated with the same formula used for hyponatremia. For example, a 70-kg man with a serum sodium of 170 mEq/liter, must receive 9 liters to lower the sodium to 140 mEq/liter. The change in osmolality is from 340 mOsm (170×2) to 280 mOsm (140×2) or 60 mOsm; at a rate of 2 mOsm/hr, this decrease would require 30 hours (19). Thus, the 9 liters of hypotonic fluid should be administered in a period of 30 hours or more. Water replacement calculated by the usual formula, plus removal of sodium with diuretic therapy and substitution of water lost with this drug, is the therapy of choice when iatrogenic hypernatremia (e.g., that caused by excessive bicarbonate infusion utilized to correct uremic acidosis) is present in acute renal failure. Of course, when a diuretic is not efficacious, dialysis is the only choice.

PATHOPHYSIOLOGY OF POTASSIUM METABOLISM

Potassium is the major cation of the body. Ninety-eight percent of potassium is located in intracellular fluid, while only 2% is extracellular. In consideration of the great difference between intra- and extracellular potassium content, factors controlling transcellular potassium distribution, such as acid-base status, pancreatic hormones, catecholamines, aldosterone, osmolality, exercise, and cellular potassium content, are of great importance in maintaining normal serum levels (44). If internal regulation plays a major role in short-term potassium homeostasis, the long-term homeostasis is governed mainly by the kidneys.

In general, potassium is freely filtered at the glomerulus; up to 90% of the filtered potassium is reabsorbed in the proximal tubule. The potassium excreted in the urine is primarily the result of secretion in the distal convolute tubule and in the collecting duct. The potassium handling by distal nephron is influenced by several factors such as potassium plasma concentration, sodium delivery and urine flow rate, transepithelial potential difference, acid-base status, and hormonal interferences by aldosterone and glucocorticoids (44).

In acute renal failure, some of the factors responsible for the potassium balance are deranged, so that in the oliguric form an increase in potassium is often present.

The most important causes of hyperkalemia are the following (19): (a) the glomerular filtration rate is often severely reduced, thereby becoming itself a limiting factor for potassium excretion; (b) distal sodium delivery and urine flow rate are markedly decreased; (c) the most common cause of acute renal failure is tubular necrosis, which results in damage of that part of the nephron primarily responsible for potassium secretion; and (d) potassium is shifted out of the cells because of acidemia and hyperosmolality. Regarding the former, it has been demonstrated that a change in blood pH of 0.1 unit results in average 0.6 mEq/liter change in plasma potassium concentration (12). For example, a reduction of 0.1 unit of pH, as observed in acidosis, is accompanied by an increase of plasma concentration of 0.6 mEq/liter. However, more recent studies indicate that this relationship is more complex and this interaction is highly variable (2).

Suppression of renin and aldosterone secretion may partly play a role for hyperkalemia in acute renal failure induced by nonsteroidal antiinflammatory drugs (14). Also angiotensin-converting enzyme inhibitors cause hypoaldosteronism and hyperkalemia by blocking the secretion of aldosterone, which is angiotensin II-mediated (35). Cyclosporine, a potent immunosuppressive drug, produces hyperkalemia not only by inducing hyporeninemic hypoaldosteronism, but also by interfering directly with tubular secretion of potassium (43).

The increase of serum potassium by mechanisms reported above, in noncatabolic patients, is about 0.5 mEq/day. Higher rates of elevation should suggest catabolism, tissue necrosis, hemolysis, or an exogenous origin, such as medications, diet, or blood transfusions.

In the oliguric phase of acute renal failure, hypokalemia may also be observed. It is caused by potassium losses through vomiting or nasogastric suction, intestinal drainage, or diarrhea. Finally, hypokalemia and potassium depletion secondary to urinary losses have been described in association with postobstructive diuresis and with diuresis in the recovery phase of acute tubular necrosis (43).

Clinical Manifestations

The signs and symptoms of hyperkalemia are cardiac and neuromuscular. The earliest cardiac sign that may be found when serum potassium is 5–6.5 mEq/liter is represented by a peaking or tenting of T waves. More severe hyperkalemia (serum potassium of 6.5–8 mEq/liter) is characterized by a flattening of P wave, prolongation of the P-R interval, and widening of QRS complex with development of deep S wave. A more severe hyperkalemia (levels >8 mEq/liter) produce a further widening of QRS. Often the S wave merges with the peaked T waves to produce a sine wave pattern, which is a prelude to ventricular fibrillation or cardiac arrest (23).

Neuromuscular manifestations include tingling and muscle weakness that may progress to symmetric ascending flaccid paralysis, often accompanied by paresthesias in the extremities (23). Neuromuscular involvement is also described in hypokalemia and potassium depletion. A mild degree of depletion may be asymptomatic, but in some patients muscular weakness, especially in the lower extremities, is present. With more severe hypokalemia and a potassium deficit, the involvement of skeletal muscles varies from deep weakness to paralysis that can also affect the respiratory muscles with consequent hypoxia, hypercapnia, and death (23). Reduced gastrointestinal tract motility, with symptoms ranging from constipation to ileus, is often observed in profound potassium depletion (45). Finally, severe hypokalemia predisposes to rhabdomyolysis (24). The typical electrocardiographic changes of hypokalemia include depression of the ST segment of 0.5 mm or more, U wave amplitude greater than 1 mm, and U wave amplitude greater than T wave amplitude in the same lead (42). Potassium depletion enhances the cardiac toxicity of digitalis, predisposing to atrial and ventricular arrhythmias.

Treatment

The treatment of hyperkalemia is directed to counteract cardiac toxicity, to shift potassium into cells, and to remove potassium from the body (Table 36.3).

The first step in treatment is obtained by the use of calcium salts (gluconate is preferable); between 10 and 30 ml of a 10% solution should be administered IV over a period of 3–4 minutes.

The second step is accomplished by two methods: (a) rapid IV infusion of 50–100 mEq/ of NaHCO₃, and (b) rapid IV infusion of 50 ml of a 50% glucose solution plus 10 units of regular insulin, followed by continuous infusion of 500 ml of 10% glucose over 30–60 minutes plus 10 units of regular insulin (23).

The definitive therapy is the removal of potassium from the body that can be accomplished with cation exchange resin (Kayexalate). Oral administration is more efficient than enemas, and each gram of resin removes 1.0 mEq of potassium. It is customary to simultaneously use cathartics such as sorbitol. In those circumstances in which resin is not efficient, dialysis is the only method to remove potassium.

In hypokalemia, when the conditions are not urgent, it is preferable to use potassium supplementation by the oral route at a dosage of 40–120 mEq/day (44). Emergencies require IV therapy; the optimal rate of infusion should be 20 mEq/hr and should not exceed 100–150 mEq/day, unless the need for more rapid infusion is demonstrated by large losses during the period of replacement therapy (23).

Potassium infusion rates greater than 40 mEq/hr should be given only for extreme potassium depletion and hypokalemia and only under close monitoring (23).

PATHOPHYSIOLOGY OF DIVALENT IONS METABOLISM

Hyperphosphatemia and hypermagnesemia are almost always present during the oliguric phase of acute renal failure (29). The retention of these ions is secondary to the inability of the kidney to excrete them. Hyperphosphatemia is usually moderate, but elevated values up to 18.0 mg/dL may be seen in rhabdomyolysis (28). Hypermagnesemia is mild, but greater values can be observed in patients ingesting medications containing magnesium. During the diuretic phase of acute renal failure, the levels of phosphorus and magnesium fall, returning to normal after the recovery of renal function.

Hypocalcemia, particularly severe in rhabdomyolysis, is invariably noted during the oliguric phase and occurs early after the onset of acute renal failure (29). Hypocalcemia usually persists during the diuretic phase and normalizes after the recovery of renal function.

Several factors contribute to hypocalcemia, including hyperphosphatemia and increased tissue deposition of calcium, particularly frequent in rhabdomyolysis, hypoalbuminemia, or alterations in calcium binding by serum protein. However, the most important factor involved in the genesis of hypocalcemia is the skeletal resistance to the calcemic action of parathormone (29), which is associated with reduced levels of 25-(OH)D (34) and 1,25-(OH)₂D (26). The low levels of 1,25-(OH)₂D, which decrease intestinal calcium absorption, may further contribute to the persistence of hypocalcemia.

Hypercalcemia can be observed in the recovery phase of acute renal failure, particularly in rhabdomyolysis. The mechanism may be related to the mobilization of

---

Table 36.3
Hyperkalemia Therapy

1. Counteraction of cardiac toxicity of potassium
   Calcium gluconate
2. Passage of potassium into cells
   Sodium bicarbonate
   Glucose and insulin
3. Removal of potassium from the body
   Cation exchange resin
   Hemodialysis

calcium previously precipitated in the damaged muscles and to the high levels of 1,25-(OH)$_2$D (26). The mechanism responsible for the elevation of 1,25-(OH)$_2$D is caused by the release from injured muscles of vitamin D that provides more substrate for the production of 1,25-(OH)$_2$D. Kidneys recovering from acute renal failure may not have regained their usual control of production of 1,25-(OH)$_2$D, so that this metabolite may be produced in greater quantities (28).

Severe hypermagnesemia is treated with an IV injection of calcium salts; in general, 100–200 mg of calcium ion are adequate to reverse symptoms (27).

Hyperphosphatemia is treated with aluminum hydroxide after meals to prevent intestinal absorption of phosphate.

Hypocalcemia rarely requires therapy. However, when associated with neuromuscular disturbances such as carpopedal spasms or tetany, or cardiac arrhythmias, treatment with IV calcium should be started. Calcium gluconate is preferred and 10–20 ml of 10% solution are administered.

It is important to mention that caution must be used in treating uremic acidosis with alkali because this therapy, by decreasing serum ionized calcium, can precipitate tetany or seizures.

Hypercalcemia that develops during the oliguric phase (this derangement may be rarely observed in acute renal failure that is induced by rhabdomyolysis), especially when the serum phosphate levels are elevated, is very dangerous because of the possibility of calcium deposition in vital organs such as lung and heart. To avoid this complication, dialysis using calcium-free dialysate or continuous arteriovenous hemofiltration (37) should be promptly instituted. The hypercalcemia of the diuretic phase, when levels of serum phosphorus are falling, is usually benign and asymptomatic. However, some patients may manifest the symptoms of hypercalcemia, such as malaise, weakness, headache, disorientation, speech defects, visual disturbances, anorexia, nausea, and hypertension. In these patients, increased urinary calcium excretion by infusion of isotonic saline and administration of furosemide (41), increased movement of calcium into bone by use of inorganic phosphate, inhibition of bone resorption by calcitonin, mytramicin, glucocorticoids, diphosphonates, and finally dialysis with a calcium-free dialysate should be carried out (30).

References

1. Adams R, Victor M, Mancall EL. Central pontine myelinolysis a hitherto undescribed disease occurring in alcoholic and malnourished patients. Arch Neurol Psychiatry 1959;81:154–172.
2. Adrogue HJ, Madias NE. Changes in plasma potassium concentration during acute acid-base disturbances. Am J Med 1981;71:456–467.
3. Anderson RJ, Schrier RV. Renal sodium excretion, edematous disorders, and diuretic use. In: Schrier RW, ed. Renal and electrolyte disorders. Boston: Little Brown, and Company, 1986:79–139.
4. Arieff AI. Hyponatremia, convulsion, respiratory arrest and permanent brain damage after elective surgery in healthy women. N Engl J Med 1986;314:1529–1535.
5. Arieff AI, Guisado R. Effects on the central nervous system of hypernatremic and hyponatremic states. Kidney Int 1976;10:104–116.
6. Arieff AI, Llach F, Massry SG. Neurological manifestations and morbidity of hyponatremia: correlation of brain water and electrolytes. Medicine (Baltimore) 1976;55:121–128.
7. Ayus CJ, Krothapalli RK, Arieff AI. Changing concepts in treatment of severe symptomatic hyponatremia. Rapid correction and possible relation to central pontine myelinolysis. Am J Med 1985;78:897–902.
8. Ayus CJ, Krothapalli RK, Arieff AI. Treatment of symptomatic hyponatremia and its relation to brain damage. A prospective study. N Engl J Med 1987;317:1190–1195.
9. Ayus JC, Olivero JJ, Frommer JP. Rapid correction of severe hyponatremia with intravenous hypertonic saline solution. Am J Med 1982;72:43–48.
10. Berl T, Anderson RJ, McDonald KM, Schrier RW. Clinical disorders of water metabolism. Kidney Int 1976;10:117–132.
11. Berl T, Schrier RV. Disorders of water metabolism. In: Schrier RW, ed. Renal and electrolyte disorders. Boston: Little Brown, and Company, 1986:1–78.
12. Burnell JM, Villamil MF, Uyeno BT, Scribner BH. The effect in humans of extracellular pH change on the relationship between serum potassium concentration and intracellular potassium. J Clin Invest 1956; 35:935–939.
13. Cheng JC, Zikos D, Skopicki HA, Peterson DR, Fisher KA. Long-term neurologic outcome in psychogenic water drinkers with severe symptomatic hyponatremia: the effect of rapid correction. Am J Med 1990;88:561–566.
14. Clive DM, Stoff JS. Renal syndromes associated with nonsteroidal anti-inflammatory drugs. N Engl J Med 1984;310:563–568.

15. Cluitmans FH, Meinders AE. Management of severe hyponatremia: rapid or slow correction? Am J Med 1990;88:161–166.
16. Covey CM, Arieff AI. Disorders of sodium and water metabolism and their effects on the central nervous system. In: Brenner BM, Stein JH, eds. Contemporary issues in nephrology. New York: Churchill Livingstone, 1978:212–241.
17. Daggett P, Deanfield J, Moss F, Reynolds D. Severe hypernatremia in adults. Br Med J 1979;1:1177–1180.
18. De Fronzo RA, Thier SO. Fluid and electrolyte disturbances. Hypo and hyperkalemia. In: Martinez-Maldonado M, ed. Handbook of renal therapeutics. New York: Plenum Medical, 1983;25–55.
19. Dixon BS, Schrier RW. Hyponatremia and Hypernatremia. In: Massry SG, Glassock RJ, eds. Textbook of nephrology. Baltimore: Williams & Wilkins, 1989:246–256.
20. Feig PU. Hypernatremia and hypertonic syndromes. Med Clin North Am 1981;65:271–290.
21. Finberg L. Fluid, electrolyte and acid-base abnormalities in pediatrics. In: Maxwell NH, Kleeman CR, eds. Clinical disorders of fluid and electrolyte metabolism. New York: McGraw-Hill, 1980:1563–1580.
22. Kassirer JP, Schwartz WB. The response of normal man to selective depletion of hydrochloric acid. Am J Med 1966;40:10–18.
23. Kassirer JP, Wish JB. Disorders of potassium metabolism. In: Suki WN, Massry SG, eds. Therapy of renal diseases and related disorders. Boston: Martinus Nijhoff, 1984:63–81.
24. Knochel JP, Schlein EM. On the mechanism of rhabdomyolysis in potassium depletion. J Clin Invest 1972;51:1750–1758.
25. Lassiter WE. Disorders of sodium metabolism. In: Earley LE, Gottschalk CV, eds. Strauss and Welt's diseases of the kidney. Boston: Little Brown, and Company, 1979:1507–1541.
26. Llach F, Felsenfeld AJ, Haussler MR. The pathophysiology of altered calcium metabolism in rhabdomyolysis-induced acute renal failure. N Engl J Med 1981;305:117–123.
27. Massry SG. Hypomagnesemia and Hypermagnesemia. In: Massry SG, Glossock RJ, eds. Textbook of nephrology. Baltimore: Williams & Wilkins, 1989:323–327.
28. Massry SG. Metabolic and endocrin abnormalities in acute renal failure. In: Massry SG, Glassock RJ, eds. Textbook of nephrology. Baltimore: Williams & Wilkins, 1989:880–888.
29. Massry SG, Arieff AI, Coburn JW, Palmieri G, Kleeman CR. Divalent ion metabolism in patients with acute renal failure: studies on the mechanism of hypocalcemia. Kidney Int 1974;5:437–445.
30. Massry SG, Kaptein EM. Hypercalcemia and hypocalcemia. In: Massry SG, Glassock RJ, eds. Textbook of nephrology. Baltimore: Williams & Wilkins, 1989:300–311.
31. Narins RG. Therapy of hyponatremia. Does haste make waste? N Engl J Med 1986;314:1573–1575.
32. Narins RG, Jones ER, Stom MC, Rudnick MR, Bastl CP. Diagnostic strategies in disorders of fluid, electrolyte and acid-base homeostasis. Am J Med 1982;72:496–520.
33. Norenberg MD, Leslie KO, Robertson AS. Association between rise in serum sodium and central pontine myelinolysis. Ann Neurol 1982;11:128–135.
34. Pietrek J, Kokot F, Kuka J. Serum 25-hydroxyvitamin D and parathyroid hormone in patients with acute renal failure. Kidney Int 1978;13:178–185.
35. Ponce SP, Jennings AE, Madias NE, Harrington JT. Drug-induced hyperkalemia. Medicine (Baltimore) 1985;64:357–370.
36. Robertson GL, Berl T. Pathophysiology of water metabolism. In: Brenner BM, Rector FC, eds. The kidney. Philadelphia: WB Saunders, 1991: 677–736.
37. Ronco C, Brendolan A, Bragantini L, et al. Continuous arteriovenous hemofiltration. Contrib Nephrol 1985;48:70–88.
38. Simmons MA, Adcock EW, Bard H, Battaglia FC. Hypernatremia and intracranial hemorrhage in neonates. N Engl J Med 1974;291:6–10.
39. Sterns RH. The treatment of hyponatremia: First, do not harm. Am J Med 1990;88:557–560.
40. Sterns RH. The management of severe hyponatremia. Semin Nephrol 1990;10:503–514.
41. Suki WN, Yium JJ, VonMinden M, Eknoyan G, Martinez-Maldonado M. Acute treatment of hypercalcemia with furosemide. N Engl J Med 1970;283:836–840.
42. Surawicz B. Electrolytes and the electrocardiogram. Postgrad Med 1974;55:123–129.
43. Tannen RL. Hypokalemia and Hyperkalemia. In: Massry SG, Glassock RJ, eds. Textbook of nephrology. Baltimore: Williams & Wilkins, 1989: 273–283.
44. Tannen RL. Disorders of potassium balance. In: Brenner BM, Rector FL, eds. The kidney. Philadelphia: WB Saunders, 1991:805–840.
45. Welt LG, Hollander W Jr, Blythe WB. The consequences of potassium depletion. J Chron Dis 1960;11:214–254.

37

Acid-Base Derangements in Acute Renal Failure

Luciano Gattinoni
Mariano Feriani

The kidney makes an indispensable contribution to the day-to-day stabilization of the acid-base equilibrium by preventing excretion of filtered bicarbonate and by promoting excretion of the strong acids generated by metabolic processes. On the other hand, since the kidney precisely modulates the excretion of excessive blood bicarbonate in the urine, in the case of metabolic alkalosis, or by enhancing net acid excretion, in the case of metabolic acidosis, an intact renal function is an essential condition for maintaining the acid-base equilibrium of the body.

When renal function abruptly declines, such as in acute renal failure (ARF), several acid-base derangements can be encountered depending on the etiology and the associated complications of ARF. In this chapter we will focus on (a) the effects of an acute impairment of kidney function on acid-base balance, (b) the effect of the kidney function impairment when associated with an additional acid load, as in the circulatory failure, or an associated impairment of respiratory function, as commonly found in the critically ill patients, and (c) the treatment of these acid-base disorders, emphasizing the use of different extracorporeal techniques. A summary on the acid-base physiology is essential to approach the complex relationship between lung and kidney in handling acid-base balance, as may be observed in critically ill patients.

ACID-BASE PHYSIOLOGY AND PHYSIOPATHOLOGY

Buffer System

Despite the daily production of approximately 16,000 mEq of hydrogen ion (H^+), the concentration of free H^+ in the extracellular compartment remains 40 nmol/liter (40×10^{-9} mol/L, or pH=7.40). The limits compatible with life are between 16 (pH=7.80) and 160 nmol/liter (pH=6.8). The extremely low free H^+ concentration in the body is made possible by the presence of buffer systems (which may capture or release H^+) minimizing the changes of free H^+.

The body buffers are primarily weak acids mixed with the salt of that acid and a strong base. At the given pH, the relative concentration of the base (able to accept H^+) and the acid (able to give up H^+) are defined by the Henderson-Hasselbalch equation:

$$pH = pK + \log \frac{\text{BASE (dissociated)}}{\text{ACID (undissociated)}} \quad (1)$$

A buffer system that, at the blood pH, is present half as base and half as acid is the most efficient in buffering an increase or a decrease of H^+ into the system. This condition occurs when the pK of a particular buffer system equals the pH (log 1 is equal to 0, pH=pK in equation 1); 80% of buffering occurs when pK is within + or − 1

Table 37.1
Characteristics of Physiologic Buffer Systems

Buffer and Normal Concentration	Base Acid	pK	Base/Acid Ratio at pH=7.4	Primary Location
Bicarbonate-carbonic acid 25 mEq/liter	$\dfrac{HCO_3^-}{H_2CO_3}$	6.1	20:1	Extracellular
Phosphate dibasic-monobasic inorganic-organic 2 mEq/liter	$\dfrac{HPO_4^{2-}}{H_2PO_4^-}$	6.8	4:1	Extracellular Intracellular Urine
Proteins 14 mEq/liter (7 g/100 ml)	$\dfrac{P^-r}{HPr}$	6.8	4:1	Intracellular
Hemoglobin 90 mEq/liter (15 g/100 ml)	$\dfrac{Hb^-}{HHb}$	6.8	4:1	Plasma

pH unit, i.e., when the base-acid ratio is within 10:1 and 1:10. As an example, a buffer with pK=3 shows buffer effect in a solution where pH is between 2 and 4. The pK of the most important buffers, their normal concentration in blood, and base-acid ratio at pH=7.40 is summarized in Table 37.1.

It is important to note that:

1. Phosphate, proteins, and hemoglobin pairs, with pK=6.8, are suitable buffers because the pK for an extracellular buffer to be biologically effective should range between 6.4 and 8.4.
2. The bicarbonate/carbonic acid buffer, due to the low pK (6.1), is per se relatively uneffective; it becomes the most important buffer of the body because HCO_3 and CO_2 are regulated independently by the kidney and the lung. The CO_2 is not an acid; however when hydrated ($CO_2 + H_2O$) becomes H_2CO_3. There is approximately one molecule of H_2CO_3 for 340 molecules of CO_2. Adding CO_2 to a solution increases the acidity through generation of H_2CO_3. The CO_2 dissolved in a solution is proportional to $Paco_2$. For each mm Hg $Paco_2$, 0.03 mmol/liter CO_2 are dissolved.
3. All other organic acids generated by intermediate metabolism have pK values too far from physiologic pH to have buffer effect. Lactic acid, as an example, with a pK of 3.9, is almost completely dissociated at pH 7.4; i.e., the base/acid ratio is 3162:1. All

these acids donate their H^+ as free H^+, which must be immediately buffered by the systems previously described. It is important to remember that "base" is the acid after the H^+ has been given up, i.e., acid = base + H^+. A base/acid ratio 3162/1 indicates, in the case of lactic acid, that at pH=7.4 for each molecule of lactic acid undissociated 3162 molecules released the H^+ as free H^+.

The Acid-Base Load

Table 37.2 summarizes the acid load in a normal 70-kg man. Two kinds of acid may be considered: volatile acids, ultimately cleared by the lung, which include carbonic acid and lactic acid, and nonvolatile acids, cleared by the kidneys. The dramatic difference in the acid load that must be cleared by the lung, which is approximately 150 times greater than the acid load cleared by the kidney, is immediately evident.

Response to an Acid-Base Load

The response to an acid or base load may be seen and analyzed in different phases: (a) closed system—extracellular and intracellular buffering; (b) open system—acute respiratory buffering; and (c) open system—chronic kidney response.

Table 37.2
Acid Load

	Input	Intermediate Metabolism	Output
Volatile CO₂ Lactate	mEq/day 15.000 1.500	Liver 60% Kidneys 30%	Lungs
Nonvolatile (from protein metabolism)			Kidneys
Phosphoric acid $H_2PO_4^-$	50	Titrable activity	
Sulphuric acid $(NH_4^+) SO_4^{2-}$ Others	100	NH_4^+	

Closed System: "The Buffers' Buffering"

Fixed Acid Load

Let us consider the effect of an acid load in a closed system, as the extracellular fluid before the blood reaches the lungs. When a fixed acid is loaded into the extracellular fluid, the buffer system reacts to capture the free H^+. The H^+ load is shared by the various buffer pairs according to the pK of the buffer and their relative concentration. At a normal blood pH of 7.40 and a Paco₂ of 40 mm Hg (1.2 nmol/liter or 40.0.03), the relative concentration of the various buffer pairs (see Table 37.1) present as base (potential acceptor of free H^+ and undissociated acid (potential donor of free H^+) are defined as follows:

$$HCO_3/CO_2 \qquad Pr^-/HPr \qquad Hb^-/HHb$$
$$pH\ 7.40 = 6.1 + \log\frac{24}{12} = 6.8 + \log\frac{11.2}{2.8} = 6.8 + \log\frac{72}{18}$$

$$HPO_4^-/H_2PO_4$$
$$= 6.8 + \log\frac{1.6}{0.4}$$

As proteinate, hemoglobin (the concentration of the buffer is the highest in the blood) and phosphate have the same pK, they may be pooled together. Thus, the buffer's equilibrium in the blood in normal conditions may be written as:

$$pH\ 7.40 = 6.1 + \log\frac{24\ (HCO_3^-)}{1.2(CO_2)} = 6.8 + \log\frac{84.8\ (A^-)}{21.2\ (AH)}$$

where A^-/AH is the sum of hemoglobin, proteins, and phosphate present as base (A^-) or acid (AH).

When a strong acid, such as HCl, or lactic acid is added in an amount L (load), it will be shared by the HCO₃/CO₂ and A^-/AH pairs. An amount X will titrate the HCO₃ (which becomes CO₂) and the remaining amount (L−X) will titrate the A (which becomes AH).

The new pH and the Paco₂ will be defined by the following identities (see appendix for details):

$$pH = 6.10 + \log\frac{HCO_3^- - X}{CO_2 + X} = 6.8 + \log\frac{A^- - (L-X)}{AH + (L-X)}$$

Adding, for example, 10 mEq/liter (L) of a strong acid in a closed system, and solving the above equation for X, the pH will decrease to 7.19, the Paco₂ will rise to 63 mm Hg, the bicarbonate will decrease from 24 to 23.3, and AH will increase from 21.2 to 30.5 mEq, while the A^- will decrease from 84.2 to 75.9. Figure 37.1 describes the relationship between the acid load and Paco₂ and pH. It is interesting to note that only 7% of the acid load is buffered by the HCO₃/CO₂ pair, while 93% is buffered by the A^-/AH pair. This is due both to the pK differences (6.1 versus 6.8) and to the concentration differences. However, the 0.7 mEq generated from the titration of HCO_3^- (which becomes $H_2CO_3 \rightarrow CO_2 + H_2O$) are sufficient to increase the Paco₂ by 23 mm Hg (0.7/0.03=23 mm Hg). The anions lost (HCO₃ and A^-) are replaced by the anions of the added acid (Cl⁻, lactate⁻, etc.). The power of the buffer system is, however, impressive: of ten million nanomoles of free H^+ added per liter, only 23 nmol/liter of H^+ are left free in the system (from pH 7.40 to 7.19 the H^+ increases from 40 to 63 nmol/liter).

Fixed Base Load

The base load is equivalent to the acid load, but with opposite sign, and the buffer system will react, sharing the base load equal to L between the buffers as follows:

$$pH = 6.10 + \log \frac{HCO_3^- + X}{CO_2 - X} = 6.8 + \log \frac{A^- + (L - X)}{AH - (L - X)}$$

For example, adding 10 mEq/liter of strong base in a closed system, the new equilibrium will be defined by a $Paco_2 = 20.5$ mm Hg and pH 7.70. Only 5.8% of the base load is buffered by the carbonic acid, which is transformed in HCO_3^- ($H_2CO_3 + OH^- \rightarrow HCO_3 + H_2O$). However, this small

decrease in CO_2 concentration (0.58 mmol/liter) causes a sharp decrease in $Paco_2$ (from 40 to 20.5 mm Hg). The relationship between the base load and the $pH - Paco_2$ changes is described in Figure 37.1.

Volatile Acid Load

Only the carbonic acid will be considered. The main difference between the nonvolatile acid load and the carbonic acid load is that the HCO_3/CO_2 pair cannot buffer the carbonic acid. In fact: $H_2O + CO_2 \leftrightarrow H_2CO_3 + HCO_3^- \leftrightarrow HCO_3^- + H_2CO_3 \leftrightarrow CO_2 + H_2O$. All the carbonic acid load must then be buffered by the A^-/AH pair buffering system (infra vide).

The main component of this system is

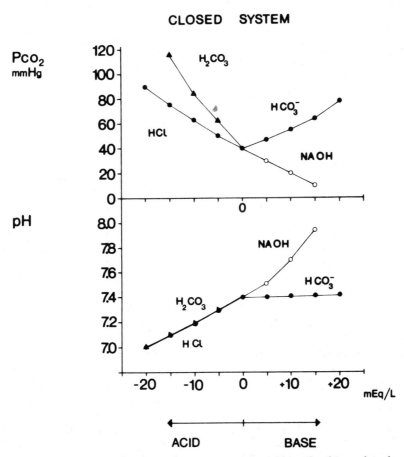

Figure 37.1. $Paco_2$ and pH changes as a function of acid and base load in a closed system. Note that both HCl, H_2CO_3 (acids) and HCO_3^- (base) cause a $Paco_2$ rise. The acid load is associated with a decrease of pH; the HCO_3^- load is associated with a pH almost unchanged.

the hemoglobin (1 gm/dL = 6 mEq/liter, which plays a major role in buffering the H_2CO_3. When H_2CO_3 is added to the system, it will titrate the A^-, which becomes AH. During this process, the H_2CO_3 will be decreased by the amount X, the A^- will be decreased by X being transformed in AH. The titration of A^- with H_2CO_3 will generate bicarbonate in amount X according to the equation: $H_2CO_3 + A^- = AH + HCO_3$ (where A^- and AH are mainly hemoglobin in the base/acid forms). Thus, the following equilibrium will be reached:

$$pH = 6.10 + \log \frac{HCO_3 + X}{CO_2 + (L-X)} = 6.8 + \log \frac{A^- - X}{AH + X}$$

For example, adding 10 mEq H_2CO_3, the new equilibrium will be defined by pH = 7.206, and $Paco_2$ = 85 mm Hg. The bicarbonate (resulting from the titration of A^-) will rise to 32.6 mEq/liter and 1.36 mmol of the 10 mEq H_2CO_3 added will stay as CO_2, causing an increase of 45 mm Hg (1.36/0.03 = 45) above the basal $Paco_2$ level of 40 mm Hg. The relationship between the H_2CO_3 load and pH and $PaCO_2$ are illustrated in Figure 37.1.

Bicarbonate Load

The bicarbonate load cannot be buffered by the HCO_3^-/CO_2 pair because the titration of carbonic acid regenerates the bicarbonate, according to the equation:

$$HCO_3^- + H_2CO_3 \rightarrow H_2CO_3 + HCO_3^-$$

The bicarbonate load must then be buffered by the other buffer pairs A^-/AH. The HCO_3^- will be buffered by AH; this reaction will generate H_2CO_3 in an amount X (i.e., $CO_2 + H_2O$) and the HCO_3^- will decrease by X while the AH decreases by the same amount, being transformed in A^-. The final equilibrium, adding an amount of HCO_3^- equal to L, will be:

$$pH = 6.1 + \log \frac{HCO_3^- + (L-X)}{CO_2 + X} = 6.8 + \log \frac{A^- + X}{AH - X}$$

Adding 10 mEq of HCO_3^- is a closed system, the pH will only rise from 7.40 to 7.41, while the $Paco_2$ will rise from 40 to 54.5 mm Hg. Then, of 10 mEq of HCO_3^- added, 9.56 mEq remain as bicarbonate

(the total concentration HCO_3^- will be 24 + 9.56 = 33.56) and only 0.44 mEq will be transformed in H_2CO_3 through the buffer action of AH. However, this small amount will cause the observed rise in $Paco_2$ (0.44/0.003 = 14.6 mm Hg). The relationship between the bicarbonate load and the pH − $Paco_2$ is illustrated in Figure 37.1.

The sharp differences in pH and $Paco_2$ changes caused by a strong base (NaOH) and bicarbonate are easily understandable; in the former case, NaOH titrates both carbonic acid (decrease in $Paco_2$) and AH, and in the latter case, $NaHCO_3$ titrates only AH, and this will generate $H_2CO_3 \rightarrow H_2O + CO_2$ (increase in $Paco_2$). Understanding this basic mechanism is important for the rational use of HCO_3^- in the treatment of acidosis.

Intracellular Buffering

So far we have only considered the extracellular buffers; it is important, however, to realize that the intracellular compartment plays a key role in buffering acid-base loads. The primary intracellular buffers are proteins and organic and inorganic phosphate. Moreover, the bone (carbonate salts) plays a substantial role, buffering up to 40% of the acid load, particularly during chronic acidosis. The classic experiments (50) in nephrectomized dogs undergoing an acute acid load (L) indicate that about 57% of the load is buffered intracellularly. The H^+ enters the cell in exchange with Na^+ (36% of the load), with K^+ (15% of the load). Anion exchange (HCO_3 into the cell and Cl out of the cell) accounts for 6% of the buffering capacity. The remaining 42% of the acid load is buffered in the extracellular fluid, according to the mechanisms described above. The intracellular buffering occurs in a few hours, while the extracellular buffering is almost immediate.

Open System: "The Respiratory Buffering"

So far we have considered the pH-$Paco_2$ variations due to different acid-base loads in a closed system. The major buffering power results from the nonvolatile buffers, while the HCO_3/CO_2 pair shows minor changes, buffering only 5% to 10% of the load. However, these changes induce great modification of $Paco_2$ and pH, which are strong physiologic signals for changing ventilatory drive. We will now discuss the modifications of the system when open, i.e., when the CO_2, through changes in ventilation, is free to leave the system at varying rates. It is important to realize that the capability to set a given $Paco_2$ depends on the condition of the subject. For example, patients with respiratory failure may have limited capacity to decrease $Paco_2$, whereas paralyzed patients on mechanical ventilatory support cannot set their own ventilation.

Fixed Acid Load and Respiratory Buffering

When a fixed acid is added to the system, the immediate resetting consists in a slight decrease of HCO_3, a decrease of A^-/AH ratio, a decrease of pH, and a rise of $Paco_2$. The magnitude of these changes depends on the load and the buffer concentrations, as previously described. The increase in $Paco_2$ increases ventilatory drive, and CO_2 (i.e., H_2CO_3) is excreted in the expired gas and is lost by the system. A new equilibrium $Paco_2$ is reached as defined by that given level of $Paco_2$; that is, the system becomes open. The following sequence of reactions takes place:

$$AH \rightarrow A^- + H^+ + HCO_3^- \rightarrow$$
$$H_2CO_3 \rightarrow H_2O + CO_2$$

The acid load, which is mainly buffered as AH, is now eliminated as CO_2, which leaves the system, until the equilibrium $Paco_2$ is reached; the equilibrium $Paco_2$ is a function of the capability of the patient to properly react to the triggers (pH and $Paco_2$) with changes in ventilation and cardiac output.

The equilibrium pH for a given $Paco_2$ is then defined by the following equation:

$$pH = 6.10 + \log \frac{HCO_3^- - X}{Paco_2 * 0.003} = 6.8 + \log \frac{A^- + X}{AH - X}$$

where X is the amount of acid load that has been eliminated as CO_2 (i.e., H_2CO_3) Figure 37.2 illustrates the relationship among $Paco_2$, pH, HCO_3^-, and acid load when the system is closed and then opened at different levels of $Paco_2$ (i.e., different ventilatory responses).

When a fixed acid is progressively loaded into the system closed, the $Paco_2$ rises and HCO_3 decreases slightly. At a load of 20 mEq of acid, the $Paco_2$ will reach 90 mm Hg and the pH will be 7.02, with HCO_3^- decreasing 1.5 mEq/liter. If the patient is able to reduce the $Paco_2$ to its original level of 40 mm Hg, the HCO_3^- would decrease to 14 mEq/liter, and the pH rises to 7.17. This indicates that 50% of the load has been cleared as CO_2 (a decrease of 10 mEq/liter HCO_3^-) while 50% of the acid load is still buffered as AH. To restore a pH of 7.40 by purely respiratory compensation (i.e., 100% load eliminated as CO_2) the $Paco_2$ would need to be as low as 6.7 mm Hg, and HCO_3^- 4 mEq/liter. These values cannot be reached clinically. However, if the acid load was less, say 10 mEq/liter, the pH 7.40 could be reached at $Paco_2 = 23.5$mm Hg, and $HCO_3 = 14$ mEq/liter. In this case, the entire acid load could be eliminated as CO_2.

A few points must be stressed.

1. The original strong acid added (e.g., HCl) has been eliminated as CO_2, with corresponding decrease of HCO_3^-
2. The power of HCO_3/CO_2 pair as a buffer is due to the possibility of eliminating the CO_2 in the expired gas
3. The final result is that the pH is restored (if the patient is able to ventilate enough), but at the expenses of decrease in HCO_3^- stores.

The decrement in HCO_3^- is then equivalent to the increment of anion of fixed acid (i.e., -10 mEq $HCO_3^- = +10$ mEq Cl^-, if the fixed acid were HCl). However, this stoichiometry is influenced by the kidney response and intracellular-extracellular exchanges of H^+, HCO_3^-, and acid anions.

Fixed Base Load and Respiratory Buffering

Loading the system with fixed base in amount X causes an immediate increase in pH and decrease in $Paco_2$ (Fig. 37.1). The respiratory response is equivalent, with opposite sign, to that observed with an

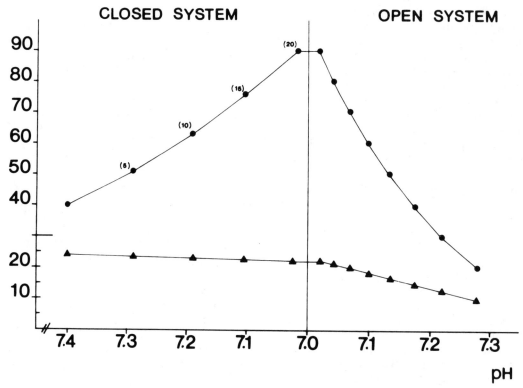

Figure 37.2. The $Paco_2$ and HCO_3^- as a function of pH in closed system *(right)* after progressive acid load *(in parentheses)*. The same relationship *(left)* when $Paco_2$ is allowed to decrease (open system).

acid load; i.e., the ventilation properly decreases and the $Paco_2$ (H_2CO_3) increases.

The equilibrium pH will depend on the patient's ability to tolerate high $Paco_2$ and will be defined by the following equation:

$$pH = 6.1 + \log \frac{HCO_3^- + X}{Paco_2*0.03} = 6.1 + \log \frac{A^- + X}{AH - X}$$

If the patient, after a load of 10 mEq of NaOH (the starting condition in a closed system is pH = 7.40, $Paco_2$ = 20.6, HCO_3 = 24.58, AH = 11.8 mEq, A^- = 94.2 mEq) is able to reduce the ventilation to reach $Paco_2$ = 56 mm Hg, then the pH will be 7.40, the A^-/AH pair will be restored to the preload values (84.8/21.2), and the HCO_3^- will rise to 33.4 mEq/liter. All the base will then be buffered by the HCO_3^-/CO_2 pair through CO_2 retention. Clearly, the limitation to this respiratory adaptation rests not in the CO_2 retention, which is physiologic, but in the associated hypoxemia.

Carbonic Acid Load and Respiratory Buffering

Carbonic acid is the major acid produced during normal metabolism. The carbonic acid load, in normal conditions, is about 15000 mEq/day, plus 1500 mEq lactic acid, which is normally metabolized to CO_2 (i.e., H_2CO_3). As previously discussed, the carbonic acid is buffered by the A^-/AH pairs (mainly the hemoglobin) and, immediately after its production by the cells (closed system), causes an increase of $Paco_2$ and a decrease in pH. This stimulates ventilatory drive (open system) and the CO_2 load is normally cleared by the lung.

The carbonic acid load is increased mainly in the following conditions: *(a)* increase of CO_2 production (increase in metabolism, hypercaloric carbohydrate parenteral feeding, etc.); *(b)* decreased elimination as in the respiratory insufficiency (decreased alveolar ventilation or elevated shunt fraction or circulatory failure). However, it is important to emphasize that the decreased elimination is a transient phenomenon (if not, the patient would not survive). If the CO_2 metabolic production is, for example, 210 ml/min, at $Paco_2 = 40$ mm Hg, 3.75 liter/min of alveolar ventilation would clear the load (i.e., 40/713*3.75 liter/min = 210 ml/min CO_2). With impaired ventilation, the CO_2 is transiently retained until a new equilibrium. This new steady state is characterized, for example, by $Paco_2$ of 80 mm Hg and half ventilation = 1.87 liter/min. In this new equilibrium the CO_2 metabolically produced would be exactly cleared as before (i.e., 80/713*1.87 liter/min = 210 ml/min CO_2). (*c*) Finally, titration of bicarbonate by fixed acid with resulting CO_2 production (i.e., H_2CO_3).

It is important to stress that a fixed acid load, as previously discussed, reduces the HCO_3^- concentration with an equivalent increase in CO_2 (i.e., H_2CO_3). The final result is that the fixed acid load is transformed into H_2CO_3 load, which must be cleared through an adequate ventilation.

Bicarbonate Load and Respiratory Buffering

The bicarbonate load in a closed system results in minimal variations of pH and in increased $Paco_2$. For the $NaHCO_3$ to increase the pH, which is the desired effect, the system must be open and ventilation-perfusion adequate to clear the CO_2 through the lung. Figure 37.3 illustrates the alkalinizing effect of bicarbonate when, starting from a closed system, the system is open at a given equilibrium $Paco_2$.

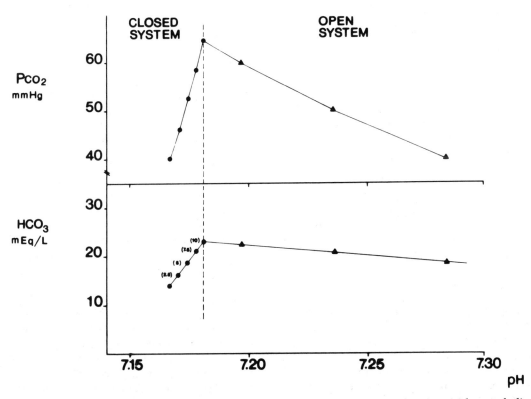

Figure 37.3. The $Paco_2$ and HCO_3^- as a function of pH in a patient starting with metabolic acidosis ($HCO_3^- = 14$ mEq, $Paco_2 = 40$ mm Hg), loaded with $NaHCO_3$. In a closed system (*left*), the $Paco_2$ rises and pH is only marginally affected (from 7.17 to 7.18). When the system is ventilated (open system, *right*) the alkalinizing effect of the $NaHCO_3$ is evident (pH from 7.18 to 7.28).

Kidney Response: "The Renal Buffering"

So far as we have discussed the first two stages of the homeostatic response to an acid-base load. For example, when an acid is loaded into the extracellular fluid, it is immediately buffered (closed system) by the buffer pairs, with a decrease of pH and an increase of $Paco_2$. Ventilation is stimulated, according to patient conditions, and the fixed acid load is cleared, as carbonic acid, through the lung. A full clearing would result in normal pH and decrease of HCO_3^- equivalent to the milliequivalent of fixed acid loaded into the system. However, during this process in normal conditions, the slight acidemia (not detectable clinically), together with a transient $Paco_2$ increase is sufficient to stimulate in the kidney tubular cells hydrolysis of water; i.e., $H_2O \rightarrow H^+ + OH^-$. The H^+ is excreted into the lumen while the OH^-, combining with intracellular CO_2, generates HCO_3^-, which is secreted into the blood. The presence of carbonic anhydrase, which catalyzes the H_2O dissociation, greatly accelerates the process.

The H_2O hydrolysis in the kidney provides two fundamental functions, bicarbonate reabsorption and net acid excretion.

Bicarbonate Reabsorption

The kidney filtrates approximately 4500 mEq HCO_3 per day, which must be reabsorbed. The HCO_3 filtered through the glomeruli combines in proximal tubular lumina with the H^+ that the tubular cells have secreted in these lumina. The reaction between the H^+ secreted and the HCO_3^- filtered produces H_2CO_3, which immediately dissociates in $H_2O + CO_2$. The CO_2 equilibrates with the cell where it combines with OH^- as HCO_3^-. The new bicarbonate that has been produced in the cell is transferred into the blood. This process takes place in the proximal tubule, where most bicarbonate lost through the glomerular filtration is reabsorbed. During this process the balance between the

HCO_3^- filtered and reabsorbed (or H^+ in and out) is equal to zero.

Net Acid Excretion

The only means to generate a really new HCO_3^- pool (able to regenerate the stores depleted by adding a fixed acid) is to produce a net acid excretion. This is possible when the H^+ is not "consumed" to reabsorb HCO_3^-. The net acid excretion is then only possible when virtually all filtered bicarbonate has been reabsorbed.

The excretion of H^+ (the normal daily production of H^+ to be excreted ranges between 5 and 10 million nanomoles) is not possible as free H^+ because the lowest urine pH in physiologic range is not lower than 4.5. The H^+ load must then be buffered during the process of urine production. It is important to realize that some organic acid, without the buffer effect at blood pH, may have important buffer effect at low urinary pH. An interesting buffer is, for example, the β-hydroxybutyrate (pK = 4.8) that allows a great increase of H^+ excretion during ketoacidosis. Titrable acidity is defined as the amount of H^+ that is buffered by the filtered buffers, as phosphate or creatinine. However, the most important buffering is due to the NH_3 produced by the tubular cells, which combines with secreted H^+ to form NH_4^+.

In normal conditions the net acid excretion is about 50–100 mEq/day; during acidosis it may increase up to 700 mEq/day, mainly through production of NH_3 by the tubular cells.

In summary, in normal conditions an acid load is buffered immediately by the extracellular buffers; in minutes the $Paco_2$ decreases due to increase in ventilation. Consequently the pH (i.e., the HCO_3^-/CO_2 ratio) is maintained near to physiologic values. Approximately 50% of the load is buffered in the intracellular compartment (hours). The kidney reacts modulating the HCO_3^- levels: (a) reabsorbing the filtered HCO_3^-, and (b) generating new bicarbonate (NH_4^+ + titrable acidity). In normal conditions the small variation of $Paco_2$ and pH caused by the dietary acid load are not detectable clinically.

Acid-Base Disorders and Compensatory Responses

From the previous discussion, it is evident that metabolic or respiratory alkalosis/acidosis may lead to severe alkalemia or acidemia when the imbalance between acid-alkali production and elimination is so severe as to overcome the compensatory responses that tends to maintain the pH in a normal range.

Metabolic Acidosis

Metabolic acidosis is characterized by a decreased HCO_3^- in plasma, and it leads to acidemia when the compensatory decrease in $Paco_2$ is not sufficient to maintain the normal HCO_3^-/CO_2 ratio of 20:1 (normal range within 22.4:1 = pH 7.45 and 17.8:1 = pH 7.35). The acidemia (pH < 7.35) is then characterized by a HCO_3^-/CO_2 ratio lower than 17.8:1. The primary disturbance, then, is an HCO_3 fall. This occurs in two broad conditions: (a) titration of HCO_3 by an increased amount of fixed acid (HCO_3^- is transformed into H_2CO_3 and then $CO_2 + H_2O$); and (b) losses of HCO_3^- as such. The fixed acid may be increased due to: (a) increased endogenous production such as lactic acidosis, uncompensated diabetes mellitus ketoacidosis, severe catabolism, and massive rhabdomyolysis; (b) exogenous ingestion of acid or acid-producing substances such as salycilate, methanol, ethylene glycol, etc; and (c) decreased elimination (renal failure). The HCO_3 losses include gastrointestinal losses, renal tubular acidosis, and possible losses of HCO_3^- through artificial devices (as with hemofiltration).

Metabolic Alkalosis

The primary disturbance in metabolic alkalosis is an increase of HCO_3^- in the plasma. This leads to alkalemia when the compensatory increase of $Paco_2$ is not sufficient to keep in the normal range the HCO_3/CO_2 ratio. The HCO_3^- increase may be due to two broad conditions:

1. The HCO_3^- administration or other base loads (as citrate$^-$ in banked blood);

2. Losses of H^+ (gastrointestinal or vomiting) or renal (use of diuretics).

The compensatory responses should be an increase of $Paco_2$ and, finally, the excretion by the kidney of the excess HCO_3^-. In normal conditions, the kidney rapidly eliminates the excess HCO_3^- (and urine becomes alkalotic), correcting the pH. In clinical settings, however, it is quite common to observe acid urine in the presence of metabolic alkalosis. This is usually due to an enhanced bicarbonate reabsorption caused by relative or absolute hypovolemia.

Respiratory Acidosis

Respiratory acidosis is characterized by the retention of H_2CO_3 due to the transient decrease of the elimination of the CO_2 produced by the metabolism. A new equilibrium is reached, defined by higher $Paco_2$ and lower pH. The higher equilibrium $Paco_2$ allows a normal CO_2 elimination. For example, if the carbonic acid retention is caused by halving the ventilation, the steady state will be reached when $Paco_2$ is doubled.

The acute load of carbonic acid may only be buffered by the A^-/AH buffer pairs, with HCO_3^- generation (slight increase in HCO_3^-). The compensatory response, however, is mainly due to a generation of new HCO_3^- by the kidney. The complete adaptive response takes 3–5 days. The titrable acidity and NH_4^+ excretion increases during this period (new HCO_3^- generation) and then, when a new steady state is reached, return toward normal baseline values.

The acute H_2CO_3 retention is then characterized by high $Paco_2$ and sharp decrease in pH, with only slight increase in HCO_3^-. The HCO_3^- rises in a few days (if the condition leading to H_2CO_3 retention persists), until a new steady state is reached, characterized by high $Paco_2$, higher HCO_3 levels, and consequently higher pH than in acute ventilatory failure.

Respiratory Alkalosis

The primary disturbance in respiratory alkalosis is a decreased $Paco_2$ (hyperventilation). The compensatory response is a decreased H^+ excretion by the kidney with consequent loss of HCO_3^-. This tends to restore a near-normal HCO_3^-/CO_2 ratio.

Compensatory Responses

To understand the possible impact of a kidney impairment on associated acid-base disorders (for example, lactic acidosis, respiratory acidosis, etc.) it is important to understand the average compensatory response in vivo. These are summarized in Table 37.3. During severe acidosis and alkalosis, the homeostatic mechanism tends to restore a normal pH. This goal, however, is not generally reached.

From Table 37.3 it also evident that kidney failure should enhance metabolic acidosis of nonrenal origin and play a significant role in patients with ventilatory failure, of whatever origin.

Impact of Acute Kidney Failure on Associated Conditions Leading to Acid-Base Derangements

Uncomplicated Renal Failure

The uncomplicated renal failure invariably leads to metabolic acidosis. This is not due to HCO_3^- losses in the urine (oliguria/anuria), but to the inability of the kidney to generate new HCO_3^-. The HCO_3^- lost through the lung as CO_2 when titrated by the fixed acid produced by the daily protein catabolism is not replaced, and this leads to progressive metabolic acidosis.

The average decrease of HCO_3^- in uncomplicated renal failure is between 1 and 2 mEq/liter/day. Assuming that the acid load is evenly buffered in the extracellular and intracellular space (60% of body weight), 1–2 mEq/liter/day HCO_3^- decrease would correspond to an acid load between 84 and 168 mEq/day. These figures agree reasonably with the 50–100 mEq/day of normal acid load.

Even in severe catabolic states, the acid load should not be excessively increased. The metabolic H^+ generation, in a literature survey (17), was shown to be equal to 0.77 times the protein catabolic rate; i.e., H^+ (millimoles per day) = 0.77 ± 0.14 mmol * protein catabolic rate (grams per day) (variability at 95% confidence $\pm$ 36%). Assuming, for example, an extreme severe catabolism of 250 g of protein per day, this would produce an acid load of 192 mEq/day (range at 95% confidence, 123–261 mEq/day). Thus, uncomplicated renal failure,

Table 37.3
Compensatory Responses to Acid-Base Derangements

		Examples of CR		pH	
	Compensatory Response (CR)	HCO_3^- (mEq)	$Paco_2$ (mmHg)	With CR	Without CR
Metabolic acidosis	1.2 mmHg decrease $Paco_2$ for 1 mEq HCO_3^-	14	28($\downarrow$)	7.32	7.168
Metabolic alkalosis	0.7 mmHg decrease $Paco_2$ for 1 mEq increase HCO_3^-	34	47($\uparrow$)	7.48	7.55
Respiratory acidosis (acute)	1 mEq increase HCO_3^- for 10 mmHg increase $Paco_2$	27($\uparrow$)	70	7.21	7.15
Respiratory acidosis (chronic)	3.5 mEq increase HCO_3^- for 10 mmHg $Paco_2$ increase (kidney act.)	34.5($\uparrow$)	70	7.31	7.15
Respiratory alkalosis (acute)	2 mEq decrease HCO_3^- for 10 mmHg $Paco_2$ decrease	21($\downarrow$)	25	7.54	7.60
Respiratory alkalosis (chronic)	5 mEq decrease HCO_3^- for 10 mmHg $Paco_2$ decrease	16.5($\downarrow$)	25	7.44	7.60

even in severe catabolic patients, does not lead to an acute severe acidosis.

However, in these patients, substantial alkali losses (i.e., diarrhea, biliary drainage, gastric suction) may contribute to worsen metabolic acidosis.

Complicated Renal Failure

Acute Renal Failure and Metabolic Acidosis

Acute renal failure may be associated with severe metabolic acidosis, as may occur with lactic acidosis or ketoacidosis. These conditions are characterized by a massive acid load that is primarily buffered by body buffers, with consequent hyperventilation, and HCO_3^- decrease. Associated acute renal failure may considerably worsen the acidosis and should not be underestimated. In fact, the kidney is able to eliminate up to 750 mEq/day of H^+ (compared to the normal of 100 mEq/day), with consequent generation of 750 mEq of new bicarbonate. The lack of this adaptive mechanism greatly enhances the HCO_3^- depletion, accelerating the pH decrease.

Acute Renal Failure and Metabolic Alkalosis

The kidney corrects a metabolic alkalosis by excreting the excess bicarbonate in the urine. The development of metabolic alkalosis requires a hypovolemic state or an impairment in renal function. An example of this is excessive alkali administration to a patient in ARF.

Loss of gastric fluid (vomiting, nasogastric suctioning) is a frequent cause of metabolic alkalosis and it can sometimes be present in ARF patients. In uremic patients, the disturbance in fluid balance and acid-base equilibrium that results from vomiting or gastric suction is totally a function of direct loss of water and HCl from the stomach, since in normal subjects the renal response to depletion of HCl is very important in shaping the final composition of body fluids. When patients with chronic hypercapnia experience a rapid reduction in $Paco_2$, such as is when they require assisted ventilation, blood pH increases abruptly, often to frankly alkalemic levels,

because the plasma HCO_3^- concentration (increased during prior adaptation to hypercapnia) remains elevated. This state is called "posthypercapnic" alkalosis. In patients with normal renal function, acid excretion will be suppressed, HCO_3^- excretion will increase, and plasma HCO_3^+ concentration will decrease toward normal. In ARF patients, these mechanisms cannot occur and metabolic alkalosis can persist.

Acute Renal Failure and Respiratory Acidosis

The kidney reacts to a respiratory acidosis, when the ventilatory failure persists for a few days, by increasing net acid excretion and generating new HCO_3^-, until a new steady state is reached. If an acute renal failure is associated to a ventilatory failure, it may have a profound impact on the pH control. As illustrated in Figure 37.4 and according to figures discussed above (i.e., the 3.5 mEq HCO_3^- increase every 10 mm Hg $Paco_2$ rise, and catabolic acid load leading per se to a decrease of 2 mEq/liter/day/HCO_3^-), a dramatic difference in response to a ventilatory failure conditioning $Paco_2$ of 60 mm Hg in a patient with and without acute renal failure. Assuming that a new steady state is reached by the fourth day, the pH in a patient with a preserved renal function should reach 7.34 with HCO_3^- equal to 31 mEq/liter; in a patient with a renal failure, the pH should be 7.07 with HCO_3^- equals 21 mEq/liter. This illustration emphasizes the major impact of renal failure on acid-base comparison when associated with ventilatory failure. This relation should be appreciated when applying new ventilatory techniques as the controlled hypoventilation (pervasive hypercapnia) (25) to prevent pulmonary barotrauma in the treatment of acute respiratory failure if the patient also has acute renal failure.

TREATMENT

Treatment for acidosis is rarely required in uncomplicated acute renal failure if periodic hemodialysis or peritoneal dialysis is employed to control the uremia. The alkali

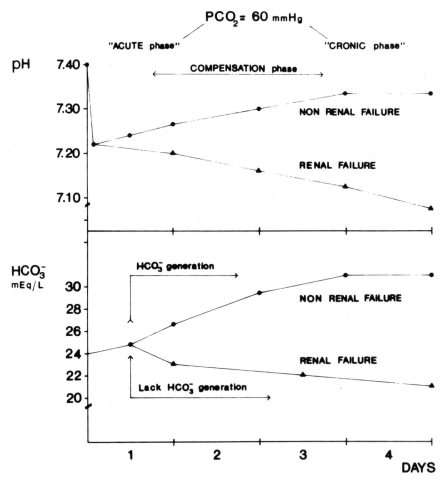

Figure 37.4. The pH and HCO_3^- behavior during ventilatory failure in acute phase (day 1) and in chronic phase (day 4) in a patient with and without renal failure. (See text for further details.)

provided by dialysis usually offsets the effect of the relatively small quantity of endogenous acid retained during the interdialytic interval. Intravenous administration of sodium bicarbonate ($NaHCO_3$) may be necessary when hypercatabolism or other factors cause severe acidosis; however, the risk of fluid overload attending alkali administration in this setting may necessitate more frequent dialysis (20).

Only limited information is available concerning the adequacy of bicarbonate reabsorption and acid excretion during the recovery phase of ARF. Marked defects in ammonium excretion were found in several patients recovering from acute oliguric renal failure (12). Although certain types

of tubular dysfunction may persist (35) for some time in patients recovering from ARF, defects in bicarbonate reabsorption or acid excretion rarely persist and generally are detectable only by acid-loading tests, not by the presence of unprovoked acidosis (9).

Mild-to-moderate metabolic alkalosis usually requires no special attention, and vigorous attempts to restore normal values of bicarbonate concentration in such patients are unwarranted unless complicating electrolyte disorders require such intervention (21). Diluted hydrochloric acid (0.1 N HCl) can be used in patients with renal failure and severe alkalosis, but dialysis per se is very effective in alkali removal if the dialysate bath contains high concentrations of Cl^- and low concentrations of buffers (51).

Hemodialysis

Buffer Kinetics

During hemodialysis, changes in plasma bicarbonate result from a passive exchange of bicarbonate or alkali precursors (acetate) across the semipermeable membrane between the dialysate and the patient. In general, dialysis corrects the metabolic acidosis characteristic of the uremic state, but both the extent of the bicarbonate change and its direction are function of several factors, including the specific dialytic method (22), the gradient for bicarbonate across the membrane, called driving force, the type and the concentration of the buffer used in the dialysate, the rates of dialysate and blood flow, the duration of dialysis, the ultrafiltration applied, the surface area of the dialyzer, and the rate of metabolism of the alkali-generating anions (36).

In hemodialysis, because diffusion is the major determinant of the small solute transport, bicarbonate flux across the membrane depends mainly on bicarbonate driving force (47). It can be noted that the gain of bicarbonate increases as the driving force increases. A high driving force can be achieved when a high bicarbonate concentration is used in the dialysate or when low plasma bicarbonate level is present. Driving force is negative and consequently a bicarbonate loss occurs when plasma bicarbonate concentration is higher than the dialysate bicarbonate concentration, or when acetate is employed in dialysate as buffer instead of bicarbonate.

From a clinical point of view, when bicarbonate is the sole source of alkali in the dialysate, if plasma bicarbonate is low (metabolic acidosis), bicarbonate is taken up substantially from dialysate. Conversely, if plasma bicarbonate is very high (severe metabolic alkalosis), passive movement of bicarbonate from patient to dialysate is favored, and the alkalosis is ameliorated.

Acetate Dialysis

Acetate transport in hemodialysis depends on its diffusibility, likewise bicarbonate, and on its metabolic conversion to CO_2 and water, which generates bicarbonate. When the acetate infusion rate is higher than acetate metabolic rate, plasma acetate levels increase and the acetate driving force decreases, resulting in a reduction of acetate gained by the patient.

Acetate Metabolism

Acetate is primarily metabolized in peripheral tissue (38), although in the past, the liver was considered the main site of its metabolism (19). Acetate thiokinase activates the reaction between acetate and CoA to form acetylCoA, and one hydrogen ion is captured in this process. AcetylCoA may enter different metabolic pathways such as decarboxylation in the Krebs cycle, condensation to ketone bodies or fatty acids, and glucose generation via gluconeogenesis. The buffering effect is concluded and the hydrogen ion is transferred to the respiratory chain only when acetylCoA is decarboxylated. When alternative pathways are entered or the decarboxylation process is not complete, the buffering effect is delayed until the intermediate products are completely decarboxylated (34).

When glucose-free dialysate is used, a remarkable increase of free fatty acids, ketone bodies, and gluconeogenesis precursors can be seen (55). Concurrently, serum insulin levels fall, suggesting a possible role of this hormone in acetate metabolism. High levels of acetoacetate and β-hydroxybutyrate can also be found in highly efficient dialysis treatments, probably depending on the large acetate load (53). These metabolites commonly dissociate in body fluids and release hydrogen ions, so their previous buffering effect vanishes. However, when not lost in the dialysate, they can still operate as buffers being reconverted to acetylCoA.

Acetate metabolism depends on an intact oxidative phosphorylation system; since Krebs cycle activity is regulated by the ATP/ADP ratio, when ATP concentration increases acetate metabolism is slowed (56). Lundquist (38) estimated the maximal rate of acetate metabolism in normal subjects to be 5 mmol/min. Such a rate seems to be lower in uremic patients (3–4 mmol/min) because of possible impairment of the Krebs cycle activity. In fact, Yamakawa et al. (57) have found that malate and citrate concentrations increase during dialysis and isocitrate becomes detectable in blood when acetate levels exceed 7 mmol/liter. In regular acetate dialysis, the acetate flux is about 3.5–4 mmol/min. The complete decarboxylation of 1 mol of acetate leads to the production of 2 mol of CO_2 and consumes 2 mol of O_2. Since 1 mol of CO_2 is consumed in the acetate-acetic acid reaction, the final CO_2/O_2 ratio is ½ (44).

$$CO_2 \text{ (consumed)} + H_2O + CH_3COONa \rightarrow NaHCO_3 + CH_3COOH$$

$$CH_3COOH + 2O_2 \text{ (consumed)} = 2O_2 \text{ (produced)} + 2H_2O$$

Therefore, if the buffer was the main source of energy, the respiratory quotient (Q_R) should be reduced, but several factors may interfere with the final value of this ratio.

From a clinical point of view, in acetate dialysis, buffer balance is the arithmetical sum of bicarbonate and acetate flux, being usually acetate-flux positive and bicarbonate-flux negative. If acetate infusion rate is lower than the metabolic rate, final balance depends on bicarbonate losses. When plasma bicarbonate is low (metabolic acidosis), acetate uptake is higher than bicarbonate losses and consequently base balance is positive. Conversely, if plasma bicarbonate is very high (severe metabolic alkalosis), passive transport of bicarbonate from patient to dialysate is enhanced, thus worsening alkalosis.

The use of acetate in dialysis may influence the patient's clinical condition both during treatment and in the interdialytic period. Specific effects on acid-base equilibrium, ventilation, cardiovascular activity, and endogenous metabolism can be observed.

Effects on Acid Base

In the first 30 min of dialysis, acetate metabolism may not be fast enough to balance bicarbonate losses and a fall of plasma bicarbonate levels and pH can be seen. This effect may even worsen the metabolic acidosis in this period (32). Subsequently, the rate of acetate utilization increases, counterbalancing bicarbonate losses. Patients, therefore, show a progressive decrease of $Paco_2$, an increase of blood pH, and a relative stability of plasma bicarbonate. Plasma acetate levels rise during the dialysis session reaching an average value of 5 mmol/liter at the end (53). After dialysis has ceased, pH and HCO_3^- rapidly increase while $Paco_2$ returns to predialytic values (Fig. 37.3) (18). These effects depend on the sudden decrease of bicarbonate losses through the dialyzer and on the complete metabolism of acetate accumulated in the body. These observations are typical of a standard dialysis session carried out with blood flow of 250 ml/min. dialysate flow of 500 ml/min, and cuprophan dialyzer for 240 min. In between two dialysis sessions, blood pH and bicarbonate progressively decrease according to the metabolic acid production rate.

Effects on Ventilation

Acetate dialysis significantly decreases Pao_2 during the entire duration of the treatment. This fall of Pao_2 occurs in about 90% of patients. The decrease in Pao_2 ranges between 5 and 35 mm Hg (average value, 14 mm Hg) (43). After the treatment Pao_2 values return to predialytic values within 1 or 2 hr. Some authors have suggested that this dialysis-induced hypoxemia might be important in the genesis of some intradialytic symptoms such as hypotension, which is particularly evident in patients with compromised cardiopulmonary function. This hypoxemia has a multifactorial origin and its pathophysiology has not yet been totally clarified.

Dialytic hypoxemia has been ascribed to a possible Bohr effect (54). The pH increase during dialysis might lead to a parallel increase in hemoglobin affinity for O_2. In this setting, although a stable Pao_2 and blood oxygen content are maintained, the O_2 delivery to the tissues decreases significantly. However, it has been pointed out that the variations of blood pH and 2,3-diphosphoglycerate inside the red cells, as well as other intracellular phosphate, are not sufficient to completely explain the dialysis-induced hypoxemia (26).

Bischel et al. (3) have suggested that hypoxemia may depend on lung microembolization due to circulating microaggregates of platelets, leukocytes, or fibrin deriving from the blood/membrane interaction. In other studies, however, the microfiltration of venous blood failed to prevent hypoxemia during dialysis (1). Craddock et al. (10) have suggested that the blood interaction with cuprophan membranes may activate the complement cascade via the alternative pathway with a consequent leukocyte agglutination and pulmonary trapping of the microaggregates and a final effect of neutropenia. This may lead to an impairment of gas diffusion in the lungs and consequent hypoxemia. Two observations, however, are against this hypothesis: hypoxemia also occurs with more biocompatible materials such as polyacrylonitrile or polysulphide in which complement activation does not take place and neutropenia is blunted (28). During isolated ultrafiltration with cellulosic membranes the neutropenic effect is present but hypoxemia does not occur (8).

Scherlock et al. (49) and Aurigemma et al. (1) have proposed that the CO_2 losses across dialysis membranes could be the main cause of hypoventilation and hypoxemia. The reduced CO_2 excretion with the increased O_2 consumption, without any alteration of A-a O_2 gradient, determines a significant fall of Q_R. The Q_R, however, is in the normal range when its calculation takes into account CO_2 losses through the dialyzer. In addition, these authors demonstrated that hypoventilation and hypoxemia can be avoided by bubbling CO_2 in the dialysate. Dolan et al. (13) have recently demonstrated the occurrence of hypoventilation-hypoxemia in acetate but not in bicarbonate dialysis where CO_2 losses do not take place. The importance of hypoventilation in inducing hypoxemia during dialysis has also been confirmed by Bouffard et al. (7). These authors have demonstrated that hypoxemia does not occur in patients with acute renal failure dialyzed during mechanical ventilatory support. A different approach to the problem has been proposed by Oh et al. (44), who

suggested that acetate metabolism might be the main cause of increased O_2 consumption and decrease of CO_2 production with a consequent RQ reduction. This reduction has been demonstrated to be proportional to the amount of administered acetate during the session (45).

In conclusion dialysis-induced hypoxemia appears to be a multifactorial phenomenon and, although it has not yet been completely clarified, two major determinants are generally considered: acetate infusion and metabolism and CO_2 losses across the dialyzer (16).

Cardiovascular Effects

When cardiovascular effects of acetate dialysis are considered, it is important to share the specific effects determined by acetate from the general effects generated by dialysis treatment. It is well known that acetate infusion in man has a vasodilatory effect (2). It has, therefore, been suggested that in some patients acetate could be the main cause of hypotension and other cardiovascular effects recorded during dialysis. Kirkendol et al. (30), studying the effects of an intravenous bolus of acetate in anesthetized dogs, concluded that acetate causes a dose-dependent reduction of myocardial performance and arterial blood pressure, thus suggesting a cardiodepressant action of the buffer. However, an increase in cardiac output and a decrease in total peripheral resistance and mean arterial pressure were recorded by the same authors in a subsequent study carried out at a constant rate of acetate infusion (31). These effects were confirmed by several studies (37, 40). Finally, in a recent study carried out in healthy volunteers treated with isovolemic acetate dialysis, Danielssonn et al. (11) demonstrated with an invasive technique that systemic vasodilation occurs during dialysis compensated by a heart rate-dependent increase of cardiac output. Thus, it has been widely demonstrated that acetate has a direct vasodilatory effect, although its pathogenesis is not clear.

A possible interaction of acetate with ionized calcium (15) or a direct vasodilatory effect induced by acetate metabolites such as adenosine or adenine nucleotides (37), have been suggested. The myocardial response to this vasodilation is an increase in cardiac output, presumably in the attempt to maintain a stable blood pressure. This response, however, may be altered during dialysis because of associated autonomic nervous system dysfunction or a borderline cardiomyopathy. Hence, dialysis-induced hypotension is probably due to several different mechanisms and factors. One of these mechanisms could be an insufficient increase in cardiac output in response to the vasodilation induced by acetate. Hypoxemia, altered serum osmolality, ultrafiltration, and hypovolemia with a consequent reduction of the vascular filling pressure may also contribute to this pathologic event during acetate dialysis (29).

Bicarbonate Dialysis

The mechanism of treatment of metabolic acidosis operating in bicarbonate dialysis differs from that of acetate dialysis. This results in different effects on acid-base balance, ventilation, and cardiovascular function.

Effects on Acid-Base Status

In bicarbonate dialysis blood pH and plasma bicarbonate progressively increase throughout the session, while $Paco_2$ shows stable values or moderate increase (18, 42). At the end of dialysis a moderate mixed metabolic and respiratory alkalosis can be observed; its degree depends on the total bicarbonate balance and on the predialytic acid-base status. Thereafter, blood pH and plasma bicarbonate progressively decrease until the subsequent dialysis. This behavior contrasts with acetate dialysis where the rapid metabolism of infused acetate in the absence of bicarbonate losses temporarily increases pH and plasma bicarbonate. Despite a slightly positive base balance in bicarbonate dialysis (4), it is still controversial whether acid-base correction with this treatment is more effective than with acetate.

Effects on Ventilation

The effects of bicarbonate dialysis on ventilation and, in particular, the possible occurrence of dialysis-induced hypoxemia are still controversial. Some authors (14) have observed no differences in patients treated alternatively with bicarbonate and acetate dialysis. Others (42) could observe hypoxemia in patients undergoing bicarbonate dialysis. This might depend on the bicarbonate concentration in the dialysate. In fact, dialysate concentration of bicarbonate higher than 37 mmol/liter might be responsible for a rapid alkalinization of the patient with a consequent compensatory hypoventilation (52).

Cardiovascular Effects

Several studies report a better clinical tolerance of bicarbonate dialysis in terms of incidence of hypotensive episodes and intradialytic symptoms such as nausea, vomiting, encephalopathy, and cramps. Unanimous agreement on this point has not yet been reached (18, 27, 41).

Patients on bicarbonate hemodialysis respond hemodynamically quite differently from those on acetate dialysis. Under similar conditions of ultrafiltration, bicarbonate dialysis achieves better stability of mean arterial pressure due to the maintenance of systemic vascular resistance, cardiac output, and heart rate within acceptable ranges (41). This hemodynamic response observed in bicarbonate dialysis may be explained by the absence of the vasodilatory effect of acetate or by a favorable effect of alkalosis on vascular reactivity (46). Furthermore, myocardial contractility and left ventricular function may be improved in this condition (23), despite a possible reduction in myocardial reactivity due to variations of ionized calcium related to alkalosis (39).

On the contrary, Mansell et al. (39), comparing acetate and bicarbonate dialysis, showed a significant increase of heart rate only in acetate, while blood pressure and peripheral resistance were similar with both dialysates. They attributed the beneficial effects of bicarbonate dialysis more to a steadiness of the $Paco_2$ during the treatment than to the absence of adverse cardiovascular effects of acetate. In addition, when high sodium dialysis solutions are used, no differences in vascular stability between acetate and bicarbonate dialysis seem to occur (5).

Hence, it is still controversial as to whether bicarbonate dialysis may directly benefit vascular stability during dialysis. Although bicarbonate dialysis cannot really eliminate some of the causes of hypotension such as ultrafiltration and vascular filling pressure reduction, this treatment should be preferred over acetate dialysis in critically ill patients.

Hemofiltration

Hemofiltration and continuous arteriovenous hemofiltration are often used in the treatment of acute renal failure mainly because convective treatments should provide a better control of cardiovascular stability during the session as compared to hemodialysis.

Few acid-base studies have been carried out in patients treated by hemofiltration (48). The net acid-base balance is obtained by the difference between the base losses in the ultrafiltrate (bicarbonate, organic anions, and part of buffer infused intravenously), and the amount of buffers administered to the patient with the substitution fluid. The buffer utilized in the substitution fluid are acetate or lactate at an average concentration of 40 mmol/liter. Similar to acetate hemodialysis, during a hemofiltration session pH and bicarbonate show a significant initial drop probably related to accumulation of lactate in the body, $Paco_2$ remains stable, while less variation of $Paco_2$ was recorded (6). Following dialysis, a significant increase in pH and serum bicarbonate levels was observed as compared to acetate hemodialysis.

Continuous arteriovenous hemofiltration is very useful in the management of acid-base derangements in acute renal failure because the separation of fluid from the bicarbonate losses permits the administration or removal of bicarbonate. Thus, in the treatment of metabolic acidosis, bicarbonate can be administered in the sub-

stitution fluid following the patient's needs, while in the metabolic alkalosis the reinfusion of a fluid without any buffer allows restoration of correct plasma bicarbonate levels (33).

Peritoneal dialysis

Although peritoneal dialysis has served for years as an alternative treatment of acute renal failure, this type of treatment has now been almost abandoned.

Bicarbonate in peritoneal lavage fluid readily diffuses down its concentration gradient across the peritoneal membrane. Lactate is widely used as buffer in peritoneal dialysis fluid and it, like bicarbonate, is absorbed from peritoneal cavity following its concentration gradient (33). In addition, bicarbonate and lactate kinetics depend on dwell time, ultrafiltration, and permeability coefficient of the membrane. The acid-base behavior during an intermittent peritoneal dialysis session is depicted in Figure 37.4. Serum bicarbonate levels and pH progressively increase during peritoneal dialysis, while $Paco_2$ and Pao_2 levels remain unchanged. Peritoneal dialysis has been reported to also be effective as acetate dialysis in the correction of metabolic acidosis. Nevertheless, its use in critically ill patients has been reduced as more efficient and tolerated extracorporeal treatment became available.

References

1. Aurigemma NM, Feldman NT, Gottlieb M, Ingram RH, Lazarus JM, Lowrie EG. Arterial oxygenation during hemodialysis. N Engl J Med 1977;297:871–875.
2. Bauer W, Richards JW. A vasodilatory acation of acetate. J Physiol 1928;66:371–384.
3. Bischel MD, Scoles BG, Mohler JG. Evidence for pulmonary microembolization during hemodialysis. Chest 1975;67:335–343.
4. Borges H, Fryd DS, Rosa AA, Kjellstrand CM. Hypotension during acetate and bicarbonate dialysis in patients with acute renal failure. Am J Nephrol 1981;1:24–31.
5. Bosh JP, Lauer A. Acid-base balance in hemofiltration. In: Henderson LW, Wuellhorst EA, Baldamus CA, Lysaght MJ, eds. Hemofiltration. Berlin: Springer Verlag, 1986:147–161.
6. Bosch JP, Ronco C. Continuous arteriovenous hemofiltration and other continuous replacement therapies: operational characteristics and clinical

use. In: Maher JF, ed. Replacement of renal function by dialysis. Dordrecht 1989;347–359.

7. Bouffard Y, Viale JP, Annat G, et al. Pulmonary gas exchange during hemodialysis. Kidney Int 1986;30:920–927.

8. Brautbar N, Shinaberger JH, Miller JH, Nachman M. Hemodialysis hypoxemia: evaluation of mechanism utilizing sequential ultrafiltration-dialysis. Nephron 1980;26:96–103.

9. Briggs JD, Kennedy AC, Young LN, et al. Renal function after acute tubular necrosis. Br Med J 1967;3:513–515.

10. Craddock PR, Fehr J, Brigham KL, Kronenberg RS, Jacob HS. Complement and leukocyte-mediated pulmonary dysfunction in hemodialysis. N Engl J Med 1977;296:770–774.

11. Danielsson A, Freyschuss U, Bergstrom J. Cardiovascular function and alveolar gas exchange during isovolemic hemodialysis with acetate in healthy man. Blood Purif 1987;5:41–50.

12. DeLuna MB, Metcalfe-Gibson A, Wrong O. Urinary excretion of hydrogen ion in acute oliguric renal failure. Nephron 1964;1:3–8.

13. Dolan KJ, Whipp BJ, Davidson WD, Weitzman RE, Wasserman K. Hypopnea associated with acetate hemodialysis: carbon dioxide flow-dependent ventilation. N Engl J Med 1981;305:72–77.

14. Eiser AR, Jayammane D, Kokseng C, Che H, Slifkin RF, Neff MS. Contrasting alterations in pulmonary gas exchange during acetate and bicarbonate hemodialysis. Am J Nephrol 1982;2:123–129.

15. Frohlic ED. Vascular effects of the Krebs intermediate metabolites. Am J Physiol 1965;208:149–156.

16. Garella S, Chang BS. Hemodialysis-associated hypoxemia. Am J Nephrol 1984;4:273–283.

17. Gotch FA, Sargent JA, Keen ML. Hydrogen ion balance in dialysis therapy. Artif Organs 1982;6:388.

18. Graefe U, Milutinovich J, Follette WC, Vizzo JB, Babb AL, Scribner BH. Less dialysis-induced morbidity and vascular instability with bicarbonate in dialysate. Ann Intern Med 1978;88:332–340.

19. Harper PV, Neal WB, Hlavacek GR. Acetate utilization in dog. Metabolism 1953;2:62–70.

20. Harrington JT, Cohen JJ. Metabolic acidosis. In: Cohen JJ, Kassirer JP, eds. Acid/Base. Boston: Little Brown, and Company, 1982:121–225.

21. Harrington JT, Kassirer JP. Metabolic Alkalosis. In: Cohen JJ, Kassirer JP, eds. Acid/Base. Boston: Little Brown, and Company, 1982:227–306.

22. Harrington JT, Kassirer JP. Dialysis, hypotermia, blood transfusion. In: Cohen JJ, Kassirer JP, eds. Acid/Base. Boston: Little Brown, and Company, 1982:391–402.

23. Henrich W, Hunt J, Nixon J. Increased ionized calcium and left ventricular contractility during hemodialysis. N Engl J Med 1983;310:19–23.

24. Henrich WL, Woodard TD, Meyer BD, Chappel TR, Rubin LJ. High sodium bicarbonate and acetate hemodialysis: double-blind crossover comparison of hemodynamic and ventilatory effects. Kidney Int 1983;24:240–248.

25. Hickling KG, Henderson SJ, Jackson R. Low mortality associated with low volume pressure limited ventilation with permissive hypercapnia in severe adult respiratory distress syndrome. Int Care Med 1990;16:372–377.

26. Hirszel P, Maher JF, Tempel GE, Mengel CE. Effect of hemodialysis on factors influencing oxygen transport. J Lab Clin Med 1975;85:978–984.

27. Iseki K, Onoyama K, Maeda T, et al. Comparison of hemodynamics induced by conventional acetate hemodialysis, bicarbonate hemodialysis and ultrafiltration. Clin Nephrol 1980;14:294–301.

28. Jacob AI, Gavellas G, Zarco R, Perez G, Bourgoignie JJ. Leucopenia, hypoxia and complement function with different hemodialysis membranes. Kidney Int 1980;18:105–112.

29. Kinet JP, Soyeur D, Balland N, Saint-Remy M, Collignon P, Godon GP. Hemodynamic study of hypotension during hemodialysis. Kidney Int 1982;21:868–874.

30. Kirkendol PL, Devia CJ, Bower JD, Holbert RD. A comparison of the cardiovascular effects of sodium acetate, sodium bicarbonate and other potential sources of fixed base in hemodialysate solutions. Trans Am Soc Artif Intern Organs 1977;23:399–403.

31. Kirkendol PL, Robie NW, Gonzales FM, Devia CJ. Cardiac and vascular effects of infused sodium acetate in dogs. Trans Am Soc Artif Intern Organs 1978;24:714–718.

32. Kveim M, Nesbakken R. Utilization of exogenous acetate during hemodialysis. Trans Am Soc Artif Intern Organs 1975;21:138–42.

33. La Greca G, Biasioli S, Chiaramonte S. Acid-base balance on peritoneal dialysis. Clin Nephrol 1981;16:1–6.

34. La Greca G, Fabris A, Feriani M, Chiramonte S, Ronco C. Acid-base homeostasis in clinical dialysis. In: Maher JF, ed. Dordrecht: Kluwer Academic Publisher, 1989:808–826.

35. Lewers DT, Mathew TH, Maher JF, Schreiner GE. Long-term follow-up of renal function and histology after acute tubular necrosis. Ann Intern Med 1970;73:523–531.

36. Lewis EJ, Tolchin N, Rpnerts JL. Estimation of the metabolic conversion of acetate to bicarbonate during hemodialysis. Kidney Int 1980;18(suppl 10):S51–S61.

37. Liang CS, Lowenstein JM. Metabolic control of the circulation effects of acetate and pyruvate. J Clin Invest 1978;62:1029–1035.

38. Ludquist F. Production and utilization of free acetate in man. Nature (London) 1962;193:579–585.

39. Mansell MA, Morgan SH, Moore R, Kong KH, Laker MF, Wing AJ. Cardiovascular and acid-base effects of acetate and bicarbonate hemodialysis. Dial Transplant 1987;1:229–237.

40. Metha BR, Fisher D, Ahmad M, Dubose TD Jr. Effects of acetate and bicarbonate hemodialysis on cardiac function in chronic dialysis patients. Kidney Int 1983;24:782–787.

41. Mitchell J, Wildenthal K, Johnson R. The effects of acid base disturbances on cardiovascular and pulmonary function. Kidney Int 1972;1:375–382.

42. Nissenson AR. Prevention of dialysis-induced

hypoxemia by bicarbonate dialysis. Trans Am Soc Artif Intern Organs 1980;26:339–344.

43. Nissenson AR, Kraut JA, Shinaberger JH. Dialysis-associated hypoxemia: pathogenesis and prevention: ASAIO Trans 1984;7:1–9.

44. Oh MS, Uribarri J, Del Monte ML, Friedman EA, Carroll HJ. Consumption of CO_2 in metabolism of acetate as an explanation for hypoventilation and hypoxemia during hemodialysis. Proc Clin Dial Transpl Forum 1970;9:226–231.

45. Raja RM, Kramer MS, Rosenbaum JL, Bolisay CG, Krug MJ. Hemodialysis associated hypoxemia. Role for acetate and pH in etiology. Trans Am Soc Artif Intern Organs 1981;27:180–183.

46. Ruder MA, Alpert MA, Van Stone J, et al. Comparative effects of acetate and bicarbonate hemodialysis on left ventricular function. Kidney Int 1985;27:768–773.

47. Sargent JA, Gotch FA. Bicarbonate and carbon dioxide transport during hemodialysis. ASAIO Trans 1979;2:61–72.

48. Schaefer K, Ryzlewics T, Sandri M, von Bernewitz S, von Herrath D. Effect of hemofiltration on acid base status and ventilation. Contrib Nephrol 1982;32:69–75.

49. Scherlock J, Ledwith J, Letteri J. Hypoventilation and hypoxemia during hemodialysis: reflex response to removal of CO_2 across the dialyser. Trans Am Soc Artif Intern Organs 1977;23:406–410.

50. Swan RC, Pitts RF. Neutralization of infused acid by nephrectomized dogs. J Clin Invest 1955;34:205.

51. Swartz RD, Jacobs JF Jr. Modified dialysis for metabolic alkalosis. Ann Intern Med 1978;88:432–440.

52. Van Stone JC. A clinical comparison of bicarbonate and acetate dialysate. Contr Dial 1980;9:25–31.

53. Vreman HJ, Assomull VM, Kaiser BA, Blaschke TF, Weiner MW. Acetate metabolism and acid-base homeostasis during hemodialysis: influence of dialyzer efficiency and rate of acetate metabolism. Kidney Int 1980;18(suppl 10):62–70.

54. Waten RL, Ferris FZ, Nagar D, Keshaviah P. An alternative explanation for dialysis-induced arterialo hypoxemia [Abstract]. Kidney Int 1978;14:689.

55. Waten RL, Keshaviah P, Hommeyer P, Cadwell K, Comty CM. The metabolic effects of hemodialysis with and without glucose in the dialysate. Am J Clin Nutr 1978;31:1870–1878.

56. Waten RL, Ward RA. Disturbances in fluid, electrolyte, and acid base in the dialysis patient. In: Massry SG, Glassock RJ, eds. Textbook of Nephrology. Vol 2. Baltimore: Williams & Wilkins 1983:98–121.

57. Yamakawa M, Yamamoto T, Kishimoto T, et al. Serum levels of acetate and TCA cycle intermediates during hemodialysis in relation to symptoms. Nephron 1982;32:155–162.

38

Management of Acute Renal Failure in the Critically Ill Patient

Claudio Ronco
Hilmar Burchardi

Acute renal failure (ARF) is a syndrome characterized by a sudden decrease of renal function (105). Several etiologies can give rise to this event and the pathophysiologic mechanisms are rather complex (140). In the early phases, when a prerenal azotemia is present, the therapy should be specifically designed to remove the dangerous condition negatively acting upon the patient's renal function (221). Moreover, when the risk of ARF is suspected, special care should be taken in order to early prevent its occurrence (168). Once ARF is established in its organic form, conservative treatment may not be sufficient to manage the patient's clinical derangements and an efficient renal replacement therapy must be undertaken (127). We must emphasize, however, that the treatment of ARF in intensive care should be adapted to the critical conditions of the patients, and these cannot be compared to those of the noncomplicated ARF commonly observed in the nephrologic setting (34).

APPROACH TO PREVENTION OF ARF

It has been demonstrated that a rapid and adequate reconstitution of extracellular and circulating plasma volumes are of great importance in preventing not only prerenal azotemia (39), but also its progression to acute tubular necrosis (170). An efficient prevention of renal insufficiency by rapid and accurate maintenance of intravascular volume has been confirmed in

patients with trauma, burns, major surgery, and all forms of renal hypoperfusion (39, 170). These pathologic events may sometimes unmask forms of underlying renal insufficiency not yet clinically evident in elderly, hypertensive, or diabetic patients. These patients are in fact characterized by a reduced renal functional reserve without significant manifest clinical or biochemical derangements (120). In these circumstances, even a transient volume depletion may represent a potential risk of progression toward acute tubular necrosis and all possible attempts must be made in order to maintain circulating plasma volume as well as systemic blood pressure (78, 128). Special care and caution must be exerted when diuretics, nonsteroidal antiinflammatory drugs, or potent vasodilators are used. In these cases an adequate hydration and volume repletion of the patient may partially overcome the potential risks and hazards related to these substances. An optimal patient's hydration may also reduce the possible impact on renal function of various substances like contrast agents, antibiotics, and toxins. It should be emphasized that in patients with suspected chronic renal insufficiency, where the best hydration will not normalize renal blood flow and where glomerular filtration rate cannot be increased in response to specific stimuli, the exposure to potentially toxic therapies or hazardous diagnostic procedures should be carefully avoided (37).

A few specific measures are available to

630

protect the kidneys from an imminent toxic exposure such as the administration of cysteamine, N-acetylcysteine, or glutathione in case of acetaminophen overdosage (189), the use of chelating agents in case of heavy metal intoxication (186), the forced diuresis in case of possible tubular obstruction due to precipitation of myoglobin, uric acid, etc. (201). Most of these conditions, however, require an early elimination of the original pathology supporting the observed clinical derangement.

Several pharmacologic agents can also be proposed in order to prevent acute tubular necrosis, to reduce its clinical severity, or to improve the outcome by shortening the oliguric phase. The use of Mannitol (16, 20, 51, 77, 157, 199) and its potential effect on ATN prevention is still matter of controversy. The beneficial effect due to increased water and solute excretion, reduction of cellular swelling, and prevention of tubular obstruction does not find an unanimous consensus. The chief benefit appears to be an increase in urine flow rather than in glomerular filtration rate (16).

Loop diuretics such as furosemide have been proposed as a possible prevention for acute tubular necrosis because of their maintenance of urine flow (14, 148), a certain vasodilation (5), and a suggested reduction of active transport and O_2 demand in the thick ascending limb (35, 36). Although some studies have demonstrated that the outcome of patients treated with diuretics is not significantly different from that of those not treated in this manner (58, 99, 146), these agents are widely used in the clinical routine. The better control of the body fluid balance permitted by them may represent a rationale for their use since, in intensive care, a high fluid turnover is often needed (e.g., for parenteral nutrition). Nevertheless, before using these diuretics, volume depletion must be excluded.

The renal vasodilatory effect of low-dose dopamine (3–5 μg/kg/min) has been utilized to prevent or attenuate acute tubular necrosis and ischemic kidney damage (48, 128, 208). However, this effect is seldom observed in the absence of an adequate cardiac output and plasma volume repletion (58, 83, 142). During mechanical ventilation, however, low-dose dopamine is often administered anyway in order to compensate the depressing effect of increased intrathoracic pressure on hemodynamics.

The intravenous administration of amino acids has been proposed for the prevention and management of acute tubular necrosis to reduce the severity of the kidney damage and to produce a beneficial effect on kidney function restoration (3, 152, 210, 212). In patients with intact residual renal function, amino acid infusion can in fact produce a significant increase in glomerular filtration rate because of a prostaglandin-mediated afferential vasodilation (32). The clinical importance of this observation is under evaluation. In conclusion, prevention of acute tubular necrosis and oliguria still represent an intriguing target that is only seldom entirely reached. Most often a slight attenuation of renal damage is probably achieved as a good result.

CONSERVATIVE MANAGEMENT OF ARF AND INITIATION OF RENAL REPLACEMENT THERAPY

Once acute renal failure is established, a conservative regimen of therapy restoring fluid balance metabolism and electrolyte equilibration must be instituted (Table 38.1).

Fluid Balance

An accurate balance of fluid intake and losses must be done to maintain a stable patient's fluid status. However, even when the patient's body weight and infusion/losses balance is accurate, it is difficult to assess the third space fluid volume, and the hemodynamic monitoring becomes critical in the final evaluation. An accurate volume repletion without causing dangerous conditions of pulmonary overload and edema can only be carried out with a parallel invasive monitoring of hemodynamic parameters such as central venous pressure, mean pulmonary artery pressure, pulmonary capillary wedge pressure, mean arterial pressure, and cardiac output. Because a possible alveolar or pulmonary

Table 38.1
Approach to Management of ARF[a]

Prevention Measures	Conservative Therapy	Substitutive Therapy

Maintain adequate volume repletion	Metabolism
	  Restrict protein intake
	    (≤0.5 g/kg/day)
		Peritoneal dialysis
		  Consider:
		  Peritoneal access

Reconstitute circulating plasma volume	Maintain caloric intake (30–50 cal/kg/day)	Tx schedule (IPD, CAPD, TPD)
Carefully check patient's hydration when administering potentially toxic substances	Provide adequate amount of carbohydrates to avoid ketosis and protein catabolism	Tx efficiency and prescription Respiratory problems Peritonitis risk

Avoid potentially hazardous and risky diagnostic procedures	Check daily nitrogen and phosphate balance	Hemodialysis
		  Consider:
		  Access to circulation

Consider the use of
  Mannitol
  Furosemide
  Dopamine
  Amino acid infusion
  All needed pharmacologic support
	Fluid balance
	  Make accurate intake/
	    output balance
	  Restrict fluid intake (if oliguria) to maintain BW
	  Intake = urine output + extrarenal losses
		Tx schedule (HD, HF, HDF)
		Tx efficiency and prescription
		Cardiovascular problems
		Poor clinical tolerance

Adjust drug dosage to GFR	Consider weight loss due to catabolism	Continuous therapies Consider:
Undertake all specific measures in case of possible toxic exposure	Monitor accurately fluid infusion rate	Access to circulation (AV or pUMP)
	Electrolyte and acid-base Prevent and treat hypo- and hypernatremia	Tx schedule (CAVH, CAVHD, CVVH, etc.)
	Prevent and treat hyperkalaemia	Tx efficiency and efficacy and prescription
	Consider body pools and distribution spaces	Extrarenal effects Good clinical tolerance
	Correct metabolic acidosis (check potassium and calcium)	
	Correct hyperphos-phatemia and hypocalcemia	
	Consider initiation and choice of the renal replacement therapy	

[a] Abbreviations: GFR, glomerular filtration rate; BW, body weight; Tx, treatment; IPD, intermittent peritoneal dialysis; CAPD, continuous ambulatory peritoneal dialysis; TPD, tidal peritoneal dialysis; HD, hemodialysis; HF, hemofiltration; HDF, hemo-diafiltration; AV, arteriovenous; CAVH, continuous arteriovenous hemofiltration; CAVHD, continuous arteriovenous hemo-dialysis; CVVH, continuous venovenous hemofiltration.

capillary damage can occur in these conditions, it is mandatory to provide the volume repletion required for an adequate kidney perfusion without causing significant fluid trapping in the lungs (24, 32, 106, 131, 229). Loop diuretics may be sufficient to solve, at least in part, a severe fluid overload (106), but in case of failure, early dialysis or ultrafiltration may be advisable (19, 63, 88, 163). Finally, for an accurate fluid balance, extrarenal losses such as intestinal, surgical drainages, and perspiration must be considered.

Metabolism

Conservative treatment is aimed at minimizing endogenous tissue breakdown and preventing starvation ketoacidosis (226). Malnourished patients suffer from increased postoperative complications, immunologic defects, and infections (49, 56, 149, 192). In most patients, endogenous fat stores are sufficient to supply caloric requirements for several days of semistarvation. If the objective is to avoid dialysis, strenuous hyperalimentation should be avoided since the water carrier for nutrients must be restricted. Daily provision of 100 g of carbohydrates is generally sufficient in the first days of ARF to avoid ketosis. Additional calories given as carbohydrates or fat do not appreciably reduce endogenous protein breakdown any further, and while the addition of sufficient exogenous protein such as amino acids may partially substitute for endogenous protein, they do not reduce the accumulation of nitrogen waste products (1). Therefore, when the excretory capacity is limited, strenuous hyperalimentation given in the attempt to reverse the catabolic effects of injury and achieve a positive nitrogen balance may, on the contrary, exacerbate the signs and symptoms of uremia. Sargent and Gotch (191) have suggested that the urea appearance rate should be measured and used to titrate individual hyperalimentation requirements. Urea generation rate can be calculated by multiplying total body water of a patient derived from clinical examination and tables, by the change in blood urea nitrogen concentration, measured over a 24-hr interval. Protein catabolic rate (PCR) can be calculated by different formulas:

$$PCR = 6.4 \times BUN \text{ generation} + 11, \text{ and}$$

$$PCR = 6.75 \times BUN \text{ generation} + 5.1.$$

When plotting PCR against caloric intake, in most patients a significant decrease in protein catabolism can be seen as the caloric intake is increased (43). It has been demonstrated (1) that hyperalimentation should be moderate in the first days and a full regimen should be instituted only after 3–4 days. Intake of 0.5 g/kg/day of essential or mixed essential/nonessential amino acids (2:1) plus histidine should be adequate to spare endogenous tissue proteins. The amount of calories should be adapted to the patient's metabolic response.

Studies have demonstrated an early recovery of renal function in patients treated with essential amino acids containing hyperalimentation solution (3). Some aspects are in favor of an enteral nutrition rather than a central venous infusion. The gastrointestinal route might, in fact, be safer and more effective if diarrhea is avoided. However, in most patients a central venous infusion permits a complete parenteral nutrition even though a strict regimen of aseptic measures must be instituted (110, 187, 188, 194). In this case, a careful monitoring of volumes and blood variables (25, 166) (electrolytes, calcium, magnesium, phosphorous, osmolality, acid-base status, lipids, liver function, coagulation factors) is mandatory as well as accurate hormonal, trace element, and vitamin replacement (insulin, iron, ascorbic acid, vitamins B, K, D, etc.) (2, 10, 13, 61, 97, 107, 124, 126, 147, 151, 169, 225). A careful daily review of medications should also be considered in relation to the variable renal and extrarenal drug clearances.

When all these measures become insufficient to maintain the patient under adequate control, substitutive techniques must be initiated and the nutritional regimen should be adapted to the new metabolic condition (59, 76, 101, 162).

Electrolyte and Acid-Base

Several derangements are observed in ARF patients, but hyperkalemia is generally the most severe and life-threatening complication (8). A detailed analysis and discussion of these problems and the relevant management is discussed in Chapter 36 (Electrolyte Derangements in Acute Renal Failure).

INITIATION OF RENAL REPLACEMENT THERAPY

Despite an urgent indication for dialysis, as may frequently occur in cases of hyperkalemia (>7 mmol/liter), severe acidosis ($HCO_3 < 15$ mmol/liter), BUN levels over 150 mg/dL, and creatinine levels over 10 mg/dL, renal replacement therapy should be started long before these concentrations occur. Electrolyte, acid-base, fluid overload, and azotemia should not progress until their severity precipitates the need for emergency dialysis. The modern trend is toward an early initiation of dialysis treatment and, in most cases, this approach presents dangerous derangements and life-threatening conditions (8, 45, 68). The temptation to define a fixed rule for dialysis initiation is, in our view, unnecessary and sometimes harmful to the patient. The complex nature of ARF syndrome requires a personalization in its treatment and management. One patient is different from one other and a rule for substitutive therapy initiation cannot be fixed. Whenever conservative measures begin to fail their objectives and potential derangements are seen in the immediate future, an early renal replacement therapy may not only produce the beneficial effects of an effective blood purification and blood equilibration, but it may also prevent the progression of potential complications related to the patient's clinical condition.

CHOICE OF THE RENAL REPLACEMENT THERAPY

Since the early clinical experience of Teschan et al. (209) during the Korean war, when the artificial kidney was first introduced, several developments have been made in this field, and the treatment of ARF in the critically ill patient can today be performed with a wide number of techniques. Among these we can identify three groups: (*a*) peritoneal dialysis; (*b*) hemodialysis; and (*c*) continuous therapies. All these techniques use a wide number of derived procedures that respond to the principles of the original stem technique.

The choice for an effective renal replacement therapy must depend on several conditions (12). The technological support and the training of the personnel is a condition sine qua non for the performance of each substitutive treatment. Some techniques require less investment in terms of machinery and personnel and they may sometimes be preferred in spite of their limited efficacy. On the other hand, precise clinical indications are today proposed for some of these techniques such as continuous therapies. We will try to define

the advantages and disadvantages of different forms of therapy, allowing the reader to make his or her own choice in personal situations. The key point, in our view, is in the definition of the critically ill patient as a patient who suffers from a form of ARF that has nothing to do with the noncomplicated ARF generally treated in the nephrologic departments. For this reason, a standard renal replacement therapy as conceived for chronic patients cannot be the answer to all clinical requirements of an acute patient in intensive care. Therefore, special care must be placed in finding a soft, gentle, but effective form of renal replacement therapy to treat such complicated patients who do not need further derangements created by the therapy itself.

REQUIREMENTS FOR AN ADEQUATE RENAL REPLACEMENT THERAPY

Once the impairment of renal function has reached a point in which conservative treatment becomes inadequate, the complex nature of ARF in the critically ill patient requires an effective substitutive therapy to achieve not only a blood purification, but also acceptable treatment of the various associated clinical derangements (Table 38.2). The clinical and technical requirements for an adequate renal replacement therapy in intensive care can be summarized in different points.

Easy Institution and Monitoring

The treatment should be easy to institute and simple to monitor. The experience can be different from one center to the other, and frequently the success of a renal replacement therapy is directly related to the training of the personnel. A complex dialysis machine may not be easy to handle, and various peritoneal dialysis techniques may not be sufficiently experienced to guarantee a safe procedure. Therefore, the choice of treatment depends more often on the clinical routine of a given department than on precise clinical indication. In any case, the chronic lack of personnel requires a simple and rapid treatment to-

Table 38.2
Technical and Clinical Requirements for an Adequate Renal Replacement Therapy in Intensive Care Patients

Rapid and easy institution and simple treatment monitoring

Efficiency and efficacy adequate to therapy prescription

Possibility of maintenance of the desired body weight

No restriction in fluid administration and hyperalimentation

Achievement of a stable and correct acid-base balance

Possibility of correction of electrolyte disorders

High biocompatibility with minimal or no interaction with blood

Optimal clinical tolerance and hemodynamic stability

Reliability and predictability in terms of blood purification

Easy adjustment of drug dosage

Minimal incidence of technical and clinical complications

Adequate costs/benefit balance

gether with optimal clinical performances requiring no significant increases in personnel demand or labor intensity.

Efficiency and Efficacy

Under these two terms, we summarize the ability of a given renal replacement therapy to quantitatively remove uremic toxins like urea, and the ability to remove waste products in a wide range of molecular weight. While the amount of urea to be removed can be easily calculated from a daily urea nitrogen balance record (29), the adequate amount to be removed has not yet been defined for other solutes (creatinine, uric acid, phosphate, chemically active mediators, β-2 microglobulin, etc.). For this reason, based on our experience in the past few years, we could suggest as adequate a replacement therapy that guarantees a daily urea clearance in liters more than or equal to the volume of total body water and a daily clearance of vitamin B_{12} (chosen as a marker molecule for larger solutes) in liter $\geq$60% of total body water. Total body water can be easily calculated

from anthropometric tables or simply as 60% of body weight.

$$\text{Urea } \frac{K \times t}{V} \geq 1 \quad \text{vitamin } B_{12} \frac{K \times t}{V} \geq 0.6$$

where K = clearance in milliliters per minute, t = time in minutes, and V = volume in liters of total body water (29, 74, 174).

This means that, in the majority of patients, even in the presence of a severe catabolic state, these parameters guarantee a satisfactory blood purification for urea and other waste products (176).

Maintenance of Patient's Body Weight

An optimal patient's hydration status must be obtained in order to avoid respiratory problems, cardiovascular overload, or symptomatic hyper- or hypotension. This may also influence the outcome of the syndrome and the process of recovery of renal function. However, fluid excess in third spaces can be misleading. Furthermore, volume loss may exist even in the presence of significant tissue edema.

Clinical Tolerance and Hemodynamic Response

A patient's correct body weight must be achieved over an adequate period of time, avoiding significant hemodynamic disturbances. The cardiac performance as well as peripheral resistances should be maintained as stable as possible or even improved by the treatment and its rate of ultrafiltration. This may be difficult, especially in cases of sepsis and multiple organ failure where the autoregulation of systemic circulation may be considerably impaired; therefore, hemodynamic stability depends not only on intravascular volume.

Correction of Electrolyte Imbalances

The treatment must guarantee an adequate correction of electrolyte derangements, not only in terms of plasma concentration but also in terms of body pool. In this case, the correct body weight of the patient must be defined and maintained in order to avoid electrolyte shifts related to states of hypo- or hyperhydration.

Correction of Acid-Base Derangements

Patients with ARF frequently present with a severe metabolic acidosis, even though this is not the rule in all patients. The treatment must be able to correct the acid-base imbalance and to maintain an adequate blood chemistry over time. For this purpose, bicarbonate is the most physiologic buffer, but other alkaline equivalents such as acetate or lactate can be used. The buffer is generally added to the dialysate bath or to the replacement fluids and, again, an accurate buffer balance must be made not only in relation to the plasma values but also in terms of mass balance and body pool.

Biocompatibility

The treatment must be carried out with materials ensuring the minimal blood/system interaction. Besides the use of sterile and pyrogen-free fluids both as dialysate and replacement solutions, the membrane utilized can be of major importance. It has been shown that while synthetic membranes like Polysulfon, Polyamide, and polyacrylonitrile produce minimal or no inflammatory effects, cellulosic membranes like cuprophan are able to stimulate monocyte activation with release of cytokines and chemical mediators. Therefore, while in the septic patient synthetic membranes may reduce the plasma concentration of several mediators by filtration and adsorption, cellulosic membranes are not only inadequate to filter these products from the blood, but may even increase their plasma levels due to a remarkable macrophage immunostimulation.

Low Rate of Complications

The treatment must be safe and free of major technical and clinical complications. The costs should be adequate to the results achieved and the treatment should not result in a significantly higher labor intensity for either doctors or nursing staff.

BASIC MECHANISMS OF WATER AND SOLUTE TRANSPORT ACROSS SEMIPERMEABLE MEMBRANES

The term dialysis comes from the Greek language where "διαλύῶ" means to "pass across." All the mechanisms involved in renal replacement therapies can therefore be summarized as a transport process of water and solutes (4, 11, 12, 18, 80–82, 108, 138).

The artificial membranes used in extracorporeal treatments belong essentially to two different groups, cellulosic (Cuprophan-Hemophan-cellulose acetate) and synthetic (Polysulfon-Polyamide-Polyacrylonitrile). The former presents low ultrafiltration capacities and are primarily used in standard dialysis, while the latter group has higher ultrafiltration coefficients and solute permeability and are specifically used in treatments with high convective component (hemofiltration). The mechanisms utilized for solute and water transport across these membranes are schematically illustrated in Figure 38.1.

Diffusion

In this mechanism, the molecules move casually in all directions and tend to achieve an equal concentration in both sides of the membrane. The concentration gradient (dc) represents the driving force, while the permeability and thickness (dx) of the membrane represents the major resistance. Diffusive transport depends directly on temperature (T), surface area of the membrane (A), and solute diffusivity (D). As the membrane thickness and solute molecular weight increase, diffusion coefficients tend to decrease and solute transport by diffusion is poor. That means that the diffusion transport process is more effective for smaller molecules. Synthetic membranes are not adequate for diffusion treatments and are better used in the convective mode because of their thickness. Diffusion clearance in a dialytic system can be calculated from the following formula:

$$Kd = \frac{Qbi \times Cbi}{Cbi} - \frac{Qbo \times Cbo}{Cbi} = \frac{Qdo \times Cdo}{Cbi} - \frac{Qdi \times Cdi}{Cbi}$$

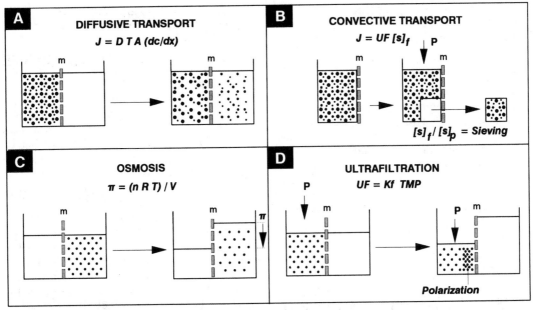

Figure 38.1. Mechanisms of solute and water transport utilized for renal replacement therapy. **A,** diffusion is directly proportional to diffusivity *(D)*, temperature *(T)*, membrane area *(A)*, and concentration gradient *(dc)*, and is inversely correlated with the membrane thickness *(dx)*. **B,** convection depends on ultrafiltration *(UF)* and membrane sieving capacity *(s)*. **C,** osmosis is mostly utilized in peritoneal dialysis. (See text for details.) **D,** ultrafiltration depends on transmembrane pressure *(TMP)*, and membrane permeability coefficient *(Kf)*.

where: Kd = diffusive clearance or dialysance, Qb = blood flow, Qd = dialysate flow, Cb = concentration of a given solute in blood, Cd = concentration of the solute in the dialysate, and i and o = inlet and outlet of the dialyzer.

Convection

In this mechanism, solutes are transported across the membrane carried by the solvent movement (ultrafiltration) that takes place in response to a certain transmembrane pressure. In this process of ultrafiltration, the permeability of the membrane (measured with solute-sieving coefficients) plays an important role. Synthetic membranes retain cells and proteins, but permit the passage of other solutes up to a given molecular size (cut-off valve) at the same concentration as in plasma water. In this case, an ultrafiltrate with the same characteristics of plasma water is achieved. In the case of membranes with lower permeability, the porosity of the membrane will regulate the passage of solutes up to a

point in which only water can cross the membrane and this is the case of reverse osmosis or hyperfiltration.

In convection, the solute transport will depend on the amount of ultrafiltrate (depending on the product pressure × permeability, or TMP × Kf), the solute concentration in plasma water, and the sieving capacity of the membrane (the sieving coefficient S is the ratio between the concentration of a solute in the ultrafiltrate and its concentration in plasma water in the absence of a gradient for diffusion). When the sieving coefficient for a given solute is 1, the solute can freely cross the membrane and its concentration in the ultrafiltrate will be the same as in plasma water. Convective clearance will therefore be calculated from the following formula:

$$Kc = Qf \times [s]p \times S = Qf \times [s]uf$$

where Kc = convective clearance, Qf = ultrafiltration rate, [s] = concentration of the solute s, p = plasma, uf = ultrafiltrate, and S = sieving coefficient. For solutes with a sieving coefficient of 1, the convective clearance will equal the ultrafiltration rate.

Osmosis

This particular mechanism is utilized in peritoneal dialysis. The relatively low rate of glucose absorption from the peritoneal cavity permits the dialysis solution to exact a certain osmotic power that generates significant amounts of water transport by osmosis. In this case in fact, a water movement proportional to the number of osmotically active particles (n) is achieved and the patient's hydration can be controlled.

Ultrafiltration

The water transport across the membrane depends on the transmembrane pressure gradient (TMP) and the hydraulic permeability coefficient of the membrane (Kf). While cellulosic membranes present a Kf = 5–6 ml/h/mm Hg/m^2, synthetic membranes may reach values of Kf up to 30–40 ml/hr/mm Hg/m^2. For this reason, synthetic membranes are used in treatments with high convective components and high ultrafiltration rates. Their use is generally reserved for machines and techniques equipped with ultrafiltration control systems or reinfusion of substitution fluids.

In conclusion, in diffusion treatments utilizing cellulosic membranes, small molecules such as urea can be adequately and efficiently removed. If a wider range of molecular weight solutes must be removed, purely convective or mixed diffusion-convective treatments utilizing synthetic membranes are definitely required.

PERITONEAL DIALYSIS

In this treatment, sterile pyrogen-free solutions are infused in the peritoneal cavity and drained in a subsequent series of cycles. Usually 2 liters of fresh dialysate are infused via a peritoneal catheter at each exchange, and several treatment schedules can be performed. In Figure 38.2 the basic mechanisms operating in peritoneal dialysis are schematically shown. Removal of solutes by diffusion is achieved because

of a concentration gradient between blood flowing in the peritoneal capillary network and the dialysate (144). Six resistances to this transport can be identified: stagnant layer of plasma, endothelium, basement membrane, interstitium, peritoneal mesothelium, and stagnant layers of dialysate (60). A convective removal of water and solutes can also be obtained by increasing dialysate osmolality (79). Standard solutions may contain 1.5%, 2.5%, and 4.25% glucose and this represents the major component of peritoneal transmembrane pressure. In the lower panels of Figure 38.2, the possible treatment schedules and the relevant performances are shown. Intermittent peritoneal dialysis consists of a series of rapid exchanges with complete drainage of fluid at any cycle (27). Continuous equilibration peritoneal dialysis utilizes long intraperitoneal dwell times in order to achieve a dialysate/plasma equilibration and reduce the amount of used fluid (165). Equilibration for urea occurs at about 4-hr dwell time. In tidal peritoneal dialysis, 1 liter of solution is maintained in the peritoneal cavity and rapid 1-liter exchanges are continuously performed (87). This schedule reduces the time in which the peritoneal cavity is empty.

Efficiency

It can be observed that intermittent peritoneal dialysis may reach remarkable clearance and ultrafiltration values even though large amounts of fluid are required and a continuous monitoring is mandatory. Continuous peritoneal dialysis requires much less dialysis solution, but its efficiency is rather low. Tidal peritoneal dialysis may offer a good compromise, although peritoneal dialysis machinery is generally required for its correct performance. In intermittent peritoneal dialysis, urea clearances up to 25 liters/day can be achieved at an average dialysate flow rate of 5 liter/hr, while with other peritoneal dialysis techniques, lower clearances are generally achieved. Despite its low efficiency in some patients, peritoneal dialysis can effectively control BUN levels because of a continuous action that guarantees a stable biochemistry and significant solute

SOLUTE DIFFUSION

ULTRAFILTRATION & CONVECTION

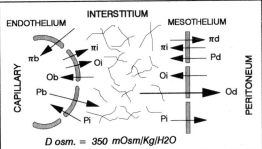

TREATMENT SCHEDULES

TREATMENT PERFORMANCE

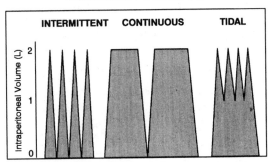

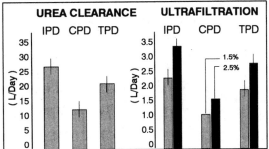

Figure 38.2. Characteristics of peritoneal dialysis function. Solutes encounter six resistances (R_1–R_6) to move by diffusion from the blood into dialysate. Convective transport is facilitated by the osmotic power of the dialysis solution (P, hydrostatic pressure, o, osmotic pressure, π, oncotic pressure, b, blood, d, dialysate, i, interstitium). Treatment schedules depend on the fluid volume exchanged and the frequency of the exchanges. (See text for details.) The efficiency of the system is shown in the lower right panel. *IPD,* intermittent peritoneal dialysis; *CPD,* continuous equilibration peritoneal dialysis; *TPD,* tidal peritoneal dialysis.

extractions (165). Moreover, the peculiar permeability of peritoneal membrane allows for remarkable clearances of larger molecules other than urea and ensures a certain removal of peptides up to 50,000 daltons (193).

Clinical Results

Intermittent peritoneal dialysis has been widely used as a treatment of ARF (42, 216). By comparison with hemodialysis, intermittent peritoneal dialysis seems to offer advantages in terms of safety and technical simplicity, no bleeding risk, excellent cardiovascular tolerance, and low risk of dialysis related disequilibrium (91). On the other hand, despite the use of large amounts of dialysate, a low efficiency is often observed and insufficient amounts

of daily ultrafiltration are produced even in the presence of remarkably high dialysate glucose concentrations (135). Furthermore, in cases of high dialysate glucose concentration, not only the ultrafiltration produced is insufficient to maintain the patient in an adequate fluid balance, but also the risk of a severe hyperglycemia and protein loss is enhanced (150). Following the large-scale use of continuous ambulatory peritoneal dialysis, continuous peritoneal dialysis has also been proposed for the treatment of ARF (165, 214). Despite the good clinical tolerance and the remarkable simplicity, the efficiency of this treatment may not be sufficient to maintain potassium, phosphate creatinine, and BUN levels under adequate control in the critically ill patient. Tidal peritoneal dialysis may be a good compromise even though the constant presence of fluid in the abdomen may also enhance the risk of respiratory problems (decrease of functional residual capacity and gas exchange deficiency) and transperitoneal leakage (87).

Complications

In all forms of peritoneal dialysis a reliable peritoneal access must be created. The percutaneous puncture of the peritoneum has been used for years, but represents a risk of bowel perforation that is today no longer acceptable (197). Therefore, a surgical insertion of a soft Tenckhoff catheter is advised, with special care to the skin exit site (158). The major risk of peritoneal dialysis is infection (205, 220). Peritonitis may worsen the patient's clinical condition and render the treatment dangerous and life-threatening (198). Peritonitis incidence in intensive care is significantly higher than that observed in chronic patients. The nonspecifically trained personnel, together with the lower host defences and the high risk of contamination may really enhance the possibility of peritoneal infection and treatment failure in the intensive care setting. In Table 38.3, the advantages and disadvantages of peritoneal dialysis are summarized along with the possible complications.

Indications

Although peritoneal dialysis has been partially abandoned in the treatment of ARF due to its high rate of complications and low efficiency, it can still represent one of the possible renal replacement therapies for a variety of clinical derangements. Peritoneal dialysis is generally preferred in cases of bleeding risk or fluid overload associated with severe cardiovascular instability (139). Before the clinical development of continuous arteriovenous hemofiltration (CAVH), peritoneal dialysis represented a unique form of treatment for extracellular volume expansion and cardiac failure (40). The high clinical tolerance and the slow continuous ultrafiltration were permitting a satisfactory correction of these derangements. In cases of acute bacterial peritonitis and acute tubular necrosis, peritoneal dialysis permits treatment of both peritoneal infection and ARF, and stimulates an early recovery of peristalsis (213). Peritoneal dialysis has also been used in cases of toxic ARF to remove the offending agent and, in particular, iodinated contrast material. In one study, peritoneal clearance of iodide was reported as high as 12 ml/min and 56% of iodide was removed over a period of 64 hr of treatment (33).

Interesting reports concerning the removal of drugs and poisons with peritoneal dialysis have been published (21, 227). Because of its low efficiency, however, peritoneal dialysis does not permit a rapid removal of poisons or drugs and there is a general agreement that, in these cases, the higher clearances achievable with hemodialysis or hemoperfusion should be

Table 38.3
Peritoneal Dialysis

Advantages	Disadvantages	Complications
Cardiovascular stability	Low efficiency	Bacterial or fungal peritonitis
Slow and gentle treatment	Low rate of ultrafiltration	Catheter malfunction
No need of machines	Need of a peritoneal access	Leakage
Easy monitoring	Respiratory problems	Pulmonary atelectasis
No need of heparin	Glucose load	Cardiac arrhythmias
Administration of nutrients	Risk of infection	Hypernatremia
Administration of drugs	Contraindicated in burns	Hyperglycemia
No need for vascular access	and recent abdominal sur-	Intestinal perforation
No risks of extracorporeal	gery	Pneumoperitoneum
circulation	Large amounts of dialysate if	Hernias
Steady state chemistry when	intermittently performed	Hydrothorax
continuously performed	Protein losses	
	Increased intraabdominal	
	pressure	

utilized for the most effective results (53). Peritoneal dialysis can effectively correct a variety of electrolyte and acid-base derangements such as hyperkalemia, hypokalemia, hyper- or hyponatremia, and metabolic acidosis. Most of the dialysis solutions use lactate as a buffer, although a recent clinical experience with bicarbonate-containing solutions has demonstrated the feasibility and the effectiveness of this newer approach (57). Hypercalcemia and hyperuricemia can also be treated with peritoneal dialysis with remarkable correction of the acute metabolic derangement. The suggested beneficial effects of peritoneal dialysis in acute pancreatitis (222) are still matters of controversy and perspective studies on this topic should be undertaken to find a final evaluation. To conclude, we must remind the reader that peritoneal membrane is a possible way to infuse drugs and nutrients in the critically ill patient. Despite a constant protein loss, it is possible to infuse glucose and amino acids in the patient, although a positive nitrogen balance is rarely achieved.

During the past decade, indications for peritoneal dialysis became less common in ARF. This presumably is the result of the multiple technological advances observed in extracorporeal dialysis. The introduction of bicarbonate dialysis with ultrafiltration control, hemofiltration and hemodiafiltration, and continuous therapies such as CAVH and continuous arteriovenous hemodialysis (CAVHD) have resulted in better cardiovascular stability and clinical tolerance to extracorporeal therapies. Temporary blood access was easily achieved with percutaneous vessels cannulation and specific double-lumen catheters. The bleeding risk of extracorporeal therapies was effectively reduced by a circuit optimization and low-dose heparinization. Furthermore, extracorporeal treatments offer the potential for higher ultrafiltration rates and facilitate an excellent control of the extracellular volume when total parenteral nutrition is required. Despite all these observations, peritoneal dialysis still maintains an important position among the different renal replacement therapies and should not be neglected. It still represents one of the possible treatment alternatives in patients with ARF.

INTERMITTENT HEMODIALYSIS

Under this heading we generally include all forms of extracorporeal treatments utilizing specific dialyzers and machines and performed intermittently for a few hours per session. These techniques require an adequate vascular access and specially trained nurses to carry out the dialysis session. Moreover, complete equipment devoted to correct performance of the treatment is required. A specific water softening and deionization is required in order to achieve pure water for the dialysate preparation. In some cases, despite the use of reverse osmosis as a water treatment system, on-line ultrafilters are needed to achieve a bacterial- and pyrogen-free dialysate. The dialysis machine must respond to the standards of reliability and safety with an adequate blood module, a precise dialysate-preparing module with adequate warming and debubbling systems, and all parts must have active alarms to avoid any possible accident. In other words, sophisticated machinery is required for this kind of treatment, and potential risks related to the techniques should not be neglected or underestimated.

Vascular Access

The access to the circulation for acute hemodialysis is generally obtained by percutaneous cannulation of the femoral, subclavian, or jugular veins (188). Intraoperative application of a Scribner shunt can also be used and it can be transformed later in arteriovenous subcutaneous fistula, in cases of patients who do not regain their renal function (47) Catheters with double lumen are easily utilized with a regular blood pump, while single-lumen catheters require a double-headed blood pump. Complications related to these procedures are the same as those observed for any kind of venous catheterization: thrombosis, pulmonary embolism, and possible hematomas. The subclavian vein catheterization is the more complicated approach and may lead to severe complications such as hemo- or pneumothorax (50). Catheters may stay in place for days and even weeks, but special care must be taken to avoid skin exit site infection and to maintain the patency with periodic lavages or internal guides when the cannula is not used for dialysis.

Anticoagulation

Continuous heparin infusion is generally provided during dialysis at the rate of 600–800 iu/hr (55). This amount guarantees a safe anticoagulation with minimal or no systemic effects. It should be noted, however, that in patients with high bleeding risk, dialysis can be carried out with lower amounts or even without heparin (89). In other cases, regional heparinization (204), low molecular weight heparin (7), or alternative anticoagulants can be used (207, 215). When a constant blood flow is provided by a well-functioning access and a calibrated blood pump, clotting of the fibers rarely occurs and minimal platelet, white and red blood cell trapping can be observed at the end of the treatment. Special care should be taken in the placement of the venous drip chamber that tends to clot much easier than the dialyzer. If heparin administration cannot be avoided in risky patients, protamine sulphate can be administered as well at the end of the session with satisfactory inhibition of the anticoagulant effect.

Techniques

In Figure 38.3 a schematic representation of the three basic therapies included under the general heading of intermittent hemodialysis is shown. Their operational characteristics are schematically summarized.

Hemodialysis

In the upper left panel of Figure 38.3, standard hemodialysis is shown. This

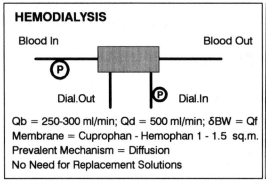

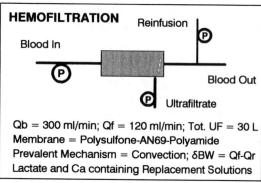

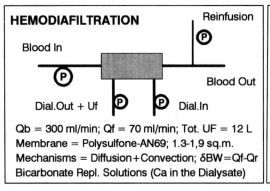

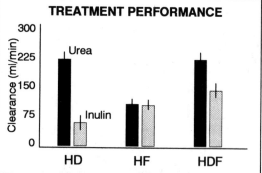

Figure 38.3. Schematic representation of three different forms of intermittent extracorporeal therapy. They are generally included under the common term of intermittent hemodialysis even though they are hemodialysis, hemofiltration, and hemodiafiltration. The performances of these treatments are reported in the lower right panel.

technique is carried out for 3–4 hr a session with an average blood flow of 250–300 ml/min. A low permeability membrane such as Cuprophan or Hemophan is utilized with an average surface area of 1–1.5 m². Dialysate flow is 500 ml/min and the rate of ultrafiltration achieved corresponds to the patient's weight loss. Hemodialysis works primarily in diffusion and small molecular weight solutes are removed faster from the body than medium-to-large-sized molecules.

Hemofiltration

In the upper right panel of Figure 38.3, mechanical hemofiltration is shown. In this technique, treatment time depends on the rate of ultrafiltration and the total amount of fluid to be exchanged. Blood flow is around 300 ml/min and no dialysate is present. A highly permeable membrane is utilized in this form of therapy and solutes are removed by convection. In Figure 38.4 the sieving coefficients of different membranes for solutes of various molecular

weight are shown. It may be noted that synthetic membranes like polysulfon present a sieving capacity near 1 for a wide spectrum of molecular weights. On the contrary, with cellulosic membranes, sieving coefficients significantly decrease, even for moderate increases of molecular weight. For this reason, synthetic membranes are used in hemofiltration where high amounts of ultrafiltrate with the same characteristics of plasma water are achieved. Ultrafiltrate is totally or partially replaced with a sterile substitution fluid and solute concentrations in plasma are lowered. The patient weight loss depends on the difference between ultrafiltration and reinfusion, and different-sized molecules are removed from the body. The standard treatment duration for a 30-liter exchange hemofiltration is 3–4 hr.

Hemodiafiltration

In the lower left panel of Figure 38.3, hemodiafiltration is shown. This technique represents a real compromise between he-

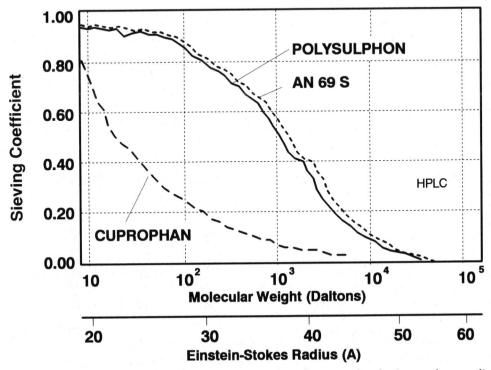

Figure 38.4. In vitro sieving coefficients for neutral dextrans. Synthetic membranes display a stable sieving value for a wide range of molecular weights, while cuprophan membrane presents a sudden decrease of the sieving value even for slight increases of molecular weight.

modialysis and hemofiltration. Highly permeable membranes are utilized and solutes of different sizes are removed both by diffusion and convection; 9–12 liters of ultrafiltrate are produced in each session and substitution fluid is reinfused according to the patient's ideal body weight or to fluid infusion requirements. Hemodiafiltration has recently been shown to guarantee better sodium and buffer balances with a remarkable cardiovascular stability and adequate treatment of metabolic acidosis (6).

Efficiency and Prescription

In the lower right panel of Figure 38.3, the relevant clearances for the three techniques are reported. Urea and inulin are taken as marker molecules for small and large molecular weight solutes. All these treatments can achieve a filtration volume/replacement volume index >1 in the single session while CAVH and CAVHD are significantly more efficient in removing solutes other than urea. The clinical meaning and toxicity of such solutes in acute patients is a matter of a continuous study and research. These techniques are characterized by a rapid decrease in solute plasma concentrations after a short time from the beginning. In this case, while the clearance value is fairly stable, the solute extraction tends to decrease and the final amount of solute removed from the body may be less in comparison with other less efficient but continuous therapies (54).

As a demonstration of this concept, a sudden urea concentration rebound is generally observed a few hours after the treatment has ceased. This means that these highly efficient intermittent techniques can remove solutes primarily from the intravascular or extracellular fluid, but they cannot achieve a complete purification of body fluids (especially intracellular ones) because of a remarkable resistance to transport solutes from the different compartments of the body. The speed of removal by dialysis is therefore faster than the capacity of equilibration between interstitial and vascular spaces and intracellular and extracellular compartments. This

phenomenon not only reduces the efficacy of the therapy, but also supports the theory that intermittent treatments are not physiological and may result in disequilibrium syndromes (6).

Dialysate Composition

Dialysate composition can be adjusted to the patient's clinical requirements. Sodium has been raised to 140 mmol/liters in recent years, and acetate has been substituted with bicarbonate (28, 125, 224). This has produced a series of beneficial effects in terms of vascular stability and acid-base balance. The potassium content can be regulated on the basis of the degree of hyperkalemia. Calcium concentrations of 1.75 mmol/liter have been shown to be adequate in acute patients for achieving a positive calcium balance. The presence of glucose in the dialysate bath is mandatory in acute patients, which presents "unphysiologic" increases of Krebs cycle intermediates in plasma with a consequent worsening of acidosis related to alkaline equivalents loss (223).

Biocompatibility

Minimal blood/membrane interactions are guaranteed by the use of synthetic membranes (85). It should be noted, however, that highly permeable membranes may lead to a risk of backfiltration of a nonsterile dialysate with a consequent transport back into the blood of endotoxin fragments that are able to stimulate complement and macrophage activation, and interleukin-1 (IL-1) production (173). This should be regulated with an adequate manometric setting of the machine that can be achieved with modern ultrafiltration control systems.

Complications

Acute hypotension is the most common complication of intermittent dialysis treatment (109). Dry body weight must be achieved in few hours and fluid withdrawal may be remarkable. In chronic patients we have observed that the frequency of hypotensive episodes during dialysis is significantly correlated with the rate of ultrafiltration (185). When ultrafiltration ex-

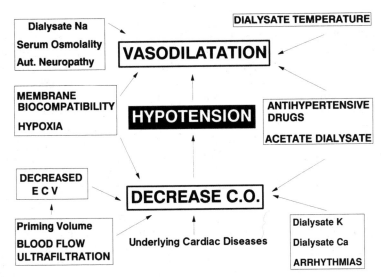

Figure 38.5. Factors causing hypotension during extracorporeal dialysis treatment. *ECV*, extracellular volume.

ceeds 0.35 ml/min/kg of body weight, the frequency of hypotension increases dramatically and may reach values of 60% for ultrafiltration rates of 0.6 ml/hr/kg. These values must even be restricted for acute patients who are severely unstable and sometimes hypotensive at the outset.

Several factors have been proposed in the pathogenesis of dialysis hypotension. In Figure 38.5 we present a summary of the factors potentially involved in the pathogenesis of dialysis-related hypotension. The acute decrease in plasma osmolality may contribute to significant fluid shifts and hypotension (100). This phenomenon is partially avoided in hemofiltration, where iso-osmotic ultrafiltration takes place. Interactions of blood components with the dialyzer may result in complement activation and increased leukocyte adherence and sequestration in the lungs (46). This partially contributes to hypoxemia and potentially to hypotension. Autonomic dysfunction may be present and will inhibit an adequate response to ultrafiltration (52). This can be the case also in patients with manifest or underlying myocardial dysfunction. Finally, septic patients are severely unstable and dialysis hypotension may occur with higher frequency. Hypoxemia can also be present because of significant losses of CO_2 in the

dialyzer and consequent hypoventilation (9, 143). This must be carefully observed and eventually corrected by changing the dialysate composition or the composition of substitution fluid.

Cardiac arrhythmias may occur during dialysis in the acutely ill patient. Remarkable electrolyte and pH shifts may significantly contribute to this complication (98). We have already mentioned possible plasma water shifts because of a differential osmolality among body compartments. This factor may also contribute to a cellular edema or to a worsening of a brain edematogenic state (116). This has been confirmed with computerized tomography studies after intermittent treatments, while it has been excluded in continuous therapies (117). Therefore, in unstable critically ill patients the use of these intermittent techniques is limited. Continuous techniques may provide much better conditions in these patients.

Bleeding episodes are rarely observed if the coagulation status is accurately monitored. The low rate of heparinization and the possible use of protamine sulfate may in fact guarantee a very low incidence of this complication. Other technical complications related to the dialysis machine or equipment are seldom observed, and the quality of today's machines is high enough

Table 38.4
Intermittent Hemodialysis in Critically Ill Patients [a]

Advantages	Disadvantages	Complications
High efficiency	Cardiovascular instability	Infections and bacteremia
Shortness of the session	High ultrafiltration time	Access malfunction
High ultrafiltration capacity	Need of a vascular access	Bleeding
Low heparinization	Postdialytic solute rebound	Hypoxemia and hypoventilation
Possibility to adjust therapy prescription	Difficult solutes balance	Cardiac arrhythmias
Clearances of drugs predictable	Extracorporeal circulation	Severe hypotension
Possibility of rapid and effective correction of hyperkalemia and other life-threatening derangements	Contraindicated in hypotensive and critically ill patients	Air embolism
	Large amounts of dialysate and replacement solutions	Disequilibrium syndrome
	Body fluid and solute shifts and possible disequilibrium among body compartments	Worsening of brain edema
	Machine required	Machine disfunction
	Complex monitoring	Circuit coagulation
		Lines disconnection

[a] In chronic patients undergoing renal replacement therapies, the relevant advantages and disadvantages may be significantly different.

Table 38.5
Problems of Hemodialysis and Peritoneal Dialysis in Intensive Care Patients with ARF

Hemodialysis	Peritoneal Dialysis
Problems	
Intermittency of treatment	Low clearances
Variable technical efficiency	Poor metabolic control
Fluid and electrolyte shifts	Hyperglycemia
Poor metabolic control	Protein loss
Fluid restriction required	Low ultrafiltration
Difficult solute balance	Infections
Cardiovascular instability	Fluid leakage
Neurologic disorders	Cardiac disturbances
Machine and personnel required	Respiratory failure
Bed scale or ultrafiltrate control system	
Contraindications	
Cardiovascular instability	Abdominal surgery
Severe hypotension	Myocardial dysfunction
Hemorrhagic risks	Respiratory problems

to guarantee a safe and reliable dialytic procedure. In Table 38.4 the advantages and disadvantages of intermittent hemodialytic techniques are summarized, along with the most common complications.

CONTINUOUS THERAPIES

Most of the patients who suffer from isolated acute renal failure are generally treated in nephrologic departments and dialysis units. The outcome of these patients with noncomplicated ARF is good in a very high percentage, and temporary intermittent hemodialysis is generally the therapy of choice. In intensive care departments, however, ARF frequently occurs in patients with medical or surgical complications and multiorgan dysfunction. Those patients have a severe prognosis and the standard renal replacement therapies might be contraindicated or present potential hazards. In Table 38.5 we have summarized the possible limitations or contraindications relevant to intermittent hemodialysis or peritoneal dialysis in the severely ill patient.

Starting from the previous experiences of Henderson et al. (81) in 1967 and Silverstein et al. (196) in 1974, who used plasma ultrafiltration as a treatment for fluid overload and azotemia, Kramer et al. (114) in 1977 first described a new method called continuous arteriovenous hemofiltration. This procedure was intended to be a continuous form of renal replacement therapy as opposed to intermittent hemodialysis or hemofiltration. Continuous arteriovenous hemofiltration was considered an alternative to other therapies and remained limited to a small group of investigators until 1983 when Lauer et al. (120) described the unique operational characteristics of the system and the enormous potential for the treatment of ARF in intensive care departments. Continuous arteriovenous hemofiltration is an extracorporeal therapy in which water, electrolytes, and other low molecular weight solutes are removed from the patient by convection over an extended period of time. Ultrafiltration takes place in a small filter by means of a hydrostatic pressure gradient across a semipermeable membrane (15, 179) (Figure 38.6).

Simultaneously, the blood volume is reconstituted by the administration of a replacement fluid with a composition similar to that of normal plasma. No blood pumps are used and the arteriovenous pressure gradient represents the driving force that moves the blood throughout the extracorporeal circuit. Continuous arteriovenous hemofiltration provides an uninterrupted renal replacement therapy for patients with ARF. The objective is to achieve 12–18 liters for every 24 hr of ultrafiltrate, which provides the equivalent of a glomular filtration rate of 8–14 ml/min. The ultrafiltrate can be totally replaced to lower solute plasma concentration, partially replaced to achieve solute concentration and volume control, or not replaced at all to achieve maximal body fluid control (159).

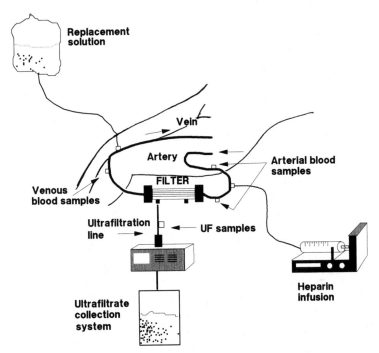

Figure 38.6. Schematic representation of continuous arteriovenous hemofiltration therapy. UF, ultrafiltration.

Continuous arteriovenous hemofiltration has been widely used in the recent years for the treatment of patients with refractory fluid overload, complicated ARF, acid-base and electrolyte derangements, and finally for those patients that could not be treated with other forms of therapy because of clinical or technical complications. While the simplicity and easy monitoring of continuous arteriovenous hemofiltration, together with the excellent clinical tolerance, were found to be the major advantages of this system, the low efficiency and the easy clotting of the filters represented the major limitation in a wider clinical application. It should be noted, however, that most of the limits and complications encountered in the past were related to the fact that materials and equipment not originally created for this purpose were utilized in continuous arteriovenous hemofiltration. On the contrary, in recent years a significant development of the techniques, equipment, and materials has taken place. New technical improvements and a better clinical understanding of continuous arteriovenous hemofiltration and derived forms of therapy have spurred a new interest in continuous therapies that are today more and more utilized in different clinical settings.

Vascular Access

Continuous hemofiltration or hemodialysis can be performed both by arteriovenous driven spontaneous circulation (continuous arteriovenous hemofiltration—CAVHD), and with a mechanical blood pump (continuous venovenous hemofiltration (CVVH)—continuous venovenous hemofiltration with dialysis (CVVHD)). In the arteriovenous setting, the vascular access should guarantee an adequate arteriovenous gradient; it must be biocompatible, clinically well-tolerated, and flexible without any reduction of the inner lumen (155, 156). Different accesses to circulation can be used (Fig. 38.7). Percutaneous cannulation of an artery and a vein provides adequate circulatory access for continuous arteriovenous hemofiltration. The femoral artery and vein are par-

ticularly suitable for the procedure (Fig. 38.7, **A** and **B**). The brachial artery and vein can also be utilized (Fig. 38.7, **C** and **D**). The catheters should guarantee an adequate arteriovenous gradient; they must be biocompatible and flexible without reduction of the inner lumen. Catheters must provide low resistance, having an adequate diameter (2 mm) and a reduced length (80–100 mm). Accordingly, the resistance of the entire extracorporeal circuit must be reduced at the minimum in order to avoid the use of large catheters with a higher bleeding risk without any specific advantage. In some cases a Scribner shunt can be used (Fig. 38.7, **E** and **F**); in these patients the arterial and venous branches of the shunt are connected to the arterial and venous lines of the extracorporeal circuit. In this access, the blood flow may be limited and possible occlusion of the branches may occur. This can be crucial not only for acute treatment, but also for later use with intermittent chronic techniques.

More and more venous-venous hemofiltration is utilized in the clinical routine with addition of a roller blood pump to the circuit. Continuous renal replacement therapy can be performed in this case with a double-lumen venous catheter, or a single-lumen venous catheter and a double-headed blood pump.

The use of the blood pump might partially reduce the advantages of the arteriovenous treatment in terms of vascular stability, no risk of air embolism, and self-limited ultrafiltration; on the other hand, it permits treatment of a patient with poor arteriovenous pressure gradient or with potential risks related to the arterial cannulation. While blood flows ranging from 50–120 ml/min are generally observed in arteriovenous-driven circulation for an average mean arterial pressure of 60–90 mm Hg, the blood flow in a pumped circuit can be adjusted at much higher values without any technical problem (118).

There has been much debate among different groups about the advantage of using one system over the other. If all requirements are met, we think that both approaches should be utilized depending on the patient's clinical conditions and re-

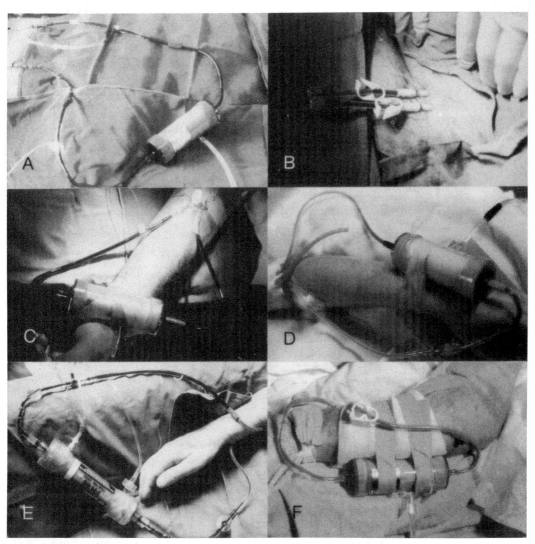

Figure 38.7. Vascular access in continuous arteriovenous hemofiltration: **A,** femoral artery and vein; **B,** femoral artery and vein (homolateral); **C,** brachial artery and cephalic vein; **D,** arteriovenous fistula; **E** and **F,** Scribner shunt.

quirements. The final decision must be made at the bedside, once all the pros and cons have been considered.

Extracorporeal Circuit

Various factors may affect blood flow rate and consequently ultrafiltration in continuous arteriovenous hemofiltration (178, 180). Five resistances are schematized in the blood circuit: arterial access; arterial line; hemofilter; venous line; and venous

access. Arterial and venous lines should be maintained as short as possible to avoid unnecessary pressure loss along the tubes (Fig. 38.8). Since low pressures are operating in the system, all the skills devoted to reduce the resistance of the circuit and to achieve its optimal performance must be undertaken in order to increase the efficiency. A reduction of the length of the arterial line would increase the hydrostatic blood pressure inside the filter. When the blood pump is utilized, these aspects lose

C.A.V.H. SYSTEM

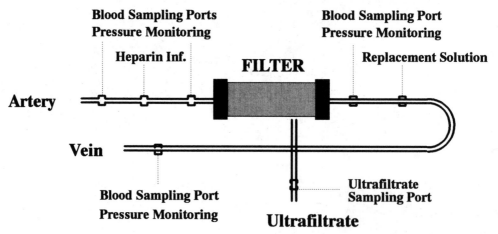

BASIC CONCEPT

Blood Flow in a Non-Pumped
Circulation strictly depends
on the A-V Pressure Gradient
and the Overall Resistance.

$$Qb = \frac{\pi r^4}{8 n l} \times \Delta P$$

TECHNICAL REQUIREMENTS

1) Short length (Low Resist.)
2) Adequate diameter
3) No kinking
4) Specific connections
5) Sampling ports
6) Pressure monitoring
7) Heparin and reinfusion

Blood Sampling Ports
Pressure Monitoring

Heparin Inf.

FILTER

Blood Sampling Port
Pressure Monitoring

Replacement Solution

Artery

Vein

Ultrafiltrate
Sampling Port

Blood Sampling Port
Pressure Monitoring

Ultrafiltrate

Figure 38.8. Detailed representation of the extracorporeal circuit for continuous arteriovenous hemofiltration (CAVH).

importance since a constant blood flow is mechanically guaranteed despite remarkable variations of the resistances in the extracorporeal circuit (Fig. 38.9).

Membranes, Ultrafiltration, and Clearances

Conventional hemodialysis membranes have insufficient hydraulic permeability to provide adequate fluid removal at the pressure available in continuous arteriovenous hemofiltration: hemodialysis membranes contain interdigitating pores of different sizes extending throughout the whole membrane thickness, resulting in a labyrinth of different diffusion distances. These membranes provide good removal of small molecules such as urea (mostly in the diffusion mode) in response to differ-

ent concentration gradients between blood and dialysate. As depicted in Figure 38.10, diffusion depends on several factors and membrane thickness is one of the most important. As the solute molecular weight increases, diffusion is no longer efficient both because of the low diffusion coefficients of medium-to-large molecules, and for the sieving effect of the membrane. Convection is essential for removing these solutes and more open membranes are required (174). In continuous arteriovenous hemofiltration (that represents a purely convective treatment), the membranes used have higher hydraulic permeability and the sieving coefficient for solutes is nearly 1 in a wide range of molecular weights, until values approach the cut-off of the membrane. These membranes are defined as asymmetric because they are

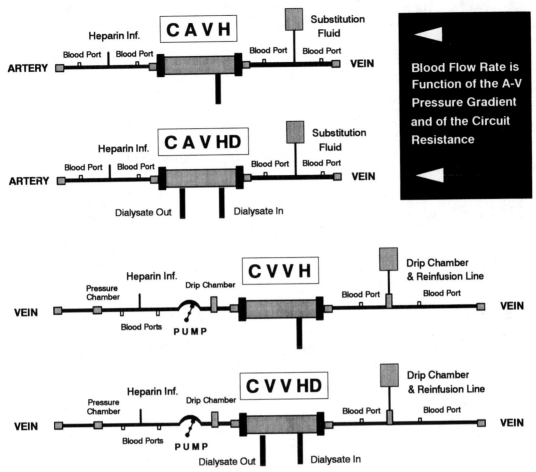

Figure 38.9. Typical circuits utilized for continuous arteriovenous hemofiltration *(CAVH)*, continuous arteriovenous hemodialysis *(CAVHD)*, continuous venovenous hemofiltration *(CVVH)*, and continuous venovenous hemodialysis *(CVVHD)*.

composite structures that present an inner skin layer with pores of the same size and length, and an external structure of macropores supporting only the mechanical integrity of the membrane. In these membranes, the solute is removed by ultrafiltration because of a solvent-drag phenomenon, and the permeability of the membrane governs the passage of the molecule (the Stavermann reflection coefficient is an intrinsic property of the membrane that leads to a certain observed sieving coefficient). In this way, if the solute is not restrained by the membrane, the ratio between the ultrafiltrate (UF) and plasma concentration (P) will be 1 and the clearance (C) will be entirely represented by the value of the ultrafiltration rate

$(C = Qf*[UF]/[P] = Qf*1 = Qf)$. The ultrafiltration rate (Qf) is proportional to the product between the permeability coefficient of the membrane and transmembrane pressure $(Kf \times TMP)$. Transmembrane pressure is calculated with the following formula:

$$TMP = Pb + Puf - \pi$$

where Pb is the hydrostatic pressure of blood, Puf is the negative pressure exerted by the ultrafiltrate column, and π is the oncotic pressure of blood. The simple hydrostatic pressure, Pb, would be insufficient to achieve significant amounts of filtration without the contribution of Puf. For this reason it is critical to place the ultrafiltrate collecting bag in the lowest position

SIZE DEPENDENT FREE DIFFUSION COEFFICIENTS
OF SOLUTES IN WATER AND VARIOUS MEMBRANES

$$J = D \, T \, A \, \delta c / \delta x$$

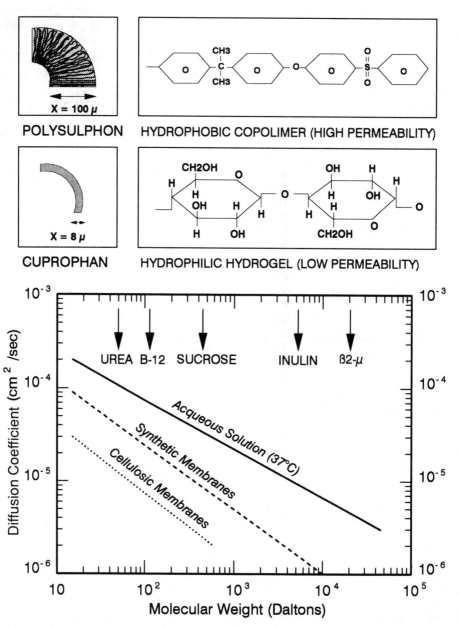

Figure 38.10. Chemical and physical structure of different membranes and solute diffusion in water and inside the membrane structure. As the molecular weight increases, diffusion decreases in all media. Although diffusion appears to be better in synthetic membranes than in cuprophan, the bigger thickness of the synthetic structure leads to a worse diffusion capacity.

C.A.V.H. SYSTEM

$$TMP = \frac{Pi + Po}{2} + Pf - \frac{\pi i + \pi o}{2}$$

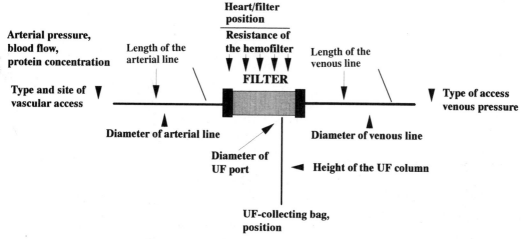

Heart/filter position

Arterial pressure, blood flow, protein concentration

Length of the arterial line

Resistance of the hemofilter

FILTER

Length of the venous line

Type and site of vascular access

Type of access venous pressure

Diameter of arterial line

Diameter of venous line

Diameter of UF port

Height of the UF column

UF-collecting bag, position

Figure 38.11. Factors affecting ultrafiltration rate in continuous arteriovenous hemofiltration. Ultrafiltration *(UF)* depends on membrane permeability and transmembrane pressure.

to maximize the ultrafiltrate flow rate. Additional suction, however, is not available because it may cause early clotting of the filter. In Figure 38.11 the factors affecting ultrafiltration rate in continuous arteriovenous hemofiltration are schematized.

In cases of treatment where diffusion and convection are used simultaneously, membranes with intermediate properties are utilized such as polyacrylonitrile or symmetric thinner Polysulphon. In this case, a compromise is achieved and solutes in a wide range of molecular weights can be removed.

Hemofilters

Continuous arteriovenous hemofiltration is a system operating under conditions of low blood flow, low regimen of pressures, and filtration pressure equilibrium (72, 161, 175, 180). These observations stress the importance of adapting the size and geometry of the hemofilter to the operational conditions. In a standard hemofilter, as the water is removed by ultrafiltration,

plasma proteins, hematocrit, and viscosity increase. The progressive decrease in hydrostatic pressure of the blood is accompanied by an increase in oncotic pressure generated by proteins; there may be a point inside the filter where ultrafiltration ceases because of the equivalence between hydrostatic and oncotic forces acting in opposite directions. Inside the filter, from this point the hemoconcentration increases the resistance to flow and therefore the risk of clotting. On the basis of these concepts, blood path geometry and design of the device have been improved (175). According to the Hagen-Poiseuille law, a shorter filter with a larger cross-sectional area should permit higher blood flows at a given arteriovenous pressure gradient and avoid filtration pressure equilibrium. The results achieved with such filters have confirmed this hypothesis and have permitted a significantly reduced heparin requirement with a longer filter life span (175). Another approach consisted of the development of new membranes with an increased inner diameter of the fibers (250 μ) that guarantees a lower resistance of the device and reduces the risk of clotting in the distal segment of the fibers (72). As an alternative, plate devices for continuous arteriovenous hemofiltration are also provided; despite the large housing of these hemofilters, the flat sheet geometry may represent a real advantage in reducing the heparin requirement during treatment (183).

Again, all these aspects may lose importance when a blood pump is added to the circuit and the extracorporeal blood flow is maintained independently on the patient's arterial pressure. On the other hand, since more and more frequently CAVHD and CVVHD are performed, all filters are now equipped with twin dialysate ports in order to permit the circulation of dialysis solution. Therefore, when highly permeable membranes are utilized, the devices should be more correctly defined as hemodiafilters instead of hemofilters. In Table 38.6 some characteristics of the commercially available filters for continuous therapies are provided. It may be noted that different membranes are employed and different surface areas and geometries are utilized. While larger devices (0.6 m^2) can be utilized for patients with stable arterial blood pressure or with a blood pump, shorter and smaller filters (0.2 m^2) with lower resistance can be very useful in patients with severe hypotension and presumably low extracorporeal blood flows. Such a policy allows for a longer filter life span with a lower heparin requirement and reduces the frequency of treatment failure for technical reasons (96, 184).

Efficiency and Quality of Treatment

The metabolic control of acute renal failure with continuous arteriovenous hemofiltration generally requires at least 15–20 liters of ultrafiltrate per day. When the classic technique cannot achieve such a result, predilution, suction, pump-assisted circulation, addition of diffusion, and other techniques can be used to maintain the

Table 38.6
Commercially Available Filters for Continuous Therapies

Company	Name	Membrane	Surface (m^2)	N of Fibers	Length (cm)	Fiber Radius (μ)
Amicon (Danvers, MA)	Diafilter 30	Polysulfon	0.60	4800	20.0	125
	Diafilter 20	Polysulfon	0.25	5000	12.7	125
	Diafilter 10	Polysulfon	0.20	6000	9.5	125
	Minifilter	Polysulfon	0.015		11.5	1100
	Minifilter Plus	Polysulfon	0.08		15.0	570
Asahi Medical (Tokyo, Japan)	Ultrafilter GS	Polyacrylonitrile	0.50	4300	19.0	100
Bellco (Mirandola, Italy)	BL 650	Polysulfon	0.20	5000	9.5	110
Fresenius (Oberursel, Germany)	AV-400	Polysulfon	0.70	4500	23.0	110
	AV-600	Polysulfon	1.35	9000	23.0	100
Gambro (Lund, Sweden)	FH 66	Polyamide	0.60	6000	18.0	100
	FH 22	Polyamide	0.15	3000	12.0	100
Hospal (Lyon, France)	Multiflow 60	AN 69S	0.60	6000	18.0	100
	PLATE	AN 69S	0.50		26.0	
Renal System (Minneapolis, MN)	HF500	Polysulfon	0.50	3000	22.0	140
	HF250	Polysulfon	0.25	3000	14.0	140
Sorin (Saluggia, Italy)	HFT 04	Polysulfon	0.45	6750	11.5	100
	HFT 02	Polysulfon	0.24	4600	9.5	100

CLEARANCE ENHANCEMENT

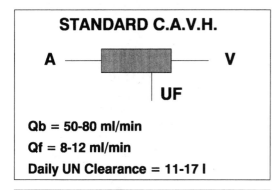

STANDARD C.A.V.H.

Qb = 50-80 ml/min

Qf = 8-12 ml/min

Daily UN Clearance = 11-17 l

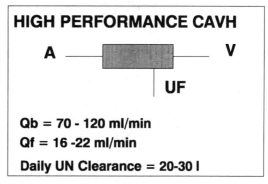

HIGH PERFORMANCE CAVH

Qb = 70 - 120 ml/min

Qf = 16 -22 ml/min

Daily UN Clearance = 20-30 l

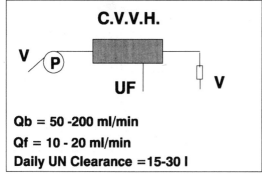

C.V.V.H.

Qb = 50 -200 ml/min

Qf = 10 - 20 ml/min

Daily UN Clearance =15-30 l

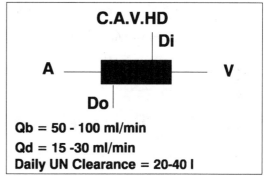

C.A.V.HD

Qb = 50 - 100 ml/min

Qd = 15 -30 ml/min

Daily UN Clearance = 20-40 l

Figure 38.12. Maximal urea clearance in different techniques.

BUN level of the patient under adequate control (Fig. 38.12) (65, 71, 92–95, 132, 133, 135, 181).

Continuous arteriovenous hemofiltration, as originally conceived, provides for a maximum of 17 liters for every 24 hours of ultrafiltrate with a pure convective transport (181).

Pure convection is also used with new highly performant continuous arteriovenous hemofiltration filters, but even a total daily clearance of 20–22 liters might sometimes not be enough. When a blood pump is utilized, the blood flow can easily be increased and an overall daily clearance of 30 liters can be achieved. In this case, however, large amounts of replacement solution must be reinfused to the patient and the fluid balance might become complicated. In recent years, several authors have described the possibility of using diffusion in addition to convection (64, 65, 160, 171, 181, 182) or diffusion alone (64) in the treatment of acute renal failure in the intensive care unit. In this case, satis-

factory clearances of small molecules are generally achieved by circulating small amounts of dialysis fluid in the ultrafiltrate compartment of the filter. In these treatments, however, the clearance of middle molecules might be remarkably low, either for the use of membrane with low hydraulic permeability or for a poor diffusion capacity of middle-sized molecules.

Therefore, if we consider that the patient in intensive care who suffers from acute renal failure complicated by sepsis, multiorgan dysfunction, and severe catabolism might produce a large amount of substances (chemical mediators, vasoactive substances, cytokines, etc.) in the middle molecular weight range (500–5,000 daltons), we can determine that an adequate treatment must achieve not only an optimized control of blood urea nitrogen levels, but also a satisfactory blood purification from other substances with higher molecular weight. In this case, a certain amount of convection is mandatory, which must be obtained with synthetic mem-

CONTINUOUS HIGH-FLUX DIALYSIS (VENO-VENOUS)
CHFD

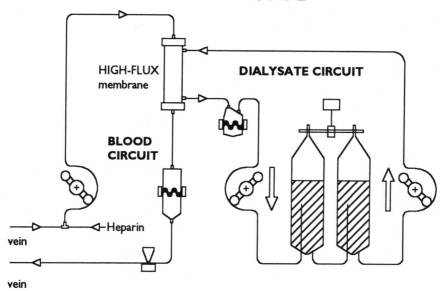

CONTINUOUS HIGH-FLUX DIALYSIS (ARTERIO-VENOUS)
CHFD

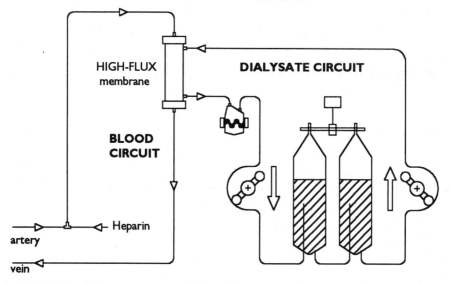

Figure 38.13. Schematic representation of the emergency care unit system for continuous high flux dialysis (CHFD). This high permeability of the hemodiafilter and the special manometric setting produce a typical pressure profile with a consequent filtration-backfiltration mechanism. In this case, fluid balance is controlled, and convection is preserved with an increased removal of larger solutes.

branes because of their higher sieving capacities.

To come up with a compromise and to meet the requirements of adequate amounts of convection and diffusion, reduced quantities of replacement solution, and easy monitoring, we have devised a new system called continuous high flux dialysis (Fig. 38.13) (174). The system consists of a circuit for continuous hemodialysis modified in order to achieve a continuous dialysate volume control. In this case, a 0.6 m^2 hemodiafilter with highly permeable membrane (Amicon D-30, Gambro FH66, Hospal Multiflow 60) is utilized and two roller pumps are applied to the dialysate circuit. Once the inlet dialysate flow has been set and provided by the first pump, the second pump applied to the dialysate outlet regulates the net ultrafiltration in response to a specific programming module. The system may operate in conditions of single pass or of dialysate recirculation.

In this system, once the patient's dry weight has been established by achieving a negative balance in the dialysate (outlet volume > inlet volume), the circuit operates at zero net filtration using a sterile dialysate at various flows 20–100 ml/min. As shown in Figure 38.14, both in the single pass condition and in the recirculation mode, the system may provide urea nitrogen clearances up to 30–40 liter every 2 hr.

This represents a very efficient blood purification, obtaining a daily clearance close to the whole area distribution space of the patient. In this case, the fractional clearance over total body water (K/V) approaches daily (t) the value of 1, which guarantees an adequate blood purification in the majority of patients. If performed continuously, the weekly Kt/V index may be in the range of 7, thus resulting in a treatment efficiency much higher than that achieved with other therapies (171, 174). On the other hand no replacement solution is utilized because the system permits operation in conditions of zero net filtration.

The clearances of larger molecules such as inulin is also satisfactory and may reach the value of 15–20 liters every 24 hr because of the special mechanism that op-

erates in the synthetic membrane. The high clearance for inulin in this case is not achieved because of diffusion, but primarily because of the convective transport that takes place in the proximal side of the filter. The zero net filtration is in fact achieved through a mechanism of proximal filtration and distal backfiltration. Therefore, inside the filter a hemodiafiltration-like process takes place wherein the ultrafiltrate is produced in the first half of the length of the fibers and the reinfusion is provided in the second half of the length of the fibers by a backfiltration of the sterile dialysate.

Figure 38.15 illustrates the mechanisms of urea and inulin removal in different treatment modalities. While CAVH or CVVH represent pure convective treatments and CAVHD-CVVHD are purely diffusive therapies, CAVHDF-CVVHDF (continuous hemodiafiltration) and CAVHFD-CVVHFD (continuous high-flux dialysis) represent a really mixed form of therapy. However, while in the hemodiafiltration setting, large amounts of replacement solution are required, in the high-flux dialysis the dialysate represents both the dialysis solution and the replacement fluid. There has been debate on the opportunity to use bicarbonate-containing dialysate instead of lactate- or acetate-containing dialysate. However, bicarbonate solutions must be freshly prepared and calcium must be added at the moment of use, creating some problems of fluid storage and purity. Since lactate can be safely utilized in the majority of patients with an adequate correction of the metabolic acidosis, we suggest the use of sterile bicarbonate dialysate only in those patients where lactate cannot be easily metabolized due to special clinical conditions. One should also monitor the "anion gap" to identify if acidosis is developing.

Treatment Monitoring and Automation

Different procedures have been proposed in the past to make the treatment of ARF simpler and easy to monitor. However, these devices or procedures have not always fulfilled the aim of simplifying the treatment and in some cases they have

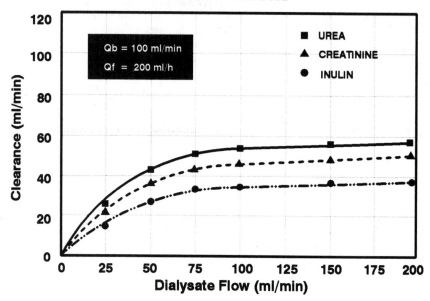

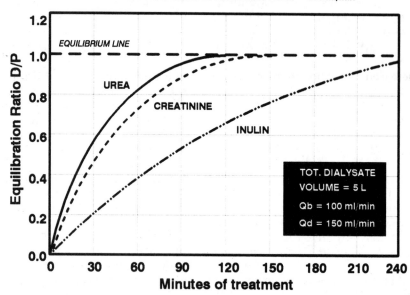

Figure 38.14. Solute clearances in continuous high flux dialysis versus dialysate flow in single-pass configuration. In the lower panel, the dialysate/plasma equilibration of various solutes is reported in recirculation configuration.

MECHANISMS OF SOLUTE REMOVAL IN ACUTE CONTINUOUS RENAL REPLACEMENT THERAPIES

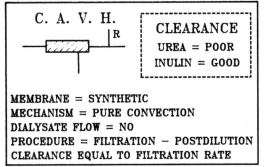

C. A. V. H.

CLEARANCE
UREA = POOR
INULIN = GOOD

MEMBRANE = SYNTHETIC
MECHANISM = PURE CONVECTION
DIALYSATE FLOW = NO
PROCEDURE = FILTRATION – POSTDILUTION
CLEARANCE EQUAL TO FILTRATION RATE

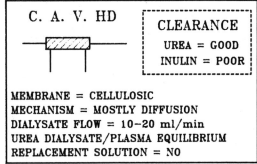

C. A. V. HD

CLEARANCE
UREA = GOOD
INULIN = POOR

MEMBRANE = CELLULOSIC
MECHANISM = MOSTLY DIFFUSION
DIALYSATE FLOW = 10–20 ml/min
UREA DIALYSATE/PLASMA EQUILIBRIUM
REPLACEMENT SOLUTION = NO

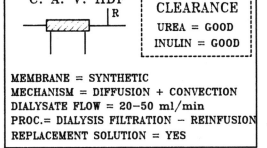

C. A. V. HDF

CLEARANCE
UREA = GOOD
INULIN = GOOD

MEMBRANE = SYNTHETIC
MECHANISM = DIFFUSION + CONVECTION
DIALYSATE FLOW = 20–50 ml/min
PROC.= DIALYSIS FILTRATION – REINFUSION
REPLACEMENT SOLUTION = YES

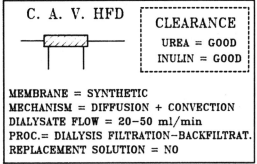

C. A. V. HFD

CLEARANCE
UREA = GOOD
INULIN = GOOD

MEMBRANE = SYNTHETIC
MECHANISM = DIFFUSION + CONVECTION
DIALYSATE FLOW = 20–50 ml/min
PROC.= DIALYSIS FILTRATION–BACKFILTRAT.
REPLACEMENT SOLUTION = NO

Figure 38.15. Mechanisms of action of the different continuous therapies.

even increased the labor intensity or the system complexity. For this reason a new generation of fluid-balancing systems has been developed (172). The Equaline balancing system created by Amicon to monitor and control the fluid balance in patients undergoing continuous therapies as CAVH or CAVHD offers some advantages in terms of simplicity. It can be carried at the bedside and works without a pump by gravity (Fig. 38.16). Other machines with volumetric ultrafiltration control systems have been provided both for the use in CAVHD and in CVVHD. A specifically oriented machine originally described by Graziani et al. (75) has been recently developed by Carex (Mirandola, Italy). The machine consists in a dialysate delivery system with an integrated ultrafiltration control apparatus. The system (continuous high flux dialysis) meets the requirements of simplicity and allows a reduction in the nurses' work load. The mechanism filtration-backfiltration can be easily regulated by the ultrafiltration control system, and

the final monitoring of the treatment becomes easy and safe. The system reproduces at different operative levels the technique of high flux dialysis recently developed for chronic patients (153). Other simple machines have been created by Hospal and Gambro groups. These simple machines consist essentially of simplified dialysate delivery systems with or without ultrafiltration control apparatus.

Anticoagulation

An effective anticoagulation can be achieved with a continuous heparin infusion during the treatment (120). The goal is the maximal anticoagulant effect inside the filter with minimal systemic effects. Patients with high hemorrhagic risk would have an advantage from a heparin-free treatment, or at least from a monitored administration of small amounts of heparin. The reduction of the heparin requirement during CAVH is strictly linked to specific procedures: (*a*) the filter must be washed before use with large quantities of heparinized

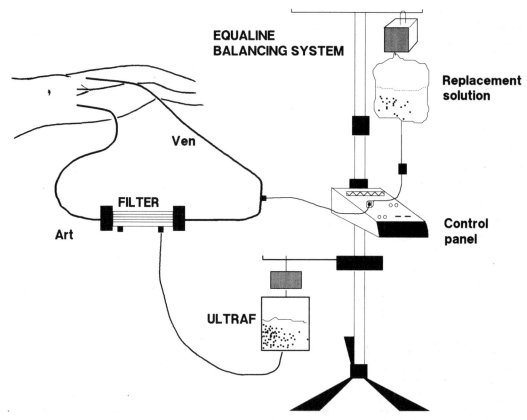

Figure 38.16. Equaline fluid balancing system. This equipment works only by gravity; no pumps are employed. The fluid balance and the programmed patient's weight balance is achieved through a continuous weight control operated on ultrafiltrate and the fluid reinfusion bag. The fluid reinfusion is fluid regulated by an electronically driven clamp.

saline solution. *(b)* The maximal blood flow allowed by the patient's blood pressure must be maintained by reducing all the unnecessary resistances of the circuit. *(c)* The optimal vascular access, blood lines, and filter geometry should be chosen to adapt the extracorporeal circuit to the patient's clinical and technical requirements. *(d)* The use of predilution when necessary (however, the fluid balance becomes more difficult). *(e)* Frequent lavages of the system by flushing the filter with saline solution. *(f)* The use of biocompatible membranes (84, 90, 136, 153, 164, 230, 231). An average infusion rate (a motor pump is recommended) of 300–600 iu/hr of heparin is the rule for safe continuous arteriovenous hemofiltration treatment. The continuous heparin infusion into the arterial line of the extracorporeal circuit offers the advantage of a certain self-regulation of the anticoagulative effect. In the case of

deceased extracorporeal flow rate, heparin concentration will increase in the extracorporeal circuit without increasing in the systemic circulation.

Some substances have also been used to coat the inner surface of the fibers in order to make them more biocompatible. The ultimate approach in reducing the risk of clotting in the fibers is the improvement of the blood path geometry of the filter in order to achieve higher blood flows and lower filtration fractions at a given arteriovenous gradient. Although the use of a blood pump can reduce the heparin requirement and may reduce the clotting of the fibers, it is a common finding that after 24 hr of use the permeability of the membrane becomes significantly reduced and the filter should be changed to avoid dangerous reductions in treatment efficiency. There are no clear demonstrations, therefore, that the venovenous pump-driven-circulation represents a real advantage in terms of filter survival. On the other hand, the arteriovenous-driven system may sometime become really cumbersome; the use of the blood pump simplifies the procedure and reduces the number of maneuvers at the bedside.

Reinfusion of Substitution Fluid

The quality of substitution fluid is based on the clinical requirements of the patient. The real improvement in recent years is seen in the use of large amounts of solutions for parenteral nutrition. An early institution of a well-balanced parenteral hyperalimentation guarantees improved clinical results because of a control of the patient's catabolism and urea nitrogen production. This leads to an amelioration of the treatment efficacy because of better metabolic control of BUN levels (113). Other specific advantages come from the manipulation of the extracellular fluid composition made possible by the continuous arteriovenous hemofiltration treatment (133). Among these, correction of metabolic acidosis and electrolyte derangements represent the most important applications for this therapy. It should be emphasized that some results obtained with convection and reinfusion of different substitution fluids cannot easily be achieved with other mixed diffusion-convective forms of therapy. The desired balance of electrolytes, buffers, and other substances can only be precisely regulated in the hemofiltration mode, reproducing the logic of the human kidney. In diffusion therapies, the balance of different substances and the shifts of solutes and water are less easily controlled, even though the final desired blood equilibration and purification can be achieved in most of the cases.

In the case of continuous high flux dialysis, the replacement solution is represented by the dialysate. Different substances could be added to the dialysate in order to meet the patient's clinical requirements.

Clinical Indications

The possible clinical indications for continuous renal replacement therapies are still

Table 38.7
Continuous Arteriovenous Hemofiltration Versus Intermittent Hemodialysis

Slow continuous therapy and fluid removal
Exclusively convective solute transport
High biocompatibility of the system
High sieving capacity of the membrane
High adsorbitive capacity of the membrane
Isotonic ultrafiltration
Good clinical tolerance and hemodynamic response
Possible manipulation of extracellular fluid composition with different substitution fluids
No rebounds in solute concentrations
Stability of the desired body hydration
Possibility of hyperalimentation

matters of discussion and controversy. The definition of continuous therapies as an alternative to standard hemodialysis appears, in our view, rather restricted. In Table 38.7 we list a series of points in which continuous hemofiltration differs from hemodialysis and we enumerate several interesting aspects of continuous therapies. Patients who are candidates to be treated with continuous therapies are entirely different from those who are generally treated in the nephrology department. Patients in intensive care are critically ill, present a series of medical and surgical complications, are severely unstable, and need a gentle and progressive renal replacement therapy (154).

From clinical experience, we are more and more inclined to propose these treatments even for patients with multiple organ failure, sepsis, and other conditions in which an early renal support, a possible removal of substances chemically active as mediators, and a real hemoequilibration might definitely help in the crucial phase of the syndrome. It is therefore still controversial whether we should start the treatment very early, when the patient is not yet oliguric, in an attempt to filtrate and adsorb special substances released in the circulation that may be responsible for bringing the patient in the "dangerous zone" of the multiple organ failure syndrome. On the other hand, as an invasive technique, it carries its own risks that must be carefully balanced against the possible benefits. At any rate, we should realize that the standard hemodialysis is not the tool we need in those patients and a specific form of renal replacement therapies should be used in those instances.

We will try to summarize, starting from the pathophysiology of the acute renal failure, some of the interesting aspects offered by the various continuous therapies in the treatment of the critically ill patient and the typical complications encountered.

Fluid Overload

Fluid overload is a common finding in critical patients; the typical condition is a wet lung with disturbed gas exchange and a hampered blood flow in the kidney circulation. The operational characteristics of continuous arteriovenous hemofiltration allow a continuous progressive fluid removal from the patient who generally responds well and avoids significant episodes of hypotension and hypoperfusion. Several factors have been proposed to explain the vascular stability during continuous arteriovenous hemofiltration (20, 38, 102, 112, 119, 130). These include the slow continuous ultrafiltration, plasma refilling due to the isosmotic composition of the ultrafiltrate, the stability of the renin-angiotensin system, and the stability of the extracellular osmolality.

In our opinion, the great advantage of continuous arteriovenous hemofiltration is that it dissociates the removal of sodium and water (30). In other words, it is possible, by changing the composition of the replacement solution, to remove sodium and water independently. For example, we can remove 2 liters of ultrafiltrate with sodium of 140 mEq/liters. In this case, the patient will have a net weight loss of 2 kg and a sodium loss of 280 mEq. In another patient, we can remove 10 liters of ultrafiltrate with sodium of 140 mEq/liters and reinfuse 8 liters of substitution fluid with sodium of 130 mEq/liters. In this case, the net weight loss of the patient will also be 2 kg but the sodium loss will be 360 mEq. This potential manipulation of the composition of body fluids may influence the hemodynamic response to fluid with-

Table 38.8
Factors Conditioning a Remarkable Vascular Stability During Continuous Hemofiltration

Continuity and graduality of the depurative treatment
Continuous slow removal of fluid
Iso-osmotic fluid removal and plasma refilling
Reduction of fluid shifts from the vascular space
Stability of the renin-angiotensin system
Maintenance of physiologic levels of dopamine β-hydroxylase
High biocompatibility with minimal or no interaction with blood
No side effects due to dialysate buffers (acetate)

drawal in continuous arteriovenous hemofiltration (Fig. 38.17). A good response to fluid withdrawal is achieved in continuous arteriovenous hemofiltration through an increase in the cardiac index in the presence of a reduction of peripheral vascular resistances. In Table 38.8 the factors potentially involved in the vascular stability achieved with continuous arteriovenous hemofiltration are summarized. Moreover, the stability of blood pressure is not the only clinical advantage of continuous therapies; further advantages are in the maintenance of constant body weight, solute concentration, and acid-base correction (Fig. 38.18). These facts make continuous hemofiltration (CAVH-CVVH) a first-choice treatment in patients with ARF associated with myocardial dysfunction and congestive heart failure, and allows an improvement of the cardiac function during therapy. In septic patients with low peripheral resistances and high cardiac output, the response can be different; studies on this topic are lacking.

Solute Removal

Despite its low depurative efficiency, continuous arteriovenous hemofiltration can be used successfully as an alternative treatment in patients with ARF who cannot be treated with other therapies because of medical or technical problems. When a severe catabolic state is present, several supporting procedures can be applied to improve the efficiency of the system in

EXAMPLE OF HEMODYNAMIC RESPONSE TO FLUID WITHDRAWAL IN C.A.V.H.

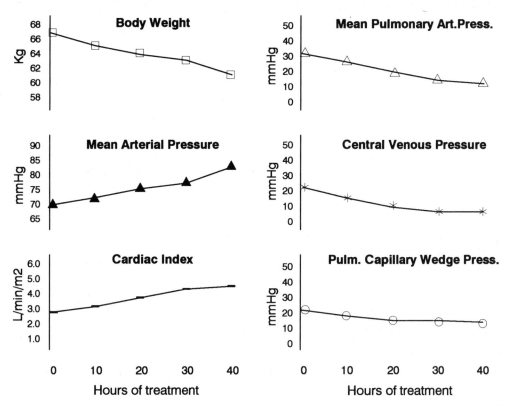

Figure 38.17. Hemodynamic response to fluid withdrawal in continuous arteriovenous hemofiltration.

removing waste products (67, 70, 195). The optimization of the extracorporeal treatment and its continuous performance added to an adequate hyperalimentation can contribute to a reduction of the protein catabolic rate and its effect on BUN concentration.

Although the new generation of hemofilters allows for ultrafiltration rates ranging between 10 and 28 ml/min, sometimes the patient's hypotension does not allow for blood flows adequate to achieve the best performance of the system, and the BUN level cannot be maintained under control. The pump-driven venovenous hemofiltration is independent from the spontaneous driving blood pressure and, thus, it proves to be much more efficient. The ultrafiltration rate can easily be in-

creased so that BUN always can be kept under control, even in high catabolic states. On the other hand, an increase in efficiency of the arteriovenous hemofiltration can be achieved by adding diffusion transport to the convective principle, using the combined method of CAVHD (66).

It should be noted, however, that some of the advantages typical of convective transport might be at least partially lost with continuous diffusion hemodialysis. We personally believe that the last described treatment, continuous high flux dialysis, should probably represent the optimal compromise between diffusion and convection and will probably become a more effective renal replacement therapy in intensive care (174). Solute concentration rebound, as that seen after intermit-

CONTINUOUS VS INTERMITTENT RENAL REPLACEMENT THERAPY
BIOCHEMICAL AND CLINICAL PROFILES

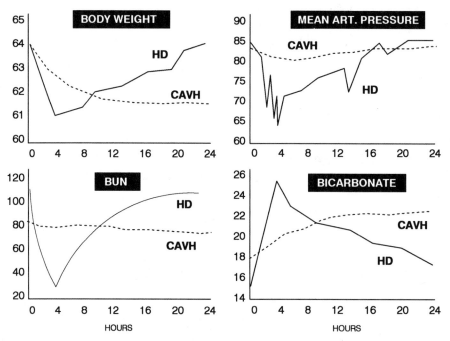

Figure 38.18. Example of biochemical and clinical profiles recorded in the same patients during intermittent and continuous treatment.

tent treatments is not observed in continuous therapies, which represent a major advantage in controlling BUN time average concentration. While in intermittent hemodialysis BUN concentrations suddenly fall after 1 hr of treatment and solute extraction becomes irrelevant showing a remarkable postdialytic rebound, BUN concentrations are steadily controlled with continuous therapies, and the average BUN concentration over time is lower (Fig. 38.18).

Electrolyte and Acid-Base Derangements

Continuous arteriovenous hemofiltration may be used to correct water and electrolyte imbalances by changing the composition of the substitution field. Hypohypernatremia can be corrected not only by achieving a normal plasma sodium concentration, but also by restoring the normal body sodium content. Hyperkalaemia can also be corrected with continuous ar-

teriovenous hemofiltration; the efficiency in removing potassium is directly related to the amount of fluid removed during the treatment and its replacement with potassium-free solutions. However, the efficiency of continuous arteriovenous hemofiltration to remove potassium is rather low and depends on the plasma potassium concentration. For example, if plasma potassium concentration is 6 mEq/liters, an ultrafiltration of 10 liters eliminates only 60 mEq of potassium.

Bicarbonate loss during continuous arteriovenous hemofiltration can easily be measured directly in the ultrafiltration or predicted by using the formula:

$$HCO_3(f) = UF \times HCO_3(s) \times 1.124$$

where $HCO_3(f)$ and $HCO_3(s)$ = bicarbonate concentration in the ultrafiltrate and in the serum, UF = total amount of ultrafiltrate, and 1.124 = average bicarbonate sieving coefficient.

When continuous arteriovenous hemofiltration is applied without fluid substitution in order to reduce the patient's fluid overload, bicarbonate losses are compensated by the reduction of the body volume distribution for the buffer, and the serum concentration does not change significantly. On the contrary, when replacement solutions are infused to maintain the body fluid balance, the same amount of bicarbonate lost in the ultrafiltrate must be administered to achieve stable serum levels of the buffer. Finally, when continuous arteriovenous hemofiltration is utilized to correct metabolic acidosis, the amount of HCO_3 in the replacement solution must exceed the amount lost in the ultrafiltrate, providing a positive balance of the buffer (167).

In continuous high flux dialysis the bicarbonate dialysate provides an adequate buffer balance, and smaller fluctuations of the acid-base status are usually observed.

Continuous Arteriovenous Hemofiltration in Newborns

A special indication for continuous arteriovenous hemofiltration is represented by the treatment of acute renal failure in newborns and small babies (177). The use of small hemofilters (minifilter) and special circuits allow for a safe renal replacement therapy in such small-sized patients.

Risks and Complications

Continuous therapy is generally well tolerated with a low rate of complications. The outcome is partially related to various factors including the severity of the illness and the presence of concomitant factors such as mechanical ventilation or artificial cardiovascular support. The number of organs involved in multiple organ failure syndrome appears to be criticial to the final outcome and the mortality rate. For example, in Table 38.9 we report a summary of the population with complicated ARF (only intensive care patients) treated at the Vicenza hospital since 1982. The rate of complication and the list of potential complications suggested by other authors are reported in Table 38.10.

As continuous hemofiltration is an in-

Table 38.9
Diagnosis and Outcome of the Treated Population

Diagnosis	Treated	Survived
Multiple organ failure	18	5
ARF polytrauma	25	15
ARF postsurgery	96	57
Hemorragic shock	12	7
Congestive heart failure	17	15
ARF in newborns	18	9
Miscellaneous	26	14
Total	212	122

Table 38.10
Complications of Continuous Therapies Recorded in a Total of 212 Patients

Complication	N	%
Bleeding	18	8.4
Hematoma	8	3.7
Access malfunction	1	0.4
Line disconnection	17	8.0
Frequent filter clotting	5	2.3
Treatment-induced hypotension	7	3.3
Cannulation site infection	2	0.9
Hypothermia	4	1.9
Hypophosphatemia	5	2.3
Vein thrombosis	1	0.4
Lactic acidosis	2	0.9
Fluid imbalance	4	1.9
Anaphylactic reaction		
Depletion		

vasive technique, certain typical risks have to be considered. The most severe complications are associated with the arterial access of the continuous arteriovenous hemofiltration procedure (111, 200). The venovenous access reduces the complication rate considerably.

Bleeding

Transcutaneous puncture and introduction of the large canula by the modified Seldinger technique may lead to bleeding and even vessel perforation. With careful technique and experience, this rarely happens. However, in the case of local atheriosclerosis, serious bleeding may occur by injury to the vessel wall and detachment of plaques. Therefore, in cases of suspected severe local artheriosclerosis, another access (preferably, e.g., venous) should definitely be used. During the course of hemofiltration, careful control of the anticoagulation (low-dose heparinization) reduces the risk of bleeding. However, at the end of the procedure, bleeding may result even from the removal of the arterial cannula. Careful and persistent compression is mandatory. If bleeding continues, the decision for surgical intervention should be made immediately. The infection of a large persistent hematoma may cause an abscess that is difficult to treat in this critical femoral region.

Thrombosis and Thromboemboli

Local thrombosis at the arterial cannula site occurs rather often (i.e., in about 10% of cases). Occasionally, this may critically restrain the perfusion of the leg; prompt surgical interference is mandatory if this happens. Therefore, frequent and regular control of perfusion (e.g., by Doppler sonography) is highly advisable. Local thrombosis becomes a considerable risk especially in severe arteriosclerosis.

Infections

Local infections at the cannula site (especially infected hematomas) are serious complications because this may threaten the arterial perfusion. Therefore, the extracorporeal circuit must be handled with extreme care by sterile handling, avoiding or reducing disconnections for blood sampling, avoiding bleeding and hematoma, etc.

Disconnection

At the high perfusion rate of the extracorporeal circuit (especially in continuous arteriovenous hemofiltration without monitoring), any accidental disconnection acutely threatens life. Therefore, always be sure that all connections are securely locked, that the whole circuit is freely visible (e.g., not covered by blankets), and that there is always continuous surveillance by a competent nurse. It is generally accepted that the risk for technical complications is inversely related to the competence and quality of nursing care.

Air Embolism

Air embolism in modern pump-driven systems is prevented by special monitoring and alarm mechanisms that are incorporated into the systems to immediately stop perfusion when air enters it. Except in cases of technical defects, this safety system excludes any air embolism. However, in the spontaneous continuous arteriovenous hemofiltration technique without any alarm systems, air embolism can indeed occur when there is a disconnection at the venous access and negative inspiratory pressures then suck air into the venous system.

Fluid Overload

Accidental fluid overload is a constant danger of the continuous hemofiltration technique, especially when a high fluid turnover is maintained. Meticulous monitoring and recording of fluid intake and output is mandatory. Everyone must be made aware of the danger of possible recording errors. Furthermore, the clinical condition of the patient must be watched closely and carefully.

Hypothermia

Hypothermia can occasionally occur when large amounts of ultrafiltrate are exchanged; a simple warming of substitution fluid may correct this inconvenience. On the other hand, continuous hemofiltration can be used effectively to reduce body temperature in case of hyperthermia.

Hypophosphatemia

Hypophosphatemia in patients undergoing continuous therapies has been reported and, as with other electrolytes or nutrients and drugs, solute imbalances can easily be avoided with frequent monitoring of the ultrafiltrate and plasma concentrations and adjustments in the replacement fluid composition.

Special Clinical Aspects

Treatment of Sepsis and Multiple Organ Failure

Acute renal failure cannot be effectively treated unless the underlying problems are solved. Sepsis seems to play the major role in the development of renal failure and multiple organ failure in critically ill patients. However, it is well known that sepsis may often be difficult to detect. This is particularly true for intraabdominal sepsis.

Source Control

Source control is an essential principle of therapy. If intraabdominal abscesses are suspected, modern imaging techniques such as ultrasonography, computerized tomographic scanning, and the like, may be helpful. However, surgical reexploration of the suspicious abdomen (repeated, if necessary) is the most effective measure. In the case of surgical infections, early, aggressive, and repeated surgical treatment (operative excision, drainage, and repeat laparotomy) still remain essential. In patients undergoing antibiotical therapy, blood cultures often remain negative. In such instances, only clinical alertness and careful examination may lead to early diagnosis or at least suspicion.

Antibiotic Therapy

For early and effective antibiotic treatment, it is important to identify the infecting pathogens accurately. Whenever possible, antibiotics should be selected only after microbiologically proven efficacy. Adequate dosage to achieve therapeutic concentrations is imperative. However, in reduced renal elimination correct dosage may be difficult to define. Guidelines for drug dosage are clearly more difficult to define during hemofiltration than in renal failure generally (190). The reason for this is that drug elimination not only depends on the impaired renal elimination but also on pharmacokinetic parameters such as plasma protein binding and the volume of drug distribution. These may indeed vary considerably in patients under hemofiltration.

The drug elimination rate by the ultrafiltration itself is governed by different variables (73). Theoretically, the simplest means to determine drug elimination rate would be to estimate drugs as a product of the sieving coefficient and filtration rate. However, these variables do not remain

constant during the hemofiltration process. Therefore, simple methods for calculating adequate drug dosages (115) may often be misleading. If exact drug monitoring in plasma (and in ultrafiltrate) is not available, creatinine clearance (mostly between 5 and 10 ml/min) will be the best landmark, combined with data from literature (17, 22). In the individual cases, drug elimination can only be exactly quantified retrospectively.

Both Gram-negative and Gram-positive organisms as well as yeasts can cause systemic infections with acute renal failure. However, until now, aerobic Gram-negative rod infections remained the major clinical and therapeutical problem, especially in immunocompromised patients. For the prevention of nosocomial Gram-negative rod infections, the new concept of intestinal gut decontamination (202) may be helpful. This has proved to be extremely effective in reducing nosocomial pneumonia in some studies (121, 145, 206, 218). However, the decrease of sepsis is less impressive and a significant reduction in mortality has only been demonstrated in a few studies (69, 121, 219). Thus, the final guarantee of effectiveness needs still further research.

Recently, monoclonal antibodies to act against endotoxin have been developed and these may improve therapy of Gram-negative sepsis (228). However, they are ineffective when the mediators cascade has already been activated. In these cases, monoclonal antibodies to act against tumor necrosis factor α have been successfully used in experimental models. Interleukin-1 receptor antagonists are under investigation as well to reduce the gravity of the septic syndrome.

Ventilatory Support

Respiratory failure can develop rapidly. Ventilatory support must be instituted early. Continuous positive airway pressure in spontaneous breathing or with some support (pressure support ventilation, intermittent mandatory ventilation) often is sufficient for oxygenation. In cases of respiratory pump failure, controlled mechanical ventilation with positive end-expiratory pressure may become necessary.

In severe respiratory failure, gas exchange may be improved considerably by inverting the inspiratory/expiratory time ratio (I/E ratio) (the so-called inversed ratio ventilation, IRV). However, heavy sedation and even muscle relaxation methods may still be necessary. Positive intrathoracic pressure during continuous positive airway pressure or ventilation with positive end expiratory pressure interferes with hemodynamics. Thus, low-dose catecholamines (1–4 Ig/kg/min dopamine infusion) may often be necessary to maintain adequate circulation.

Hemodynamics and Fluid Balance

Early shock treatment, especially with sufficient volume loading (crystalloids as well as colloids and blood), is mandatory for preventing renal failure. This is particularly true in polytrauma patients where effective emergency therapy (rescue systems, competent clinical interdisciplinary emergency treatment) have reduced complications and mortality significantly. However, during the later course of intensive care, especially in septic patients, a generalized capillary leak syndrome may have developed. Then, the lung competes with the kidneys for optimal fluid supply. Even a small degree of fluid overload will deteriorate pulmonary gas exchange. Therefore, a close and very careful fluid balance monitoring system is mandatory. The aim of this is to keep patients in fluid balance (or in a slightly negative balance).

Even a short-term fluid overload must be avoided. However, this does not mean "to dry the patient out," which leads to the development of prerenal oliguria and considerably increases the risks resulting from nephrotoxins. We tend to maintain an increased fluid turnover (excretion and delivery) by improving diuresis with catecholamines (dopamine) and diuretics (furosemide or mannitol or both). If this conservative treatment becomes ineffective, hemofiltration offers a valuable replacement therapy. In any case, the effects of forced diuresis or hemofiltration have to be monitored carefully by such methods as watching for changes in physical signs, pulmonary gas exchange, and chest x-ray.

Nevertheless, the diagnosis of an adequate fluid balance is extremely difficult in critically ill patients. It must be considered that even peripheral edema does not exclude a considerable deficit in blood volume. In the case of persistent unstable hemodynamics, the early administration of catecholamines and vasopressors (adrenaline or noradrenaline, depending on the systemic vascular resistance) is advisable in order to maintain renal perfusion.

Nutrition

Adequate nutritional support in patients with multiple organ failure is extremely important. However, even in severe sepsis, metabolic rates of more than 2500 kcal/day are uncommon. A number of metabolic disturbances have been associated with acute renal failure, although they may also be connected to the underlying diseases such as glucose intolerance, insulin resistance, impaired fatty acid metabolism, and increased protein degradation. There have been some promising studies on the positive effects of the administration of amino acids; however, in a review, Toback (211) concluded that amino acid treatment has not yet been shown to improve survival in severely ill patients. Thus, in severely ill patients on the ICU, it seems not necessary to modify the nutritional management considerably because of the acute renal failure. As a guideline, these patients may require about 30–40 nonprotein kcal/kg/day and 0.2–0.4 g kg/day of nitrogen, either from carbohydrate alone or combined with fat (not more than 20–30% of the daily calories). Nitrogen is administered in the form of conventional amino acid solutions (23).

OUTCOME OF ACUTE RENAL FAILURE

Isolated acute renal failure as the result of the insufficiency of a single organ (e.g., caused by nephrotoxins, infections, and other renal diseases) generally has a good prognosis. Mortality is considered to be below 10% (41). However, in critically ill patients ARF is usually part of a multiple organ failure arising during the hospital stay and the intensive care treatment, often

Table 38.11
Temporal Relation Between Clinical Onset of Sepsis and Onset of Organ Failure[a]

Organ System Failure	Average Number of Days Postoperatively
Onset of sepsis	2.4
Pulmonary failure	2.3
Hepatic failure	5.9
Stress bleeding	9.5
Renal failure	11.6

[a] From Fry DE, Pearlstein L, Fulton RL, Pohl HC Jr. Multiple system organ failure. The role of uncontrolled infection. Arch Surg 1980; 115:136.

following complicated surgery and connected to sepsis (Table 38.11). Here, mortality still remains extremely high, depending on the number of other failing organs. In these cases, mortality cannot be directly connected to the renal failure, but is rather the result of the multiple organ failure as a whole (62, 141). Coratelli et al. (44) found that sepsis is the major cause of death in up to 70% of patients with acute renal failure. Once the multiple organ failure syndrome is established, the respiratory and cardiovasculatory support and the development of coma, liver, and coagulation failure play a key role and renal failure becomes only one of many problems. Therefore, it seems rather pointless to assign the mortality to the acute renal failure alone.

Consequently, neither can the positive effects of the renal support therapies be exclusively compared and measured by mortality. The fact that mortality of ARF in critically ill patients could not be significantly improved has often been used as an argument against the continuous renal support therapies. However, this does not seem appropriate. For a true comparison we need reliable methods for comparing the severity of illness of the patients involved. Measuring the severity of illness, for instance, by APACHE II or III (103), simplified acute physiological score (122), mortality probability monitoring or organ systems failure may help to prove the effect of renal support therapies. But, even then, all measures of the intensive care treatment of the multiple organ failure will contribute to the final outcome. In a large

study of 5677 patients from an intensive care unit, including 2719 with well-defined organ system failure, the strong correlation between the number of failing organ systems and mortality was again demonstrated. A two-organ failure for more than 1 day increased the death rate to 60%; a three-organ failure for more than 3 days had a mortality of 92% (104). In a multidisciplinary study (26) involving 38 intensive care units, ARF was found in 685 (18.8%) of 3647 patients. Patients with ARF were older (67% were over age 50) than those without ARF (47% over age 50); mortality was higher in patients with ARF (44.9% versus 18.5%). The factors influencing poor prognosis were the severity of illness (increased simplified acute physiological score), poor previous health status, necessary mechanical ventilation, and the presence of oliguria.

Certainly, scoring systems are a necessary tool for measuring the severity of illness in controlled clinical trials. However, scores should not be used in making the decision of therapeutic interventions in individual patients. In individual cases, prediction of outcome cannot be made from the severity of illness alone. These indexes are not a substitute for experienced clinical judgment.

CONCLUSION

The use of the above-mentioned procedures renders CAVH and derived therapies reliable and efficient techniques for the treatment of patients with ARF. Some specific advantages such as simplicity, easy monitoring, and easy institution make this technique a first-choice treatment in several clinical conditions. For patients with severe cardiovascular instability, multiple organ failure, or polytraumatia, continuous therapies are today more than a simple alternative treatment to hemodialysis.

One of the main features of continuous renal replacement therapy is the flexibility of the utilized materials. Machines and devices can be utilized both for exclusively convective therapies and for treatments combining diffusion and convection without any complication. The circuit can be used with a blood pump or in arteriovenous-driven mode. The choice of the technique and materials will depend on the patient's clinical requirements, the hospital facilities, and the knowledge and training of the nursing staff. The institution of the above-described procedures and the use of new devices and materials will override the classic limits of low depurative efficiency or frequent clotting of the filters; continuous arteriovenous hemofiltration and related techniques will be used more in the treatment of critically ill patients in the future.

References

1. Abel RM. Acute renal failure, role of parenteral nutrition. Contemp Surg 1978;13:21.
2. Abel RM, Abbott WM, Beck CH Jr, et al. Essential L-amino acids for hyperalimentation in patient with disordered nitrogen metabolism. Am J Surg 1974;128:317.
3. Abel RM, Beck CH, Abbott WM, Ryan JA, Barnett GO, Fisher JE. Improved survival from acute renal failure after treatment with intravenous essential L-amino acids and glucose. Results of a prospective double-blind study. N Engl J Med 1973;288:695.
4. Alwall N. On the artificial kidney. I. Apparatus for dialysis of blood in vivo. Acta Med Scand 1947;128:317–321.
5. Anderson CC, Shahvari MBG, Zimmerman JE. The treatment of pulmonary edema in the absence of renal function—a role for sorbitol and furosemide. JAMA 1979;241:1008.
6. Arieff AI, Lazarowitz, VC, Guisado R. Experimental dialysis disequilibrium syndrome: prevention with glycerol. Kidney Int 1978;14:270.
7. Armstrong VW, Kandt M, Kstering H, Quellhorst E. Low molecular weight heparin in hemodialysis and hemofiltration patients. Kidney Int 1985;28:823.
8. Asbach HW, Stoeckel H, Schuler HW, et al. The treatment of hypercatabolic acute renal failure by adequate nutrition and haemodialysis. Acta Anaesthesiol Scand 1974;18:255.
9. Aurigemma NM, Feldman NT, Gottlieb M, Ingran RH, Lazarus JM, Lowrie EG. Arterial oxygenation during hemodialysis. N Engl J Med 1977;297:871.
10. Ayus JC, Oliviero JJ, Adrogue HJ. Alkalemia associated with renal failure. Arch Intern Med 1980;140:513.
11. Babb AL, Farrell PC, Uvelli DA, Scribner BH. Hemodialyzer evaluation by examination of solute molecular spectra. Trans Am Soc Artif Intern Organs 1972;18:98–105.
12. Babb AL, Strand MJ, Uvelli DA, Milutinovich J, Scribner BH. Quantitative description of dialysis treatment: a dialysis index. Kidney Int 1975;7(suppl 2):23–28.
13. Baek SM, Makabali GG, Bryan-Brown CW, et al. The influence of parenteral nutrition on the course of acute renal failure. Surg Gynecol Obstet 1975;141:405.
14. Bailey RR, Natale R, Turnbull DI, Linton AL. Protective effect of furosemide in acute tubular necrosis and acute renal failure. Clin Sci Mol Med 1973;45:1.
15. Bartlett R, Bosch JP, Paganini EA, Geronemus R, Ronco C. Continuous arterio-venous hemofiltration. Trans Am Soc Artif Intern Organs 1987;38:345.
16. Beall AC Jr, Hall CW, Morris GC Jr, DeBakey ME. Mannitol induced osmotic diuresis during vascular surgery. Arch Surg 1963;86:34.
17. Bennett WM. Guide to drug dosage in renal failure. Clin Pharm 1988;15:326.
18. Bergstrm J. Ultrafiltration without dialysis for removal of fluid and solutes in uremia. Clin Nephrol 1978;9:156–161.
19. Bergstrm J, Asaba H, Frst P, Oules R. Dialysis, ultrafiltration, and blood pressure. Proc Eur Dialysis Trans Assoc 1976;13:293.
20. Berman LB, Smith LL, Chisolm GD, Weston RE. Mannitol and renal function in cardiovascular surgery. Ann Surg 1964;88:239.
21. Berman LB, Vogelsang P. Removal rates for barbiturates using two types of peritoneal dialysis. N Engl J Med 1964;270:77.
22. Bickley SK. Drug dosing during continuous arteriovenous hemofiltration. Clin Pharm 1988;7:198.
23. Bihari DJ. The prevention of severe combined acute respiratory and renal failure in the intensive therapy unit. In: Bihari D, Neild G, eds. Acute renal failure in the intensive therapy unit. Heidelberg: Springer-Verlag 1990:359.
24. Bland R, Shoemaker WC, Shabot MM. Physiologic monitoring goals for the critically ill patient. Surg Gynecol Obstet 1978;147:833.
25. Bluemle LW Jr, Potter HP, Elkinton JR. Changes in body composition in acute renal failure. J Clin Invest 1951;35:1094.
26. Bobrie G, Patois E. Facteurs prognostiques de l'insuffisance renale aigue en réanimation multidisciplinaire [Abstract]. Ran Soins Intens Med Urg (Paris) 1987;3:284.
27. Bomar JB, Decherd JF, Hlavinka DJ, Moncrief JW, Popovich RP. The elucidation of maximum efficiency—minimum cost peritoneal dialysis protocols. Trans Am Soc Artif Intern Organs 1974;20:120.
28. Boquin E, Parnell S, Grondin G, et al. Crossover study of the effects of different dialysate sodium concentrations in large surface area, short-term dialysis. Proc Clin Dial Transplant Forum 1977;7:48.
29. Borah MF, Schoenfeld PY, Gotch FA, et al. Nitrogen balance during intermittent dialysis therapy of uremia. Kidney Int 1978;14:491.
30. Bosch JP, Ronco C. Continuous arterio venous hemofiltration. In: Maher JF, ed. Replacement of renal function by dialysis. Dordrecht: Kluwer Academic Publishers, 1989;15:347.
31. Bosch JP, von Albertini B, Ronco C. Hemofiltration and hemodiafiltration. In: Glassock RJ, ed. Current therapy in nephrology and hypertension. Toronto: BC Decker Inc, 1987:258–263.
32. Brenner BM, Meyer TW, Hostetter TH. Dietary protein intake and the progressive nature of kidney disease. The role of hemodynamically me-

diated injury in the pathogenesis of progressive glomerular sclerosis in aging, renal ablation and intrinsic renal disease. N Engl J Med 1982;307:652.

33. Brooks MH, Barry KG. Removal of iodinated material by peritoneal dialysis. Nephron 1973;12:10.

34. Brown R, Babcock R, Tablert J, Gruenberg J, Czurak C, Campbell M. Renal function in critically ill postoperative patients: sequential assessment of creatinine, osmolar and free water clearance. Crit Care Med 1980;8:68.

35. Brezis M, Rosen S, Silva P, Epstein FH. Selective vulnerability of the medullary thick ascending limb to anoxia in the isolated perfused rat kidney. J Clin Invest 1984;73:182.

36. Brezis M, Rosen S, Spokes K, Silva P, Epstein FH. Transport-dependent anoxic cells injury in the isolated perfused rat kidney. Am J Pathol 1984;116:327–341.

37. Bullock ML, Umen AJ, Finkelstein M, Keane WF. The assessment of risk factors in 462 patients with acute renal failure. Am J Kidney Dis 1985;5:97.

38. Burchardi H. Die kontinuierliche arterio-vense Hemofiltration (CAVH). Intensivmed Notfallmed Ansthes 1987;62:51.

39. Bush HL, Huse JB, Johnson WC, O'Hara ET, Nabseth DC. Prevention of renal insufficiency after abdominal aortic aneurysm resection by optimal volume loading. Arch Surg 1981;116:1517–1524.

40. Cairns KB, Porter GA, Kloster FE, Bristow JD, Griswold HE. Clinical and hemodynamic results of peritoneal dialysis for severe cardiac failure. Am Heart J 1968;76:227.

41. Cameron JS. Acute renal failure in the intensive care unit today. Intensive Care Med 1986;12:64.

42. Cameron JS, Ogg C, Trounce JR. Peritoneal dialysis in hypercatabolic acute renal failure. Lancet 1967;1:1118.

43. Cerra FB. Hypermetabolism, organ failure, and metabolic support. Surgery 1987;1:1.

44. Coratelli P, Passaranti G, Giannattasio M, Amerio A. Acute renal failure after septic shock. Adv Exp Med Biol 1987;212:233.

45. Corwin HL, Teplick RS, Schreibner MJ, Fang LST, Bonventre JV, Coggings CH. Prediction of outcome in acute renal failure. Am J Nephrol 1987;7:8.

46. Craddock PR, Fehr J, Daimasso AP, Brigham KL, Jacob HS. Haemodialysis leukopenia: pulmonary vascular leukostasis resulting from complement activation by dialyzer cellophane membranes. J Clin Invest 1977;59:879.

47. Davin TD, Lynch RE, Hodson EH, Simmons RL, Najarian JS, Kjellstrand CM. Fistulization of shunt vasculature: a unique approach to fistula development. Br J Med 1977;2:933.

48. Davis RF, Lappas DG, Kirklin JK, Buckley MJ, Lowenstein E. Acute oliguria after cardio-pulmonary bypass: renal improvement with low dose dopamine infusion. Crit Care Med 1982;10:852.

49. Dionigi R, Zonta A, Dominoni L, Gnes F, Ballabio A. The effects of total parenteral nutrition on immunodepression due to malnutrition. Ann Surg 1977;185:467.

50. El-Nachef, Rashed F, Ricanati ES. Occlusion of the subclavian vein: a complication of indwelling subclavian venous catheters for hemodialysis. Clin Nephrol 1985;24:42.

51. Etheredge EE, Levitin H, Nakamura K, Glenn WW. Effect of mannitol on renal function during open heart surgery. Ann Surg 1965;161:53.

52. Ewing DJ, Winney R. Autonomic function in patients with chronic renal failure on intermittent haemodialysis. Nephron 1975;15:424.

53. Exaire E, Trevino-Becerra A, Monteon F. An overview of treatment with peritoneal dialysis in drug poisoning. Contr Nephrol 1979;17:39.

54. Fabris A, La Greca G, Chiaramonte S, et al. Total solute extraction versus clearance in the evaluation of standard and shot hemodialysis. Trans Am Soc Artif Intern Organs 1988;34:627.

55. Farrell PC, Ward RA, Schindhelm K, Gotch FA. Precise anticoagulation for routine hemodialysis. J Lab Clin Med 1978;92:164.

56. Feinstein EI, Blumenkranz MJ, Healy M, et al. Clinical and metabolic responses to parenteral nutrition in acute renal failure. Medicine (Baltimore) 1981;60:124.

57. Feriani M, Biasioli S, Borin D, et al. Bicarbonate buffer for CAPD solution. Trans Am Soc Artif Intern Organs 1985;31:668.

58. Fink M. Are diuretic useful in the treatment or prevention of acute renal failure? South Med J 1982;75:329.

59. Fischer RP, Griffin WO, Resiser M, Clark DS. Early dialysis in the treatment of acute renal failure. Trans Am Soc Artif Intern Organs 1964;10:200–206.

60. Flessner MF, Dedrick RL, Schultz JS. A distributed model of peritoneal-plasma transport: theoretical considerations. Am J Physiol 1984;246:R597.

61. Freud H, Harmian S, Fischer JE. Comparative studies of parenteral nutrition in renal failure using essential and non-essential amino acid containing solutions. Surg Gynecol Ostet 1980;151:652.

62. Fry DE, Pearlstein L, Fulton RL, Pohl HC Jr. Multiple system organ failure. The role of uncontrolled infection. Arch Surg 1980;115:136.

63. Gerhardt RE, Abdulla AM, Mach SJ, Hudson JB. Isolated ultrafiltration in the treatment of fluid overload in cardiogenic shock. Arch Intern Med 1979;139:358.

64. Geronemus R, Schneider N. Continuous arteriovenous hemodialysis. In: Paganini E, Geronemus R, eds. Proceedings of the Third International Symposium on Acute Continuous Renal Replacement Therapy. Ft. Lauderdale, 1987:77.

65. Geronemus R, Schneider N. Continuous arteriovenous hemodialysis: a new modality for treatment of acute renal failure. Trans Am Soc Artif Intern Organs 1984;30:610–613.

66. Geronemus RP, Schneider NS, Epstein M. Survival in patients treated with continuous arteriovenous hemodialysis for acute renal failure and chronic renal failure. Contrib Nephrol 1991;93:29–31.

67. Geronemus R, von Albertini B, Glabman S, Lysaght M, Kahn T, Bosch JP. Enhanced molecular clearance in hemofiltration. Proc Clin Dial Transplant Forum 1978;8:147.

68. Gillum DM, Dixon BS, Yanover MJ, et al. The role of intensive dialysis in acute renal failure. Clin Nephrol 1986;5:249.

69. Godard J, Guillaume C, Reverdy ME, et al. Intestinam decontamination in a polyvalent ICU. A doubleblind study. Intensive Care Med 1990;16:307.

70. Golper TA. Continuous arteriovenous hemofiltration in acute renal failure. Am J Kidney Dis 1985;6:373.

71. Golper TA, Kaplan AA, Narasimhan N, Leone M. Transmembrane pressures generated by filtrate line suction maneuvers and predilution fluid replacement during in vitro continuous arteriovenous hemofiltration. Int J Artif Organs 1987;10:41–46.

72. Golper TA, Roncom C, Kaplan AA: Continuous arteriovenous hemofiltration: improvements, modifications and future directions. Semin Dialysis 1988;1:50–54.

73. Golper TA, Wedel SK, Kaplan AA, Saad AM, Donta ST, Paganini EP. Drug removal during continuous arteriovenous hemofiltration: theory and clinical observations. Int J Artif Organs 1985;8:307.

74. Gotch FA, Sargent JA. A mechanistic analysis of the National Cooperative Dialysis Study. Kidney Int 1989;28:526.

75. Graziani G, Casati S, Ponticelli C. CAVH e CAVHD nel paziente acuto ipercatabolico. Nefrologia Dialisi e Trapianto 1986;31:235.

76. Hall JW, Johnson WJ, Maher FT, Hunt JC. Immediate and long-term prognosis in acute renal failure. Ann Intern Med 1970;73:515–521.

77. Hayes DM, Cvitkovic E, Golbey RB, et al. High dose cisplatinum diammine dichloride. Amelioration of renal toxicity by mannitol diuresis. Cancer 1977;39:1372.

78. Henderson IS, Beattie TJ, Kennedy AC. Dopamine hydrochloride in oliguric states. Lancet 1980;2:827.

79. Henderson LW. Peritoneal ultrafiltration dialysis: enhanced urea transfer using hypertonic dialysis fluid. J Clin Invest 1966;49:950.

80. Henderson LW. Biophysics of ultrafiltration and hemofiltration. In: Maher JF, ed. Replacement of renal function by dialysis. A textbook of dialysis. 3rd ed. Dozdrecht: Kluwer Academic Publishers, 1989:300–326.

81. Henderson LW, Besarab A, Michaels A, Bluemle LW Jr. Blood purification by ultrafiltration and fluid replacement (diafiltration). Trans Am Soc Artif Intern Organs 1967;17:216–221.

82. Henderson LW, Colton CK, Ford C. Kinetics of haemodiafiltration. II Clinical characterization of a new blood cleansing modality. J Lab Clin Med 1975;85:372–375.

83. Hilberman M, Derby G, Spencer RJ, Stinson EB. Effect of the intra aortic balloon pump upon postoperative renal function in man. Crit Car Med 1981;9:85.

84. Hirsch J, Ofosu F, Buchanan M. Rationale behind the development of low molecular weight heparin derivates. Semin Thromb Hemost 1985;11:13.

85. Hoenich NA, Levett D, Fawcett S, Woffindin C, Kerr DNS. Biocompatibility of haemodialysis membrane. J Biomed Eng 1986;8:3.

86. Holliday RL, Doris PJ. Monitoring the critically ill surgical patient. Can Med Assoc J 1979;121:931.

87. Indrapasit S, Taramas W, Panparde O. Complete dialysate drainage: an unnecessary step in intermittent peritoneal dialysis. Peritoneal Dial Bull 1985;5:233.

88. Ing TS, Ashbach DL, Kanter A, Oyama JH, Armbruster KFW, Merkel FK. Fluid removal with negative-pressure hydrostatic ultrafiltration using a partial vaccum. Nephron 1975;14:451.

89. Ivanovich P, Xu CG, Kwaan HC, Hathiwala S. Studies of coagulation and platelet functions I, heparin-free hemodialysis. Nephron 1983;33:116.

90. Josefowicz M, Josefowicz J. New approaches to anticoagulation with heparin-like biomaterials. Am Soc Artif Intern Organs J 1985;8:218.

91. Kanter A, Nadler N, Vertel RM, Pollak VE. Peritoneal dialysis: indications and technique in the surgical patient. Surg Clin North Am 1968;48:47.

92. Kaplan AA. The effect of predilution during continuous arterio-venous hemofiltration [Abstract]. Am Soc Nephrol 1984:66A.

93. Kaplan AA. Predilution vs postdilution for continuous arteriovenous hemofiltration. Trans Am Soc Artif Intern Organs 1985;31:28–31.

94. Kaplan AA. Clinical trials with predilution and vacuum suction: enhancing the efficiency of the CAVH treatment. Trans Am Soc Artif Intern Organs 1986;32:49–51.

95. Kaplan AA, Longnecker RE, Folkert VW. Suction assisted continuous arterio-venous hemofiltration. Trans Am Soc Artif Intern Organs, 1983;29:408–412.

96. Kaplan A, Longnecker RE, Folkert VW: Continuous arteriovenous hemofiltration. Ann Intern Med 1984;100:358–364.

97. Kaptein EM, Levitan K, Feinstein EI, Nicoloff JT, Massry SG. Alterations of thyroid hormone indices in acute renal failure and in acute illness with and without acute renal failure. Am J Nephrol 1981;1:138–143.

98. Keshaviah P, Ilstrup K, Costantini E, Berkseth R, Shapiro F. The influence of ultrafiltration and diffusion on cardiovascular parameters. Trans Am Soc Artif Intern Organs 1980;26:328.

99. Kjellstrand CM. Ethacrynic acid in acute tubular necrosis. Indications and effect on the natural course. Nephron 1972;9:337.

100. Kjellstrand CM, Rosa AA, Shidemann JR. Hypotension during hemodialysis: osmolality fall is an important pathogenic factor. Am Soc Artif Intern Organs J 1980;3:11.

101. Kleinknecht D, Jungers P, Channard J, Barbanel C, Ganeval D. Uremic and non-uremic complications in acute renal failure: evaluation of early and frequent dialysis on prognosis. Kidney Int 1972;1:190–196.

102. Knaus WA, Draper EA, Wagner DP, et al. APACHE II—A severity of disease classification. Crit Care Med 1985;13:818.

103. Knaus WA, Draper EA, Wagner DP, Zimmerman JE. Prognosis in acute organ-system failure. Ann Surg 1985;202:685.

104. Knaus WA, Zimmerman JE. Prediction of outcome from critical illness. In: Ledingham IMA, ed. Recent advances in critical care medicine. 3rd ed. Edinburgh: Churchill Livingstone, 1988:1.

105. Knochel J. Biochemical, electrolyte and acid-base disturbances in acute renal failure. In: Brenner BM, Lazarus JM, eds. Acute renal failure. Philadelphia: WB Saunders Co, 1983:568–585.

106. Kohen JA, Opsahl JA, Kjellstrand CM. Deceptive patterns of uremic pulmonary edema. Am J Kidney Dis 1986;7:456.

107. Kokor F, Kuska J. The endocrine system in patients with acute renal insufficiency. Kidney Int 1976;10:526–531.

108. Kolff WJ. First clinical experience with the artificial kidney. Ann Intern Med 1965;62:608–612.

109. Korchik WP, Brown DC, DeMaster EG. Hemodialysis induced hypotension. Int J Artif Organs 1978;1:151.

110. Kornhall S. Acute renal failure in surgical disease with special regard to neglected complications. Acta Chir Scand 1971;419:3.

111. Kramer P. Limitations and pitfalls of continuous arteriovenous hemofiltration. In: Kramer P, ed. Arteriovenous hemofiltration. Heidelberg: Springer Verlag, 1985:206.

112. Kramer P, Bhler J, Kehr A, et al. Intensive care potential of continuous arteriovenous hemodialysis. Trans Am Soc Artif Intern Organs 1982;28:28–32.

113. Kramer P, Schrader J, Bohnsack W, Grieben G, Grone HJ, Scheler F. Continuous arteriovenous hemofiltration: a new kidney replacement therapy. Proc Eur Dialysis Trans Assoc 1981;18:743.

114. Kramer P, Wigger W, Rieger J, Matthaei D, Scheler F. Arteriovenous hemofiltration: a new and simple method for treatment of overhydrated patients resistant to diuretics. Klin Wschr 1977;55:1121.

115. Kroh U, Hofmann W, Dehne M, El Abed K, Lennartz H. Dosisanpassung von Pharmaka whrend kontinuierlicher Hemofiltration. Anaesthesist 1989;38:225.

116. La Greca G, Dettori P, Blasioli S, et al. Brain density changes during hemodialysis. Lancet 1980;2:582.

117. La Greca G, Dettori P, Biasioli S, et al. Study on morphological and densitometrical changes in the brain after hemodialysis and peritoneal dialysis. Trans Am Soc Artif Intern Organs 1981;27:40–44.

118. La Greca G, Fabris A, Ronco C. CAVH Proceedings of the International Symposium on Continuous Arteriovenous Hemofiltration. Vicenza 1986. Milano: Wichtig editor, 1986.

119. Lauer A, Alvis R, Beal A, Avram M. Hemodynamic consequences of continuous arteriovenous hemofiltration in intractable fluid overload [Abstract]. Kidney Int 1986;29:218.

120. Lauer A, Saccaggi A, Ronco C, et al. Continuous arteriovenous hemofiltration in the critically ill patient. Ann Intern Med 1983;99:455–460.

121. Ledingham IMcA, Alcock SR, Eastaway AT, McDonald JC, McKay IC, Ramsay G. Triple regimen of selective decontamination of the digestive tract, systemic cefotaxime, and microbiological surveillance for prevention of acquired infection in intensive care. Lancet 1988;1:785.

122. Le Gall JR, Loirat P, Alperovitch A, et al. A simplified acute physiology score for ICU patients. Crit Care Med 1984;12:975.

123. Lemeshow S, Teres D, Avrunin JS, et al. Refining intensive care unit outcome prediction by using changing probabilities of mortality. Crit Care Med 1988;16:470.

124. Leonard CD, Luke RG, Siegel RR. Parenteral essential amino acids in acute renal failure. Urology 1975;6:154.

125. Leunissen KML, Hoorntje SJ, Fiers HA, Dekkers WT, Mulder AW. Acetate versus bicarbonate hemodialysis in critically ill patients. Nephron 1986;42:146.

126. Levitan D, Moser S, Goldstein DA, Kletzky O, Massry SG. Disturbances in the function of the hypothalamicpituitary gonadal (H-P-G) axis during acute renal failure. Kidney Int 1981;19:131.

127. Lien J, Chan V. Risk factors influencing survival in acute renal failure treated by hemodialysis. Arch Intern Med 1985;145:2067.

128. Lindner A. Synergism of dopamine and furosemide in diuretic-resistant, oliguric acute renal failure. Nephron 1983;33:121.

129. Lindner A, Cutler RE, Goodman WG. Synergism of dopamine plus furosemide in preventing acute renal failure in the dog. Kidney Int 1979;16:158.

130. Little RA, Campbell IT, Green CJ, Kishen R, Waldek S. Nutritional support in acute renal failure in the critically ill. In: Bihari D, Neild G, eds. Acute renal failure in the intensive therapy unit. Heidelberg: Springer Verlag, 1990:347.

131. Lucas CE, Ledgerwood AM, Shier MR, Bradley VE. The renal factor in the post-traumatic 'fluid overload' syndrome. J Trauma 1977;17:667.

132. Lysaght MJ. Hemodialysis membranes in transition. Contribution to nephrology. Basel: Karger Verlag, 1988;61:1–17.

133. Lysaght MJ, Boggs D. Transport in continuous arteriovenous hemofiltration and slow continuous ultrafiltration, In: Paganini E, ed. Acute continuous renal replacement therapy. Boston: Martinus-Nijhof, 1986;43–50.

134. Lysaght MJ, Schmidt B, Gurland HJ. Mass transfer in arteriovenous hemofiltration. In: Kramer P, ed. Arteriovenous hemofiltration. Berlin: Springer-Verlag, 1985:3–13.

135. Maher JF, Chakrabarti E. Ultrafiltration by hyperosmotic peritoneal dialysis fluid excludes intracellular solutes. Am J Nephrol 1984;4:169.

136. Maher JF, Lapierre L, Schreiner GE, Geoger M, Westervelt FB. Regional heparinization for hemodialysis. N Engl J Med 1963;268:451.

137. Maher JF, Schreiner GE. Cause of death in acute renal failure. Arch Intern Med 1962;110:493.

138. Maher JF, Schreiner GE, Waters TJ. Successful intermittent haemodialysis—longest reported maintenance of life in true oliguria (181 days). Trans Am Soc Artif Intern Organs 1960;6:123–126.

139. Mailloux LU, Swartz CD, Onesti G, Heider C,

Ramirez O, Brest AN. Peritoneal dialysis for refractory congestive heart failure. JAMA 1967;199:873.

140. Mann HJ, Fuhs DW, Hemstrom CA. Acute renal failure. Drug Intell Clin Pharm 1986;20:421.

141. Manship L, McMillin RD, Brown JJ. The influence of sepsis and multisystem organ failure on mortality in the surgical intensive care unit. Am J Surg 1984;50:94.

142. Maseda J, Hilberman M, Derby G, Spencer RJ, Stinson EB, Myers BD. The renal effects of sodium nitroprusside in postoperative cardiac surgical patients. Anesthesiology 1981;54:284.

143. Mault JR, Dechert RE, Bartlett RH, Swartz RD, Ferguson SK. Oxygen consumption during hemodialysis for acute renal failure. Trans Am Soc Artif Intern Organs 1982;28:510.

144. Maxwell MH, Rockney RE, Kleeman CR, Twiss MR. Peritoneal dialysis. I. Technique and application. JAMA 1959;170:917.

145. McClelland, Murray AE, Williams PS, Saene HKF van, et al. Reducing sepsis in severe combined acute renal and respiratory failure by selective decontamination of the digestive tract. Crit Care Med 1990;18:935.

146. Minuth AN, Terrell JB, Suki WN. Acute renal failure: a study of the course and prognosis of 104 patients and of the role of furosemide. Am J Med Sci 1976;271:317.

147. Mondon CE, Dokas CB, Reaven GM. The site of insulin resistance in acute uremia. Diabetes 1978;27:571–576.

148. Montoreano R, Cunarro J, Mouzet MT, Ruiz-Guinazu A. Prevention of the initial oliguria of acute renal failure by administration of furosemide. Postgrad Med J 1971;47(suppl):7.

149. Mullen JL, Buzby GP, Matthews DC, Smale BF, Rosato EF. Reduction of operative morbidity and mortality by combined preoperative and postoperative nutritional support. Ann Surg 1980;192:604.

150. Nolph KD, Rosenfield PS, Powell JT, Danforth E Jr. Peritoneal glucose transport and hyperglycemia during peritoneal dialysis. Am J Med Sci 1970;259:272.

151. Nordstrom H, Lennquist S, Lindell B, Sjberg HE. Hypophosphataemia in severe burns. Acta Chir Scand 1977;143:395.

152. Oken DE, Sprinkel FM, Kirschbaum BB, Landwehr DM. Amino acid therapy in the treatment of experimental acute renal failure in the rat. Kidney Int 1980;17:14.

153. Olbricht CJ, Hebel U, Frei U, Koch KM. High performance CAVH without pumps, suction and predilution. Blood Purif 1986;4:222.

154. Olbricht C, Mueller C, Schurek HJ. Treatment of acute renal failure in patients with multiple organ failure by continuous spontaneous hemofiltration. Trans Am Soc Artif Intern Organs 1982;28:33–37.

155. Olbricht CJ, Schurek HJ, Stolte H, Koch KM. The influence of vascular access modes on the efficiency of CAVH. In: Sieberth HG, Mann H, eds. Continuous arteriovenous hemofiltration. Basel: Karger, 1985:14–24.

156. Olbricht CJ, Schurek HJ, Tytul S, Muller C, Stolte H. Comparison between Scribner shunt and femoral catheters as vascular access for continuous arteriovenous hemofiltration. In: Kramer P, ed. Arteriovenous hemofiltration. Berlin: Springer Verlag, 1985:57–66.

157. Olivero JJ, Lozano-Mendez J, Ghafary EM, et al. Mitigation of amphotericin B nephrotoxicity by mannitol. Br J Med 1975;1:550.

158. Oreopoulos DG, Helfrich GB, Khanna R, et al. Peritoneal catheters and exit-site practices. Perit Dial Bull 1987;7:130.

159. Paganini EP. Acute continuous renal replacement therapy. Boston: Martinus Nijhoff, 1986.

160. Paganini EP, Fouad F, Tarazi RC, Bravo EL, Nakamoto S. Hemodynamics of isolated ultrafiltration in chronic hemodialysis patients. Trans Am Soc Artif Intern Organs 1979;25:422–425.

161. Pallone TL, Peterson J. Continuous arteriovenous hemofiltration, an in vivo simulation. Trans Am Soc Artif Intern Organs 1987;33:304–308.

162. Parsons FM, Hobson SM, Blagg CR, et al. Optimum time for dialysis in acute reversible renal failure. Lancet 1961;1:129–134.

163. Pierides AM, Kurts SB, Johnson WJ. Ultrafiltration followed by hemodialysis. A longterm trial and acute studies. J Dial 1978;2:325.

164. Pinnick RV, Wiegmann TB, Diederich DA. Regional citrate anticoagulation for hemodialysis in patients at high risk for bleeding. N Engl J Med 1983;308:258.

165. Posen GA, Luiselto J. Continuous equilibration peritoneal dialysis in the treatment of acute and chronic renal failure. Proc Clin Dial Transplant Forum 1979;9:50.

166. Radtke HW, Claussener A, Erbes PM, Scheuermann EH, Schoeppe W, Koch KM. Serum erythropoietin concentration in chronic renal failure: relationship to degree of anemia and excretory renal function. Blood 1979;54:877.

167. Raimondi F, Bianchi T, Emmi V. Use of continuous arteriovenous hemofiltration (CAVH) in lactic acidosis: A case report. In: La Greca G, Fabris A, Ronco C, eds. CAVH. Milan: Wichtig Editore, 1986:135.

168. Rasmussen HH, Pitt EA, Ibels LS, McNeil DR. Prediction of outcome in acute renal failure by discriminant analysis of clinical variables. Arch Intern Med 1985;145:2015.

169. Rodrigo R, Shideman J, McHugh R, Buselmeier T, Kjellstrand CM. Osmolality changes during hemodialysis. Natural history, clinical correlations, and influence of dialysate glucose and intravenous mannitol. Ann Intern Med 1977;86:554.

170. Ron D, Traitelman U, Michaelson M, et al. Prevention of acute renal failure in traumatic rhabdomyolysis. Arch Intern Med 1984;144:277–280.

171. Ronco C. Arterio-venous hemodiafiltration (AVHDF): a possible way to increase urea removal during CAVH. Int J Artif Organs 1985;8:61–62.

172. Ronco C. Continuous arterio-venous hemofiltration: optimization of technical procedures and

new directions. In: Horl WH, Schollmeyer P, eds. New perspectives in hemodialysis, peritoneal dialysis, arteriovenous hemofiltration and plasmapheresis. New York: Plenum Press, 1989:167.

173. Ronco C. Backfiltration in clinical dialysis: nature of the phenomenon, mechanisms and possible solutions. Int J Artif Organs 1990;13:11–21.

174. Ronco C. Continuous renal replacement therapies in intensive care patients. Clin Nephrol 1992 (in press).

175. Ronco C, Bosch JP, Lew S, et al. Technical and clinical evaluation of a new hemofilter for CAVH; theoretical concepts and practical applications of a different blood flow geometry. In: La Greca G, Fabris A, Ronco C, eds. Proceedings of the International Symposium on CAVH, Vicenza 1986. Milan: Wichtig Editor, 1986:55.

176. Ronco C, Bragantini L, Brendolan A, et al. Arteriovenous hemofiltration (AVHDF) combined with continuous arteriovenous hemofiltration (CAVH). Trans Am Soc Artif Intern Organs 1985;31:349.

177. Ronco C, Brendolan A, Borin D, et al. Continuous arteriovenous hemofiltration in newborns. In: Continuous arteriovenous hemofiltration. Sieberth H, Mann H, eds. Basel: Karger, 1984:76–79.

178. Ronco C, Brendolan A, Bragantini L, et al. Self limited dehydration during CAVH. Blood Purif 1984;2:88.

179. Ronco C, Brendolan A Bragantini L, et al. Continuous arterio-venou hemofiltration. Contrib Nephrol 1985;48:70–78.

180. Ronco C, Brendolan A, Bragantini L, et al. Studies on blood flow dynamic and ultrafiltration kinetics during continuous arteriovenous hemofiltration. Blood Purif 1986;4:220.

181. Ronco C, Brendolan A, Bragantini L, et al. Arteriovenous hemodiafiltration associated with continuous arteriovenous hemofiltration. A combined therapy in the hypercatabolic patient. In: La Greca G, Fabris A, Ronco C, eds. Proceedings of the International Symposium on Continuous Arteriovenous Hemofiltration, Venice 1986. Milan: Wichtig Editor, 1986:171–183.

182. Ronco C, Brendolan A, Bragantini L, et al. Solute and water transport during continuous arterio-venous hemofiltration. Int J Artif Organs 1987;10:179–184.

183. Ronco C, Brendolan A, Bragantini L, et al. Continuous arteriovenous hemofiltration with AN69S membrane; procedures and experience. Kidney Int 1988;33(suppl 24):150–153.

184. Ronco C, Brendolan A, Bragantini L, et al. Technical and clinical evaluation of a new polyamide hollow fiber hemofilter for CAVH. Int J Artif Organs 1988;11:33–38.

185. Ronco C, Fabris A, Chiaramonte S, et al. Comparison of four different short dialysis techniques. Int J Artif Organs 1988;3:169–174.

186. Rosa RM, Brown RS. Acute renal failure associated with heavy metals and organic solvents.

In: Brenner BM, Lazarus JM, eds. Acute renal failure. Philadelphia: WB Saunders Co, 1983:321–332.

187. Rowley KM, Clubb KS, Walker Smith GJ, Cabin HS. Right-sided infective endocarditis as a consequence of flow-directed pulmonary-artery catheterization. N Engl J Med 1984;311:1152.

188. Rozsival V, Bastecka D, Fixa P, Kozak J, Herout V. Long-term experience with the technique of subclavian and femoral vein cannulation in hemodialysis. Artif Organs 1979; 3:241.

189. Rumack BH, Meredith TJ, Peterson RG, Prescott LF, Vale JA. Management acetaminophen overdose. Arch Intern Med 1981;141:401–403.

190. Rumpf KW, Kramer P. Drug dosage in patients on continuous arteriovenous hemofiltration. In: Kramer P, ed. A arteriovenous hemofiltration. Heidelberg: Springer Verlag, 1985:158–163.

191. Sargent JA, Gotch FA. Nutrition and treatment of the acutely ill patient using urea kinetics. Dial Transplant 1981;10:314.

192. Schrimshaw NS. An analysis of past and present recommended dietary allowances for protein in health and disease. N Engl J Med 1976;294:136.

193. Scribner BH, Giordano C, Oreopoulos DG, et al. Long term peritoneal dialysis. Proc Eur Dialysis Trans Assoc 1975;12:131.

194. Sherertz RJ, Falk RJ, Huffman KA, Thoman CA, Mattern WD. Infections associated with subclavian Uldall catheters. Arch Intern Med 1983;143:52.

195. Sigler M, Teehan BP. Solute transport in slow continuous arteriovenous hemodialysis: an improved method for treating acute renal failure. Proceedings of the Third International Symposium on Acute Continuous Renal Replacement Therapy. Fort Lauderdale, FL:1987;3:78.

196. Silverstein ME, Ford CA, Lysaght MT, Henderson LW. Treatment of severe fluid overload by ultrafiltration. N Engl J Med 1974;291:747.

197. Simkin EP, Wright FK. Perforating injuries of the bowel complicating peritoneal catheter insertion. Lancet 1968;1:64.

198. Singh S, Wadhwa N. Peritonitis, pancreatitis, and infected pseudocyst in a continuous ambulatory peritoneal dialysis patient. Am J Kidney Dis 1987;9:84.

199. Stokes JB, Averon J. Prevention of organ damage in massive ethyleneglycol ingestion. JAMA 1980;243:2065.

200. Stokke T, Kettler D. Komplikationen der kontinuierlichen arteriovensen Hmofiltration. Anaesthesist 1985;34:528.

201. Stone WJ, Knepshield JH. Post-traumatic acute renal insufficiency in Vietnam. Clin Nephrol 1974;2:186.

202. Stoutenbeek CP, Saene HKF van, Miranda DR, Zandstra DF. The effect of selective decontamination of the digestive tract on colonization and infection rate in multiple trauma patients. Intensive Care Med 1984;10:185.

203. Sumpio BE, Chaudry IH, Baue AE. Reduction of the drug-induced nephrotoxicity by ATP-MgC12. 1. Effects on the cis-diamminedichlo-

roplatinum-treated isolated perfused kidneys. J Surg Res 1985;38:429.

204. Swartz RD, Port FK. Preventing hemorrhage in high-risk hemodialysis regional versus low-dose heparin. Kidney Int 1979;16:513.

205. Swartz RD, Valk TW, Brain AJP, Hsu CH. Complications of hemodialysis and peritoneal dialysis in acute renal failure. Am Soc Artif Intern Organs J 1980;3:98.

206. Sydow M, Burchardi H, Crozier TA, Rchel R, Busse C, Seyde WC. Einfluß der selektiven Dekontamination auf nosokomiale Infektionen, Erregerspektrum und Antibiotikaresistenz bei langzeitbeatmeten Intensivpatienten. Ansth Intensivther Notfallmed 1990;25:416.

207. Taenaka O, Shimada Y, Hirata T, Nishijima A, Yoshiya I. New approach to regional anticoagulation in hemodialysis using gabexate mesilate (FOY). Crit Care Med 1982;10:773.

208. Talley RC, Forland M, Beller B. Reversal of acute renal failure with a combination of intravenous dopamine and diuretics. Clin Res 1970;18:518.

209. Teschan PE, Baxter CR, O'Brian TE, et al. Prophylactic haemodialysis in the treatment of acute renal failure. Ann Intern Med 1960;53:992–1016.

210. Toback FG. Amino acid enhancement of renal regeneration after acute tubular necrosis. Kidney Int 1977;12:193.

211. Toback FG. Amino acid treatment of acute renal failure, In: Brenner BM, Stein JH, eds. Acute renal failure. Contemporary issues in nephrology. Vol 6. Edinburgh: Churchill Livingstone, 1985:202–213.

212. Toback FG, Teegarden DE, Havener LJ. Amino acid-mediated stimulation of renal phospholipid biosynthesis after acute tubular necrosis. Kidney Int 1979;15:542.

213. Tolhurst Cleaver CL, Hopkins AD, Kee Kwong KG NG, Rafiery AT. The effect of postoperative peritoneal lavage on survival, peritoneal wound healing and adhesion formation following fecal peritonitis: an experimental study in the rat. Br J Surg 1974;61:601.

214. Trevino-Becerra A, Munoz P, Avilez C, Maimone MAS, Lopez MLE. Equilibrium peritoneal dialysis in acute renal failure secondary to rhabdomyolysis. Perit Dial Bull 1987;7:244.

215. Turney JH, Williams LC, Fewell MR, Parsons V, Weston MJ. Platelet protection and heparin sparing with prostacyclin during regular dialysis therapy. Lancet 1980;2:219.

216. Tzamaloukas AH, Garella S, Chazan JA. Peritoneal dialysis for acute renal failure after major abdominal surgery. Arch Surg 1973;106:639.

217. Ufferman RC, Jaenike JR, Freeman RB, Pabico RC. Effect of furosemide on low-dose mercuric chloride acute renal failure in the rat. Kidney Int 1975;8:362.

218. Unertl K, Ruckdeschel G, Selbmann HK, et al. Prevention of colonization and respiratory infections in long-term ventilated patients by local antimicrobial prophylaxis. Intensive Care Med 1987;13:106.

219. Ulrich C, Harinck-de Weerd JE, Bakker NC, Jacz K, Doornbos L, de Ridder VA. Selective decontamination of the digestive tract with norfloxacin in the prevention of ICU-acquired infections: a prognostive randomized study. Intensive Care Med 1989;15:424.

220. Vas SI. Peritonitis. In: Nolph KD, ed. Peritoneal dialysis. 2nd ed. Boston: Martinus Nijhoff, 1985:411.

221. Wagner DP, Knaus WA, Draper EA. Physiologic abnormalities and outcome from acute disease. Arch Intern Med 1986;146:1389.

222. Wall AJ. Peritoneal dialysis in the treatment of severe acute pancreatitis. Med J Austr 1965;52:481.

223. Wathen R, Keshaviah P, Hommeyer P, Cadwell K, Comty C. Role of dialysate glucose in preventing gluconeogenesis during hemodialysis. Trans Am Soc Artif Intern Organs 1977;23:393.

224. Wehle B, Asaba H, Castenfors J, et al. The influence of dialysis fluid composition on the blood pressure response during dialysis. Clin Nephrol 1978;12:62.

225. Weinrauch LA, Healy RW, Leland OS Jr, et al. Decreased insulin requirement in acute renal failure in diabetic nephropathy. Arch Intern Med 1978;138:399.

226. Wesson DE, Mitch WE, Wilmore DW. Nutritional considerations in the treatment of acute renal failure. In: Brenner BM, Lazarus JM, eds. Acute renal failure. Philadelphia: WB Saunders, 1983:618–642.

227. Winchester JF, Gelfand MC, Knepshield JH, Shreiner GE. Dialysis and hemoperfusion of poison and drugs—update. Trans Am Soc Artif Intern Organs 1977;23:762.

228. Ziegler EJ, Fisher CJ, Sprung CL, Straube RC, et al. Treatment of Gram-negative bacteremia and septic shock with Ha-1A human monoclonal antibody against endotoxin. A randomized, double-blind, placebo-controlled trial. N Engl J Med 1991; 324:429.

229. Zimmerman JE. Respiratory failure complicating post-traumatic acute renal failure: etiology, clinical features and management. Ann Surg 1971;174:12.

230. Zobel G, Trop M, Muntean W, Ring E, Gleispach H. Anticoagulation for continuous arteriovenous hemofiltration in children. Blood Purif 1988;6:90–95.

231. Zusman RM, Rubin RH, Cato A. Hemodialysis using prostacyclin instead of heparin as the sole antithrombotic agent. N Engl J Med 1981;304:934.

39

Acute Complications in Patients with Chronic Renal Failure

Hans G. Sieberth
Helmut Mann
Horst Kierdorf

CLINICAL PICTURE OF END-STAGE RENAL FAILURE

Azotemia is generally understood as a rise in plasma concentrations of the substances usually eliminated with the urine, while the term uremia covers the multitude of clinical manifestations in the stage of decompensated renal failure.

"In the entire discipline of medicine there is no systemic disease, which shows such a variety of symptoms as the disease of the uropoietic system of the kidneys" (13).

Symptoms and results in Vollhard's detailed description date from a time before the availability of dialysis treatment and kidney transplantation, and are familiar to only a very few physicians today, just as the complete picture of uremia can be seen today only if patients are admitted too late or if uremic complications occur in chronically intermittent dialysis treatment. For this reason, the physician must still be familiar with the clinical picture. Table 39.1 gives the principal signs and participating organs as well as important diagnostic and therapeutic measures.

This chapter will describe those diseases relevant to intensive care that have come about during the past few years in the course of dialysis treatment and kidney transplantation. To begin with, the basic principles, which also lead to the uremic manifestations, will be discussed. Following this, organic disorders caused by uremia as well as hematologic changes and sepsis, and finally complications due to dialysis treatment and kidney transplantation will be discussed.

BASIC PROBLEMS IN UREMIA

Azotemia

With progressing renal insufficiency, an increase in a multitude of retention values of substances in the serum is observed, of which urea and creatinine are the most important indicators for implementation of the daily routine. As the glomerular filtrate decreases, the retention values rise exponentially; i.e., in the final stage, a minor reduction of the clearance leads to a considerable increase of the retention values. An increase in protein intake as well as in catabolism (aggression syndrome after trauma or surgery, serious infections, the appplication of glucocorticosteroids or tetracycline) leads to an additional increase of the retention values (3).

The elimination of drugs is equally reduced with increasing renal insufficiency. If the pharmacokinetics of certain substances are disregarded, the clinical picture is frequently superimposed by drug intoxication, which may at times be difficult to distinguish from the uremic symptoms. The therapeutic measures to influence uremia have been compiled in Tables 39.1–39.3 and overall therapy for specific problems summarized in Table 39.4 later on.

Hypervolemia

In the final stage of renal insufficiency and, even more often, in dialysis patients, hypervolemia occurs either because of incorrect infusions or through excessive drinking due to imperative thirst. Depend-

Table 39.1
Clinical Picture of End-Stage Renal Failure

Organ	Diagnosis	Symptoms and Signs	Laboratory Findings	X-ray and ECG	Causes	Prophylaxis	Therapy
Lungs	Fluid lung	Physical examination of lungs within normal limits	Hypoxemia	Perihilar shadows	Uremia, unadapted fluid intake	Proper fluid balance	Fluid removal, ultrafiltration, vasodilation
	Pulmonary edema	Crepitations	Hypoxemia	Clouding of peripheral lung fields	Left heart failure, hypertension, fluid overload	Proper fluid balance, control of hypertension, digitalis, ACE-blocker	Fluid removal, control of hypertension, digitalis, hyperbaric ventilation
	Pneumonia	Localized physical findings	Hypoxemia, leukocytosis fever	Infiltrations	Pulmonary edema, immunosuppression infection	Prophylaxis of infections	Appropriate dose of antibiotics
Circulatory system	Hypotension, collapse, shock	Tachycardia, hypotension	Low venous pressure	Elevation of CPK, LDH, SGPT, evidence of infarction in ECG, see etiology in case of myocardial infarction	Hypovolemia, bleeding, loss of fluids, hyponatremia, hyperkalemia, hypokalemia, acidosis, myocardial infarction	Proper fluid and electrolyte balance, replenishment of blood volume, management of acidosis, adequate dialysis	Volume and electrolyte substitution, management of shock and underlying disease
	Hypertension	Tachycardia, hypertension	Elevated venous pressure, hypernatremia	Enlargement of heart size, shadow	Fluid overload, hypernatremia, renal artery stenosis, disequilibrium syndrome	Control of fluid status, proper electrolyte balance, normal saline	Antihypertensive therapy, dehydration, restriction of sodium intake
Heart	Heart failure	Bradycardia, tachycardia, shortness of breath	Elevated venous pressure, low cardiac output	Widened cardiac shadow, ST-segment depression in hyperkalemia pseudonormal T, echocardiography, reduced cardiac contraction	Fluid overload, hyperkalemia, acidosis, azotemia, hypertension	Fluid and electrolyte balance, careful digitalization in view of altered pharmacokinetics	Removal of fluid overload, vasodilation, digitoxin

Rhythm disturbance	Irregular pulse rate	Electrolyte disturbance, esp. potassium	Beginning of extrasystoles of varying origin	Preceeding potassium, compartimentation, disturbance (acidosis), digitalis, overdosage	Control of acidosis, normalization of potassium, evaluate the dose of digitalis	Bicarbonate in acidosis and hyperkalemia, administration of Ca^{2+}, and Na^+, ion exchange, in digitalis overdosage potassium administration, phenytoin, hemodialysis
Pericarditis	Friction rub over sternum and lingula	Azotemia, signs of inadequate dialysis	No typical radiologic findings, echo: pericardial and effusion	Azotemia, inadequate dialysis	Adequate dialysis	Daily dialysis, careful heparinization in view of hemorrhagic pericardial effusion
Pericardial effusion	Muffled heart sounds, obstruction to venous return, pulsus paradoxus	Azotemia, inadequate dialysis	Often cannot be differentiated from cardiac dilatation, echocardiography, computer tomography	Pericarditis, uremic bleeding, heparinization	Adequate dialysis	Daily dialysis, occasionally in hemorrhagic effusion, pericardiocentesis, pericardial window or pericardectomy may be required
Gastrointestinal tract						
Diarrhea	Water or mucous stools	Low potassium, hypotension, observe bacteriologic findings of stool cultures	Signs of electrolyte disturbance	Viral bacterial, azetomia, antibiotics, pseudomembraneous colitis (*C. difficile*)	Adequate dialysis	Symptomatic: loperamide charcoal or silicid acid, selected antibiotic administration with paromomycin, neomycin sulfate, vancomycin orally
Peritonitis, paralytic ileus	Tender, distended abdomen, rarely fever	In periotoneal dialysis, turbid dialysate with many leukocytes	Multiple fluid levels	Underlying disease, azotemia, peritoneal dialysis, endogenous toxins	In toxic states, intestinal disinfection (Gut sterilization), in ileus do not begin peritoneal dialysis; danger of perforation	Antibiotics, prostigmine and panthenol, when peritonitis occurs during chronic ambulatory peritoneal dialysis further dialysis with antibiotics
Bleeding	Circulatory collapse and shock, coffeeground emesis, melena, hematozechia	Fall in hematocrit or hemoglobin	Gastroscopy, angiography with contrast material	Shock, artificial ventilation, azotemia, heparinization, impaired thrombocyte function	Antacids, adequate dialysis	Antacids (hemostyptics), blood transfusion, peritoneal dialysis, when hemodialysis cannot be avoided low heparin or prostacyclin analogs

Table 39.1 (*continued*)

Organ	Diagnosis	Symptoms and Signs	Laboratory Findings	X-ray and ECG	Causes	Prophylaxis	Therapy
Central nervous system	Brain edema	Headache, muscular twitchings, photophobia, meningismus, disorientation, convulsions, coma, papilledema	Minimal changes in CSF, increased CSF pressure	Cranium normal, CT: evidence of brain edema	Fluid overload, azotemia-induced permeability disturbance, hypoxia, hypernatremia, hypertension, sudden decrease in sodium concentration	Fluid and electrolyte balance, slow correction of hypernatremia, disequilibrium, control of hypertension	Dehydration through furosemide, not to use osmotically acting substances in view of elimination disturbance, in convulsions: barbitrates, phenytoin, diazepam
Blood	Anemia	Fatigue, relative decrease in hematocrit	Fall in hemoglobin level	None	Hemolysis, reduced erythropoiesis, low ferritin	Adequate dialysis	Transfusion (on clinical grounds only), iron substitution, erythropoietin
	Bleeding	Acute blood loss	Platelet dysfunction, thrombocytopenia, disturbance of plasma coagulation factors, vascular defect	None	Azotemia, sepsis, shock	Adequate dialysis, identify consumptive coagulopathy due to underlying disease	Peritoneal dialysis, in case of hemodialysis prostacyclin or its analogs and low-dose heparin or heparin-free dialysis

**Table 39.2
How to Treat Azotemia and Uremia**

Improve hemodynamics
1. Correct heart failure
2. Improve renal perfusion
3. Raise blood pressure
4. Perform angioplasty on renal artery stenosis
5. Remove thrombus occluding renal artery

Improve excretion
1. Increase administration of fluids
2. Eliminate causes of hyponatremia (salt-losing kidney)
3. Administer potent diuretics, e.g., furosemide
4. Reduce administration of proteins
5. Correct or reduce hypercatabolism

Dialysis therapy, the first line of approach in all life-threatening conditions

---

ing on the degree of severity, edema, hypertension, left ventricular insufficiency, lung edema, and hypoxia with repercussions on heart and brain will follow as alarming consequences. Parallel to this, brain edema with convulsions and coma may develop. The fastest way to improve this potentially fatal state is by means of hemofiltration, which should be administered as continuous arteriovenous filtration if an appropriate device is unavailable. It should be noted, however, that too rapid hemofiltration without insufficient refilling from tissue may cause hypovolemia with tachycardia and a drop in blood pressure. Potent diuretics are mainly effective only in the predialysis stage or at the onset of dialysis treatment, and should be applied alone only in less potentially fatal cases.

Acidosis

Concurrently with azotemia, most patients develop a metabolic acidosis. However, in the final stage of renal insufficiency, in particular in interstitial tubular renal disease when acidosis is most pronounced, patients have adapted to it rather well. Therefore, metabolic acidosis in chronic renal insufficiency is rarely a reason for intensive care. It is frequently intensified by other metabolic disturbances, such as diabetes mellitus or circulatory distur-

bances as, for instance, gut ischemia with resulting lactacidosis (9).

Metabolic acidosis can be balanced by oral or intravenous application of bicarbonate, with the fastest correction being possible by a bicarbonate dialysis. In the case of hypervolemia with pulmonary disturbances, acidosis may be intensified through the absence of respiratory compensation or even through an additional respiratory acidosis.

Electrolyte Imbalance

Sodium

Hyponatremia is frequently observed in salt-losing kidneys. In these cases it often causes a rapid deterioration of renal function, which can be balanced in time by an adequate application of salt. In renal insufficiency, an increased oral salt intake leads to hypervolemia and a rise in blood pressure and, occasionally, to a hypertensive crisis due to the almost always concurrent fluid intake. Excessive hypernatremia is usually only observed in cases of incorrect infusion therapy (9).

During dialysis treatment, both hypo- as well as hypernatremia may occur due to incorrect dialysis fluid management. Acute hyponatremia is often accompanied by hemolysis, as is hypernatremia by severe neurologic disturbances. As soon as this has been detected, the patients have to undergo dialysis with a normal dialyzing fluid composition until the disturbance has largely receded. Cases of death due to acute hypernatremia have been reported. However, such complications seldom occur when modern dialysis machines, which measure conductivity, are being used. Neurologic disturbances, on the other hand, take more time to regress when hypernatremia has persisted for a longer time. It must be pointed out that slowly developing hypo- or hypernatremia should be corrected equally slowly in order to avoid neurologic disturbances; the daily balance is approximately 5 mmol/liter of serum.

Potassium

Hyperkalemia is one of the most serious complications that dialysis patients face. It occurs mainly after dietary lapses, particularly after excessive fruit intake. Patients with renal insufficiency but sufficient diuresis rarely develop hyperkalemia because of their still-functioning potassium clearance. However, it is observed in cases of advanced renal insufficiency, particularly after incorrect application of potassium-saving saluretics such as amiloride, triamterene, and aldosterone antagonists. Due to acidosis, potassium is discharged from the cells and hyperkalemia is thus intensified (9, 10).

In the end stage of renal insufficiency, hypokalemia is rarely observed, even when saluretics are being given. Hypokalemia may occur in the diarrheal state and may even reach potentially dangerous manifestations. There are also incidences of dysrhythmia, especially in patients treated with digoxin or digitoxin, when, during dialysis, the serum potassium level is rapidly reduced. In those cases, arrhythmias may even occur in the presence of a low normal potassium level and may call for the administration of potassium.

SINGLE ORGAN FAILURE IN END-STAGE RENAL FAILURE

Neurologic Complications

Uremic Encephalopathy

Uremic encephalopathy is an organic brain syndrome occurring in patients with severely impaired renal function and ressembles other metabolic or toxic encephalopathies. It may be modified by the presence of acidosis, hypoxia, hypo- and hyperosmolality, and other biochemical alterations that occur in renal failure. The clinical features do not correlate well with the degree of uremia. They are more pronounced in patients with acute renal failure. The symptoms include malaise, irritability, difficulty in concentration, fatigue, insomnia, and apathy. More specific symptoms are dysarthria, rapid irregular tremors, asterixis and myoclonus. Seizures and coma are late manifestations of uremia. Hypertensive encephalopathy is associated with retinopathy and often is accompanied by focal signs (6).

Uremic Neuropathy

Neuropathy in uremia involves peripheral nerves and the autonomous nervous system. The manifestations of peripheral uremic neuropathy are similar to those with other metabolic disorders. Usually it is a symmetrical, distal, mixed motor, and sensory polyneuropathy. As a typical manifestation, restless leg syndrome occurs, which is an irresistible compulsion of the patients to move their legs. Loss of deep tendon reflexes, mainly in the lower extremities, is an early physical sign of uremic neuropathy. The vibration sense especially is impaired very early. Pathogenetically, uremic neuropathy seems to result from axonal damage caused by the cumulative effects of various neurotoxins (6).

Autonomic neuropathy is defined as an abnormal Valsalva response, reduced baroreceptor sensitivity, an abnormal response of heart rate to atropine, and ultrafiltration during dialysis therapy. Since cold pressor test shows normal increase in noradrenaline but abnormal response in blood pressure, the end-organ responsiveness seems to be diminished.

Cerebral Hemorrhage

Intracerebral bleeding is a fatal complication in uremics. It primarily appears as a massive hemorrhage into the brain. It is primarily caused by hypertension and anticoagulation during therapy. Symptoms occur acutely and include severe headache, nausea, vomiting, meningeal signs, hemiparesis, coma, and death.

Dialysis Dementia

Dialysis dementia is a progressive, in most cases fatal, neurologic disorder occurring in dialysis patients due to accumulation of aluminum from the dialysis fluid or longtime phosphate binding therapy with aluminum hydroxide. It is characterized by dysarthria, dyspraxia, and speech arrests. This may be followed by difficulty in swallowing. Development of dementia, myoclonus, and seizures are late signs. In these patients, a high concentration of aluminum is found in the grey matter of the brain (10).

Cardiovascular Complications

Coronary Heart Disease and Myocardial Infarction

In about 50–60% of all dialysis patients, who are over 50 years old, a severe coronary stenosis must be taken into account, with an even higher probability if the patient also suffers from diabetes mellitus. Unlike patients with normal renal function, almost half of these patients show no symptoms, although ischemia can already be identified in the resting electrocardiogram (autonomous polyneuropathy) (3). Therefore, whenever a dialysis patient having hemodialysis therapy is affected by a collapse of unknown origin, a coronary heart disease, possibly previously unnoticed, or a coronary infarction has to be taken into consideration. Immediate electrocardiogram and specific laboratory studies will yield a precise diagnosis.

According to the statistics of the European Dialysis and Transplantation Association in 1990, more than 60% of patients with end-stage renal failure die of cardiovascular complications. In spite of this, acute myocardial infarction during dialysis therapy remains a rarity. This is possibly due to the complete anticoagulation, which is mandatory as part of the extracorporal treatment. In patients with a relapse of typical angina pectoris symptoms during hemodialysis therapy or recurring drops in blood pressure during treatment, alternative methods of treatment, as, for instance, continuous ambulatory peritoneal dialysis or hemofiltration, should be discussed. Drug therapy for coronary disease in dialysis patients does not differ from that of patients with normal renal function (10).

Pericarditis and Pericardial Tamponade

Uremic pericarditis is a rare but typical complication of the decompensated renal insufficiency. Normally, a comprehensive hemodialysis therapy should succeed in avoiding this complication, but especially when intercurrent diseases such as a virus infection occur, metabolic deterioration and a concurrent pericarditis may develop.

Typically, these patients complain about symptoms similar to those in angina pectoris, with or without radiation in arms and neck. Neither the electrocardiogram, laboratory tests, x-rays of the thorax nor the ultrasound cardiogram prove to be of directive value. Instead, the diagnosis will be confirmed on the basis of the auscultatory result (systolic/diastolic friction murmur over sternum and lingula of the left lobe of the lung).

In patients with uremic pericarditis, a daily hemodialysis therapy is indicated. It should be borne in mind, however, that the inevitable anticoagulation has to be administered with utmost care in case a hemorrhagic pericardial effusion develops. Such an event could ultimately lead to a pericardial tamponade with cardiac shock. Frequently such a dramatic clinical occurrence develops in patients with pericarditis after a period with almost no complaints because patients are primarily without pain after a pericardial effusion has developed. The pericardial tamponade is characterized by an upper functional blockage, in the possible absence of other clinical signs such as silent heart sounds or the apex beat. The diagnosis will be confirmed by means of echocardiography, which will also provide a monitoring for a possibly needed relieving puncture. Surgical interventions as, for instance, pericardial fenestration or pericardectomy are rarely needed today.

Arrhythmias

In a number of collective statistics the incidence of extrasystoles in hemodialysis patients is, on average, 30%, of which another 20–25% were more complex arrhythmias of the Lown classes III–V (2, 11). Apart from a coronary heart disease and earlier medication (digitalis, calcium antagonists), changes in the electrolyte concentrations are mainly responsible. Thus, during the initial hours of hemodialysis therapy, tachyarrhythmia is frequently observed, possibly as a result of the reduction of potassium and calcium concentration in serum. By contrast, the incidence of bradyarrhythmia in the presence of hemodialysis therapy is rather rare. However, during a dialysis-free interval, the reverse is true. The indication for therapy of arrhythmias corresponds to that of patients with normal renal fuanction; the dosage, however, must be reduced for several arrhythmia drugs (see "Drug Dosage"). Many cases, on the other hand, do not call for an antiarrhythmic therapy, but rather for no such medication because 30–50% of all arrhythmias in dialysis patients can be traced to an overdosage of digitalis (11).

Hypotension

The most frequent complication in hemodialysis therapy is the sudden drop in blood pressure (5, 12). Apart from heart disease and drugs, such as β-blockers, and dialysis-induced variables as, for instance, acetate-dialysis or an overreduced sodium concentration, a pronounced ultrafiltration (net fluid loss) resulting from a high weight increase during the dialysis-free interval must be held responsible. In all cases, pronounced gastrointestinal bleeding with corresponding hemoglobin decrease or a hypovolemia of some other cause must be excluded.

In the presence of recurrent hypotonic episodes without high ultrafiltration, increasing serum osmolarity by an increase of sodium concentration in the dialysate is recommended as therapy (5, 6).

Hypertension

In dialysis patients the combination of renal hypertension and hyperhydration may rapidly turn into a hypertensive crisis. Its clinical manifestations are likely to be cerebral or cardiac symptoms, similar to those of patients with normal renal function. The treatment of these patients is guided by the clinical findings but frequently, apart from medication, a rapid dehydration is necessary, especially in the presence of cerebral symptoms. Medication during a hypertensive crisis does not differ from that of patients with normal renal function (see "Drug Dosage"). During hospital treatment the parenteral application of nifedipine or urapidil and, alternatively, the administration of dihydralazine and clonidine have been proven useful. Dosage is

primarily based on the clinical picture and the extent of rise in blood pressure, with the aim of rapidly lowering the pressure, while keeping in mind a corresponding dose adjustment in antihypertensive medication at a later point (see "Drug Dosage").

Pulmonary Complications

Hyperhydration and Fluid Lung

Accumulation of fluid in the lungs is one of the most frequent complications in patients with end-stage renal failure. In most cases, the reason for this is an excessive fluid intake, which, as a rule, further induces a deterioration in the stabilization of the patient's renal hypertension (1, 4, 9). Concurrently, only a moderately stabilized cardiac insufficiency may deteriorate, in some cases developing into a pronounced lung edema (Table 39.1). This is also true in cases of an excessive infusion therapy within the scope of surgery or intensive care monitoring of patients with end-stage renal disease.

Many patients recognize the early stage of this situation (fluid lung I–II) and feel motivated to visit the dialysis center whenever dyspnea or a gain in body weight occurs. On the other hand, this clinical picture may also deteriorate rather rapidly (fluid lung III–IV). At this stage an increasing pulmonary fluid accumulation will always result in hypoxemia owing to alveolar flooding. As a result, the peripherally restricted oxygen supply will soon lead to an intensified acidosis, which in turn can trigger a serious hyperkalemia.

In the case of a pronounced dyspnea, the clinical picture presents the lack of auscultatory or percussion findings. An x-ray of the lung, however, will provide information as it is characterized, even at this early stage, by butterfly-shaped densification areas close to the hila (Table 39.1). Histologically it correlates with an edema in the interstice, with initially only a slight involvement of the alveoli. An early hemodialysis treatment in the stages I–III will quickly show positive effects, and radiologic signs of water accumulation may disappear within a few hours.

If in the clinical picture the lung edema

is predominant, with symmetrical moist rales and radiologically noticeable, rather peripheral shadows, a reduction in blood pressure and treatment of the (left) cardiac insufficiency are imperative, apart from the treatment of the hyperhydration. In even more serious clinical pictures, mechanical ventilation with positive end-expiratory pressure—as in patients with normal renal function—must be initiated.

Pneumonia

Recurrent accumulations of fluid in the lungs, chronic cardiac insufficiency, and an increased rate of infections are responsible for a higher rate of pneumonia in dialysis patients when compared to patients with normal renal function. (3)

The incidence of infections in end-stage renal disease is shown in Table 39.3. Patients with end-stage renal disease definitely suffer from infections more frequently than patients with healthy kidneys. Next to coronary circulation diseases, these represent the main causes for morbidity and death. One of the reasons is defects in the immune resistance, as has been clearly demonstrated for some lympho-cyte- and granulyte-functions.

The clinical diagnosis of pneumonia in end-stage renal failure patients is frequently made difficult because there may be no classic symptoms such as coughing or a high temperature. This leads to the fact that in patients with concurrent hypervolemia or a compensated cardiac insufficiency on record, the diagnosis of pneumonia can be missed because of the partly poor auscultatory findings. The diagnosis can be proved by an x-ray of the lungs.

The changes described in the immune pathogen system of the patients account for the variety in the spectrum of pneumonia of these patients when compared to patients with normal renal function. Thus, it seems that the percentage of interstitial pneumonia, with up to 20–40%, is markedly increased. Even some rarer pathogenic microorganisms as, for instance, legionellae, mycobacteriae, and also fungi are observed more frequently than in patients with normal renal function. In

Table 39.3
Intensive Care Treatment of Patients with End-Stage Renal Failure in a 2-Year Period[a]

Treatment For:	N	%
1. Overhydration and fluid lung	36	19.5
2. Uremia	10	5.4
3. Hypokalemia	1	0.5
4. Hyperkalemia	12	6.5
5. Arrhythmia	7	3.8
6. Myocardial infarction and coronary heart disease	16	8.6
7. CAPD-associated peritonitis[b]	8	4.3
8. Complications after transplantation	13	7.1
9. Bleeding after transplant puncture	2	1.1
10. Occlusion of fistula	18	8.6
11. Infection of fistula	11	5.4
12. Complications of fistula (total)	29	14.1
13. Neurologic complications	6	3.2
14. Hypertension	7	3.2
15. Pneumonia (mechanical ventilation)	6	3.2
16. Endocarditis	2	1.1
17. Other infections	4	2.1
18. Gastrointestinal bleeding	15	8.1
19. Ileus and peritonitis	2	1.1
20. Pancreatitis	2	1.1
21. Bleeding	1	0.5
22. Thrombosis	1	0.5
23. Desiccation	1	0.5
24. Suicide	1	0.5
25. Diabetes	3	1.8
Total	185	100

[a]Total number in group = 600.
[b]CAPD, chronic ambulatory peritoneal dialysis.

particular, because of the relatively high incidence of legionella pneumonia (5–20%), the primary administration of erythromycin is highly recommended, especially for community-acquired pneumonia, as it is not necessary to adapt the dosage to the degree of renal insufficiency. With regard to the possible pathogens, the risk of a staphylococcal pneumonia has to be borne in mind, which may be due to septic, shunt-induced emboli.

Abdominal Complications

Intestinal Bleeding

Bleeding of ulcers is the most frequent of all types of intestinal bleeding. All bleeding must be clarified by endoscopy. Local endoscopic procedures (while injecting) and the administration of antacids are of prime importance, and accurate diagnosis is imperative for surgery.

In the presence of uremic gastritis, serious bleeding may develop from erosion of the mucosa. This complication, which is fairly infrequent today, is most likely to occur in the presence of high retention values. Besides treatment with antacids, a daily dialysis therapy with rapid reduction of the retention values is essential, in which case surgery will not be necessary.

Bleedings from other parts of the intestines have not been frequently observed in patients with end-stage renal failure. Patients in the dialysis program who suffer from diarrhea are likely to develop hypovolemic states because they observe their restrictions on fluid and electrolyte intake while the diarrhea continues. Therefore close-meshed monitoring of body weight and electrolytic levels is necessary. In case of frequently recurring diarrhea, a chronic intestinal disease has to be considered as well as an amyloidosis. In immune-suppressed patients who are treated with antibiotics for a long time, the occurrence of diarrhea should also call for a consideration of the rather serious pseudomembranous endocolitis by *Clostridium difficile* (rectoscopy and bacteriologic tests; when suspected vancomycin should be administered; 0.5 g p.o. every 4 hr).

Uremic Pancreatitis

A number of authors have reported a high incidence of pancreatitis. It should be noted, in this context, that most certainly amylase and most likely also lipase will have a reduced excretion or will be broken down by the impaired kidney. From our experience, mild pancreatitis is relatively frequent, whereas necrotizing pancreatitis does not often occur in patients with chronic renal insufficiency.

Peritonitis

The accepted general diagnostic and therapeutic recommendations are also applicable to peritonitis and ileus. Four individual forms, however, have to be given special consideration whenever patients with end-stage renal failure are concerned.

Uremic Pseudoperitonitis

In the end stage of renal disease, particularly in the presence of very high retention values, the full clinical picture of peritonitis with ileus may develop, which leads to the fact that these patients undergo an inappropriate laparatomy. In most cases, the symptoms will recede within a few hours if a sufficient dialysis therapy is administered. The diagnosis can then be made in retrospect. If, however, the symptoms do not recede, a laparotomy must be carried out.

Ileus and Electrolyte Disturbances

In the presence of serious electrolyte disturbances, particularly in the case of hypokalemia, a paralytic ileus may develop. The symptoms will recede after the condition has been normalized.

Diverticulitis and Enterocolitis

A high incidence of diverticulosis in dialysis patients must be assumed. In these diverticula enteroliths may form, especially during antacid treatment, which may lead to diverticulitis with perforation and peritonitis. An immediate surgical intervention is imperative in these cases.

Peritonitis in Peritoneal Dialysis

In peritoneal dialysis, a form of the iatrogenic peritonitis is observed. The earliest indication is a rise of the number of leukocytes in the dialysate (normal is up to 100 per m^3) and later on its clouding. Further symptoms are pain, an indication of ileus, and a high temperature. If a peritonitis is suspected, the dialysate must immediately be tested bacteriologically. At first nonspecific, but later specifically bacteriologic treatment must be administered. If a peritonitis is recurrent at short intervals, the peritoneal catheter must be removed and be reimplanted after normalization. The exclusion of other causes for peritonitis is often difficult while a peritoneal dialysis is being carried out. Appendicitis, adenitis, and cholecystitis should be kept in mind.

Hemostatic Complications

Bleeding Complications

Bleeding complications in dialysis patients are frequently an indication for admission to special intensive care treatment. (Table 39.3). In the majority of cases, bleeding occurs in the upper gastrointestinal tract (erosive gastritis, petechial hemorrhage, ulcer bleeding). There is a general tendency for dialysis patients to show a markedly higher incidence of bleeding. The cause of this tendency is a disturbed thrombocyte function, in the presence of a normal or slightly reduced total number of thrombocytes. Normally, no plasma clotting disturbances are recorded; however, an increased prostacyclin binding in the small vessels has been reported. Moreover, additional factors such as postoperative stress situations or medication (anticoagulation, nonsteroidal antiinflammatory drugs, glucocorticoids, etc.) can enhance the bleeding tendency in dialysis patients. In the case of a manifest upper gastrointestinal bleeding, the extracorporal therapy has to be carried out without anticoagulation. Consequently, a peritoneal or heparin-free dialysis has to be initiated (Table 39.1).

Thrombosis

In dialysis patients the rate of thrombosis seems to be fairly low. This is possibly due to the bleeding tendency and the recurrent complete anticoagulation in the scope of extracorporal treatment. Table 39.3 shows that only one of our patients had to be treated for a thrombosis in a 2-year period. It is necessary, however, to differentiate in this context thrombotic events that develop as ascending or progressing thromboses following shunt punctures or shunt-induced complications. The same holds true for thromboses in the area of the upper vena cava, resulting from long-term cannulation by a Sheldon catheter.

Infections

Sepsis

Apart from acute shunt infections, the dialysis patient is also exposed to danger of chronic asymptomatic shunt infection, which may lead to septic emboli. Due to the immune deficiency in the patient (see above), this can also lead to isolated organ inflammations as, for instance, to pneumonia or to the full clinical situation of sepsis. In a large number of cases the primary nidus in the shunt will be asymptomatic. The only clinical sign of this condition will be recurrent attacks of fever without positive blood cultures. In many cases and at a rather early stage, the cardiac valves (see below) are involved, which determines the clinical picture in later stages of the disease.

Aside from the Brescia Cimino fistula, a septicemia can also result from a Sheldon catheter placed in the upper vena cava. After shunt complications or in the presence of shunt infections, such a catheter is frequently needed for hemodialysis therapy during a longer period of time. Next to the risk of clot formation in the cannulated vena, the risk of a catheter sepsis exists at all times.

Staphylococcus aureus is the most frequent agent in septicemias in the hemodialysis patient. Only in shunt infections that have persisted for a long period of time, must an involvement of streptococci be considered. Antibiotic therapy must therefore always include a staphylococcal-effective substance. In terminal renal insufficiency, the application of 1–1.5 g of vancomycin once a week has been proven effective. With this dosage, a reduction in the plasma levels of the antibiotic to subtherapeutic values occurs only after 8 days, in spite of a continuation of hemodialysis.

Endocarditis

Patients with end-stage renal failure have a high risk for developing endocarditis. Impaired immune resistance and the recurrent shunt punctures are predisposing factors. Due to a hypertension of long duration, valve ring sclerosis is frequently

Table 39.4
Electrolyte Imbalance in Chronic Renal Failure

	Leading Symptoms	Clinical Findings	Laboratory Findings	Therapy
Hyperhydration	Dyspnea, dry cough	Edema, hypertension, increased jugular venous pressure crepitations, hepatomegaly	Fluid lung, pulmonary edema, ECG: p-pulmonale ST-depression	Potent diuretics, furosemide, hemofiltration, hyperbaric ventilation
Metabolic acidosis	Kussmaul's breathing	Lethargy	Acid-base status	Bicarbonate infusion, bicarbonate hemodialysis
Hypernatremia	Thirst, seizures, coma		Sodium >150 ml/liter	Slow dilution with sodium-free infusions, attention: cerebral edema
Hyponatremia	Muscle cramps, headache, seizures, coma	Increased intracranial pressure papilledema	Sodium <130 ml/liter	Oral or parenteral substitution with sodium chloride
Hyperkalemia	Paraesthesia (esp. perioral), muscle weakness, periodic paralysis	Bradycardia, hypotonic paralysis	ECG: peaking T-wave, PQ-prolongation, QT-shortening, bundle branch block	Ion exchange resin orally or as retention enema, hemodialysis with low potassium dialysate, insulin-glucose infusion, calcium gluconate, salbutamol (β_2-adrenotropic)
Hypokalemia	Apathy, muscle weakness, nausea	Muscular atony, muscular fasciculation on tapping, ileus rhythm disturbance	ECG: PQ-shortening, ST-depression, fusion of U-wave	Cautious potassium substitution especially in rhythm disturbances, control of acid-base status

observed, particularly at the aortic valve, as well as changes in the mitral valve, which are due to cardiac insufficiency.

In the absence of further risk factors, a staphylococcal endocarditis will usually be diagnosed. The echocardiogram will locate the vegetations on the mitral or the aortic valve. In the presence of sclerosis, however, the detection is frequently difficult. Likewise, the clinical diagnosis is just as difficult because, in general, patients notice only a slight reduction in their well-being, as septicemia with shivering attacks is rare. In the majority of cases, patients complain only of a rise in temperature and of night sweats.

The therapeutic spectrum for endocarditis in dialysis patients does not differ from that for patients with normal renal function; the different spectrum of agents (Staphylococcus), however, must be considered. In case the echocardiography of the heart or a heart catheter examination reveals an increasing valve insufficiency, the indication for valve replacement must be decided on fairly early because, as a rule, the valve infection in a dialysis patient will completely heal either not at all or only over a very long period of time.

DIALYSIS TREATMENT-INDUCED COMPLICATIONS

Treatment of end-stage renal failure using intermittent hemodialysis or hemofiltration and continuous ambulatory peritoneal dialysis is affected with some typical complications that are due to the mode of treatment itself. The incidence of these complications is especially high when the patient undergoes dialysis treatment for the first time.

Osmotic Disequilibrium Syndrome

Osmotic disequilibrium syndrome is a constellation of transient central nervous symptoms that starts after at least 2 hr of hemodialysis. Manifestations include headache, nausea, increase in blood pressure, and, in severe cases, coma and seizures. These signs also may occur after termination of dialysis treatment. They disappear slowly clearing within 12 hours.

Osmotic disequilibrium syndrome is mainly related to highly efficient and low-sodium dialysis treatment. It is caused by a rapid decrease in plasma sodium concentration of the patient (8). By removal of sodium chloride from plasma, osmotic pressure in the extracellular compartment decreases (decrease of plasma sodium concentration by 10 mmol/liter = decrease in extracellular osmolarity by 18 mOsmol/liter). The consequence of this is a fluid shift into the intracellular space, which in the central nervous system induces an increase in intracranial pressure.

Osmotic disequilibrium syndrome can be avoided by using a dialysate sodium concentration slightly higher (2–4 mmol/liter) than plasma sodium concentration. Treatment of symptoms of disequilibrium is symptomatic.

Hard Water Syndrome

Dialysis fluid is usually prepared continuously by the dialysis machine adding deionized water to a salt concentration in the proportion of 1:34. Control of general dialysis fluid composition is done by measuring conductivity. If there is failure of the tap water deionizing system (reverse osmosis), the patient may have dialysis with too high a calcium and magnesium concentration without any change of conductivity. In such cases, dialysis fluid calcium levels of >14.0 mg/dl have been reported causing acute symptoms like hypertension, nausea, vomiting, with progressing lethargy and weakness. Today, hard water syndrome is very rare, but its probability should be kept in mind (10).

Pyrogenic Reactions

Febrile reactions during dialysis may be caused by pyrogenic contamination or bacterial infection. Fever due to infection most likely occurs early after the start of treatment, while fever and chills that develop during the course of treatment are more likely due to a pyrogenic reaction with endotoxinemia. Infection should be verified by blood cultures and treated with antibiotics. Pyrogenic reactions are treated symptomatically.

Acetate Intolerance

To achieve a buffer balance by hemodialysis, acetate or bicarbonate is used in dialysis fluid. Acetate has the advantage of low cost, bacteriostatic effect in the solution, and easy handling by the dialysis equipment. There is instantaneous equimolar conversion of acetate to bicarbonate in the patient. The velocity of acetate metabolism depends on liver function, muscle mass, and age. Especially in older patients, it may happen that acetate concentration in plasma increases up to more than 5–8 mmol/liter because mass transfer of acetate through the dialyzer membrane exceeds maximal metabolic capacity. Clinical symptoms of acetate intolerance are weakness and hypotension by a decrease of peripheral vascular resistance, decrease in arterial Po_2, and incomplete correction of metabolic acidosis. Because of loss of bicarbonate through the dialyzer, acidosis may even increase during dialysis. If bicarbonate dialysis is not available, in cases of acetate intolerance, mass transfer through the dialyzer should be decreased using blood flows less than 150 ml/min.

On the other hand, when bicarbonate is used in the dialysis fluid, blood flows more than 200 ml/min may be used, but the correct bicarbonate concentration in dialysis fluid should be chosen to prevent alkalosis at the end of dialysis. In lactic acidosis, bicarbonate should be used exclusively (10).

Muscle Cramps

Muscle cramps induced by dialysis are painful. They occur primarily when sodium concentration decreases during dialysis and when too much fluid is removed. Symptomatic therapy is best done with intravenous bolus injections of 2 g of hypertonic (10–20%) sodium chloride or 40% glucose.

SHUNT-INDUCED COMPLICATIONS

Shunt Complications

The most common shunt complication is shunt occlusion due to thrombi, stenoses, and occasionally to hematomas, which compress the vessel. Intensive care may become necessary following less common complications, such as massive bleeding and infection.

Massive bleeding generally occurs from shunt veins that have become dilated due to aneurysm. Such bleeding may be life-threatening, particularly if it occurs unnoticed during sleep. Bleeding can usually be arrested easily by compression, but often necessitates surgical intervention.

Shunt infections require special attention because of the serious complications they entail. Most commonly, the infections in question are caused by staphylococci or streptococci. In addition to local measures, early antibiotic treatment is indicated: 1–2 g of vancomycin per week for staphylococcal infections, and 3 million units of penicillin per day for streptococcal infections. Prophylactic antibiotic therapy is indicated in patients with a history of endocarditis or a severe valvular sclerosis.

Chills, fever, shock, and consumption coagulopathy signal septic complications as a result of massive invasion of pathogens into the bloodstream. In such circumstances, shunt infection may behave like bacterial endocarditis. Immediate shutdown of shunt flow is indicated in such cases. Antibiotic therapy should then be prescribed initially toward the incidence and sensitivity of particular pathogens at the site, with a later switch to specific antibiotic therapy once the results of blood cultures are known. Plastic prostheses must be removed immediately in the event of septic complications.

EMERGENCIES FOLLOWING RENAL TRANSPLANTATION

A number of different emergencies may occur following renal transplantation:

1. Ruptured kidney, bleeding from vascular anastomoses, acute pyelonephritis, hypertension due to renal artery thrombosis, ureteral leaks, ureterocele.
2. Rejection reactions (due to humoral or lymphotic rejection of the graft by the host).
3. Infection and toxic damage to the transplant organ.
4. Infection in the recipient due to immunosuppression.

5. Toxic effects of immunosuppressant drugs on the recipient.

A basic knowledge of certain complications that may necessitate intensive care has become essential in view of the growing number of patients undergoing transplant surgery. Definite treatment should be the special preserve of the transplant centers; the measures necessary in the center will not be detailed here.

Ruptured Kidney

During the first weeks after transplant surgery, this condition is noted by pain in the vicinity of the graft, fall in diuresis, macrohematuria, graft enlarged on palpation and ultrasound, and fall in blood pressure that is usually only mild and gradual. There is good prognosis after immediate oversuturing. Thus, one never removes the kidney immediately if the diagnosis is rupture.

Bleeding from the vascular anastomoses (which may occur weeks to a few months after transplant surgery) is noted by sudden pain in the transplant bed and shock. There is no hematuria. Treat the patient for shock and institute immediate surgical repair.

Acute pyelonephritis is noted by sudden outflow obstruction from the transplanted kidney due to preexisting urinary tract infection. There is high fever, oliguria, and few local symptoms. Outflow obstruction is seen on ultrasound or in IV pyelogram. The most dangerous condition is septic shock. General antibiotic therapy should be started immediately. Surgical correction of the outflow disturbance should be done; often the graft kidney has to be removed.

Acute exacerbation of pyelonephritis of the native kidney is noted by high fever and pain in the native renal bed. Treatment is nephrectomy of the native kidney.

Rejection

Acute rejection is associated with a rapid fall in diuresis and a rise in retention values. Fever and pain in the transplant region are further clinical signs. Rejection is mitigated during treatment with cyclosporine. However, cyclosporine may also cause a deterioration in renal function.

Differentiation from rejection is extremely difficult and can only be performed in a transplant center.

Complications Due to Immunosuppression

Infections

Immunosuppression and granulocytopenia (due to azathioprine, in particular) may encourage infections caused by viruses, bacteria, and fungi. High fever and relative (or absolute) leukopenia are characteristic.

Common infections are atypical pneumonia (especially *Pneumocystis carinii*, mycoplasmas, viral infections, fungal infections, and tuberculosis also possible), endocarditis, esophagitis due to fungal infection, herpes simplex with the risk of herpes encephalitis, and meningoencephalitis.

Discontinue immunosuppressant therapy immediately; admit the patient at once to a transplant center for further specific therapy.

Side Effects of Immunosuppressant Drugs

Mention will be made only of those complications that may necessitate intensive care:

Glucocorticosteroids

1. Bleeding from the upper intestinal tract.
2. Diabetes mellitus.

Azathioprine

1. Bone marrow depression (especially in various combinations with allopurinol). Simultaneous administration of allopurinol is contraindicated.
2. Liver damage.

Cyclosporin A

1. Renal damage, probably only following overdose.
2. Fluid retention, hypertension, convulsions (rare).

OKT3

1. Pulmonary edema.

SPECIAL INTENSIVE CARE TREATMENT

Blood Access

In patients without existing blood access who have to be dialyzed, the quickest way to obtain a blood flow of 150–200 ml/min as temporary blood access is puncture of the subclavian or jugular vein using a catheter. If there is no other vein for return of the blood to the patient, a single-needle technique also can be applied. Subclavian vein catheters can be used repeatedly for weeks or even months until a functioning Brescia-Cimino fistula is available. Complications of subclavian vein puncture are infection, septicemia, and stenosis by thrombus formation. Therefore, scrupulous catheter and skin care is mandatory. If continuous treatment is necessary, as in continuous hemofiltration the same blood access can be utilized but blood flow has to be maintained using a blood pump (continuous venovenous pump-assisted hemofiltration). Puncture of the femoral artery seems unnecessary. It is more dangerous because of bleeding complications. When puncture of the femoral or subclavian veins are contraindicated, external shunts such as the Quinton-Scribner shunt may be chosen. The Quinton-Scribner shunt is comprised of two silastic tubes that, under local anesthesia, are inserted into a peripheral artery (arteria radialis, arteria tibialis posterior) and an adjacent vein. When the shunt is not in use, both tubes are connected outside the skin by a Teflon connector.

Parenteral Nutrition

As a rule, patients with end-stage renal failure who are in need of intensive care treatment will show the typical metabolic changes of a hypermetabolism syndrome. This syndrome develops following major surgery and also for a number of internal diseases, such as myocardial infarction, acute pancreatitis, and decompensated heart failure, it causes an increased energy consumption as well as a pronounced catabolism. Patients are at risk due to these metabolic processes, independent of their primary disease. If the energy carrier and proteins are not sufficiently substituted, the mortality of the patients increases. In this context, loss of body weight of more than 10% can lead to a mortality of 100%.

This signifies that patients with chronic renal disease must be appropriately nourished when faced with additional acute diseases or surgery. In this situation, for instance, a limited amino acid administration would be contraindicated. Patients in need of dialysis should receive approximately 1.5 g/kg per body weight per day of protein, which takes into account that, per dialysis treatment, approximately 15–30 g of amino acids are lost. The solution should contain 50% essential (25–30% branched-chain amino acids) and 50% nonessential amino acids. The total calorie administration for these patients should amount to in between 30 and 35 kcal/kg per body weight per day, the main energy carrier being glucose (5–6 g/kg per body weight per day). The maximum fat intake should not exceed 1.5 g/kg per body weight per day (Table 39.5). If a pronounced hyperlipidemia exists, as often occurs in chronic renal failure, a regular control of the triglycerides and of the cholesterol is necessary. Fat must not be administered if the serum concentration is already increased before surgery or if concentrations are markedly increased during fat application.

Oral nutrition is preferred. Alternatively, an enteral application via a thin-walled jejunal catheter is possible. Most important, however, is the early start of the nutritional therapy.

The early phase of an intensive care treatment frequently necessitates parenteral nutrition via a central vein, especially in comatose or precomatose conditions, in decompensated heart failure, or in gastrointestinal disturbances. In order to be able to infuse a sufficient amount of energy carriers and amino acids, a fluid administration of more than 1.5 liters per day is normally needed. This necessitates a daily dialysis for all critically ill patients with end-stage renal failure.

The administration of electrolytes should follow the daily balance and the currently measured serum levels. In critically ill patients, special consideration needs to be

Table 39.5
Total Parenteral Nutrition in Critically Ill Patients with End-Stage Renal Failure

Nutrient	Amount	Compounds
Energy	35 kcal/kg bw	glucose: maximum 6 g/kg bw fat: maximum 1.5 g/kg bw
Amino acids (AA)	1.5 g/kg bw	50% essential AA (25–30% branched-chain AA) 50% nonessential AA
Electrolytes	Daily balance, adapted to serum concentration	
Vitamin and trace elements	Water-soluble vitamins daily, lipid-soluble vitamins twice a week, trace elements on demand	

given to the organic phosphate, which may decrease in these patients in spite of the existing secondary hyperthyroidism.

Water-soluble vitamins should be given daily; fat-soluble vitamins should be added two to three times per week. Special attention must also be given to the substitution of trace elements in parenteral nutrition.

Drug Dosage

Many drugs or their effective metabolites are subject to a retarded excretion. Therefore it is necessary to adapt the dose and dose interval to renal function. The overview presented here will only consider the dosage of drugs for patients in need of dialysis and within the scope of intensive care treatment (Table 39.6). For many substances that play an important role in intensive care medicine, precise dosages cannot be recommended. On the other hand, close intensive care monitoring allows for a relatively early measurement of the effectiveness of certain drugs such as antihypertonics or insulin. Thus, a precise dosage need not be detailed. (7)

Analgetics

Morphine, pentazosine, tilidine, and various other morphine derivates do not have a cumulating effect, which will only occur in their predominantly ineffective metabolites. Generally, the substances mentioned, including acetaminophen, can be administered in the usual dosage without any disadvantage if therapy continues for only a limited time.

Antibiotics

The three major groups of antibiotics (β-lactam antibiotics, aminoglycosides, and quinolones) are mainly effective in their applied form. Correspondingly, the half-life period in end-stage renal failure is generally 10 to 20 times that of patients with normal renal function. Simultaneously, the therapeutic safety of the β-lactam antibiotics, in contrast to the aminoglycosides, should be considered. Aminoglycosides, even when only slightly overdosed, show an oto- or vestibular toxicity. A determination of plasma levels of applied aminoglycosides is mandatory in intensive care treatment, with lowest and highest levels recorded.

Quinolones, which in most cases are renally excreted, must also be reduced in their dosage in order to avoid severe cerebral side effects. In this context, ciprofloxazin with a renal elimination of only 50% seems to be of advantage, but prolongs the half-life of theophylline.

All the antibiotics mentioned are suitable for dialysis; i.e., by dialysis, their plasma level is reduced. Sufficiently documented reports on the precise influence of individual hemodialysis treatment are still missing for practical advice. It is therefore recommended to administer the calculated dose of an antibiotic after hemodialysis treatment.

When facing staphylococcal infections in dialysis patients, vancomycin has been proven as a therapeutic agent of first choice. The half-life in end-stage renal failure is great prolonged; i.e., a single application of 1–1.5 g of vancomycin after a hemodialysis treatment will be sufficient in order to ensure sufficient plasma levels for a week following hemodialysis therapy.

Antihypertensive Agents

Drugs frequently used in intensive care medicine such as nifedipine and nitrendipine, verapamil, dihydralazine, or hydralazine usually either do not have a cumulative effect or only a slight one; i.e., the dosage of these substances can orientate itself by their effect.

Antiarrhythmics

Due to a predominantly extrarenal excretion, dosage of the following drugs can remain unchanged: amiodarone, aprindine, calcium, lidocaine, mexiletine, phenytoin, and propafenone. However, active metabolites such as chinidine and verapamil can have a cumulative effect. Disopyramide, procainamide, and lorcainide must be adjusted to renal function. Hemodialysis patients receive about one fourth of the usual dose of these drugs. From the group of digitalis drugs, digitoxin should be given preference because it has no cumulative effect, whereas other drugs such as digoxin can have a strong cumulative effect in end-stage renal disease.

Diuretics

While in some patients with chronic renal disease the application of furosemide in doses between 0.5 and 2 g per day resulted in an increase of the diuresis, all other

Table 39.6

Half-life of Antibiotics in Patients with Normal Renal Function Compared with Half-life and Dosage Interval in Patients with End-Stage Renal Failure

| Antibiotic | Half-life (hr) | | Dosage Interval in End-Stage Renal Failure + <10 |
	Normal Renal Function	End-Stage Renal Failure	
Penicillin G	0.65	7–10	12
Oxacillin	0.4	2	8
Flucloxacillin	0.75	8	12
Ampicillin	1.0	8.5	12–24
Ticarcillin	1.1	16	12–24
Azlocillin	1.25	8–10	12–24
Mezlocillin	0.8	6–14	12–24
Piperacillin	1.0	6–10	12–24
Cephalotine	0.65	3–18	8
Cephaloline	1.5	5–20	24–48
Cefuroxime	1.2	5–20	24–48
Cefoxitin	0.75	5–10	24
Cefotaxime	1.0	14	12
Cefoperazone	2.0	5–10	12
Latamoxef	2.0	5–20	24
Cephalexin	1.0	30	24–48
Cefaclor	1.0	6–10	12
Gentamicin-tobramycin	2	60	48
Amikacin	2.3	72–96	72–96
Vancomycin	6	216	240
Tetracycline	8–9	30–128	72–96
Lincomycine	5	10–13	12
Clindamycin	3	3–5	12
Trimethoprim and sulfamethoxazole	10 bzw. 12	12–24	—
Flucytosine	3–4	6–12	24–48
Metronidazole	7	8–12	24

nonloop diuretics are contraindicated or ineffective.

Plasma Expanders

Dextran and gelatine have a cumulative effect in end-stage renal failure. Thus, the half-life period of dextran 40 amounts to 4200 min in such patients as compared to 500 min in patients with normal renal function. The maximum dose of this drug is therefore 300–500 ml per week. More frequent application may lead to higher dextran concentrations, which would result in a reduction of blood coagulation. Hydroxyethyl starch also has a cumulative effect in renal failure. A recurrent high dosage application can therefore not be recommmended. In addition, an increase of pancreas enzymes in serum may occur while this substance is being given in end-stage renal failure.

Sedatives

The majority of sedatives available have a cumulative effect in patients with end-stage renal failure. Only the benzodiazepines are transformed in the liver partly into ineffective and partly into only slightly effective metabolites. Therefore, a cumulative effect of these drugs is not to be expected, particularly because, as a rule, their sedative effect can be easily monitored during intensive care treatment.

Contrast Media Containing Iodine

Contrast media containing iodine have a cumulative effect in end-stage renal failure. In parenteral application of only a minor dose of a commercially available x-ray contrast medium, cerebral side effects may result. After such an application in which a dose of 50–100 ml was exceeded, a 3-hr hemodialysis must be carried out which, as a rule, will lead to a sufficient reduction of the plasma level of the contrast material.

References

1. Bell D, Nicoll J, Jackson M, Millar A, Winney RJ, Muir AL. Altered lung vascular permeability during intermittent hemodialysis. Nephrol Dial Transplant 1988; 3:426.
2. Blumberg A, Häutermann M. Strub B, Jenzer HR: Cardiac arrhythmias in patients on maintenance hemodialysis. Nephron 1983;33:91.
3. Brenner BM, Rector FC, eds. The kidney. 4th ed. ·WB Saunders, Philadelphia: WB Saunders Co, 1991.
4. Cardoso M, Vinay P, Vinent P, Leveillee M, Prudhomme M, Tejedor A, Coureau M, Gongoux A, St. Louis G, Lapierre L, Piette Y. Hypoxemia during hemodialysis: a critical review of facts. Am J Kidney Dis 1988;11:281.
5. Daul AE, Wang XL, Michel MC, Brodde OE. Arterial hypotension in chronic hemodialyzed patients. Kidney Int 1987;32:728.
6. Friedmann, EA, ed. Strategy in renal failure. New York: John Wiley & Sons, 1978.
7. Goodman LS, Gilman A, ed. The pharmacological basis of therapeutics. New York: Macmillan Publishing Co, 1990.
8. Gürich W, Mann H, Stiller S. Sodium elimination and changes in the EEG during dialysis. Artif Org 1980;3(suppl):94.
9. Klahr S. ed. The kidney and body fluids in health and disease. New York: Plenum, 1984.
10. Maher JF, ed. Replacement of renal function by dialysis. Dodrecht: Kluwer Academic Publishers, 1989.
11. Marzegalli M, Bernansconi M, Potenza S, Caprari M, Regalia F, Fiorista F, Vendemia F. Incidence, prognosis and therapy of cardiac arrhythmias in dialysis patients. Contrib Nephrol 1988;61:199.
12. Swartz RD, Somermeyer MG, Hsu CH. Preservation of plasma volume during hemodialysis depends on dialysate osmolality. Am J Nephrol 1982;2:189.
13. Vollhard F. Vierenerkrankungen und Hochdruck. Leipzig: JA Barth, 1942:63.

40

Esophageal Problems

Jacques Belghiti
Y. Panis

ESOPHAGITIS: INFECTION VERSUS INFLAMMATION

Esophageal Infection

Esophageal infections are more common in immunocompromised patients and have specific endoscopic and biopsy features.

Candida Esophagitis

The most common fungal infection of the esophagus is due to *Candida*. *Candida* is usually not a pathogen in humans; it is a commensal organism that is found almost universally in the gastrointestinal tract of healthy persons. Although antibiotic therapy can increase susceptibility to *Candida*, the esophagus is predominantly affected when host defenses are altered, such as with the acquired immunodeficiency state, lymphoma, or leukemia. This infection principally affects the oropharynx and esophagus. The most common symptom of candidiasis is odynophagia followed by dysphagia (11). Hematemesis has been reported in some patients. Oral lesions may be absent. A barium swallow may indicate thick exudate and mucosal ulcerations and rarely strictures. The standard diagnostic test is esophagoscopy showing white plaques adhering to a friable mucosa. Cytologic examination of the exudate reveals mycelia. Esophageal biopsy demonstrates mycelia invading the mucosa.

Topical therapy with nystatin (Mycostatin) can be used as treatment or as prophylaxis. Systemic therapy can be per-formed in necrotizing *Candida* esophagitis using amphotericin B (Fungizone), 5-fluorocytosine (Ancotil), or ketoconazole (Nizoral). Repeating the esophagogram can be considered as a good method for evaluating a patient's response to therapy (10).

Herpetic Esophagitis

Acute ulcerative esophagitis due to Herpes simplex viruses (HSV) is generally found in patients immunosuppressed. Esophagitis may result from the direct extension of oral-pharyngeal HSV infection into the esophagus or may occur by reactivation of HSV. The predominant symptoms are odynophagia, dysphagia, substernal pain, and weight loss. Esophagoscopy can show multiple ulcerations on erythematous mucosa with or without pseudomembrane. The distal esophagus is most commonly involved. Endoscopic examination and barium examination show similar features than observed in the case of candidiasis. Cytologic examination and culture provide the most accurate material for diagnosis. Although the efficacy of therapy is not established, the risk for potential dissemination of HSV infection leads to the treatment of some patients with systemic antiviral chemotherapy (3).

Caustic Esophagitis

Accidental or intentional swallowing of caustic substances may result in serious burns with an acute necrotic phase during the first days after injury followed by strictures some months later. The degree of injury depends on the nature of the caustic, its concentration, and the amount ingested. Alkalis produce deep lesions because the tissue is dissolved, where as acids result in more superficial injury because the normal squamous epithelium of the esophagus is resistant to acid. Alkalis injure the esophagus more than they do the stomach. During the first days, caustic substances produce intense inflammation and hemorrhage. Necrotic tissue with ulceration is followed by the formation of granulation tissue. Stricture formation ensues after 2 or 3 weeks or later. The submucosa and muscular layers are replaced by fibrous tissue.

The initial symptoms of caustic ingestion are oral and retrosternal pain, associated with dysphagia. Stridor and wheezing are signs of possible injury to the supraglottic or glottic regions. Oral burns may be present, but there is no relation to the degree of esophageal burn (5). Fever is frequently present and bleeding may occur. Ingestion of acid can produce systemic acidosis with renal failure.

The assessment of injury degree and location during initial evaluation is established by early endoscopy. In addition, findings during endoscopy correlate with eventual esophageal stricture formation, in that patients with low grade of injury have a low risk of stricture.

Initial management of caustic esophagitis included intubation or tracheostomy if upper airway obstruction is present and oral suctioning in order to prevent pulmonary infection. There is great controversy regarding the administration of neutralizing substances, the use of steroids, and the use of a nasogastric tube to reduce the incidence of esophageal stricture (4, 5).

Patients with severe lesions should be given nothing orally, a routine barium swallow is useful 2–3 weeks after the injury to assess the degree of stricture. Patients with evidence of gastric necrosis or esophageal perforation require urgent surgical intervention with resection and staged reconstruction. Esophageal resection can be performed by abdominal and cervical approach without thoracotomy (8).

PERFORATION

Perforation of the esophagus can occur spontaneously (Boerhaave's syndrome) but is iatrogenic in more than half the cases: after instrumental manipulation (i.e., endoscopy, dilatations of achalasia) or less frequently during surgery (i.e., truncal vagotomy, hiatus hernia repair). Rarely, perforation is secondary to ingestion of a foreign body (i.e., fish bone), carcinoma, caustic ingestion, Mallory-Weiss syndrome or penetrating trauma (12). Contamination of the mediastinum with corrosive fluids, food, and bacteria leads to severe sepsis with cardiorespiratory embarrassment, shock, and major fluid losses.

Pathogenesis of Boerhaave's syndrome associates two factors: rapid distension of the esophagus (i.e., during vomiting) and the presence of an anatomical weakness, in the majority of cases, on the left lateral wall of the distal esophagus. Mucosal and muscular laceration of up to 20 cm of esophagus with inflammation due to regurgitated gastric secretions induces edema and inflammation on the edges of perforation, making suture closure difficult in perforations not treated within 24 hr of injury. Extrusion of gastric juice results in severe mediastinitis; the pleural outpouring of fluid in response to contamination may amount to several liters in only a few hours, leading to hypovolemic shock (9).

Iatrogenic perforations are most often seen in the cricopharyngeal region, followed by the lower end of the esophagus (during achalasia's dilatation). A rigid endoscope is associated with a perforation rate of 0.11–0.4%, and a flexible scope with a 0.03% perforation rate; however, extensive manipulation increases this risk, which is: 8% for intubation, 0.25% for dilatation, and 4% for achalasia (1, 12).

Characteristic presentation of Boerhaave's syndrome includes forceful vomiting followed by acute, severe pain on the retrosternal area and/or epigastric pain; later, fever and dyspnea, followed by hemodynamic shock may be observed. At examination, epigastric tenderness and abdominal resistance are observed. Mediastinal emphysema can be found, frequently later in the evolution of the syndrome. The sequence of vomiting before pain is important in considering this rare disorder. In the case of cervical perforation, neck pain exacerbated by swallowing is observed and associated with subcutaneous emphysema in two thirds of the cases (9, 12). Chest x-ray shows mediastinal widening, mediastinal or subcutaneous emphysema, and pleural effusion; a gastrograffin esophagogram usually confirms the diagnosis, showing a leak.

Emergency resuscitative measures must be started prior to operation, including broad-spectrum antibiotics (for both Gram-positive and -negative organisms), nasogastric decompression, and fluid resuscitation. In case of cervical perforation, through a left cervicotomy, primary repair of the perforation is usually associated with cervical drainage. In the case of thoracic perforation, the incision is guided by the presence of pleural effusion, or if not, through a left thoracotomy (1, 6). If operation is begun within 48 hr after perforation, a primary repair of the mucosa and muscular layer, (facilitated by an opposite myotomy) can be associated with a flap coverage (with pleura, pericardium, or muscle) and both mediastinal and pleural drainage (1, 6, 7). In case of delayed diagnosis, if primary closure is not possible, both cervical and abdominal exclusion of the esophagus must be performed with multiple mediastinal drainage; some authors associate a T-tube drainage through the perforation (2). Primary closure of inflammatory mucosa (peptic or caustic) increases the risk of postoperative leakage. When perforation occurs in an abnormal esophagus, definitive operation for the underlying disease should be performed: esophagectomy in case of carcinoma, cardiomyotomy for achalasia, and resection

for severe esophagitis. In very critically ill patients, Celestin tube intubation with drainage may help to control infection (7).

Nonoperative "conservative" treatment has been suggested in some cases of iatrogenic perforation recognized early, with minimal signs; however, reported experience is very limited (1).

References

1. Bladergroen MR, Lowe JE, Postelthwait RW. Diagnosis and recommended management of esophageal perforation and rupture. Ann Thorac Surg 1986;42:235–239.
2. Brewer LA, Carter R, Mulder GA, Stiles QR. Options in the management of perforations of the esophagus. Am J Surg 1986;152:62–69.
3. Corey L, Spear PG. Infection with herpes simplex viruses. N Engl J Med 1986;314:686–691.
4. DiCostanzo J, Noirclerc M, Jouglard J, et al. New therapeutic approach to corrosive burns of the upper gastrointestinal tract. Gut 1980;21:370–375.
5. Ferguson MK, Migliore M, Staszak VM, Little AG. Early evaluation and therapy for caustic esophageal injury. Am J Surg 1989;157:116–120.
6. Flynn AE, Verrier ED, Way LW, Thomas AN, Pellegrini CA. Esophageal perforation. Arch Surg 1989;124:1211–1215.
7. Gayet B, Breil P, Fékété F. Mechanical sutures in perforation of the thoracic esophagus as a safe procedure in patients seen late. Surg Gynecol Obstet 1991;172:125–128.
8. Gossot D, Sarfati E, Célerier M. Early blunt esophagectomy in severe caustic burns of the upper digestive tract. J Thorac Cardiovasc Surg 1987;94:188–191.
9. Justicz AG, Symbas PN. Spontaneous rupture of the esophagus: immediate and late results. Am Surg 1991;57:4–7.
10. Kodsi BE, Wickremesinghe PC, Kozinn PJ, Iswar K, Goldberg PK. Candida esophagitis, a prospective study of 27 cases. Gastroenterology 1976;71:715–719.
11. Mathieson R, Dutta SK. Candida esophagitis. Dig Dis Sci 1983;28:365–370.
12. Sharp KW, Sawyers JL. Caustic and traumatic injury of the esophagus. In: Moody F, et al, eds. Surgical treatment of digestive disease. Chicago: Year Book, 1988:171–184.

41

Stress Ulcer Prophylaxis

Deborah J. Cook
Thomas A. Raffin

PATHOPHYSIOLOGY OF STRESS ULCERATION

Critically ill patients are at increased risk of bleeding from the proximal gastrointestinal tract due to stress ulceration. The pathogenesis of stress ulceration involves disruption of the usual mechanisms of gastric mucosal integrity. Hypotension and systemic acidosis decrease gastric blood flow, resulting in impaired turnover of gastric epithelium, loss of the protective mucous and bicarbonate barriers, and back diffusion of hydrogen ions across the gastric mucosa (30). Therefore, the development of stress ulceration is a complex interplay of both local and systemic factors.

The occurrence of upper gastrointestinal bleeding due to acute ulceration of the gastric or duodenal mucosa was described in association with severe burns almost 150 years ago (17). Since then, gastroesophageal endoscopy has demonstrated that gastroduodenal mucosal lesions occur in almost all seriously ill patients (97). Serial endoscopic studies have shown that within 24 hr of admission to the intensive care unit (ICU), areas of extensive gastric mucosal hyperemia can progress to discrete, shallow erosions, which may enlarge, increase in number, or bleed.

STRESS ULCER PROPHYLAXIS

Prophylactic therapy against stress ulceration has focused on neutralization of gastric acid (with antacid therapy), reduction of gastric acid secretion (with histamine-2-receptor antagonists), or cytoprotection (with sucralfate). The generally positive results of randomized trials in stress ulcer prophylaxis have led to recommendations that prophylaxis be administered to a large proportion of critically ill patients (3, 25, 68, 98). As such, control of gastric pH has been described as standard practice in intensive care units in North America and Europe (65).

DEFINITIONS OF BLEEDING

Although stress ulceration may be demonstrated endoscopically in many ICU patients, clinical signs or symptoms of bleeding may or may not be evident. In the trials of stress ulcer prophylaxis, diverse criteria for the outcome of bleeding have been employed. Stress ulceration can result in occult, overt, or clinically important gastrointestinal bleeding.

Occult bleeding is microscopic, usually inconsequential, and occurs in 20–40% of ICU patients. Occult bleeding is defined as a positive guaiac test of either gastric contents or stool. Many trials have included occult bleeding in their definition of stress ulcer bleeding, which may be problematic. In studies using a guaiac-positive nasogastric aspirate as a criterion for stress ulceration, evidence of bleeding is counted in each group, then the difference in bleeding incidence between groups may be entirely attributed to the suppression of bleeding due to stress ulcers. This approach may overestimate the incidence of bleeding from stress ulceration because of inclusion of bleeding due to other causes, such as trauma from a nasogastric tube. In addition, results of guaiac testing are nonspecific (53); cimetidine itself may produce a false-positive occult blood test (38, 64, 77). Moreover, occult bleeding, even in the absence of prophylactic therapy, rarely

Table 41.1
Risk Factors for Gastrointestinal Bleeding

Author (Ref)	Number of Subjects	Definition of Bleeding	Risk Factors Evaluated	Relative Risk Quantified	Independent Contribution to Risk Assessed	Result
Skillman (80)	150	"Massive bleeding"	Sepsis, respiratory failure, peritonitis, hypotension, jaundice	No	No	All 8 who bled had sepsis, hypotension, respiratory failure, 6/8 also had jaundice and peritonitis
Kamada (45)	433 with head injury	Hematemesis, melena, or bloody gastric aspirate	Type of head injury, shock, oxygenation, steroid treatment	No	No	72 patients bled, type of head injury, presence of shock predictors
Schuster (78)	179	Occult and overt (hematemesis, coffee grounds appearance, or melena)	Coagulopathy, respiratory failure, ventilation, COPD, sepsis, hypotension, shock[a]	No	Yes	Need for mechanical ventilation and coagulopathy only, independent risk factors
Hastings (37)	100	Bloody or guaiac-positive nasogastric aspirate	Respiratory failure, sepsis, peritonitis jaundice, renal failure, hypotension	No	No 0–1 risk factor: no bleeds in antacid group, 9.1% in control group 2 risk factors: no bleeds in antacid group, 20% in control group 3 risk factors: 10.5% in antacid group, 40% in control group	

				No	No	
Van den Berg (93)	28	Blood loss of >15 ml	Respiratory failure, sepsis, shock, jaundice, renal failure, peritonitis	No	No	All patients with bleeding had at least 3 risk factors
Basso (3)	116	Hematemesis or blood nasogastric aspirate or melena or decrease in hemoglobin	Respiratory failure, sepsis, acute renal failure, multiple trauma, hypotension, neurosurgery, head injury, burns	No	No	Risk associated with highest bleeding incidence was renal failure
Priebe (71)	75	Bloody nasogastric aspirate or guaiac-positive aspirate on three occasions	Major operation, respiratory failure, sepsis, peritonitis multiple trauma, renal failure, hypotension, jaundice	No	No	2 risk factors: 18.2% on antacids, 0 on cimetidine 3 or more: 45.4% cimetidine, 0 antacids
Groll (32)	221	Hematemesis or blood nasogastric aspirate or melena with endoscopy	Major operation, respiratory failure, shock, trauma, coma, renal failure, jaundice, sepsis	No	No	No correlation between number and risk factors and risk of hemorrhage
Tryba (87)	100	Hematemesis or blood nasogastric aspirate	Total risk score from previous study (89)	No	No	Coagulopathy, sepsis, and pancreatitis were risk factors with the highest incidence of bleeding
Tryba (90)	100	Hematemesis or bloody nasogastric aspirate or melena	Total risk score from previous study (89)	No	No	Risk score less than 20: 0 Risk score 20–29: 2.9% Risk score >29: 12.5% (difference in risk nonsignificant)

[a]COPD, chronic obstructive pulmonary disease.

progresses to overt bleeding (68), or is clinically important (50, 87, 95) and is therefore of questionable significance.

Other studies have considered overt bleeding as the outcome of interest. Overt bleeding includes hematemesis, altered blood (coffee grounds), bloody gastric aspirate, or melena. It is generally agreed that overt bleeding does not, in most instances, progress to clinically important bleeding associated with morbidity.

The truly relevant outcome, clinically important bleeding, is defined as overt bleeding associated with hemodynamic instability, a significant decrease in hemoglobin, or the need for blood transfusion. Specifically, clinically important bleeding (13) has been defined as overt bleeding plus one of the following:

1. A spontaneous drop of systolic or diastolic blood pressure of 20 mm Hg or more within 24 hr of upper gastrointestinal bleeding (in the absence of other causes);
2. A decrease in hemoglobin of 3 g/liter in 24 hr (in the absence of other causes);
3. Transfusion of more than 2 units of packed red blood cells in 24 hr.

However, no single study of stress ulcer prophylaxis has been large enough to address the question of the impact of stress ulcer prophylaxis on clinically important bleeding.

RISK FACTORS FOR BLEEDING

Ideally, the evidence regarding the risk of bleeding from stress ulceration would be found in large prospective studies or randomized trials in which various risk factors were assessed. A relative risk would be reported for each factor, and a regression equation would be constructed to determine which factors were independent contributors to the risk assessment. Finally, confidence intervals around the risk estimates would be provided.

The first five factors for massive gastrointestinal hemorrhage were identified in a series of eight patients by Skillman et al. and included sepsis, hypotension, respiratory failure, jaundice, and peritonitis (80). A number of similar studies have since been published which suffered from methodologic limitations. These included

retrospective chart reviews without documentation of reproducibility (36, 89) and two studies describing patients who bled, without comparison to a control group (23, 29).

The most valuable information comes from three prospective cohort studies (45, 78, 80) and seven randomized trials (3, 32, 37, 71, 87, 91, 93) summarized in Table 41.1. A number of issues arising from these data deserve emphasis. First, most studies examined the ability of risk factors to predict either occult or overt bleeding. Therefore, these are of questionable relevance to the prediction of clinically important bleeding. Second, the relative risk associated with individual variables was not quantified in any of these studies. Third, in only one of them was the independent contribution of risk factors explored (78). Finally, in most cases, the risk factors presented were the ones chosen by the authors on the basis of previous work, rather than factors generated from their own study. While this increases our confidence that the factors previously identified have some predictive power, it is not at all certain that if each group of investigators had looked at all possible risk factors they would have found the same set of predictors.

These issues limit the inferences that can be made from these studies. Nevertheless, it appears that a number of conditions increase the risk of bleeding from stress ulceration. These conditions include: respiratory failure, sepsis, hypotension, coagulopathy, renal failure, hepatic failure, burns, and head injury. The strongest single independent risk factor for bleeding in one prospective study of 100 ventilated patients was the presence of coagulopathy (12). In this study, the odds ratio associated with the presence of coagulopathy was 12 ($p < 0.001$), suggesting that critically ill patients are 12 times more likely to experience gastrointestinal bleeding than age-matched controls.

THE EFFICACY OF STRESS ULCER PROPHYLAXIS
Previous Descriptive Reviews

Several descriptive review articles of stress ulcer prophylaxis have been published (31, 39, 71, 97). One overview combined the data from 16 randomized trials to evaluate the efficacy of antacid and cimetidine therapy (79). Both agents were more effective than placebo in preventing overall, occult and overt bleeding ($p < 0.05$). When data were pooled from trials using occult blood as the minimum criterion for bleeding, antacids appeared to have a prophylactic advantage over cimetidine ($p < 0.003$). However, when detection of overt bleeding was used as the minimum criterion for bleeding, these drugs appeared equally efficacious. A subsequent quantitative review of studies evaluating antacids and cimetidine in the overall incidence of bleeding produced congruent results with respect to their equivalence (common odds ratio of 1.61, 95% confidence interval (CI) 0.97–2.65) and superiority over placebo (51).

None of these reviews have examined the differential effect of prophylaxis on clinically important bleeding in critically ill patients. To examine the differential effect of prophylaxis on overt and clinically important bleeding in critically ill patients, and to ascertain the relative impact of different therapies, a meta-analysis of the results of 42 randomized clinical trials of stress ulcer prophylaxis was performed.

A Critical Appraisal: The Efficacy of Stress Ulcer Prophylaxis

Meta-analysis entails critically reviewing and statistically combining the results of independent studies, thereby increasing statistical power and improving both the precision and accuracy of the estimate of treatment effect. Meta-analysis takes a more structured approach to data synthesis than does a traditional narrative review. The search for relevant literature in this overview was comprehensive; an extensive search of both published and unpublished literature was performed, and experts and governing agents were contacted to minimize the possibility of a publication bias. The study selection criteria were well defined, and quality assessment of the primary studies was performed by two reviewers blinded to the study results. The techniques of statistical analysis used in this meta-analysis were among those that have become standard for scientific overviews (4).

The focus of this discussion will be on the three most commonly prescribed classes of drug: antacids, histamine-2-receptor antagonists, and sucralfate. Thirty-four trials involved comparisons of antacids, histamine-2-receptor antagonists, and sucralfate with each other or with placebo. However, other agents have been evaluated. Prostaglandins were compared with antacids in two trials (81, 99) and with placebo in another (94). The anticholinergic pirenzepine was compared with histamine-2-receptor antagonists in three additional studies (41, 61, 91), and with placebo in another (57) and one study compared meciadanol, a histadine decarboxylase inhibitor, with antacids and sucralfate (62).

Of the 28 trials evaluating antacids, 21 titrated therapy to maintain a pH of 3.5–7.0 (5–9, 21, 43, 55, 56, 58, 59, 65, 68, 69, 71, 81, 95, 98, 99). Twenty-four of 29 trials evaluating histamine-2-receptor antagonists used cimetidine (five of these in continuous infusion form) (46, 48, 50, 90, 93). Five others employed ranitidine (61, 65, 72, 73, 90, 91). Therapy was titrated to maintain a pH of 3.5–5.0 in 11 of these studies. The dosage of cimetidine ranged from 300 to 1200 mg/day, the dose of ranitidine ranged from 200 to 600 mg/day, and the dose of sucralfate ranged from 4 to 6 g/day.

A total of 4409 subjects with a wide spectrum of medical and surgical illnesses were studied. Some trials enrolled only particular subgroups of critically ill patients, such as those with head injury, burns, and hepatic failure, or those patients who are ventilated or are status postabdominal aortic surgery. Populations were drawn from medical and surgical intensive care units, respiratory care units, neurosurgery units, burn units, a coronary care unit, pediatric intensive care unit, and a liver failure unit.

The effect of prophylaxis on overt bleeding derived from the 32 trials that allowed ascertainment of this endpoint are displayed in Table 41.2. The common odds ratio of 0.40 (95% CI 0.20–0.79) comparing antacids with placebo, and the common odds ratio of 0.29 (95% CI 0.17–0.45) comparing histamine-2-receptor antagonists to placebo, indicate that these two forms of

Table 41.2
Meta-analysis of Randomized Trials of Stress Ulcer Prophylaxis

Comparison	N^a	Odds Ratio (95% CI)
Antacids versus placebo control		
Overt bleeding	5	0.40 (0.20–0.79)
Clinically important bleeding	3	0.35 (0.08–1.33)
Mortality	6	1.06 (0.67–1.66)
Histamine-2-receptor antagonists versus placebo/control		
Overt bleeding	9	0.29 (0.17–0.45)[b]
Clinically important bleeding	6	0.35 (0.15–0.76)
Mortality	9	0.80 (0.54–1.18)
Antacids versus sucralfate		
Overt bleeding	9	1.19 (0.62–2.29)
Clinically important bleeding	5	0.65 (0.16–2.49)
Mortality	8	1.22 (0.83–1.79)
Antacids versus prostaglandins		
Overt bleeding	1	0.99 (0–22, 026.00)
Clinically important bleeding	2	1.04 (0.03–38.86)
Mortality	2	0.80 (0.39–1.79)
Histamine-2-receptor antagonists versus antacids		
Overt bleeding	13	0.56 (0.33–0.97)
Clinically important bleeding	9	0.84 (0.45–1.56)
Mortality	14	1.16 (0.83–1.61)
Histamine-2-receptor antagonists versus sucralfate		
Overt bleeding	4	1.77 (0.78–3.96)
Clinically important bleeding	1	0.95 (0.06–15.40)
Mortality	3	1.25 (0.61–2.58)

[a] Abbreviations used are: *N*, number of trials included in analysis; 95% CI, 95% confidence interval.
[b] Statistical heterogeneity.

prophylaxis significantly reduce overt gastrointestinal bleeding. Analysis of the nine trials allowing direct comparison of histamine-2-receptor antagonists and antacids yields a common odds ratio of 0.56 (95% CI 0.33–0.97), suggesting a benefit of histamine-2-receptor antagonists over antacids with regard to the outcome of overt bleeding. In the three trials directly comparing histamine-2-receptor antagonists to pirenzepine, the common odds ratio of 3.78 (1.33–14.45) suggests a benefit of pirenzepine over histamine-2-receptor antagonists. This anticholinergic is used in Europe, but infrequently in North America.

Next, information was abstracted from the 26 trials in which it was possible to identify the incidence of clinically important bleeding. Comparison of the prophy-

lactic agents are recorded in Table 41.2. The common odds ratio of 0.35 (95% CI 0.15–0.76) comparing histamine-2-receptor antagonists to no therapy confirms the efficacy of histamine-2-receptor antagonists in reducing the incidence of both clinically important as well as overt bleeding. The common odds ratio of 0.35 (95% CI 0.08–1.33) comparing antacid to no treatment is identical, though the effect is not statistically significant. The confidence interval around this estimate is wide because only three trials comparing antacids and no treatment are available. Therefore, when histamine-2-antagonists and antacids are compared indirectly (odds ratio for histamine-2-antagonists versus control compared to odds ratio for antacids versus control), the odds ratios are similar. Direct comparison of histamine-2-receptor antagonists with antacids for the outcome of clinically important bleeding (common odds ratio 0.84, 95% CI 0.45–1.56) suggests their equivalence.

When antacids are compared with sucralfate, the common odds ratio of 1.19 (95% CI 0.62–2.29) for overt bleeding and 0.65 (95% CI 0.16–2.49) for clinically important bleeding indicates that these two modes of prophylaxis are equally efficacious. There are only four trials comparing histamine-2-receptor antagonists with sucralfate, from which information on overt bleeding is extractable. The limited power of these trials notwithstanding, there is no significant difference between histamine-2-receptor antagonists and sucralfate with respect to clinically important bleeding (odds ratio 1.77, 95% CI 0.78–3.96).

Comparison of various prophylactic drugs in trials from which mortality rates are available (Table 41.2) shows that all of the 95% confidence intervals include unity (an odds ratio of one suggesting no treatment effect). Therefore, mortality does not appear to be reduced by stress ulcer prophylactic drugs.

These results confirm previous findings that stress ulcer prophylaxis with antacids, histamine-2-receptor antagonists, or sucralfate is associated with a 60–70% reduction in the risk of bleeding in the critically ill population. For a final decision on which agent to use, however, the costs and adverse effects of these agents must also be considered.

THE DISADVANTAGES OF STRESS ULCER PROPHYLAXIS

Adverse Effects: Histamine-2-receptor Antagonists

Numerous adverse reactions have been attributed to histamine-2-receptor antagonists. Published studies report a side effect rate of 4.5 to 17% (24). The most frequent reactions involve the gastrointestinal tract (nausea, vomiting, diarrhea, and constipation in 2.1% of cases) and central nervous system (confusion, lethargy, headache, and seizures in 1.2% of cases). Central nervous system toxicity appears to be more common in the young and the elderly and in patients with hepatic or renal disease.

Interstitial nephritis, hepatotoxicity, gynecomastia, and blood dyscrasias have been described. In addition, cimetidine inhibits the cytochrome P-450 enzyme system, thereby reducing the clearance of several drugs, including warfarin, diazepam, chlordiazepoxide, phenytoin, theophylline, and propranolol.

Case reports of bradycardia, atrioventricular block, and hypotension following infusion of histamine-2-receptor antagonists prompted randomized controlled trials designed to examine adverse hemodynamic sequelae of these agents. Although intravenous cimetidine (40) but not ranitidine (28, 66) has been associated with a significant decrease in mean arterial pressure when compared with control, randomized trials have not suggested clinically important changes in cardiac output, central venous pressure, or pulmonary artery wedge pressure (60).

Adverse Effects: Antacids

The complication rate associated with antacid administration is reportedly very low, although the frequency of adverse reactions was 36% in one study (25). The most frequent side effects associated with antacid use are altered gastrointestinal motility; magnesium-containing antacids may produce diarrhea while aluminum salts may cause constipation. The use of antacids containing aluminum, calcium, or magnesium salts can lead to small but significant increases in plasma levels of these elements, which may be of importance, particularly in patients with renal impairment. Metabolic alkalosis is a rare complication reported in less than 1% of patients enrolled in stress ulcer prophylaxis trials. However, the adverse effect rate has not been established with certainty in the critically ill population.

Adverse Effects: Sucralfate

In patients receiving sucralfate, side effects are unusual, reportedly occurring in approximately 3.6% of patients (26). The most common symptoms include constipation (2.2%) and xerostomia (0.7%), which are of little significance in most critically ill patients.

Summary of Side Effects of Stress Ulcer Prophylaxis

The side effect rate of stress ulcer prophylactic drugs has been noted primarily in the ambulatory population. Therefore, the incidence of adverse events due to stress ulcer prophylaxis in the critically ill population has not been established with certainty. Pharmacokinetics and pharmacodynamics may be altered in the critically ill due to multisystem disease. In addition, polypharmacy is common in the ICU. These problems make the identification of adverse events due to specific medications most difficult.

STRESS ULCER PROPHYLAXIS AND NOSOCOMIAL PNEUMONIA

Nosocomial Pneumonia: The Role of Gastric pH

Nosocomial pneumonia occurs in 0.5–5.0% of all hospital admissions (85). The incidence in mechanically ventilated patients is 4–21 times higher than in patients not requiring assisted ventilation (10, 16, 35). Pneumonia remains the leading cause of death from nosocomial infection (3, 25), with an associated mortality rate in ventilated patients approaching 50–60% (14, 15, 33, 83).

Colonization of the upper respiratory tract with Gram-negative bacteria is a major risk factor for the development of nosocomial pneumonia (42). Factors believed to predispose to colonization include lung disease, endotracheal intubation, diabetes, malnutrition, antibiotic therapy, and gastric acid neutralization (63).

Acid pH maintains the sterility of the stomach in the fasting state. However, in critically ill patients receiving stress ulcer prophylaxis with drugs that suppress (histamine-2-receptor antagonists) or neutralize (antacids) gastric acid, growth of intragastric Gram-negative bacteria is common (19, 20, 22, 75). Transmission of these organisms from the stomach to the respiratory tract has been well documented (2, 19, 22, 27, 44). Therefore, in patients receiving stress ulcer prophylaxis, the stomach is a potential reservoir of pathogenic bacteria that may colonize the lower respiratory tract. Aspiration of these organisms is believed to be an important mechanism in the development of nosocomial pneumonia. Furthermore, the presence of an endotracheal tube does not afford complete protection; the rate of passive aspiration may be as high as 20% (82).

Gastric pH and Pulmonary Infections

The role of gastric colonization in the development of pulmonary infection is supported by a prospective study of risk factors for pneumonia in ventilated patients (15), which showed that gastrointestinal bleeding prophylaxis using histamine-2-receptor antagonists with or without antacids was independently associated with the development of pneumonia. In another series of ventilated patients receiving stress ulcer prophylaxis with pH-altering drugs, the rate of pneumonia directly correlated with increasing gastric pH ($p < 0.025$); the incidence of pneumonia was 41% in patients whose gastric pH was less than 3.4, whereas the rate was 69% in patients whose pH was greater than 5.0 (19). This, however, could reflect the fact that the more severely ill patients were the ones receiving prophylaxis. Moreover, many critically ill patients have an increased gastric pH without prophylactic therapy. This study was limited in that its design was uncontrolled, and its small sample size was associated with wide confidence intervals.

A number of randomized controlled trials have been performed that examine the extent to which various prophylactic agents are associated with nosocomial pneumonia. Some of these have evaluated sucralfate, an agent that has cytoprotective properties but does not appreciably increase pH. Sucralfate is also efficacious in the prevention of bleeding due to stress ulceration (6, 8, 90). Although a number of these trials have been recently reviewed (96), no attempt has been made to synthesize these data in a formal quantitative manner.

A Critical Appraisal: The Association between Stress Ulcer Prophylaxis and Pneumonia

We performed a meta-analysis of the results of eight randomized clinical trials of gastrointestinal bleeding prophylaxis to evaluate the differential effect of preventive agents on the rate of nosocomial pneumonia.

Four of the eight remaining studies were published in peer-reviewed journals (21, 49, 52, 72); one of those published in peer-reviewed journals was reported in two parts. Of the other four trials, one was presented in a symposium. The remaining three studies were published in abstract form (46, 47, 76); data sets were made available to the authors in one case (R. Karlstadt, personal communication). These trials are summarized in Table 41.3.

To examine the role of gastric pH in the development of nosocomial pneumonia, we evaluated trial results according to whether or not treatment altered gastric pH. Patients receiving histamine-2-receptor antagonists or antacids showed a trend toward an increased incidence of pneumonia in three of the eight trials (21, 49, 52), and a significantly greater incidence in the fourth study (87). The remaining trials showed a trend toward (47, 72, 76) and significant decrease (46) in the rate of pneumonia with pH-altering drugs. There were systematic differences between results of these studies that bring into question the validity of aggregating data; therefore, the results of these eight studies cannot be combined.

To test the first hypothesis that titration of prophylactic therapy to achieve a specific gastric pH alters the incidence of nosocomial pneumonia, an analysis was performed examining only the three trials in which pH-altering therapy was titrated to a gastric pH of 3.5 or greater. The individual study odds ratios and common odds ratio of 0.63 (95% confidence interval 0.24–1.62) are displayed in Figure 41.1. The confidence interval crosses the odds ratio

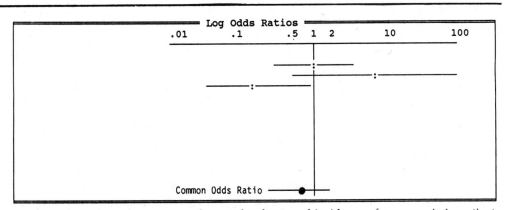

Prophylaxis Titrated to Gastric pH vs No Titration

Author	Year	Exper. Obs	Tot	Control Obs	Tot	Odds Ratio	95% CI Lo	Hi
Reusser	1989	7	19	8	21	0.95	0.27	3.37
Laggner	1989	2	16	0	16	7.90	0.47	99.99
Karlstadt	1989	0	45	6	49	0.13	0.03	0.69
Typical odds ratio and 95% CI						0.63	0.24	1.62

Figure 41.1. These data suggest a trend toward a decreased incidence of pneumonia in patients receiving stress ulcer prophylaxis that is titrated to achieve a gastric pH of 4.0 or greater. *CI*, confidence interval.

Table 41.3
Populations and Interventions of the Eight Randomized Controlled Trials of Stress Ulcer Prophylaxis that Evaluate the Outcome of Nosocomial Pneumonia

Study (year)	Driks (1987)	Tryba (1987)	Reusser (1988)	Karlstadt (1989)
No. patients and type of ICU	69 medical/surgical	100 medical/surgical	40 surgical	104 medical/surgical
Proportion ventilated	1.0	1.0	1.0	0.44
Treatment	1 g sucralfate q6h NG	1 g sucralfate q4h NG	150–200 mg i.v. ranitidine ± antacids to achieve pH >4.0	300 mg cimetidine then 50 mg/hr to achieve pH >4.0
	vs	vs	vs	vs
	Standard regimens of antacid and histamine receptor antagonists sometimes titrated to pH	10 ml antacid q2h NG	Control	Placebo

of unity (which corresponds to no beneficial or adverse treatment effect). Thus, there is no significant effect on the rate of pneumonia in patients receiving prophylactic therapy titrated to gastric pH of 3.5 or greater. It should be noted, however, that the extent to which a pH of 3.5 is achieved in these trials is uncertain. Gastric pH was significantly higher in the cimetidine group than in the placebo group in one trial (72), significantly higher in the ranitidine group than in the sucralfate group in another (52), but not explicitly reported in the third trial (46).

To examine the second hypothesis that sucralfate differs from pH-altering drugs in its effect on the incidence of pneumonia, trials comparing drugs that alter gastric pH with placebo or control were compared (Fig. 41.2). The individual odds ratios and the common odds ratio of 0.42 (95% confidence interval 0.16–10) are displayed in Figure 41.2. Although there is a trend toward a decreased rate of pneumonia in patients receiving pH-altering drugs, these results do not reach statistical significance.

Next, having established no significant difference in the incidence of pneumonia when comparing placebo/control with pH-altering drugs, trials comparing sucralfate with antacid and/or histamine-2-receptor

antagonist therapy were evaluated (Fig. 41.3). The common odds ratio associated with the use of sucralfate was 0.55 (0.28–1.06), indicating a trend toward a reduced rate of pneumonia with the prophylactic use of sucralfate as compared with pH-altering drugs.

In summary, there was no increase in the incidence of pneumonia with pH-altering drugs in comparison to placebo or no-treatment control. However, the comparison of pH-altering drugs to sucralfate revealed a significant reduction in the incidence of nosocomial pneumonia in patients receiving sucralfate. The bacteriostatic effect of sucralfate on Gram-negative organisms, which has been demonstrated in vitro, may partly explain these results (19, 88).

For a number of reasons, these findings cannot be considered conclusive. First, only eight of 48 trials evaluating stress ulcer prophylaxis either recorded or reported the outcome of nosocomial pneumonia. Thus, a publication bias may affect the results of this analysis. Examination of the methodologic quality of the individual trials reveals several other possible sources of bias. For example, although patient characteristics were similar between groups in the majority of cases, in three of the trials,

Laggner (1989)	Karlstadt (1990)	Ryan (1990)	Karlstadt (1990)
32 medical/surgical	87 medical/surgical	90 medical/surgical	13 medical/surgical
1.0	0.21	1.0	?
50 mg ranitidine q4h i.v. to achieve pH >3.5	300 mg cimetidine then 50 mg/hr	Cimetidine 900 mg/hr	300 mg cimetidine then 50–100 mg/hr
vs Sucralfate 1 g NG q4h	vs Placebo	vs Sucralfate 1 g q6h	vs Placebo

pH-altering Drugs versus Placebo/Control

Author	Year	Exper. Obs	Tot	Control Obs	Tot	Odds Ratio	95% CI Lo	Hi
Reusser	1989	7	19	8	21	0.95	0.27	3.37
Karlstadt	1989	0	45	6	49	0.13	0.03	0.68
Karlstadt	1990	1	54	0	33	5.01	0.09	99.99
Karlstadt	1990	0	56	4	61	0.12	0.00	1.92
Typical odds ratio and 95% CI						0.42	0.16	1.10

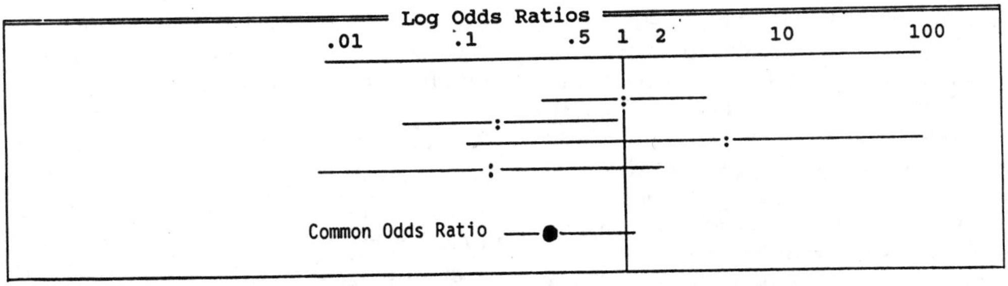

Figure 41.2. These data suggest a trend toward a decreased incidence of pneumonia in patients receiving stress ulcer prophylaxis that alters gastric pH as compared with no prophylaxis.

the patients were selected (39, 91, 93). It may be that characteristics that led patients to be selected in these trials are systematically related to the differential risk of pneumonia in patients treated with, and without, pH-altering agents. Moreover, confounding factors that could influence the incidence of pneumonia such as diabetes, immunosuppression, and chronic endotracheal intubation were always not

Sucralfate versus pH-altering Drugs

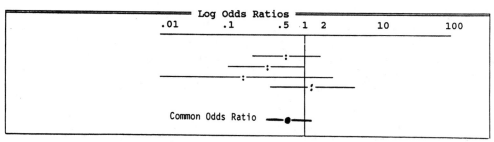

Author	Year	Exper. Obs	Tot	Control Obs	Tot	Odds Ratio	95% CI Lo	Hi
Driks	1987	7	29	16	40	0.49	0.18	1.35
Tryba	1987	3	29	11	32	0.26	0.08	0.86
Laggner	1989	0	16	2	16	0.13	0.01	2.12
Ryan	1990	8	45	6	45	1.41	0.39	5.13
Typical odds ratio and 95% CI						0.55	0.28	1.06

Figure 41.3. These data suggest a trend toward a decreased incidence of pneumonia in patients receiving sucralfate as compared with stress ulcer prophylactic drugs that increase gastric pH.

described. Perhaps more plausibly related to outcome is the fact that, in diagnosing pneumonia, blinding of the radiologist and the clinician to the treatment group was not performed in any of the trials. This lack of blinding may result in considerable bias in these studies, given the difficulty in accurately diagnosing nosocomial pneumonia in critically ill patients (1).

The proportion of patients included in this analysis with a nasogastric tube, an important risk factor for pulmonary infection (11, 63), is very high. In five of the studies, all patients had nasogastric tubes inserted; in three studies (47, 52, 72, 73), the proportion is not specifically stated but it is likely close to 1.0. Because the proportion is so high in these studies, differences in the rate of nasogastric tube placement cannot explain differences in the rate of pneumonia. Aspiration is infrequent when enteral feeding is administered through a small bore nasoenteral feeding tube (60, 86), nasogastric size was reported in only one trial (87). The location of the tip of the feeding tubes was not recorded in any of the trials. Finally, enteral feeding, which increases intragastric volume, alters gastric pH (74, 92), and increases

isolation of gastric Gram-negative bacteria (67), was not controlled in these studies.

The fact that only eight of 42 randomized trials of gastrointestinal bleeding prophylaxis provided data on the incidence of pneumonia, and the methodologic deficiencies of these studies limit the strength of the inferences that can be made from these data. A large methodologically sound prospective randomized trial examining the different approaches to stress ulcer prophylaxis while controlling for confounding risk factors for nosocomial pneumonia therefore remains warranted.

POLICY RECOMMENDATIONS

In generating clinical recommendations for the prevention of bleeding due to stress ulceration in the critically ill, the large body of literature on stress ulcer prophylaxis must be considered.

Which Agent to Use?

Antacids, histamine-2-receptor antagonists, and sucralfate all appear to decrease the incidence of clinically important gastrointestinal bleeding. The risk reduction for these three classes of drug is comparable and is approximately 60–70%. Therefore, considering only the issue of efficacy, stress ulcer prophylaxis in the crically ill patient using either antacids, histamine-2-receptor antagonists, or sucralfate is recommended.

Taking into account side effects, sucralfate has the lowest incidence of adverse reactions of all the stress ulcer prophylactic drugs. The most serious potential adverse effect of stress ulcer prophylaxis is the development of nosocomial pneumonia, which has a high morbidity and mortality rate in the critically ill. Meta-analysis of the studies available does not support the biologic rationale that patients receiving stress ulcer prophylaxis with gastric pH altering agents (antacids or histamine-2-receptor antagonists) have a higher incidence of pneumonia than those patients receiving no prophylaxis. However, there is a trend toward a decreased incidence of pneumonia with the use of sucralfate as compared to histamine-2-receptor antagonists, suggesting that sucralfate is the preferred agent in most situations. Nevertheless, the recommendation to prescribe sucralfate to the critically ill for the prevention of bleeding must be interpreted with caution because of methodologic problems in these studies and the possibility of publication bias.

There are several reasons why the widespread use of stress ulcer prophylactic agents may not be in patients' best interests. First, diverse definitions of bleeding have been employed in the trials of stress ulcer prophylaxis, ranging from bleeding that is insignificant to life threatening. The truly relevant outcome, the clinically important gastrointestinal bleeding, has not been established with certainty. Moreover, it has been suggested that the incidence of bleeding has decreased over the last decade.

What Is the Incidence of Gastrointestinal Bleeding?

Before policy implications can be discussed, the incidence of clinically important gastrointestinal bleeding must be addressed. Stress ulceration is seen endoscopically in the majority of seriously ill hospitalized patients (18, 54). Although minor upper gastrointestinal hemorrhage due to stress ulceration is a common occurrence in the critically ill patient (79), the incidence of overt bleeding is approximately 10% (34, 78).

However, the true incidence of clinically important gastrointestinal bleeding, which is accompanied by morbidity and mortality, is uncertain. Moreover, many investigators feel that the incidence of clinically important gastrointestinal bleeding, has, independent of the use of prophylaxis, decreased considerably in the last decade (69, 78). Factors responsible may include improved methods of ventilatory support, more aggressive shock management, early attention to nutrition in the critically ill, control of bleeding diatheses, and the decreasing use of steroids in septic shock.

The best evidence in support of a decrease in the incidence of clinically significant bleeding over time would come from one center in which this outcome was repeatedly evaluated over many years. No such data exist. However, information can be obtained from the 26 relevant randomized trials of prophylaxis evaluating antacids, histamine-2-receptor antagonists, and no treatment, published before and after 1980. (Sucralfate was not studied prior to 1981.) The incidence of clinically important bleeding in patients receiving no treatment was 9/75 (12.0%) before 1980 and 15/322 (4.7%) after 1980 ($p = 0.03$). Thus, clinically important bleeding in untreated patients does appear to have decreased in the last decade and is approximately 5%.

Who Should Receive Prophylaxis?

Risk factors for acute gastrointestinal ulceration in the critically ill have been derived from studies that are methodologically limited. However, it is reasonable to prophylax patients with a coagulopathy (the most important risk factor), sepsis, prolonged hypotension, chronic mechanical ventilation, hepatic failure, renal failure, burns, and central nervous system disease, and those patients with a history of upper gastrointestinal sign or symptoms of bleeding.

If a low risk group of patients were

identifiable (for example, a group with a baseline risk of less than 1%), then consideration could be made to withhold prophylaxis from this group. However, classification of ICU patients into groups with a negligible and appreciable risk of clinically important bleeding is difficult. It is probably reasonable not to prophylax patients with an anticipated short ICU stay if no risk factors for bleeding exist. Unfortunately, the characteristics of patients with a negligible risk of bleeding have not been forthcoming from the literature.

FUTURE RESEARCH

Given the declining incidence of clinically important bleeding due to stress ulceration, further studies of stress ulcer prophylaxis are needed to identify the true incidence. The characteristics of patients at low risk for gastrointestinal bleeding need to be defined, and the effect of withholding prophylaxis from this subgroup needs to be evaluated. A large multicenter natural history study of the Canadian Critical Care Trials Group addressing this issue is nearing completion.

The other trial needed in this area is a large methodologically rigorous randomized double-blind study comparing the effect of sucralfate and histamine-2-receptor antagonists on the incidence of nosocomial pneumonia. Consideration should be given to the use of the more specific and sensitive protected brush catheter for the diagnosis of nosocomial pneumonia in future trials. Assuming a baseline incidence of nosocomial pneumonia in the critically ill of 20%, a trial of 450 patients per group would be required to detect a 33% risk reduction with 80% power.

We must await the results of such a trial with interest.

References

1. Andrews CP, Coalson JJ, Smith JD, Johanson WG Jr. Diagnosis of nosocomial bacterial pneumonia in acute, diffuse lung injury. Chest 1981;80:254–258.
2. Atherton ST, White DJ. Stomach as a source of bacteria colonizing respiratory tract during artificial ventilation. Lancet 1978;ii:968–969.
3. Basso N, Baragani M, Materia A, et al. Cimetidine and antacid prophylaxis of acute upper gastrointestinal bleeding in high risk patients. Am J Surg 1981;141:339–341.
4. Boissel JP, Blanchard J, Panak E, et al. Considerations for the meta-analysis of randomized clinical trials. Controlled Clin Trials 1989;10:254–281.
5. Borrero E, Margolis IB, Bank S. Antacid versus sucralfate in preventing acute gastrointestinal bleeding. Am J Surg 1984;148:809–812.
6. Borrero E, Bank S, Margolis IB, et al. Comparison of antacid and sucralfate in the prevention of gastrointestinal bleeding in patients who are critically ill. Am J Med 1985;79(2C):62–64.
7. Borrero E, Ciervo J, Chang JB. Antacid versus sucralfate in preventing acute gastrointestinal tract bleeding in abdominal-aortic surgery. Arch Surg 1986;121:810–812.
8. Bresalier RS, Grendell JH, Cello, JP et al. Sucralfate suspension versus titrated antacids in the prophylaxis of acute stress-related gastrointestinal hemorrhage in critically ill patients. Am J Med 1987;83(3B):110–116.
9. Cannon LA, Heiselman DE, Gardner WG, et al. Prophylaxis of upper gastrointestinal tract bleeding in mechanically ventilated patients. Arch Intern Med 1987;147:2101–2106.
10. Celis R, Torres A, Gatell JM, Almella M, Rodriguez-Roisin R, Agusti-Vidal A. Nosocomial pneumonia: a multivariate analysis of risk and prognosis. Chest 1988;93:318–324.
11. Cheadle WG, Vitale GC, Mackie CR, Cushieri A. Prophylactic postoperative nasogastric decompression. Ann Surg 1985;202:361–365.
12. Cook DJ, Cook RJ, Pearl RG, Guyatt GH. The incidence of clinically important bleeding due to stress ulceration in the critically ill. J Intens Care Med (in press).
13. Cook DJ, Witt LG, Cook RJ, Guyatt GH. Stress ulcer prophylaxis in the critically ill—a meta-analysis. Am J Med 1991;91:519–527.
14. Craven DE, Driks MR. Nosocomial pneumonia in the intubated patient. Semin Respir Infect 1987;21(1):20–33.
15. Craven DE, Kunches LM, Kilinsky V, Lichtenberg DA, Make BJ, McCabe WR. Risk factors for pneumonia and fatality in patients receiving continuous mechanical ventilation. Am Rev Respir Dis 1986;133:792–796.
16. Cross AS, Roup B. Role of respiratory assistance devices in endemic nosocomial pneumonia. Am J Med 1981;70:681–685.
17. Curling TB. On acute ulceration of duodenum in cases of burn. Medico-Chirurgical Transactions London 1842;25:260.
18. Czaja AJ, McAlhany JC, Pruitt BA. Acute gastroduodenal disease after thermal injury: an endoscopic evaluation of incidence and natural history. N Engl J Med 1974;291:925–929.
19. Daschner F, Kappstein I, Engles I, Reuschenbach K, Pfisterer J, Kreig N, et al. Stress ulcer prophylaxis and ventilation pneumonia: prevention by antibacterial cytoprotective agents. Infect Control Hosp Epidemiol 1988;9:59–65.
20. Donowitz LG, Page MC, Mileur BL, Guenthner SH. Alteration of normal gastric flora in critical care patients receiving antacid and cimetidine therapy. Infect Control 1986;7:23–26.

21. Driks MR, Craven DE, Celli BR, et al. Nosocomial pneumonia in intubated patients given sucralfate as compared with antacids or histamine type 2 blockers. N Engl J Med 1987;317(22):1376–1382.

22. du Moulin GC, Paterson DG, Hedley-Whyte J, Lisbon A. Aspiration of gastric bacteria in antacid-treated patients: a frequent cause of postoperative colonization of the airway. Lancet 1982;i:242–245.

23. Fogelman MJ, Garvey JM. Acute gastrointestinal ulceration incident to surgery and disease: analysis and review of eighty-eight cases. Am J Surg 1966;112:651–656.

24. Freston JW. Cimetidine: adverse reactions and patterns of use. Ann Intern Med 1982;97:728–734.

25. Friedman CJ, Oblinger MJ, Surrat PM, et al. Prophylaxis of upper gastrointestinal hemorrhage in patients requiring mechanical ventilation. Crit Care Med 1982;10:316–319.

26. Garnett WR. Sucralfate—alternative therapy for peptic ulcer disease. Clin Pharm 1982;1:307–314.

27. Garvey BM, McCambley JA, Tuxen DV. Effects of gastric alkalinization on bacterial colonization in critically ill patients. Crit Care Med 1989;17:211–216.

28. Goelzer SL, Farin-Rush C, Coursin DB. Ranitidine produces minimal hemodynamic depression in stable intensive care unit patients: a double-blind prospective study. Crit Care Med 1988; 16(1):8–10.

29. Goodman AA, Frey CF. Massive upper gastrointestinal hemorrhage following surgical operation. Ann Surg 1968;167:180–184.

30. Gottlieb JE, Menashe PI, Cruz E. Gastrointestinal complications in critically ill patients: the intensivist's overview. Am J Gastroenterol 1986; 81(4):227–238.

31. Greene WL, Bollinger RR. Cimetidine for stress-ulcer prophylaxis. Crit Care Med 1984;12(7):571–575.

32. Groll A, Simon JB, Wigle RD, et al. Cimetidine prophylaxis for gastrointestinal bleeding in an intensive care unit. Gut 1986;27:135–140.

33. Gross PA, Neu HC, Aswapokee P, Van Antwerpen C, Aswapokee N. Deaths from nosocomial infection: experience in a university hospital and a community hospital. Am J Med 1980;68:219–223.

34. Gurman G, Samri M, Bearman JE, et al. The rate of gastrointestinal bleeding in a general ICU population: a retrospective study. Intensive Care Med 1990;16:44–49.

35. Haley RW, Hooton TM, Culver DH, Stanley RC, Emori JG, Hardison CD, et al. Nosocomial infections in U.S. hospitals, 1975–1976: estimated frequency by selected characteristics of patients. Am J Med 1981;70:947–959.

36. Harris SK, Bone RC, Ruth WE. Gastrointestinal hemorrhage in patients in a respiratory care unit. Chest 1977;72:301–304.

37. Hastings PR, Skillman JJ, Bushnell LS, et al. Antacid titration in the prevention of acute gastrointestinal bleeding. N Engl J Med 1978;298:1041–1045.

38. Hauser A, Quigley L, Driever CW, et al. More on false positive "hemoccult" reaction with cimetidine [Letter]. N Engl J Med 1981;304:847.

39. Hillman K. Acute stress ulceration. Anaesth Intensive Care 1985;13:230.

40. Iberti TJ, Paulch TA, Helmer L, et al. The hemodynamic effects of intravenous cimetidine in intensive care units: a double-blind prospective study. Anesthesiology 1986;64:87.

41. Jmelnitzky AC, Moday MC, Gallardo EA, et al. Prophylaxis of acute gastric hemorrhage from stress induced lesions—comparison of pirenzipine and cimetidine in intensive care units [Abstract]. Dig Dis Sci 1986;31(10):A814.

42. Johanson WG, Pierce AK, Sanford JP, Thomas GD. Nosocomial respiratory infections with gram negative bacilli: the significance of colonization of the respiratory tract. Ann Intern Med 1982; 77:701–706.

43. Kahn F, Parekh A, Chitkara R, et al. Results of gastric neutralization with hourly antacids and cimetidine in 320 intubated patients with respiratory failure. Chest 1981;79:409–412.

44. Kahn RJ, Serruys-Schoutens E, Brimioulle S, Vincent J-L. Influence of antacid treatment on the tracheal flora in mechanically ventilated patients [Abstract]. Crit Care Med 1982;10:A:229.

45. Kamada T, Fusamoti H, Kawano S, et al. Gastrointestinal bleeding following head injury: a clinical study of 433 cases. J Trauma 1977;17:44–47.

46. Karlstadt R, Herson J, Palmer R, et al. Cimetidine reduces upper gastrointestinal bleeding and nosocomial pneumonia in intensive care unit patients [Abstract]. Am J Gastroenterol 1989; 84(9):A93.

47. Karlstadt R, D'Ambrosio C, McCafferty J, Palmer R, Rockhold F, Fox M. Cimetidine is effective prophylaxis against upper gastrointestinal bleeding in the intensive care unit. World Congress of Gastroenterology, Sydney, Australia, September 1990.

48. Karlstadt R, Frank W, Palmer R, et al. Comparison of cimetidine and placebo in the prophylaxis of stress bleeding. J Intensive Care Med 1990; 5:226–232.

49. Karlstadt RG, Iberti TJ, Silverstein J, Lindenberg L, Bright-Asare P, Rockhold F, et al. Comparison of cimetidine and placebo for the prophylaxis of upper gastrointestinal bleeding due to stress-related gastric mucosal damage in the intensive care unit. J Intensive Care Med 1990;5:226–232.

50. Kingsley AN. Prophylaxis for acute stress ulcers: antacids or cimetidine. Am Surg 1985;51(9):545–547.

51. Lacroix J, Infante-Rivard C, Gauthier M, et al. Upper gastrointestinal tract bleeding acquired in a pediatric intensive care unit: prophylaxis trial with cimetidine. J Pediatr 1986:108:1015–1018.

52. Laggner AN, Lenz K, Base W, Drume W, Schneeweiss B, Grimm G. Prevention of upper gastrointestinal bleeding in long term ventilated patients: sucralfate versus ranitidine. Am J Med 1989;86(suppl 6A):81–84.

53. Layne EA, Mellow MH, Lipman TO. Insensitivity

to guaiac slide tests for detection of blood in gastric juice. Ann Intern Med 1981;94:774–776.

54. Lucas CE, Sugawa C, Riddel J, et al. Natural history and surgical dilemma of stress gastric bleeding. Arch Surg 1971;102:266.

55. MacDougall BRD, Bailey RJ, Williams R. Histamine-2-receptor antagonists and antacids in the prevention of acute gastrointestinal hemorrhage in fulminant hepatic failure. Lancet 1977;1:617–619.

56. Martin LF, Max MH, Polk HC. Failure of gastric pH control by antacids or cimetidine in the critically ill: a valid sign of sepsis. Surgery 1980;88(1):59–68.

57. Mattes P, Peros S, Belohlavek D, et al. Stresulkus-prophylaxe mit pirenzipin—eine kontrollierte studie. Z Gastroenterologie 1980;18:325–327.

58. McAlhany JC, Czaja AJ, Pruitt B. Antacid control of complications from acute gastrointestinal disease after burns. J Trauma 1976;16:645–649.

59. McElwee HP, Sirinek KR, Levine BA. Cimetidine affords protection equal to antacids in prevention of stress ulceration following thermal injury. Surgery 1979;86(4):620–626.

60. Metheny NA, Eisenberg P, Spies M. Aspiration pneumonia in patients fed through nasoenteral tubes. Heart and Lung 1986;15:256–261.

61. More DG, Raper RF, Watson CJ, et al. Combination therapy with ranitidine and pirenzepine for control of intragastric pH in the critically ill. Crit Care Med 1985;13:651–655.

62. Mundinger GH, Hays A, Allo M, et al. Effect of meciadanol and sucralfate as compared with antacid titration regimen on prevention of acute gastrointestinal hemorrhage in post-operative intensive care patients. Surg Forum 1985;36:121–123.

63. Niederman MS, Craven DE, Fein AM, Schultz DE. Pneumonia in the critically ill hospitalized patient. Chest 1990;97(1):170–181.

64. Norfleet RG, Rhodes RA, Saviage K. False positive "hemoccult" reaction with cimetidine. N Engl J Med 1980;302:467.

65. Noseworthy TRW, Shustack A, Johnston RG, et al. A randomized clinical trial comparing ranitidine and antacids in critically ill patients. Crit Care Med 1987;15(9):817–819.

66. Onofrey D, Kelly KM, Gentili DR, et al. The hemodynamic effects of intravenous ranitidine in intensive care unit patients: a double blind prospective study. J Clin Pharmacol 1988;28:1098–1100.

67. Pingleton SK, Hinthorn D, Lui C. Enteral nutrition in patients receiving mechanical ventilation. Am J Med 1986;80:827–832.

68. Pinilla JC, Oleniuk FH, Reed D, et al. Does antacid prophylaxis prevent upper gastrointestinal bleeding in critically ill patients? Crit Care Med 1985;13:646–650.

69. Polesky H, Spanier AH. Cimetidine versus antacids in the prevention of stress erosions in critically ill patients. Am J Gastroenterol 1986;81(2):107–111.

70. Preibe HJ, Skillman JJ. Methods of prophylaxis in stress ulcer disease. World J Surg 1981;5:223–233.

71. Preibe HJ, Skillmann JJ, Bushnell LS, et al. Antacid versus cimetidine in preventing acute gastrointestinal bleeding. N Engl J Med 1980;302:425–427.

72. Reusser P, Gyr K, Scheidegger D, et al. A randomized controlled endoscopic study of ranitidine and antacids for the prevention of gastroduodenal stress lesions and bleeding in critically ill patients. Gastroenterology 1988;94(5):Part 2,A:373.

73. Reusser P, Zimmerli W, Scheidegger D, et al. Role of gastric colonization in nosocomial infections and endotoxemia: a prospective study in neurosurgical patients on mechanical ventilation. J Infect Dis 1989;160(3):414–421.

74. Rigaud D, Chastre J, Accary JP, Bonfils S, Gibert C, Hance AJ. Intragastric pH profile during acute respiratory failure in patients with chronic obstructive pulmonary disease. Chest 1986;90:58–62.

75. Ruddell WSJ, Axon ATR. Effect of cimetidine on the gastric bacterial flora. Lancet 1980;672–674.

76. Ryan P, Dawson J, Teres D, Navab F. Continuous infusion of cimetidine versus sucralfate: incidence of pneumonia and bleeding compared. Crit Care Med 1990;18(4)(suppl):S253.

77. Schentag JJ. False positive "hemoccult" reaction with cimetidine. N Engl J Med 1980;303:110.

78. Schuster DP, Rowley H, Feinstein S, et al. Prospective evaluation of the risk of upper gastrointestinal bleeding after admission to a medical intensive care unit. Am J Med 1984;76:623–630.

79. Shuman RB, Schuster DP, Zuckermann GR. Prophylactic therapy for stress ulcer bleeding: a reappraisal. Ann Intern Med 1987;106:562–567.

80. Skillman JJ, Bushnell LS, Goldman H et al. Respiratory failure, hypotension, sepsis and jaundice: a clinical syndrome associated with lethal hemorrhage from acute stress ulceration of the stomach. Am J Surg 1969;117:523–530.

81. Skillman JJ, Lisbon A, Long PC, et al. 15(R)-15-methyl prostaglandin E2 does not prevent gastrointestinal bleeding in seriously ill patients. Am J Surg 1984;147:451–455.

82. Spray SB, Zuidema GD, Cameron JL. Aspiration pneumonia: incidence of aspiration with endotracheal tubes. Am J Surg 1976;131:701–703.

83. Stevens RM, Teres D, Skillman JJ, Feingold DS. Pneumonia in an intensive care unit: a thirty month experience. Arch Intern Med 1974;134:106–111.

84. Stothert JC, Siminowitz DA, Dellinger EP, et al. Randomized prospective evaluation of cimetidine and antacid control of gastric pH in the critically ill. Ann Surg 1980;192:169–173.

85. Tobin MJ, Grenvik A. Nosocomial lung infection and its diagnosis. Crit Care Med 1984;12(3):191–199.

86. Treolar DM, Stechmiller J. Pulmonary aspiration in tube-fed patients with artificial airways. Heart Lung 1984;13:667–671.

87. Tryba M. Risk of acute stress bleeding and nosocomial pneumonia in ventilated intensive care unit patients: sucralfate versus antacids. Am J Med 1987;83:117–124.

88. Tryba M, Mantey-Stiers F. Antibacterial activity of sucralfate in human gastric juice. Am J Med 1987;83(suppl 3B):125–127.

89. Tryba M, Hurchzermeyer H, Torok M, et al. Single-drug and combined medication with cimetidine, antacids and pirenzipine in the prophylaxis of acute upper gastrointestinal bleeding. Hepatogastroenterology 1983;20:154.

90. Tryba M, Zevounou F, Torok M, et al. Prevention of acute stress bleeding with sucralfate, antacids or cimetidine. Am J Med 1985:79(2C):55–61.

91. Tryba M, Zevounou F, Wruck. Stresblutungen und postoperative pneumonien bei intensivpatienten unter ranitidin oder pirenzepin. Dtsch Med Wschr 1988;113(21):930–936.

92. Valentine RJ, Turner WW, Borman DR, Weigelt JA. Does nasoenteral feeding afford adequate gastroduodenal stress prophylaxis? Crit Care Med 1986;14:599–601.

93. Van den Berg B, Van Blankenstein M. Prevention of stress-induced gastrointestinal bleeding by cimetidine in patients on assisted ventilation. Digestion 1985:31:1–8.

94. Van Essen HA, Van Blankenstein M, Wilson P, et al. Intragastric prostaglandin E2 and the prevention of gastrointestinal hemorrhage in ICU patients. Crit Care Med 1985;13(11):957–960.

95. Weigelt LA, Aurbakken CM, Geweitz BL, et al. Cimetidine versus antacid in prophylaxis for stress ulceration. Arch Surg 1981;116–597–601.

96. Wenzel RP. Hospital-acquired pneumonia: overview of the current state of the art for prevention and control. Eur J Clin Microbiol Infect Dis 1989;8(1):56–60.

97. Wilcox CM, Spenney JG. Stress ulcer prophylaxis in medical patients: who, what and how much? Am J Gastroenterol 1988;83:1199–1211.

98. Zinner MJ, Zuidema GD, Smith PL, et al. The prevention of upper gastrointestinal tract bleeding in patients in an intensive care unit. Surg Gynecol Obstet 1981:153:214–220.

99. Zinner MJ, Rypins EB, Martin L, et al. Misoprostol versus antacid titration for preventing stress ulcers in postoperative surgical ICU patients. Ann Surg 1989;210(5):590–595.

42

Acute Abdominal Processes

Jacques Belghiti
Y. Panis

MECHANICAL OBSTRUCTION OF THE INTESTINES

Paralytic ileus may develop in patients with inflammatory process of abdominal viscera, in patients with obstruction of both small intestine or large bowel, but also in some patients without any obstruction. In this latter case, intestinal pseudoobstruction can be due to abnormal reflex mechanisms that impair intestinal contractility and that result from temporary local or distant disorders, such as pancreatitis, acute cholecystitis, renal colic, sepsis, acute respiratory failure, or myocardial infarction. It may also follow general abdominal surgery. Acute pseudoobstruction is self-limited and is resolved when the inciting event disappears. The purpose of this chapter is to discuss only mechanical intestinal obstruction.

Acute Small Intestinal Obstruction

Pathophysiology

Once the small bowel occlusion is completed, gas (due not only to air swallowing but also to sugar fermentation, blood diffusion, and produced CO_2) and fluid begin to collect, leading to bowel distension. Later, increase of bowel lumen pressure compromises the capillary system leading to alteration of fluid reabsorption by the small bowel; furthermore, secretion into the lumen is increased. Transudation of fluids into the peritoneal cavity causes a reduction of the extracellular fluid volume with potential hypovolemia, oliguria, and more rarely shock. Vomiting contributes to increased depletion of extracellular vol-

ume. Biochemical abnormalities are uncommon, because electrolyte concentrations are the same in both intestinal and extracelular fluid, except in the case of duodenal obstruction, which leads to a hypokalemic alkalosis (60).

Necrosis of the affected segment may occur very early in the case of strangulation obstruction (where vascularization is primarily altered), but not in other cases (lumen obstruction or external compression), where blood supply is not primarily altered.

Acute small intestinal obstruction in adults is caused most commonly by postoperative adhesion, followed by external hernia, carcinoma, internal hernia, intussusception, and volvulus (32).

Clinical, Biological, and Radiological Features

Symptoms include abdominal pain, vomiting, abdominal distension, and absence of spontaneous evacuation of flatus or stool. Symptoms depend on the anatomical site and the degree (complete or not) of obstruction.

The pain is relatively sudden in onset, severe, and intermittent. Pain and vomiting are more severe if the site of obstruction is high. In some patients the initial response to acute obstruction is to expel intestinal contents beyond the point of obstruction. Temperature, pulse rate, and respiratory rate are normal in the early stages and become altered when there is significant reduction of extracellular volume. The abdomen must be examined for the presence of scars of a previous operation or injury. The inguinal and femoral areas must be examined for the presence of a hernia. Abdominal distension is variable; auscultation may reveal increased bowel sounds. An elevated white blood cell count is common and the hematocrit may increase when vomiting has led to significant loss of extracellular fluid.

Roentgenographic study of the abdomen is important for the diagnosis of intestinal obstruction demonstrating an abnormal pattern of gas within the small bowel with air-fluid levels visible when the patient is examined in an upright position and the absence of gas in the large bowel.

Treatment
Initial Medical Treatment

Medical treatment prepares the patient for operation; it includes electrolyte and fluid correction and intestinal decompression by nasogastric intubation.

Surgical Treatment

Laparotomy is mandatory in the majority of cases. Surgical treatment depends on the etiology; however, complete small bowel exploration must be performed and all the adhesions must be lysed. After careful evaluation of small bowel viability, partial resection must be done if necessary. Retrograde decompression of the bowel through nasogastric intubation is done to facilitate abdominal wall closure.

Large Bowel Obstruction
Pathophysiology

Obstruction of the large intestine is caused in most patients by carcinoma of the distal portion of the colon (up to 80% of the cases). Other causes included volvulus of the colon, sigmoid diverticulitis, and fecal impaction (60).

Large bowel dilatations by air and fluid sequestration occur but extracellular fluid reduction (and its consequences) seen in acute small bowel obstruction is observed only in neglected cases. If the ileocecal valve remains competent, progressive colonic dilatation ultimately can cause cecal "diastatic" perforation.

Clinical and Radiological Features

Symptoms include abdominal pain, abdominal distention, and obstipation and later vomiting. Sigmoid volvulus presents an acute problem with sudden pain, acute and marked abdominal distension and failure to pass either gas or stools. On the other hand, when colon carcinoma or diverticulitis is the cause of obstruction, the patient gives a history of progressive constipation, and after a few days of failure to defecate, the patient complains of distension. Nausea and vomiting are present in patients with large bowel obstruction but are less prominent than in small bowel obstruction. The chief feature of examination of the patient is distension of the abdomen.

Roentgenographic study of the abdomen shows distension of the colon down to the point of obstruction with little or no small bowel dilatation (or major small bowel dilatation, which can be due not only to an incompetent ileocecal valve, but also due to associated ileus obstruction or ileus adherence to the colonic disease). A barium enema will clarify the site and cause of obstruction. In the case of sigmoid volvulus, a massive distended portion of large bowel centrally located is observed.

Treatment
Initial Medical Treatment

Medical treatment prepares the patient for operation; it includes electrolyte and fluid correction and intestinal decompression by nasogastric intubation.

Surgical Treatment

In the case of sigmoid volvulus, passage of a soft rubber tube relieves the obstruction and allows preparation for elective surgery. In other cases, laparotomy is mandatory and a variety of operations can be performed according to the type and site of obstruction: primary cecostomy or colostomy without resection (as the first step of a "staged" procedure), and colonic resection with or without anastomosis.

ACUTE CHOLECYSTITIS AND CHOLANGITIS

Acute Cholecystitis

Pathology and Clinical Features

Inflammation of the gallbladder can be acute or chronic. It can be associated with stones (calculous cholecystitis) or occur in their absence (acalculous). This chapter deals only with acute cholecystitis.

Acute Calculous Cholecystitis

Acute obstructive cholecystitis (calculous) results from cystic duct obstruction by a stone impacted in the cystic duct, or more often in Hartman's pouch. However, the clinical observation that chronic cystic duct obstruction leads to hydrops of the gallbladder rather than to acute cholecystitis suggests that factors other than obstruction are critical in the pathogenesis of calculous cholecystitis (22). The mechanism by which cholecystitis develops in patients with gallstones is probably due to distension of the gallbladder with edema and impairment of venous return, with the possibility of developing ischemia. Other factors such as alteration in gallbladder biliary lipid composition (i.e., cholesterol saturated bile) and local release of inflammatory agents (i.e., lysolecithin, leukocytic substances) contribute to the pathogenesis of acute cholecystitis (15). The gallbladder becomes acutely inflamed, due rather to chemical phenomen (i.e., phospholipase, prostaglandins) than to bacterial origin. Infected gallbladder bile is encountered later on, during the second week of the disease, and approximately half of the patients have positive bile cultures (15). The most common organisms found, of intestinal origin, are *Escherichia coli*, *Streptococcus faecalis*, and *Klebsiella pneumoniae*. Rarely anaerobes are observed: *Bacteroides fragilis* and *Clostridium perfringens* (29). Clinical signs and symptoms of acute cholecystitis are variable and nonspecific. Acute presentation can be preceded by chronic right hypochondrium pain over several months to years. Typically, acute presentation includes persistent right upper-quadrant or epigastric pain that may radiate to the back, fever, nausea, and vomiting. Physical examination reveals localized tenderness in the right upper quadrant associated with guarding and rebound. Mild jaundice may be present in up to 20% of the patients. Laboratory findings include raised leukocyte levels, and in somes cases, raised transaminase levels. Mildly elevated serum bilirubin level and/or serum alkaline phosphatase can be due to associated common bile duct stones and/or to infectious hepatic dysfunction (58). At ultrasound examination, in the presence of gallstones, with a thickened gallbladder wall, 3 mm or more in thickness, and/or Murphy sign, the positive predictive value for acute cholecystitis exceeds 90% (7). However, such wall thickening is nonspecific and can be observed in cases of ascites, portal hypertension, or hepatitis. (59).

Other clinical forms include acute emphysematous, gangrenous suppurative, and perforated cholecystitis. Acute emphysematous cholecystitis is a severe fulminant form caused by a mixed infection including gas-forming organisms (which can be outlined by plain x-ray). It is usually, but not always, acalculous. It is more often observed in males (70%) and diabetics (38). Marked deterioration in the general condition and peripheral circulatory failure are the most common features (15). The gallbladder is usually gangrenous at laparotomy. Bile cultures are positive in 90% of cases with clostridial organisms in 50%, and mortality exceeds 20%. Gangrene and/or localized perforation of the gallbladder with pericholecystic collection and abscess are seen in 5–10% of the patients. Grangrene is more often seen in the elderly and debilitated. Empyema (suppurtative cholecystitis) is rare, seen in 2% of the patients, particuarly in elderly patients; aerobic cultures of the gallbladder contents are positive in 80%. Generalized peritonitis by free perforation is less frequently encountered, approximately in 2% of the patients, and carries a high mortality rate of 30–50% in the reported series (15).

Acute Acalculous Cholecystitis

Acute inflammation can occur without stones in up to 15% of acute cholecystitis (14). Patients at risk are critically ill patients (i.e., multiple trauma, burns, severe sepsis, major surgery) (14). In these patients, dehydratation, prolonged fasting, and narcotic analgesic administration contributed to bile stasis, gallbladder distension, mucosal injury, and vascular occlusion, leading to acute inflammation of the gallbladder. Other factors include: prolonged intravenous hyperalimentation, multiple blood transfusions, mechanical ventilation with positive end-expiratory pressure, and hypersensitivity reaction to some antibiotics (42). Clinical presentation is often insidious: fever, right upper quadrant pain, tenderness, and leukocytosis are the most common features (15). Jaundice and abnormal liver functions test (i.e., raised in alkaline phosphatase, transaminases) are observed in up to 50% of cases (14). Organisms found on bile culture are the same as those found for calculous cholecystitis (16). Ultrasound seems to be superior to scintigraphy and CT for diagnosis of acalculous cholecystitis (39). Ultrasound signs include gallbladder distension, sludge, wall thickening, pericholecystic fluid, and subserosal edema. Reported mortality ranged between 6.5% and 44% due to delayed diagnosis and treatment in debilitated patients (39).

Specific Clinical Settings

In elderly patients, the disease is often diagnosed late because of minimal signs and is associated with a high complication rate (empyema, perforation) carrying a high mortality rate (18). In cirrhotic patients, despite a higher incidence of cholelithiasis, cholecystitis is a very rare situation and often misdiagnosed with others causes of sepsis and jaundice in cirrhotic patients. Inapproprite cholecystectomy carries a very high mortality rate in these patients (2). In diabetic patients, acute cholecystitis is associated with a higher incidence of infection-related complications and supports the need for aggressive treatment in terms of antibiotics coverage and early operation (15). In children, cholecystitis is uncommon and hemolytic diseases (spherocytosis, sickle cell anemia) are encountered in up to 30% of cases (27, 144). In patients with acquired immunodeficiency syndrome, acalculous cholecystitis is fre-

quently associated with cholangitis; however, its pathogenesis remains unknown (30).

Treatment

Initial Medical Treatment

In all patients, medical treatment is begun with parenteral antibiotics. The choice of antibiotics depends on the severity and the clinical setting. At the present time, we use, as do many other centers, a third generation cephalosporin (i.e., cefotaxime, 3 g/day) or a new generation of penicillin (Augmentin, 3 g/day). In cases of severe infection, particularly in elderly patients and in patients with presumed gangrenous cholecystitis, metronidazole (1 g/day) is added to cephalosporin.

Surgical Treatment

At the present time, conventional cholecystectomy through subcostal incision remains the treatment of choice for acute cholecystitits. However, recent studies reported somes cases of laparoscopic cholecystectomies for acute cholecystitis, and intraoperative conversion from laparoscopic to conventional open cholecystectomy due to inflammatory process was reported in only 5% of the cases; however, this new procedure must be carefully evaluated, especially in acute cholecystitis, because of the 0.5% reported risk of bile duct injury during laparoscopic surgery, slightly higher than during conventional surgery (54).

The optimal timing for cholecystectomy in acute cholecystitis remains controversial. Urgent cholecystectomoy is mandatory in the case of progressive/life-threatening disease: deterioration in the general condition, no improvement after 24 hr of medical management, signs of biliary peritonitis, and gas in the gallbladder. Complete cholecystectomy and operative cholangiography is performed only if identification of the cystic duct is easy; otherwise, only the gallbladder fundus is removed and Hartmann's pouch is left in place, drained by Petzer's drain. In very high risk patients with acalculous cholecystitis, percutaneous cholecystostomy is sometimes the only treatment.

In other cases, early cholecystectomy is the treatment of choice. The patient is operated on after 48–72 hr of parenteral antibiotics, after the onset of their symptoms. Several studies have demonstrated the benefit from this procedure compared to delayed cholecystectomy (after 2 or 3 months of latency), which increased the risk of further acute attack up to 24% (15, 33). During operation, a high incidence of associated common bile duct stones requires intraoperative cholangiography. After cholecystectomy, the need for subhepatic drainage remains controversial. Several reports have clearly demonstrated that drainage after cholecystectomy increases postoperative infections and length of hospital stay (15). In recent reports, operative mortality ranged from 2 to 3%, and morbidity from 5 to 15% (especially wound infections) (47).

Cholangitis
Pathology and Clinical Features

Cholangitis is defined as infection of both the extra- and intrahepatic biliary tree. This infection is usually the result of partial obstruction of the bile duct by calculi, malignant lesions, and parasites. Increased causes of cholangitis are due to stenosis of bilioenteric anastomosis, biliary percutaneous or endoscopic exploration, and biliary drainage catheters. The pathophysiology of the sepsis is believed to be an ascending invasion of the partially obstructed common bile duct. Complete obstruction by a malignant lesion of the biliary tree is much less likely to be associated with cholangitis than are stones or endoprotheses (52). Important factors in the pathogenesis of cholangitis are increased intraductal pressure and the presence of bacteria in bile. Infection of stagnant bile may occur by way of direct ascent from the gut, from portal venous blood, or by way of lymphatics. Reflux of infected bile into lymphatics and hepatic sinusoids results in bacteriema. As a consequence of infection, liver microabscesses may occur. Commonly encountered bacteria in cholangitis are enteric and often polymicrobial. These include *E. coli, S. faecalis* (enterococcus), and *Klebsiella* species. Anaerobes are rarely observed (23, 29).

Clinically, patients with cholangitis present with fever and chills, right upper quadrant pain, and jaundice. The typical triad of associated pain, fever, and jaundice, appearing within 48 hr, is present in 50–70% of cases (6). In somes cases, early diagnosis can be difficult when one or two symptoms are predominant. Severe sepsis can be associated with mental obtundation, hypotension, renal failure, thrombocytopenia, hypoglycemia, and liver abscess (48). Laboratory findings include raised leukocyte levels and abnormal liver function tests. Blood cultures are positive in 40% of cases.

Treatment

Standard therapy for cholangitis includes fluid resuscitation, parenteral antibiotics, and biliary drainage.

Because severe cholangitis can be life-threatening, fluid resuscitation should be monitored and proper choice of antibiotics (after blood cultures are performed) is important. The choice of antibiotics depends on factors including antibacterial spectrum, toxicity, and biliary excretion. Although some antibiotics are preferentially excreted into bile, those that achieved adequate tissue levels are preferred (31). As many patients with cholangitis are already at increased risk of developing renal problems, aminoglycoside administration is unwarranted. A third generation cephalosporin (i.e., cefotaxime, 3 g/day) or a new generation of penicillin (3 g/day) are effective in most cases. If concomitant anaerobic infection is suspected (malignant diseases, endoprotheses, and in elderly patients), metronidazole (1 g/day) is added (29). For the infrequent patient who does not respond to the initial medical treatment, emergency measures are indicated to decompress the biliary tree. Endoscopic sphincterotomy is the treatment of choice for patients with common duct stones and in some with ampullary carcinoma. Percutaneous drainage is indicated in patients with bilioenteric anastomosis and if endoscopic sphincterotomy is not feasible. Failure to accomplish nonoperative drainage indicates the need for an emergency surgical procedure with biliary T-tube drainage (without removal of calculi in very high risk patients) or bilioenteric anastomosis. (9).

Most patients presenting with acute cholangitis will respond to antibiotics within 24–48 hr (52). Diagnostic studies and operation must be delayed 48 hr after the onset of sepsis (9). Then the etiological treatment of cholangitis can be performed electively.

PERITONITIS AND ABDOMINAL ABSCESSES

The peritoneal cavity normally contains less than 100 ml of fluid, which has a lubricating function. Peritonitis is an inflammation of the peritoneum and can be divided into primary, secondary, and tertiary peritonitis. The most frequently encountered type is an acute bacterial inflammation of the peritoneum secondary to contamination. Abscesses are well-defined collections of pus, which are walled off from the rest of the peritoneal cavity.

Peritonitis

Primary Peritonitis

Primary peritonitis is defined as a diffuse peritoneal infection without an apparent intraabdominal source. It occurs in young girls, in cirrhotic patients, and in patients with continuous ambulatory dialysis.

Primary peritonitis in young girls occurs predominantly in childhood between the fifth and the ninth years and is caused by *Streptococcus penumoniae* (28). Possible routes of infection are ascending infection via the genital tract. Chills and vomiting develop abruptly with a fever of 39–40°C. The abdomen is diffusely tender and moderately distended. The white blood cell count is markedly elevated, often with a count over 30,000 cells/mm^2. The diagnosis is made by culture of the peritoneal fluid obtained by paracentesis. The most important consideration in the differential diagnosis is a perforation of acute appendicitis. If a Gram-negative organism is found, a surgically correctable lesion could not be excluded, and a diagnostic exploratory laparotomy is usually performed. Antibiotic therapy through systemic administration should be directed at the isolated organism. Penicillin or ampicillin plus one aminoglycoside could be used as empirical therapy until the return of bacteriological samples.

Primary peritonitis in cirrhotic patients is a common complication in patients with chronic liver disease and ascites. Deficiencies in the host defense mechanisms of cirrhotic patients that predispose to bacterial infection are impairment of Kuppfer cell function, impaired leukocyte chemotaxis and cell-mediated immunity, low serum level of complement, and defective opsonization (1). The ascitic fluid protein content in patients who developed spontaneous peritonitis was significantly lower than in those patients with sterile ascites (51). Ascitic fluid is probably infected by hematogenous seeding from the urinary and respiratory tract. A single organism is cultured form 90% of cases, especially Gram-negative enteric pathogens (i.e., *E. coli*). Gram-positive cocci appears in up to 30% of cases, whereas anaerobes are unfrequently isolated.

Although fever and abdominal pain and tenderness in patients with chronic liver disease and ascites should always suggest a primary peritonitis, clinical presentation is often atypical and the diagnosis should always be considered in the presence of deteriorating renal or hepatic function and worsening encephalopathy.

Definitive diagnosis is based on a positive culture of ascitic fluid, but it requires at least 24 hr. Because suspected infection must be promptly treated, therapy must be started on the basis of preliminary laboratory analysis (51). Numerous methods of immediate diagnosis have been evaluated including ascitic fluid lactate and pH but the polymorphonuclear leukocyte count (with a cutoff of 250 cells/mm^3) remains the single best test (51).

Patients should have systemic antibiotic therapy with cefotaxim rather than with aminoglycosides, which are responsible for renal toxicity in some patients (20). Antimicrobial therapy should be adjusted when the results of culture and sensitivity testing become available. There is no specific indication for peritoneal dialysis in these patients since parenterally administered antibiotics achieve adequate levels in ascitic fluid.

Primary peritonitis in dialysis patients, as

in patients with cirrhosis, presents with clinical manifestations that are often vague: mild pain, low-grade fever, and mild tenderness. Peritonitis can be assumed to be present when the dialysate drainage fluid contains more than 100 leukocytes/mm^3. Gram's stain is positive in about half the cases and culture usually reveals a single organism, in most cases *Staphylococcus epidermidis,* followed by *Staphylococcus aureus, Streptococcus,* and then Gram-negative enteric organisms (55).

In patients on continous ambulatory periotoneal dialysis, initial therapy commonly used includes intraperitoneal antibiotics. Empiric therapy including tobramycin plus cephalothin is used and adjusted depending on the culture and sensitivity data at each institution. Therapy is usually continued for a week after the last positive culture. The catheter should be removed when there is a persistent or recurrent infection with the same organism (49).

When peritoneal fluid contains multiple enteric organisms, a laparotomy is indicated. This infection, occurring 24–48 hr after insertion of a catheter, can be due to a perforation of intestine. When the infection occurs in patients on chronic peritoneal dialysis, the infection can be also caused by underlying gastrointestinal pathology such as appendicitis, perforated diverticulitis, or perforated ulcer (55).

Secondary Peritonitis

The common etiological causes of secondary peritonitis are rupture of viscus such as appendicitis, gastric or duodenal peptic ulcers, and diverticulitis of the colon. Other causes include: (a) ulcerated lesions from ulcerative colitis, typhoid, or necrotizing enterocolitis and (b) ischemic necrotic bowel due to vascular insufficiency, incarcerated hernias, volvulus, or cancer. Pelvic inflammatory disease, including salpingitis and endometritis, can produce a localized lower abdominal peritonitis indistinguishable from appendicitis. Postoperative peritonitis is generally due to anastomotic disruption.

The diagnosis of secondary peritonitis usually is not difficult. Symptoms can be grouped into two classes, reflex and toxic. Reflex symptoms include localized or generalized pain, vomiting, and muscular rigidity. Toxic symptoms are due to accumulation of bacterial toxins and exudates with intestinal distension, paresis, general toxemia, and bacteremia. Laboratory tests showing leukocytosis, mildly abnormal liver function, and a slight elevation of serum amylase serve to support the diagnosis. The roentgenographic examination of the abdomen may reveal air under the diaphragm in the cases of ruptured viscus, paralytic ileus, or volvulus. There are several clinical circumstances in which history taking and physical examination may not be reliably applied to the diagnosis of secondary peritonitis. These include patients with a decreased level of consciousness, patients receiving immunosuppressive drugs such as steroids, and some elderly patients. In these patients, diagnostic peritoneal lavage, with a presence of more than 500 white blood cells/mm^3, appears to be a safe and accurate method of determining the presence of peritonitis requiring surgery (36).

Differential diagnosis of peritonitis includes several diseases such as Mediterranean fever, porphyria, granulomatous peritonitis (tuberculosis, starch), ulcerative colitis and regional enteritis, acute hemorrhagic pancreatitis, ruptured ectopic pregnancy or torsion of an ovary, and retroperitoneal hemmorrhage. The Fitz-Hugh and Curtis syndrome results from perihepatitis in the upper part of the abdomen due to gonococcal infection (28). Some nonabdominal diseases that can mimic peritoneal pain by referral are pleuropneumonia, acute myocardial infarction, and pericarditis.

Bacterial peritonitis typically is caused by multiple organisms. Upper gastrointestinal perforations usually release predominantly Gram-positive organisms; however, patients receiving antacids or H$_2$-antagonists have a greater number of Gram-negative bacilli in their stomach prior to perforation (50). Perforation of the distal small bowel or colon results in the release of hundreds of bacterial species but a few remain in the peritoneal cavity. These infections are almost always polymicrobial, containing a mixture of aerobic and anaerobic bacteria. *E. coli* is the predominant facultative aerobic organism, followed by group D streptococcus (49). Anaerobic organisms include *B. fragilis, Clostridium,* and anaerobic *Streptococcus pyogenes* (37). The Gram-negative aerobic bacteria exert their pathogenic potential mainly through endotoxin, which acts by way of mediators, causing systemic septic response. The main virulence factor of anaerobic bacteria are exoenzymes and capsular polysaccharides. Peritoneal infections are truly synergistic, including protection against host defense and creation of a suitable environment by one member of the flora for another. Aside from bacteria, certain adjuvant substances, i.e., bile, gastric juice, blood, and necrotic tissue, play a role in the pathogenesis of peritonitis. The peritoneum deals with infection in three ways: first, the direct absorption of bacteria into the lymphatics via the diaphragmatic peritoneum; second, the local destruction of bacteria through phagocytosis by macrophages or polymorphonuclear granulocytes attracted to the peritoneal cavity; and third, the localization of the infection in the form of an abscess (26).

Emergency resuscitative measures must be started prior to operation, including nasogastric decompression and fluid resuscitation. Systemic antibiotics to cover coliforms and anaerobes should be started before surgery and continued as early as the fourth postoperative day. Surgical management of peritonitis should first eliminate the source of peritonitis: appendicitis is treated by appendicectomy; perforation of the duodenum due to peptic ulcer is safely treated by primary closure; and a perforated gastric ulcer is included in a distal gastric resection with a gastrojejunal anastomosis. For colonic pathology, the surgical treatment includes resection of the perforated segment with exteriorization of the proximal end as an end-colostomy. Primary anastomosis in this setting is at high risk of dehiscence. The risk associated with primary anastomosis of the small intestine following resection is much lower unless peritoneal soiling is particularly extensive (19).

The second goal of the surgical management is to prevent recurrent or persistent sepsis. After débridement of the entire peritoneal cavity, all purulent exudates and debris should be aspirated. Intraoperative lavage reduces bacterial numbers and removes adjuvant substances such as blood, fecal matter, and necrotic tissue (19). Removal of contamined fluid and of necrotic material through intraperitoneally placed drains is still a matter of controversy. The use of a drain after surgical treatment of peritonitis is indicated if the drain is placed into a well-defined abscess cavity or to establish a controlled fistula (49). In order to reduce the morbidity and mortality of diffuse peritonitis, especially postoperative peritonitis, other perioperative techniques can be used, including continuous postoperative peritoneal lavage with or without antibiotics in the peritoneal lavage and open peritoneal drainage. An efficacy of a continous postoperative peritoneal lavage for 48–72 hr or until the effluent is clear was found by some authors (34). However, this technique requires intensive care unit monitoring and is not demonstrated by well-performed prospective randomized trials. The use of antibiotics in peritoneal lavage solution has obtained little support from clinical studies. This technique did not reduce intraabdominal abscess formation and overall mortality rate (41). The aim of leaving the abdomen open is to remove recurrent localized collections as necessary. Although several authors have supported this approach by demonstrating reduced mortality associated with its use, the procedure is not without complications (19). These include prolonged mechanical ventilation, fistula formation, continued fluid and protein loss, and late abdominal wall hernias.

Tertiary Peritonitis

Some patients with imparied host defense mechanisms are unable to contain infection and they develop persistent diffuse peritonitis, so-called "tertiary peritonitis" (49). Infection tends to be diffuse and poorly localized collections containing serosanguineous fluid. Despite aggressive surgical management, these patients develop progressive multiple system organ failure. The microbiology of tertiary peritonitis shows that *S. epidermidis* and *Pseudomonas* and *Candida* species are the predominant organisms recovered from these patients (10). An immunocompromised host appears to contribute to the pathogenicity of these microorganisms. Innovative techniques such as selective decontamination or enhancing the integrity of the mucosal barrier may improve survival in this high-risk patient population (21).

Intraabdominal Abscesses

Abscesses may occur in the peritoneal cavity, in abdominal viscera, or in the retroperitoneum. Nonvisceral abscesses may follow resolution of diffuse peritonitis or may be due to a perforation of a viscus successfully walled off by peritoneal defense mechanisms. Postoperative gastric, colonic, and biliary tract surgery are sources of abscess formation. Visceral abscesses (i.e., liver or spleen) are more commonly due to hematogenous or lymphatic spread of bacteria to the organ. Retroperitoneal abscesses may originate through perforation of the gastrointestinal tract into the retroperitoneum or by hematogenous or lymphatic spread to retroperitoneal organs. Most abscesses are found to have multiple species both of aerobic and anaerobic bacteria. Diagnosis is based on clinical suspicion of fever and chills, which are present in a great majority of patients. Pain is helpful in localization of the abscess in some cases, although subphrenic abscesses may be painless. Abscesses always should be considered in the postoperative patient who develops a fever several days to weeks after the surgery. Ultrasound and CT scanning are clearly the examinations of choice for the diagnosis. (49).

Treatment includes antibiotic therapy and drainage of the abscess. Drainage has the primary role. Antibiotics are used primarily to prevent metastatic infection from bacteremia and to treat nondrainable cellulitis around the abscess. Percutaneous drainage is the treatment of choice in the management of single, well-defined intraabdominal abscess (24). CT scanning has greatly simplified the elective percutaneous approach to subphrenic, subhe-patic, and pelvic abscesses. Laparotomy is necessary when abscesses are on the interloop or when multiple abscesses are present, particularly in the early postoperative period (19).

ACUTE PANCREATITIS

Acute pancreatitis presents a wide variety of pancreatic inflammatory conditions. It includes pancreatic edema and interstitial inflammation as well as frank pancreatic necrosis or hemorrhage. Although necrotizing pancreatitis represents approximately 20% of acute pancreatitis, mortality still remains high, from 10 to 50% (45). These patients have a high risk of infection with severe general and local complications; they require surgery in the evolution of the disease. On the other hand, acute pancreatitis will subside in the majority of patients with conservative treatment.

Acute necrotizing pancreatitis is characterized by two phases: (a) the initial phase, with systemic consequences of local inflammation and release of toxic substances in the circulation; during this phase, treatment should prevent and treat systemic manifestations and detect local infections; and (b) the second phase, beginning usually 1 week later, is related to local evolution of pancreatic necrosis, which requires in most cases surgical treatment.

Pathology

The pathophysiologic evolution of necrotizing pancreatitis begins with parenchymal necrosis and ductal and capsular rupture, with leakage of active enzymes into the retroperitoneum, which is progressively digested, as well as into the peripancreatic tissue, producing collections of fluid and necrotic tissue. Toxins formed are reabsorbed into the bloodstream and produce systemic effects due to the releases of active proteases, phospholipase A2, vasoactives substances, complement activation and oxygen free radicals. Peritoneal and retroperitoneal fluid sequestration is associated with ileus and vomiting. Systemic consequences of acute pancreatitis included circulatory shock, pulmonary complications, renal failure, and mental obnubilation. Circulatory shock is secondary to hypovolemia and vasoactive substances; pulmonary complications with acute respiratory distress syndrome can be due to the association of alterations of the alveolocapillary membrane, atelectasis, and pleural effusions; renal failure is mainly due to hypovolemia but other associated factors are vasopressor release and intravascular coagulation. Many other metabolic disturbances have been observed in acute pancreatitis: hyperglycemia, hypocalcemia, hyperlipidemia and metabolic acidosis (56).

The second phase of the pathophysiologic evolution of necrotizing pancreatitis is due to the local evolution of pancreatic and peripancreatic necrosis. Necrosis and its superinfection can induce colonic complications (necrosis, perforation, and hemorrhage).

Several etiologies of acute pancreatitis are described, but in France most pancreatitis is due to chronic alcohol consumption and biliary gallstone. Other causes include endoscopic retrograde cholangiography, trauma, postoperative hyperlipidemia, medicament, hyperparathyroidism, and pancreas divisum. In patients with chronic alcohol consumption, acute pancreatitis arises in a pancreatic parenchyma with fibrosis, whereas acute pancreatitis from other causes arises without underlying pancreatic disease (56).

Clinical, Biological, and Radiological Features

Clinical Presentation

The major symptom is epigastric pain, which typically radiates to the back. Other signs less frequently observed initially include: nausea and vomiting, fever, arterial hypotension, jaundice, and respiratory failure. At examination, epigastric tenderness or even guarding is observed (3).

Laboratory Findings

According to the severity and the etiological factor of pancreatitis, several biological disturbances can be observed, but they are nonspecific as well, as in other critical ill patients. Serum and urinary amylase levels remain the most accurate test for diagnosis of acute pancreatitis. Serum amylase levels are elevated in 95% of patients with acute pancreatitis. On the other hand, in patients with high serum amylase levels, 75% have acute pancreatitis. Increased serum lipase levels are frequently observed. Other laboratory findings includes hypoglycemia and hypocalcemia, which are features of severe acute pancreatitis (35).

Radiological Findings

Plain abdominal x-ray can show segmental bowel ileus in the left upper abdominal quadrant and mild dilatation of the tranverse colon.

Ultrasonography is of limited value for determining the presence or absence of acute pancreatitis because marked gaseous distension of the bowel interferes with examination; however, it can be useful for early diagnosis of associated gallbladder gallstones.

Computed tomography (CT) is the most important imaging procedure in suspected acute pancreatitis. The most frequent findings are: diffuse pancreatic enlargement, obliteration of the peripancreatic fat planes, inflammation of the left anterior pararenal spaces, and peripancreatic fluid collections. Contrast-enhanced CT evaluates the presence and extension of necrosis (46). The evaluation of the severity of the pancreatitis by CT, according to pancreatic enlargement and the extent of fluid collection, is correlated to the number of prognostic signs as described by Ranson (13).

Prognostic Assessment

Using an experience analysis, Ranson et al. have proposed 11 early signs correlated to the severity of the pancreatitis (Table 42.1). Several studies have confirmed that a relationship exists between the number of early prognostic signs and morbidity and mortality. Other multiple parameter systems have also found a similar predictive accuracy of only 60–70% (5, 17). Pancreatitis is judged to be mild if three or fewer signs are present, and severe if more than three are present. Mortality reaches 100% if seven or more signs are present (13). Mortality rate is related to the clinical

Table 42.1
Prognosis Signs Used by Ranson et al. (45)
Correlated to the Severity of Pancreatitis

At admission
  Age >55 years
  White blood cell count $>16 \times 10^9$/liter
  Blood glucose >11 mmol/liter
  Serum lactic dehydrogenase >350 IU/liter
  SGOT >250 IU/liter[a]
During initial 48 hr
  Hematocrit fall >10 percentage points
  Urea rise >1.7 mmol/liter
  Serum calcium level <2 mmol/liter
  Arterial Po_2 <60 mm Hg
  Base deficit >4 mmol/liter
  Estimated fluid sequestration >6,000 ml

[a]SGOT, serum glutamic oxaloacetic transaminase.

setting rather than to the etiology of the pancreatitis.

Treatment of Severe Acute Pancreatitis

Early Medical Treatment

Goals of initial treatment are relief of pain and correction of hydroelectrolytic, hemodynamic, and respiratory disturbances. The intravascular volume of the patient must be carefully restored and monitored, and an adequate hydration must be maintained. Fluid resuscitation includes crystalloid and colloid administration. Major antalgics are given in case of severe pain. In severe acute pancreatitis, nasogastric suction is helpful for reducing vomiting and abdominal distension, and oral findings should be interrupted until the onset of pain. Nasogastric suction may also decrease pancreatic secretion. Other treatment modalities that inhibit pancreatic secretion (i.e., glucagon, anticholinergic drugs, atropine) or inhibit the action of proteolytic enzymes, such as the use of aprotinin, have been no more effective than placebo plus nasogastric suction (7). To prevent upper gastrointestinal hemorrhage from acute ulceration, antacids are given. Nutritional support by intravenous alimentation is started in order to prevent nutritional depletion. No study has demonstrated that antibioprophylaxis prevents local infections, and antibiotics are given

only in proven infections (43). Respiratory failure may require endotracheal intubation with positive end-expiratory pressure and pleural effusion drainage.

Peritoneal lavage may be a valuable treatment in acute pancreatitis. It can remove toxic substances released from the pancreas that are thought to be responsible for systemic complications. Results of this method showed a prompt improvement of cardiovascular and respiratory status in some patients but the outcome in patients with severe pancreatitis is not affected by peritoneal lavage (8).

Surgical Treatment

Once pancreatic necrosis has been identified by CT scan, how should it be managed? Indications for surgery and the timing and extent of operations are still debated (45, 53).

Early removal of necrosis has been used in order to enhance the chances of recovery by extirpation of the disease. However, this approach overestimates the amount of pancreatic necrosis, leading to extensive pancreatectomy with high mortality rate, and surprisingly does not prevent the septic complications (53). Furthermore, it has been demonstrated that débridement of sterile necrosis is associated with a higher superinfection rate of necrosis (12). The timing of resection is also controversial. Delayed excision of necrosis is justified by studies showing that bacterial invasion of necrotic tissues rarely occurs within the first week (53). Pancreatic necrosis by itself, even associated with systemic complications, is not an absolute indication for surgery. On the other hand sterile pancreatic necrosis of limited extent must be managed conservatively (53).

Conversely, infected necrosis requires prompt drainage. Several reports have shown a significantly higher mortality rate for patients with infected necrosis compared with those with sterile necrosis (45). Percutaneous puncture under CT is now the most accurate procedure for early diagnosis of infection (53).

When infected necrosis has been demonstrated, how should it be managed? Percutaneous drainage can be used favorably in some cases with fluid collections and minimal necrotic debris, but this technique has a high failure rate and infected pancreatic necrosis requires surgical débridement. Surgical drainage after débridement of necrosis can be performed through a direct retroperitoneal approach or through a laparotomy with either a closed or an open drainage following débridement (45, 53).

Pancreatitis associated with gallstones should be managed in two steps: first, to eliminate the risk of recurrent attacks of pancreatitis; second, to manage necrosis and its consequences. Many studies have clearly demonstrated that early removal of gallstones, even impacted gallstones, does not ameliorate the progression of pancreatitis, and operative mortality is high (12, 57). In order to prevent recurrent acute pancreatitis in patients with gallstones, surgery including cholecystectomy and common duct exploration within the first week must be performed. In patients with severe necrotic pancreatitis, we advocate early endoscopic papillotomy, eliminating the risk of recurrence. The time of surgery should be delayed until a few days later for drainage of eventual infected necrosis (4, 40).

References

1. Akalin HE, Laleli Y, Telatar H. Bactericidal and apsonic activity of ascitic fluid from cirrhotic and non cirrhotic patients. J Infect Dis 1983;147:1011.
2. Aranha GV, Sontag SJ, Greenlee HB. Cholecystectomy in cirrhotic patients: a formidable operation. Am J Surg 1982;163:55.
3. Banks PA. Acute pancreatitis: clinical presentation. In: Go VLW, Gardner JD, Brooks FP, Lebenthal E, Di Magno EP, Scheele GA, eds. The exocrine pancreas. New York: Raven Press, 1986:475–479.
4. Belghiti J, Kleinman P, Cherqui D, Perniceni T, Bernades P, Fékété F. Traitement précoce de la lithiase biliaire au cours des pancréatites biliaires. Gastroenterol Clin Biol 1987;11:786–789.
5. Blamey SC, Imrie CW, O'Neil J, Gimourw H, Carter DC. Prognostic factors in acute pancreatitis. Gut 1984;25:1340–1346.
6. Boey JH, Way LW. Acute cholangitis. Ann Surg 1980;191;264–270.
7. Bradley EL. Antibiotics in acute pancreatitis. Current status and future directions. Am J Surg 1989;158:472–478.
8. Bradley EL, Allen K. A prospective longitudinal study of observation versus surgical intervention in the management of necrotizing pancreatitis. Am J Surg 1991;161:19–25.
9. Cameron JL, Pitt HA. Biliary sepsis and suppurative cholangitis. In: Moody F, et al, eds. Surgical treatment of digestive disease. Chicago: Year Book, 1988:359–374.
10. Carrico CJ, Meakins JL, Marshall JC. Multiple organ failure syndrome: the gatrointestinal tract— the motor of "MOF." Arch Surg 1986;121:197.
11. Carroll BA. Preferred imaging techniques for the diagnosis of cholecystitis and cholelithiasis. Ann Surg 1989;210:112.
12. Carter DC. Pancreatitis and the biliary tree: The continuing problem. Am J Surg 1988;155:10–17.
13. Corfield AP, Williamson RCN, Mac Mahon MJ, Shearer MG, Looper MJ, Mayer AD, Dickson AP, Imrie CW. Prediction of severity in acute pancreatitis: prospective comparison of three prognostic indices. Lancet 1985;ii:403–407.
14. Cornwell EE III, Rodriguez A, Mirvis SE, Shorr RM. Acute acalculous cholecystitis in critically injured patients. Ann Surg 1989;210:52–55.
15. Cuschieri A. Acute cholecystis. In: Blumgart LH, ed. Surgery of the liver and the biliary tract. Edinburgh: Churchill Livingstone, 1988:531–539.
16. Devine RM, Farnell MB, Mucha P. Acute cholecystitis as a complication in surgical patients. Arch Surg 1984;119:1389–1393.
17. Di Magno EP. What is appropriate nonoperative treatment of acute pancreatitis? Dig Dis Sci 1979;24:337–338.
18. Edlund G., Ljungdhal M. Acute cholecystitis in the elderly. Am J Surg 1990;159:414–416.
19. Farthmann EH, Schöffel U. Principles and limitations of operative management of intra abdominal infections. World J Surg 1990;14:210–217.
20. Felisant J, Rimola A, Arroyo V. Cefotaxime is more effective than is ampicillin-tobramycin in cirrhotics with severe infections. Hepatology 1985;5:457.
21. Fry DE. Multiple system organ failure. Surg Clin North Am 1988;68:107.
22. Gambill EE, Hodgson JR, Priestley JT. Painless obstructive cholecystopathy. Arch Intern Med 1962;110:442.
23. Gigot JF, Leese T, Dereme T, Coutinho J, Castaing D, Bismuth H. Acute cholangitis. Multivariate analysis of risk factors. Ann Surg 1989;209:435–438.
24. Haaga JR. Imaging intra abdominal abscesses and nonoperative drainage procedures. World J Surg 1990;14:204–209.
25. Harken AH, Schochat SJ. Gram positive peritonitis in children. Am J Surg 1973;125;769.
26. Hau T. Bacteria, toxins and the peritoneum. World J Surg 1990;14:167–175.
27. Holcomb GW Jr, O'Neill JA, Holcomb GW III. Cholecystitis, cholelithiasis and common duct stenosis in children and adolescents. Ann Surg 1980;191:502–505.
28. Holdstock G, Balasegaram M, Millward-Sadler GH, et al. The liver in infection. In: Alberti et al, eds. Liver and biliary disease. Philadelphia: WB Saunders, 1985:1077–1079.
29. Hruska JF. Gastrointestinal and intra-abdominal infections. In: Reese RE, Douglas RG, eds. A

practical approach to infectious diseases. Boston: Little, Brown, 1986:284–326.

30. Iannuzzi C, Belghiti J, Erlinger S, Menu Y, Fékété F. Cholangitis associated with cholecystitis in patients with acquired immunodeficiency syndrome. Arch Surg 1990;125:1211–1213.

31. Keighley M, Flinn R, Alexander-Williams J. Multivariate analysis of clinical and operative findings associated with biliary sepsis. Br J Surg 1976;63:528–534.

32. Kudchadkar A, Pauwaa MC, Wilder JR. Acute intestinal obstruction. Mt Sinai J Med 1979;46:247–250.

33. Lahtinen J, Alhava EM, Aukee S. Acute cholecystitis treated by early and delayed surgery. A controlled clinical trial. Scand J Gastroenterol 1978;13;673.

34. Leiboff AR, Soroff HS. The treatment of generalized peritonitis by closed postoperative peritoneal lavage, a critical review of the literature. Arch Surg 1987;122:1005.

35. Levitt MD, Eckfeldt JH. Diagnosis of acute pancreatitis. In: Go VLW, Gardner JD, Brooks FP, Lebenthal E, Di Magno EP, Scheele GA, eds. The exocrine pancreas. New York: Raven Press, 1986:481–502.

36. Lobbato V, Cioroiu M, LaRaja RD. Peritoneal lavage as an aid to diagosis of peritonitis in debilitated and elderly patients. Am Surg 1985;51:508.

37. Lorber B, Swenson RM. The bacteriology of intra abdominal infections. Surg Clin North Am 1975;55:1349.

38. Mentzer RM, Golden GT, Chandler JG. A comparative appraisal of emphysematous cholecystitis. Am J Surg 1975;129:10–15.

39. Mirvis SE, Vainright JR, Nelson AW. The diagnosis of acute acalculous cholecystitis: a comparison of sonography, scintigraphy and CT. AJR 1986;147:1171–1175.

40. Neoptolemos JP, London N, Slater ND, Carr-Locke DC, Fossard DP, Moosa AR. A prospective study of ERCP and endoscopic sphincterotomy in the diagnosis and treatment of gallstone acute pancreatitis. Arch Surg 1986;121:697–702.

41. Nomikos IN, Katsouyanni K, Papaioannou AN. Washing with or without chloramphenicol in the teatment of peritonitis: a prospective clinical trial. Surgery 1986;99:20.

42. Parry SW, Pelias ME, Browder W. Acalculous hypersensitivity cholecystitis: hypothesis of a new clinicopathologic entity. Surgery 1988;140:911–916.

43. Pellegrini CA. The treatment of acute pancreatitis: a continuing challenge. N Engl J Med 1985;312:436–438.

44. Pierreti R, Auldist AW, Stephens CA. Acute cholecystitis in children. Surg Cynecol Obstet 1975;140:16–18.

45. Ranson JHC. Acute pancreatitis: surgical management. In: Go VLW, Gardner JD, Brooks FP, Lebenthal E, Di Magno EP, Scheele GA, eds. The exocrine pancreas. New York: Raven Press, 1986:503–511.

46. Ranson JHC, Rifkind KM, Roses D, Fink SD, Eng K, Spencer FC. Prognostic signs and the role of operative management in acute pancreatitis. Surg Gynecol Obstet 1974;139:69–81.

47. Reiss R, Nudelman I, Gutman C, Deutsch A. Changing trends in surgery for acute cholecystitis. World J Surg 1990;14:567–571.

48. Reynolds BM, Dargan EL. Acute obstructive cholangitis. A distinctive clinical syndrome. Ann Surg 1959;150:299–303.

49. Rotstein OD, Meakins JL. Diagnostic and therapeutic challenges of intra abdominal infections. World J Surg 1990;14;159–166.

50. Ruddell WSJ, Axon ATR, Findlay JM. Effect of cimetidine on the gastric flora. Lancet 1980;1:672.

51. Runyon BA. Spontaneous bacterial peritonitis: an explosion of information. Hepatology 1988;8:171–175.

52. Sievert W, Vakyl NB. Emergencies of the biliary tract. Gastroenterol Clin North Am 1988;17:245–264.

53. Smadja C, Bismuth H. Pancreatic debridment in acute necrotizing pancreatitis: an obsolete procedure? Br J Surg 1985;73;408–410.

54. The Southern Surgeons Club. A prospective analysis of 1518 laparoscopic cholecystectomies. N Engl J Med 1991;324:1073–1078.

55. Spence PA, Mathews RE, Khanna R, Oreopoulos DG. Indications for operation where peritonitis occurs in patients on chronic ambulatory peritoneal dialysis. Surg Gynecol Obstet 1985;161:450.

56. Steer ML. Etiology and pathophysiology of acute pancreatitis: surgical management. In: Go VLW, Gardner JD, Brooks FP, Lebenthal E, Di Magno EP, Scheele GA, eds. The exocrine pancreas. New York: Raven Press, 1986:465–474.

57. Stone HH, Fabian TC, Dunlop WE. Gallstone pancreatitis. Biliary tract pathology in relation to time of operation. Ann Surg 1981;195:305–312.

58. Stryker SJ, Beal JM. Acute cholecystitis and common duct calculi. Arch Surg 1983;118:1063–1064.

59. Wegener M, Borsch G, Schneider J. Gallbladder wall thickening: a frequent finding in various nonbiliary disorders. A prospective ultrasonographic study. J Clin Ultrasound 1987;15:307–312.

60. Welch JP. Mechanical obstruction of the small and large intestines. In: Moody F, et al, eds. Surgical treatment of digestive disease. Chicago: Year Book, 1988:766–785.

43

Severe Diarrhea

Emmanuel Rene

Diarrhea is a common complication in critically ill patients. One prospective study found that 41% of patients in a general intensive care unit (ICU) had diarrhea, defined as the passage of three to four liquid stools per day (6). The adverse effects of diarrhea in critically ill patients, especially in AIDS patients, are many and affect all aspects of the patient's care.

Conversely, such severe diarrhea may be a life-threatening condition by itself. In the western world, although acute travellers's diarrhea may occasionally require hospitalization for parenteral rehydration, severe acute colitis, defined as an acute dilatation of the colon associated with systemic toxicity, though a rare event, constitutes the most severe, life-threatening complication of ulcerative colitis.

PATHOPHYSIOLOGY

Normal persons from developed countries excrete no more than 200 g of stool per day, of which no more than 75% is fluid (2). Diarrhea, therefore, can be defined as intestinal malabsorption of certain cations and water.

Intestinal Absorption

Seven to nine liters of fluid enter the upper intestine during a normal day in nutritive solutions as well as from salivary, gastric, pancreatic, and biliary secretions. The major part of this fluid is absorbed in the small bowel, and no more than 1.5 liters enters the colon. Thus, the normal small bowel has a large capacity for absorption, whereas the large bowel has a greater efficiency but a smaller total capacity (5). When fluid volume entering the cecum from the small bowel exceeds 5 liters, fecal fluid losses increase (4). Digestion of nutrients derived from the diet tends to produce osmotic forces that move water from interstitial fluid into the lumen across the semipermeable intestine. Simple diffusion down concentration gradients equilibrate differences in ionic concentrations in lumen and plasma. As products of digestion of nutrients are absorbed in the upper intestine, luminal fluid becomes hypotonic and water is absorbed along with solute (4). A large proportion of luminal sodium, chloride, and potassium is absorbed in the jejunum by passive processes, and the movement of water through the permeable intercellular junctions of the jejunum moves salts by solvent drag. Intestinal permeability is greatly reduced in the distal ileum and colon, and the lower permeability in these regions prevents water from leaking back into the lumen. In these regions of the distal bowel, active absorption of salt is the main driving force for water absorption (5). The active-transport processes by which sodium can enter the enterocyte (5) are localized in the basolateral membrane of the enterocyte. Hydrolysis of ATP catalyzed by Na-K-ATPase exchanges Na^+ for K^+, thereby establishing a steep electrochemical gradient for entry of Na^+ from the lumen. Potassium absorption occurs in exchange for hydrogen but may also utilize an energy-dependent process—perhaps a ouabain-insensitive, K-activated ATPase in the colon.

Intestinal Secretion

A distinct electrolyte secretory mechanism is now recognized to exist in both the small and the large bowel (7). It normally functions at a low basal rate and is particularly located in crypt cells, whereas absorptive processes are largely restricted to the villus surface. The Cl^- secretory mechanism is similar to that in other epithelia; it is dependent on Na^+. The driving force for the movement of Cl^- from the apical cell membrane after the channel is opened by any particular secretory stimulus is the Cl^- electrochemical gradient. The gradient depends on energy derived from coupled NaCl entry at the basolateral membrane.

Pathogenetic Mechanisms for Diarrhea

Diarrhea results from disturbances of the normal processes by which salt and water are absorbed from the intestinal lumen and from distinct intestinal secretory and motility disorders.

Osmotic diarrhea results from the presence within the intestinal lumen of unabsorbed solute, which causes water to be retained in the bowel lumen to maintain isotonicity (1). It is recognized that this process accounts for the diarrhea induced by osmotic laxatives such as magnesium sulfate, which contains poorly absorbed cation and anion components. Lactose ingestion in lactase-deficient subjects causes diarrhea that depends on the load of the unabsorbed solute, the rate of its transit, and the capacity of the colon to absorb the metabolic products. (Lactic acid is a relatively poorly absorbed short-chain fatty acid). During and after postinfectious diarrhea, a number of other nutrients may also be absorbed poorly and thus contribute to dietary-induced diarrhea by increasing the osmotic load.

Secretory diarrhea is the recognized causative factor in several enterotoxigenic infectious diseases, traveler's diarrhea in particular.

A reduced absorptive capacity through reduction of mucosal absorptive surface area may be a factor in the diarrhea associated with short-bowel syndrome or with generalized disorders of the mucosa of the small intestine, such as celiac disease and tropical sprue.

Increased rapidity of intestinal transit may be an important factor in the diarrhea associated with thyrotoxicosis. However, in other motility disorders (e.g., those associated with intestinal pseudoobstruction or systemic sclerosis), factors such as bacterial overgrowth may also contribute to impaired transport of intestinal fluid (1).

Mechanisms for diarrhea in invasive diarrheal disorders are usually multifactorial; bacteria-derived toxins and inflammatory products increase secretion of intestinal fluid and cause mucosal damage as well as direct bacterial or viral invasion of tissue, a process that can also reduce the absorptive capacity of small-bowel or colonic mucosa. Some bacterial exotoxins (e.g., cholera toxin, heat-stable and heat-labile enterotoxins of *Escherichia coli*) are well-defined direct stimuli to active intestinal fluid secretion. In several instances, the membrane receptors for these exotoxins have been characterized and the mode of action through activation of cyclic nucleotide second messengers has been defined in great detail (5). Other bacterial infections that cause diarrhea may be associated with both the production of enterotoxin and the capacity of the organism to invade the mucosa. Toxins derived from these organisms may be both cytotoxic and enterotoxic (3). The exact mode of action of these toxins upon release into the bowel lumen or within the invaded enterocyte is less well defined than the action of enterotoxins.

Localized tumors comprise collections of neuropeptide-secreting cells that secrete vasoactive intestinal polypeptide. Substance P, serotonin, prostaglandins, histamine, and others secreting the gastrointestinal hormones gastrin and enteroglucagon have been associated with diarrheal disorders (5). Several different intracellular mechanisms may account for the diarrheal processes in which systemic release of these specific chemical agents from the tumor results in disordered fluid homeostasis. Eicosanoids of both the cyclooxygenase and lipoxygenase series are recognized as enhancing fluid secretion in pharmacologic doses, but their role in the physiologic control of intestinal fluid remains speculative. Elevated levels of both series of eicosanoids can be identified in luminal fluid and tissue in various diarrheal states associated with inflammation in the bowel wall. Nevertheless, their exact role in causing fluid secretion remains unclear. Inhibitors of prostaglandin synthesis have had only a limited role in the treatment of these disease processes, and the correlation of antidiarrheal effects with reduced production of eicosanoids has still not been defined.

Products of Inflammation and Diarrheal Disorders

Many products of the inflammatory response that are derived from neutrophils, immune cell products, mast cells, and phagocytic cells may all induce fluid secretion under various experimental conditions. Their action may be endocrine or paracrine in nature. For instance, cholecystokinin (CCK), which is released from CCK cells in the jejunal mucosa as a gastrointestinal hormone, is also present as a neurotransmitter in the central and enteric nervous sytems. Receptors for CCK are present on monocytes, and CCK may also act as a chemoattractant. During an inflammatory response in the bowel wall, release of interleukin-1 (IL-1)—such as might occur with an invasive diarrheal disorder—from lymphocytes may act directly on ileal cells or indirectly via an effect on enteric neurons. IL-1 has been shown to have other paracrine and hormonal effects, with actions targeted on macrophages, lymphocytes, the CNS, and the liver. Moreover, various neuropeptides (such as CCK) that are present in the intestine modulate immune function through their release from the autonomic system. Other neuropeptides act specifically on monocytes to modulate their release of inflammatory cytokines and kinins. Intensive studies will be required to characterize these types of interactions in the bowel wall during both enterotoxigenic and invasive diarrheal disease. It is likely that greater understanding of pathophysiology will clarify the causes of not only the diarrheal fluid production but also the severe symptomatic complaints that develop in many patients with travelers' diarrhea and invasive diarrheal disease. The contribution of the gut-brain axis to these debilitating symptom complexes, the types of gastrointestinal hormones involved, and the role of cytokines, neuropeptides, and products of inflammation released from the bowel wall are at present unknown for many acute infectious diarrheal states that affect the traveler. Systemic symptoms such as fever, sleep disturbances, and myalgia during infectious processes have been clearly ascribed to release of the cytokine polypeptide IL-1.

ACUTE DIARRHEAL DISEASE

This terminology includes a wide range of situations covering mainly infectious involvement of the gut.

This is a worldwide problem but of much greater magnitude in developing countries. A recent estimation (9) showed that children younger than 5 years in Africa, South America, and Asia (excluding China) suffer from between 744 and 1000 million episodes annually (an average of 2.2 episodes per child) and that 4.6 million of these children die yearly. Mortality is mainly in children of lower socioeconomic groups and could be reduced by up to 80% by widespread use of oral rehydration supplements. In surviving patients, acute diarrheal disease has a significant morbidity due to secondary malnutrition in children and loss of productivity in adults.

Viral and bacterial infections are the main causes and are cosmopolitan in distribution. Protozoal infections, notably amebiasis and giardiasis, are less often responsible and helminth infections seldom cause acute diarrhea. Diarrhea is also a common event during other infections, notably malaria and measles, and contributes to their mortality. In tropical areas, visitors are more susceptible to diarrheal diseases and usually the risk is inversely related to the poverty of the region. Individual protection relies on common sense precautions with food and water hygiene except where effective immunization is available. The variety of causes limits the efficacy of chemoprophylaxis (8). In Dacca, the causes of acute diarrhea in children younger than 2 years are different from those in older children and adults, and other developing countries have similar etiology. Even with the facilities at the International Centre for

Diarrhoeal Disease Research, Bangladesh, no pathogen was found in 36% of patients (10), but infections with more than one organism are common. Antibiotics are ineffective against a number of the causative organisms and the emphasis in management is on control of dehydration.

TOXIC MEGACOLON
Causes and Lesions

Although the syndrome may occasionally complicate other forms of infectious colitis, including amebic colitis, bacillary dysentery, typhoid fever, and pseudomembranous colitis, acute dilatation of the colon associated with systemic toxicity is probably the most severe, life-threatening complication of ulcerative colitis. Data from large retrospective studies have reported its occurrence in 1.6–13% of patients with ulcerative colitis. Histologic examination of colons removed at surgery or autopsy from patients with toxic megacolon show extensive deep ulceration and acute inflammation involving all muscle layers, often with extension of the inflammatory process to the serosa. The depth and extent of the colonic inflammatory process of these patients are usually more marked than in the resected colon specimens of patients with severe or fulminant ulcerative colitis without colonic dilatation. Presumably, the presence of widespread inflammation involving all layers of the colon accounts for both the systemic toxicity (fever, tachycardia, abdominal pain and tenderness, leukocytosis) and the apparent loss of colonic muscular tone, resulting in dilatation of the colon. Evidence of inflammation can be found in small arterioles (vasculitis) and myenteric or submucosal nerve plexuses. However, these latter findings are variable, and probably vasculitis and inflammation and destruction of the myenteric or submucosal plexuses are secondary phenomena in this syndrome.

In addition to widespread inflammation and destruction of the colonic musculature, other factors that tend to promote high intraluminal pressures or decrease colonic muscular tone are thought to contribute to colonic dilatation. These factors include excessive use of opiates or anticholinergic drugs and hypokalemia.

The association between barium enema and toxic megacolon is uncertain. Although many patients with toxic megacolon have undergone barium enema examinations, a high proportion of the examinations were done several days prior to the development of toxic dilatation of the colon. Nevertheless, barium enema studies in patients affected with ulcerative colitis still hold a risk for toxic complications and must be avoided in patients who are acutely ill.

Clinical Picture and Diagnosis

As the name implies, the patient with toxic megacolon usually is severely ill. Fever, abdominal pain and distension, and fatigue are prominent complaints. Occasionally, a patient with active colitis and bloody diarrhea will experience a sudden decrease in frequency of bowel movements as a heralding symptom of a toxic megacolon. This decrease in stool frequency reflects diminished colonic evacuation rather than an improvement in the patient's status. Misinterpretation may be avoided by patient examination, which often reveals a toxic appearance, with fever, dehydration, tachycardia, diminished bowel sounds, tympany, abdominal distension, and local or diffuse rebound tenderness. Patients receiving corticosteroids may display attenuated signs and symptoms that should not be underestimated.

Leukocytosis (often greater than 20,000 cells/mm^3), anemia, and hypoalbuminemia are common laboratory findings. A plain radiography of the abdomen shows dilatation extended to the entire colon or limited to the transverse colon. Although dilatation of the transverse colon (usually greater than 7 cm in diameter) on plain supine abdominal radiography is the most conspicuous finding, it is not indicative of a special severity of the disease in this segment of the colon, but rather is determined by the anterior position of the transverse colon. Repositioning the patient prone, for example, redistributes gas to the more posterior descending colon and dramatically decreases gas distension of the transverse colon. Irregular colonic mucosa, occasionally with intramural air silhouetted against the gas in the colon, may also be discerned on flat film. An upright abdominal film may reveal free air under the diaphragm if colonic perforation has already occurred.

Perforation is a common complication of toxic megacolon, occurring most often in the transverse and sigmoid colon. Perforation (both free and scaled off) complicates toxic megacolon in approximately 35% of patients. Free perforation may be dramatic in its suddenness, and shock may be irreversible. The occurrence of perforation has by far the greatest impact on mortality rate, regardless of whether the perforation is free or sealed off. The appearance of free colonic perforation may be associated with a marked increase in abdominal distension and obliteration of hepatic percussion dullness by free air. Peritonitis and septicemia closely follow fecal contamination of the intraperitoneal space.

The diagnosis of ulcerative colitis may be difficult when toxic megacolon is the initial clinical presentation. Toxic megacolon may develop so rapidly that a history of previous rectal bleeding and diarrhea may be obscured. In this setting, the condition may be confused with acute diverticulitis and pericolic abscess, carcinoma (presenting with lower quadrant pain, fever, and colonic dilatation), ischemic colitis (which may be associated with colonic dilatation proximal to the vascular insult), or colonic volvulus. The correct diagnosis may be established by a plain film of the abdomen and sigmoidoscopy. The latter, which should be carried out despite the severe illness and the obvious discomfort to the patient, can be done in the left lateral position, in bed if necessary, without colonic preparation. The sigmoidoscope needs to be inserted over only a short distance without air insufflation for, in most of individuals affected by ulcerative colitis complicated by toxic megacolon, the rectosigmoid mucosa exhibits lesions characteristic of inflammatory bowel disease.

Treatment

Therapy for toxic megacolon includes (a) initial resuscitative and supportive measures and (b) medical or surgical treatment aimed at the underlying necrotic process ongoing in the colon. Although there is general agreement on early therapy, the role of early surgical intervention versus prolonged medical treatment remains controversial.

Careful correction of fluid and electrolyte deficits requires immediate attention, as severe hypovolemia and hypokalemia may be present on initial presentation, owing to antecedent diarrhea, vomiting, and loss of fluid into the dilated colon. Not uncommonly, 80–100 mEq of potassium chloride within the first 24 hr are needed. Blood transfusions are indicated when significant colonic bleeding is responsible for anemia and hypovolemia. Prednisolone, 100–200 mg (or an equivalent dose of hydrocortisone), should be administered intravenously in divided doses throughout the day. Large doses of corticosteroids are given not only to improve the inflammatory process in the colon but also to avoid relative adrenal insufficiency in patients who have received lower doses of steroids prior to the superimposed stress of toxic megacolon.

Nasogastric suction aims to remove swallowed air and thereby to reduce the passage of air and fluid into the colon. A long peroral intestinal tube may further facilitate decompression of bowel gas. Additional decompression of the colon may be obtained by repositioning the patient prone for a period of time. This allows gas redistribution to the more posterior descending colon.

Anticholinergic drugs and opiates should be withdrawn if the patient had been receiving them previously. Usually, abdominal pain is not severe enough to require opiate analgesics. In view of the transmural, and often serosal, inflammation in patients with toxic megacolon, frank perforation is a constant danger. To limit the consequences of these perforations, intravenous antibiotics are recommended. Broad-spectrum coverage aimed at enteric Gram-negative and anaerobic pathogens, as well as at the enterococci, should be provided. Several regimens are acceptable: intravenous ampicillin, 1.5–2.0 g every 4 hr, with gentamicin or tobramycin, 1.0–1.5 mg/kg every 8 hr, and either clindamycin, 600 mg every 6 hr, or metronidazole, 500 mg every 6 hr, all given intravenously.

The patient's response to treatment must be monitored carefully in an intensive care unit. Abdominal girth should be measured and recorded two to three times daily. The physician should examine the patient at frequent intervals to ascertain whether bowel sounds are returning, whether an area of localized tenderness or rebound tenderness has developed, whether signs of perforation are present, and whether cardiovascular complications associated with bacterial sepsis have appeared. Adequacy of fluid and electrolyte repletion must be recorded; in difficult situations, monitoring of central venous pressure and pulmonary wedge pressure is required, in addition to standard intake and output balance sheets. Frequent radiographs of the abdomen are mandatory during the acute phase.

When clinical or radiographic evidence of colonic perforation is present, or if perforation is strongly suspected, early emergent colectomy with ileostomy is clearly necessary. Most of the recent literature includes patients with toxic megacolon complicating both ulcerative colitis and Crohn's colitis but demonstrates a similar outcome in both groups. Roughly 70–80% of patients with toxic megacolon will require surgery during their initial hospitalization for documented or suspected perforation or for fulminant colitis. Many surgeons favor early laparotomy because of mortality rates approaching 40–50% in the presence of perforation, regardless of whether they are free or contained. Several authors reported a much lower incidence of perforation and postoperative mortality by adopting a policy of early surgery for toxic megacolon.

The outlook for patients who initially respond to medical therapy adds additional support for surgical intervention for toxic megacolon. Up to 60% of this subgroup require subsequent hospitalization for fulminant colitis or recurrent toxic megacolon during periods of follow-up lasting up to 2 years after the initial episode. Unfortunately, there are nondiscriminating factors that can predict the likelihood of recurrence in a particular patient.

Mortality rates for surgery in patients with toxic megacolon are highest during the first few days after presentation and when operations are delayed for more than a month. The optimum timing for surgery is between 1 and 4 weeks after diagnosis—that is, after initial medical management has improved the activity of the necrotizing colitis. Mortality rates during this period are expected to be as low as 5–10%.

Subtotal colectomy with ileostomy, and proctocolectomy with ileostomy, remain the procedures of choice depending on the overall medical condition of the patient. During surgery and for 3–4 days postoperatively, the patient should be continued on high-dose corticosteroids to prevent relative adrenal insufficiency. Thereafter, the dose is tapered and the drug may be withdrawn by several weeks after surgery if the patient has recovered. At surgery, technical difficulties, as well as the extensively, inflamed, dilated, "paper-thin" colonic wall, may result in peritoneal contamination with bacteria; postoperative intraabdominal abscess formation is common and may be masked by continued administration of corticosteroids. Therefore, it is recommended that antibiotics be given for 2 weeks after corticosteroids have been discontinued. If a postoperative intraabdominal abscess develops, it should be treated by surgical or percutaneous drainage; again, in the event of this complication, the patient must be observed carefully for signs of relative adrenal insufficiency.

DIARRHEA IN THE CRITICALLY ILL

This situation includes a wide heterogenous set of causes involving both the small bowel and the colon.

Causes

Potential causes of diarrhea such as the residual effects of purgatives given before admission to the ICU, preceeding diarrheal illness, diarrhea associated with AIDS, and spurious diarrhea should be recognized from the patient's history and physical examination, which should always include a rectal examination. In patients who have undergone recent abdominal surgery, this will also help to exclude pelvic abscess. However, these causes account for only a minority of the diarrhea in the ICU.

More often, diarrhea is a side effect of treatment. Up to 25% of general ward patients develop diarrhea while on nasogastric feeds and the incidence is at least twice as high in the critically ill (6). The diarrhea associated with enteral feeds has been ascribed to their high osmolality and to lactose intolerance in patients with disaccharidase deficiency or bacterial contamination. Newer lactose-free formulas, which are approximately iso-osmolar with plasma, together with closed delivery systems, should have minimized these problems, though osmolality may increase rapidly once gut enzymes begin to digest the feed.

The sudden change from a high residue to a low residue diet is another potential cause for diarrhea. Some preparations containing dietary fibers are now available. Alternatively, it has been suggested that methylcellulose or a mucilaginous bulk laxative added to nasogastric feeds may reduce diarrhea. However, the efficacy of fecal bulking agents has not been assessed yet in a controlled trial.

The way in which nasogastric feeds are given may also affect the incidence of diarrhea. Constant gravity-assisted infusion of feeds seems to be associated with less diarrhea than bolus feeds. If diarrhea persists, controlling the infusion rate with a pump may cause it to resolve, perhaps by lowering the rate at which the osmotic load is delivered. Feeds given straight from the refrigerator have been said to be more likely to cause diarrhea than feeds at room temperature.

Many ICU patients have had a period of fasting or inadequate feeding before their admission to the ICU or a period of intravenous nutrition before starting enteral feeds. In these patients, malabsorption caused by villous atrophy may result in diarrhea. Animal models have shown a decrease in both villous height and cell proliferation in the mucosal clefts after periods of fasting or intravenous feeding.

Diarrhea may still occur in patients enterally fed. In these patients, malabsorption alone seems unlikely to be responsible for all the increased incidence of diarrhea. In critically ill patients, colonization with lactose-fermenting organisms or coliforms occurred when H_2 histamine receptor antagonists were used to increase the pH of gastric aspirate above 4. Moreover, a raised gastric pH is associated with an increase in jejunal bacterial content. Although a clinical syndrome of diarrhea and malabsorption caused by bacterial overgrowth has not been demonstrated in normal bowel, severe diarrhea ascribed to H_2 histamine receptor antagonists has been reported. Since bacterial overgrowth appears to be pH dependent, the effect of antacids is likely to be similar with added purgative effects from magnesium-containing antacids.

Some studies have suggested that antibiotics, especially when given orally, are the major cause of diarrhea occurring during enteral feeding by altering the normal bowel flora. However, antibiotics do not appear to increase the incidence of diarrhea in critically ill patients (6), perhaps because they are nearly always given parenterally. The potentially serious complication of pseudomembranous colitis should always be considered as a cause for diarrhea in patients receiving antibiotics. Nearly all except vancomycin and parenteral aminoglycosides can predispose to the growth of *Clostridium difficile*, the organism that produces the toxin responsible for pseudomembranous colitis. The infection may occur with both oral and parenteral antibiotics.

Finally, and likely underestimated, is diarrhea as a manifestation of multiple organ failure. Gastric dilatation and ileus frequently accompany critical illness, but some patients respond to severe illness—particularly during the early stages of sepsis and shock—with diarrhea. Diarrhea as a nonspecific manifestation of serious illness is well recognized in children, but less well documented in adults. Possible causes include malabsorption caused by diversion of blood flow from the intestinal mucosa during shock or by exogenous catecholamines, failure to absorb sodium and water from the colon against high electrochemical and concentration gradients, and perhaps changes to bile acid metabolism. Even minor changes to the enterohepatic circulation of bile salts result in diarrhea.

Management

Management of the critically ill patient is greatly compromised by diarrhea. A major commitment must be made for maintaining cleanliness and dignity. This is difficult to achieve when a continuous flow of liquid feces continues for more than a short time. Under these circumstances, a soft-walled rectal tube may provide temporary relief. However, its use may be risky, particularly if the bowel is inflamed, and should be reserved for the most difficult cases. It is usual to stop, or to reduce the amount of, nasogastric feeds. Samples of them may be sent for culture, though the yield from this should be very low if modern feed delivery practices are followed. The administration of other medicines should be reviewed. In addition to laxatives, antacids and H_2 receptor antagonists, many other drugs may cause diarrhea. Accordingly, all except essential drugs should be stopped.

Stools are often sent for culture but recognized intestinal pathogens are rarely isolated (6). Nevertheless, *Salmonella* species, *Shigella* species, *Campylobacter* species, *Yersinia enterocolitica*, enterotoxigenic *E. coli*, and *C. difficile* should be excluded and, when the fecal supernatant is positive for *C. difficile* or its toxin, the patient should be treated with oral vancomycin, 250–500 mg 6 hourly, or metronidazole. This is because of the hazards of pseudomembranous colitis to the critically ill and also the risk of cross-infection for other patients in the ICU, many of whom are likely to be on antibiotic therapy. Simple isolation procedures also reduce the risk of cross-infection and should be continued until the stool has been shown to be cleared of *C. difficile* after 10 days of treatment. Relapse occurs in 10–15% of patients after treatment.

Other investigations may be indicated by the patient's history or clinical examination. For example, amebic dysentery or giardiasis may present during intercurrent illness, diseases such as ulcerative colitis may recur, and the symptoms caused by a previously undiagnosed carcinoma of the colon may not have been sought or volunteered in a patient affected by acute trauma or severe illness caused by disease in another sytem.

Adequate replacement of water and electrolytes together with nutritional support is essential. During profuse diarrhea, daily fluid losses may exceed 3 or 4 liters. Depending on the cause of diarrhea, almost any combination of acid base and electrolyte disturbances can occur. The main losses are of water, sodium, potassium, bicarbonate, and chloride but unless renal function is normal and diarrhea only moderate, metabolic imbalance can be avoided only by frequent measurements. Greater than normal amounts of magnesium, zinc, and copper may also be lost. Replacement fluid is usually given intravenously. The effect of oral glucose/electrolyte solutions, such as those used successfully during the management of infant diarrhea, has not been assessed.

There are many proposed symptomatic remedies but few comparative or controlled trials to guide treatment. Fecal bulking agents such as methylcellulose, Metamucil, or Fybogel may be of some help. Mixtures containing kaolin or chalk are often said to act by absorbing "toxins" from the gut, but there is little evidence for this. The small amounts of opiates that are sometimes included in these mixtures are unlikely to have much effect. On the other hand, larger doses, such as codeine phosphate 30–60 mg 4–6 hourly, do seem to be effective in some patients.

Diphenoxylate with atropine (Lomotil) seems to enjoy an undeserved popularity. It is a central nervous system depressant and interacts with other sedative drugs and does not seem to have any advantage over codeine phosphate.

Loperamide is a newer antidiarrheal agent with fewer side effects but its efficacy has not been assessed in this context.

Lactobacillus acidophilus tablets, live yogurt, and *Saccharomyces boulardii* have been suggested as means of restoring the normal bowel flora when diarrhea is thought to be caused by antibiotics.

References

1. Banwell JG. Pathophysiology of diarrhea. In: Gorbach BL, ed. Infectious diarrhea. Boston: Blackwell Scientific Publications, 1986:1–15.
2. Binder HT. Pathophysiology of bile acid and fatty acid induced diarrhea. In: Field M, Fodtran JS, Schultz SG, eds. Secretory diarrhea. Baltimore: American Physiological Society, 1977:159.
3. Cooke HJ. Neurobiology of the intestinal mucosa. Gastroenterology 1988;90:1057–1081.
4. Debongnie JC, Phillips SF. Capacity of the human colon to absorb fluid. Gastroenterology 1978;74;698–703.
5. Fondacaro J. Intestinal ion transport and diarrhea disease. Am J. Physiol 1986;47;88–90.
6. Kelly WJ, Patrick MR, Hillman KM. Study of diarrhea in critically ill patients. Crit Care Med 1983;11:7.
7. Powell DW. Intestinal water and electrolyte transport. In: Johnson LA, Christenson J, Jacobsson ED, Jackson MJ, Walsh JH, eds. Physiology of the gastrointestinal tract. New York: Raven Press, 1986:1267–1307.
8. Rohde JE. Selective primary health care: strategies for control of disease in the developing world. XV. Acute diarrhoea. Rev Infect Dis 1984;6:840.
9. Snyder JD, Merson MH. The magnitude of the global problem of acute diarrhoeal disease: a review of active surveillance data. Bull WHO 1982;60:605.
10. Stoll BJ, Glass RI, Banu H, Huq MI, Khan MU, Ahmed M. Value of stool examination in patients with diarrhoea. Br Med J 1983;286:2037.

44

Pathophysiologic Mechanisms of Brain Injury

Deborah A. Hayek
Christopher Veremakis

The final outcome following a central nervous system (CNS) insult depends on the extent of brain injury during the initial event, as well as on deleterious sequelae that develop during the recuperative process. CNS injury may be classified as primary or secondary. Primary injury is the initial insult and, by definition, is complete at the time of clinical presentation. Secondary injury is a dynamic process that results from perpetuation of the primary pathologic process, or from the cascade of harmful events triggered by the primary injury. Secondary injury can succeed the primary event within minutes, hours, or days. Prevention or amelioration of secondary injury following a CNS insult is the goal of brain resuscitation. Optimal clinical management requires cognizance of the pathophysiologic principles underlying secondary brain injury. This article reviews these principles, and the therapeutic aspects of brain resuscitation is discussed in the succeeding chapter.

MECHANISMS OF TISSUE INJURY

In all forms of CNS injury, tissue ischemia is the final common pathway to irreversible cellular damage. Brain tissue ischemia results from an imbalance between oxygen supply and demand, which may occur when cerebral oxygen delivery is decreased, cerebral oxygen consumption is increased, or tissue oxygen uptake is impaired. Global cerebral oxygen delivery is the product of cerebral blood flow and systemic arterial oxygen content (CaO_2) (Table 44.1). Abrupt cessation of cerebral blood flow results in a loss of consciousness with 5–10 sec. Compared to other organs, the brain is especially sensitive to ischemia because of a high resting energy requirement and lack of oxygen reserves (57). The brain extracts more oxygen from systemic blood than do most organs. Consequently, cerebral venous oxygen saturation is lower than that of systemic venous blood (Table 44.1).

The complex mechanism by which cerebral ischemia progresses to neuronal damage and death involves multifactorial interactions at the cellular level and is not completely elucidated (22, 25, 47, 57, 54). Oxygen deprivation causes a rapid depletion of ATP stores and other high energy substrates, anaerobic metabolism, and termination of all energy-requiring reactions (47, 57). Lactic acid production increases and intracellular pH declines. The ATP-dependent Na^+/K^+ pump fails with subsequent breakdown of cellular ionic gradients. As K^+ leaks into the extracellular space, Na^+, water, and Ca^{2+} diffuse into the cytoplasm. Increased release of the

Table 44.1
Cerebral Oxygen Delivery and Consumption (Approximate Values) [a]

Cerebral blood flow (CBF)	50 ml/100 g/min
Systemic arterial oxygen content (Cao_2)	20 ml/100 ml
Jugular venous oxygen content ($Cjvo_2$)	13 ml/100 ml
Jugular venous oxygen saturation ($Sjvo_2$)	65%
Cerebral arteriovenous oxygen content difference ($CAVo_2 = Cao_2 - Cjvo_2$)	6.3–7.0 ml/100 ml
Cerebral oxygen delivery ($\dot{C}Do_2 = CBF \times Cao_2$)	10 ml/100 g/min
Cerebral oxygen consumption ($\dot{C}Vo_2 = CBF \times CAVo_2$)	3.5 ml/100 g/min

[a] Data from Refs. 34, 37, 39, and 44.

excitatory neurotransmitters glutamate and aspartate into the extracellular space may contribute to the loss of ionic homeostasis and increase neuronal excitability, boosting the metabolic requirements of tissue already compromised by ischemia. These events promote cell membrane degradation and the intracellular breakdown of proteins, nucleic acids, and lipids. This cellular catabolism may, in turn, stimulate the formation of toxic products (e.g., oxygen free radicals, eicosanoids), which further accelerate cellular death (22, 25, 47, 54). The massive calcium influx is especially detrimental and has been linked to membrane disruption, formation of toxic products, excitatory neurotransmitter activity, postischemic hypoperfusion, and vasospasm (25, 47, 57).

Reperfusion following cerebral ischemia may exacerbate further neuronal damage. The reintroduction of oxygen into an ischemic environment can result in the formation of injurious free radicals such as the superoxide and hydroxyl species. These highly reactive oxygen free radicals accelerate tissue destruction by causing membrane lipid peroxidation, protein and nucleic acid damage, and have also been implicated in the pathogenesis of vasogenic edema, vasospasm, and loss of autoregulation (22, 54). The formation of oxygen radicals during reperfusion may occur through several pathways. With ischemia, ATP is irreversibly degraded to hypoxanthine, a product which is usually metabolized to xanthine and uric acid in the presence of xanthine dehydrogenase. Under ischemic conditions, however, xanthine dehydrogenase is converted to xanthine oxidase. When oxygen is reintroduced after ischemia, the metabolism of hypoxanthine

by xanthine oxidase generates large amounts of hydroxyl and superoxide radicals. Oxygen free radicals may also be generated as a consequence of impaired mitochondrial respiration, neutrophil activation, auto-oxidation of catecholamines, and metabolism of arachidonic acid released from the cell membrane (22, 54). Reperfusion can also result in the conversion of liberated arachidonic acid to vasoconstricting leukotrienes and prostaglandins. Lipid peroxidation and further cell damage are accelerated in an acidotic environment. Lactic acid accumulation following ischemia is enhanced by premorbid hyperglycemia, which may subsequently potentiate reperfusion injury (47, 57, 74). Reperfusion may account for a large portion of the overall damage that ensues following the primary ischemic insult. Likewise, severe prolonged partial ischemia may actually cause more injury than brief complete ischemia, because the persistent "trickle" of flow may accelerate the production of toxic products (57).

The degree of brain injury after a cerebral insult is related to both duration and severity of ischemia, and also to regional variations in the ischemic vulnerability of brain tissue. Highly metabolic regions such as the hippocampus, cerebral cortex, and basal ganglia are most susceptible to ischemic injury (25). Neurologic recovery after cardiac arrest is influenced by the duration of the arrest and subsequent resuscitation (1). However, the traditional concept that after 5 min of complete ischemia, metabolic activity ceases and neurologic damage is irreversible has been questioned. Recovery of neurologic function may occur after 10–20 min of complete global ischemia in primates and humans (51). It has recently been shown that mitochondrial function and cellular metabolism can completely recover after even longer periods of ischemia (25, 47, 57).

The progressive damage and loss of function that results from decremental reduction of cerebral blood flow (CBF) is shown in Figure 44.1. Electroencephalographic silence and cessation of synaptic transmission occur when the flow *threshold of electrical failure* is reached at 15–20 ml/100 g/min (4, 62, 63). With a further decrease to 6–10 ml/100 g/min, the *threshold of membrane failure*, ionic disequilibrium and depletion of energy stores occurs (4, 57, 63). Tissue receiving CBF between these two thresholds is described by the concept of the ischemic penumbra (4); such tissue is electrically silent and nonfunctional, yet viable. This potentially salvageable tissue within the zone of penumbra provides a rationale for aggressive brain resuscitation to minimize secondary injury.

MAINTENANCE OF CEREBRAL BLOOD FLOW

The brain receives 15% of the cardiac output and utilizes up to 20% of total body oxygen consumption. Global cerebral blood flow is approximately 50–55 ml/100 g/min but can vary regionally from 20 to 80 ml/100 g/min. The cerebral blood volume occupies 10% of the intracranial space and

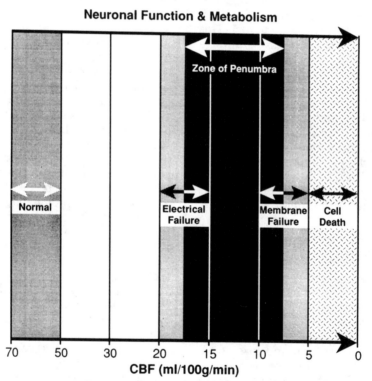

Figure 44.1. Schematic representation of flow thresholds for cerebral function and metabolism. As cerebral blood flow *(CBF)* is reduced below 30 ml/100 g/min, cognitive disfunction, alterations in consciousness, and EEG abnormalities develop. With further reductions to 15–20 ml/100 g/min, the *threshold of electrical failure* is reached, characterized by an isoelectric EEG, evoked response failure, and cessation of synaptic transmission. When CBF decreases to 6–10 ml/100 g/min the *threshold of membrane failure* is reached and ionic gradients deteriorate, energy metabolism is disrupted, and cellular function and integrity become impaired. The *zone of penumbra* describes brain tissue with flows between the upper limit of the electrical failure threshold and the lower limit of the membrane failure threshold (4, 57, 62, 63).

the majority of this volume is contained within the venous capacitance vessels.

Regulation of CBF

The major factors that regulate cerebral flood flow are Pao_2, $Paco_2$, pressure autoregulation, and cerebral metabolic activity. Cerebral blood flow is closely coupled or matched to metabolic needs, which in turn, are dependent on the level of neuronal stimulation. Hypoxia and hypercarbia produce cerebral vasodilation and increase cerebral blood flow (see Fig. 44.2). Although cerebral blood flow does not increase significantly until the partial pressure of oxygen falls to less than 50 torr, flow is very sensitive to changes in the partial pressure of carbon dioxide. Within the physiologic range of $Paco_2$, a fluctuation of 1 torr effects a 3–4% change in cerebral blood flow and a 0.04 ml/100 g change in cerebral blood volume. Both the vasoconstrictive and vasodilating effects of CO_2 are mediated by alterations in extracellular fluid pH. The marked influence of $Paco_2$ on cerebral blood flow and cerebral blood volume is of major clinical significance when intracranial compliance is compromised. When the mechanisms that compensate for elevated intracranial pressure and volume are exhausted, hypoventilation may precipitate massive secondary damage through an increase in cerebral blood volume and intracranial pressure (ICP) (Fig. 44.3). In contrast, therapeutic hyperventilation in the same setting can be dramatically beneficial.

Autoregulation accounts for the constancy of cerebral blood flow in spite of variations in mean arterial pressure from 50 to 150 mm Hg (Fig. 44.2). Outside of this range, cerebral blood flow is linearly related to mean arterial pressure. The upper and lower autoregulatory limits are shifted upward in chronically hypertensive patients, because of morphologic changes in the cerebral resistance vessels (6, 42). Cerebral autoregulation is postulated to be mediated by either a direct myogenic arterial response, or through the local action of a vasodilator metabolite (27).

Cerebral perfusion pressure (CPP) is the true driving force of cerebral blood flow and is defined as the difference between mean arterial pressure and cerebral ve-

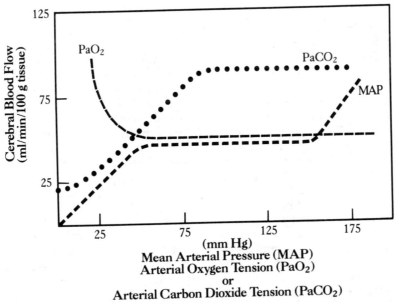

Figure 44.2. Changes in cerebral blood flow *(CBF)* in response to changes in mean arterial pressure *(MAP)*, arterial oxygen tension *(PaO₂)*, or arterial carbon dioxide tension *(PaCO₂)*. CBF remains constant as MAP varies between 50 and 150 mm Hg, as long as autoregulation is intact.

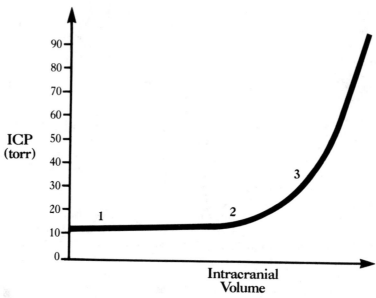

Figure 44.3. Compliance characteristics of the intracranial compartment. The flat portion of the curve *(1 → 2)* reflects the extent of compensatory mechanisms that operate when intracranial pressure *(ICP)* rises. When these compensatory mechanisms are exhausted, further small increases in intracranial volume can produce rapid and dangerous ICP elevation *(2 → 3)*.

nous pressure. With intracranial hypertension, ICP becomes the limiting downstream pressure, and cerebral perfusion pressure equals the mean arterial pressure minus the ICP. Therefore, a rising ICP may result in reduced cerebral blood flow in spite of adequate systemic blood pressure. Global cerebral blood flow is markedly compromised below a CPP of 40 mm Hg.

Many types of acute brain injury can cause regional or global impairment of autoregulation (27, 37). In the absence of autoregulation, blood flow to damaged areas becomes linearly related to cerebral perfusion pressure and directly dependent on mean arterial pressure and ICP. Nevertheless, it is difficult to predict the overall effect of raising mean arterial pressure in these circumstances. Elevation of mean arterial pressure could increase cerebral perfusion pressure and increase perfusion to ischemic tissue, or it could increase cerebral blood volume and precipitate edema formation, thus promoting secondary injury. Similarly, regional loss of the vasoconstrictor response to hypocarbia may also occur following brain injury, although

global loss of CO_2 reactivity is much less frequent (35, 39). Some arteries and arterioles in ischemic areas may be characterized by *vasomotor paralysis:* such vessels have lost the capacity to autoregulate flow, cannot couple flow to metabolism, respond abnormally to CO_2 changes, and become maximally vasodilated (27). Consequently, when intact brain responds appropriately to vasodilatory stimuli (such as hypercarbia) with regional increases in cerebral blood flow, blood can be shunted away from "vasoparalyzed" zones, producing an "intracerebral steal syndrome." Conversely, stimuli that increase cerebral vascular resistance in intact areas (e.g., hypocarbia) may shunt blood flow into vasoparalyzed zones, producing an "inverse steal" (4, 27, 63). In summary, after cerebral injury, multiple pathophysiologic events may compromise regional cerebral blood flow, even when cerebral perfusion pressure or global cerebral blood flow are adequate. The extent to which such regional flow impairments exacerbate secondary injury, and the influence of therapeutic manipulation of mean arterial pressure and $Paco_2$ on regional flow variations in specific disease states, remain to be determined.

Measurement of Cerebral Blood Flow

The currently available techniques for quantitation of cerebral blood flow are not easily implemented at the bedside to routinely assess and monitor ICU patients, although some methods are more practical than others. The most common technique employed clinically utilizes scintigraphic detection of the rate of clearance of inhaled or intravenous radioactive xenon from the brain (37). Much of the data that describes cerebral blood flow alterations in brain injury has been gathered with this method. Quantitative measurement of regional cerebral blood flow can also be derived from sequential CT scanning combined with the inhalation of nonradioactive xenon (xenon-enhanced CT) (20, 27). Positron emission tomography (PET) is a good method for quantitation of regional and global cerebral blood flow, but is expensive and cumbersome (43). Single photon emission computed tomography (SPECT) is more easily applied in the clinical setting, but less accurate for assessment of cerebral blood flow than is PET (27, 43). Transcranial Doppler ultrasound is a noninvasive method that evaluates the velocity of flow in the large intracranial arteries (9). This technique does not provide quantitative CBF estimates, but may allow qualitative identification and serial assessment of vasospasm, vascular constriction or stenosis, cerebral perfusion pressure reduction, and impaired autoregulation. Transcranial Doppler ultrasound is applicable at the bedside for continuous or repetitive testing. Near-infrared spectroscopy (niroscopy) can be used to continuously monitor cerebrovascular hemoglobin saturation; this noninvasive technique allows qualitative estimation of brain oxygenation and cerebral circulatory reserve (44, 59). Niroscopy is feasible for use in the ICU but at the present time has not been extensively tested. Advances in the diagnostic and therapeutic aspects of cerebral resuscitation would be greatly facilitated by the refinement of technologies that allow bedside quantification and continuous monitoring of regional cerebral blood flow.

Disorders of Cerebral Blood Flow

Regional and global cerebral hypoperfusion are the primary consequences of ischemic stroke and cardiac arrest, respectively. However, generalized and focal decreases in cerebral blood flow also develop after subarachnoid hemorrhage, traumatic head injury, and severe meningitis (37, 64, 68). Normalization of blood flow after cerebral insult occurs, to a greater or lesser extent, over time. During the first few days after acute stroke, global and regional cerebral blood flow decreases, and then increases, over the next few weeks (8, 20). The degree to which such reductions in cerebral blood flow adversely influence ultimate neurologic outcome after brain injury is not known.

When the circulation is restored after cardiac arrest lasting longer than 5 min, four succeeding forms of cerebral reperfusion abnormalities have been described (51). (*a*) Immediately after global ischemia, there is a multifocal absence of cerebral perfusion, termed the *no reflow* phenomenon, which may resolve spontaneously or persist in scattered areas of brain. The extent of no reflow depends on the duration and severity of the ischemic insult and the adequacy of subsequent reperfusion. No reflow is the pathophysiologic basis for irreversible damage resulting from the primary ischemic injury and is attributed to microcirculatory obstruction at the capillary level, local alterations in blood viscosity, or focal edema (19). (*b*) Global hyperemia follows in the first 20 min after recirculation and is transient (15–30 min) (51). (*c*) Delayed global hypoperfusion subsequently develops and persists for hours (19, 51). Postischemic hypoperfusion has also been observed after focal ischemia and incomplete global ischemia. This phenomenon is ascribed to increased arterial tone and vasoconstriction. (*d*) The last reperfusion abnormality involves either resolution of flow, continued hypoperfusion and/or hyperemia, or cessation of flow and brain death (51).

Vasospasm is severe arterial constriction,

which can result in cerebral ischemia and infarction. Vasospasm is the leading cause of postadmission morbidity and mortality following subarachnoid hemorrhage (2, 23). Vasospasm usually develops 3–10 days after subarachnoid bleeding, frequently involves multiple arteries near the hemorrhage, and can last days to weeks. Vasospasm occurs in some patients with severe head injury (37) and has also been observed during bacterial meningitis (21), although the pathophysiologic relevance in these disorders is not clearly delineated. The pathogenesis of vasospasm is poorly understood, but the presence of blood in the subarachnoid space is a necessary prerequisite (2). The activation or lysis of subarachnoid clot components (platelets, mast cells, neutrophils, erythrocytes) may initiate an inflammatory response in blood vessels or may promote the release of vasoactive mediators, which constrict smooth muscle or cause endothelial damage. The vascular narrowing is also related to morphologic changes in the arterial wall, which have been observed postmortem. Severe angiographic vasospasm may be present without clinical symptoms of ischemia. Clinical features include a gradual onset of confusion or decreased level of consciousness, focal hemispheric motor and speech impairments, or more nonspecific signs (fever, leukocytosis, malaise, drowsiness). The presence on admission CT scan of large, thick collections of blood in the subarachnoid space is the best predictor of vasospasm after subarachnoid hemorrhage (2).

Hyperemia or *luxury perfusion* can occur after acute brain injury. This abnormality of blood flow in excess of metabolic need is attributed to impaired autoregulation and vasomotor paralysis (27) and may be present with increased cerebral blood flow (absolute hyperemia) or decreased or normal cerebral blood flow (relative hyperemia). Hyperemia is characterized by a narrowed cerebral arteriovenous oxygen content difference and decreased cerebral oxygen extraction since flow is uncoupled to metabolism (39) (Table 44.2). Hyperemia can cause secondary brain injury by disruption of the blood brain barrier with edema and elevated ICP as consequences. Absolute and relative hyperemia may occur after head injury, stroke, and cardiac arrest (11, 20, 37, 51). Hyperemia after cardiac arrest is associated with a worsened prognosis (11). Although more common in pediatric patients, hyperemia occurs in up to 55% of severely head-injured adults and is associated with an increased incidence of intracranial hypertension in this setting (37, 39).

INTRACRANIAL PRESSURE

Regulation of Intracranial Pressure and Compliance

The volume of the intracranial cavity is comprised of brain (80%), cerebrospinal fluid (CSF) (10%), and blood (10%). Because the cranium is nondistensible, the total volume of the intracranial cavity is fixed. Consequently, when the volume of one component increases, the volume of the other components must decrease or pressure within the cranium will rise. This principle is known as the Monroe-Kellie doctrine. The pressure-volume relationship (i.e., functional compliance) of the intracranial cavity is depicted in Figure 44.3. Since the brain is basically noncompressible, an augmentation of intracranial

Table 44.2
Interrelationship of CBF, $C\dot{V}O_2$, and $CA\dot{V}O_2$ in Brain Injury

	CBF	$C\dot{V}O_2$	$CA\dot{V}O_2$
Normal (N)	N	N	N
Compensatory flow-metabolism coupling	↓	↓	N
Compensatory flow-metabolism coupling	↑	↑	N
Ischemia	↓	N	↑
Infarction	↓	↓	↑
Hyperemia	↑/N	↓	↓

volume initially causes a compensatory decrease of blood or CSF volume. Normal ICP is maintained through displacement of CSF into the spinal subarachnoid space and by venoconstriction so that cerebral venous blood is shifted into the jugular system (Fig. 44.3, *1 → 2*). When these compensatory mechanisms have reached their limits, further small increases in intracranial volume can produce rapid and dangerous ICP elevation (Fig. 44.3 *2 → 3*).

Intracranial hypertension causes secondary brain injury by compromising cerebral blood flow and/or by producing brain shift. ICP elevation results in decreased cerebral perfusion pressure, which may, in turn, compromise cerebral blood flow if cerebral perfusion pressure falls to less than 50 mm Hg (or at perfusion pressures even higher if autoregulation is impaired). A rise in pressure gradients across the intracranial compartments causes distortion of brain tissue and obstruction and tearing of small blood vessels, and in the extreme case, the brain is displaced from one cranial compartment into another, initiating a herniation syndrome. The extent of injury and subsequent neurologic deficit is a function of the failure of normal compensatory mechanisms and the rate of rise of ICP rather than the actual level of ICP. If an elevated pressure is equally distributed throughout the brain and autoregulation of cerebral blood flow is intact, high pressures may not be associated with functional neurologic impairment. Slow progressive volume expansion (as occurs with tumors or benign intracranial hypertension) is often well tolerated since time allows for greater CSF reduction, and brain tissue itself may atrophy. Acute brain injury, however, usually produces rapid ICP elevations, as well as impairment of autoregulation. Intracranial pressure-volume decompensation is most frequently associated with contusions, intracranial hematomas, edema, and tumors. A normal ICP is 0–10 mm Hg, and elevations above 15–20 mm Hg are considered to be clinically significant.

Most of the clinical information regarding the detrimental effect of increased ICP derives from the study of traumatic brain injury. Significant ICP elevation occurs in up to approximately 55% of patients with severe head injury, usually develops over the first 72 hr postinjury, and is associated with both increased neurologic morbidity and mortality (36, 38). Persistent uncontrollable ICP elevation is present in approximately 15% of head-injured patients and is usually fatal (31, 36, 38). Aggressive treatment of intracranial hypertension improves prognosis and survival in head trauma (26, 36, 53).

Increased ICP following cardiac arrest may develop in association with diffused cerebral edema, but sustained elevations are uncommon in the absence of underlying cranial pathology or seizures (52). Intracranial hypertension can also complicate massive strokes, severe CNS infections, and the toxic-metabolic encephalopathies associated with Reye's syndrome, fulminant acute hepatic failure, diabetic ketoacidosis, or hyponatremia and is adversely related to outcome in these syndromes (49, 56, 64). Therapy to reduce ICP improves outcome in Reye's syndrome (56), but evidence of a beneficial effect of therapy following global hypoxic injury and massive stroke is less conclusive (46, 49, 72).

Monitoring Intracranial Pressure

ICP can be measured at the bedside through devices placed in the epidural, subdural, subarachnoid, ventricular, or intraparenchymal space (66, 69). Intraventricular catheters provide the most accurate pressure readings and have the additional advantage of enabling drainage of CSF to reduce ICP. The major drawback of this technique is the significant incidence of intracranial infection, including ventriculitis (7–21%) (5, 66). Additionally, intraventricular monitors are difficult to insert if the ventricles are small or distorted, and there is a risk of hemorrhage during insertion. In general, devices placed in the subarachnoid, subdural, and epidural spaces are more easily inserted and associated with lower infection rates (1–15%) but are more inaccurate (5, 66, 69). As with all invasive devices, infection risk soars when ICP monitors are in place more than 4–5 days (5). A fiberoptic, transducer-tipped catheter has been recently developed, which may allow improved ICP measurement; it can be placed in subarachnoid or intraparenchymal sites (66, 69).

Although treatment of intracranial hypertension improves outcome and is clearly indicated in many forms of brain injury, the necessity of continuous invasive ICP measurement to administer efficacious therapy is debatable. Clinical data support the premise that therapeutic regimens that employ ICP monitoring improve survival in head injury and Reye's syndrome (7, 56), but several studies have demonstrated that empiric therapy for intracranial hypertension delivered without actual ICP measurement appeared as effective as monitor-titrated therapy (60, 61). Nonetheless, advocates of ICP monitoring argue that, since raised ICP strongly correlates with worsened morbidity and mortality, recognition of changes in ICP are difficult to appreciate by clinical examination, and since monitoring permits early recognition of intracranial hypertension and precise titration of therapy, ICP should be measured in patients with severe brain injury (36). The benefits of therapy guided by invasive ICP measurements must be weighed against the risk of complications. Until further data is available, indications for ICP monitoring remain controversial and are frequently a matter of individual philosophy and judgment. ICP monitoring should be considered when there is a strong probability of significantly increased ICP, and (a) measures to lower ICP are likely to improve outcome or (b) sequential neurologic examination will not be informative, as for example, patients in deep coma or who require the use of neuromuscular paralyzing agents.

Brain Edema

Injured brain swells when it is damaged. Brain edema is defined as the abnormal accumulation of intracranial fluid associated with volumetric enlargement of brain tissue. As in the lung, brain edema can form as a general response to a variety of primary injuries and may also complicate systemic illnesses such as acute fulminant hepatic failure, diabetic ketoacidosis, and fat emboli. Secondary injury is produced as edema develops, at first from focal encroachment on blood vessels and regional flow impairment, then from ICP elevation and compromise of global perfusion, and finally from compression and herniation of brain tissue.

There are three types of brain edema (13, 24). *Cytotoxic edema* is the intracellular fluid accumulation that occurs with cell membrane dysfunction and loss of the normal ionic and osmolar gradients between the intracellular and interstitial compartments. Cytotoxic edema is precipitated by hypoxia, ischemia, hyposmolar states, meningitis and other severe CNS infections, and toxins that impair cellular respiration. *Vasogenic edema* develops from extravasation of protein-rich fluid from the intravascular to the interstitial space following injury to the vascular endothelium and blood-brain barrier. This form of edema is seen with brain tumor or abscess, contusion, hemorrhage, infarction, lead intoxication, and meningitis. *Interstitial edema* is most commonly associated with obstructive hydrocephalus and results from CSF outflow obstruction, which causes fluid to shift from the ventricles into the periventricular interstitium.

Ischemic brain edema is comprised of both cytotoxic and vasogenic edema (24, 63). The magnitude of edema depends on the severity of the ischemic insult. Ischemic brain edema evolves over several days and reaches maximum severity within 48–72 hr of the initial insult.

CEREBRAL METABOLISM IN THE NORMAL AND INJURED BRAIN

The brain consumes between 15 and 20% of the total body oxygen consumption. Global cerebral oxygen consumption is the product of cerebral blood flow and the cerebral arteriojugular venous oxygen content difference. Normal values for cerebral oxygen consumption and delivery are shown in Table 44.1

Cerebral Metabolic Monitoring

Cerebral arteriovenous oxygen content difference is measured clinically by simultaneous sampling of systemic arterial and jugular bulb venous blood. Venous blood from the jugular bulb, which represents the "mixed-venous" blood from the brain, is obtained by cannulation of the jugular vein and passage of the catheter upward to the level of the jugular bulb (15, 37, 39). Continuous monitoring of jugular venous oxygen saturation ($SjvO_2$) can be accomplished with standard oximetry catheters, thus enabling titration of therapy based on estimates of cerebral oxygen utilization, in a manner similar to the use of the mixed-venous oxygen saturation in systemic hemodynamic management. Interpretation of $SjvO_2$ data is limited by the fact that low saturations are only suggestive is ischemia, and normal saturations are not absolute proof of adequate cerebral perfusion (44). Noninvasive monitoring of combined arteriovenous cerebral hemoglobin saturation is possible with near-infrared spectroscopy, which also provides another means of assessing cerebral oxygen utilization (44, 59).

Positron emission tomography can be used to determine global and regional cerebral oxygen consumption, oxygen extraction, and glucose metabolism (43). Magnetic resonance spectroscopy can also provide information about cerebral metabolism by identifying abnormalities in ATP, phosphocreatine, and lactate, for example (45). These methods are presently employed as investigational tools to study the effects of ischemia on cerebral energy metabolism.

Regulation of Cerebral Metabolism

Global cerebral oxygen consumption increases with neuronal stimulation, hyperthermia, seizures, and elevated systemic oxygen consumption. Hypothermia reduces cerebral oxygen consumption: when temperature is reduced from 37 to 27°C, cerebral oxygen consumption is halved (34). Pharmacologic agents that decrease cerebral oxygen consumption include the volatile anesthetics, barbiturates, and benzodiazepines (33, 34). In the nonpathologic state, cerebral blood flow is closely coupled to cerebral oxygen con-

sumption, adjusting in parallel to match changes in metabolism, so that the cerebral arteriovenous oxygen content difference remains constant over a wide range of cerebral metabolic activity (27). Flow-metabolism coupling may be mediated by changes in the concentrations of ions (H^+, K^+, Ca_2^+) or adenosine in the extravascular fluid (27). PET studies have demonstrated that flow-metabolism coupling normally results in a uniform value for the cerebral oxygen extraction fraction of approximately 0.33 (43).

When cerebral blood flow declines, cerebral oxygen consumption is maintained by increased oxygen extraction (indicated by a drop in $SjvO_2$ and widening of the cerebral arteriovenous oxygen content difference), up to a certain point. A further decline in cerebral blood flow exhausts compensatory mechanisms, and cerebral oxygen consumption decreases as ischemia, cellular disruption, and infarction develop (43). During acute stroke, there is an initial period when both regional cerebral blood flow and cerebral oxygen consumption are low and oxygen extraction in the affected area is high (71). The progression from an increased to a decreased regional oxygen extraction may signify the progression from ischemia to irreversible infarction, since infarcted tissue does not utilize oxygen. The presence of elevated oxygen extraction in ischemic regions may indicate the presence of marginal perfusion in nonfunctioning, but still viable, brain tissue. Improved regional oxygen delivery could potentially rescue such tissue, which corresponds to the *ischemic penumbra* (43). In irreversibly damaged brain, oxygen extraction and metabolism are minimal, and cerebral blood flow and cerebral oxygen consumption are uncoupled, i.e., regional flow exceeds the metabolic needs of the tissue.

Cerebral oxygen consumption is often decreased after primary brain injury; such reductions have been observed after head injury and subarachnoid hemorrhage, as well as after ischemic stroke (18, 37, 39, 68, 71). Decreased cerebral blood flow may be a consequence of the primary injury, but may also develop as a regulatory response to depressed cerebral oxygen consumption, as occurs, for example, during general anesthesia. When concurrent reductions in cerebral blood flow and cerebral oxygen consumption reflect intact flow-metabolism coupling rather than ischemia, cerebral arteriovenous oxygen content difference is normal (Table 44.2). When this coupling is not compromised, therapeutic maneuvers to reduce cerebral oxygen consumption may be beneficial if cerebral blood flow is pathologically decreased and cerebral arteriovenous oxygen content difference is increased. Conversely, increased cerebral metabolic demand could precipitate tissue ischemia if either cerebral oxygen delivery or flow-metabolism coupling is impaired.

CNS INFECTIONS

The potential for secondary injury that exists when the brain in invaded by microorganisms is an important consideration during cerebral resuscitation. The most frequent CNS infections seen in the ICU are bacterial meningitis or meningeoencephalitis, viral encephalitis, and brain abscess.

Bacterial invasion of the meninges initiates a pathophysiologic cycle of replication and inflammation that is often associated with cerebral edema, hypoperfusion, and vascular occlusion. Bacterial cell wall components and endotoxin interact with endothelial cells and macrophages to produce cytokines and complement activation, resulting in vascular adhesion of neutrophils and their passage into the subarachnoid space, as well as further endothelial cell injury (64). Several consequences of subarachnoid space inflammation, thought to be mediated by the action of inflammatory cytokines and humoral factors such as antibodies and complement, produce secondary brain injury (64). Ongoing neutrophil activation causes the release of toxic substances, which produce further neuronal cell damage and cytotoxic edema. Endothelial cell damage may result in thrombosis of arteriolar, venular, and capillary beds, producing ischemic cellular injury, cytotoxic edema, and hypoperfusion (21, 73). Injury to the choroid plexus epithelium and microvascular endothelium results in altered blood-brain barrier permeability and vasogenic edema. Persisting inflammation may cause obstruction of CSF outflow and interstitial edema which can result in hydrocephalus (21). Cytotoxic, vasogenic, and interstitial edema result in ICP elevation and subsequent cerebral hypoperfusion.

The diagnostic and therapeutic approach to CNS infections has been reviewed in depth (10, 64, 70) and is beyond the scope of this chapter. Empiric antibiotic therapy for bacterial meningitis is based on pathogen probability and status of underlying host-defense mechanisms. In the neonate, the most likely pathogens are *Escherichia coli, Listeria monocytogenes,* and group B streptococci, while in infancy and childhood the most common pathogens are *Haemophilus influenzae, Neisseria meningitidis,* and *Streptococcus pneumoniae.* Adult bacterial meningitis is usually caused by *S. pneumoniae* and *N. meningitidis;* in older debilitated patients or those with compromised immunity, Gram-negative bacilli, *L. monocytogenes,* the yeast *Cryptococcus neoformans,* and other opportunistic organisms become important pathogens. When meningitis develops in the postoperative neurosurgical patient, Gram-negative bacilli and *Staphylococcus aureus* should be considered. Meningitis following cranial trauma is most frequently caused by *S. pneumoniae;* however, antimicrobial prophylaxis is ineffective and not routinely indicated after blunt head injury.

The use of antibiotics to halt bacterial replication is the cornerstone of therapy for bacterial CNS infections. However, destruction of microorganisms may transiently increase the release of toxic bacterial wall products, thus briefly intensifying inflammatory mechanisms, which aggravate cellular damage. Consequently, the adjunctive use of antiinflammatory agents has been proposed as a strategy to reduce secondary brain injury (32, 64). In three clinical trials, dexamethasone administered concomitantly with the initiation of antibiotic treatment (0.15 mg/kg i.v. q6h×4 days) has been prospectively shown to reduce the incidence of sensorineural hearing loss and other neurologic sequelae (seizures, paresis, ataxia) of pediatric bacterial meningitis predominately caused by

H. influenzae (28, 32, 40). In another prospective study, adjunctive therapy with dexamethasone (8–12 mg q12h × 3 days) was associated with improved survival and fewer adverse neurologic sequelae (i.e., impaired hearing and paresis) in both adults and children with pneumococcal meningitis (14). An improvement in several acute pathologic parameters (i.e., fever duration, CSF glucose, protein and lactate) has been noted in some studies (28, 32, 40). The beneficial effects of dexamethasone presumably result from reduction of inflammatory mediators (e.g., tumor necrosis factor, platelet-activating factor, interleukin-1) in the CSF (32, 40). Although the preliminary evidence is encouraging, the routine use of dexamethasone in bacterial meningitis has been challenged on the basis of limited clinical data and the potential for adverse effects (17), and therefore remains a matter of individual clinical judgment (3).

The potential efficacy of other antiinflammatory agents such as inhibitors of arachidonic acid metabolism in bacterial meningitis is investigational, as is adjunctive therapy with specific monoclonal antibodies (64, 65). Supplementary steriod therapy for brain abscess remains controversial (10, 55). The potential benefits and/or drawbacks of antiinflammatory agents such as corticosteriods in the treatment of viral encephalitis have not been clarified.

BRAIN DEATH

Over the last decade, an international consensus has recognized whole brain criteria in addition to the traditional cardiopulmonary criteria as a medical basis for the determination of death (16). Following the medical lead, most governmental bodies have adjusted their legal statutes to include whole brain criteria for certification of legal death. An individual is dead when either of the following is established: (a) irreversible cessation of circulatory and respiratory function or (b) irreversible cessation of function of the entire brain (including the brainstem). Cessation of brain function is determined when examination reveals both absent cerebral as well as brainstem function. Irreversibility is determined by confirmation of a clear-cut structural or metabolic etiology for the coma, exclusion of the possibility of recovery, and persistence of the absence of total brain function for an appropriate period of time (16). Certification of brain death is based primarily on clinical examination and exclusion of reversible etiologies of CNS depression (Table 44.3). Confirmatory tests such as an isoelectric EEG or cerebral blood flow studies are not required unless a complete examination cannot be performed or the clinical findings are obscured by a complicating factor such as drug or metabolic intoxications or hypothermia. It must be verified that the patient is in deep coma, is unresponsive to painful stimuli, and has no brainstem reflexes. Spinal cord reflexes may persist after brain death and do not preclude the diagnosis (29, 48). Nonfunction of the respiratory center is established by the apnea test (30, 41, 50). This study consists of hyperoxygenation followed by withdrawal of mechanical ventilation and the subsequent demonstration of apnea in the presence of hypercarbia. It is very important to perform this test correctly, since a severely brain-injured patient who is not brain dead may have function of the medullary center. Although brain death criteria are objective and unambiguous, frequent clinical variations require the participation of a physician experienced in the brain death certification process. The false-positive diagnosis of brain death must never occur.

Donors who have fulfilled brain death criteria provide the majority of transplanted organs, and care of the brain dead organ donor presents multiple clinical challenges. The somatic pathology manifested by the brain dead patient includes hypotension, cardiac dysfunction, electrolyte and endocrinologic abnormalities, and hypothermia (12, 67). Consequently, optimal management of the potential donor often begins during the later stages of brain death certification. A sensitive balance must be achieved between the certification process and concurrent somatic donor maintenance on the one hand and consideration of patient integrity and family sensibilities on the other hand.

Table 44.3
Clinical Criteria for Brain Death Certification[a]

Exclusion of reversible CNS depression
  Absence of hypothermia
  Absence of drugs (e.g., ethanol, barbiturates)
  Absence of metabolic perturbations that could potentiate CNS depression (e.g., abnormalities
    in electrolytes, osmolarity, serum ammonia, creatinine, hypercarbia, hypoxemia)
Absent cortical function
  Unresponsiveness to painful stimuli
  No spontaneous muscular movements (in the absence of muscle relaxants)
  No posturing, shivering, or seizure activity (in the absence of muscle relaxants)
Absent brainstem function
  Pupils nonreactive and fixed to light
  No corneal reflexes
  No gag or cough reflexes
  No oculocephalic reflexes
  No oculovestibular reflexes
Documentation of apnea
  Absence of spontaneous breathing for 30 sec after $Paco_2$ >50 torr with pH <7.35 at end of
    apnea test
  Patients dependent on hypoxic drive should have Pao_2 <50 torr
Additional confirmatory studies (optional)
  Cerebral blood flow study (radionuclide imaging or four-vessel angiogram)
  Electroencephalogram
  Evoked potentials

[a] Data from Ref. 16.

CONCLUSION

Primary and secondary brain injury causes irreversible CNS damage through the final common pathway of cellular ischemia. Disruption of the balance between CNS oxygen supply and demand results from pathologic changes in cerebral blood flow and intracranial pressure, which decrease cerebral oxygen delivery, or from pathologic alterations in cerebral metabolism, which modify cerebral oxygen consumption. Ischemic cellular dysfunction initiates mechanisms such as calcium-mediated cell damage, the production of free radicals or other toxic mediators, and intracellular acidosis. At the tissue level, the initial CNS insult can trigger a series of events that result in impaired cerebral perfusion and aberrant regulation of intracranial impaired cerebral perfusion and aberrant regulation of intracranial volume, thus overwhelming normal compensatory mechanisms and producing secondary brain injury. The pathophysiologic mechanisms of secondary brain injury include cerebral hypoperfusion, vasospasm, hyperemia, edema, intracranial hypertension, seizures, and the formation of toxic metabolites. The extent that these various forms of secondary brain injury are manifest depends on the type and severity of the primary injury. The purpose of the brain resuscitation is to limit the development of secondary injury.

Acknowledgment. The authors gratefully acknowledge the assistance of Carolyn Linenbroker, Jacklyn O'Brien, and Marie Wolinski in the preparation of this manuscript.

References

1. Abramson NS, Safar P, Detre KM, et al. Neurologic recovery after cardiac arrest: effect of duration of ischemia. Crit Care Med 1985;13:930–931.
2. Adams HP, Kassell NF, Torner JC, et al. Predicting cerebral ischemia after aneurysmal subarachnoid hemorrhage: influence of clinical condition, CT results, and antifibrinolytic therapy. Neurology 1987;37:1586–1591.
3. American academy of pediatrics. Committee on infectious diseases. Dexamethasone therapy for bacterial meningitis in infants and children. Pediatrics 1990;86(1):130–133.
4. Astrup J. Energy-requiring cell functions in the ischemic brain. J Neurosurg 1982;56:482–497.

5. Aucoin PJ, Kotilainen HR, Gantz NM, et al. Intracranial pressure monitors. Epidemiologic study of risk factors and infections. Am J Med 1986;80:369–376.

6. Bertel O, Marx B, Conen D. Effects of antihypertensive treatment on cerebral perfusion. Am J Med 1987;82(suppl 3B):29–36.

7. Bowers SA, Marshall LF. Outcome in 200 consecutive cases of severe head injury treated in San Diego county: a prospective analysis. Neurosurgery 1980;6:237–242.

8. Burke AM, Younkin D, Gordon J, et al. Changes in cerebral blood flow and recovery from acute stroke. Stroke 1986;17:173–178.

9. Caplan LR, Brass LM, DeWitt LD, et al. Transcranial Doppler Ultrasound: present status. Neurology 1990;40:696–700.

10. Chun CH, Johnson JD, Hofstetter M, et al. Brain abscess. A study of 45 consecutive cases. Medicine 1986;65:415–431.

11. Cohan SL, Mun SK, Petite J, et al. Cerebral blood flow in humans following resuscitation from cardiac arrest. Stroke 1989;20:761–765.

12. Darby JM, Stein K, Grenvik A, Stuart SA. Approach to management of the heartbeating "brain dead" organ donor. JAMA 1989;261:2222–2228.

13. Fishman RA. Brain edema. N Engl J Med 1975;14:706–711.

14. Girgis NI, Farid Z, Mikhail I, et al. Dexamethasone treatment for bacterial meningitis in children and adults. Pediatr Infect Dis J 1989;8:848–851.

15. Goetting MG, Preston G. Jugular bulb catheterization: experience with 123 patients. Crit Care Med 1990;18:1220–1223.

16. Guidelines for the determination of death. Report of the medical consultants on the diagnosis of death to the President's Commission for the study of ethical problems in medicine and biomedical and behavioral research. Crit Care Med 1982;10:62–64.

17. Havens PL, Wendelberger KJ, Hoffman GM, et al. Corticosteriods as adjunctive therapy in bacterial meningitis. A meta-analysis of clinical trials. Am J Dis Child 1989;143:1051–1055.

18. Hino A, Mizukawa N, Tenjin H, et al. Postoperative hemodynamic and metabolic changes in patients with subarachnoid hemorrhage. Stroke 1989;20:1594–1510.

19. Hossman KA. Hemodynamics of postischemic reperfusion of the brain. In: Weinstein PR, Faden AI, eds. Protection of the brain from ischemia. Baltimore: Williams & Wilkins, 1990:21–36.

20. Hughes RL, Yonas H, Gur D, et al. Cerebral blood flow determination within the first 8 hours of cerebral infarction using stable xenon-enhanced computed tomography. Stroke 1989;20:754–760.

21. Igarashi M, Gilmartin RC, Gerald B, et al. Cerebral arteritis and bacterial meningitis. Arch Neurol 1984;41:531–535.

22. Ikeda Y, Long DM. The molecular basis of brain injury and brain edema: the role of oxygen free radicals. Neurosurgery 1990;27:1–11.

23. Kassell NF, Sasaki T, Colohan AR, et al. Cerebral vascular spasm following aneurysmal subarachnoid hemorrhage. Stroke 1985;16:562–572.

24. Klatzo I. Brain oedema following brain ischaemia and the influence of therapy. Br J Anaesth 1985;57:18–22.

25. Kochanel PM. Novel pharmacologic approaches to brain resuscitation after cardiorespiratory arrest in the pediatric patient. Crit Care Clin 1988;4:661–677.

26. Langfitt TW, Gennarelli TA. Can the outcome from head injury be improved? J Neurosurg 1982;56:19–25.

27. Lassen NA, Astrup J. Cerebral blood flow: normal regulation and ischemic thresholds. In: Weinstein PR, Faden AL eds. Protection of the brain from ischemia. Baltimore: Williams & Wilkins, 1990:7–19.

28. Lebel MH, Freij BJ, Syrogiannopoulos GA. Dexamethasone therapy for bacterial meningitis. Results of two double-blind, placebo-controlled trials. N Engl J Med 1988;319:964–971.

29. Mandel S, Arenas A, Scasta D. Spinal automatism in cerebral death. N Engl J Med 1982;307:501.

30. Marks SJ, Zisfein J. Apneic oxygenation in apnea tests for brain death. A controlled trial. Arch Neurol 1990;47:1066–1068.

31. Marshall LF, Smith RW, Shapiro HM. The outcome with aggressive treatment in severe head injuries. Part II: acute and chronic barbiturate administration in the management of head injury. J Neurosurg 1979;50:26–30.

32. McCracken GH Jr, Lebel MH. Dexamethasone therapy for bacterial meningitis in infants and children. Am J Dis Child 1989;143:287–289.

33. McPherson RW, Kirsch JR, Traystman RJ. Optimal anesthetic techniques for patients at risk of cerebral ischemia. In: Weinstein PR, Faden AI, eds. Protection of the brain from ischemia. Baltimore: Williams & Wilkins, 1990:237–252.

34. Michenfelder JD. Anesthesia and the brain. New York: Churchill Livingstone 1988.

35. Miller JD. Head injury and brain ischaemia—implications for therapy. Br J Anaesth 1985;57:120–129.

36. Miller JD, Butterworth JF, Gudeman SK, et al. Further experience in the management of severe head injury. J Neurosurg 1981;54:289–299.

37. Muizelaar JP. Cerebral bood flow, cerebral bood volume, and cerebral metabolism after severe head injury. In: Becker DP, Gudeman SK, eds. Textbook of head injury. Philadelphia: WB Saunders, 1989:221–240.

38. Narayan RK, Kishore PR, Becker DP, et al. Intracranial pressure: to monitor or not to monitor? J Neurosurg 1982;56:650–659.

39. Obrist WD, Langfitt TW, Jaggi JL, et al. Cerebral blood flow and metabolism in comatose patients with acute head injury. J Neurosurg 1984;61:241–253.

40. Odio CM, Faingezicht I, Paris M, et al. The beneficial effects of early dexamethasone administration in infants and children with bacterial meningitis. N Engl J Med 1991;324:1525–1531.

41. Oikkonen M, Aittomaki J, Saari M. Apnoeic Oxygenation of brain-dead patient. Lancet 1987;2:908–909.

42. Paulson OB, Waldemar G, Schmidt JF, et al. Cerebral circulation under normal and pathological conditions. Am J Cardiol 1989;63:2C–5C.

43. Powers WJ. Positron emission tomography. In: Weinstein PR, Faden AI eds. Protection of the brain from ischemia. Baltimore: Williams & Wilkins, 1990:99–110.

44. Prough DS. Brain monitoring. In: Taylor RB, Shoemaker WC eds. Critical care state of the art. Vol 12. Fullerton, CA: Society of Critical Care Medicine, 1991:157–196.

45. Ramadan NM, Deveshwar R, Levine SR. Magnetic resonance and clinical cerebrovascular disease. An update. Stroke 1989;20:1279–1283.

46. Rockoff MA, Marshall LF, Shapiro HM. High dose barbiturate therapy in humans: a clinical review of 60 patients. Ann Neurol 1979;6:194–199.

47. Rolfsen ML, David WR. Cerebral function and preservation during cardiac arrest. Crit Care Med 1989;17:283–292.

48. Ropper AH. Unusual spontaneous movements in brain-dead patients. Neurology 1984;34:1089–1092.

49. Ropper AH, Shafran BL. Brain edema after stroke. Clinical syndrome and intracranial pressure. Arch Neurol 1984;41:26–29.

50. Robber AH, Kennedy SK, Russell L. Apnea testing in the diagnosis of brain death. J Neurosurg 1981;55:942–946.

51. Safar P. Resuscitation from clinical death: pathophysiologic limits and therapeutic potentials. Crit Care Med 1988;16:923–941.

52. Sakabe T, Tateishi A, Miyauchi Y, et al. Intracranial pressure following cardiopulmonary resuscitation. Intensive Care Med 1987;13:256–259.

53. Saul TG, Ducker TB. Effect of intracranial pressure monitoring and aggressive treatment on mortality in severe head injury. J Neurosurg 1982;56:498–503.

54. Schmidley JW. Free radicals in central nervous system ischemia. Stroke 1990;21:1086–1090.

55. Scully RE, Mark EJ, McNeely WF, et al. Case records of the Massachusetts General Hospital. Case 16-1990. N Engl J Med 1990;322:1139–1148.

56. Shaywitz BA, Rothstein P, Venes JL. Monitoring and management of increased intracranial pressure in Reye Syndrome: results in 29 children. Pediatrics 1980;66:198–204.

57. Siesjö, BK. Mechanisms of ischemic brain damage. Crit Care Med 1988;16:954–963.

58. Deleted in proof.

59. Smith DS, Levy W, Maris M, et al. Reperfusion hyperoxia in brain after circulatory arrest in humans. Anesthesiology 1990;73:12–19.

60. Smith HP, Kelly DL, McWhorter JM, et al Comparison of mannitol regimens in patients with severe head injury undergoing intracranial monitoring. J Neurosurg 1986;65:820–824.

61. Stuart GG, Merry GS, Smith JA, et al. Severe head injury managed without intracranial pressure monitoring. J Neurosurg 1983;59:601–605.

62. Sundt TM Jr, Sharbrough FW, Piepgras DG, et al. Correlation of cerebral blood flow and electroencephalographic changes during carotid endarterectomy. Mayo Clin Proc 1981;56:533–543.

63. Symon L. Flow thresholds in brain ischaemia and the effects of drugs. Br J Anaesth 1985;57:34–43.

64. Tunkel AR, Wispelwey B, Scheld WM. Bacterial meningitis: recent advances in pathophysiology and treatment. Ann Intern Med 1990;112:610–623.

65. Tuomanen E, Hengstler B, Rich R, et al. Nonsteroidal anti-inflammatory agents in the therapy for experimental pneomococcal meningitis. J Infect Dis 1987;155:985–990.

66. Unwin DH, Giller CA, Kopitnik TA. Central nervous system monitoring. What helps, what does not. Surg Clin North Am 1991;71:733–747.

67. Veremakis C, Hayek DA, Mallory DL. Brain death evaluation and management of potential organ donors. Problems in Critical Care 1991;5:308–327.

68. Voldby B, Enevoldsen EM, Jensen, FT. Regional CBF, intraventricular pressure, and cerebral metabolism in patients with ruptured intracranial aneurysms. J Neurosurg 1985;62:48–58.

69. Ward JD. Intracranial pressure monitoring. In: Fuhrman BP, Shoemaker WC eds. Critical care state of the art. Vol 10. Fullerton, CA: Society of Critical Care Medicine, 1989:173–185.

70. Whitley RJ. Viral encephalitis. N Engl J Med 1990;323:242–250.

71. Wise RJ, Bernardi S, Frackowiak RS, et al. Serial observations on the pathophysiology of acute stroke. Brain 1983;106:197–222.

72. Woodcock J, Ropper A, Kennedy SK. High dose barbiturates in non-traumatic brain swelling: ICP reduction and effect on outcome. Stroke 1982;13:785–787.

73. Yamashina T, Kashihara K, Ikeda K, et al. Three phases of cerebral arteriopathy in meningitis: vasospasm and vasodilatation followed by organic stenosis. Neurosurgery 1985;16:546–553.

74. Yatsu FM. Cardiopulmonary arrest and intravenous glucose. J Crit Care 1987;2:1–3

45

Cerebral Resuscitation

Deborah A. Hayek
Christopher Veremakis

Successful cerebral resuscitation acts to interrupt the pathophysiologic mechanisms that are set in motion after an acute neurologic insult and allows healing process to commence. Aggressive management in the emergency room and then in the intensive care unit may improve not only survival but also functional recovery. This chapter reviews the physiologic basis for current therapeutic regimens employed in brain resuscitation. Since brain injury also disturbs somatic physiology, which may in turn precipitate additional neurologic damage, the systemic impact of brain injury will also be addressed. Therapeutic interventions will be discussed in the context of the pathophysiologic process toward which treatment is directed.

Minimization of secondary injury requires that general resuscitative and supportive measures are instituted immediately following the initial insult. These interventions include the correction of hypoxemia, hypercarbia, acidosis, anemia, hypotension, and electrolyte abnormalities. Thereafter, the specific aspects of cerebral resuscitation focus on (*a*) restoration of the balance between CNS oxygen supply and demand through manipulation of cerebral oxygen consumption or improvement of cerebral oxygen delivery (e.g., increasing cerebral blood flow, decreasing intracranial pressure), and (*b*) enhancing cellular protection against further ischemia.

THERAPEUTIC STRATEGIES IN CEREBRAL RESUSCITATION

The major pathophysiologic mechanisms of secondary injury that complicate the most common primary brain injuries are presented in Table 45.1. Management strategies for each disease entity are directed toward reversing the deleterious sequelae associated with the initial insult and ameliorating further secondary impairment. Therapeutic modalities with established or potential efficacy in cerebral resuscitation are described in Tables 45.2 and 45.3

Therapeutic Measures That Decrease Intracranial Pressure

Elevated ICP is often a final common pathway to the production of secondary brain injury. Nonsurgical treatment of intracranial hypertension is focused on the reduction of intracranial volume through manipulation of cerebral blood volume, CSF volume, or tissue fluid content (edema).

Effects of Head Position on Intracranial Pressure

Cerebral venous return and ICP can be altered by head position when intracranial compliance is compromised. The vasculature draining the CNS does not have venous valves, and consequently a rise in central venous pressure may increase intracranial venous pressure and volume. Lowering of the head below the heart may impede cerebral venous drainage, and head elevation to 30° helps to promote it (128). It has been suggested that head elevation will facilitate reduction of ICP and blunt the increased ICP response during positive pressure ventilation (46, 128). However, several studies suggest that head elevation does not improve ICP in all patients and may actually elevate it in some cases (28,

Table 45.1
Pathophysiologic Mechanisms of Secondary Ischemic Injury

Disease	Pathophysiology
Traumatic head injury	Expanding intracranial mass lesion Edema ↑ ICP Hyperemia Vasospasm Seizures
Subarachnoid hemorrhage	Rebleed Vasospasm Hydrocephalus ↑ ICP Seizures
Ischemic stroke	Regional hypoperfusion Hyperemia Edema and ↑ ICP in massive strokes Reperfusion injury Seizures
Cardiac arrest	Hyperemia Reperfusion injury Delayed global hypoperfusion Seizures
CNS infection	↑ ICP Edema Hydrocephalus Vasospasm Cerebrovascular thrombosis Seizures
Brain tumor	Compressive effect of mass lesion Vasogenic edema Elevated ICP Seizures
Metabolic encephalopathy, *e.g.*, Reye's syndrome, fulminant hepatic failure	Toxins Edema Elevated ICP Seizures

Table 45.2
General Treatment Goals of Brain Resuscitation

Increase cerebral oxygen delivery	
Improve arterial oxygen content	Avoid hypoxemia Control airway Correct anemia

Improve cerebral blood flow	Establish hemodynamic stability
	Establish normovolemia
	Reduce ICP
	  Minimize cerebral venous pressure
	  Minimize intrathoracic pressure
	  Avoid agitation

Reduce cerebral metabolic rate	Control hyperthermia Control seizures Control pain Avoid agitation, excessive stimulation, shivering

Table 45.3
Specific Medical Treatment Options during Brain Resuscitation

	Established	Adjunctive/Possibly Beneficial	Investigational/Promising	Not Beneficial
ICP elevation	Hyperventilation Osmotic agents CSF drainage	Furosemide Barbiturates for refractory ↑ ICP	Oncodiuretic therapy Iatrogenic hypertension	Steroids
Edema Ischemic Peritumor Interstitial	Osmotic diuretics Steroids	Furosemide Acetazolamide ?Steroids for inflammatory etiology	Oncodiuretic therapy	Steroids
Vasospasm	Iatrogenic hypertension Normovolemia/hypervolemia Calcium channel blockers	Hemodilution	Perfluorocarbons Tissue plasminogen activator (intracisternal)	Nitroglycerin Nitroprusside
Focal ischemia	Supportive care	Hemodilution ?Anticoagulation in some cases (e.g., embolic stroke, stroke in evolution)	Calcium channel blockers Magnesium Pentoxifylline Tissue plasminogen activator Naloxone Mannitol Perfluorocarbons	Barbiturates Prostacyclin
Global ischemia	Supportive care		Calcium channel blockers Magnesium Hemodilution Hypothermia	Barbiturates

113a). Furthermore, head elevation can produce a fall in cerebral perfusion pressure to dangerously low levels (28, 116). Consequently, the effects of head elevation should be individually determined in each patient.

Hyperventilation

Iatrogenic hyperventilation is a mainstay in the treatment of increased ICP. Hyperventilation to a $Paco_2$ of 25 torr causes cerebral vasoconstriction resulting in decreased cerebral blood volume and ICP within minutes (60). Many brain-injured patients will spontaneously hyperventilate to a $Paco_2$ of 30 torr or less. The effectiveness of hyperventilation is most pronounced when cerebral blood flow is hyperemic but is also present with low cerebral blood flow (94). Hypocarbia-induced ICP reduction is mediated by changes in extracellular fluid pH. The therapeutic benefit of hyperventilation is considered to last only 24–48 hr since thereafter compensatory mechanisms restore normal CSF pH. However, some clinical data suggest a more prolonged effect of hyperventilation in brain-injured patients (52, 94).

$Paco_2$ should not be reduced below 20 torr since extreme hypocarbia may cause vasoconstriction severe enough to compromise tissue oxygen supply and precipitate ischemia (66). Therapeutic levels of hyperventilation have been associated with reduced regional cerebral blood flow and a widened cerebral arteriovenous oxygen content difference in some brain-injured patients (19, 94). Therefore, in the absence of ICP monitoring, hyperventilation should be employed only in diseases frequently characterized by an elevated ICP (e.g., traumatic head injury, Reye's syndrome, fulminant hepatic failure). Hyperventilation after stroke can potentially worsen ischemia through vasoconstriction of collateral flow channels. Hyperventilation has no role in the management of global ischemia or subarachnoid hemorrhage, where further cerebral blood flow reductions may aggravate the damage caused by vasospasm and postarrest hypoperfusion. Jugular venous blood sampling and tracking of cerebral arteriovenous oxygen content

difference in conjunction with ICP monitoring may help to define subsets of patients who are likely to be harmed from iatrogenic hyperventilation. Another consideration is the avoidance of extreme respiratory alkalosis, which may precipitate hypocalcemic symptoms and lower the seizure threshold (46). Hyperventilation should be withdrawn gradually over 24–48 hr, since rapid $Paco_2$ increases may result in cerebral vasodilation and rebound ICP elevation (52).

Osmotic and Nonosmotic Diuresis

Osmotic diuretics are routinely administered to control ICP. These agents create an osmotic gradient between the brain and blood stream and draw fluid from brain tissue. An intact blood-brain barrier is necessary to maintain this gradient and therefore dehydration occurs primarily in normal brain rather than in edematous tissue. The effect of a single drug bolus lasts 4–6 hr, since the osmotic gradient narrows as blood levels dwindle. Repeated doses (or continuous infusion) may be necessary if ICP is difficult to control. However, chronic osmotherapy beyond 48–72 hr is not advisable since the brain adapts to serum hyperosmolality by increasing intracellular osmolality, and osmotic agents will gradually enter edematous tissue; consequently, rebound ICP elevation may occur with prolonged use (42, 140).

Mannitol (20% solution) is the most frequently prescribed osmotic agent. Single doses of 0.25–1 g/kg i.v. (or continuous infusion of 0.05–0.1 g/kg/hr) reduce ICP with the maximal effect apparent after 20 min (77, 82). In addition to an osmotic diuretic effect, mannitol decreases viscosity and consequently may improve flow to marginally perfused injured areas (85, 87). The major complication associated with osmotic agents is hyperosmolality with hypernatremia. Serum osmolality should not exceed 320 mosm or additional neuronal injury, rebound edema, and renal failure may develop (77).

Cerebrospinal fluid is formed at a rate of 500 ml/day. Cerebrospinal fluid production is decreased by furosemide (40–80 mg) or acetazolamide (250 mg bid/qid) (42).

In brain-injured patients, furosemide alone decreases ICP without affecting cerebral perfusion pressure (53) and in combination with mannitol produces greater brain shrinkage and more sustained ICP reduction than either agent alone (122).

Corticosteroids

The theoretical bases for steroid administration following acute brain injury include reduction of vasogenic edema through cell membrane stabilization and preservation of blood-brain barrier integrity, as well as inhibition of arachidonic acid release. There is also a rationale for steroid use in inflammatory CNS disorders where the host immunologic response is responsible for secondary tissue injury. There is no basis for a steroid effect on cytotoxic edema (42).

Several prospective, randomized clinical investigations have consistently demonstrated that steroids are not beneficial in the treatment of ischemic or traumatic brain injury. Steroid treatment does not reduce the mean ICP or improve neurologic outcome or mortality after severe head injury (31, 119), intracerebral hemorrhage, or ischemic cerebral infarction (92, 105). On the other hand, corticosteroid administration during brain resuscitation causes additional morbidity from systemic complications such as infection, sepsis, and hyperglycemia (29, 105).

Steroids have been used to treat the peritumor edema associated with primary and metastatic brain tumors for more than 25 years, and their efficacy in this setting is established (42). Early treatment with methylprednisolone after spinal cord injury has recently been reported to improve neurologic outcome (9). Adjunctive dexamethasone therapy reduces the incidence of hearing loss complicating pediatric bacterial meningitis, although additional beneficial effects on long-term neurologic outcome have not yet been conclusively demonstrated (4).

Therapeutic Measures That Increase Cerebral Blood Flow and Cerebral Oxygen Delivery

The restoration of impaired regional cerebral blood flow (CBF) in acute ischemic stroke is an important therapeutic strategy in cerebral resuscitation. Some of the earliest clinical investigations in this area examined the efficacy of anticoagulation on stroke morbidity. Clinical trials have failed to conclusively demonstrate any benefit of heparin or antiplatelet therapy in thrombotic stroke (35, 38, 48). Early work with thrombolytic agents in stroke revealed an unacceptably high risk-to-benefit ratio, but more recent studies with tissue plasminogen activator have suggested a potential therapeutic benefit, which is as yet unsubstantiated (30).

Despite advantageous results generated by laboratory models of ischemia, clinical trials with multiple other agents (including vasodilators) have proven ineffective in altering the course of acute stroke. Prospective clinical studies of focal ischemic injury treated with prostacyclin (a prostaglandin with vasodilator and antiplatelet aggregation effects) (57) and pentoxifylline (a hemorheologic agent that reduces blood viscosity) (100) have not demonstrated any sustained neurologic benefits. Preliminary results with calcium antagonists will be discussed in conjunction with cytoprotective measures.

Iatrogenic Hypertension and Hemodilution

In pathologic conditions where global or regional ischemia occur in the absence of significant ICP elevation, manipulation of mean arterial pressure to increase cerebral perfusion pressure has theoretical merit. When autoregulation is impaired, raising cerebral perfusion pressure may increase cerebral blood flow. This approach in conjunction with intravascular volume loading has been applied with considerable success in the treatment of vasospasm following subarachnoid hemorrhage (6, 64, 86). Phenylephrine, dopamine, and other vasopressors have been successfully administered to increase cerebral blood flow and reverse neurologic deficits in this clinical setting. The role of iatrogenic hypertension in the treatment of acute stroke has not been defined.

When ICP is elevated, traditional thinking has cautioned against raising mean arterial pressure or volume loading since an increase in cerebral perfusion pressure could worsen edema formation, increase cerebral blood volume, and aggravate the ischemic process. This caveat has recently been challenged in patients with traumatic head injury (117), and a management protocol that targets a cerebral perfusion pressure of 70–80 mm Hg has been advocated. Aggressive treatment of ICP with cerebrospinal fluid (CSF) drainage and mannitol is combined with volume loading and vasopressors to elevate mean arterial pressure and maintain a high cerebral perfusion pressure. Initial results with this approach are encouraging (117) and are supported by other reports that induced hypertension is effective in the treatment of ischemia associated with head injury (85).

Hemodilution with and without volume loading has been employed to increase cerebral blood flow during ischemic stroke and vasospasm. Blood flow increases as blood viscosity decreases. Hematocrit is a major determinant of blood viscosity, especially in the microcirculation or in areas of low flow (148). Evidence suggests that a hematocrit of 30–33% is optimal for maintaining a balance between improved blood flow and the decreased Cao_2 resulting from a drop in hematocrit. Hemodilution can be accomplished in several ways (55). Phlebotomy produces hypovolemic hemodilution, which has little clinical applicability. Isovolemic hemodilution combines phlebotomy and volume replacement to maintain euvolemia. Hypervolemic hemodilution is achieved by volume expansion with asanguinous fluids (crystalloid or colloid). Cardiac failure and ICP elevation are common complications that argue for prophylactic hemodynamic monitoring when this modality is employed.

The rationale that hemodilution may salvage marginal tissue by improving blood flow to ischemic areas following stroke has been studied in several clinical trials. A therapeutic benefit using iso- or hypervolemic hemodilution in stroke management was suggested initially by a few small clinical studies (132, 147). However, several large, prospective, randomized, multicenter studies have subsequently demonstrated minimal or no improvement in long-term neurologic outcome or mortality with hemodilution (54, 59, 120, 121). These trials have been criticized with regard to study design and patient selection, and since some positive trends were apparent, it is argued that subsets of stroke patients who may benefit from hemodilution remain to be defined (54, 55).

Therapeutic Measures That Decrease Cerebral Metabolic Demand

Cerebral metabolism is frequently reduced following acute brain injury (85, 94, 139, 146), but seizures, hyperthermia, a hypermetabolic state, excess motor activity, and pain all increase cerebral oxygen consumption and may precipitate further brain injury. Even when global cerebral blood flow is adequate, vascular obstruction may prevent a regional increase of cerebral blood flow in response to increased metabolic needs. General therapeutic measures to prevent increased cerebral oxygen consumption in the brain-injured patient include adequate analgesia, sedation, and prevention of postoperative shivering.

Temperature Alterations

Fever often occurs in brain-injured patients in the absence of an infectious etiology and may be mediated by increased release of interleukin-1 (98). A rise in temperature of 1°C above normal can increase cerebral oxygen consumption by 10–15% (95). Temperature elevations should be aggressively controlled with antipyretics and cooling blankets, if necessary. Mild hypothermia to lower cerebral oxygen consumption is probably beneficial to the injured brain (60, 118), although induced extreme hypothermia is difficult to implement and may cause hemodynamic instability, shivering, and metabolic acidosis.

Seizures

Seizures greatly increase cerebral oxygen consumption. Ischemic brain damage is a recognized sequela of prolonged seizure activity (24, 80). Furthermore, an increase in cerebral blood flow in response to elevated cerebral oxygen consumption may worsen ICP if intracranial compliance is reduced. If focal or generalized seizures occur following acute brain injury, immediate treatment is necessary. An intravenous benzodiazepine should be administered in incremental doses (diazepam, 5–40 mg, or lorazepam, 2–8 mg) sufficient to terminate all seizure activity. Subsequently, a full loading dose of phenytoin (15–20 mg/kg i.v.) should be administered and followed by maintenance therapy (300 mg/day) to prevent seizure recurrence. The evaluation and therapy of status epilepticus and chronic seizures is beyond the scope of this text and has been recently reviewed elsewhere (44, 123). It should be kept in mind that akinetic seizures may be a cause of persisting or unexplained coma.

Seizures are a common acute complication and chronic sequela of meningitis, encephalitis, and brain abscess. Seizures may also occur after traumatic head injury, intracranial hemorrhage, cerebral ischemia, or in association with CNS tumors and metabolic encephalopathies (Table 45.1). Anticonvulsant prophylaxis is recommended in head injury, subarachnoid hemorrhage, brain tumor, and cerebral abscess (33, 135). The indications for anticonvulsant prophylaxis following stroke and global ischemia are not as clearly delineated. However, early seizures may develop after successful resuscitation in approximately 20% of cardiac arrest patients (10, 72). The benefit of prophylactic phenytoin therapy must always be weighed against the risk of serious adverse reactions (ranging from rash to anaphylaxis), which occur in up to 15% of patients (33).

Barbiturates

Barbiturates depress neuronal function, suppress seizure activity, and lower cerebral oxygen consumption (79). The concomitant decreases in cerebral blood flow and cerebral blood volume act to lower ICP (81). The combined benefit of reduced cerebral oxygen consumption and ICP make high dose barbiturate therapy a theoretically attractive strategy for cerebral resuscitation. However, clinical investigations have failed to identify extensive clinical benefits.

Two prospective, randomized clinical trials did not show a beneficial effect of barbiturates when given as initial rather than second-line treatment in severe head injury (125, 142). Similarly, barbiturate treatment of elevated ICP in association with stroke has not been shown to improve outcome (111, 149). A prospective, randomized multicenter trial of thiopental (30 mg/kg i.v.) administered immediately after resuscitation from cardiac arrest demonstrated no difference in long-term mortality or neurologic outcome after barbiturate therapy (10).

Barbiturates may be of moderate use as an adjunctive, last-line measure to treat uncontrollable ICP elevations, which are associated with a very high mortality. Several clinical trials have employed barbiturate loading after standard measures failed to reduce ICP in patients with head injury and nontraumatic brain injury (37, 109, 149). In this setting, barbiturate coma can produce sustained ICP reduction in up to 50% of patients, with improvement in mortality, but not necessarily functional recovery. Pentobarbital coma is induced by a loading dose of 3–10 mg/kg followed by maintenance infusion of 1–3 mg/kg/hr, to maintain serum barbiturate levels of 2.5–4 mg % (37, 142). Barbiturate coma should not be considered a benign therapeutic maneuver. Because of respiratory depression, mechanical support of ventilation is mandatory. Hypotension occurs frequently (10, 142) since these drugs produce systemic vasodilation and myocardial depression. Hemodynamic monitoring for titration of volume administration and inotropic agents is also necessary. The potential efficacy of barbiturate therapy in providing cellular protection during incomplete (focal) ischemia is currently being evaluated in the experimental (81) and clinical settings (93).

Therapeutic Strategies to Protect and Preserve the Neuronal Environment

Cytoprotective agents function to maintain cellular structure and function following an ischemic insult. The potential applicability and efficacy of these agents in cerebral resuscitation is currently under intense investigation (118, 129) but conclusive therapeutic benefits remain to be demonstrated. The excitotoxic hypothesis of neuronal damage suggests that increased release and availability of glutamate, aspartate, and other excitatory neurotransmitters during ischemic injury alter transmembrane fluxes of sodium and calcium and propagate the degenerative metabolic cascade that leads to cell dissolution. The ability of n-methyl-D-aspartate antagonists (e.g., dextromethorphan) to block excitatory receptors and antagonize these actions is under study (20). Naloxone and other opioid antagonists inhibit the action of endogenous opioids and may exert several cytoprotective actions, although results from clinical trials are inconclusive (39, 96). Another pharmacologic approach involves inhibition of free radical formation and free radical-mediated injury with the free radical scavengers (e.g., superoxide dismutase, catalase, allopurinol, ascorbic acid, α-tocopherol), iron chelators, and 21-aminosteroids (58, 68, 124). Prevention of eicosanoid effects with cyclooxygenase and lipoxygenase blockers and antithromboxane agents represents another area of investigation (113, 118). Other promising therapeutic agents include the cell membrane precursors CDP choline and GM$_1$ ganglioside, which potentially confer cytoprotection by accelerating phospholipid synthesis, inhibiting release of free fatty acids, or promoting neuronal regeneration (5, 134). The putative benefits of phenytoin and lidocaine on brain ischemia are attributed to modulation of cellular metabolism and membrane stabilization (81, 113, 118).

Calcium Channel Blockers

The concentration of extracellular free calcium is 10,000 times greater than that of intracellular calcium. This concentration gradient is maintained by energy-dependent calcium channels in the cell membrane. When severe ischemia produces ATP depletion and disruption of energy metabolism, calcium floods the cell, initiating a pathologic sequence involving the activa-

tion of proteases and phospholipases, generation of free radicals and eicosanoids, and excitatory neurotransmitter release, all of which promote irreversible cell damage (68, 129, 151). In smooth muscle, increased calcium availability may mediate ischemic vasoconstriction or vasospasm. The potential efficacy of calcium antagonists in brain resuscitation is predicated on (a) improvement of cerebral oxygen delivery through reversal of vasospasm or optimization of flow through small collateral vessels and (b) amelioration of adverse sequelae resulting from intracellular calcium overload (2, 131, 151). The "cerebrospecific" calcium antagonists cross the blood-brain barrier and act preferentially on cerebral vessels and cells rather than on the myocardium or peripheral vasculature. These agents include the dihydropyridines (nimodipine, nicardipine, nilvadipine) and the diphenylalkylamines (flunarizine, cinnarizine).

Several prospective, randomized, placebo-controlled clinical trials have demonstrated the modest efficacy of prophylactic oral nimodipine (60–90 mg every 4 hr) in ameliorating neurologic morbidity from vasospasm-induced cerebral ischemia following subarachnoid hemorrhage (1, 101, 102, 103). However, nimodipine does not alter the incidence of symptomatic or angiographic vasospasm or overall mortality in these patients and is of no value when given after symptoms of vasospasm develop. Nicardipine, which is available in an intravenous preparation, is currently being evaluated for the prevention and reversal of vasospasm (65). Preliminary investigation of nimodipine and nicardipine in the treatment of stroke has produced encouraging, but inconclusive, results (45, 70). Current data do not support the use of calcium antagonists to improve neurologic outcome after cardiac arrest (11, 43).

SOMATIC RESUSCITATION AND GENERAL THERAPEUTIC CONSIDERATIONS AFTER CEREBRAL INJURY

Following a primary brain injury, regardless of the specific etiology, there are certain general considerations and extracerebral aspects of patient management that should be addressed in the prevention and treatment of secondary brain injury.

Initial Evaluation and Management Following Neurologic Injury

Cerebral resuscitation begins with the establishment of adequate cardiopulmonary function and acceptable systemic oxygen delivery. The comatose patient should receive both 50% dextrose (50 ml i.v.) and thiamine (50–100 mg i.m.). Naloxone (0.4 mg i.v., which can be repeated every 5 min) should be administered if opiate overdose is suspected. If injury to the neck or spinal cord is a consideration, the cervical spine should be stabilized and x-rays of the cervical spine reviewed before further manipulation of the neck. Routine laboratory studies including arterial blood gases, serum electrolytes, coagulation parameters, and a drug screen should also be obtained.

Any patient who has sustained a significant head injury or been rendered temporarily unconscious should be observed carefully for at least 8–12 hr, even in the absence of neurologic signs. With a history of altered consciousness and head trauma or the presumption of brain injury, CT scan is the initial diagnostic procedure of choice. CT scan characterizes the extent of primary injury, differentiates hemorrhagic from nonhemorrhagic lesions, and identifies the need for emergent surgical intervention. The presence of a mass lesion (e.g., intracranial hematoma or tumor) accompanied by significant brain shift is an indication for surgical removal. Rapid identification and definitive treatment of expanding mass lesions is critically important. Morbidity and mortality significantly improve if subdural hematomas, for example, are evacuated within 4 hr of presentation (126). Intracranial hematomas are often associated with head trauma, but should also be considered when there is a history of recent neurologic surgery, anticoagulant therapy, ethanol abuse, and chronic hypertension. When an expanding mass lesion is suspected, medical therapy to reduce ICP should begin prior to and during CT scanning, and these patients should be continuously attended by a physician. Temporizing measures pending surgery include intubation, hyperventilation, and osmotic diuresis.

Neurologic Examination and Serial Assessment

A patient who on presentation is unconscious or uncommunicative, has focal neurologic defects, or a deteriorating neurologic examination, should be considered to have ongoing secondary brain injury. The initial neurologic assessment of the stuporous or comatose patient should establish whether brainstem function is intact. This entails a rapid but systematic examination to determine the level of consciousness, breathing pattern, pupillary size and reactivity, presence and characteristics of eye movements, as well as delineation of purposeful or reflex motor activity.

Consciousness is characterized by the presence of awareness (mediated by the activity of the cerebral cortex and subcortical nuclei) and arousal (which depends on the integrity of the reticular activating system). Coma, or complete unresponsiveness, is caused by either bilateral hemispheric or brainstem lesions. The spectrum of mental status between full consciousness and coma includes delirium (primarily an abnormality of cognitive functions), obtundation (reduced alertness), and stupor (unresponsiveness with the ability to be aroused by intense stimuli) (104).

Pupillary size and responsiveness provides important diagnostic information in coma evaluation (104). Preservation of the light reflex serves to distinguish toxic-metabolic from structural etiologies. In general, symmetric, small, reactive pupils are seen with bilateral cortical lesions and toxic-metabolic pathologies (overdoses of atropine, scopolamine, and glutethimide are the exceptions). With midbrain lesions, the pupils are midposition, fixed, and nonreactive (as occurs in transtentorial herniation). When the third nerve or its nucleus in the midbrain is compressed, as occurs in uncal herniation, the pupil on the side of the lesion is dilated and poorly reactive to light. After cardiac arrest the pupils may be wide, fixed, and nonreactive; the latter finding and its persistence are associated with poor outcome (72). Hypothermia can also be associated with fixed pupils. With pontine lesions such as pontine hemorrhage, pupils are pinpoint with the light reflex preserved. In opiate intoxication, pupils are pinpoint and reactive (although this may be difficult to appreciate), resembling pontine hemorrhage.

The existence of spontaneous or roving eye movements signifies intact brainstem function. Conjugate deviation of the eyes is associated with an ipsilateral hemispheric or contralateral pontine lesion (104). Asymmetric oculomotor abnormalities are more usual with structural versus toxic-metabolic forms of brain injury. The presence of a bilateral corneal response implies brainstem integrity. The doll's head maneuver and cold calorics, which test the oculocephalic and oculovestibular reflexes, respectively, are used to identify brainstem dysfunction. These reflexes are subserved by the oculomotor and vestibular cranial nerve nuclei and their interconnecting pathways, which include the medial longitudinal fasciculus. In the comatose patient, the presence of the dolls' eye reflex—consisting of conjugate eye movement in the opposite direction to that of brisk head turning—implies an intact brainstem and suggests a bilateral supratentorial or toxic-metabolic etiology (Fig. 45.1). Similarly, cold caloric testing (which is a stronger stimulus than head turning) elicits tonic conjugate eye deviation toward the irrigated ear in the unconscious patient with an intact brainstem. After damage to the mid to upper brainstem, with both maneuvers the eye that should deviate laterally moves appropriately, but the eye that should adduct medially moves only to the midline (Fig. 45.1). Cold caloric and doll's eye testing elicit no eye movements when there is a low brainstem lesion. However, the absence of oculocephalic and oculovestibular reflexes is not always synonymous with brainstem dysfunction, since severe intoxication from certain drugs (sedatives, tricyclics, dilantin, aminoglycosides, and neuromuscular blockers) can also block these oculovestibular responses (104).

Assessment should include observation of the presence or absence of purposeful

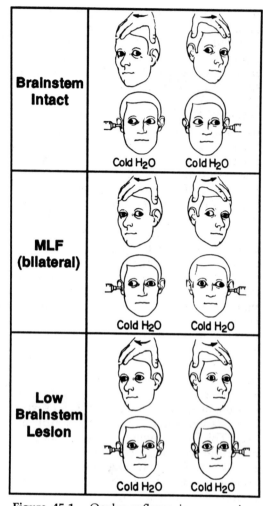

Figure 45.1. Ocular reflexes in unconscious patients. The *top panel* shows oculecephalic *(above)* and oculovestibular *(below)* reflexes in a comatose patient whose brainstem ocular pathways are intact. Lateral conjugate eye movements to head turning are full and opposite in direction to the movement of the face. Irrigation of the tympanic membranes with cold water is a stronger stimulus. There is tonic conjugate deviation of both eyes toward this stimulus. In the *middle panel*, the effects of bilateral medial longitudinal fasciculus *(MLF)* lesions on ocular reflexes are shown. Oculocephalic or oculovestibular stimulation deviates the appropriate eye laterally and brings the eye that would normally deviate medially, only to the midline. The *bottom panel* illustrates the effects of low brainstem lesion. Neither head turning nor cold water irrigation causes lateral deviation of the eyes (adapted from Plum F, Posner JB. The diagnosis of stupor and coma. 3rd ed. Philadelphia: FA Davis, 1980:55.)

or semipurposeful movements. When there is no spontaneous movement, the patient may still respond to noxious stimuli with a purposeful withdrawal from pain or with reflex posturing. Decorticate posturing (flexion of the arms and extension of the legs) is usually consistent with hemispheric lesions or toxic-metabolic pathology. Decerebrate posturing (extension and internal rotation of the arms and legs) is seen with midbrain and pontine damage and severe metabolic disease (hepatic coma, hypoglycemia, anoxic injury) and may also occur with massive bilateral forebrain injury.

An additional concern with protracted coma or coma of obscure etiology is akinetic seizures. Nonconvulsive status epilepticus is a cause of altered consciousness and should be considered when no obvious metabolic or structural etiology of coma is apparent (36). Electroencephalographic studies are necessary to confirm the diagnosis.

The Glasgow Coma Scale can be used for serial assessment of the brain-injured patient and provides accurate prediction of outcome when used to follow neurologic status over the first week postinjury (61). This scale, which is easily obtained and recorded, consists of points assigned for eye opening, verbal, and motor responses (Table 45.4). The possible scores obtainable, ranging from worst to best, are 3–15.

Serial neurologic evaluation should also address potential changes from the initial baseline examination findings, as well alterations in vital signs, ventilatory pattern, and bowel and bladder continence. In the first 24 hr after brain injury, the standard "q 1 hr neuro check" is generally inadequate, and serial examinations may be needed every 15–30 min in order to monitor the development of secondary injury. The frequency of assessment should be guided by knowledge of the specific disease entity and the rapidity of deterioration that may be expected. Serial assessment after a cerebral insult may also be facilitated by monitoring modalities such as continuous jugular venous oxygen saturation measurements, niroscopy, and ICP monitors (106, 137, 141).

Table 45.4
The Glasgow Coma Scale[a]

Clinical Parameter	Points
Eye opening	
Spontaneous	4
Response to speech	3
Response to pain	2
No response	1
Verbal response	
Oriented and appropriate	5
Disoriented and confused	4
Inappropriate words	3
Incomprehensible sounds	2
No response	1
Best motor response	
Obeys commands	6
Localizes pain	5
Withdraws from pain	4
Flexor response	3
Extensor response	2
No response	1

Glasgow Coma Score (GCS) = (1) + (2) + (3)

Best Possible GCS = 15,
Worst Possible GCS = 3

[a]Modified from Jennet B, Teasdale G. Management of head injuries. Philadelphia: FA Davis, 1981:78.

Diagnostic Considerations and Prognostic Considerations

The CT scan can provide information relating to the probability of intracranial hypertension after head trauma. When the admission CT scan is normal, the risk of sustained ICP elevations is relatively low (approximately 15–30%) (74, 89), while contusions or hematomas (with or without midline shift) are associated with increased ICP in more than 50% of patients (83, 89). However, significant ICP elevations may develop in the absence of focal lesions or midline shift on initial scan (83, 89). Abnormal ventricles (small, absent, or enlarged) are also associated with the later development of significant ICP elevations (67, 83), while up to 50% of patients with "low density" CT lesions may also develop increased ICP (89). Since up to one third of patients with normal admission CT scans may develop new abnormalities (generalized brain swelling, delayed hematoma) over the first week posttrauma, it is reasonable to obtain a follow-up CT scan in a few days, or at the first sign of clinical deterioration (74, 89).

Magnetic resonance imaging (MRI) is a noninvasive technique that may be superior to CT in identifying several types of brain injury, particularly with regard to ischemic cerebrovascular disease. MRI is more sensitive than CT for detecting ischemic tissue changes, early brain edema, vascular malformations, blood vessel morphology, and gross flow characteristics (107). MRI may be more sensitive than CT for detecting cerebral venous thrombosis and also provides better resolution of the posterior fossa. Brain abnormalities in patients with transient ishcemic attacks are more frequently identified with MRI than with CT, and MRI is a very sensitive modality for the evaluation of stroke in the subacute to chronic stages, especially in the case of lacunar infarction. However, CT is still the optimal study to exclude acute brain hemorrhage. The application of MRI to ICU patients presents several practical disadvantages: it is difficult to implement, the imaging procedure is more prolonged than CT, and the patient is deep inside a magnet and more difficult to monitor during scanning.

Sensory evoked potentials provide another modality for neurologic assessment and trend monitoring (15, 106). Frequent repetitive sensory stimuli are presented and the transmitted neural response is measured by electrodes and evaluated by analysis of waveforms generated and displayed as voltage signals over time. These evoked potentials reflect the integrated activity of incoming and outgoing neural pathways and the interposed CNS structures that process the stimuli. Several types of evoked potentials can be measured including somatosensory evoked responses, visual evoked responses, and brainstem auditory evoked responses. Evoked potentials are distorted by traumatic and ischemic cerebral insults. Although evoked responses are altered by anesthetic, narcotic, and sedative drugs, they are relatively unaffected by muscle relaxants, hypothermia, and barbiturate therapy and may be used for neurologic assessment during barbiturate coma.

Evoked potential monitoring is often employed during neurosurgery to identify evolving ischemia and neuronal dysfunction. The diagnostic and prognostic value of this modality has been demonstrated in head trauma, but may also be applicable to ischemic brain injury (15, 106). Modification of evoked responses may be helpful in predicting an unfavorable prognosis in coma. The disappearance of various evoked responses can also be employed in the assessment of impending brain death. Evoked potential are very accurate prognostic indicators after head injury, superior to both initial CT or ICP data, enhancing the prognostic accuracy of clinical data alone, and equal or superior to the Glasgow Coma Scale with regard to prediction of long-term outcome (62, 73, 88). The presence of abnormal evoked responses can be used to facilitate clinical management decisions in traumatic brain injury (62). In head-injured patients with normal admission CT scans, the presence of abnormal multimodality evoked responses is a good indicator of subsequent ICP elevation, while intracranial hypertension develops infrequently when evoked responses are normal (89). The clinical response to therapeutic interventions can also be assessed by changes in evoked potentials.

The utility of evoked potentials monitoring is restricted by the fact that this technique is both time- and labor-intensive (requiring expensive equipment, skilled technicians to perform the monitoring, and specialized knowledge in recognizing and interpreting pattern changes) as well as having limited applicability for serial assessment (106). Evoked potential monitoring may have the greatest values in clinical evaluation during situations where physical examination is difficult or inaccurate, as is the case with barbiturate coma, muscular paralysis, or hypothermia.

Pharmacologic Considerations during Cerebral Resuscitation

A variety of pharmacologic agents used in the operative and intensive care settings can alter cerebral oxygen consumption, as well as cerebral blood flow, cerebral blood volume, and consequently, ICP (79, 81). The effects of some of the more commonly used drugs are summarized in Table 45.5. Among the volatile anesthetics, halothane produces the most marked increases in cerebral blood flow and ICP. The dissociative anesthetic ketamine increases cerebral blood flow and ICP and is consequently not recommended for use in patients with intracranial pathology. Cerebral effects of narcotics are variable, but in general these agents do not significantly change cerebral blood flow and cerebral oxygen consumption or worsen ICP. Changes in neurologic status may be masked by pharmacologic sedation, so the use of short-acting agents is preferable. When muscular paralysis is necessary, succinylcholine should be avoided since it has been reported to increase ICP during laryngoscopy and intubation and may also cause hyperkalemia in severely traumatized patients (79).

Most evidence suggests that adrenergic pressor agents, including dopamine in moderate doses, do not cross an intact blood-brain barrier, and thus do not directly affect cerebral vessels or cerebral blood flow (69, 79, 81). However, any agent that increases mean arterial pressure will indirectly alter cerebral blood flow and cerebral blood volume when autoregulation is impaired. During cardiopulmonary resuscitation, epinephrine improves cerebral blood flow by causing systemic vasoconstriction and increasing mean arterial pressure and cerebral perfusion pressure, without concurrent cerebral vasoconstriction (69, 112).

Cardiovascular Concerns during Cerebral Resuscitation

Cardiac Abnormalities Associated with CNS Injury

Primary brain injury may directly result in myocardial damage and arrhythmias, as well as alterations in hemodynamics and vasomotor tone. Evidence suggests that these abnormalities are pathophysiologically related to compromise of CNS centers, which control parasympathetic and sympathetic function, as well as to elevation of circulating catecholamines. Furthermore, the presence of underlying cardiovascular disease (common in cerebrovascular occlusive disorders (130)) can

Table 45.5
Clinical Effects of Pharmacologic Agents on Cerebral Blood Flow (CBF) and Cerebral Oxygen Consumption (C$\dot{\text{V}}$o$_2$) (7, 8, 79, 81)

	CBF	C$\dot{\text{V}}$o$_2$
Inhalational anesthetics		
Halothane, enflurane, isoflurane	↑ [a]	↓
Nitrous oxide	↑	0?
Ketamine	↑	0/ ↑ ?
Barbiturates	↓	↓
Narcotics	0/ ↓ ?	0/ ↓ ?
Benzodiazepines	↓	↓
Muscle relaxants		
Depolarizing: succinylcholine	↑	0
Nondepolarizing: pancuronium, vecuronium,		
atracurium	0	0
Adrenergic pressors	0	0
Antihypertensive drugs		
Nitroprusside	↑	0/ ↓ ?
Nitroglycerin	↑	?
Hydralazine	↑	?
Calcium antagonists	↑	0
α- and β-blockers	0	0

[a] ↑, increases; ↓, decreases; 0, no major clinical effect; ?, equivocal or conflicting effects have been reported, or effects are not well characterized.

be exacerbated by the strain that cerebral injury imposes on the cardiovascular system.

The CNS centers and pathways involved in cardiovascular regulation are those that modulate autonomic tone and neuroendocrine function. A cerebral insult involving any of these anatomic locations could potentially impact on cardiovascular control mechanisms. Experimental data suggest that brain injury results in an abrupt, transient sympathetic discharge that is accompanied by an appreciable catecholamine release that has been linked to electrocardiographic and myocardial abnormalities (133). Elevated circulating catecholamine levels have been observed in patients after several types of cerebral insult, but have been best documented in patients with subarachnoid hemorrhage (76, 90) and severe head injury (18, 25).

A hyperdynamic hemodynamic pattern is present after head trauma, with elevated cardiac index, increased heart rate, hypertension, normal or decreased systemic vascular resistance, and increased systemic oxygen consumption (18). The increase in cardiac index is associated with a normal or increased left ventricular function curve and dependent on adequate preload. All of the cardiovascular variables except systemic vascular resistance correlate significantly with increased blood levels of epinephrine and norepinephrine (18).

Myocardial damage in the absence of coronary artery disease may occur after brain injury. Myocardial microhemorrhages and infarctions have been documented postmortem in patients with traumatic head injury, subarachnoid hemorrhage, and cerebrovascular accidents (25, 76, 90, 133). The myocardial damage has been found in association with increased catecholamine levels (25, 78, 90), and the creatine kinase myocardial isoenzyme fraction may be elevated even in the absence of electrocardiographic evidence of transmural myocardial infarction (25, 49). It is speculated that the mechanism of myocardial injury involves hypercatecholaminergic effects such as increased myocardial oxygen demand, transient coronary vasoconstriction, or direct myocardial toxicity (25, 49, 78, 133).

Electrocardiographic (ECG) abnormalities frequently accompany brain injury. The ECG changes most commonly seen with CNS disease include prolonged QT interval, depressed ST segments, flattened/inverted T waves, and U waves. Tall peaked T waves, notched T waves, elevated ST segments, and Q waves can also occur (133). These abnormalities can be present in the absence of appreciable myocardial injury, and the ECG usually normalizes several weeks after the primary brain injury. Combinations of these ECG changes are reported with varying incidence in subarachnoid and intracerebral hemorrhage, stroke, head trauma, meningitis and brain tumor (49, 76, 133).

Cardiac arrhythmias may occur after cerebral injury, ranging from nonsustained ventricular ectopy and various supraventricular tachycardias to ventricular tachycardia, flutter, and fibrillation (133). Insults that produce intracranial blood and epileptogenic foci are most frequently associated with these arrhythmias. Bradycardia can develop within seconds of an acute brain injury, but is transient. The onset of bradycardia is often a sign of medullary compromise and impending herniation. When arrhythmias occur, contributing factors such as abnormal levels of potassium, calcium, magnesium, or drug toxicities should be investigated and appropriately treated. Although prophylactic antiarrhythmic therapy is not indicated after brain injury, arrhythmias that cause hemodynamic compromise should be managed in the standard fashion. Since hyperadrenergic tone may be the underlying cause of the arrhythmias, β-blockade is the best therapy for nonventricular tachyarrhythmias. Prospective treatment with atenolol after head injury has been demonstrated to reduce the occurrence of supraventricular tachycardia, creatine kinase elevation, and ECG abnormalities (25, 90). Bradyarrhythmias can be controlled with atropine or β-agonists

Although in hospital mortality after a cerebral insult is rarely due to cardiac pathology, the extent to which myocardial injury and arrhythmias contribute to morbidity is not yet fully defined. Since cardiac abnormalities are not infrequent and the potential for increased morbidity exists, continuous rhythm monitoring and a high index of clinical suspicion are warranted.

Hypertension

Hypertension is very common after cerebral injury. The substantial sympathetic discharge and hyperadrenergic state that follow brain insults can cause de novo blood pressure elevation or exacerbate preexisting essential hypertension. *Cushing's response* describes an acute rise in blood pressure associated with a significant ICP increase and is caused by distortion of the medulla or vasomotor centers in the floor of the fourth ventricle. Vagally mediated bradycardia may precede or accompany the hypertension. *Cushing's triad* of bradypnea, bradycardia, and hypertension is often a preterminal event associated with herniation.

Aggressive control of hypertension is indicated with intracranial hemorrhage or hypertensive encephalopathy; treatment of hypertension in other forms of brain injury remains controversial. When autoregulation is impaired, elevated perfusion pressure may benefit areas of segmental ischemia, and lowered blood pressure could aggravate ischemic lesions. In chronic hypertension the autoregulatory limits are shifted upward, so that the brain's tolerance to acute mean arterial pressure elevations is improved, but tolerance to hypotension is impaired (99). Rapid control of blood pressure in this setting can precipitate global cerebral ischemia at a "normal" mean arterial pressure. Conversely, when intracranial compliance is decreased, even moderate rise in mean arterial pressure can increase cerebral blood volume and ICP. In addition, when autoregulation is compromised or the blood-brain barrier is damaged, mean arterial pressure elevation can produce vascular fluid extravasation, which worsens intracranial bleeding and vasogenic edema, resulting in increased ICP and further ischemia.

When antihypertensive therapy is necessary, the choice of drug is problematic since many effective agents are vasodilators (Table 45.5) (79, 81). Cerebral vasodilators can increase cerebral blood volume, promote vasogenic edema, and increase ICP while decreasing mean arterial pressure (and cerebral perfusion pressure) (7, 138). Vasodilation in intact regions of brain may also cause a steal of flow from injured, vasoparalyzed areas (8). Nitroprusside, nitroglycerin, hydralazine, and nifedipine are cerebral vasodilators, and ICP elevation has been observed in patients with compromised intracranial compliance after treatment with these agents (53, 81, 138). Since a hyperadrenergic state is partially responsible for hypertension after cerebral injury, α- or β-blockade may be the treatment of choice (41). Adrenergic blockade does not directly alter cerebral blood flow or ICP except through effects on mean arterial pressure (7, 8, 138). Propranolol, labetalol, and the α-blocker urapidil do not worsen ICP in brain-injured patients (18, 97, 138).

In summary, it is difficult to ascertain the ideal blood pressure in brain injury. Therapy should be individualized. Transient hypertension after brain injury often responds to simple sedation or adequate analgesia (18). Iatrogenic hypotension is invariably worse than persistent mild or moderate hypertension. In patients with occlusive cerebrovascular disease or chronic hypertension, it is reasonable to maintain a systolic blood pressure between 150 and 180 mm Hg. When ICP is not monitored, aggressive treatment of hypertension should be instituted only when systolic pressure exceeds 200 mm Hg. Control of hypertension should be achieved in a conservative, nonprecipitous fashion. When ICP is elevated, cerebral vasodilators may produce neurologic deterioration; adrenergic blockade is the best option for control of hypertension in this setting.

Hypotension and Fluid Resuscitation

Hypotension is not a usual consequence of cerebral injury unless the medulla is damaged, although it is a common complication of brain death and spinal cord injury. Traumatic brain injury, however, is frequently associated with systemic trauma and hypovolemic hypotension.

Hypotension and anemia may be catastrophic and should be vigorously corrected in order to maximize cerebral perfusion pressure and cerebral oxygen delivery. With severe head injury, a systolic blood pressure less than 90 mm Hg is associated with worsened morbidity and mortality (83). Hypotension in the first 24 hr after head injury is a significant risk factor for the later development of increased ICP (67), even when the admission CT scan is normal (89).

The standard principles of shock resuscitation are applicable to the brain-injured patient. Pressor agents should not be administered until hypovolemia is corrected. The optimal choice of fluids for the treatment of shock after cerebral insults has been a subject of intense study (127). The argument that in the damaged brain, where autoregulation and the blood-brain barrier are impaired, isotonic crystalliod resuscitation will increase brain edema and ICP to a greater extent than colliod, remains unresolved. Is is reasoned that colliod, or hypertonic crystalloid, will establish favorable oncotic and osmotic gradients in the brain, shifting water from the parenchyma to the intravascular space. Current evidence suggests that colloids provide no clear advantage over crystalloid in reducing cerebral complications, are more expensive, and may be associated with increased bleeding (127).

In the absence of shock, conventional fluid management after brain injury includes isotonic fluids to maintain euvolemia or mild dehydration. Experimental evidence suggests that fluid restriction is not required and that normovolemia does not worsen cerebral edema (18, 84, 127). Furthermore, volume depletion may precipitate hypotension or exacerbate reductions in cerebral perfusion pressure secondary to positive end-expiratory pressure (PEEP) or head elevation.

Patients with decreased intracranial compliance should not be placed in the Trendelenburg position for central venous line insertion, because cerebral venous return may be compromised and ICP elevation may result (128). When intracranial hypertension is present, cerebral perfusion pressure is maximal in the horizontal position (116). The head should be maintained in the midline position since head and neck rotation occlude jugular venous flow, which may precipitate ICP increases (128). Venous access via the internal jugular vein is not contraindicated in brain-injured patients and appears to be relatively safe even when intracranial hypertension is present (47, 94), although there is a potential risk of venous occlusion.

Pulmonary Aspect of Cerebral Resuscitation

Brain injury can be associated with a variety of pulmonary abnormalities, which may be compounded by the presence of concurrent chest trauma. Furthermore, therapy to improve pulmonary dysfunction may worsen intracranial hypertension.

Abnormalities/Problems of Ventilation and Gas Exchange

Several abnormal ventilatory patterns can occur in association with brain injury (104), and their presence may provide diagnostic and prognostic information, although the correlation of these patterns with anatomic localization of damage is not precise. Cheyne-Stokes respiration is a cyclical breathing pattern where periods of crescendo-decrescendo variation in tidal volume alternate with briefer periods of apnea or hypopnea. It may occur with bilateral hemispheric or subcortical lesions, hypertensive encephalopathy, and other toxic metabolic causes of coma. True central neurogenic hyperventilation, manifested by sustained hyperpnea, is associated with damage of the lower midbrain to upper pons and may also be present in hepatic coma. The much more common tachypnea seen in comatose patients may reflect compensation for additional nonneurologic factors including increased pulmonary shunt, stimulation of intrapulmonary afferent receptors, and systemic acidosis. Apneustic breathing with sustained inspiratory pauses is seen with mid to low pontine lesions, such as pontine infarction, and may also occur with progressive transtentorial herniation, severe meningitis, and hypoglycemia. Low pontine to high medullary damage can result in cluster breathing, in which clusters of breaths are irregularly separated by respiratory pauses. Ataxic breathing is an irregular and random combination of deep and shallow breaths with intermittent apnea; it is due to medullary disease and posterior fossa lesions that compress the medulla and is frequently an agonal rhythm. Sedative and narcotic drug toxicity can produce a gradual medullary depression, which results in complete ventilatory failure.

Provision of supplemental oxygen is essential during cerebral resuscitation. Hypoxemia should be avoided and quickly corrected. Hypoxemia and increased venous admixture are often present in brain-injured patients on admission, in the absence of pulmonary lesions. These abnormalities, best studied in head trauma, are associated with poor outcome (46, 83). Compromised oxygenation may be caused by several factors, including transient apnea at the time of the initial cerebral insult, microatelectasis, ventilation-perfusion abnormalities, and increased pulmonary capillary permeability.

Severe CNS injury can precipitate neurogenic pulmonary edema. The pathophysiology of this form of noncardiogenic pulmonary edema is thought to be due to a transient massive sympathetic discharge leading to systemic vasoconstriction. The subsequent rise in venous return and pulmonary vasoconstriction are postulated to cause elevation of capillary hydrostatic pressures and endothelial damage, resulting in increased pulmonary microvascular permeability. Treatment is supportive and directed at maintaining oxygenation and cardiac output, in conjunction with measures to decrease ICP in order to minimize brain ischemia. Catecholaminergic blockade is a potentially beneficial therapeutic approach, but without established efficacy (32), moderate increases in extravascular lung water with normal pulmonary artery occlusion pressure may be common (75), suggesting that subclinical edema may

contribute to pulmonary dysfunction following brain injury.

Spontaneous hyperventilation and hypocarbia are frequently observed after brain injury. Hypercarbia and hypoventilation are less common on presentation, but may occur secondary to low brainstem damage, aspiration due to depressed cough and gag reflexes or partial airway obstruction from failure to control the tongue. If the stuporous or comatose patient is unable to maintain the upper airway without assistance, intubation is required. Some recommend intubation and mechanical ventilation if the Glasgow coma score is 8 or less (46).

Intubation and Mechanical Ventilation

Intubation and mechanical ventilation may be necessary to deliver therapeutic hyperventilation for intracranial hypertension or to correct abnormalities in gas exchange. The pharyngeal and laryngeal stimulation during intubation produces a catecholaminergic discharge that causes hypertension and a rise in central venous pressure. The subsequent abrupt increase in cerebral perfusion pressure can have a deleterious effect on injured brain, and if intracranial compliance is low, severe ICP elevations can be precipitated. Pretreatment with rapidly acting sedative and narcotics such as fentanyl (3–8 μg/kg), droperidol (150 μg/kg), or thiopental (200 mg) may help prevent ICP elevation during intubation, but can also cause hypotension (138). Intravenous lidocaine (1.5 mg/kg) attenuates ICP elevation during intubation (51, 138). β-Blockade with labetalol (20 mg i.v.) or esmolol infusion (300–500 μg/kg/min) prior to intubation may prevent tachycardia and systemic and intracranial hypertension (26, 138). Nondepolarizing agents are preferable for muscular paralysis (Table 45.5).

Positive pressure ventilation and positive end-expiratory pressure can elevate ICP by several mechanisms. Mechanical ventilation increases intrathoracic pressure and impedes cerebral venous return. In addition, increases in intrathoracic and intraabdominal pressure may be transmitted to the epidural veins producing venous engorgement, compression of the spinal subarachnoid space, and subsequent translocation of CSF intracranially. Suctioning, coughing, straining, nasogastric tube placement, and routine nursing measures also increase ICP by these mechanisms. Furthermore, PEEP can cause reductions in cerebral perfusion pressure by increasing ICP and/or decreasing systemic venous return, which may lower blood pressure. Clinical studies suggest, however, that moderate amounts of PEEP may be employed in brain-injured patients, when absolutely necessary. The adverse effect of PEEP on ICP are least pronounced when pulmonary compliance is low, since only small amounts of pressure are transmitted to the mediastinum, minimizing the effect on cerebral venous pressure and ICP (13). In head-injured patients with low intracranial compliance, PEEP of up to 15 cm H_2O applied with the head elevated did not produce clinically significant ICP elevations or neurologic deterioration (23, 46). When PEEP is used in the setting of suspected or established intracranial hypertension, it should be applied and withdrawn slowly, hypovolemia should be corrected, and ICP monitoring is crucial with levels above 15 cm H_2O. Although high frequency ventilation is associated with lower peak airway pressures than conventional ventilation, no clear-cut advantage with regard to ICP elevation has been demonstrated in the brain-injured patient (46).

Transient hypercarbia during suctioning or intubation may worsen ICP by causing cerebral vasodilation. Severe impairment of cerebral venous drainage may result when patients "fight" the ventilator, and sedation or muscle relaxants may be necessary to prevent raised ICP. Elevation of the head 30° and keeping the head in the midline position both maximize cerebral venous drainage and may help to blunt ICP responses during positive pressure ventilation and routine pulmonary care (46, 128). Intratracheal lidocaine provokes the cough reflex and initially increases ICP, but does attenuate ICP changes with suctioning (143). Neuromuscular blockade di-minishes the ICP response to suctioning (143).

Delayed Pulmonary Complications

Pulmonary infection is an important cause of delayed morbidity and mortality in the brain-injured patient (22, 32). Aspiration and atelectasis contribute to morbidity. Maintenance of good pulmonary toilet and clinical vigilance constitute the preventative approach to nosocomial pneumonia; prophylactic antibiotics should be avoided. Pulmonary embolism is another source of late morbidity in brain injury. Intermittent pneumatic leg compression is the recommended prophylaxis for deep vein thrombosis in patients with traumatic lesions or hemorrhagic stroke; nonhemorrhagic stroke may be prophylaxed with low dose heparin (21).

Metabolic and Endocrinologic Concerns during Cerebral Resuscitation

Systemic and Intracerebral Acidosis

A constant CSF pH is maintained in intact brain even with major systemic acid-base disturbances. Although the cerebral blood vessels are sensitive to alterations in extracellular pH, responding to acidosis with dilation and to alkalosis with constriction, intracranial buffering mechanisms operate to preserve the acid-base balance of the brain when systemic pH changes, (as long as ventilation is not impaired). The administration of sodium bicarbonate does not improve brain pH during ischemia (69). Exogenous bicarbonate does not cross the blood-brain barrier as rapidly as CO_2, and increased CO_2 production in response to bicarbonate-induced alkalemia may result in paradoxical CNS acidosis.

Although adequate ventilation and oxygenation minimize the effect of systemic acidosis on the injured brain, cerebral intracellular acidosis is less easily controlled. Tromethamine is an intracellular alkalinizing agent that crosses the blood-brain barrier and potentially may reverse intracellular acidosis. In spite of promising results with this agent in experimental brain injury (115), tromethamine administration to head-injured patients did not improve outcome even though a beneficial effect on control of ICP was apparent (71).

Hyperglycemia

Lactate accumulation during cerebral ischemia is a major cause of brain acidosis, and hyperglycemia worsens intracerebral lactate production and acidosis during experimental brain injury, presumably because of increased availability of substrate for anaerobic glycolysis (129). Hyperglycemia is associated with more pronounced brain edema and poorer neurologic outcome in animal models of brain ischemia (27, 129, 152). Clinical investigations have also suggested that hyperglycemia during a cerebral insult may have deleterious effects on neurologic outcome (14, 152), but the consequences of glucose administration subsequent to a completed brain injury are not well clarified. In the absence of hypoglycemia, glucose-containing infusions should be minimized during resuscitation from neurologic injury (152). Hyperglycemia in brain-injured patients should be corrected with the administration of short-acting insulin.

Hypermetabolism and Nutritional Support

Acute brain injury is associated with a hypermetabolic state, similar to that seen with systemic trauma, and characterized by increases in systemic oxygen consumption, resting energy expenditure, carbon dioxide production, and nitrogen wasting. This augmented systemic metabolism, which contrasts with the reduction in cerebral oxygen consumption frequently observed after cerebral insult, has been best studied in severe head injury and subarachnoid and intracerebral hemorrhage (17, 18, 136). The hypermetabolism, like the hyperdynamic cardiovascular state, is related to the excessive sympathetic discharge and increased catecholamine release that follows primary brain injury (17a, 18).

After head trauma, the resting energy expenditure is moderately increased up to 50% greater than predicted, and this change is most pronounced in the first few days after injury (17, 18, 136). Consumption of protein and fat is elevated, while carbohydrate consumption is reduced, and nitrogen balance is difficult to maintain (136, 154). A negative nitrogen balance may be sustained for long periods in spite of protein and calorie replacement based on basal requirements (18, 154). Severity of neurologic injury appears to be an important determinant of hypercaloric requirements and nitrogen wasting, which both worsen as Glasgow Coma Score diminishes (18). Abnormal motor posturing is associated with marked increases in resting metabolic expenditure in head-injured patients (17, 154).

Serum cortisol and glucagon are increased after brain injury and may mediate the augmented protein catabolism. There is also evidence of an inflammatory acute phase response, manifested by increased serum ceruloplasmin, copper, and C-reactive protein, and hypozincemia (98). The cytokine interleukin-1, which may mediate several aspects of the acute phase response as well as accelerate muscle catabolism, is elevated in head-injured patients (98).

Nutritional support may contribute to improved outcome after acute brain injury, but this has not been conclusively demonstrated (108). As in other critically ill patients, early and aggressive nutritional support is likely to improve immunocompetence and wound healing and to reduce the potential for late complications such as sepsis. Cell-mediated immunity and T-cell function are depressed immediately after severe head injury (56, 153). General guidelines for nutritional support following brain injury have not been clearly established, but may be extrapolated from recommendations used for multiple trauma patients. Adequate protein replacement (1.5–2.0 g/kg/day) adjusted to nitrogen excretion is important, with nonprotein calories calculated at approximately 1.5 times the resting energy expenditure and comprised of 40–50% fat (to a maximum of 2.5

g/kg/day) and 50–60% carbohydrate (to a maximum of 5–7 g/kg/day) (154).

Gastrointestinal Bleeding

Acute brain injury predisposes to superficial erosive gastritis. The association between cerebral insults and gastrointestinal mucosal lesions was first described by Cushing in neurosurgical patients. In an early clinical study, gastrointestinal bleeding due to erosive gastritis occurred early after head injury in over 50% of patients and correlated with severity of injury (63). The stress ulceration is attributed to increased gastric acid secretion. Initial investigations indicated that H_2-blocker prophylaxis limited the severity but not the incidence of gastric mucosal lesions (50). More recent clinical data suggest that, although stress erosions are indeed common after acute brain injury, progression to ulcers and overt bleeding are infrequent (12, 110) and the benefits of acid-reducing prophylaxis in this setting have been questioned (110). Consequently, routine stress ulcer prophylaxis may not be necessary and may increase bacterial overgrowth and the risk of nosocomial pulmonary infection.

Endocrine Abnormalities

Dysfunction of the hypothalamic-pituitary axis and abnormalities of pituitary function are common after a cerebral insult (16). Even though ACTH is not elevated (16, 40), cortisol secretion is increased after acute brain injury (17a, 40) and the increase is associated with intracranial hypertension (40). Decreased thyroxine and triiodothyronine levels have been observed after head injury, and are associated with a lower Glasgow Coma Score and poor outcome, as well as with increased catecholamine levels, suggesting that sympathetic activation may partially mediate endocrine dysfunction (150).

Hyponatremia is often associated with acute neurologic injury and may aggravate cerebral edema. Hyponatremic hypoosmolar syndromes have been reported in patients with head injury, subarachnoid hemorrhage, tumors, pituitary surgery, and intracranial infections (34, 91, 145). There appear to be two hyponatremic syndromes in patients with neurologic disease: the syndrome of inappropriate antidiuretic hormone secretion (SIADH) and the syndrome of cerebral salt wasting (34, 91, 144). Both entities are characterized by hyponatremia, hypotonic serum, inappropriately concentrated urine, and elevated urine sodium excretion. Patients with SIADH are euvolemic or slightly hypervolemic, have a dilutional hyponatremia because of an inability to excrete water, and retain the capability of conserving sodium chloride. Fluid restriction alone usually corrects the serum sodium and is considered the treatment of choice. Demeclocycline, which blocks the renal action of antidiuretic hormone, is rarely required as an adjunctive therapy. In contrast, patients with cerebral salt wasting are often intravascularly volume depleted. This condition results from persistent inappropriate natriuresis despite volume contraction and is related to a renal rather than neurohypophyseal lesion. It is theorized that this syndrome is caused by release of natriuretic hormones or abnormal neural input to the kidney although clinical studies have not consistently demonstrated abnormal levels of atrial natriuretic factor, antidiuretic hormone, or aldosterone (3, 114). Distinguishing SIADH from cerebral salt wasting is clinically important since patients with cerebral salt wasting will develop progressive hyponatremia, volume contraction, and hypotension if subjected to fluid restriction. The appropriate therapy is salt and volume loading (34, 91, 144).

CONCLUSION

Primary brain injury produces tissue ischemia, which is the final common pathway to irreversible cell damage. Cellular and tissue ischemia initiate a cascade of pathophysiologic events that promote secondary injury. Secondary injury results from further abnormalities of cerebral blood and metabolism, intracranial hypertension, and brain edema. These processes assume more or less prominence depending on the specific initiating disease entity (Table 45.1). Furthermore, systemic factors and extracranial organ dysfunction frequently complicate neurologic injury and may worsen an already complex pathophysiologic interaction. The increased sympathetic activation following an acute cerebral insult underlies much of the associated somatic pathophysiology, which is manifested as abnormalities of the cardiovascular, pulmonary gastrointestinal, and endocrine systems.

The goals of cerebral resuscitation are to limit the damage caused by primary brain injury, prevent or ameliorate secondary injury, and promote healing. The primary therapeutic objective is to reestablish a favorable balance between cerebral oxygen supply and demand by improving cerebral oxygen delivery and minimizing elevations in cerebral oxygen consumption (Table 45.2). Various therapeutic measures have established efficacy in the treatment of elevated ICP, edema, vasospasm, and CNS infection, while treatments that directly reverse cellular ischemia are under current investigation (Table 45.3). The application of these therapies is dictated by the specific etiology of the primary brain injury. Successful cerebral resuscitation results in improved neurologic outcome with an enhanced quality of survival.

Acknowledgments. The authors gratefully acknowledge the assistance of Carolyn Linenbroker, Jacklyn O'Brien, and Marie Wolinski in the preparation of this manuscript.

References

1. Allen GS, Ahn HS, Preziosi TJ, et al. Cerebral arterial spasm—a controlled trial of nimodipine in patients with subarachnoid hemorrhage. N Engl J Med 1983;308:619–624.
2. Allen GS. Role of calcium antagonists in cerebral arterial spasm. Am J Cardiol 985;55:149B–153B.
3. Al-mufti H, Arieff A. Hyponatremia due to cerebral salt wasting syndrome. Combined cerebral and distal tubular lesion. Am J Med 1984;77:740–745.
4. American Academy of Pediatrics. Committee on Infectious Diseases. Dexamethasone therapy for bacterial meningitis in infants and children. Pediatrics 1990;86(1):130–133.
5. Argentino C, Sacchetti ML, Toni D, et al. The Italian acute stroke study. GM1 gaglioside therapy in acute ischemic stroke. Stroke 1989;20:1143–1149.
6. Awad IA, Carter P, Spetzler RF, et al. Clinical vasospasm after subarachnoid hemorrhage: response to hypervolemic hemodilution and arterial hypertension. Stroke 1987;18:365–372.
7. Barry DI. Cerebrovascular aspects of antihypertensive treatment. Am J Cardiol 1989;63:14C–18C.
8. Bertel O, Marx B, Conen D. Effects of antihypertensive treatment on cerebral perfusion. Am J Med 1987;82(suppl 3B):29–36.
9. Bracken MB, Shepard MJ, Collins WF, et al. A randomized, controlled trial of methylprednisolone or naloxone in the treatment of acute spinal-cord injury. Results of the second national acute spinal cord injury study. N Engl J Med 1990;322:1405–1422.
10. Brain Resuscitation Clinical Trial I Study Group. Randomized clinical study of thiopental loading in comatose survivors of cardiac arrest. N Engl J Med 1986;314:397–403.
11. Brain Resuscitation Clinical Trial II Study Group. A randomized clinical study of a calcium-entry blocker (lidoflazine) in the treatment of comatose survivors of cardiac arrest. N Engl J Med 1991;324:1224–1231.
12. Brown TH, Davidson PF, Larson GM. Acute gastritis occurring within 24 hours of severe head injury. Gastrointest Endosc 1989;35(1):37–40.
13. Burchiel KJ, Steeg TD, Wylar AR. Intracranial pressure changes in brain-injured patients requiring positive end-expiratory pressure ventilation. Neurosurgery 1981;8:443–449.
14. Candelise L, Landi G, Orazio EN, et al. Prognostic significance of hyperglycemia in acute stroke. Arch Neurol 1985;42:661–663.
15. Cascino GD. Neurophysiological monitoring in the intensive care unit. J Intensive Care Med 1988;3:215–223.
16. Chioléro RL, Lemarchand TH, Schutz Y, et al. Plasma pituitary hormone levels in severe trauma with or without head injury. J Trauma 1988;28:1368–1374.
17. Chioléro RL, Breitenstein E, Thorin D, et al. Effects of propranolol on resting metabolic rate after severe head injury. Crit Care Med 1989;17:328–334.
17a. Chioléro RL, Schutz Y, Lemarchand TH, et al. Hormonal and metabolic changes following severe head injury or noncranial injury. J Parenter Enteral Nutr 1989;13:5–12.
18. Clifton GL, Robertson CS, Grossman RG. Management of the cardiovascular and metabolic responses to severe head injury. In: Becker DP, Povlishock JT, eds. Central nervous system trauma status report. Bethesda: National Institutes of Health, NIH/NINCDS, 1985:139–159.
19. Cold GE. Does acute hyperventilation provoke cerebral oligaemia in comatose patients after acute head injury? Acta Neurochir 1989;96:100–106.
20. Collins RC, Dobkin BH, Choi DW. Selective vulnerability of the brain: new insights into the pathophysiology of stroke. Ann Inter Med 1989;110:992–1000.
21. Consensus conference. Prevention of venous thrombosis and pulmonary embolism. JAMA 1986;256:744–749.
22. Cooper KR. Respiratory complications in patients with serious head injuries. In: Becker DP, Gudeman SK, eds. Textbook of head injury. Philadelphia: WB Saunders, 1989:255–264.

23. Cooper KR, Boswell PA, Choi SC. Safe use of PEEP in patients with severe head injury. J Neurosurg 1985;63:552–555.

24. Corsellis J, Banton C. Neuropathology of status epilepticus in humans. Adv Neurol 1983;34:129–139.

25. Cruickshank JM, Degaute JP, Kuurne T, et al. Reduction of stress/catecholamine-induced cardiac necrosis by beta-selective blockade. Lancet 1987;585–589.

26. Cucchiara RF, Benefiel DJ, Matteo RS, et al. Evaluation of esmolol in controlling increases in heart rate and blood pressure during endotracheal intubation in patients undergoing carotid endarterectomy. Anesthesiology 1986;65:528–531.

27. D'Alecy LG, Lundy EF, Barton KJ, et al. Dextrose containing intravenous fluid impairs outcome and increases death after eight minutes of cardiac arrest and resuscitation in dogs. Surgery 1986;100:505–511.

28. Davenport A, Will EJ, Davison AM. Effect of posture on intracranial pressure and cerebral perfusion pressure in patients with fulminant hepatic and renal failure after acetaminophen self-poisoning. Crit Care Med 1990;18:286–289.

29. De Maria EF, Reichman W, Kenney PR, et al. Septic complications of corticosteroid administration after central nervous system trauma. Ann Surg 1985;202:248–252.

30. Del Zoppe CJ. Thrombolytic therapy in cerebrovascular disease. Stroke 1988;19:1174–1179.

31. Dearden NM, Gibson JS, McDowall DG, et al. Effect of high-dose dexamethasone on outcome from severe head injury. J Neurosurg 1986;64:81–88.

32. Demling R, Riessen R. Pulmonary dysfunction after cerebral injury. Crit Care Med 1990;18:768–774.

33. Deutschman CS, Haines SJ. Anticonvulsant prophylaxis in neurological surgery. Neurosurgery 1985;17:510–517.

34. Diringer M, Ladenson PW, Borel C, et al. Sodium and water regulation in a patient with cerebral salt wasting. Arch Neurol 1989;46:928–930.

35. Duke RJ, Bloch RF, Turfie AG, et al. Intravenous heparin for the prevention of stroke progression in acute partial stable stroke. Ann Intern Med 1986;105:825–828.

36. Dunne J, Summer Q, Stewart-Wynne E. Nonconvulsive status epilepticus: a prospective study in an adult general hospital. Q J Med 1987;62:117–126.

37. Eisenberg HM, Frankowski RF, Contant CF, et al. High dose barbiturate control of elevated intracranial pressure in patients with severe head injury. J Neurosurg 1988;69:15–23.

38. Estol CJ, Pessin MS. Anticoagulation: is there still a role in atherothrombotic stroke? Stroke 1990;21(5):820–824.

39. Faden AI. Role of opiate antagonists in the treatment of stroke. In: Weinstein PR, Faden AI eds. Protection of the brain from ischemia. Baltimore: Williams & Wilkins, 1990:265–271.

40. Feibel J, Kelly M, Lee L, Woolf P. Loss of adrenocortical suppression after acute brain injury:

41. Feibel JH, Baldwin CA, Joynt RJ. Catecholamine-associated refractory hypertension following acute intracranial hemorrhage: control with propranolol. Ann Neurol 1981;9:340–343.

42. Fishman RA. Brain edema. N Engl J Med 1975;14:706–711.

43. Forsman M, Aarseth HP, Nordby HK, et al. Effects of nimodipine on cerebral blood flow and cerebrospinal fluid pressure after cardiac arrest: correlation with neurologic outcome. Anesth Analg 1989;68:436–443.

44. Frere RC. Status epilepticus. Problems in Critical Care 1991;5:269–278.

45. Gelmers HJ, Gorter K, De Weerdt CJ, et al. A controlled trail of nimodipine in acute ischemic stroke. N Engl J Med 1988;318:203–207.

46. Gildenberg PL, Frost EA. Respiratory care in head trauma. In: Becker DP, Povlishock JT, eds. Central nervous system trauma status report. Bethesda: National Institutes of Health, NIH/NINCDS, 1985:161–176.

47. Goetting MG, Preston G. Jugular bulb catheterization: experience with 123 patients. Crit Care Med 1990;18:1220–1223.

48. Grotta JC. Current medical and surgical therapy for cerebrovascular disease. N Engl J Med 1987;317:1505–1516.

49. Hackenberry LE, Miner ME, Rea GL, et al. Biochemical evidence of myocardial injury after severe head trauma. Crit Care Med 1982;10(10):641–644.

50. Halloran LG, Zfass AM, Gayle WE, et al. Prevention of acute gastrointestinal complications after severe head injury: a controlled trial of cimetidine prophylaxis. Am J Surg 1980;139:44–48.

51. Hamill JF, Bedford RF, Weaner DC, et al. Lidocaine before endotracheal intubation: intravenous or laryngotracheal? Anesthesiology 1981;55:578–581.

52. Havill JH. Prolonged hyperventilation and intracranial pressure. Crit Care Med 1984;12:72–74.

53. Hayashi M, Kobayashi H, Kawano H, et al. Treatment of systemic hypertension and intracranial hypertension in cases of brain hemorrhage. Stroke 1988;19:314–321.

54. Hemodilution in Stroke Study Group. Hypervolemic hemodilution treatment of acute stroke. Results of a randomized multicenter trial using pentastarch. Stroke 1989;20:317–323.

55. Heros RC, Korosue K. Hemodilution for cerebral ischemia. Stroke 1989;20:423–427.

56. Hoyt DB, Ozkan AN, Hansbrough JF, et al. Head injury: an immunologic deficit in T-cell activation. J Trauma 1990;30(7):759–767.

57. Hsu CY, Faught RE, Furlan AJ, Coull BM, et al. Intravenous prostacyclin in acute nonhemorrhagic stroke: a placebo-controlled double-blind trial. Stroke 1987;18(2):352–358.

58. Ikeda Y, Long DM. The molecular basis of brain injury and brain edema: the role of oxygen free radicals. Neurosurgery 1990;27:1–11.

role of increased intracranial pressure and brain stem function. J Clin Endocrinol Metab 1983;57:1245–1249.

59. Italian Acute Stroke Study Group. Haemodilution in acute stroke: results of the Italian haemodilution trial. Lancet 1988;1:318–321.

60. James HE, Langfitt TW, Kumar VS, et al. Treatment of intracranial hypertension. Analysis of 105 consecutive, continuous recordings of intracranial pressure. Acta Neurochir 1977;36:189–200.

61. Jennet B, Teasdale G. Management of head injuries. Philadelphia: FA Davis, 1981:78, 317–332.

62. Judson JA, Cant BR, Shaw NA. Early prediction of outcome from cerebral trauma by somatosensory evoked potentials. Crit Care Med 1990;18:363–368.

63. Kamada T, Fusamoto H, Kawano S, et al. Gastrointestinal bleeding following head injury: a clinical study of 433 cases. J Trauma 1977;17(1):44–47.

64. Kassell NF, Peerless SJ, Durward QJ, et al. Treatment of ischemic deficits from vasospasm with intravascular volume expansion and induced arterial hypertension. Neurosurgery 1982;11:337–343.

65. Kassell NF, Haley EC, Torner JC, et al. Nicardipine and angiographic vasospasm [Abstract]. J Neurosurg 1991;74:341A.

66. Kennealy JA, McLennan JE, Loudon RG, et al. Hyperventilation-induced cerebral hypoxia. Am Rev Respir Dis 1980;122:407–411.

67. Klauber MR, Toutant SM, Marshall LF. A model for predicting delayed intracranial hypertension following severe head injury. J Neurosurg 1984;61:695–699.

68. Kochanek PM. Novel pharmacologic approaches to brain resuscitation after cardiorespiratory arrest in the pediatric patient. Crit Care Clin 1988;4:661–677.

69. Koehler RC, Traystman RJ. Preservation of cerebral blood flow during cardiopulmonary resuscitation. In: Taylor RB, Shoemaker WC, eds. Critical care state of the art. Vol 12. Fullerton, CA: Society of Critical Care Medicine, 1991:569–594.

70. Kramer G, Tettenborn B, Rothacher B, et al. Nimodipine German Austrian stroke trial [Abstract]. Neurology 1990;40(suppl 1):415.

71. Levi L, Wolf AL, Ward JD, Marmarou A, et al. Failure of THAM to improve outcome in patients with severe head injury: a two-center randomized study [Abstract]. J Neurosurg 1991;74:365A.

72. Levy DE, Caronna JJ, Singer BH, et al. Predicting outcome from hypoxic-ischemic coma. JAMA 1985;253:1420–1426.

73. Lindsay K, Pasaoglu A, Hirst D, et al. Somatosensory and auditory brain stem conduction after head injury: a comparison with clinical features in prediction of outcome. Neurosurgery 1990;26:278–285.

74. Lobato RD, Sarabia R, Rivas JJ. Normal computerized tomography scans in severe head injury. J Neurosurg 1986;65:784–789.

75. Mackersie RC, Christensen JM, Pitts LH, et al. Pulmonary extravascular fluid accumulation following intracranial injury. J Trauma 1983;23:968–974.

76. Marion DW, Segal R, Thompson ME. Subarachnoid hemorrhage and the heart. Neurosurgery 1986;18(1):101–106.

77. McGillicuddy JE. Cerebral protection: pathophysiology and treatment of increased intracranial pressure. Chest 1985;87:85–93.

78. McLeod AA, Dwyer GN, Meyer CH, Richardson PL, et al. Cardiac sequelae of acute head injury. Br Heart J 1982;47:221–226.

79. McPherson RW, Kirsch JR, Traystman RJ. Optimal anesthetic techniques for patients at risk of cerebral ischemia. In: Weinstein PR, Faden AI, eds. Protection of the brain from ischemia. Baltimore: Williams & Wilkins, 1990:237–252.

80. Meldrum BS. Metabolic factors during prolonged seizures and their relation to nerve cell death. Adv Neurol 1983;34:261–275.

81. Michenfelder JD. Anesthesia and the brain. New York: Churchill Livingstone, 1988l.

82. Miller JD. Head injury and brain ischaemia—implications for therapy. Br J Anaesth 1985;57:120–129.

83. Miller JD, Butterworth JF, Gudeman SK, et al. Further experience in the management of severe head injury. J Neurosurg 1981;54:289–299.

84. Morse ML, Milstein JM, Haas JE, et al. Effect of hydration on experimentally induced cerebral edema. Crit Care Med 1985;13:563–565.

85. Muizelaar JP. Cerebral blood flow, cerebral blood volume, and cerebral metabolism after severe head injury. In: Becker DP, Gudeman SK, eds. Textbook of head injury. Philadelphia: WB Saunders, 1989:221–240.

86. Muizelaar JP, Becker DP. Induced hypertension for the treatment of cerebral ischemia after subarachnoid hemorrhage. Direct effect on cerebral blood flow. Surg Neurol 1986;25:317–325.

87. Muizelaar JP, Lutz HA III, Becker DP. Effect of mannitol on ICP and CBF correlation with pressure autoregulation in severely head-injured patients. J Neurosurg 1984;61:700–706.

88. Narayan RK, Greenberg RP, Miller JD, et al. Improved confidence of outcome prediction in severe head injury. J Neurosurg 1981;54:751–762.

89. Narayan RK, Kishore PR, Becker DP, et al. Intracranial pressure: to monitor or not to monitor? J Neurosurg 1982;56:650–659.

90. Neil-Dwyer G, Cruickshank JM, Doshi R. The stress response in subarachnoid haemorrhage and head injury. Acta Neurochir 1990;47:102–110.

91. Nelson PB, Seif SM, Maroon JC, Robinson AG. Hyponatremia in intracranial disease: perhaps not the syndrome of inappropriate secretion of antidiuretic hormone (SIADH). J Neurosurg 1981;55:938–941.

92. Norris JW, Hachinski VC. High dose steroid treatment in cerebral infarction. Br Med J 1986;292:21–23.

93. Nussmeier NA, Arlund C, Slogoff S. Neuropsychiatric complications after cardiopulmonary bypass: cerebral protection by a barbiturate. Anesthesiology 1986;64:165–170.

94. Obrist WD, Langfitt TW, Jaggi JL, et al. Cerebral blood flow and metabolism in comatose patients with acute head injury. J Neurosurg 1984;61:241–253.

95. Olesen WD. Cerebral function, metabolism, and blood flow. Acta Neurol Scand 1974;57:38–43.

96. Olinger CP, Adams HF, Brott TG, et al. High dose intravenous naloxone for the treatment of acute ischemic stroke. Stroke 1990;21:721–725.

97. Orlowski JP, Shiesley D, Vidt DG, et al. Labetalol to control blood pressure after cerebrovascular surgery. Crit Care Med 1988;16:765–768.

98. Ott L, Young B, McClain C. The metabolic response to brain injury. J Parenter Enteral Nutr 1987;11(5):488–493.

99. Paulson OB, Waldemar G, Schmidt JF, et al. Cerebral circulation under normal and pathological conditions. Am J Cardiol 1989;63:2C–5C.

100. The Pentoxifylline Study Group. Pentoxifylline in acute non-hemorrhagic stroke. Stroke 1988; 19:716–722.

101. Petruk KC, West M, Mohr G, et al. Nimodipine treatment in poor grade aneurysm patients. Results of a multicenter double-blind placebo-controlled trial. J Neurosurg 1988;68:505–517.

102. Philippon J, Grob R, Dagreau F, et al. Prevention of vasospasm in subarachnoid hemorrhage. A controlled study with nimodipine. Acta Neurochir 1986;82:110–114.

103. Pickard JD, Murray GD, Illingworth R, et al. Effect of oral nimodipine on cerebral infarction and outcome after subarachnoid hemorrhage: British aneurysm nimodipine trial. Br Med J 1989;298:636–642.

104. Plum F, Posner JB. The diagnosis of stupor and coma. 3rd ed. Philadelphia: FA Davis, 1980:1–86.

105. Poungvarin N, Bhoopat W, Viriyavejakul A, et al. Effects of dexamethasone in primary supratentorial intracerebral hemorrhage. N Engl J Med 1987;316:1229–1233.

106. Prough DS. Brain monitoring. In: Taylor RB, Shoemaker WC, eds. Critical care state of the art. Vol. 12. Fullerton, CA: Society of Critical Care Medicine, 1991:157–196.

107. Ramadan NM, Deveshwar R, Levine SR. Magnetic resonance and clinical cerebrovascular disease. An update. Stroke 1989;20:1279–1283.

108. Rapp RP, Young B, Twyman D, et al. The favorable effect of early parenteral feeding on survival in head-injured patients. J Neurosurg 1983;58:906–912.

109. Rea GL, Rockswold GL. Barbiturate therapy in uncontrolled intracranial hypertension. Neurosurgery 1983;12:401–404.

110. Reusser P, Gyr K, Scheidegger D, Buchmann B, et al. Prospective endoscopic study of stress erosions and ulcers in critically ill neurosurgical patients: current incidence and effect of acid-reducing prophylaxis. Crit Care Med 1990; 18(3):270–274.

111. Rockoff MA, Marshall LF, Shapiro HM. High dose barbiturate therapy in humans: a clinical review of 60 patients. Ann Neurol 1979;6:194–199.

112. Rogers MC. The physiology of cardiopulmonary resuscitation. Intensive Care Med 1989;15:55–58.

113. Rolfsen ML, Davis WR. Cerebral function and preservation during cardiac arrest. Crit Care Med 1989;17:283–292.

113a. Ropper AH, O'Rourke DO, Kennedy SK. Head position, intracranial pressure, and compliance. Neurology 1982;32:1288–1291.

114. Rosenfeld JV, Barnett GH, Sila CA, et al. The effect of subarachnoid hemorrhage on blood and CSF atrial natriuretic factor. J Neurosurg 1989;71:32–37.

115. Rosner MJ, Becker DP. Experimental brain injury: successful therapy with the weak base, tromethamine. J Neurosurg 1984;60:961–971.

116. Rosner MJ, Coley IB. Cerebral perfusion pressure, intracranial pressure, and head elevation. J Neurosurg 1986;65:636–641.

117. Rosner MJ, Daughton S. Cerebral perfusion pressure management in head injury. J Trauma 1990;30(8):933–941.

118. Safar P. Resuscitation from clinical death: pathophysiologic limits and therapeutic potentials. Crit Care Med 1988;16:923–941.

119. Saul TG, Ducker TB, Salcman M, et al. Steroids in severe head injury. A prospective randomized clinical trial. J Neurosurg 1981;54:596–600.

120. Scandinavian Stroke Study Group. Multicenter trial of hemodilution in acute ischemic stroke: I. Results in the total patient population. Stroke 1987;18:691–699.

121. Scandinavian Stroke Study Group. multicenter trial of hemodilution in acute ischemic stroke: results of subgroup analyses. Stroke 1988;19:464–471.

122. Schettini A, Stahurski B, Young H. Osmotic and osmotic-loop diuresis in brain surgery. J Neurosurg 1982;56:679–684.

123. Scheuer ML, Pedley TA. The evaluation and treatment of seizures. N Engl J Med 1990; 323:1468–1474.

124. Schmidley JW. Free radicals in central nervous system ischemia. Stroke 1990;21:1086–1090.

125. Schwartz ML, Tator CH, Rowed DW, et al. The University of Toronto head injury treatment study: a prospective, randomized comparison of pentobarbital and mannitol. Can J Neurol Sci 1984;11:434–440.

126. Seelig JM, Marshall LF, Toutant SM, et al. Traumatic acute subdural hematoma. Major mortality reduction in comatose patients treated within four hours. N Engl J Med 1981;304:1511–1518.

127. Shackford SR. Fluid resuscitation in head injury. J Intensive Care Med 1990;5:59–68.

128. Shapiro HM. Intracranial hypertension: therapeutic and anesthetic considerations. Anesthesiology 1975;43:445–471.

129. Siesjö, BK. Mechanisms of ischemic brain damage. Crit Care Med 1988;16:954–963.

130. Sirna S, Biller J, Skorton DJ, et al. Cardiac evaluation of the patient with stroke. Stroke 1990; 21:14–23.

131. Steen PA, Gisvold SE, Milde JH, et al. Nimodipine improves outcome when given after complete cerebral ischemia in primates. Anesthesiology 1985;62:406–414.

132. Strand T, Asplund K, Eriksson S, et al. A ran-

domized controlled trial of hemodilution therapy in acute ischemic stroke. Stroke 1984;15:980–989.

133. Talman WT. Cardiovascular regulation and lesions of the central nervous system. Ann Neurol 1985;18:1–12.

134. Tazaki Y, Sakai F, Otomo E, et al. Treatment of acute cerebral infarction with a choline precursor. Stroke 1988;19:211–216.

135. Temkin NR. Dikmen SS, Wilensky AJ, et al. A randomized, double-blind study of phenytoin for the prevention of post-traumatic seizures. N Engl J Med 1990;323:497–502.

136. Touho H, Karasawa J, Shishido H, et al. Hypermetabolism in the acute stage of hemorrhagic cerebrovascular disease. J Neurosurg 1990;72:710–714.

137. Unwin DH, Giller CA, Kopitnik TA. Central nervous system monitoring. What helps, what does not. Surg Clin North Am 1991;71:733–747.

138. Van Aken H, Cottrell JE, Anger C, et al. Treatment of intraoperative hypertensive emergencies in patients with intracranial disease. Am J Cardiol 1989;63:43C–47C.

139. Voldby B, Enevoldsen EM, Jensen, FT. Regional CBF, intraventricular pressure, and cerebral metabolism in patients with ruptured intracranial aneurysms. J Neurosurg 1985;62:48–58.

140. Wald SL, McLaurin RL. Oral glycerol for the treatment of traumatic intracranial hypertension. J Neurosurg 1982;56:323–331.

141. Ward JD. Intracranial pressure monitoring. In: Fuhrman BP, Shoemaker WC, eds. Critical care state of the art. Vol 10. Fullerton, CA: Society of Critical Care Medicine, 1989:173–185.

142. Ward JD, Becker DP, Miller JD, et al. Failure of prophylactic barbiturate coma in the treatment of severe head injury. J Neurosurg 1985;62:383–388.

143. White PF, Schlobohm RM, Pitts LH, et al. A randomized study of drugs for preventing increases in intracranial pressure during endotra-

cheal suctioning. Anesthesiology 1982;57:242–244.

144. Wijdicks EFM, Vermeulen M, Hijdra A, et al. Hyponatremia and cerebral infarction in patients with ruptured intracranial aneurysms: is fluid restriction harmful? Ann Neurol 1985;17:137–140.

145. Wijdicks EFM, Vermeulen M, ten Haaf JA, et al. Volume depletion and natriuresis in patients with a ruptured intracranial aneurysm. Ann Neurol 1985;18:211–216.

146. Wise RJ, Bernardi S, Frackowiak RS, et al. Serial observations on the pathophysiology of acute stroke. Brain 1983;106:197–222.

147. Wood J, Fleischer A. Observations during hypervolemic hemodilution of patients with acute focal cerebral ischemia. JAMA 1982;248:2999–3004.

148. Wood JH, Kee DB Jr. Hemorheology of the cerebral circulation in stroke. Stroke 1985;16:765–772.

149. Woodcock J, Ropper A, Kennedy SK. High dose barbiturates in non-traumatic brain swelling: ICP reduction and effect on outcome. Stroke 1982;13:785–787.

150. Woolf PD, Lee LA, Hamill RW, et al. Thyroid test abnormalities in traumatic brain injury: correlation with neurologic impairment and sympathetic nervous system activation. Am J Med 1988;84:201–208.

151. Wong MC, Haley EC Jr. Calcium antagonists: stroke therapy coming of age. Stroke 1990;21:494–501.

152. Yatsu FM. Cardiopulmonary arrest and intravenous glucose. J Crit Care 1987;2:1–3.

153. Young AB, Ott LG, Thompson JS, et al. The cellular immune depression of non-steroid treated severely head-injured patients [Abstract]. Neurosurgery 1985;16:725.

154. Young B, Ott L, Norton J, et al. Metabolic and nutritional sequelae in the non-steroid treated head-injury patient. Neurosurgery 1985;17:784–791.

46

Neuromuscular Disease

Marc D. Malkoff

Neuromuscular dysfunction can lead to respiratory failure and disturbances of autonomic regulation. Ventilatory failure may ensue from either bulbar or diaphragmatic weakness. Autonomic dysregulation may occur from alteration of vagal tone or sympathetic nerve output. The pathophysiology and abnormalities encountered dictate the treatment of these entities.

Motor control begins in the cerebral cortex, where cell bodies send their axons caudally in the corticospinal and corticobulbar tracts. These axons synapse directly and indirectly (via internuncial neurons) upon anterior horn cells in the ventral part of the spinal gray matter. In the brainstem, cells with these roles are found in the motor nuclei of the cranial nerves. These anterior horn cells send off heavily myelinated axons, which may ramify to supply one to several hundred muscle fibers. The axon terminal releases acetylcholine, which, upon binding to receptors on the muscle, initiates depolarization and contraction (Fig. 46.1 and Table 46.1).

Clinical symptoms from disruption of this system primarily consist of weakness. The pattern of weakness, the accompanying clinical picture, and other neurologic signs will often suggest the site and/or the cause of the dysfunction. Dysfunction of one corticobulbar or cortical spinal tract may cause unilateral weakness and spasticity and hyperactive reflexes, but does not lead to respiratory dysfunction. Bilateral dysfunction may lead to aspiration. Since the anterior horn cells of the phrenic nerve receive bilateral innervation, unilateral tract dysfunction does not often cause diaphragmatic dysfunction. Dysfunction of the internuncial neurons leads to marked rigidity.

Disease at or distal to the anterior horn cell will present with weakness and/or flaccidity and hyporeflexia in varying patterns. Primary muscle disease (myopathy) tends to present with proximal muscle (deltoid, hip flexors) weakness. Since axonal dysfunction (or death) and demyelination tend to be more obvious in the longest nerves, distal weakness is seen. Axonal death, either directly or indirectly via anterior horn cell death, will cause muscle fiber irritability, seen grossly as fasciculations, after 10–20 days of the loss of the axon terminal at the neuromuscular junction. Reinnervation from nearby healthy axons may occur (45). Sensory loss or symptoms often accompany demyelination. Weakness in disorders of neuromuscular junction disease tends to occur in those areas of relatively rapid rates of axonal firing.

The dysfunctions that usually lead to intensive care admission are secondary to autonomic disturbances and ventilatory failure. Autonomic dysfunction may occur from either demyelination or axonal dysfunction of the vagus or sympathetic hyperstimulation leading to relatively unopposed sympathetic activity (31).

Neuromuscular diseases induce ventilatory failure by impairing the activity of respiratory processes requiring muscle function. Muscular effort is required for inspiratory ventilatory effort, forced expiratory effort (cough), and airway maintenance. Inspiration is accomplished by muscular contraction of the diaphragm with help from accessory muscles, such as the internal intercostals, sternocleidomastoid, trapezius, and pectorals. Since the diaphragm is the major muscle involved in inspiration, weakness of this muscle will lead to poor tidal volumes. The compensatory response of tachypnea may aggra-

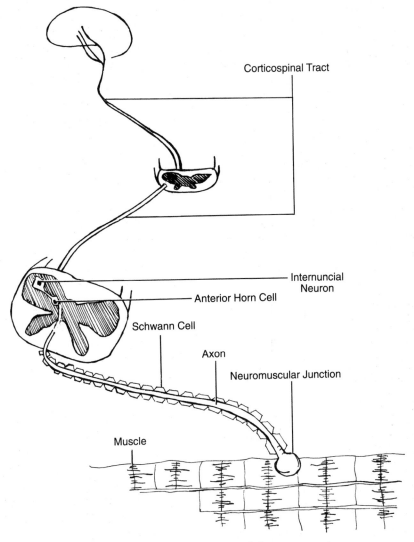

Figure 46.1. Schematic diagram of the motor system.

vate the situation by increasing muscle fatigue (23). This occurs because the diaphragm is perfused only during expiration (48). As a result, minute ventilatory volume may be impaired, which would lead to hypercarbia and a relatively high dead space to tidal volume ratio. In addition, this decrease in minute ventilatory volume may be inadequate to compensate for increases in metabolic demand in conditions such as sepsis, fever, and starvation refeeding. In conditions of tachypnea, the total amount of time spent in inspiration increases proportionately.

Expiration is generally a passive process resulting from the elastic recoil of the chest wall and diaphragm. Forced expiration (coughing) is crucial to clear secretions and foreign objects from the respiratory tract. The musculature involved is primarily the external intercostals and the abdominals. Glottic muscles, however, are necessary to occlude the airway long enough for thoracic pressure to rise so that air can be forcefully expelled. Weakness of these muscles causes an impaired cough. The subsequent retention of secretions leads to atelectasis in the dependent portion of the

Table 46.1
Common Neurological Diseases Causing Weakness

Corticospinal Tract	Internuncial Neuron	Anterior Horn Cell	Schwann Cell	Axon	Neuromuscular Junction	Muscle
Stroke and trauma Motor neuron disease	Stiff-man syndrome Tetanus	Motor neuron disease (amyotrophic lateral sclerosis, spinal muscular atrophies) Polio	Acute inflammatory demyelinating polyneuropathy (or Guillain-Barré syndrome) Chronic immune demyelinating polyneuropathy	Motor neuropathy Motor neuron disease (spinal muscular atrophy)	Myasthenia gravis Eaton-Lambert myasthenic syndrome	Acid maltase deficiency Polymyositis Starvation Rhabdomyolysis Myopathies

lungs. The resulting increase in dead space continues to be perfused, leading to less efficient gas exchange.

Upper airway dysfunction is caused primarily by weakness of the laryngeal and glottic muscles and may be clinically evident by difficulty swallowing, chewing, or speaking. The subsequent weakness of these muscles will lead to aspiration and further aggravate any problems the weak cough may entail (22).

Clinical manifestations of respiratory failure are generally seen with tachypnea and alternate patterns of respiratory breathing, including contractures and alternation between diaphragmatic and accessory muscle breathing. These conditions may occur even at the expense of decreased tidal volume and carbon dioxide excretion (11, 49). As a result, the normal ventilatory response may become blunted, and altered ventilatory drive will occur (3, 27).

Monitoring of these patients is primarily restricted to various methods of strength testing. Manual testing of muscle strength is not often uniform between examinations and examiners and often does not correlate with respiratory muscle dysfunction (25) (Table 46.2). Since the neck flexors are innervated by the same nerve roots as the phrenic nerve, their strength may provide some correlation with diaphragmatic strength. Although diaphragmatic pressure (Pdimax) may be a better indication of respiratory muscle strength, it is awkward to measure (8). Most clinicians measure forced vital capacity, negative inspiratory force and/or flow volume loops (9, 40, 47, 52, 53, 55). Other respiratory monitoring is covered elsewhere in this book and in Table 46.3. Nerve conduction velocities and electromyography are useful as diagnostic tools and provide prognostic information in Guillain-Barré syndrome but are otherwise of little value (12) (Figs. 46.2 and Table 46.4).

MYASTHENIA GRAVIS

Myasthenia gravis is an autoimmune disorder whose symptoms manifest due to antiacetylcholine receptor antibody acting at the neuromuscular junction. Intensive care admission usually occurs due to "myasthenic crisis" (respiratory failure) and

Table 46.2
Medical Research Council Muscle Power Grading Scale[a]

0 No movement
1 Muscle contracts, flicker of movement
2 Joint moves with gravity eliminated
3 Resists gravity
4 Offers resistance, but not normal strength
5 Normal power

[a]Adapted from Medical Research Council. Aids to the examination of the peripheral nervous system. Memorandum No. 45. 3rd ed. Eastbourne: Baillière-Tindall, 1986.

Table 46.3
Criteria for Ventilatory Failure in Patients with Neuromuscular Disease

	Normal	Borderline	Failure
Forced vital capacity	>15 ml/kg	10–15 ml/kg	<10 ml/kg
Negative inspiratory force	> – 40 mm Hg	– 25–40 mm Hg	< – 25 mm Hg
Airway integrity	Eats, drinks normally; no difficulty articulating	Cannot handle fluids well, manages with oral suctioning; noticeable impairment of speech	Obstruction of airway in certain positions; intermittent aspiration of secretion
Chest x-ray	Absence of atelectasis	Presences of subsegmental atelectasis	Major atelectasis or infiltrate

[a]Notes to chart on respiratory failure: Decision to intubate should also be based upon clinical criteria of respiratory distress, including respiratory rate, paradoxical movement of the abdomen and rib cage, hypoxia, and hypercarbia. The negative respiratory forces are values less than atmosphere.

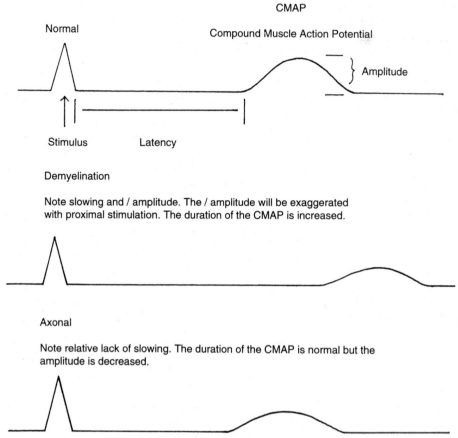

Figure 46.2. *Nerve conduction velocities* give information on the speed of propagation of electrical signals along the nerve by latencies (the length of time it takes to travel a set distance) and in the amplitude of the signal transmitted. The amplitudes may be taken from a sensory nerve or from the muscle stimulated by the nerve. In axonal disease, the latency is only mildly prolonged but the motor action potential may be quite low, whereas, in demyelinating disease, the latency will be markedly prolonged, i.e., marked slowing, and the motor action potential may be relatively normal in amplitude. *EMG* is a way of measuring muscular irritability and recruitment of motor units. In myopathies, recruitment occurs relatively quickly and the motor units may appear small or normal. In central disorders, there is diminished recruitment. In conditions of reinnervation, the motor units appear much larger and more complex than normally. In conditions of denervation, signs of muscular irritability such as fibrillations and fasciculations may be seen.

postoperatively (most commonly from thymectomy). Treatment goals are to reduce antibody production and/or to increase the effect of exiting free acetylcholine receptors.

Classically, myasthenia presents with ptosis, then bulbar weakness, and finally global weakness in a myopathic pattern (proximal muscles). Fatigue is common. Respiratory dysfunction and symptoms often do not correlate with skeletal muscle strength. Respiratory drive may not be normal and CO_2 retention can occur (9).

The diagnosis is made by history and confirmed by at least one of three tests: edrophonium (Tensilon) test, antiacetylcholine receptor antibody test (in reference laboratories), and electromyography (EMG) (50). The Tensilon test consists of blind administration of 1–2 mg of edrophonium, a cholinesterase inhibitor, and then placebo followed by the remainder of the 10

Table 46.4
Common Neuromuscular Causes of
Respiratory Failure

Acute inflammatory demyelinating
 polyneuropathy (Guillain-Barré syndrome)
Myasthenia gravis
Chronic immune demyelinating
 polyneuropathy
Motor neuron disease
Acid maltase deficiency
Periodic paralysis (rare)
Muscular dystrophies (rare in adults)
Polymyositis (rare)
Polyneuropathy of critical illness

Table 46.5
Common Physical Examination Maneuvers in
Myasthenia Gravis

Ptosis time
 Have the patient look up and observe
 patient's upper eyelid in reference to the
 pupil. The patient should not blink. The
 length of time it takes the eyelid to droop
 to approach the pupil without having the
 patient blink or look down is the ptosis
 time. This should normally be greater than
 2 minutes.
Arm adduction time
 The patient adducts the arms and holds
 them out in front of him/her, much like a
 policeman directing traffic. The length of
 time the patient is able to keep his/her arms
 off the bed and in a horizontal position
 without support is the arm adduction time.
 Normally this should be greater than 2
 minutes.

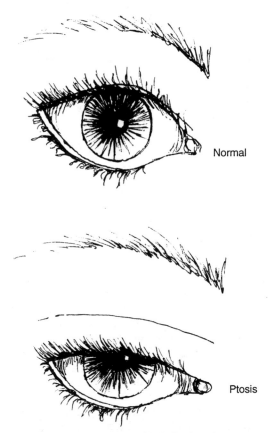

Figure 46.3. Example of lid changes in myasthenia gravis.

mg of edrophonium and then placebo. Strength, particularly arm adduction time, ptosis time, and phonation are tested (Figs. 46.3 and Table 46.5). Myasthenics often improve with edrophonium (1). Since bradycardia, bronchospasm, and asystole may

occur, atropine should be coadministered or nearby. The antibody test is positive about 90% of the time and probably should be obtained in all patients (50). EMG can also confirm the diagnosis by a decrease in compound motor action potentials on repetitive stimulation or single-fiber EMG (1, 41, 50).

Clinical management of the myasthenic patient consists of pharmacologic therapy. Exacerbation of weakness from aminoglycosides or calcium channel blockers may reverse with calcium. Anticholinesterase agents such as pyridostigmine are increased until bulbar or systemic weakness is minimized or side effects of increased vagal tone, such as abdominal cramps, bronchorrhea, sialorrhea, and bradycardia are not manageable even with atropine or related compounds, such as glycopyrrolate. Immunosuppressive therapy, such as steroids, or thymectomy are done if necessary (1, 50).

Myasthenic crises are precipitated by one of five general reasons (Table 46.6). Management strategy consists of determining and correcting the cause, providing supportive respiratory care and monitoring, optimizing myasthenic treatment, and addressing other concurrent medical problems. Intubation should be performed

Table 46.6
Causes of Myasthenia Crisis

Undertreatment
    Includes nonrecognition of myasthenia
Overtreatment
    Often called "cholinergic crisis"; symptoms
    include sialorrhea, bronchorrhea, broncho-
    spasm, diarrhea, and fasciculation
Recent steroid use
    May occur in days 7–21 during the initia-
    tion of steroid therapy
Coexisting primary pulmonary disease
    Examples: Pneumonia
                    Atelectasis
                    Bronchospasm
Serious medical illness

for the usual indications, realizing that the duration of action of neuromuscular blocking agents will be increased. A clinical determination of cholinergic status (over or under) should be made and the dosage of the anticholinesterase adjusted. This determination may be aided by a Tensilon test described earlier. Worsening with edrophonium implies there is no benefit with an increased dose. Patients requiring more medication usually feel weak just before taking their dose and improve with edrophonium. If a determination of cholinergic status cannot be made, discontinuation of these medications for 48–72 hr and restarting at 30 mg of pyridostigmine every 4 hr with titration is recommended. Neostigmine may be given as a parenteral substitute for pyridostigmine at 1 mg of neostigmine for 60 mg of Mestinon as a drip and the dose adjusted. (Conversion values range from 1:15 to 1:180 in my experience (18). In any event, secretions should be dried with glycopyrrolate or atropine.

Most patients will also need adjustment or initiation of immunosuppressive therapy. Plasmapheresis, which decreases antibody load, usually causes a dramatic but relatively short (1–2 month) improvement in muscle weakness within five or six exchanges (28, 43). Prednisone is often started or increased to 80 mg/day and usually begins to work in 1–3 weeks. About 1/3 of the patients may initially weaken on steroids, precipitating respiratory failure (19)—thus, the attractiveness of both pheresis

and steroids used together. Tapering of steroids should be slow. Other immunosuppressives, such as cyclophosphamide or azathioprine, are generally too toxic or slow for the ICU (29). Administration of IgG, which suppresses endogenous IgG production, has been used in some centers (6).

Weaning should take place after respiratory muscle function and bulbar strength return, as demonstrated by examination and monitoring. CO_2 retention must be avoided and the patient's other pulmonary and medical problems should be addressed prior to extubation. Atelectasis can be avoided by encouraging coughing, sighing, and chest physical therapy. Some authorities use intermittent positive pressure breathing (22).

GUILLAIN-BARRÉ SYNDROME

Guillain-Barré Syndrome (GBS), also known as Landry-Guillain-Barré syndrome and acute inflammatory demyelinating polyneuropathy, is a syndrome of acute peripheral nerve demyelination. This usually presents as an ascending paralysis, usually affecting the legs (longest nerves), often with accompanying paresthesias. Deep tendon reflexes are usually, but not necessarily, lost around the time of presentation. The paralysis may ascend to the point of respiratory compromise, bulbar weakness, and "locked-in state". Patients also may complain of neuropathic or muscular pain. Clinical variants include a descending paralysis starting with bulbar involvement (the "Miller-Fisher variant") and patterns of diffuse weakness (5, 15, 30).

The process classically begins 1–3 weeks after a flu-like (usually GI) illness. The diagnosis is made primarily by the demonstration of abnormalities in cerebrospinal fluid (CSF) and nerve conduction velocity and by ruling out other mimics. The CSF typically shows an increased protein with few (<10/ml) or no white blood cells ("albuminocytologic dissociation"). CSF may be normal initially but will generally show the typical pattern 7–10 days after symptoms begin (15, 34). Nerve conduction studies will show evidence of demyelination (Fig. 46.3) and may be used to establish overall prognosis (5, 12). Other diseases that need to be considered in these patients include tick paralysis, polio, diphtheria, botulism, heavy metal poisoning, and porphyria. Human immunodeficiency virus infection can also present with a severe demyelinating neuropathy similar to Guillain-Barré syndrome (although pleocytosis may be present) (35). Primary therapy in Guillain-Barré syndrome is usually plasmapheresis with five or six exchanges of 30–45 ml/kg plasma (total 250 ml/kg) and has been shown to decrease the average duration of ventilator dependence from 60 to 30 days if done within 2 weeks of the onset of symptoms (16, 17, 24). Fluid shifts and third spacing of fluids are common during pheresis and may necessitate invasive hemodynamic monitoring (36). Intravenous γ-globulin has also been used (20, 37). The therapies are thought to decrease antimyelin antibodies present in serum (17). These methods are thought to reduce the length of stay on a ventilator and increase the speed of recovery (24).

Autonomic failure usually manifests as cardiovascular instability. Inappropriate sinus tachycardia with variation of R-R interval is common (32). Usual causes of sinus tachycardia will also produce exaggerated responses (44, 57). This sinus tachycardia increases caloric requirements in a manner similar to fever (39). Vascular tone may also increase, leading to hypertension, or decrease, leading to hypotension (4, 54, 56). This complicates pheresis-based fluid shifts. Treatment of both disorders should be gradual since the autonomic fluctuations can be severe.

Autonomic failure also can cause gastrointestinal and other systemic disturbances. Ileus is common but can be surmounted at times by administration of elemental duodenal feedings. This technique of delivery may also help avoid the consequences of gastroparesis. The syndrome of inappropriate antidiuretic hormone secretion (SIADH) is also common (26). Fever with and without hyperhidrosis has occasionally been blamed on dysautonomia, but is usually due to inflammatory or infectious causes (33). Hy-

perhidrosis is seen alone and is of uncertain clinical significance.

Since the average duration of mechanical ventilation is approximately 30 days for patients having pheresis and 60 days without (16), attention must be paid to prevention of pulmonary emboli, stress ulcers, and contractures. The usual measures such as subcutaneous heparin or pneumatic compression stockings and sucralfate usually suffice.

MOTOR NEURON DISEASE

Motoe neuron disease is a British term for a general group of disorders that involve the lateral corticospinal tracts and the anterior horn cells. In the American literature, these diseases are often called by names such as amyotrophic lateral sclerosis in adults, spinal muscular atrophies, which are most commonly seen in children, and a variety of hereditary motor and sensory neuropathies. In general, only amyotrophic lateral sclerosis will be seen in adult intensive care units. This is a name given to a syndrome consisting of degeneration of the lateral corticospinal tracts and the anterior horn cells, as described above. This manifests as diffuse weakness with or without spasticity. Fasciculations may be seen. Clinically, the patients will present with diffuse weakness, including bulbar signs and respiratory muscle weakness. Tongue fasciculations are a common feature (2).

In general, most varieties of motor neuron disease are very slowly progressive and, at the present time, there is little direct treatment for the root cause of the disorder. There are, however, several other entities that may mimic motor neuron disease that are eminently treatable. These include motor neuropathies associated with lymphoma and paraproteinemias, compressive myelopathies, syringomyelia and syringobulbia, and rare forms of heavy metal intoxication. As such, it is therefore incumbent to make certain of the diagnosis. Direct management of amyotrophic lateral sclerosis is limited to a variety of experimental therapies, which, at this point, show limited promise.

The primary clinical symptom that brings

the patient to the intensive care unit is respiratory failure. This occurs usually secondary to bulbar and respiratory muscle weakness, leading to aspiration and atelectasis, much as described in preceding sections. Symptomatic treatment for this is primarily limited to supportive respiratory care with intermittent positive pressure breathing and chest physical therapy, treatment of any underlying pulmonary disease, and anticholinergics to eliminate hypersalivation and dry up secretions (2, 10, 21, 42). Occasional patients may benefit from cricopharyngeal myotomy (21).

Since motor neuron disease is usually a chronic condition, CO_2 retention is common in these patients (10, 21, 42). Therefore, dyspnea is often a late symptom in the ventilatory muscle weakness and will often occur only when the forced vital capacity drops below 1.5 liters or when coexisting lung disease is present (2, 21). There is some indication that inspiratory muscle training by exercise may improve ventilatory functioning in these patients. The decision to initiate ventilatory support, including intubation, should be made with respect of the patient's wishes (2). Initiation of mechanical ventilation need not be a long-term process, if a coexistent lung disease is the primary cause for the respiratory failure. Home ventilation is common in patients with motor neuron disease and can be arranged in association with tracheostomy. It should be noted, however, that this should be discussed with the patient long in advance of a crisis situation.

ACID MALTASE DEFICIENCY

Acid maltase deficiency is a disorder that may present in adults primarily with respiratory failure (14, 38). The disease was originally described by Pompe and is often known by his name and was usually considered fatal in infancy. However, milder forms of acid maltase deficiency have been noted in adults and occasionally have presented with respiratory failure. The symptoms usually begin with those of a slowly progressive myopathy, which involves the proximal muscles of the shoulder and hip.

At times, however, the patient may not present until frank respiratory failure occurs. Unlike the infantile forms, heart and liver enlargement do not occur. Enzymes of the muscle origin such as creatinine phosphokinase and serum glutamic oxaloacetic transaminase are increased in this condition. EMG findings will indicate a myopathy and the diagnosis is then usually made by muscle biopsy (51). Treatment with a low carbohydrate diet has been attempted and found to be somewhat successful in improving muscle strength (46). Nonetheless, most of these patients will need chronic ventilatory support.

POLYNEUROPATHY OF CRITICAL ILLNESS

The polyneuropathy of critical illness, also known as critical illness of polyneuropathy in some texts, is an axonal polyneuropathy of unknown origin, which often complicates critical illness. It is most commonly seen in patients who are intubated and having sepsis and/or multiple organ failure. It usually manifests as areflexia and failure of weaning mechanical ventilation. Limb weakness and muscle wasting may also be present, as well as sensory loss in the stocking-glove distribution. The diagnosis is most commonly suggested on the basis of EMG and nerve conduction velocity findings (7). The latter are consistent with an axonopathy. Therefore, distal latencies are prolonged, but dispersion of the compound muscle action potentials are not seen. In addition, the EMG often shows signs of marked denervation. Failure to wean is caused by pathologic characteristics in the phrenic nerve, which can be demonstrated by phrenic nerve stimulation. Autopsy studies of this condition have shown axonal degeneration of motor and sensory fibers with extensive denervation of both limb and respiratory muscles. Recovery from critical illness of polyneuropathy has been suggested to generally occur over 1–6 months, implying a primarily distal or axonal degeneration problem. As in acute inflammatory demyelinating polyneuropathy, recovery is often incomplete (7). Recently, others have suggested the existence of a myopathy of critical illness causing prolonged mechanical ventilation (13).

References

1. Adams R, Victor M. Myasthenia gravis in episodic forms of muscular weakness. In: Principles of Neurology. 4th ed. New York: McGraw Hill 1989:1150–1161.
2. Adams RD, Victor M. Principles of neurology. 4th ed. Edinburgh: Churchill Livingstone. 1989:953–958.
3. Aldrich T. Respiratory muscle fatigue. Clin Chest Med 1988;9:225–236.
4. Appenzeller O, Marshall J. Vasomotor disturbance in Landry-Guillian-Barré syndrome. Arch Neurol 1963;9:368–372.
5. Asbury A, Cornblath DR. Assessment of current diagnostic criteria for Guillain-Barré syndrome. Ann Neurol 1990;27:S21–24.
6. Asura E, Bick A, Brunner N, Grob D. The effects of repeated doses of intravenous immunoglobulin in myasthenia gravis. Am J Med Sci 1988;295:438–443.
7. Bolton CF, Laverty DA, et al. Critically ill polyneuropathy: electrophysiological studies in differentiation from Guillain-Barré syndrome. J Neurol Neurosurg Psychiatry 1986;49:563–573.
8. Borel CO, Malkoff MD, Hanley DF. Acute ventilatory failure in neuromuscular disease. In: Johnson RT, ed. Current therapy in neurological disease. 3rd ed. Philadelphia: BC Decker, 1991:391–395.
9. Borel CO, Tilford C, Nichols DG, Hanley DF, Treystman RJ. Diaphragmatic performance during recovery from acute ventilatory failure in Guillain-Barré syndrome and myasthenia gravis. Chest 1991;99:444–451.
10. Braun S. Respiratory system in amyotrophic lateral sclerosis. In: Brooks BR, Ed. Neurologic Clinics 1987;5:9–32.
11. Cohen C, Zagelbaum G, Groves D, et al. Clinical manifestations of inspiratory fatigue. Am J Med 1982;73:308–316.
12. Cornblath DR, Meltis ED, Griffin JW, et al. Motor conduction studies in the Guillain-Barré syndrome: description and prognostic value. Ann Neurol 1988;23:354–359.
13. Douglass JA, Tuxen DB, Horn EM, et al. Acute myopathy following treatment of severe life threatening asthma. Am Rev Respir Dis 1990;141:S83–97.
14. Engel AE. Metabolic and endocrine myopathies. In: Walton JE Sir, ed. Disorders of voluntary muscle. 5th ed. Edinburgh: Churchill Livingstone, 1988:819–822.
15. England J. Guillain-Barré syndrome. Annu Rev Med 1990;41:73–121.
16. Epstein M, Sladky J. The role of plasmapheresis in childhood Guillain-Barré syndrome. Ann Neurol 1990;28:65–69.
17. Griffin JW, Braine HG, McKhann GM, Cornblath DR. Plasmapheresis in Guillain-Barré syndrome. Crit Care Rep 1989;1:164–167.
18. Havard CWH, Fonseca V. New treatment approaches to myasthenia gravis. Drugs 1990;39:66–73.
19. Johns TR. Long term corticosteroid treatment of myasthenia gravis. In: Drachman D, ed. Myasthenia gravis biology and treatment. Ann NY Acad Sci 1987;505:568–583.
20. Kleyweg LP, van der Meche FGA, Meulste J. Treatment of Guillain-Barré syndrome with high dose gamma globulin. Neurology 1989;38:1639–1641.
21. Kuncl RW, Clawson LL. Amyotrophic lateral sclerosis. In: Johnson RT, ed. Current therapy in neurological disease. 3rd ed. Philadelphia: BC Decker, 1991:291–300.
22. Malkoff MD, Borel CO. Patients with neuromuscular disease, ventilatory support and weaning. Crit Care Rep 1989;1:100–109.
23. Marini JJ. Weaning from mechanical ventilation. N Engl J Med 1991;324:1496–1498.
24. McKhann GM, Griffin JW, Cornblath DR, et al. Plasmapheresis in Guillain-Barré syndrome: analysis of prognostic factors and the effect of plasmapheresis. Ann Neurol 1988;23:347–353.
25. Mier-Jedrezejowicz AK, Brophy C, Green M. Respiratory muscle function in myasthenia gravis. Am Rev Respir Dis 1988;138:867–873.
26. Moore T, James O. Guillain-Barré syndrome: incidents, management and outcome of major complications. Crit Care Med 1981;9:549–555.
27. Newsom-Davis J, Goldman M, Loh L, Casson M. Diaphragmatic function and alveolar hyperventilation. Q J Med 1976;45:87.
28. Newsom-Davis H, Wilson SG, Vincent A, Ward CD. Long term effects of repeated plasma exchange in myasthenia gravis. Lancet 1979;1:464–468.
29. Nyberg-Hansen R, Jerstad L. Immunopharmacological treatment in myasthenia gravis. Transplant Proc 1988;20(3)(suppl 4):201–210.
30. Ropper AH, Wijdicks GFM, Truax B. Guillain-Barré Syndrome. Philadelphia: FA Davis, 1991:73–121.
31. Ropper AH, Wijdicks GFM, Truax B. Guillain-Barré Syndrome. Philadelphia: FA Davis, 1991:95–105.
32. Ropper AH, Wijdicks GFM, Truax B. Guillain-Barré Syndrome. Philadelphia: FA Davis, 1991:99–102.
33. Ropper AH, Wijdicks GFM, Truax B. Guillain-Barré Syndrome. Philadelphia: FA Davis, 1991:104–105.
34. Ropper AH, Wijdicks GFM, Truax B. Guillain-Barré Syndrome. Philadelphia: FA Davis, 1991:155–160.
35. Ropper AH, Wijdicks GFM, Truax B. Guillain-Barré Syndrome. Philadelphia: FA Davis, 1991:175–225.
36. Ropper AH, Wijdicks GFM, Truax B. Guillain-Barré Syndrome. Philadelphia: FA Davis, 1991:232.
37. Ropper AH, Wijdicks GFM, Truax B. Guillain-Barré Syndrome. Philadelphia: FA Davis, 1991:235–236.

38. Rosenow EC, Engel AE. Acid maltase deficiency in adults presenting as respiratory failure. Am J Med 1978;64:45.

39. Rouebenoff R. Personal communication. Formerly dietitian, Johns Hopkins Hospital, Neurosciences Critical Care Unit.

40. Sahn S, Lakishminarayan S. Bedside criteria for discontinuation of mechanical ventilation. Chest 1973;63:1002–1005.

41. Sanders D. The electrodiagnosis of myasthenia gravis. In: Drachman D, ed. Myasthenia gravis biology and treatment. Ann NY Acad Sci 1987;505:539–565.

42. Serisierd E, Mastagliaph L, Gibson GJ. Respiratory muscle function in ventilatory control: in patients with motor neuron disease and in patients with myotonic dystrophy Q J Med 1982;202:205–226.

43. Seybold M. Plasmapheresis in myasthenia gravis. In: Drachman D, ed. Myasthenia gravis biology and treatment. Ann NY Acad Sci 1987;505:584–587.

44. Singh, NK, Jaiswal AK, Misra S, Srivastava PK. Assessment of autonomic dysfunction in Guillain-Barré syndrome and its prognostic implications. Acta Neurol Scand 1987;73:101–105.

45. Slater CR, Harris JB. The anatomy and physiology of the motor unit. In: Walton J Sir ed. Disorders of voluntary muscle. 5th ed, Edinburgh: Churchill Livingstone, 1988:1–26.

46. Slonim AE, Coleman IA, McElligat MA, et al. Improvement of muscle function in acid maltase deficiency by high protein therapy. Neurology 1983;33:34–39.

47. Tobin MJ. Respiratory monitoring in the intensive care unit. Am Rev Respir Dis 1988;138:1625–1642.

48. Tobin MJ. Respiratory muscle and disease. Clin Chest Med 1988;9:363–386.

49. Tobin MJ, Perez W, Guenther SM. Pattern of breathing during successful and unsuccesful trials of weaning from mechanical ventilation. Am Rev Respir Dis 1986;134:1111–1118.

50. Toyka K. Myasthenia gravis. In: Johnson RT, ed. Current therapy in neurological disease. 3rd ed. Philadelphia: BC Decker, 1991:385–391.

51. Trend PSJ, Wilees CM, Spencer GT, et al. Acid maltase deficiency in adults: diagnosis and management in five cases. Brain 1985;108:845–860.

52. Truwit JD, Marini JJ. Evaluation of thoracic mechanics in the ventilated patient. I. Primary measurements. J Crit Care 1988;3:133–150.

53. Truwit JD, Marini JJ. Evaluation of thoracic mechanics in the ventilated patient. II. Applied mechanics. J Crit Care 1988;3:199–213.

54. Tuck RR, McLeod JG. Autonomic dysfunction in the Landry-Guillain-Barré syndrome. Clin Exp Neurol 1978;15:197–203.

55. Vincken WG, Elleker MG, Kosio MG. Flow-volume loop changes reflecting respiratory weakness in chronic neuromuscular disorders. Am J Med 1987;83:673–680.

56. Weintraub MI. Autonomic failure in Guillain-Barré syndrome—value of Swan-Ganz catheterization. JAMA 1979;242:513–514.

57. Winner JB, Hughes IC. Identifications of patients at risk of arrhythmia in Guillain-Barré syndrome. Q J Med 1988;68:635–639.

47

Trauma Critical Care

David P. Strum

The impact of trauma on society and the practice of medicine is immense. Trauma ranks as the third largest killer in the United States, after cancer and heart disease. Trauma is the largest source of morbidity and mortality among the youth (first three decades of life) in this country. In terms of working years lost, trauma is the single most expensive disease that afflicts society. Worse still, if current trends continue, we may experience a period where trauma becomes the leading cause of death overall. Trauma-related morbidity and mortality are preventable, but unfortunately their causes are intertwined in the social, economic, and cultural fabric of society and, therefore, are resistant to traditional medical therapies. In the short term, physicians contribute to the war on trauma by developing effective techniques for acute management and rapid rehabilitation. In the long term, physicians must contribute to the prevention of trauma by actively campaigning against the industrial and societal causes of violence and trauma.

The typical trauma victim is male, in his third decade of life, and living in a rural or suburban community. He has suffered severe multiple injuries as a result of *blunt* trauma. The most frequent source of these injuries is high-speed motor vehicle accidents in the urban areas surrounding major cities. He is employed in a labor-intensive vocation and has a history of risk-taking behavior. He probably will be unable to return to work, especially if he has sustained head injury. Poor education, low socioeconomic status, and residual orthopaedic injury may also impede his return to productive work.

THE TRAUMA SYSTEM

In order to restore trauma patients to productive lives, trauma care must be well organized, multidisciplinary, well funded, and comprehensive. A support system that treats the patients from the time of injury until their return to work is characteristic of modern trauma centers. This continuum of care encompasses three major phases: resuscitation, definitive care, and rehabilitation.

Resuscitation

The medical treatment a patient receives from the time of initial entry into the trauma system until initial stabilization defines the resuscitation period. Resuscitation assets include paramedical staff, land and air transportation, communication facilities, and the acute care trauma team. A paramedical emergency response team treats the patient at the scene and expedites transportation to the trauma center. Hospital care begins in the emergency room or triage area, where an integrated team of specialists assesses and resuscitates the patient. The American College of Surgeons Advanced Trauma Life Support Courses (2) provide a systemized approach to initial trauma resuscitation for the physician's guidance. This system is the model used to define the trauma management detailed in this chapter.

Definitive Care

Surgical intervention and convalescence from acute trauma characterizes the period of definitive care. Definitive care assets include radiology assets, operating rooms, intrahospital transport teams, intensive care units, primary care wards, and rehabilitation facilities together with their necessary staff. Early definitive care improves survival and reduces the length of hospital convalescence (8). Rapid transport to the operating room for immediate surgery is the only means of controlling hemorrhage in some patients.

Rehabilitation

Medical and social support of the patient and family through an often prolonged convalescence characterizes the rehabilitation period. Trauma patients, particularly those with head injuries, may require prolonged hospitalization, physical rehabilitation, and job retraining. The expense incurred by these requirements may overburden family resources during a period

Table 47.1
The Trauma Score: A Simple Physiological Measure of Injury Severity

	Value	Points	Score
Respiratory rate (breaths/min)	10–24	4	
	24–35	3	
	>35	2	
	<10	1	
	0	0	A. ____
Respiratory expansion	Normal	1	
	Shallow	0	B. ____
Systolic blood pressure	>90	4	
	70–90	3	
	50–69	2	
	0–49	1	
	No pulse	0	C. ____
Capillary refill	<2 sec	2	
	>2 sec	1	
	No refill	0	D. ____

Glasgow Coma Scale (GCS)		Total GCS points	Score
1. Eye opening			
Spontaneous	4	14–15	5
To voice	3	11–13	4
To Pain	2	8–10	3
None	1	5–7	2
		3–4	1	E. ____
2. Best verbal response			
Oriented	5		
Confused	4		
Inappropriate words	3		
Incomprehensible words	2		
None	1		
3. Motor response			
Obeys commands	6		
Purposeful movement	5		
Withdraws to pain	4		
Flexion to pain	3		
Extension to pain	2		
None	1		

Total GCS points (1 + 2 + 3) ____

Trauma Score ____
(Total A + B + C + D + E)

when the family often has lost its major source of income. This is an important problem when one considers that most trauma victims come from lower socioeconomic groups.

Scoring of Injuries

Injury scoring is used as a means to triage patients, to compare care in a trauma facility with its own past performance and with that in other facilities, and to analyze patient populations for the purpose of allocating resources. The most widely used scoring system is the trauma score (4). This physiological scoring system is used to evaluate the respiratory, cardiovascular, and neurological systems as a single compound index. Specifically, the Glasgow Coma Scale score is added to points assigned for respiratory rate and depth, systolic blood pressure, and capillary refill (Table 47.1). This score is widely used in emergency situations requiring rapid triage on a large scale. One such triage scheme is shown in Table 47.2 and is useful in

Table 47.2
Triage Guidelines[a,b]

Mechanisms of blunt trauma
    Patients involved in high speed (>25 km/hr)
        motor vehicle accidents.
    Pedestrians struck by motor vehicles at high
        speed (>10–15 km/hr)
    Patients thrown from motor vehicles
    Patients falling from heights greater than
        6 m
Location of penetrating trauma
    Patients with penetrating injury to head,
        neck, chest, abdomen, pelvis, or groin
Location of blunt injury
    Blunt injury; single systems; significant
        involvement of head, neck, chest,
        abdomen, or pelvis
    Any combination of two or more of the
        above
    Two or more proximal long bone fractures
Physiological distress
    A degree of respiratory distress, shock, or
        coma that results in a Trauma Score of 12
        or less or a Coma Score of 10 or less

[a]Patients who meet the above criteria following traumatic injury are best referred to a regional trauma center for definitive care.
[b]From McMurtry RY, McLellan BA, eds. Management of blunt trauma. 1st ed. Baltimore: Williams & Wilkins, 1990.

Table 47.3
The Probability of Survival for Trauma Score Values

Admitting Trauma Score	% Survival
1	2.3
2	6.1
3	6.2
4	14.3
5	21.6
6	31.7
7	38.3
8	52.2
9	61.7
10	66.7
11	75.2
12	80.4
13	90.7
14	95.0
15	97.6
16	99.1

[a]From Stene JK, Grande CM, eds. Trauma anesthesia. 1st ed. Baltimore: Williams & Wilkins, 1991.

deciding when patients must be referred to a regional trauma center. Table 47.3 illustrates that the Trauma Score is also useful in predicting the probability of survival following trauma.

THE TRAUMA TEAM

The trauma team is the medical team that receives, assesses, and resuscitates the patient upon admission to the hospital or trauma center. The size of the teams ranges from two-person physician-nurse teams at small hospitals to large multidisciplinary teams found in large university trauma centers. A typical large trauma team consists of a trauma team leader, anesthesiologist, general surgeon, orthopedic surgeon, neurosurgeon, circulating nurse(s), recording nurse, x-ray technician, respiratory technician, and chaplain or social worker. In most university centers, the physician members of the team are physicians in training. The most influential member of the trauma team is the leader, who is responsible for the larger picture, the overall success of the resuscitation. The trauma team leader is often a general surgeon, but may be selected from any trauma-related specialty: anesthesia, emergency medicine, or any surgical subspecialty (7). It is important that the trauma team leader be experienced and capable of assuming the responsibilities of any other team member in an emergency. The team leader must have sufficient prestige to lead, and at times overrule, other members of the team in the best interest of the patient. In addition to the many surgical subspecialists who attend trauma resuscitations, trauma nurses also play a central role in resuscitation. Together with many other important tasks, they manage inventory, administer medications, record vital signs, and document the resuscitation. A radiography technician and a respiratory technologist should be available to process x-rays rapidly and be immediately available to the trauma team to assist with mechanical ventilation. A chaplain or social worker should be on call for the benefit of the distraught family.

Ideally, when good communications exist, the entire trauma team can be assembled and awaiting a new arrival in the emergency room. Team members proceed to simultaneously assess and resuscitate each patient. Each subspecialist is assigned a primary task according to specialty; anesthesiologists manage the airway, general surgeons the chest and abdomen, neurosurgeons the cranium and spine, etc. Each team member has joint responsibility for overall patient care, and task assignments are flexible. Under circumstances when the general surgeon is delayed, the neurosurgeon or anesthesiologist may need to insert the chest tubes. Each member of the team reports his or her assessment to the team leader and documents these findings meticulously. The redundancy inherent in parallel assessment and treatment of the trauma patient is a major contributor to team confidence, morale, and quality. A well-coordinated trauma team produces quality patient care in an exciting and rewarding milieu.

BLUNT TRAUMA

Primary Survey and Resuscitation

There are four phases of acute trauma management (Table 47.4). The major concern during the primary survey is the

Table 47.4
Initial Priorities in Acute Trauma Resuscitation

The four phases of acute trauma resuscitation
  The primary survey (ABCs of initial trauma assessment)
  The resuscitation phase (simultaneous with primary survey)
  Secondary survey (a complete head to toe examination)
  Definitive care (includes transportation to suitable facility)
The ABCs of initial trauma assessment
  Airway with cervical spine
  Breathing
  Circulation
  Disability (neurological assessment)
  Exposure (undress the patient)

"ABCs" of trauma assessment and resuscitation. The main methods of investigation are the classic tetrad of inspection, auscultation, percussion, and palpation. The airway is examined, and airway obstruction is relieved with manual maneuvers or intubation. Emphasis is placed on preventing damage to the cervical spine while securing the airway.

Next, the chest is examined for life-threatening conditions such as tension pneumothorax. Large chest tubes are inserted as necessary. If intubated, most patients benefit from assisted ventilation. A minimum of two large-bore intravenous catheters are inserted and blood is drawn for grouping and cross-matching, electrolytes, hemoglobin, and drug screen. Cardiovascular variables are examined to detect shock. Hypotension associated with delayed capillary refill (>3 sec) is indicative of serious tissue perfusion deficits requiring immediate intervention. Monitoring is established with an electrocardiograph and pulse oximeter.

A rapid neurological examination is performed. The best motor and verbal response to a noxious stimulus is recorded and the pupillary reflexes are evaluated. The examining physician assesses the level of consciousness and inspects the patient for evidence of focal neurological deficits, which might indicate the need for an immediate craniotomy. The spinal cord is examined for signs of injury and is then immobilized. The patient is then completely disrobed to expose any previously unnoticed injury. All immediately life-threatening injuries should have been detected and dealt with by this time. When the primary survey is completed, x-rays of the cervical spine, chest, and pelvis are initiated so that they can be available for assessment during the secondary survey.

Secondary Survey

The secondary survey consists of a systematic examination "from head to toe" in order to detect and document all the patient's remaining injuries. Injuries first identified during the primary survey are checked and rechecked when the secondary survey is performed. Beginning with the head, the facial bones and skull are examined for lacerations and fractures. The mouth and pharynx are examined to detect dislodged teeth. The thorax is reinspected for subtle conditions such as cardiac tamponade, fractured ribs, flail segments, hemothorax, and pneumothorax. The cervical spine and chest radiographs are examined in detail.

The abdomen is examined, x-ray films of the pelvis are acquired, and a rectal examination is performed. A retrograde urethrogram is performed if there is evidence of urethral discontinuity; a urinary catheter is inserted if there is not. An intravenous pyelogram is performed if renal injury is suspected. The limbs are inspected for evidence of fracture or laceration. Neurological and vascular continuity in the limbs is assessed to detect potential compartment syndromes. X-rays of the extremities are taken and evaluated, and injured extremities are immobilized to prevent further damage. Finally, a detailed neurological examination is performed, and the Glasgow Coma Scale is determined.

Definitive Care

Initial plans for treatment of the trauma patient are made in the trauma room during a meeting of the trauma team members presided over by the trauma team leader. The specialists in the team present those portions of the examination relevant to their specialty together with their recommendations for definitive care. The trauma team leader determines the priority of treatment for each injury and helps the team arrive at a pragmatic plan of definitive care. This initial plan is continually reevaluated by the subspecialty surgeons and consultants who will eventually assume responsibility for the patient.

Difficulties with intrahospital transport of unstable trauma patients are common. Long distances, elevators, and outdated transport equipment often make transport difficult and dangerous. The most difficult patients to transport are those with head, chest, and abdominal injuries, especially if accompanied by intracranial hypertension, hemodynamic instability, or patient agitation. Without team vigilance, patients may suffer additional injury during transport (3) or during radiographic investigation preceding surgery. Most of these injuries are preventable when a trauma-trained nurse and physician team transport the patient. Medical services that may be required by the patient during intrahospital transport include analgesia, sedation, invasive monitoring, resuscitation, ventilation, and airway management.

Computerized Axial Tomography Scan versus Peritoneal Lavage

A quandary is presented by patients with significant simultaneous abdominal and head injuries. A decision must be made whether to proceed first with a computed tomography (CT) scan of the head or to proceed first with a peritoneal lavage. As a rule, if the patient is unconscious or deteriorating neurologically, but hemodynamically stable, then a CT scan should be performed first. Alternatively, if the patient is neurologically stable but hemodynamically deteriorating, then a peritoneal lavage should be performed first. If the patient is deteriorating both neurologically and hemodynamically, then an abbreviated CT scan should be performed while resuscitation continues, and then the patient should be transported expeditiously to the operating room for celiotomy and any indicated neurosurgery.

Aortogram

A widened mediastinum is commonly found in radiographs of trauma patients. Whenever this radiographic finding is associated with thoracic trauma, a traumatic thoracic aortic tear may be present. As a general rule, such patients should receive an arch aortogram before transport to the operating room. Only when the patient is neurologically or hemodynamically unstable should definitive therapy be provided before this investigation. Early detection of traumatic aortic injury enables surgical repair under controlled circumstances and thereby increases the likelihood of a good outcome.

Cervical Spine Evaluation

Because classical airway intubation maneuvers may threaten the integrity of a damaged spine, the cervical spine should be examined prior to intubation. Cervical spine injury is present in 10–15% of patients with head injuries. Anteroposterior and lateral radiographs of the cervical spine should be obtained as soon as the patient arrives in the emergency department. Whenever possible, intubation is postponed until these radiographs are interpreted and the clinical neurological examination is completed.

The important features of the lateral cervical spine evaluation are listed in Table 47.5. Greater than 90% of cervical injuries may be detected with lateral cervical radiography alone. If cervical injury is de-

Table 47.5
Important Features to Evaluate in the Lateral Cervical Spine Radiograph

Alignment of the anterior vertebral bodies
Alignment of the posterior vertebral bodies
Preodontoid space less than 3 mm
Swelling in the prevertebral space
Presence of a normal lordotic curvature
Alignment of the spinolaminal lines
Symmetry of adjacent vertebral structures
  Diarthrodial joint spaces
  Spinous processes
  Vertebral bodies
  Laminae and pedicles
Integrity of the odontoid process

tected clinically or radiographically, the cervical spine must be immobilized until further investigations can be undertaken. Additional investigations that may be indicated include oblique radiography, swimmer's and odontoid views, cervical spine tomography, a cervical CT scan, and flexion-extension radiography. Postponing intubation until after the cervical spine has been evaluated has two advantages: (*a*) it reduces the likelihood of inadvertent injury to the spine, and (*b*) it allows a full neurological examination to be completed before intubation and paralysis (if required).

AIRWAY MANAGEMENT

Good airway management is important in successful trauma resuscitations (6). The majority of trauma patients benefit from an increased inspired-oxygen tension and assisted ventilation. Properly trained airway managers can safely maintain an airway and provide effective ventilation with a bag, mask, and cricoid pressure for prolonged periods. Where possible, instrumentation of the airway is avoided until conditions are favorable for both the patient and the airway manager. If patient safety is threatened, however, the trachea is intubated expeditiously.

Intubation is an act of commission with substantial potential for risk to the patient. Possible complications include cervical spine injury, aspiration, esophageal intubation, loss of airway control, cardiac arrest, and death, to mention only a few. Before intubating a patient, the questions *why, when, how, where,* and by *whom* intubation should be performed must be considered. It is important that the intubating physician address these important questions before every intubation if morbidity caused by errors in airway management are to be avoided.

Why, the reason for intubation, is determined first. Intubation is indicated for either therapy or resuscitation. The exact indication should be determined objectively according to each patient's conditions. Table 47.6 lists life-threatening disturbances in physiology that require emergent or urgent intubation for the pur-

Table 47.6
Life-Threatening Indications for Emergency
Intubation

Unprotected airway
  No gag reflex
  Loss of consciousness (GCS<9)[a]
Inadequate respiratory gas exchange
  $Q_s/Q_t > 30\%$
  $V_d/V_t/ > 60\%$
  $Pao_2 < 50$ mm Hg
  $Paco_2 > 50$ mm Hg
  Respiratory rate>35 breaths/min)
Inability to cough effectively
  Negative inspiratory force < -25 cm H_2O
  Vital capacity <10–15 mg/kg
Cardiovascular instability
  Mean arterial pressure <60 mm Hg
  Presence of major arrhythmias
    (V fib or V tach)
  Cardiac index <2.2 liters/min/m²

[a] GCS, Glasgow Coma Scale.

poses of resuscitation. Unprotected airway is the most common indication for intubation in the trauma patient. Loss of consciousness due to head injury or hypotension are the common reasons for inability to protect the airway. More subtle indications for intubation such as inability to cough and clear secretions may be seen with flail chest, chronic bronchitis, and high spinal cord injuries. Therapeutic indications including surgery, bronchoscopy, or radiological investigation are not life-threatening and therefore the urgency of the therapy decides the relative urgency of the intubation.

When, the degree of urgency, is considered second. This decision ultimately determines how, where, and by whom intubation is performed. The time frame is decided according to one of three grades: emergent, urgent, or elective. Emergent intubations are performed for life-threatening disturbances in physiology and require immediate action. Urgent intubations, by contrast, are usually performed to support a therapeutic intervention such as surgery or bronchoscopy that may yield a better therapeutic result if undertaken in a timely fashion. The airway manager may choose to delay intubation in this situation to optimize safety, but only to the extent that the delay does not result in a suboptimal surgical result. An elective intubation is at the discretion of the intubating physician and should not be undertaken until conditions for the procedure are optimal.

How, the method of airway management, is chosen from among several techniques in current use. The precise choice of methods depends on the particular clinical situation and the relative skills of the operator.

Stabilized Oral Endotracheal Intubation

The preferred method of emergent intubation of trauma patients involves stabilization of the head and neck in the neutral position by an assistant (Fig. 47.1) while an oral endotracheal tube is inserted without flexion or extension of the neck. The neck is not placed in the "sniffing" position, making this technique more difficult than routine orotracheal intubation. The main advantage of this technique is more success in inexperienced hands than blind nasal intubation. It is the preferred method of intubation for urgent and emergent intubations while the status of the cervical spine is undetermined. The disadvantages of this technique include the need for adjuvant medications to sedate the patient before intubation and the blind insertion of some endotracheal tubes necessitated by the anterior position of the larynx, which increases the risk of esophageal intubation.

Nasotracheal Intubation

This is the classic method for intubating a trauma patient with known cervical spine injury. The technique involves the insertion of a 7.0-mm inner diameter (in men) or 6.0-mm inner diameter (in women) soft endotracheal tube through either nasal passage without flexion or extension of the neck. This technique is difficult but persists in clinical use in trauma because it offers excellent protection for the cervical spine. Success with this technique improves when an Endotrol tube (Fig. 47.2) is manually directed into the larynx using

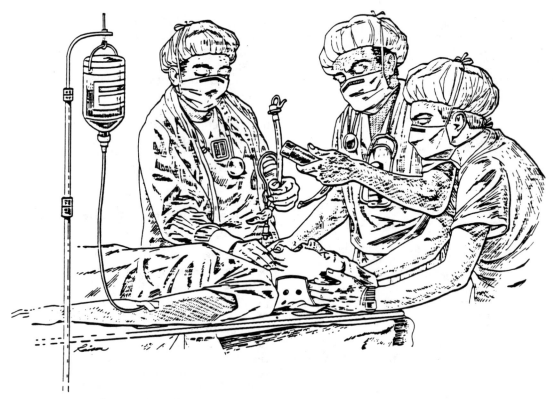

Figure 47.1. Illustrated technique of stabilized orotracheal intubation.

a finger ring and cord system to aim the tip of the endotracheal tube as it is advanced. Active or passive tongue extrusion may also be helpful (1). The method has a high rate of success and low complication rate when undertaken with good technique and gentle persistence. Blind orotracheal intubation is indicated mainly for urgent intubation of patients with known injury to the cervical spine that cannot await the time-consuming preparations for fiberoptic intubation. The disadvantages include a low rate (65%) of success after an average of four attempts and a high incidence (69%) of complications such as epistaxis, soft-tissue trauma, and turbinate fractures in inexperienced hands (5). Blind nasal intubation is contraindicated in the presence of nasal obstruction, apnea, and fractures of the face or larynx.

Fiberoptic Intubation

The surest and safest method available when the cervical spine is known to be injured and sufficient time is available is fiberoptic intubation (9). The cervical spine has excellent protection because the neck is immobilized in the neutral position. This technique requires extensive topical anesthesia and is best performed by a team of two experienced airway managers. The disadvantages include prolonged preparation and performance times and frequent failure of the technique whenever blood or copious secretions fill the airway and complicate the clinical presentation.

Standard Oral Intubation

The preferred method of intubation when the cervical spine is known not to be injured is standard oral intubation. With this procedure, the neck is flexed and the head is extended into the sniffing position. This technique is rarely indicated in the acute trauma scenario because of the difficulties in reliably ruling out cervical spine injury prior to intubation.

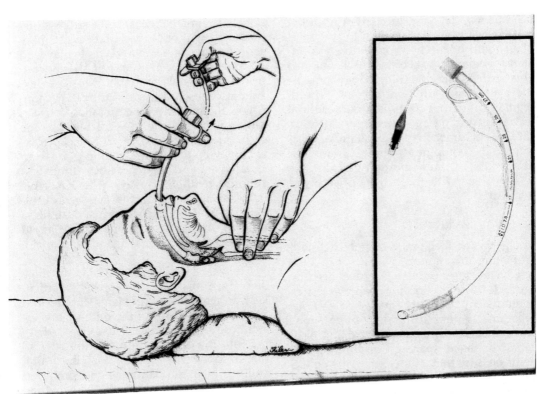

Figure 47.2. An Endotrol tube with manually fixed distal tip greatly assists nasotracheal intubation.

Cricothyrotomy

The preferred surgical management of the airway is cricothyrotomy. The procedure can be performed with minimal equipment: a scalpel with a No. 11.0 blade and a small 6.0-mm inner diameter endotracheal tube or tracheostomy tube. This technique is indicated in emergency situations whenever nonsurgical methods of intubation fail and in urgent circumstances when severe facial or laryngeal trauma are present. While cricothyrotomy is used for emergent and urgent indications of surgical airway instrumentation, it has not yet supplanted tracheostomy in elective use. The only exception to this rule is in children where needle cricothyrotomy is preferred over surgical cricothyroidotomy due to the possibility of injuring the developing larynx and disrupting its maturation.

Who, the airway manager, is decided next. Management of the trauma airway is difficult and requires training and experi-ence. Anesthesiologists are generally the best trained in such skills, but critical care physicians, emergency medicine physicians, and ear, nose, and throat surgeons frequently also possess the necessary skills. Because of the degree of difficulty associated with trauma intubations, experienced physicians must be involved in airway management. These physicians should be adept at stabilized oral intubation, blind nasal intubation, oral and nasal fiberoptic intubation, and surgical cricothyrotomy. They should be knowledgeable about sedation, muscle relaxants, and cervical spina cord injuries.

Where, the best location, is determined last. An environment that is optimal for the operator is important to safe trauma airway management. Anesthesiologists, intensivists, respiratory technologists, operating room or intensive care nurses, and anesthesia technicians should be available immediately. Whereas emergency airway management should be performed as the need arises, delaying intubation until the patient has been transported to the operating room or intensive care area is preferable whenever possible. A well-equipped area such as the operating room contains the necessary equipment for any type of regular or fiberoptic intubation or artificial airway including, if necessary, cricothyrotomy or tracheostomy. Familiar surroundings, equipment, and personnel diminish anxiety and improve performance if difficulties with the airway arise unexpectedly.

Narcotic Sedation

Analgesia and facilitation of stabilized oral intubation in trauma patients are best achieved using narcotics. An ideal narcotic agent for use in trauma patients offers hemodynamic stability, analgesia without sedation, minimal respiratory depression, rapid onset, and ready reversibility. Narcotics are used sparingly in trauma patients because they often exacerbate potential underlying hypovolemia (patients may be too unstable to receive sedation until after they have been hemodynamically resuscitated). All trauma patients should be considered hypovolemic until proven otherwise, and for this reason, the dose used to facilitate endotracheal intubation routinely is reduced to a "stun dose," about one-fifth that of an anesthetic induction dose. This small dose administered as a rapid bolus briefly obtunds the patient's reflexes, facilitates intubation, and increases the subsequent acceptance of the endotracheal tube. Narcotics are preferred over sedative-hypnotic agents for this purpose because analgesia is desirable, the neurological examination is minimally affected, and the endotracheal tube is subsequently well tolerated in conscious patients. Nonnarcotic sedatives such as the benzodiazepines are relatively contraindicated because they are not analgesic and may produce confusion and agitation while obfuscating the neurological examination.

Muscle Relaxants

These potent medications are relatively contraindicated in the tumultuous milieu of the acute trauma resuscitation. Most, if not all, trauma patients can be successfully intubated without muscle relaxants. Inappropriate use of muscle relaxants may lead to apnea, inadvertent loss of airway control, and possible mortality. Muscle relaxants also obscure the neurological examination and prevent communication between the patient and the medical team in the event of a critical problem. Muscle relaxants may be used with caution to relax an agitated patient after previous intubation attempts without muscle relaxants have failed or after the trachea has been intubated. Muscle relaxants for use in trauma patients should be nondepolarizing, rapid in onset, readily reversed, and offer hemodynamic stability.

Complex facial fractures (Le Fort's maxillary fractures I to III) represent particularly difficult airway problems. If bony and muscular structures of the midface are anatomically distorted, profuse hemorrhaging into the airway from fracture sites in the nasopharynx occurs. Stabilized oral endotracheal intubation is the preferred technique in this situation but this method may be impossible if profuse bleeding obscures the anatomic landmarks. Under these conditions, many physicians would proceed directly to surgical cricothyrotomy. Nasal intubation is contraindicated because the bony structure of the nose is disrupted, and endotracheal tubes inserted nasally may pass into false lumens or entrain blood clot or tissue into the lungs.

HEMORRHAGE AND TRANSFUSION THERAPY

What quantity and type of blood products should be administered to resuscitate the trauma patient? Transfusion therapy is based on the trauma patient's initial hemodynamic response to two rapid fluid challenges with crystalloid (10 ml/kg of Ringer's lactate per bolus). Patients are classified according to their response to fluid challenge as "responder," "transient responder," or "nonresponder." If the heart rate and blood pressure return to normal and remain that way after the fluid challenge, then the patient is considered to be a *responder*, and it is presumed that infusion of crystalloid is sufficient for resuscitation. The need for additional blood transfusion is ascertained by laboratory determination of the hematocrit. If the vital signs return to normal only transiently after each bolus, then deteriorate again, the patient is considered to be a *transient responder*, and blood transfusion is warranted. Depending on clinical indications, the physician may decide to transfuse either type-specific blood or fully cross-matched blood. If there is no transient improvement in vital signs following either of the two consecutive fluid boluses, the patient is classified as a *nonresponder*. These patients are in severe shock and require immediate transfusion with type O universal-donor blood. Female patients of childbearing years receive only type O negative blood in order to prevent subsequent Rh sensitization. Patients who fail to respond after transfusion of 6 units of whole blood require a central venous line in order to rule out a cardiac problem such as myocardial infarction or tamponade. Positive inotropes are rarely used to resuscitate trauma patients because they may exacerbate already inadequate tissue perfusion. Transient responders and nonresponders may be assumed to have continuing hemorrhage into a major body capacitance such as the chest, abdomen, retroperitoneum, or thigh.

THORACIC TRAUMA

Serious thoracic injuries may be divided into two categories: those that are immediately life-threatening and those that are potentially life-threatening. There are six classic immediately life-threatening injuries: airway obstruction, tension pneumothorax, open pneumothorax, flail chest, cardiac tamponade, and pulmonary contusion. The surgical skills necessary for resuscitation of patients with thoracic trauma are venous cutdown, tube thoracostomy, pericardiocentesis, surgical cricothyrotomy, oral and nasal intubation, and subclavian catheter insertion. Management of immediately life-threatening injuries is focused first on restoring ventilation and then on maintaining adequate systemic perfusion. An immediate, meticulous physical examination and chest radiograph are the only means necessary initially to identify these immediately life-threatening injuries. Hemothorax or pneumothorax are immediately decompressed with chest tubes because they impair respiration and venous return to the heart. If tension pneumothorax creates hemodynamic instability, it may be necessary to insert a chest tube without waiting for a chest radiograph. Pulmonary contusions and flail chest injuries are dangerous because they may produce hypoxemia, requiring intubation, ventilation, and positive end-expiratory pressure.

The classic potentially life-threatening injuries are ruptured aortic aneurysm, myocardial contusion, diaphragmatic hernia, ruptured esophagus, and tracheobronchial disruption. These injuries must be identified and corrected promptly. Esophageal perforation, tracheobronchial disruption, and diaphragmatic rupture are presumptively diagnosed with chest radiographs (Table 47.7) and subsequently are confirmed with endoscopy or a barium meal. Arrhythmias and changes in the electrocardiograph that indicate myocardial contusion may be confirmed by measuring the level of CPK-MB or creatine phosphokinase MB isoenzyme in the blood. Patients with myocardial contusion must

Table 47.7
Radiographic Signs

Radiographic signs of potentially life-threatening thoracic injuries
  Subcutaneous air or emphysema
  Pneumothorax
  Fallen lung sign
  Hydrothorax
  Pneumomediastinum
  Continued large air leak
Radiographic signs of potential aortic disruption
  Mediastinal widening (sensitive but not specific)
  Loss of aortic contour
  Left apical cap
  Rightward deviation of the nasogastric tube at the level of the aortic isthmus
  Fractured 1st or 2nd ribs at the thoracic inlet
  Rightward shift of the tracheobronchial tree

be monitored for arrhythmias but usually require only conservative management. Aortic or tracheobronchial disruptions usually require definitive corrective surgery. Aortic disruptions are fatal at the scene of the accident in 70–80% of such cases. Those few patients who reach the hospital have already demonstrated an ability to survive, but require urgent, aggressive medical attention if they are to sustain a good outcome. A chest radiograph indicating a widened mediastinum combined with any other single radiographic sign of potential aortic disruption listed in Table 47.7 indicates the need for an arteriogram. Whereas an aortogram remains the "gold standard" for the diagnosis of a ruptured thoracic aneurysm, a contrast-enhanced CT scan or transesophageal echocardiogram may also help make the diagnosis. Whether the repair of a thoracic aortic aneurysm is undertaken on an immediate basis or should be delayed by several days has been extensively debated; the final decision remains with the individual surgeon.

ABDOMINAL TRAUMA

Traumatic abdominal injuries are difficult diagnostic dilemmas. Abdominal examination yields false-positive and false-negative results that are difficult to interpret, particularly in the context of the unconscious patient. In many instances, a laparotomy is required to reliably diagnose the extent of abdominal injury. The mechanism of traumatic injury often predicts the site and extent of injury. For example, seat belts may fracture the lower ribs and lead to laceration of the liver or spleen. Free air on abdominal radiographs indicates injury to the bowel. With severe trauma, the pancreas and duodenum may be injured, and retroperitoneal hematomas may occur. A nasogastric tube is inserted because ileus and emesis occur commonly in trauma patients. Blood aspirated from the nasogastric tube may indicate gastric injury. A vaginal examination should be performed to look for uterine bleeding or vaginal lacerations. Trauma to the uterus and ovaries is common but very difficult to detect on direct examination. Definitive treatment of

abdominal injuries involves surgery, and the rule is that any abdominal pathology that cannot be verified to be benign should be explored. If examination of the abdomen is equivocal, a peritoneal lavage may be performed. Often the examination is frankly positive, and celiotomy and a definitive surgical repair are performed without the need for an intermediate peritoneal lavage.

Retroperitoneal Injuries

Trauma to the retroperitoneal area is more difficult to detect than that to the intraabdominal area. A rectal examination is performed in all trauma patients as part of the investigation for these types of injuries. Blood in the rectum may indicate bowel injury, whereas blood at the urethral meatus and a floating prostate may indicate urethral disruption. If the urethra is normal, the bladder is catheterized to monitor urine production. Hematuria may indicate renal or bladder injury. If the urethra is injured, a retrograde cystourethrogram is performed before proceeding with urinary catheterization. If the contrast medium extravasates from the urethra, then a suprapubic urinary catheter must be inserted to decompress the bladder and prevent further urethral damage. Renal injury may be detected by loss of the psoas shadow on a radiograph of the kidney and upper bladder. An intravenous pyelogram is performed when renal injury is suspected. Serial radiographs at 0, 1, 5, and 15 min after injection of the contrast medium will detect ureteric extravasation of the contrast medium or delayed asymmetric renal dye excretion, indicating one kidney with either vascular injury or partial urinary obstruction. Renal injuries are explored to prevent permanent renal injury.

Peritoneal Lavage

Trauma patients who have no absolute indication for exploratory laparotomy but who may have equivocal or false-negative clinical abdominal examinations should undergo peritoneal lavage. In general, this includes patients with decreased consciousness and continued hypovolemia of unknown etiology and those patients with

Table 47.8
Positive Laboratory Findings from Diagnostic
Peritoneal Lavage

>500 white blood cells/mm³ (uncentrifuged
  sample)
>100,000 red blood cells/mm³ (uncentrifuged
  sample)
Hematocrit >2% (centrifuged sample)
Presence of bile, bacteria, or feces

negative abdominal examinations who will
be unavailable for continued reevaluation.
Peritoneal lavage is contraindicated in the
presence of indications for laparotomy,
multiple previous abdominal operations,
or a gravid uterus. Ten milliliters of aspirate is collected from a periumbilical incision and the lavage fluid is analyzed. Any
of the findings listed in Table 47.8 indicate
a need for urgent exploratory laparotomy.
It is important to be aware that retroperitoneal injury or bleeding can go totally
undetected by diagnostic peritoneal lavage.

Pelvic Fractures

Commonly associated with seat belt trauma
and extreme force, pelvic fractures are a
very serious injury. Primary fractures to
the pelvic ring are usually accompanied by
a compensating contralateral fracture. Anterior pelvic fractures are more benign than
posterior fractures and are not accompanied by retroperitoneal hemorrhage. Posterior pelvic fractures are often associated
with severe retroperitoneal hemorrhage,
which can worsen if this space is surgically
decompressed, leading to fatal exsanguination. For this reason, surgical exploration
is discouraged, and retroperitoneal hemorrhage is usually controlled by external
fixation of the fractures and angiography
with embolization of the source. Arterial
injuries associated with diminished pulses
in the lower limbs are an exception, however, and require surgical repair. Anterior
pelvic fractures, unlike posterior fractures,
are usually unstable and require either external or internal fixation for patient comfort and nursing expediency. All pelvic
fractures are associated with a high rate of
pulmonary embolization.

SPINAL CORD INJURY

One of the major causes of years of productive life lost in the United States is
spinal cord injury. Initially, it often presents as partial paresis accompanied by
hypotension. The spinal cord becomes unstable when any two of the four columns
of support are disrupted. Anteroposterior
and lateral radiographs of the cervical, thoracic, and lumbar spine should be examined for the features listed in Table 47.9.
Partial neurological deficits and "sacral
sparing" indicate incomplete cord injury,
which is believed more responsive to therapy than complete cord injury. Management consists of hemodynamic stabilization of the patient and meticulous
documentation of the neurological status.
Unstable spinal injuries are initially immobilized using a "spine board" or "halo
traction." Definitive stabilization often requires surgical decompression and fusion.
Patients with incomplete spinal cord injury and neurological deterioration require
immediate surgical decompression. Patients with neurological deficit or radiological evidence of an unstable fracture
should be transferred immediately to an
appropriate definitive care facility.

High spinal cord injuries leave the victim tragically impaired. Not only is voluntary movement curtailed, but cardiovascular and respiratory function are also
severely compromised. Cord lesions above
the cardioaccelerator center (T1-4) decrease the tone of the sympathetic nervous

Table 47.9
Radiographic Features Indicative of Serious
Spinal Cord Injury

Unusual anteroposterior diameter of the
  spinal cord
Misalignment and unusual contour of the
  vertebral bodies
Displacement of bone fragments into the
  spinal canal
Linear or comminuted fractures of the
  laminae, pedicles, or arches
Swelling of the soft tissues anterior to the
  cervical cord
Override of adjacent vertebral bodies of more
  than 3.5 mm

system, causing hemodynamic instability. Although fluids usually are sufficient, atropine and inotropic agents may be needed to support the circulation until recovery from spinal shock. As the spine recovers from shock, somatic hyperreflexia and "mass reflexes" emerge that require medical management.

Patients with cervical cord injuries at or above the phrenic nerve outflow (C3-5) often exhibit severe respiratory dysfunction. Paralysis of the intercostal musculature and diaphragm increases the work of breathing, decreases the functional residual capacity, and reduces inspiratory force. These patients are prone to atelectasis, hypoventilation, and retention of secretions. Patients who have a negative inspiratory force of less than 15 cm H_2O or a vital capacity less than 10–15 ml/kg will usually require elective intubation. Elective fiberoptic intubation by a skilled operator is preferred to crisis management in this situation.

HEAD TRAUMA

Head injury is common in trauma victims, with as many as 70% of patients having sustained a significant injury. Long-term disability related to head trauma is a major source of lost productivity in our society (10). While the initial management of head injuries is based on clinical assessment, definitive care is planned after examination by a CT scan. The trauma team must distinguish between cerebral contusion, which produces a stable neurological deficit, and expanding intracranial hematomas, which produce progressive neurological deterioration. Cerebral contusions are usually treated with conservative medical management. Intracerebral hematomas, on the other hand, are inherently unstable and require urgent neurosurgical decompression. A unilateral blown pupil that dilates during medical management is an ominous sign. A burr hole may need to be drilled while the patient is being prepared for emergent surgery. Once the intracranial pressure is relieved, the burr hole may be enlarged to a craniotomy for definitive treatment of the intracranial hematoma.

Depressed skull fractures usually re-

quire neurosurgical intervention. If the fracture segment is depressed below the inner table of the skull, it should be surgically elevated. If the depressed skull fracture is compound, surgery must proceed urgently to prevent infection. Any patient with a Glasgow Coma Scale score (Table 47.10) of less than 7 should have invasive monitoring of intracranial pressure using an intracranial bolt or intraventricular catheter.

Whether a CT scan of the head is necessary before going to surgery is a frequently encountered decision. As a general rule, conscious patients without focal neurological deficits do not require preoperative computerized tomography. However, a CT scan often is performed on patients with a history of loss of consciousness, who require prolonged general anesthesia, or who will endure a period where neurological monitoring will be difficult or impossible. The CT scan is performed to detect intracranial bleeding that might oth-

Table 47.10
Glasgow Coma Scale [a]

	Points
Best verbal response	
Oriented with respect to person, place, and time	5
Confused with respect to person, place, and time	4
Verbalizes spontaneously—disorganized	3
Verbalizes incomprehensibly—unintelligible	2
No verbal responses	1
Best motor response	
Obeys simple commands	6
Localizes noxious stimuli	5
Withdraws from noxious stimuli—flexion	4
Withdraws from noxious stimuli—extension	3
Abnormal extension—spontaneous	2
No motor response	1
Eye opening	
Spontaneous	4
To verbal challenge	3
To noxious stimulus	2
No response	1

[a] A score of 11 or less indicates a significant head injury.

erwise progress unnoticed under general anesthesia. Intracerebral edema may be detected by CT scan, which may be considered an indication for intracranial pressure monitoring prior to prolonged anesthesia and surgery in some patients with a Glasgow Coma Scale score of >9.

ORTHOPAEDIC TRAUMA

Although musculoskeletal injury receives less attention than injuries to the vital organs, the importance of these injuries must not be minimized. Aggressive management of surgical fractures has been shown to improve outcome, decrease the length of stay in the ICU, and decrease morbidity and mortality associated with musculoskeletal trauma (8). Operative fracture management, such as débridement, and internal fixation have replaced closed management, immobilization, and traction in modern orthopaedic management. Compound fractures are urgent injuries that should be dealt with within 6 hr. These fractures are considered infected and require surgical débridement and internal fixation. Prophylactic antibiotics are administered, and the wound is closed. Injuries that penetrate joint capsules are serious and should be explored and debrided at the earliest opportunity.

Compartment syndromes are serious complications resulting from vascular or crush injury to a limb. Neurovascular and muscular function of the limb must be documented meticulously and the limb serially reexamined at intervals. Decreased motor function, decreased perfusion, and increasing neuropathy indicate the urgent need for decompression fasciotomy.

Isolated neurovascular injuries threaten the functional recovery of limbs. Isolated neurological disruptions (neurotemesis) should be surgically reapproximated on an urgent basis. Arterial injuries are particularly threatening and also must be repaired on an urgent basis. Limb perfusion may be confirmed by Doppler measurement whenever arterial injury is suspected. An arteriogram is usually performed to document the position and extent of vascular injury before vascular repair.

A severed limb is a catastrophic injury.

Recent progress has made successful limb reimplantation feasible. The limb should be salvaged, packed in ice (but never frozen), and transported along with the patient to a definitive care center within 4–6 hr of the injury. Injuries that compromise both vascular and neurological function can be considered functional amputations. Vascular and neurological repair and reimplantation are indicated immediately. The viability rate of limb reimplants approaches 75–80%. Patients prefer reimplantation to prosthetic devices, even when functional results are poor. The long-term success of reimplantation depends on the degree of recovery of neurological function. Aggressive management of fractures and reimplantation of limbs helps return trauma patients to a productive and independent life.

PENETRATING TRAUMA

The management principles for penetrating trauma are similar to those for blunt trauma. Whereas blunt trauma is usually diffuse, penetrating trauma is usually localized. From this perspective, examinations of areas remote from the site of penetration can often be performed more expeditiously than with blunt trauma. Penetrating wounds to major body cavities generally must be surgically explored. An exception is penetrating trauma to the lungs, which is managed conservatively whenever possible. Arteriography is indicated whenever wounds penetrate the neck. Exploratory laparotomy is indicated for all penetrating injuries to the abdomen. Penetrating trauma is associated with laceration of major vessels or solid organs or perforation of a hollow organ such as the bowel or bladder. In the presence of internal hemorrhage, survival may depend upon timely exploratory laparotomy. Penetrating objects such as knives often tamponade internal bleeding and should not be removed until laparotomy to avoid inadvertent exsanguination.

Trauma is a disease that affects the young and productive members of our society during the prime of their lives. Seriously injured patients should be transported to regional trauma centers where they are resuscitated, assessed, and provided the necessary definitive surgical care. Convalescence and rehabilitation can be prolonged and expensive, especially when neurological injuries are involved. Current medical efforts to combat trauma are aimed primarily at treatment of acute trauma by providing organized, aggressive, acute care trauma management by teams of dedicated, multidisciplinary specialists based in regional trauma centers. Future efforts, however, may be the most cost-effective and humane if they aim to decrease trauma-related morbidity and mortality through prevention.

References

1. Adams AL, Cane RD, Shapiro BA. Tongue extrusion as an aid to blind nasal intubation. Crit Care Med 1982;10:335–336.
2. Advanced Trauma Life Support Course for Physicians, Student Manual, Chicago: American College of Surgeons, 1989.
3. Andrews PJ, Piper IR, Dearden NM, Miller JD. Secondary insults during intrahospital transport of head-injured patients. Lancet 1990;335:327–330.
4. Champion HR, Sacco WJ, Carnazzo AJ, Copes W, Fouty WJ. Trauma Score. Crit Care Med 1981;9:672–676.
5. Dronen SC, Merigan KS, Hedges JR, Hoekstra JW, Borron SW. A comparison of blind nasotracheal and succinylcholine-assisted intubation in the poisoned patient. Ann Emerg Med 1987;16:75–77.
6. Grande CM, Stene JK, Bernhard WN. Airway management: considerations in the trauma patient. Crit Care Clin 1990;6:37–59.
7. McMurtry RY, McLellan BA, eds. Management of blunt trauma. 1st ed. Baltimore: Williams & Wilkins, 1990.
8. McMurtry RY, Nelson WR. The intensive care unit as a relative indication for open reduction and internal fixation. 1st Pan-American Congress on Critical Care Medicine, Mexico City, September 1979. Amsterdam: Exerpta Medica 1979; 499: 502–511.
9. Raj PP, Forestner J, Watson TD, Morris RE, Jenkins MT. Techniques for fiberoptic laryngoscopy in anesthesia. Anesth Analg 1974;53:708–714.
10. Scheerzer BP. Rehabilitation following severe head trauma: results of a three-year review. Arch Phys Med Rehabil 1986;67:366–374.

48

Coagulation Abnormalities: Bleeding and Thrombosis

Franklin A. Bontempo

Problems in hemostasis frequently arise in critically ill patients and are often complex due to the various effects of sepsis, multiple organ failure, indwelling catheters, implanted devices, and the simultaneous administration of multiple drugs. What follows is a clinical approach to the hemostatic problems frequently encountered in these patients.

BASIC COAGULATION

Three components are necessary for normal clot formation: (*a*) intact vascular wall endothelium, (*b*) a normal clotting cascade, and (*c*) platelets of adequate number and function. Although none of these portions of the clotting system works in isolation, most clotting disorders affect specific parts of one of these three components.

While abnormalities of the vascular wall do result in clinical coagulation disorders, they are rare and not usually of concern in critical care disorders. Therefore, physicians in intensive care settings most often face disorders of the clotting cascade or platelet number or function. Most physicians who are not required to confront coagulation problems on a routine basis are unlikely to be comfortable referring to the clotting cascade when analyzing clinical problems; however, the classical clotting cascade, shown in Figure 48.1, does provide information that is useful at the bedside.

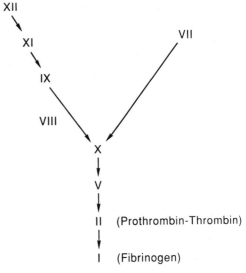

Figure 48.1. Classical clotting cascade.

The left side of the cascade, known as the intrinsic pathway, begins with factor XII and ends with the breakdown of fibrinogen, which is also known as factor I. A more useful way to remember this is to refer to this part of the cascade as the PTT system since the activated partial thromboplastin time (PTT) is a measure of its function.

The right side of the cascade, known as the extrinsic pathway, is activated at factor VII and proceeds also through the clotting of fibrinogen. This part of the cascade may be thought of as the PT system since the

805

prothrombin time (PT) is a measure of its function.

Notice should be taken that the portion of the cascade from factor X through fibrinogen is common to both pathways and is referred to as the common pathway. Additional clinical insights are gained by the knowledge that factor VII is only in the PT pathway and factors XII, XI, IX, and VIII are only in the PTT pathway. Consequently, anything that decreases the level of one of the clotting factors beneath a critical value or inhibits one of the steps in the cascade will slow the corresponding pathway or pathways and therefore prolong the PT and/or the PTT depending on whether the factor or step involved is in the extrinsic pathway (PT prolonged), intrinsic pathway (PTT prolonged), or common pathway (PT and PTT prolonged). A second way for prolongation of the PT and PTT to occur is if two factors, one in each arm of the cascade above the common pathway, are similarly affected.

Platelets also are involved in a complicated biochemical reaction sequence that causes platelet adhesion, aggregation, and plug formation to occur in association with the clotting cascade and the vascular endothelium. Receptors for several of the clotting factors are found on the surface of platelets; von Willebrand factor, produced in vascular endothelial cells, is important for platelet adhesion, and fibrinogen is necessary to form a stable platelet plug. Despite this, most platelet problems in critical care are due to thrombocytopenia, and platelet dysfunction is a much less frequent problem. Therefore, for evaluation of platelet problems a simple platelet count is the most useful test. For platelet function abnormalities, platelet adhesion and platelet aggregation tests can be obtained, but a template bleeding time in our experience, despite recent statements questioning its validity, still provides useful information when applied in appropriate clinical settings and if done by trained personnel.

APPROACH TO BLEEDING

General

When bleeding occurs, a PT, PTT, and platelet count usually are obtained as an initial workup. Just as important is an evaluation of the patient's clinical situation and history to avoid requesting unnecessary, and more costly, sophisticated clotting tests. Obviously if the patient has had recent surgery or trauma, anatomic bleeding must be considered. In some cases other structural lesions may also be bleeding, such as an ulcer or tumor, and need to be considered before assuming that a coagulopathy is present. When a history is taken, asking a patient or the family general questions concerning any past bleeding problems will usually be fruitless. Specific questions concerning intraoperative or postoperative bleeding with special attention to dental extractions and tonsillectomy are much more helpful and may result in positive findings when patients have previously denied bleeding problems. A history of menorrhagia or easy bruising may also be helpful although many persons report a history of these problems without having a coagulation defect.

Clotting Factor Analysis

In analyzing PT and PTT results, most patients' problems fit into categories that can easily be recognized with a basic understanding of the coagulation cascade as outlined above.

Causes of a prolonged PT only are:

1. Early Vitamin K deficiency
2. Recent Coumadin initiation
3. Mild liver disease
4. Congenital deficiency of factor VII (rare)

Finding the PT to be prolonged and the PTT to be normal points to a deficiency of factor VII since it is the only factor in the PT system not in the PTT system. Vitamin K-dependent factor VII has a half-life of only about 6 hr and in critically ill patients frequently reaches low levels rapidly when there has been poor oral intake, there are antibiotics destroying vitamin K-producing bowel flora, and there has been no parenteral administration of vitamin K.

When Coumadin has been started, the factor VII tends to be the first factor level to fall and therefore may cause only a PT prolongation until the other vitamin K-dependent factors II, IX, and X are depressed. At that point the PTT will also be prolonged since the latter factors are in the

PTT system. Thus despite the fact that the PT is used to monitor Coumadin therapy, the additional finding of a long PTT does not by itself indicate that a coagulopathy is present. Early liver disease may prolong the PT, but in liver disease of any severity a loss of factor V production should soon prolong the PTT as well.

Congenital deficiency of factor VII is a rare disorder, which is included to make the point that when only factor VII is absent, the PT is long and the PTT should be normal.

Causes of a prolonged PTT only are:

1. Blocking inhibitor
    a. Lupus anticoagulant type
    b. Acquired anti-factor VIII antibody
2. Heparin therapy
3. von Willebrand's disease
4. Hemophilia A or B
5. Deficiency of factors XI or XII (rare)

Of interest on the above list is that only two of the disorders are common and two of them are almost never associated with bleeding.

One of the most common problems is the blocking inhibitor of the lupus type, popularly referred to as a lupus anticoagulant. The latter name is a misnomer since most patients who have lupus do not have a lupus anticoagulant, most patients with lupus anticoagulants do not have lupus, and lupus anticoagulants are almost never associated with bleeding. Paradoxically, they are associated with thrombosis (10). Performing a PTT on a mixture of patient and normal plasma with failure of the PTT to correct is how the diagnosis is usually made although a host of other tests such as the tissue thromboplastin inhibition index (TTI), dilute Russell viper venom (dRVV) time and mix, platelet neutralization procedure, antiphospholipid antibody, anticardiolipin antibody, and depressed levels of other clotting factor levels are also used to confirm the diagnosis.

The current understanding of the defect in a lupus anticoagulant is an antiphospholipid antibody (13) which interferes with the clotting cascade at the sites where phospholipid is required, most prominent in the PTT system, thereby usually prolonging the PTT rather than the PT. Rare cases of bleeding with a lupus anticoagulant have been described when factor II levels are low but the experience in our laboratory where at least three lupus anticoagulants are seen per week and fewer than five have caused bleeding in over 9 years indicates how common this entity is and how infrequently bleeding occurs. Because of their association with thrombosis, lupus anticoagulants will be discussed further below.

Of greater clinical concern under blocking inhibitors is the acquired anti-factor VIII antibody, which is an autoantibody against the patient's own factor VIII molecule. These antibodies usually develop in elderly patients or in patients with autoimmune disorders and essentially cause an acquired form of factor VIII deficiency, which can lead to life-threatening bleeding. Both males and females are affected, which is in contrast to congenital factor VIII deficiency (hemophilia A) in which usually only males are affected. Acquired factor VIII inhibitors usually require treatment with intravenous γ-globulin, clotting factor concentrates, or immunosuppressive agents.

Again, factor VIII is located in the PTT pathway only and a deficiency of this factor does not prolong the PT. A further example of this is shown in patients with von Willebrand's disease (11), the most common congential coagulation defect, where the carrier portion of the factor VIII molecule is deficient or defective causing the functional part of the molecule to be degraded more rapidly, lowering the factor VIII level less severely than in hemophilia A but not prolonging the PT.

Deficiencies of factors IX (hemophilia B, Christmas disease), XI, or XII also cause an isolated prolongation of the PTT since they too are located in the PTT pathway only. Of note, however, despite frequently causing a markedly long PTT, factor XII deficiency is not associated with a bleeding disorder but paradoxically with thrombosis.

Lastly, heparin is a frequent cause of a long PTT without a prolongation of the PT. The mechanism for the action of heparin is to enhance the inactivation of thrombin (factor II) and inhibit factor X. These actions should cause a prolongation of the PT since factors II and X are in the common pathway; in practice, however, a long PT is rarely encountered.

Causes of prolonged PT and PTT are:

1. Liver disease
2. Disseminated intravascular coagulation
3. Renal disease
4. Coumadin
5. Primary fibrinolysis
6. Congenital deficiencies of factors I, II, V, or X (rare)

In analyzing the causes of a prolonged PT and PTT, one would expect to find that diseases that affect the common pathway clotting factors would primarily be responsible. The above list is largely in accord with that premise.

The liver plays a central role in hemostasis since it is the site of synthesis of most of the clotting factors; and diseases of the liver usually lower levels of multiple clotting factors (8). Early in liver disease, factor V, which has a half-life of about 12 hr and is not vitamin K dependent, is frequently low thereby prolonging the PT and PTT. While an isolated prolongation of the PT could occur in very mild or early liver disease from the lowering of only factor VII, most patients with liver disease have depressed levels of both factors V and VII resulting in a prolongation of the PT and PTT. Moreover, in a patient with only factor VII depressed and a normal PTT, vitamin K deficiency is probably more likely to be present than liver disease and replacement of vitamin K may be beneficial. Alternatively, if both factors V and VII are low and PT and PTT are abnormal, liver disease is more likely and a good response to vitamin K therapy should not be anticipated.

Disseminated intravascular coagulation (DIC), which causes the inappropriate activation of clotting, with resultant deposition of fibrin and consumption of platelets and numerous clotting factors (12), is probably the second most frequent cause of a long PT and PTT.

Clinical settings for DIC are:

1. Sepsis, especially meningococcemia
2. Surgery
3. Obstetric complications
4. Neoplasia, especially acute promyelocytic leukemia
5. Liver disease

6. LeVeen shunt
7. Snakebite

Diagnostic criteria also include fibrin split products, schistocytes on peripheral smear, and to a lesser degree the fibrinogen level, which as an acute phase reactant is more often normal than frequently presumed, possibly due to high pre-DIC levels.

Renal disease also causes a prolonged PT and PTT but for unclear reasons. Clotting factor levels are not always depressed but the abnormalities of the plasma milieu in these patients may lead to poor clotting function, which may be amenable to dialysis.

Coumadin after the initial period of therapy should normally prolong both PT and PTT due to later inactivation of the longer-lived factors II, IX, and X. Often downward dose adjustments are made in this period as the overall anticoagulant effect is increased.

Primary fibrinolysis is a relatively rare disorder that may cause explosive hemorrhage due to the destruction of factor V, factor VIII, fibrin, and sometimes fibrinogen through the unchecked actions of plasmin and plasminogen activators and the anticoagulant effects of fibrin degradation products.

Clinical settings for primary fibrinolysis are:

1. Urinary tract surgery or disease
2. Liver trauma or surgery
3. Cardiac bypass
4. Oral cavity trauma or surgery

If uncontrolled bleeding occurs due to primary fibrinolysis, consideration should be given to the use of the antifibrinolytic agents ϵ-aminocaproic acid (Amicar) or tranexamic acid. Extreme caution must be taken, however, to ensure that an underlying disorder such as DIC is not present, which could be worsened by the prothrombotic effect of these drugs.

Congenital deficiencies of common pathway factors are rare disorders but are listed as causes of a prolonged PT and PTT for completeness.

Platelets

Platelet disorders cause bleeding due to either low platelet number or poor platelet function. Disorders of either may be congenital or acquired. Congenital thrombocytopenias are very rare and not usually germane to a critical care discussion. Acquired thrombocytopenia is one of the most frequently faced problems in critical care settings.

Causes of thrombocytopenia are:

1. Dilution effect from massive RBC transfusion without platelets
2. DIC
3. Sepsis
4. Liver disease
5. Heparin-induced thrombocytopenia
6. Drug-induced thrombocytopenia
7. Primary autoimmune idiopathic thrombocytopenic purpura
8. Secondary to known autoimmune disorder
9. Thrombotic thrombocytopenic purpura
10. Hemolytic-uremic syndrome
11. Allograft rejection
12. Infiltrative diseases of bone marrow
13. Radiation
14. Direct marrow toxins including alcohol
15. Prosthetic cardiac valves
16. Pregnancy
17. Posttransfusion purpura
18. Neonatal alloimmune thrombocytopenic purpura

The differential in the list above covers most of the causes of thrombocytopenia in critical care patients. In general, the pathophysiologic basis of thrombocytopenia is either increased peripheral destruction of platelets or decreased bone marrow production with the former mechanism accounting for the majority of cases.

Exceptions to the above are the dilutional effect from massive transfusion, where neither mechanism is the cause, and liver disease, where splenic sequestration plays a role in addition to a production defect. DIC has associated thrombocytopenia with such high frequency (96%) (12) that its absence makes the diagnosis extremely doubtful. In addition, sepsis without DIC can cause thrombocytopenia and is well documented (14).

The statement is often made that essentially any drug can cause thrombocytopenia. While this is probably true, in critical care settings, certain drugs deserve special mention. Those that may be frequent offenders in a search for causes of thrombocytopenia include ranitidine, quinidine, heroin, zidovudine (AZT), trimethoprim-sulfamethoxazole, procainamide, gold salts, a variety of chemotherapeutic agents, and heparin.

Heparin-induced thrombocytopenia (5, 6) is given a separate listing due to its unique pathophysiology, which includes antibody mediation and thrombosis. This process may cause thrombocytopenia in as many as 5% of patients receiving heparin in the first 5–7 days after the initiation of therapy and even the small amounts of heparin used to flush indwelling intravenous or arterial lines or the heparin given with dialysis may trigger it. Most reports of heparin-induced thrombocytopenia have been with the use of beef heparin rather than porcine heparin. Occasionally, switching from one type of heparin to another may be beneficial but frequently the need to stop heparin therapy leads to difficult management decisions in an attempt to anticoagulate the patient for the original thrombotic condition. Some laboratories can perform testing of platelets to confirm the presence of heparin-induced thrombocytopenia although a sensitive and specific test has not come into widespread use.

Autoimmune thrombocytopenia may be subdivided into primary and secondary forms. The primary form is still usually referred to as idiopathic thrombocytopenic purpura (ITP) and is characterized by low platelet counts and increased megakaryocytes in the bone marrow without known cause (1). The secondary form is similar except that a known process such as systemic lupus erythematosus, rheumatoid arthritis, lymphoma, chronic lymphocytic leukemia, or acquired immune deficiency syndrome is present. Thrombotic thrombocytopenic purpura (TTP) and hemolytic-uremic syndrome (HUS) are similar disorders that may represent clinical spectra of the same process. Various combinations of fever, neurologic and renal dysfunction, microangiopathic hemolytic anemia, and thrombocytopenia occur due to microvascular thrombosis. HUS has been associated with the remote use of the chemotherapeutic drug mitomycin C. Plasmapheresis has been the mainstay of treatment for both of these disorders although less success has been noted with HUS. Rejection of renal and hepatic allografts has also been associated with thrombocytopenia although the mechanism is not clear. In settings where large numbers of transplants are performed, this possibility should be considered. Infiltrative diseases of the bone marrow including tuberculosis, lymphoma, or metastatic carcinoma may be an unsuspected cause of thrombocytopenia, which can be diagnosed by bone marrow biopsy. Some patients who have undergone radiotherapy to bone marrow-producing areas of the body will frequently have permanently depressed platelet counts due to reduced bone marrow function and fibrosis. In addition, a variety of chemical agents may be marrow toxins. Ethanol is a commonly used substance that exerts a direct marrow toxic effect in large doses and is separate from its effects on the liver that also lead to thrombocytopenia.

Prosthetic cardiac valves, especially those used in earlier years, cause thrombocytopenia by direct damage to platelets in the circulation.

Women during pregnancy or the peripartum period frequently become thrombocytopenic, probably for a variety of reasons. In some cases, the thrombocytopenia resolves shortly after delivery, but in others it is associated with complicated pregnancies, recurs with future deliveries and requires treatment similar to that for TTP.

A final cause of adult thrombocytopenia is posttransfusion purpura where sudden profound thrombocytopenia is seen about 1 week after platelet transfusion, usually in patients whose platelet membranes lack certain antigens. These patients usually have developed antibodies in their plasma against these platelet membrane antigens from prior platelet transfusion; later when random donor platelets are infused, destruction of their own platelets is seen, due to an unclear mechanism, causing thrombocytopenia. About 90% of the patients with this diagnosis have been found to be negative for the PLA1 antigen when platelet typing is performed. This is significant since about 98% of the general population have platelets that are positive for this antigen. Thus, in settings where a large number of patients are transfused with multiple units of platelets, consideration of this as a cause of thrombocytopenia

may be reasonable. Removal of the antibody with plasmapheresis is most often effective. Similar in pathophysiology is the thrombocytopenia in newborn infants, frequently but not exclusively in the firstborn, where lack of a platelet membrane antigen, again usually PLA1, on the mother's platelets leads to the development of antibodies that destroy the infant's platelets soon after delivery. If bleeding occurs, the standard treatment is to phlebotomize the mother and transfuse her washed and irradiated platelets (to avoid graft versus host disease) into the infant. Conceptually, this is similar to the incompatibility seen with Rh disease except that here the infant's platelets are the target rather than the red blood cells.

Congenital causes of platelet dysfunction other than von Willebrand's disease are very rare and need not be considered here. Again, however, acquired disorders are very common in critical care situations.

Causes of platelet dysfunction are:

1. Aspirin
2. Nonsteroidal antiinflammatory drugs
3. β-Lactam antibiotics
4. Dipyridamole
5. L-asparaginase
6. Dextran
7. Alcohol
8. Heparin
9. Renal failure
10. Liver disease
11. Cardiopulmonary bypass
12. Myeloproliferative disorders
13. von Willebrand's disease

Commonly used drugs which may cause platelet dysfunction are listed above. Importantly, aspirin and nonsteroidal antiinflammatory drug (NSAID) use may be present but, unless specifically sought, may go undetected. In addition, the aspirin defect is usually permanent and lasts for the life of the platelet (about 10 days) whereas the NSAID defect is reversible if the drug is stopped for several days. Low molecular weight dextran is occasionally used for its antiplatelet effect when heparin-induced thrombocytopenia is present. Again, while alcohol is marrow toxic, it also causes platelet dysfunction as does heparin in addition to its anticoagulant effect (4).

Renal disease, as is well known, causes

a long bleeding time, which may respond to D-amino-D-arginine vasopressin (desmopressin, DDAVP) which is a vasopressin analog. The platelet defects in liver disease, after cardiopulmonary bypass, in myeloproliferative disorders (9) such as polycythemia vera or essential thrombocytosis, or in von Willebrand's disease also often may respond to DDAVP at the standard dose of 0.3 µg/kg i.v., usually given in 50 ml of normal saline over 30 min.

APPROACH TO THROMBOSIS

General

An expanded view of the coagulation cascade, as shown in Figure 48.2, is necessary to appreciate the newer concepts in thrombosis. Note that the *left side* of the diagram is essentially the fibrinolytic system, which has plasminogen as its major component. A useful view is that the prothrombotic classical cascade exists in balance with the antithrombotic fibrinolytic system. There-

fore, anything that enhances the clotting cascade or inhibits the fibrinolytic system promotes thrombosis. Alternatively, anything enhancing the fibrinolytic system or inhibiting the clotting cascade promotes bleeding.

Modulating the balance between these two systems are true circulating anticoagulants such as antithrombin III and the vitamin K-dependent protein C system, which includes protein S as its activator (2, 3). Antithrombin III largely acts through inactivation of thrombin, also known as the active form of factor II, but also has lesser actions against other factors including the inhibition of factor X. Protein C, with the help of protein S activation, inhibits the clotting cascade by inactivating factors V and VIII and probably enhances fibrinolysis by inhibiting plasminogen activator inhibitor as shown in the diagram, thereby stimulating fibrinolysis. Other recently described proteins are also involved but they are presently of lesser clinical significance.

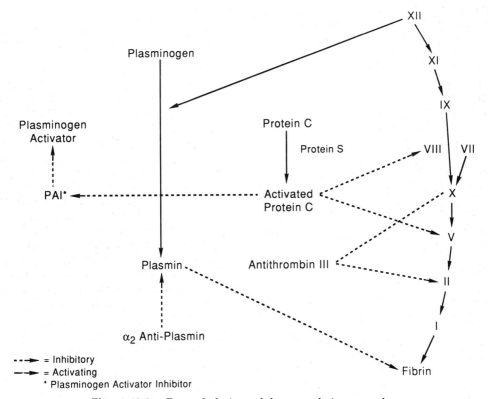

Figure 48.2. Expanded view of the coagulation cascade.

Thrombosis is a common clinical problem for which an underlying cause is found in only a small percentage of cases. However, certain clinical findings should prompt further laboratory investigation, and other predisposing conditions should prompt prophylactic measures to be undertaken.

Primary Thrombotic Disorders

Primary thrombotic disorders are in general rare congenital abnormalities. In critical care settings the three listed below are probably of greatest interest.

Congenital causes of thrombosis are:

1. Antithrombin III deficiency
2. Protein C deficiency
3. Protein S deficiency

Patients with these disorders tend to have a family history of thrombosis, thromboses at unusual sites, recurrent thrombosis, and a personal history of thromboses at an early age. Periods of immobilization after trauma or surgery, obesity, smoking, or the use of oral contraceptives may cause previously asymptomatic patients to develop thromboses, especially if they are heterozygotic for one of the above disorders.

Antithrombin III deficiency is the deficiency that has had a readily available assay in existence for the longest period. Occasionally, patients with this disorder are discovered after having a thrombotic event and being found to be difficult to anticoagulate with heparin since the presence of antithrombin III is necessary for the action of heparin against thrombin. A pooled concentrate of antithrombin III has been released recently for use in patients with congenital antithrombin III deficiency who are undergoing surgery or who are pregnant. The use of this concentrate should obviate the need for heparin treatment in these settings.

Patients with a homozygous deficiency of protein C usually die of diffuse thrombosis soon after birth; therefore, the usual clinical problem encountered is a heterozygously deficient patient who develops a thrombosis spontaneously at a young age or during a period of immobilization such as after surgery or trauma.

Because protein C is vitamin K dependent, as are clotting factors II, VII, IX, and X, when these patients are initially placed on Coumadin, the gap between the levels of protein C and factor VII may actually widen leaving the patient paradoxically hypercoagulable. This usually occurs during the first 2–3 days of Coumadin therapy and may result in an area of necrosis of the skin (7), which initially appears to be a bruise but progressively becomes necrotic. The presumed mechanism is thrombosis of an arteriole supplying the overlying skin, although pathologically this is not always supportable; the breast, buttocks, and extremities are the most frequently reported sites of occurrence.

Protein S is also vitamin K dependent but does not require activation. It serves as a catalyst for protein C activation and, when deficient, causes a hypercoagulable state clinically similar to protein C deficiency. In addition, Coumadin necrosis of the skin has also been recently described in patients with a deficiency of protein S.

In an attempt to avoid the possibility of skin necrosis, keeping the patient fully heparinized until the patient has reached a stable dose of Coumadin is usually recommended. This is based on the concept of allowing inactivation of all four of the vitamin K-dependent clotting factors before stopping heparin, although following this course does not insure that Coumadin necrosis will be avoided. In addition, the occurrence of this phenomenon does not preclude the future use of Coumadin, as skin necrosis occurs sporadically, even in the same patient, and may depend on a variety of factors at the time oral anticoagulation is begun.

Secondary Thrombotic Disorders

Most patients with definable causes of thrombosis have an acquired abnormality or an underlying condition that predisposes them to clot formation secondarily.

Acquired or secondary causes of thrombosis are:

1. Lupus anticoagulant
2. Nephrotic syndrome

3. Homocystinuria (rare)
4. Sickle cell anemia
5. Paroxysmal nocturnal hemoglobinuria
6. Myeloproliferative disorders
7. Heparin-induced thrombocytopenia
8. Malignancy
9. Factor IX concentrate therapy
10. Oral contraceptives
11. Stasis
12. Artificial surfaces
13. Pregnancy
14. Vasculitis
15. DIC

As mentioned above, a lupus anticoagulant frequently causes a long PTT but paradoxically is associated with a thrombotic tendency. The incidence of thrombosis in patients with lupus anticoagulants is difficult to specify but probably ranges from 5 to 20% depending upon how the lupus anticoagulant is defined. A complicating factor is that many lupus anticoagulants occur in the elderly who are at an inherently higher risk for thrombosis, making a causative differentiation difficult.

In addition, while numerous drugs, listed below, have been clearly associated with lupus anticoagulants, many reports indicate that the drug-induced type are not associated with thrombosis.

Drugs commonly associated with lupus anticoagulants are:

1. Procainamide
2. Hydralazine
3. Isoniazid
4. Diphenylhydantoin
5. Phenothiazines
6. Haloperidol
7. Quinidine

Lupus anticoagulants with thrombosis are sometimes considered part of an antiphospholipid antibody syndrome with recurrent clot formation at numerous sites, which are largely refractory to therapy and lead to progressive deterioration and even death. As testing for lupus anticoagulants has become more widely available, the association of these inhibitors, especially with strokes and recurrent first-trimester miscarriages, has been well documented. With time, the full extent of their morbidity will be recognized.

Nephrotic syndrome has been shown to predispose to venous thrombosis by causing the loss of antithrombin III in the urine and has been especially linked to renal vein thrombosis.

Homocystinuria is a rare congenital disorder that is unusual in causing both arterial and venous thrombosis, probably due to abnormalities in the vessel wall. Screening tests for this disorder are presently available and should be considered in young adults, especially with recurrent arterial thromboses.

Patients with sickle cell anemia are at increased risk of cerebrovascular accidents, especially those of younger ages. Other thrombotic events may also be seen.

Paroxysmal nocturnal hemoglobinuria is associated with intraabdominal thrombosis and especially Budd-Chiari syndrome. The mechanism for the thrombotic tendency is unclear. Myeloproliferative disorders are associated with thrombosis as well as with bleeding with a particular prevalence for thrombosis in polycythemia vera (9). Of special interest, some recent reports have indicated that seemingly idiopathic Budd-Chiari syndrome may be due more often than previously thought to undiagnosed myeloproliferative disorders.

Heparin-induced thrombocytopenia is discussed in the section on thrombocytopenia but, again, is associated with thrombosis rather than bleeding.

Underlying malignancy is always a consideration when a patient presents with the new onset of thrombosis. Migratory thrombophlebitis (Trousseau's syndrome) is the classic description of the thrombosis seen with a variety of malignancies, and mucinous adenocarcinoma is the cell type most often linked clinically with a hypercoagulable state. Clinical judgment must be exercised to determine when an exhaustive search for malignancy should be undertaken.

Factor IX concentrate, usually used for patients with hemophilia B or hemophilia A with an antibody to factor VIII, is associated with thrombosis, especially when used for extended periods or in high doses. This is in contrast to factor VIII where no such association is reported. Newer factor IX concentrated products currently being licensed appear to be free of this complication, but further evaluation in a large number of patients will be necessary before this is certain.

Newer oral contraceptives, despite a lowering of the amount of estrogen per dose, continue to be associated with a reduced but increased risk of thrombosis.

Numerous studies have documented the increased risk of thrombosis in patients who have static blood flow while immobilized, even those with no underlying predisposition to hypercoagulability. In patients in intensive care settings who have no bleeding tendency, the use of prophylactic low dose heparin, especially in those over the age of 40 with malignancy, cerebral infarcts, or congestive heart failure, can be supported but is not always customary.

Artificial surfaces such as indwelling catheters, intraaortic balloon pumps, or artificial cardiac devices are clearly a cause of thrombogenicity, and discontinuation needs to be considered when thrombosis has occurred.

Pregnancy is associated with an increased risk of thrombosis, although whether this is due to stasis in the lower body to true hypercoagulability is not entirely clear. While clotting factor levels and red blood cell mass are increased during pregnancy, other changes may mediate these physiologic changes. Vasculitides are associated with thromboses, possibly due to activation of clotting after endothelial cell damage occurs. Therapy for the vasculitis may prevent thrombosis in occasional patients with a wide variety of disorders in which vascular wall damage is a feature.

DIC, which is usually thought of as a bleeding disorder despite its pathophysiology, is much less often associated with large vessel thrombosis. This may respond to the therapy for the underlying disorder, although the recommendation for the use of heparin is logically stronger.

References

1. Burns TR, Saleem A. Idiopathic thrombocytopenic purpura. Am J Med 1983;75:1001–1007.
2. Clouse LH, Comp PC. The regulation of hemostasis: the protein C system. N Engl J Med 1986;314:1298–1304.
3. Esmon CT. Protein C: biochemistry, physiology, and clinical implications. Blood 1983;62:1155–1158.
4. George JN, Shattil SJ. The clinical importance of acquired abnormalities of platelet function. N Engl J Med 1991;324:27–29.
5. Kelton JB. Heparin-induced thrombocytopenia. Haemostasis 1986;16:173–186.
6. Kelton JG, Sheridan D, et al. Heparin-induced thrombocytopenia: laboratory studies. Blood 1988;72:925–930.
7. McGehee WG, et al. Coumadin necrosis associated with hereditary protein C deficiency. Ann Intern Med 1984;100:59–60.
8. Ratnoff OD. Disordered hemostasis in hepatic disease. In: Shiff L. Diseases of the Liver. 6th ed. Philadelphia: JB Lippincott, 1987:187–207.
9. Schafer AI. Bleeding and thrombosis in the myeloproliferative disorders. Blood 1984;64:1–12.
10. Schafer AL. The hypercoagulable states. Ann Intern Med 1985;102:814–828.
11. Smith P. von Willebrands pathophysiology, diagnosis and treatment. In: Hilgartner M, Pochedly C, eds. Hemophilia in the Child and Adult. New York: Raven Press, 1989:275–295.
12. Spero JA, Lewis JH, Hasiba U. Disseminated intravascular coagulation: findings in 346 patients. Thromb Haemost 1980;1:28–33.
13. Triplett DA, Brandt JT, Musgrave KA, Orr CA. The relationship between lupus anticoagulants and antibodies to phospholipids. JAMA 1988;259:550–564.
14. Wilson JJ, Neame PB, Kelton JG. Infection-induced thrombocytopenia. Semin Thromb Hemostasis 1982;8:217–233.

49

General Hematology and Transfusion

Franklin A. Bontempo

A wide variety of general hematologic problems occurs in eutrophils, which normally include mostly segmented and band forms and make up the large majority of granulocytes, usually circulating in the peripheral blood for only about 6 hr. A second marginal pool of noncirculating neutrophils, which is about equal in size to the circulating pool and is available to the circulation under specific stimuli such as stress or inflammation, adheres to the walls of small vessels. This may account for rapid shifts in circulating neutrophil count.

Eosinophils and basophils have life spans in the peripheral blood similar to neutrophils but their kinetics are less well understood.

Monocytes circulate for approximately 3 or 4 days and lymphocytes for from several hours to as long as 5 years. In general, monocytes and lymphocytes are the cells that mediate subacute or chronic inflammation.

In addition, lymphocytes are subclassified into different types, the largest numbers of which are T and B cells. T cells are mediators of delayed hypersensitivity and cell-mediated cytotoxicity and produce lymphokines, which regulate B cells. B cells are responsible for humoral immunity and the production of immunoglobulins. Small numbers of other lymphocyte cell types are present in peripheral blood and this may account for the wide variation in lymphocyte life span. In normal individuals the largest proportion of circulating lymphocytes are T cells, up to 75%, while approximately 25% are B cells. Some reports indicate that older patients have a smaller percentage of circulating T cells.

WHITE BLOOD CELLS

Clinical Approach to White Blood Cell Abnormalities

Obviously, to determine the presence of an abnormality of white blood cells, an analysis of the white blood cell count and differential count must be done, preferably with visualization of the peripheral smear.

While elevated or depressed levels of any of the white blood cell types may be considered an abnormality, the most frequent problems encountered in critical care are neutrophilia, neutropenia, and eosinophilia.

Causes of neutrophilia are:

1. Infection
2. Inflammation
3. Surgery
4. Stress
5. Smoking
6. Tumors
7. Chronic myelogenous leukemia
8. Glucocorticoids
9. Granulocyte colony stimulating factor
10. Lithium

Neutrophilia, while commonly encountered in the conditions listed above, rarely causes clinical symptoms. Infection and physical, emotional, or surgical stress may acutely lead to neutrophilia, but unless the white blood count is exceedingly high to the degree most often seen in chronic myelogenous leukemia, no therapy for the white count itself is necessary. In the case of neurologic compromise from the high white count in chronic myelogenous leukemia, leukapheresis for rapid decrease in the white count or treatment with hydroxyurea may be necessary.

In addition, neutrophilia often occurs in patients after administration of glucocorticoids, probably due to the release of granulocytes from the bone marrow and decreased flow of neutrophils into tissues. This effect may be responsible for as much as a doubling of the neutrophil count. Granulocyte colony stimulating factor may also lead to an elevated neutrophil count several days after its administration for neutropenia. Interestingly, patients receiving chronic lithium treatment for psychiatric disorders may have neutrophilia due to increases in levels of colony stimulating factor (2).

Causes of neutropenia are:

1. Drug effects
2. Chemotherapy
3. Bacterial infections
4. Viral infections
5. Hypersplenism
6. Autoimmune disorders
7. Bone marrow infiltration

Neutropenia is extremely common in acute care settings and frequently requires careful analysis and clinical intervention to prevent untoward infectious sequelae. The most common causes of neutropenia are listed above. Neutropenia as an unexpected side effect of drug treatment is often a vexing problem, which requires cessation of a series of drugs to determine the cause. While the potential list of drugs causing neutropenia is long, certain ones deserve special mention in critical care and are listed below.

Commonly used drugs causing neutropenia are:

1. Trimethoprim-sulfamethoxazole
2. Cimetidine
3. Ranitidine
4. Piperacillin
5. Captopril
6. Enalopril
7. Hydralazine
8. Procainamide
9. Quinidine
10. Allopurinol
11. Ganciclovir
12. Zidovudine

When one of these drugs is being used in a patient who becomes neutropenic, a judgment must be made regarding the relative necessity of that drug and whether another drug can be substituted for it compared to the risk from the degree of neutropenia. If more than one suspected drug is being used, further judgment must be used as to which of them should be stopped initially to observe whether the neutropenia resolves, keeping in mind that if multiple drugs are discontinued and the neutrophil count rises, the offending drug will not be specifically identified.

Usually, cessation of a drug for at least 1 week is helpful to determine if that drug has caused the neutropenia. When more than one drug has been discontinued and the neutropenia resolves, one of the drugs may be restarted to observe its effect if its use is still deemed necessary.

While this process may seem cumbersome, specific antineutrophil antibody assays are not available for general clinical use, making this approach necessary.

In the above list, chemotherapeutic agents are listed separately due to the neutropenia often occurring after they have been discontinued and because it is frequently an expected effect of their use.

Bacterial infections may cause neutropenia by increasing neutrophil utilization at the site of infection. Both bacterial and virus infections may cause increased neutrophil adherence to endothelial cells or bone marrow suppression, resulting in decreased neutrophil counts. Infections with cytomegalovirus and hepatitis B, Epstein-Barr, and human immunodeficiency viruses may act additionally by directly infecting neutrophils or neutrophil precursors. Hypersplenism in patients with liver disease and portal hypertension and a wide variety of autoimmune disorders are common causes of mildly depressed neutrophil counts. Other causes of neutropenia may make the neutropenia associated with these disorders severe enough to become clinically significant.

Infiltration of the bone marrow by metastatic tumor, lymphoma, posttransplant lymphoproliferative disease, unrecognized leukemia, or granulomas may be a cause of neutropenia. Diagnosis usually requires bone marrow aspiration and biopsy, which should be performed when neutropenia is unexplained. Eosinophilia is commonly encountered in hospitalized patients. While many conditions may be causative, parasitic diseases, allergic disorders, and hypersensitivity reactions to drugs are probably the most frequently found reasons for eosinophilia to be present in the critical care setting with treatment consisting of that for the underlying disorder or cessation of an offending drug.

RED BLOOD CELLS

General

The primary function of red blood cells is the delivery of oxygen to tissues. Red cells have a life expectancy approximately 120 days in the circulation and red cell production is regulated by the effects of erythropoietin, a humoral substance produced by the kidney.

The interior of red cells contains hemoglobin, which is responsible for oxygen transport as well as enzymes for the metabolism of glucose, glycogen, and carbon dioxide. The red cell membrane is a lipid bilayer normally in the shape of a deformable biconcave disc, characteristics which aid in oxygen transport. Normal red cell destruction occurs in the reticuloendothelial cells of the spleen, although in conditions with increased rates of destruction, reticuloendothelial cells in the liver and bone marrow also play a role.

Clinical Approach to Red Blood Cell Abnormalities

Abnormalities of the hematocrit are the most common problems of red cells in critical care. While anemia is clearly more frequently encountered, occasional patients have elevations in hematocrit due to conditions listed below.

Causes of elevated hematocrit are:

1. Dehydration
2. Chronic pulmonary disease
3. High altitude polycythemia
4. Cyanotic heart disease
5. Chronic carbon monoxide poisoning
6. Polycythemia vera
7. Abnormal hemoglobins
8. Erythropoietin-producing tumor
9. Autotransfusion

Dehydration in the critically ill is a frequent cause of a mild elevation of hematocrit, which is easily correctible.

Because of tissue hypoxia, conditions such as chronic pulmonary disease, cyanotic heart disease, life at high altitudes with low atmospheric pressure, and chronic carbon monoxide poisoning all may lead to an increased hematocrit. Smoking is related to chronically elevated blood levels of carbon monoxide, as well as chronic pulmonary disease, and is therefore associated with an elevated hematocrit.

Polycythemia vera is the classic hematologic disease associated with an increase in red cell mass but is relatively rare and is often associated with an increase in white cells and platelets as well as red blood cells. Other rare hematologic causes of an increased hematocrit include certain abnormal hemoglobins and erythropoietin-producing tumors.

Autotransfusion or "blood doping" by athletes may also be an unrecognized cause of an increased hematocrit in the appropriate setting.

Causes of anemia are:

1. Blood loss
2. Decreased red cell production
3. Increased red cell destruction

When approaching a patient with a low hematocrit in a critical care situation, the general approach outlined above is useful.

Consideration should always be given to the possibility that blood loss may be due not only to bleeding from the gastrointestinal or genitourinary tracts, or from trauma, surgical, or indwelling catheter sites, but also from the effects of repeated phlebotomy, especially in patients in intensive care units. After the exclusion of blood loss, abnormalities of red cell production or destruction should be considered.

Causes of decreased red cell production are:

1. Nutritional deficiency
2. Iron deficiency
3. Alcoholism
4. Anemia of chronic disease
5. Chronic renal failure
6. Lead poisoning
7. Bone marrow infiltration

8. Myelodysplastic anemia
9. Virus-induced red cell aplasia
10. Sideroblastic anemia

Poor oral intake may cause critical care patients to become deficient in vitamin B_{12}, folic acid, or other vitamins. Women of childbearing age who have had recent pregnancies or regular menstruation are notoriously iron deficient as are other patients with a history of significant recent blood loss. Alcoholism may also contribute to nutritional deficiencies but alcohol itself is a direct bone marrow toxin.

The anemia of chronic disease is a common normochromic normocytic or hypochromic microcytic anemia associated with low serum iron and iron binding capacity, shortened red cell survival, a decreased responsiveness to erythropoietin, increased bone marrow storage iron, and a defect in iron utilization. It is seen in many chronic diseases. Treatment at present is aimed at that for the underlying disease. Patients with chronic renal failure have anemia due to the failure of the kidney to produce sufficient erythropoietin. Many patients are now successfully treated for this type of anemia with injectable recombinant human erythropoietin.

Lead poisoning causes an insidious hypochromic microcytic anemia, which is associated with the ingestion of lead-based paint. Infiltration of the bone marrow with metastatic tumor, lymphoma, or leukemic cells may also cause red cell production to be decreased. The infiltration of plasma cells in multiple myeloma is commonly associated with a significant anemia, as is the myelodysplastic syndrome, which is felt to be a precursor to overt leukemia in older adults.

Pure red cell aplasia has been clearly described in association with parvovirus infections due to infection of bone marrow progenitor cells. This has responded to therapy with intravenous γ-globulin, making a search for this viral agent more fruitful (3,4).

Sideroblastic anemia is another cause of anemia that is often due to specific drugs or alcoholism. It may be responsive to pyridoxine or to cessation of the offending

drug. Bone marrow aspirate is necessary to confirm the diagnosis.

Hemolysis of red cells as a cause of anemia may occur extravascularly due to uptake by macrophages in the reticuloendothelial system or intravascularly with direct discharge of the contents of the red cells into the circulation. While numerous methods exist for classifying hemolytic anemias, none is entirely satisfactory for a discussion here. Certain problems are of specific interest in the critical care setting and are listed below.

Causes of increased red cell destruction are:

1. Transfusion reaction
2. Warm reacting antibodies
3. Cold reacting antibodies
4. Drugs
5. Infectious agents
6. Hypotonicity
7. Elevated inorganic copper
8. Hemodialysis
9. Hypophosphatemia
10. Mechanical trauma to red cells
11. Thermal injury
12. Insect venoms
13. Thrombotic thrombocytopenic purpura
14. Hemolytic uremic syndrome
15. Disseminated intravascular coagulation
16. Unstable hemoglobins
17. Enzyme abnormalities
18. Paroxysmal nocturnal hemoglobinuria

The first three causes of hemolysis listed above are due to immune mechanisms. Transfusion reactions are the classic examples of alloimmune destruction of red cells and are most often due to patient misidentification or an error in the handling of red cell units, often at the bedside (8). In addition, minor transfusion reactions occasionally leading to hemolysis also may occur in patients receiving large numbers of red cell units or ABO-unmatched allografts.

Approximately 20% of patients with chronic lymphocytic leukemia and many patients with systemic lupus erythematosis develop an autoimmune hemolytic anemia that reacts at body temperature. Less commonly, patients may hemolyze from an antibody that acts only at cold temperatures, i.e., below body temperature. This may be seen in cold agglutinin disease and rarely in other conditions. Occasionally, an unrecognized cold antibody will cause hemolysis after collection in blood specimen tubes, where the temperature is below body temperature, and give falsely abnormal laboratory values. This may require keeping the specimen tubes warm until they reach the clinical laboratory.

Drug-induced hemolysis may be either immune or nonimmune. Examples of immune drug-induced hemolysis include that associated with α-methyldopa where the direct antiglobulin (Coomb's) test may be abnormal, the hapten type seen occasionally with large IV doses of penicillin, or the innocent bystander type with quinidine, or sulfa drugs. Nonimmune hemolysis theoretically may occur with nitroprusside in large doses, although the main observed clinical effect is usually methemoglobinemia or cyanide toxicity. The antirejection and immunosuppressive agent FK 506 has also been associated with hemolysis in occasional patients by an unclear mechanism (1).

A number of infectious agents have been reported to be associated with hemolysis. Important among these are *Clostridium perfringens* septicemia, malaria, and bartonellosis, a disease limited to South America. While the mechanisms in the latter two diseases are poorly understood, with *Clostridium perfringens (welchii)* sepsis, the α exotoxin, a lecithinase and one of the many toxins produced by clostridial organisms, appears to mediate the often massive hemolytic response; it is probably most often seen in septic abortions.

Occasionally, red cells lyse when infused through an intravenous line with concomitant 0.45 normal saline because of the flow of water into the red cell due to the osmotic gradient created by the hypotonic fluid. Normal red cell populations begin to lyse in tonic environments slightly above 0.45 normal and the introduction of stored red cells into hypotonic fluid can cause cells to lyse prior to entering the circulation. While red cell transfusions are usually recommended to be administered through a separate intravenous line, if concomitant fluid must be given, normal saline is least likely to cause this problem.

In patients with Wilson's disease or copper sulfate ingestion, elevated levels of inorganic copper have caused hemolysis. In Wilson's disease this usually occurs in severe cases, and attempts to remove the copper with plasmapheresis have been successful.

Hemodialysis may rarely cause hemolysis by a variety of mechanisms including direct destruction in the apparatus, destruction in an arterial fistula, or by dialysis against an errant dialysate.

Debilitated patients with low phosphorus levels or those taking large doses of phosphate binders may develop hemolysis due to low intracellular ATP levels and resultant decreased red cell deformability; the hemolysis may respond to phosphate repletion and cessation of phosphate binders.

Mechanical trauma to red cells from older type prosthetic valves, excessive exercise or field marches, or bongo playing may be responsible for mild hemolysis. Thermal injury may cause lysis of red cells in the area of the thermal injury usually in the first 24 hr after the burn occurs.

Insect bites, usually with the brown recluse spiders *Loxosceles reclusus* or *Loxosceles laeta*, and less commonly with bee and wasp stings may lead to hemolysis. Thrombotic thrombocytopenic purpura, hemolytic uremic syndrome, and disseminated intravascular coagulation are causes of microangiopathic hemolytic anemia and are discussed more thoroughly in the chapter on coagulation.

A large number of rare congenital hemoglobinopathies and intracellular red cell enzyme defects cause hemolysis but these are of more concern for hematologists than for critical care physicians. Paroxysmal nocturnal hemoglobinuria is a condition that causes hemolysis due to the presence of a complement sensitive clone of red cells, which may periodically lyse and lead to hemoglobinuria; patients with paroxysmal nocturnal hemoglobinuria are also predisposed to thrombosis.

In making a diagnosis of a hemolytic state, several tests are almost always indicated and include looking at the peripheral smear for the presence of fragmented red cells, a reticulocyte count to assess enchanced red cell production, and lactic dehydrogenase, haptoglobin, and bilirubin levels. When immune hemolysis is considered a possibility, a direct antiglobulin (Coomb's) test, and determination of antinuclear antibody, and complement levels may be helpful. Patients with paroxysmal nocturnal hemoglobinuria may have a positive acidified-serum lysis (Ham's) test or a sucrose hemolysis test. Other diagnostic tests are indicated for specific conditions.

PRINCIPLES OF TRANSFUSION

There are a number of different blood products currently available for transfusion in the care of critically ill patients. They include:

1. Whole blood
2. Modified whole blood
3. Packed red blood cells
4. Leukocyte-reduced red blood cells
5. Washed red blood cells
6. Fresh frozen plasma
7. Cryoprecipitate
8. Platelets
9. Granulocytes
10. Factor VIII concentrate
11. Factor IX concentrate
12. Antithrombin III concentrate

Whole blood is usually not recommended. It could conceivably be used appropriately in an exsanguinating trauma patient with the coagulopathy of liver disease where oxygen carrying capacity, volume expansion, clotting factor replacement, and platelets were all needed emergently; but as a rule, component therapy for specific indications is superior to the use of whole blood.

Modified whole blood is whole blood with the platelets removed. Some blood banks may supply this product for procedures such as liver transplants, where predictable use of high volumes of red blood cells and fresh frozen plasma occurs frequently enough to warrant its preparation in an attempt to lower the number of patient donor exposures.

Packed red blood cells, the standard product for increasing hematocrit and oxygen carrying capacity, usually come in a volume of approximately 250 ml/unit. Packed cells should not be used for vol-

ume expansion or for mild anemia due to iron or vitamin deficiencies. In addition, the use of erythropoietin may obviate the need for transfusion with this product in some cases.

Leukocyte-reduced and washed red blood cells may be used for repeated allergic and febrile transfusion reactions with regular packed red cells. Leukocyte-reduced red cells are prepared by filtering packed cells to remove white cells, which may be inducing the reaction. Washing red cells, which removes plasma, may be helpful when plasma proteins or antibodies are the cause of reactions such as in hereditary IgA deficiency. Washed red cells are also sometimes used for ABO-mismatched bone marrow transplants after transplantation. Frozen red blood cells are not generally recommended for transfusion reactions, but are reserved for long-term storage of donor units with rare blood types (5).

Units of fresh frozen plasma (FFP) contain, as a practical approximation, 10% of the average adult's total complement of clotting factors in a volume of about 225 ml. As a result, their use should be reserved for patients with known deficiencies of clotting factors; other uses are usually not appropriate (6).

Specifically, FFP should not be used for volume expansion. In bleeding patients, accurate dosing with FFP is approximated by giving 10 ml/kg. This means that most patients will usually require a starting dose of at least 3 or 4 units of FFP with further dosing dependent on the response in prothrombin time and partial thromboplastin time. Cryoprecipitate is prepared by precipitating plasma at cold temperatures. It contains fibrinogen (factor I), factor VIII (including the von Willebrand portion of the molecule), factor XIII, and fibronectin, a glycoprotein that promotes opsonic activity. Cryoprecipitate is an excellent source of concentrated fibrinogen due to its low volume of approximately 15 ml per donor bag, although in some blood banks, multiple donor bags are pooled for more efficient clinical use. In patients with isolated decreased fibrinogen levels, cryoprecipitate should be the product of choice rather than FFP in which the concentration of fibrinogen may be as much as five times lower than cryoprecipitate. Cryoprecipitate is rarely indicated today for patients with hemophilia A (hereditary factor VIII deficiency) in part due to the inability to inactivate the human immunodeficiency virus in this product. It is indicated for patients with von Willebrand's disease who fail to respond to desmopressin or the rare type IIb von Willebrand's disease where desmopressin is contraindicated due to the propensity for platelet aggregation. Cryoprecipitate is also indicated for factor XIII deficiency; in patients with sepsis, burns, and trauma, it will also raise depressed fibronectin levels, but the clinical benefit of this effect is speculative.

Platelets are indicated for the control or prevention of bleeding in patients with abnormalities of platelet number or function. There is general acceptance that platelet transfusion is effective in bleeding patients with platelet counts less than 50,000/ml and for the prevention of spontaneous hemorrhage in nonbleeding patients with platelet counts of less than 10,000/ml.

Stable patients with immune thrombocytopenia, however, may not require repeated platelet transfusions even at levels as low as 10,000/ml. In these patients, 1- or 2-hr postinfusion platelet counts should be performed to determine if any significant elevation in platelet count is obtained. Some patients with immune thrombocytopenia of less than 10,000/ml do obtain a clinical response without significant rise in platelet count, but unless there is active bleeding, the use of repeated transfusion is not usually recommended since the risk of making the patient refractory to platelets is enhanced. In addition, trials of prednisone, intravenous immunoglobulins, or vincristine may be much more beneficial.

The critical platelet count above which platelet transfusion should be deemed inappropriate is controversial. However, a reasonable judgment in this regard depends on whether or not the thrombocytopenia is accompanied by platelet dysfunction due to liver disease, uremia, or drug effects, and possibly on the results of a bleeding time or other tests of platelet function. Platelets can almost never be rec-

ommended for patients with normal platelet function and platelet counts greater than 100,000/ml; even at 75,000, the likelihood of clinical benefit is usually low. Furthermore, platelet function defects due to an abnormal plasma milieu may be better corrected by desmopressin infusion than platelet transfusion.

Platelet dosing has come under increased scrutiny in recent years, and current recommendations suggest giving 1 unit of platelets for each 10 kg of patient body weight rather than one 8- or 10-unit dose for all patients regardless of weight. A normal response is an increase of 5,000–10,000/ml in the platelet count for each unit of platelets transfused (7). Patients who have become refractory to platelet transfusions due to alloimmunization from repeated exposure to donor blood cells may be treated with single donor platelets. One single donor platelet product is the equivalent of about 5 to 8 random donor units; in addition, single donor units may be human lymphocyte antigen-matched, i.e., chosen on the basis of which donor human lymphocyte antigens type is most likely to lead to a successful transfusion.

Granulocyte transfusion has undergone a marked reduction in use in the past decade due to improvements in the care of neutropenic patients. They continue to be used most often in the febrile neutropenic infant where a greater increment in white blood cell count can be shown. Recent technological advances in the collection of granulocytes should make similar increments attainable in febrile neutropenic adults, which may make them more clearly efficacious.

Factor concentrates are extremely low volume products made from large number of donors ranging from 5,000 to 20,000, which have undergone repeated changes since the advent of human immunodeficiency virus (HIV) infection. Factor VIII concentrate is the treatment of choice for hemophilia A, and factor IX concentrate is the treatment of choice for hemophilia B (hereditary factor IX deficiency) and for most patients with anti-factor VIII antibodies. Some factor IX concentrates may also contain various amounts of other clotting factors, especially the vitamin K-dependent factors II, VII, and X. Rarely, patients with Coumadin overdose and life-threatening intracranial hemorrhage and volume overload may benefit from factor IX concentrate despite FFP being the usual recommendation.

Antithrombin III concentrate is indicated for patients with congenital deficiency of antithrombin III and a history of thrombosis who must cease anticoagulation for surgery or pregnancy. In general, the rapid changes in concentrates, their high cost, and potential for inappropriate use dictates that a hematologist familiar with their use be consulted before administering them.

References

1. Abu-Elmagd KM, Bronsther O, Kobayashi M, Yagihashi A, Iwaki Y, Fung J, Alessiani M, Bon-
   tempo F. Acute hemolytic anemia in liver and bone marrow transplant patients under FK 506 therapy. Transplant Proc 1991;23(6):3190–3192.
2. Joyce RA. Sequential effects of lithium on haematopoiesis. Br J Haematol 1984;56:307.
3. Kurtzman G, Ozawa K, Cohen B, Hanson G, Oseas R, Young NS. Chronic bone marrow failure due to persistent B19 parvovirus infection. N Engl J Med 1987;317(5):287–294.
4. Kurtzman G, Frickhofen N, Kimball J, Jenkins DW, Nienhuis AW, Young NS. Pure red-cell aplasia of 10 years' duration due to persistent parvovirus B19 infection and its cure with immunoglobulin therapy. N Engl J Med 1989;519–523.
5. Meryman HT. Frozen red cells. Transfusion Med Rev 1989;3(2):121–127.
6. Office of medical applications of research. National Institute of Health. Fresh frozen plasma; indication and risks. JAMA 1985;253(4):551–553.
7. Office of Medical Applications of Research. National Institutes of Health. Platelet Transfusion Therapy. JAMA 1987;257(13):1777–1780.
8. Sazama K. Reports of 355 transfusion-associated deaths: 1976–1985. Transplantation 1990;30:583–590.

50

Management of the Immunocompromised Host

Peter Linden

Over the past several decades the proliferation of both aggressive medical and surgical modes of treatment for potentially lethal oncologic disease, kidney, liver and cardiac end-organ failure and autoimmune disease has improved both short- and long-term prognosis for many patients. A natural consequence however has been the evolution of both acute and chronic immunocompromised patient populations with exceptional vulnerability to both opportunistic and nonopportunistic infection due to single or multiple deficits in their host defenses. This trend is grossly reflected by the rising incidence of septic shock and sepsis related mortality over the previous fifty years despite sophisticated hemodynamic monitoring, broad spectrum antibiotics, and extensive metabolic support (36, 71–73). The serious and/or life-threatening sequelae to infection in these hosts often culminates in single or multiple system organ failure which requires critical care intervention.

The primary goal of this chapter will be to provide a brief and basic outline of the constituents of normal host defense against infectious challenge and to present a rational, succinct, and contemporaneous approach to the immunocompromised patient in the critical care setting. The pattern of opportunistic infection and its clinical management will be discussed for two major categories of immunocompromised hosts: granulocytopenia due to hematologic malignancy or solid tumor chemotherapy and cell-mediated deficiency associated with solid organ transplantation, ie., kidney, liver, heart, and heart/lung recipients.

HOST DEFENSE MECHANISM

A comprehensive discussion of the immune system is well beyond the intent and scope of this chapter. Rather, information on those aspects of host defense that are most frequently deficient due to the native disease and its therapy, or to interventions in the critical care setting and the types of infections associated with each category of immunodeficiency is of the most relevance in formulating a preventative, diagnostic, and therapeutic approach.

Anatomic Barriers to Infection

Host defense mechanisms are conventionally divided into a "first line" consisting of an intact integument of skin and the mucosa of the respiratory, gastrointestinal, and genitourinary systems (Table 50.1). The skin is adapted to provide a mechanical, biochemical, and microbiologic barrier to colonization by potential pathogens or actual invasion. Antibacterial properties include surface dryness, an acidic pH due to resident flora synthesis of lactic acid and short chain fatty acids, and the normal desquamation of surface cells (11, 99). The mucosa also constitutes a physical barrier, albeit less impervious than the intact skin. Specialized functions at the mucosal level amplify its ability to defend the host. Air filtration and particulate trapping by humidification of inspired air and the mucociliary blanket in the upper respiratory airways impair the progression of microorganisms or spores into the distal airways (85, 86). The normal acidification of

Table 50.1
Anatomic Host Defense and Normal Colonizing Flora

Site	Specialized Mechanisms	Colonizing Flora
Skin	Acidic pH Dryness Cell shedding	Coagulase negative Staphylococcus Corynebacteria
Respiratory	Particle filtration Humidification Ciliary clearance Coughing	Streptococci Anaerobes
Alimentary	Gastric acid barrier Motility Bile acids	Anaerobes Enterococci Enteric Gram-negatives
Genitourinary	Bladder emptying Intact urethra Urine composition	Sterile

the stomach, inhibitory action of the biliary secretions in the proximal small intestines, and gastrointestinal motility all limit the quantity and pathogenic potential of organisms in the gastrointestinal tract (10, 26). Genitourinary host defenses include the bacteriostatic properties of urine (urea, hyperosmolality, ammonia, pH) coupled with periodic bladder emptying (47, 56). Intact urethral anatomy which also plays a critical role in preventing bladder colonization and more serious infectious sequelae. Finally, secretory IgA bolsters antibacterial defenses at the mucosal level in all sites by impairing bacterial motility and adherence to potential mucosal receptors (106).

The normal endogenous colonizing microflora which occupy skin and mucosal surfaces exert a resistance to colonization by exogenous potential pathogens, particularly the aerobic Gram-negative bacilli and fungi (108). The composition of the normal flora according to anatomic site is shown in Table 50.1. Preferential colonization, accordingly, is determined by specific binding properties of the bacteria for epithelial or mucosal sites modulated partially by secretory IgA and fibronectin, substrate competition, and the synthesis of chemical inhibitors or bacteriocins that retard the proliferation of competing microorganisms. Susceptibility to colonization with

Gram-negative bacilli is clearly associated with increasing debility and illness of the host (53, 54). This incorporates many contributing variables including prolonged time of hospitalization which increases the period of exposure to exogenous pathogens, antimicrobial suppression of indigenous flora, bladder catheterization and intubation which bypass anatomic defenses, and obstruction and stasis in visceral organs as well as other primary less well-understood changes in the critically ill host. The clinically relevant consequences of an altered colonizing microflora include the following: (a) The majority of patients with certain nosocomial infections have documented antecedent colonization with the same organism. Thus surveillance culturing may have prospective value in some subsets of profoundly immunocompromised patients in guiding prophylactic and empiric antibiotic regimens. (b) Acquired microorganisms have a higher probability of multidrug resistance due to prior antibiotic selection pressure; (c) Breech of anatomic integrity automatically exposes the compromised host to a more virulent inoculum; (d) High density colonization due to uncontrolled overgrowth of aerobic Gram-negative bacilli and *Candida* in the gastrointestinal tract may result in translocation across an otherwise intact mucosa and account for primary bacteremia and fungemia in the immunocompromised hosts.

Cellular and Humoral-Mediated Host Defenses

The three major constituents of systemic host resistance are the circulating and organ-bound leukocytes with phagocytic function, lymphocyte-directed cell-mediated immunity, and humoral functions imparted by immunoglobulins and serum complement. The circulating pool of phagocytes include the neutrophil, eosinophil, and the monocyte. Engulfment and killing of most bacteria and fungi is primarily accomplished by the neutrophil. A complex system of target selection is mediated by the generation of bacterial products, cytokines, and activated complement components. Granulocytopenia, defined by counts less than 1000/mm³ and usually induced by cytotoxic chemotherapy, accounts for the vast majority of infections though acquired and congenital qualitative neutrophil defects also culminate in severe infections. Common infectious etiologies include the aerobic Gram-negative bacilli including the species, *Escherichia coli, Klebsiella pneumoniae, Enterobacter, Pseudomonas aeruginosa* and Gram-positive species *Staphylococcus aureus* and *S. epidermidis*. Additionally, *Candida, Aspergillus*, and the *Mucoraceae* account for the majority of opportunistic fungal infections though sporadic infections caused by the filamentous fungi *Trichosporon, Fusarium*, and *Pseudallescheria boydii* are more frequently recognized as invasive pathogens in this population (12, 43, 113, 123).

The circulating monocyte and tissue bound macrophages in the alveolar lining of the lung, lymph nodes, liver, and spleen are collectively termed the reticuloendothelial system (RES). Primary functions include scavenger activity against cellular debris and foreign antigens, engulfment and killing of a broad range of intracellular pathogens, and modulation of both cell-mediated and humoral immunity by macrophage antigen processing and presentation to both T and B lymphocytes. Common examples of compromised RES function with serious infectious sequelae include patients with anatomic or functional asplenia, i.e., sickle cell disease, thalassemia major, and end-stage liver disease.

Cell-mediated immunity is dependent on a qualitatively and quantitatively intact line of T-helper, T-suppressor and effector lymphocytes. Lymphokines in the form of macrophage-derived interleukin-1 (IL-1) and lymphocyte derived interleukin-2 (IL-2) function as nonspecific and specific activators respectively to promote growth and differentiation of T-helper lymphocytes. Either lymphocyte dysfunction or depletion may result in defective immunity against an extraordinarily wide range of microorganisms including many intracellular bacteria (*Legionella, Listeria monocytogenes, Salmonella, Nocardia asteroides*, and the mycobacteria), viruses (varicella-zoster (VZV), herpes simplex (HSV), cytomegalovirus (CMV), and Epstein-Barr virus (EBV)), fungi (*Cryptococcus, Histoplasmosis, Aspergillus*), protozoa (*Pneumocystis carinii* and *Toxoplasma gondii*), and other parasitic forms such as *Strongyloides stercoralis*. For reasons which remain unknown, particular disease- or immunosuppression-defined categories of patients with cell-mediated deficiencies have disproportionately higher incidence rates of specific infections: *Pneumocystis* and disseminated *Mycobacterium-avian intracellulare* (MAI) in acquired immunodeficiency syndrome (AIDS) patients; *Listeria* and varicella-zoster in Hodgkin's disease; and nocardiosis in renal and heart-lung transplant recipients.

Humoral immunity is principally mediated by B-lymphocyte-directed antibody synthesis, serum complement and an intact spleen for the production of specific opsonizing antibodies. Common predisposing conditions include lymphoproliferative diseases, i.e., multiple myeloma, lymphoma, chronic lymphocytic leukemia (CLL), and the postsplenectomy state. Fulminant or relapsing infections with encapsulated bacteria including *Streptococcus pneumoniae, Hemophilus influenza*, and *Neisseria meningitidis* are the classic offending pathogens.

The major categories of systemic immunodeficiency and the associated predisposing native disease or immunosuppression common to intensive care practice are shown in Table 50.2. Though such classification serves as an epidemiologic and pathophysiologic rationale for the kinds of infection that occur and assists preventative, diagnostic, and therapeutic strategies, most immunocompromised patients have either concomitant or serial immune defects, i.e., granulocytopenia and cell-

Table 50.2
Major Categories of Immunocompromised Host Defense

Granulocytopenia
  Hematologic malignancies
    Acute leukemias
      Acute nonlymphocytic leukemia
        (ANLL)
      Acute lymphocytic leukemia (ALL)
    Chronic leukemias
      Chronic nonlymphocytic leukemia
        (CNLL)
  Cytotoxic chemotherapy
  Radiation (therapeutic and accidental
    exposure)
  Aplastic anemias
    Idiopathic
    Idiosyncratic drug reaction
  Drug-induced neutropenia
Cell-mediated immune defects
  Lymphoproliferative malignancy
    Hodgkin's disease
    Non-Hodgkin's lymphoma
    Hairy cell leukemia
    Acute nonlymphocytic leukemia
  Bone marrow transplantation
  Antirejection therapy post solid-organ
    transplant
    Cyclosporine
    Antilymphocyte globulin
    Anti-CD4 lymphocyte monoclonal anti-
      body (OKT3)
    Azathioprine
  Corticosteroid therapy
  Radiation
  Cytotoxic drugs
  Acquired immunodeficiency syndrome
Humoral immune defects
  Chronic lymphocytic leukemia
  Multiple myeloma
  Postsplenectomy state
  Sickle cell disease

mediated dysfunction secondary to chemotherapy which predisposes the host to a wider spectrum of opportunistic infections.

GENERAL DIAGNOSTIC APPROACH TO THE CRITICALLY ILL IMMUNOCOMPROMISED PATIENT

Though immunocompromised patients are frequently admitted to an intensive care unit with noninfectious complications such as fluid overload, renal failure, or hemorrhage due to the underlying disease or its therapy, infection-related complications are most frequently the sole or major component of their clinical presentation. Common clinical scenarios include de novo fever with or without sepsis syndrome or frank shock, respiratory failure due to a pneumonitis, and central nervous system dysfunction either due to CNS or extra-CNS infection. Often, these patients have clinically deteriorated despite an accurate diagnosis and appropriate therapy instituted prior to ICU admission or have developed a superinfection following a favorable initial response to therapy. On occasion the immunocompromised host may even present with more than one active infectious process due to the diverse nature of their immunologic defects.

In no other area of medicine is there a greater necessity for a concise and comprehensive method when establishing a database on a critically ill immunocompromised patient requiring admission to the intensive care unit. Many transplant and oncologic centers now maintain a bedside wall chart visible to the primary critical care team as well as visiting consultants with a daily listing of prior immunosuppression and antimicrobial therapy, significant culture results, serology and pathology results, commonly required laboratory values, and any major radiologic or nuclear imaging tests. This condensed format of information, if properly maintained, should greatly facilitate data gathering and prevent unnecessary delay in formulating a diagnostic and therapeutic plan. Evaluation of these patients is naturally tailored to the clinical syndrome, however, certain significant features merit routine emphasis (Table 50.3). An assessment of the predominant and secondary type and degree of immunosuppression should be undertaken. Relevant data includes any recent cytotoxic chemotherapy, corticosteroids or recent abrupt withdrawal of corticosteroids, antilymphocyte globulin (ALG) or OKT3

Table 50.3
Database for the Initial Evaluation of the Immunocompromised Patient

Assessment of primary immune defect(s)
  Underlying disease
  Granulocytopenia
  Prior immunosuppressive chemotherapy
  Prior radiation therapy
  Postsplenectomy status
  Invasive devices, i.e., catheters, prosthetics
  Prior surgery (duration and site)
  Miscellaneous factors, i.e., cirrhosis, diabetes, uremia
Stage of underlying disease
  Duration of granulocytopenia
  Time interval from organ transplantation
Prior significant infections and culture
  Fever
  Clinically defined microorganism and/or site
    Bacteremia or fungemia
    Urinary tract
    Pneumonia
    Soft tissue
    Intravenous device
  Surveillance cultures
    Pseudomonas
    Methicillin-resistant *S. aureus*
    Candida
    Aspergillus
Epidemiologic exposure
  Native origin
  Travel to areas of endemic disease
  Recently ill close contacts
  Viral serology (HSV, CMV, VZV, hepatitis B, -C, HIV)
  Other serology (toxoplasmosis, *Legionella*)
  PPD skin testing
  Stool ova and parasites
Prior chemoprophylaxis
  Acyclovir
  TMP/SMX or aerosolized pentamidine
  Amantadine
  Selective enteral decontamination
  Oral nystatin, fluconazole, or amphotericin β

monoclonal antibody, azathioprine, cyclosporine A and FK506, total radiation dose and body site, previous splenectomy, and evidence of recent primary CMV disease which may have secondary immunosuppressive effects (15, 95).

Data pertaining to the stage of the underlying disease and the duration of a particular immune deficit may assist in narrowing the differential diagnosis of opportunistic infection. Thus, the etiology of a pneumonitis occurring early in the period of profound granulocytopenia in a patient with a hemotologic malignancy is more likely secondary to a Gram-negative bacteria or herpes simplex than an invasive fungal or protozoan infection. Conversely, a longer cumulative period of cell-mediated immunosuppression due, for instance, to repetitive cycles of antirejection therapy in solid-organ recipients or corticosteroid based chemotherapy widens the differential diagnosis to include less common opportunistic infections.

Knowledge of prior documented clinically-defined site(s) of infection and the antibiotic(s) utilized can direct subsequent diagnostic evaluation and the empiric therapy chosen. A common pattern in patients with protracted profound granulocytopenia may be a relapse of fever and other signs of clinical deterioration, after a favorable response to empiric therapy, due to the selection of resistant organisms or fungal superinfection. Consequently, the clinician should establish what chemoprophylaxis and/or selective decontamination the patient had received prior to ICU admission as it may impart added valuable clinical insight: *(a)* Prophylaxis with trimethoprim/sulfamethoxazole (TMP/SMX) has so dramatically reduced the incidence of *Pneumocystis pneumonia* in well-defined oncologic and transplant recipients with impaired cell-mediated immunity (50, 122), that its consideration in the differential diagnosis of a pneumonitis is significantly diminished. Notably however, the diagnosis of breakthrough *P. pneumonia* in the setting of active TMP/SMX prophylaxis may require more invasive procedures due to the diminished yield of bronchial lavage. *(b)* TMP/SMX prophylaxis appears to have lowered the incidence of opportunistic infection due to sensitive pathogens such as *Nocardia*, *Legionella*, and *Listeria*. (c) Enteral decontamination regimens directed at aerobic Gram-negative bacilli (colistin/gentamicin) have shown a reciprocal increase in Gram-positive infections, i.e., *Staphylococci* and enterococci (118). (d) Patients receiving systematically absorbed prophylactic agents, usually TMP/SMX or a quinolone such as norfloxacin or ciprofloxacin, have a greater incidence of infections with pathogens resistant to the prophylactic agent, i.e., multiresistant *Enterobactieceae*, *Pseudomonas*, *Candida*, and *Aspergillus* (22, 109, 111). (e) Antiviral prophylaxis with high dose acyclovir (3200 mg/day) may modify the timing and clinical presentation of CMV-related disease and the diagnostic yield of viral cultures.

Any history of antibiotic induced toxicity, severe side effects or allergic reactions should also be elicited since rechallenge with the offending drug may have life-threatening sequelae including anaphylaxis or Stevens-Johnson syndrome.

The historical database should encompass the epidemiologic exposure of the immunocompromised patient. Information that may occasionally uncover significant past epidemiological exposure includes the patient's native origin or travel to geographic areas with specific endemic disease i.e., *Histoplasmosis* and *Coccidiomycosis* in the midwest and southwest regions of United States respectively, disseminated *Strongyloidiasis* in patients from the southern United States and tropical climates, and exposure to close contacts who have recently sustained illness.

Most immunocompromised patients are admitted directly from either the same or a referring hospital and thus already have a modified endogenous flora depending on the pattern of multiresistant bacteria and the type and degree of prior antibiotic exposure. If available, prior surveillance cultures positive for methicillin-resistant *S. aureus* (128), *Pseudomonas* (92), *Candida tropicalis* (120), *Torulopsis glabrata* (1), and *Aspergillus* (2, 129) correlate positively with the probability of active or subsequent infection in select immunocompromised groups. Additionally, the results of tuberculous skin testing may be of value in assessing the risk for reactivated disease though cutaneous anergy contributes to a high incidence of false-negative results and prior BCG vaccination may cause false-positive testing. Results of prior herpesvirus serology may allow detection of seroconversion, i.e., patients with previously negative antibody titer who are now positive. Serial serologic information is the only method of distinguishing a primary from reactivated CMV infection. Since both the incidence and severity of CMV related disease in bone marrow and solid-organ recipients is greater after primary infection, this information may contribute significant diagnostic value. An account of the symptoms the patient experienced prior to intensive care admission should be elicited. Symptoms including any localized pain or irritation, dyspnea, cough, dysuria, diarrhea, nausea or vomiting, odynophagia, headache, delirium or altered cognitive abilities, and visual deterioration may direct the search for a localized or disseminated infection. The potential significance of the presence of these symptoms as it corresponds to the anatomic site and type of opportunistic pathogen are listed in Table 50.4.

The physical examination should be both expeditious and directed to the major clinical syndrome precipitating admission to the ICU, and yet still screen for any signs of infection in those organ systems most commonly affected by opportunistic infection in the immunocompromised. Pertinent areas to be covered within the physical examination include:

1. Skin examination for abscesses, vesicles, nodules, ulcers, infarcts, and any types of rash. Concealed areas in the intertriginous folds and perirectal area bear special emphasis.
2. Oropharyngeal exam for evidence of candidiasis, ulcers, gingivitis, or advanced dental disease.
3. Fundoscopic examination to screen for retinal findings consistent with endopthalmitis (bacterial, fungal) or chorioretinitis (CMV, toxoplasmosis).
4. Examination of lymph node bearing areas; submandibular, pre and post auricular, cervical, axillary, epitrochlear, and inguinal areas.
5. Direct palpation of the frontal and maxil-

Table 50.4
Symptoms of Common Infectious Etiologies in the Immunocompromised Patient

Symptom	Possible Infectious Etiology
Localized pain	
Dermatomal distribution	Herpes zoster (prodromal phase)
Overlying vertebrae	Epidural abscess, osteomyelitis
Right lower quadrant	Typhlitis
Perineal	Perirectal abscess or cellulitis
Retrosternal	Esophagitis (HSV, CMV, *Candida*)
Retroocular, sinus	*Aspergillus, Mucor*
Headache[a]	Diffuse of focal CNS infection
	Listeria monocytogenes
	Nocardia asteroides
	Aspergillus
	Candida
	Toxoplasmosis gondii
Visual deterioration	Retinitis (CMV, toxoplasmosis)
	Bacterial or fungal endopthalmitis
Nausea, emesis	Gastroduodenitis (CMV, HSV)
Diarrhea	Enteritis, colitis
	CMV, HSV
	Cryptosporidia
	S. stercoralis
	C. difficile
Dysuria	Cystitis
	Bacteria
	Candida
Dyspnea	Pneumonitis
	Aerobic Gram-negative bacilli
	S. aureus
	Legionella
	Aspergillus
	CMV, HSV, VZV
	P. carinii
	S. stercoralis

[a]With or without focal neurologic signs.

lary sinuses to elicit tenderness suggestive of occult sinus infection.

6. Auscultation of the lungs and heart.
7. Abdominal examination for localized tenderness, rebound or guarding, and hepatosplenomegaly.
8. Inspection of the perirectal area for localized erythema, induration, or frank abscess.
9. Exit site and tunnel space of any indwelling catheters or drains for purulence, erythema, warmth, or induration.
10. Neurologic examination for abnormalities in mental status (cognitive function and sensorium), meningeal signs, cranial nerve dysfunction, and the presence of upper motor neuron signs or lateralizing deficits in somatic motor and sensory functions. A complete neurologic examination is fre-

quently limited by the critical illness itself or prior sedative or neuromuscular blocking agents. Deferring use of these drugs until completion of a neurologic exam, if possible, is obviously preferable.

Baseline laboratory tests should screen for preexisting end-organ insufficiency due either to the underlying disease, infection or drug and radiation toxicity. A suggested list of screening tests are shown in Table 50.5. Nonlocalizing abnormalities in these tests such as lactic acidosis, disseminated intravascular coagulation, eosinophilia or elevations in lactic dehydrogenase (LDH) may be the only initial evidence of an otherwise occult infectious process. The practical value of such studies in directing

Table 50.5
Screening Laboratory Tests for Immunocompromised Patients Requiring ICU Admission

White blood cell count + differential
Hematocrit
Platelet count
Serum electrolytes and glucose
BUN
Creatinine
24-hr urine collection for creatinine clearance
Liver-associated enzymes
Bilirubin
Lactate dehydrogenase
Prothrombin time
Partial thromboplastin time
DIC screen: thrombin time, fibrin split products, D-dimer
Lactate
Amylase
Creatine phosphokinase
Albumin
Arterial blood gases
Urinalysis

management may include antibiotic selection and dosing based on renal or hepatic failure, directing imaging and/or invasive techniques to workup unexplained liver-associated enzyme abnormalities (CT scan or liver biopsy) or pancytopenia (bone marrow biopsy). Additionally, prompt identification of significant abnormalities of hemostasis due either to coagulopathy, thrombocytopenia or platelet dysfunction, or renal function will allow expeditious prophylactic interventions to minimize the risk of procedure related complication, i.e., fresh frozen plasma, cryoprecipitate or platelet replacement prior to visceral biopsy, or aggressive intravenous saline loading and mannitol prior to infusion of radiographic contrast.

An initial chest roentgenogram is mandatory both to detect ongoing parenchymal or pleural disease and to establish a baseline to provide for serial comparison since the appearance of infiltrates may lag due to both poor inflammatory response and hypovolemia.

Appropriate specimens for cultures in all immunocompromised patients with signs or symptoms compatible with infection include blood, sputum and urine.

Catheters which are removed should have the intradermal segment sent for semiquantitative culture in addition to culture of any discharge from the exit site. Suspicious lesions present on skin or mucosa should be evaluated by either routine swab, needle aspiration, or biopsy and sent for routine and special stains and cultures (fungal, viral, modified acid-fast, acid-fast). Cultures should be obtained expeditiously to avoid undue delay in initiating empiric antibiotic coverage if indicated. Information obtained from Gram's stain, acid-fast stain and wet mounts may provide the best available early information to guide the choice of antibiotics. The absence of inflammatory cells in sputum, urine, and wound drainage specimens does not eliminate this site as a source of fever or sepsis in the granulocytopenic or cell-mediated immunosuppressed individual. Conversely, the appearance of abundant inflammatory cells without visible organisms on conventional staining may suggest infections due to nonstaining organisms, i.e., *Legionella, Mycoplasma, Pneumocystis carinii,* and viruses under the appropriate circumstances.

Two or three sets of blood cultures, each comprised of one aerobic bottle and one anaerobic bottle, obtained by peripheral venipuncture, are adequate in most circumstances. Obtaining additional blood cultures at the time of initial workup does not boost the sensitivity for the detection of bacteremia or fungemia (35).

Obtaining the optimal quantity of blood per culture bottle does influence the sensitivity; blood:broth ratios of 1:10 or 10 ml of blood/100 ml of broth bottle provide sufficient bacterial inoculum and dilutes any antibiotics to subinhibitory levels to promote in vitro growth if bacteremia is present (117). Blood cultures obtained via indwelling central venous catheters or arterial lines are associated with a higher incidence of false positives (35, 107). Though convenient, this practice should be avoided unless the microbiology laboratory will perform quantitative cultures on both the peripheral and catheter-obtained specimens to distinguish catheter-related from noncatheter-related bacteremia (119).

Diminished sensitivity of blood cultures in immunocompromised patients may occur due either to recent or concurrent antibiotics which suppress in vitro recovery or occasionally due to the fastidious nature of the pathogen. There are several available adjunctive measures that may enhance or expedite the isolation of a blood pathogen in these circumstances. Antimicrobial-inactivating resin-containing blood culture bottles have been shown to modestly increase the isolation rate of bacteria, particularly Gram-positive species. Blood obtained in special isolator tubes available from the microbiology laboratory are processed via sequential centrifugation to partition a leukocyte-concentrated specimen followed by chemical lysis. This method enhances recovery of intracellular phagocytosed organisms such as *Candida* and

Gram-negatives (9, 45). Another method termed "blind subculturing" consists of plating broth from apparently negative blood culture bottles onto routine or enriched media. Earlier isolation for such organisms as *Pseudomonas* and meningococci with this method has been shown (105). The full range of supplemental diagnostic procedures potentially useful in the evaluation of the critically ill immunocompromised patient is shown in Table 50.6. Utilization of these tests requires close communication and coordination with the relevant laboratory to insure meaningful and accurate results.

Evaluation of Fever and Pulmonary Infiltrates

A reasonable initial differential diagnosis can be constructed based on the previ-

Table 50.6
Microbiologic, Immunologic and Pathologic Tests Utilized for the Diagnosis of Infection in the Immunocompromised Host

Detection of microbemia or microbial products
  Isolator tube blood cultures (bacteria, fungi, and mycobacteria)
  Antimicrobial inactivating resin bottles
  Blind subcultures
  Buffy coat Gram's stain
  Endotoxin assay (limulus-lysate)
  Counterimmunoelectrophoresis
  Cryptococcal antigen (serum, CSF)
Respiratory specimens

Stains	*Organisms*
Gram's	Bacteria, Fungi, *Nocardia*
Potassium hydroxide	Fungi
Acid-fast	Mycobacteria
Modified acid-fast	*Nocardia, L. micdadei*
Grocott	Fungi, *P. carinii*
Direct fluorescent antibody	*Legionella*
Papanicolaou or Wright	Viral inclusions

  Cultures
    Routine
    Quantitative (lavage or protected brush)
    Fungal
    Mycobacteria
    Nocardia
    Legionella
    Viral (routine and rapid shell vial)
Miscellaneous
  Semiquantitative cultures (intradermal catheter segment)
  Stool for ova and parasites
  Duodenal aspirate (Giemsa or wet mount for *S. stercoralis*)
  Clostridia difficile toxin assay

ously outlined information detailing epidemiologic exposure, recent clinical history, and the nature and duration of the host's immune deficits. The chest film is invaluable in further refining the differential diagnosis. The poor inflammatory response in immunocompromised hosts notoriously alters the radiographic appearance in some infections. Nevertheless, there are fundamental categories of radiographic progression and abnormality that may direct the clinician's evaluation and therapy (Table 50.7).

Obtaining an adequate sputum sample without oropharyngeal contamination is quite problematic in the immunosuppressed population as there is often only scanty production of secretions even with concomitant pneumonia. Though sputum induction with nebulized hypertonic saline may improve the diagnostic yield for some pathogens, such as *P. carinii*, there are a variety of other confounding problems. The high prevalence of upper airway colonization with potential pathogens invariably results in low specificity and diagnostic uncertainty (7, 55). Additionally, some pneumonic etiologies such as *Aspergillus* are not consistently manifested in

Table 50.7
Radiographic Presentation of Common Infectious Etiologies in Immunocompromised Hosts

Diffuse interstitial and/or alveolar pattern
  P. carinii
  Viral pneumonitis (HSV, VSV, CMV, adenovirus)
  Disseminated fungal
  Nocardia
  S. stercoralis
Focal consolidation
  Bacteria (including *Legionella*)
  Aspergillus, Mucor
  Primary tuberculosis
  Nocardia
Nodule(s)
  Fungi
  Nocardia
Cavitary
  Bacteria (*Pseudomonas, Klebsiella, S. aureus*)
  Aspergillus
  Tuberculosis
  Nocardia

the sputum by either staining or culture. Finally, the wide array of noninfectious pulmonary processes such as adult respiratory distress syndrome (ARDS), embolic phenomena, alveolar hemorrhage, and simple hydrostatic edema are not reliably distinguished from a true infectious etiology or they may even coexist. Despite all stated disadvantages of sputum analysis it is essential to perform basic and special staining (Gram's stain, KOH prep, modified and nonmodified acid-fast) if a quality specimen can be obtained. For instance, the appearance of Gram-positive beaded, branching filaments compatible with *Nocardia* or the abundance of a single morphologic bacteria with intracellular forms are helpful early information in guiding antimicrobial therapy.

Invasive alternatives for the diagnosis of pneumonia in immunocompromised individuals include flexible fiberoptic bronchoscopy with either single or combined use of transbronchial biopsy, protected bronchial brushing, or bronchoalveolar lavage. Each of these provides excellent diagnostic capabilities in the immunocompromised population. With occasional exceptions, protected brushing with or without lavage has become the procedure of choice for the diagnosis of suspected bacterial, viral, and *Pneumocystis* pneumonitis. Reasons for this include the significantly lower complication rate compared with transbronchial biopsy and the rapid advancement of laboratory techniques for the diagnosis of *Pneumocystis*, viral, and *Legionella* pneumonitis. Additionally, focal or diffuse infiltrates attributable to bacterial pneumonia may be evaluated with either bronchial lavage and/or protected brush technique and subsequent quantitative culture processing. Colony counts greater than 10^5/ml of lavage specimen or 10^4/ml of a brush specimen have correlated with "gold standard" evidence for invasive bacterial pneumonia, i.e., blood and pleural fluid cultures and lung biopsy (67, 104). However, a higher rate of both false-positive and false-negative results occurred in the setting of recent or ongoing antibiotic therapy which is often the situation in empirically treated immunocompromised patients. Open lung biopsy remains indicated for either local or diffuse infiltrates which defy diagnosis by less invasive means and fail to respond adequately to well chosen empiric therapy, and in instances where contraindications (severe hypoxemia, coagulopathy) to other techniques exist. Despite its radical nature, complication rates have been remarkably low (<3%) and diagnostic sensitivity quite impressive (34, 66). More controversial however, is whether achieving diagnostic certainty by any invasive means results in meaningful therapeutic changes that translate into improved survival in certain subsets of immunocompromised patients with pulmonary disease. At the current time, a rational, individualized approach that considers the type of infiltrate, rapidity of progression, risks of empiric therapy versus the risk of the procedure, and whether the underlying disease process is reversible seems the most prudent course.

Evaluation and Empiric Therapy of Suspected CNS Infection

Infection of the CNS has many protean manifestations in the immunocompromised host ranging from nonlocalizing symptoms, i.e., headache, confusion or obtundation to focal motor and sensory deficits, true meningismus, or frank seizure activity. Despite the nonspecificity of many of these signs and symptoms, a low threshold for the initiation of a diagnostic CNS workup is essential. High risk categories for CNS infection include impaired cell-mediated immunity secondary to the underlying disease (Hodgkin's, non-Hodgkin's lymphoma, acute lymphocytic leukemia) or therapeutic agents (corticosteroids, cyclosporine and antilymphocyte globulin) and humoral deficient states. Severe granulocytopenia does not significantly predispose the patient to bacterial CNS infection except those due to contamination following an invasive CNS procedure. Recognition of the operative immune defect(s) may narrow the differential diagnosis and guide parts of the diagnostic workup and the initial empiric therapy (Table 50.8).

Diagnostic lumbar puncture (LP) should be performed immediately if no contraindications exist. Signs or symptoms suggestive of elevated intracranial pressure such as papilledema, pupil asymmetry, cranial nerve dysfunction, and a decreased level of consciousness require evaluation with a contrast enhanced head CT prior to performing an LP to avoid LP-associated cerebral herniation. Significant thrombocytopenia with a platelet count below 50,000/mm^3 heightens the risk of puncture-induced hemorrhage and spinal cord compression. Platelet transfusions should be initiated immediately prior to and during the lumbar puncture to insure obtaining peak platelet activity when the risk of hemorrhage is the highest. If technical difficulties are encountered due to poor or altered anatomical landmarks then either a fluoroscopic guided or cisternal approach may be utilized. Initial CSF studies in all patients include cell count and differential, glucose, protein, cryptococcal antigen, a cytocentrifuged specimen of 10 ml of CSF for Gram's stain, India ink and acid-fast stains, and cultures for bacteria, fungi, and mycobacteria. Notably, the diagnostic sensitivity for staining of centrifuged specimens is increased with a greater volume of CSF due to the small microbial inoculum present.

Other clinically useful tests in select circumstances include latex agglutination for the capsular antigens of the common CNS encapsulated bacterial pathogens, i.e., *S. pneumoniae, Neisseria meningitidis,* and *Hemophilus influenza*), cytologic analysis for neoplastic cells and viral culture studies.

Unless a positive CSF stain provides a definitive early diagnosis, the decision to initiate empiric antimicrobial therapy should be based on the nature of the immune deficit, spinal fluid cell counts and chemistry, special imaging procedures, and the presence of other suspected or documented systemic infection known to be associated with CNS involvement. Occasionally, there may be convincing evidence that a noninfectious etiology is responsible for an aseptic meningitis clinical presentation. Common in such categories are drug-induced meningitis that has been described following administration of OKT3, azathioprine, trimethoprim-sulfamethoxasole, and ibuprofen (14, 24, 52,

Table 50.8
Categories of Immunocompromised Host Defense and Infections of the Central Nervous System

Host Defect and Organism(s)	Primary Therapy[a]
Granulocytopenia	
Gram-negative bacilli	Piperacillin or ceftazidime
	+ tobramycin
	+ intrathecal tobramycin[b]
S. aureus	Nafcillin, 12 g/day
	Vancomycin indicated for β-lactam allergy or
	methicillin-resistant Staphylococcus
Fungi	Amphotericin B, 1 mg/kg/day,
	+ 5-FC, 150 mg/kg/day p.o.
Cell-mediated defect	
L. monocytogenes	Ampicillin, 200 mg/kg/day
Nocardia	Sulfadiazine, 6–8 g/day i.v./p.o.
Cryptococcus	Amphotericin B, 0.6 mg/kg/day,
	+ 5-FC, 150 mg/kg/day p.o.
Aspergillus	Amphotericin B, 1 mg/kg/day
	+ Rifampin, 600 mg/day p.o.
	+ 5-FC, 150 mg/kg/day p.o.
S. stercoralis	Thiabendazole, 50 mg/kg/day p.o. × 10–14 days
T. gondii	Sulfadiazine, 6–8 g/day i.v./p.o.
	+ Pyramethamine, 25–50 mg/kg/day p.o.
Humoral deficiency	
N. meningitidis	Penicillin G, 24 million units/day
S. pneumoniae	Penicillin G, 24 million units/day
H. influenza	Ampicillin, 200 mg/kg/day

[a]Intravenous route unless specified.
[b]0.1–0.2 mg/day intrathecally.

64) and carcinomatous meningitis in patients with hematologic malignancy. However, unless a strong temporal relationship exists to support a drug-induced meningitis or a positive cytology is immediately available, then empiric therapy is still completely justified. Empiric antimicrobial recommendations based on the best available early clinical and laboratory evidence are shown in Table 50.9.

SPECIFIC ISSUES IN THE MANAGEMENT OF THE GRANULOCYTOPENIC PATIENT

Granulocytopenia, occurring secondary to an underlying hematologic malignancy or cytotoxic chemotherapy, is the most common cause of life-threatening infection in cancer patients. Moreover, cancer patients who require critical care intervention commonly have had protracted and compli-

cated periods of granulocytopenia and longer durations of prior antibiotic therapy predisposing them to infection with multiresistant bacteria and fungi. Management of these profoundly immunocompromised patients thus requires both expeditious and aggressive diagnostic and therapeutic interventions to favorably affect outcome. The most common bacterial pathogens are the aerobic Gram-negative bacilli (E. coli, Klebsiella pneumoniae, Enterobacter and Pseudomonas aeruginosa) and Gram-positive organisms (methicillin susceptible and resistant Staphylococcus aureus, coagulase negative Staphylococci, enterococci and Corynebacteria JK). Prior series demonstrate that septic episodes due to Gram-negative bacteremia had significantly higher mortality than Gram-positive bacteremia sepsis (57, 97, 127). Amongst all Gram-negative bacilli, Pseudomonas infections are associated with the highest case fatality rates (126). Notably, the past

Table 50.9
Empiric Antibiotic Therapy for the Granulocytopenic Patient Admitted to the Intensive Care Unit

Clinical considerations
  Duration of granulcytopenia
  Broad Gram-negative spectrum
  Evidence supporting a Gram-positive source
  Evidence supporting an anaerobic source
  Evidence supporting a fungal source
  Susceptibility pattern of endemic ICU flora
  Recent documented infections
  Prior recent surveillance cultures
  Bactericidal activity
  Synergism
  Allergic history
  Toxicity
Empiric antibiotic regimens
  β-Lactam/aminoglycoside
    Piperacillin[a]/tobramycin[b]
    Ceftazidime/tobramycin[b]
    Imipenem-cilastatin/tobramycin[b]
  Double β-lactam
    Piperacillin[a]/aztreonam
  Monotherapy
    Imipenem-cilastatin
    ceftazidime

[a]Mezlocillin or azlocillin may be substituted.
[b]Gentamicin or amikacin may be substituted.

decade has seen Gram-positive organisms, particularly *S. aureus*, *S. epidermidis* and the enterococci, comprise a greater proportion of all infection in the granulocytopenic population (17, 110, 130). This trend is undoubtedly secondary to the frequent use of long-term indwelling central venous access lines (Hickman, Broviac catheters (77, 84) as well as systemic and enteral antibiotic(s) whose greater Gram-negative activity favors the selection of Gram-positive flora.

The fungi constitute the other major category of microbial pathogens in the granulocytopenic host. *Candida* (49, 69) and *Aspergillus* (38, 87) species represent the overwhelming majority of these isolates with *Mucor* and other filamentious fungi such as *Fusarium*, *Trichosporon*, and *Pseudoallescheria boydii* occasionally causing tissue invasive disease (12, 43, 113, 123).

Prior series have clearly demonstrated that greater than 80% of the microbial isolates responsible for infection in the gran-

ulocytopenic host originate from the endogenous flora (94). A significant portion of this flora has been modified by the acquisition of nosocomial pathogens during the period of prior hospitalization. This epidemiologic pattern can be exploited to guide empiric antibiotic selection or a change in antibiotic therapy for granulocytopenic patients requiring ICU admission with fever and or sepsis. Previously obtained surveillance cultures from cutaneous, upper respiratory and rectal sites prior to ICU admission may demonstrate the prevalent colonizing microflora and antibiotic susceptibility pattern. However, the positive predictive value of surveillance culturing depends in part on the intrinsic invasiveness of the organism isolated. For example, Schimpff (94), reported that colonization with *Pseudomonas aeuroginosa* ultimately precedes clinical infection with this organism in 55% of cases with lower predictive rates for *Klebsiella pneumoniae* and *Escherichia coli* in granulocytopenic patients.

Prior isolation of certain fungi also has predictive value for subsequent invasive disease; isolation of *Aspergillus flavus* and *A. fumigatus* in nasal or respiratory specimens of acute leukemic patients frequently predicted subsequent invasive aspergillosis during prolonged granulocytopenia (2, 129). Additionally, colonization with *Candida tropicalis* was associated proportionally with a higher rate of subsequent invasive disease in patients colonized with this species than *Candida albicans*, the far more prevalent species (120). A clear limitation to information from prior surveillance cultures is that they reflect microorganism acquisition from a different environment, i.e., oncology ward, and fail to predict the new epidemiologic pattern of secondary endogenous colonization which commences in the intensive care unit. Thus, knowledge of the endemic pattern of bacterial species and their respective antibiotic susceptibility pattern in the ICU may supercede the value of prior cultures for any granulocytopenic patient who remains refractory or has further clinical deterioration after 48 hr in the ICU.

The net benefit of surveillance culturing in the setting of granulocytopenia, in terms of antibiotic management and cost efficacy, still remains controversial as other studies have not shown them to be efficacious (59).

The cumulative risk of infection in the granulocytopenic host increases with progressive fall in the absolute neutrophil count (ANC) below a level of 1000/mm³ with notable increases in rate and severity at an ANC of 500/mm³ and 100/mm³ respectively (40, 65, 81). In addition, a rapid rate of decline in the number of circulating granulocytes as well as the cumulative duration of granulocytopenia contribute independently to the probability and severity of infection (65).

Fever is the most common sign of documented or occult infection in the granulocytopenic host though sepsis syndrome or shock, respiratory failure, metabolic acidosis, and a consumptive coagulopathy signal more advanced deterioration. This latter subset of patients comprises to a large degree those granulocytopenic patients requiring critical care intervention. Rarely, fever may not be present in debilitated or cachectic patients, uremia or advanced liver disease, and with concurrent steroid therapy. The level of granulocytopenia at the onset of fever remains the overwhelming determinant for the stratification of infectious risk. Approximately 80% of granulocytopenic patients with fever are felt to have an infectious source. This group is comprised by those with microbiologically and/or clinically documented infection and patients who defervesce to institution of empiric antibiotic therapy. Due to the use of selective enteral decontamination, systemic antibiotic prophylaxis, and early empiric antibiotic intervention with fever, the proportion of granulocytopenic patients with microbiologic documentation of infection has decreased significantly. This epidemiologic trend clearly influences the diagnostic and therapeutic decision making of the ICU clinician who will more often encounter the previously complicated and antibiotic-treated granulocytopenic patient rather than patients with de novo fever. Two common scenarios include refractory or recrudescent fever culminating in sepsis syndrome or shock with profound granulocytopenia (ANC <100/mm³) despite prior aggressive antibiotic therapy and a pneumonitis which has failed to respond to empiric antimicrobial coverage.

Classic signs of inflammation at local sites of infection are notoriously diminished or absent in the granulocytopenic host (91). Nevertheless, a complete physical examination with special emphasis on cutaneous and mucosal (rectal, oropharyngeal) surfaces should be undertaken as approximately 20% of febrile granulocytopenic patients will have a clinically evident focus of infection. The most frequent local sites of incipient infection are: (*a*) gastrointestinal tract including orogingival and pharyngoesophageal disease, infection of the cecum (typhlitis), and perirectal/anal cellulitis; (*b*) the upper and lower respiratory tree and the paranasal sinuses; and (*c*) cutaneous entry sites of either recently-removed or indwelling central and peripheral catheters.

GUIDELINES FOR EMPIRIC ANTIBIOTIC THERAPY

Early institution of appropriate antibiotic therapy for febrile (T>38.5°C) granulocytopenic patients, with or without localizing signs of infection, has decreased early mortality and lowered the rates of progression to bacteremia and localized infection (77, 93). The basic principles which should guide empiric antibiotic selection and suggested empiric regimens are shown in Table 50.9. A great deal of emphasis should be placed on what constitutes the endemic pattern of ICU flora as well as the antibiotic susceptibility profile. Failure to cover the predominant pathogens present in the ICU will invariably result in a higher rate of clinical failures for that empiric regimen. Major controversy still exists regarding the relative efficacy of monotherapy, i.e., ceftazidime (82) or imipenemcilastatin (13) compared to combination therapy usually with a penicillinase resistant semisynthetic β-lactam agent and an aminoglycoside or double beta β-lactam combinations (121). The apparent advantages of utilizing combination therapy include a wider spectrum of microbial coverage, greater bactericidal activity due to antibiotic synergism (125), and perhaps lower rates of secondary emergence of resistance (29). The higher prevalence of multiresistant Gram-negative bacilli and the advanced clinical deterioration in the critically ill patient favors the utilization of combination empiric therapy. Recent investigation indicates no clinical advantage for the empiric utilization of vancomycin (89), however, if there is a high ICU prevalence of methicillin-resistant *S. aureus* or the clinical findings are suggestive of a Gram-positive infection, then vancomycin should be part of the initial therapy. Modification of initial therapy should be based either on the presence of unrelenting fever, lack of improvement at a clinically defined site of infection, or the new appearance of clinical or microbiologic evidence of infection.

Empiric addition of antifungal coverage with amphotericin B between the fifth and seventh day of refractory or recrudescent fever despite broad spectrum antibiotics has been shown to reduce the rate of invasive fungal infection and overall mortality (21, 48, 101). This established practice stems from the observation that both early and advanced mycotic infections infrequently manifest specific clinical symptoms or signs enabling the clinician to make a prompt tissue diagnosis. Moreover, no more than 50% of granulocytopenic patients with autopsy proven disseminated candidiasis had positive antemortem blood cultures for candida (51, 60). Contrary to standard practice for many years, amphotericin can be safely initiated at full therapeutic doses of 0.6 mg/kg/day up to 1.0 mg/kg/day for suspected infection with *Aspergillus* or *Mucor* within 24 hr of initiating therapy following a 1-mg test dose. Empiric antifungal therapy with less toxic alternatives to amphotericin B, such as ketoconazole and fluconazole, are not acceptable alternatives due to their lack of activity against *Aspergillus* and certain species of *Candida* (32).

Recommendations for the modification of the initial empiric antibiotics based on clinical and/or microbiologic-defined sites of infection are summarized in Table 50.10. The presence of bacteremia through antibiotic therapy may be secondary to simple "breakthrough" with bacteria resistant to the original antibiotics or associated with a catheter infection. Exit site infection due to coagulase negative *Staphylococcus, S. aureus,* or *Corynebacterium* may respond to vancomycin combined with either gentamicin and/or rifampin without requiring removal of the catheter (79). However, persistent fever, bacteremia, catheter infections due to *Pseudomonas* or other multiresistant Gram-negative rods, *Bacillus, Candida,* and all tunnel infections are clear indications for early catheter removal. Addition of anaerobic coverage with clindamycin is appropriate for necrotizing mucogingivitis and clindamycin or metronidazole for perirectal cellulitis and abdominal signs compatible with typhlitis (cecitis).

The new appearance or progression of chest x-ray infiltrates coupled with respiratory deterioration should be aggressively pursued with the appropriate invasive procedure. Additionally, concurrent empiric modification of the previous antimicrobial regimen should be instituted early since delayed or inappropriate therapy of pneumonitis in the setting of granulocytopenia is associated with an extremely high rate of mortality.

The duration of empiric antibiotic therapy can be based on a stratification of risk which has been demonstrated in several illustrative studies (78, 80). Rapid recovery of the granulocyte count to levels greater than $500/mm^3$ within 7 days of initiating antibiotic therapy permits cessation of antibiotics at that time without excess mortality or morbidity. Patients who initially defervesced to empiric antibiotics but remained granulocytopenic beyond 7 days constitute a high risk subset that merits a minimum antibiotic course of 14 days. Continuation of antibiotic(s) beyond 14 days with persistent granulocytopenia seems prudent though it is as yet unproven. A second high risk subset are those patients with persistent fever through the first week of empiric antibiotics who have a high rate of sepsis when antibiotics are discontinued. These patients deserve both empiric addition of amphotericin as well as the continuation of their empiric antibacterial coverage until the ANC recovers to a level over $500/mm^3$.

Table 50.10
Clinical Events Necessitating Modification of Empiric Antibiotic Therapy in the Granulocytopenic Host

Clinical Event/Etiology	Modification(s)
Persistent fever	Amphotericin B
Primary bacteremia	
MRSA, *S. epidermidis*	Vancomycin
Corynebacteria, Enterococcus	
Bacillus	
Gram-negative bacilli	Antipseudomonal penicillin[a] + aminoglycoside
Catheter infection	
Staph. sp., *Corynebacteria*	Add vancomycin and remove catheter if fever or bacteremia persists
Enterococcus	
Bacillus sp.	Remove catheter/add vancomycin
Gram-negative/*Pseudomonas*	Remove catheter + β-lactam/tobramycin
Candida	Remove catheter/add amphotericin B
Tunnel infection	Remove catheter + antibiotic(s) based on susceptibility testing
Pneumonitis	
Focal infiltrate(s)	Add amphotericin B
	Consider diagnostic bronchoscopy or open lung biopsy
Diffuse infiltrate	Add amphotericin B
	Add TMP/SMX for *P. carinii* if with cell-mediated defect
	Consider diagnostic bronchoscopy or open lung biopsy
Orogingival stomatitis	
Anaerobes	Add clindamycin
Herpes simplex	Add i.v. acyclovir
Candida	Amphotericin B or fluconazole
Esophagitis	
Herpes simplex	Add i.v. acyclovir
Candida	Amphotericin B
Typhlitis (cecitis)	Clindamycin or metronidazole
Perirectal cellulitis	Clindamycin or metronidazole

[a]Piperacillin, mezlocillin, or azlocillin.

Recently, there have been two innovative therapeutic drugs approved by the FDA which may have a significant impact on the management of the critically ill granulocytopenic patient. Recombinant granulocyte colony stimulating factor (G-CSF) has significantly shortened the duration of granulocytopenia in both leukemic and solid tumor populations with lower infection-related morbidity and mortality (131). Adjunctive treatment of Gram-negative sepsis with human monoclonal antiendotoxin antibody (HA-1A) has significantly reduced sepsis-related mortality and

morbidity in patients with Gram-negative bacteremia in a recently published multicenter trial (19). Similar efficacy in a large granulocytopenic population still has yet to be demonstrated in a prospective trial.

INFECTIONS IN THE SOLID-ORGAN TRANSPLANT RECIPIENT

Kidney, liver, heart, and heart-lung allograft recipients are immunocompromised primarily from the multidrug immunosuppressive therapy required to attenuate the normal lymphocyte-mediated host response to the transplanted allogeneic graft tissue. The introduction of cyclosporine (CsA) in 1981 has increased both graft and patient survival in the four major transplant categories and also allowed development of a more balanced, steroid-sparing immunosuppressive regimen. Addition of monoclonal anti-CD3 lymphocyte antibody therapy and more recently FK 506 to the immunosuppressive armamentarium has continued this trend. Nevertheless, the majority of deaths in solid-organ recipients are still associated with opportunistic and nonopportunistic infections. Other contributing factors are the type and severity of underlying disease prior to transplant such as cirrhosis, uremia, or diabetes that culminated in organ failure, the visceral trauma of the transplant surgery itself, reactivation of endogenous latent pathogens, and acquisition of exogenous pathogens either from the allograft, transfused blood products, or the nosocomial environment. These many variables contribute to the wide variety of observed infectious etiologies including bacteria, fungi, viruses, protozoa, and other parasites.

Solid-organ transplant recipients have a lifelong enhanced risk for infection, however the period of highest risk is within the first several months of transplantation followed by a period of decreasing but still substantial risk out to six months. Intensive care management is thus commonly required during this vulnerable period most often for the diagnosis and treatment of infection. Many infections following all types of solid-organ transplantation occur within relatively distinctive time periods, which may aid the clinician in formulating a differential diagnosis in the febrile organ recipient. Table 50.11 demonstrates the general timetable of infections following solid-organ transplantation on a cyclosporine- and corticosteroid-based immunosuppressive regimen. Significant departures in the anticipated timing of certain infections may be secondary to the effects of chemoprophylaxis, i.e., abrupt withdrawal of TMP/SMX for the prevention of *Pneumocystis* or an unrecognized nosocomial hazard such as airborne *Aspergillus*

Table 50.11
Infections Following Solid Organ Transplantation

Infections within 1 month
  Common to all solid organ recipients
    Mucocutaneous and visceral herpes simplex
    Wound infections
    Bacterial pneumonia
    Urinary tract infection
    Catheter infections
  Kidney recipients
    Pyelonephritis
    Perinephric and parenchymal abscess
  Liver recipients
    Cholangitis
    Peritonitis
    Hepatic abscess
  Heart and heart-lung recipients
    Sternal wound infection
    Mediastinitis
    Empyema
Infections during months 2–6

Bacteria	*Fungi*
L. monocytogenes	Candida
Legionella	Cryptococcus
Nocardia asteroides	Aspergillus
Virus	*Protozoa*
Cytomegalovirus	P. carinii
Herpes zoster	T. gondii
Epstein-Barr	
Adenovirus	

spores or the presence of *Legionella* in the aqueous environment.

Early Infections in the Posttransplant Period

Infections occurring within one month after transplantation are predominantly due to nosocomial bacteria and endogenous fungi. Not unexpectedly, the site of infection is closely associated with the kind of organ transplant due to either contamination of the surgical site or donor organ, hematoma formation, and visceral leaks compounded by diminished inflammatory and wound healing response from early heavy immunosuppression.

Kidney transplant recipients have a predictably high incidence of upper and lower urinary tract infection most commonly due to Gram-negative enteric organisms, or *Enterococci* which usually respond to 10–

14 day courses of antimicrobials. Persistent fever, sepsis, or flank pain may indicate renal parenchymal or perinephric abscess requiring either percutaneous or open drainage.

Intraabdominal infections, including peritonitis, cholangitis, and hepatic abscess, represent the majority of early infection in the liver recipient. Commonly, these major infections are secondary to a mechanical complication including a biliary leak or obstruction, or vascular insufficiency due to a thrombosed hepatic arterial or portal venous anastomosis to the allograft. Clinical presentations of these major intraabdominal infections may vary from relapsing bacteremia without localizing signs, to frank peritonitis, and to fever with unexplained liver enzyme abnormalities. Clinical management includes early institution of appropriate antibiotic(s) based on clinical suspicion and cultures, imaging techniques to evaluate the anatomic integrity (Doppler ultrasound, percutaneous cholangiography, and/or mesenteric angiography), and prompt surgical drainage or correction of any underlying biliary or vascular abnormalities. Liver retransplantation may be required when either severe cholestasis or ischemia compromises hepatic function beyond recovery.

Heart and heart-lung recipients most commonly develop pneumonia or other infections within the thoracic space, i.e., empyema and mediastinitis, during this early period. Both the frequency and severity of infections are higher in the combined heart-lung recipient population.

Localized or systemic reactivated herpes simplex infections in seropositive recipients usually develop within several weeks of transplantation (4). Common sites of involvement include the oropharynx, esophagus, and genitalia. The classic lesions are painful and vesicular though unroofed, and coalesced lesions may appear ulcerative. Less commonly, disseminated cutaneous or visceral herpetic infection (hepatitis, pneumonitis) occurs in the early posttransplant period. Rare instances of transmission of HSV via the allograft with subsequent reactivation and disease from the identical strain in the early posttransplant period have been reported (27).

Mucocutaneous lesions are often diagnosed accurately based on their typical appearance. Both herpetic tracheobronchitis and esophagitis may be diagnosed via bronchoscopic or endoscopic examination. All visceral disease requires tissue specimens for diagnosis. Definitive diagnosis requires the demonstration of typical multinucleated giant cells on either cytologic or histologic specimens. Other methods include viral culture (usually positive within 24–48 hr) and immunofluorescent staining for HSV antigens. Acyclovir effectively alleviates symptoms, and shortens the time for healing and viral shedding (16). Intravenous dosing (15 mg/kg/day) is recommended for cases with documented or suspected visceral involvement and severe or widespread cutaneous disease. Crystalluria-induced nephrotoxicity may be prevented with maintenance of adequate intravenous hydration. Oral acyclovir provides effective chemoprophylaxis of HSV infection at relatively low doses, i.e., 200 mg every 6 hr.

Opportunistic Infections Following Solid-Organ Transplantation

The period between the second and extending to the sixth month following organ transplantation contains the highest incidence of opportunistic bacterial, viral, fungal, and protozoan infection. The risk of developing these infections as well as their timing, severity, and outcome are determined in part by the type of transplant recipient, type and magnitude immunosuppression, inherent host immunity (CMV), exogenous exposure (*Aspergillus, Nocardia, Listeria*), and still as yet undetermined factors.

Bacterial Infections

Nocardia

These organisms are true bacteria present ubiquitously in the natural environment. Their microscopic appearance is that of thin, irregularly branching beaded filaments which stain Gram-positive and are weakly acid fast. The majority of clinical infections are due to the species, *N. asteroides*. Though generally a sporadic infection, the highest incidence of nocardiosis has been reported in heart-lung recipients (96). Nocardiosis usually has an indolent tuberculosis-like onset characterized by weeks to months of fevers, constitutional symptoms, and weight loss. Pulmonary involvement is the primary focus of disease in the majority of cases. A diverse range of radiographic presentations including single or multiple nodules, lobar infiltrates, or frank abscesses are seen (6). Systemic involvement due to hematogenous spread is common in immunosuppressed individuals and most often presents as either abscess formation in the brain or subcutaneous and cutaneous tissues. The presence of nocardia by either modified acid-fast or Gram's stain of a respiratory specimen should qualify as presumptive evidence of invasive disease in an immunosuppressed transplant recipient though colonization states are rarely recognized in this population. The diagnostic microbiology laboratory should be informed that *Nocardia* is clinically suspected due to their slow growth characteristics even on special media. Principal first line antimicrobial therapy is with oral sulfadiazine (4–8 g/day), however, TMP/SMX is an adequate alternative when oral dosing is not feasible (112). Sulfa allergic individuals can be treated with minocycline with favorable results (75). Indications for surgical resection usually include poorly responding lung, brain, and cutaneous lesions. There is a significant tendency for late recurrences of infection either in the original site or at distant locations. Thus, a minimum period treatment duration of 3 months is usually required.

Listeria monocytogenes

Listeria is an opportunistic Gram-positive rod associated with either a meningitis with or without cerebritis or a primary bacteremic sepsis syndrome (100). The organism is acquired via ingestion with asymptomatic establishment of gastrointestinal colonization. Cell-mediated immunosuppression, usually due to prior corticosteroid therapy, predisposes the host to dissemination and systemic disease.

Meningitis is the most common clinical manifestation of infection with *Listeria*

monocytogenes. Onset of symptoms is most frequently subacute with fever and headache, though meningismus is not consistently present. Focal neurologic signs may be secondary to meningeal inflammation or cerebral abscess, which occurs in approximately 10% of all cases. Cerebrospinal fluid findings may be compatible with a florid bacterial meningitis including a neutrophilic pleocytosis, hypoglycorrachia, and protein elevation over 500 mg/dl, though both a lymphocytic pleocytosis and normal CSF chemistries are not uncommon (3). The diagnostic sensitivity of a centrifuged Gram's stain is poor with only 10–25% of culture-positive CSF specimens staining positive. Definitive diagnosis is most frequently established by CSF cultures which are usually positive within 48 hr. Since *Listeria* bacteremia is present in over 60% of CNS infections, blood cultures should be obtained prior to empiric antibiotic therapy.

Ampicillin (200/mg/kg/day) remains the therapeutic agent of first choice for the treatment of either *Listeria* meningitis or bacteremia due to its predictable in vitro and clinical efficacy. Gentamicin adds synergistic activity in combination with ampicillin (70), however improved clinical outcome has not been demonstrated and its poor CNS penetrating ability necessitates both intrathecal and systemic administration. Alternative therapies with proven effectiveness include TMP/SMX or tetracycline and erythromycin in combination. Treatment duration should be at least 21 days since shorter courses have been associated with higher rates of relapse.

Legionella

Legionella are a family of aerobic bacilli with Gram-neutral or occasionally Gram-negative staining properties. Transplant recipients constitute a major target since *Legionella* establish a facultative intracellular existence and resist ultimate destruction in the setting of an impaired T lymphocyte response. The species *L. pneumophila* comprises the overwhelming majority of clinical isolates with *L. micdadei* and other species accounting for the remainder. *Legionella* are universally present in the aqueous environment and have been epidemiologically linked to several noso-comial outbreaks of infection (102). The incidence of *Legionella*-related infection has declined recently due to the control of environmental aqueous contamination with hyperchlorination. Some also speculate that the use of TMP/SMX for *Pneumocystis* pro-phylaxis in solid-organ recipients also has provided *Legionella* prophylaxis activity.

The clinical presentation of pneumonia due to *L. pneumophila* usually occurs in acute fashion with the universal presence of a high grade fever and constitutional symptoms. A cough is usually present, however, often there is only minimal spu-tum production. Both headache and diar-rhea are present in approximately 50% of documented cases. Additionally, an ence-phalitic syndrome with altered conscious-ness or cognitive ability may be present. Multivisceral involvement may be re-flected in the laboratory workup and in-cludes azotemia, proteinuria, active uri-nary sediment, elevated transaminases, and hyperamylassemia. Radiographic changes most frequently appear as unilobar alveo-lar infiltration progressing to consolidation (33). Multilobar involvement and para-pneumonic effusions occur in a significant percent of cases, however, cavitation, ab-scess, and empyema are uncommon se-quelae (41).

A definitive diagnosis of pneumonia due to *L. pneumophila* can be established early in the clinical course by the demonstration of the organism by either direct fluorescent antibody (DFA) or gene probe technique on either sputum, tracheal aspirate, or bronchial lavage and brush specimens. *L. micdadei* may be diagnosed by its property of staining with modified acid-fast tech-nique. Other clinical clues suggestive of *Legionella* pneumonia include respiratory secretions with abundant neutrophils and no staining organisms and failure to achieve a clinical response to empirically chosen antibiotics. Since both the DFA and gene probe rapid techniques have a maximum sensitivity of only 50–70%, a significant fraction of actual cases of *Legionella* pneu-monia elude early diagnosis by such meth-ods. Serologic diagnosis with immunoflu-orescent antibody titer determinations are rarely helpful for acute diagnosis in the

immunosuppressed organ recipient. Iso-lation of *Legionella* on specialized culture media remains the diagnostic gold stan-dard (132). The diagnostic microbiology laboratory must be informed of the clinical suspicion of legionellosis to initiate appro-priate isolation methods. Culture growth usually requires a period of 3–5 days. In-travenous erythromycin (4 g/day) is the antibiotic of first choice due to its proven clinical efficacy. Supplementation with oral rifampin (600–1200 mg/day) is recom-mended for advanced or poorly respond-ing cases (90). Favorable clinical experi-ence with TMP/SMX, doxycycline, and ciprofloxacin has been reported however there are no prospective comparative clin-ical trials against erythromycin.

Viral Infection

Cytomegalovirus (CMV)

CMV remains the most common infectious pathogen in all organ transplant popula-tions with infection rates as high as 90% in some series (28, 88). Infection may be classified as primary (seronegative recipi-ent who receives a CMV positive organ or blood transfusion), secondary (reactiva-tion of the recipient's latent CMV strain), or superinfection (CMV positive recipient infected with a different CMV strain from the donor organ or transfused blood). Clinical involvement ranges from asymp-tomatic infection manifesting only as ser-oconversion or viral shedding in the blood, urine, or saliva, to a febrile mononucleo-sis-like syndrome and frank tissue inva-sive disease. Risk factors for symptomatic disease include pretransplant seronegative status (103) and the utilization of either antilymphocyte globulin or OKT3 (76, 98). CMV-related morbidity and mortality also appears to be greater in the heart-lung and liver transplant populations. Common presentations include pneumonia (fever, diffuse infiltrates, and hypoxemia), hepa-titis (fever, constitutional symptoms, and either elevated transaminase or canalicular enzymes), and enteritis (fever, diarrhea or gastrointestinal hemorrhage). Pneumonia and disseminated disease are associated with the highest mortality rates. Accurate diagnosis depends on the histologic demonstration of cytopathic effect (CMV intranuclear and intracytoplasmic inclusion bodies), positive immunoperoxidase staining, or positive rapid shell viral replication testing with a compatible clinical picture. Reliance on seroconversion and routine viral culture methods which may require up to 4 weeks are too slow to rely on and have little value in guiding acute management.

Ganciclovir, a guanosine analogue with in vitro CMV activity, now constitutes first line therapy for serious CMV disease in solid-organ transplant recipients (30). Its principal toxicity is leukopenia which is related to the cumulative dose. Dosing must be adjusted for renal insufficiency. Trisodium phosphonoformate (Foscarnet), has recently been approved by the FDA as a therapeutic option for patients who cannot tolerate ganciclovir therapy or with ganciclovir resistant strains of CMV (58). Additionally, the immunosuppression should be judiciously tapered if possible, without precipitating allograft rejection. Prophylactic high dose oral acyclovir (3200 mg/day) effectively lowered the incidence and severity of serious CMV disease in kidney recipients (5). Hyperimmune CMV globulin therapy is now undergoing clinical investigation to determine its efficacy for both the prevention and adjunctive treatment of CMV disease in solid-organ transplant recipients.

Fungal Pathogens

Candida

Many factors following solid-organ transplantation predispose to serious *Candida* infection including broad spectrum antibiotic therapy for prophylaxis and perioperative bacterial infection, immunosuppression, visceral disruption due to surgery, parenteral nutrition, and the use of long-term central venous access lines. Liver transplant recipients have the highest rates of documented invasive candidiasis with one series demonstrating an incidence of 16% (61). Operative disruption of the biliary tree and proximal small intestines allowing local peritoneal inoculation no doubt plays a major role since the probability of *Candida* infection increases with total operative time (61).

Disseminated candidiasis usually presents with nonspecific clinical findings ranging from fever and constitutional symptoms to full blown sepsis and shock. Specific physical findings such as retinal exudates or nodular skin lesions are pathognomonic but are only present in a small minority. Suggestive laboratory features are elevations in the canalicular liver enzymes or unexplained renal insufficiency due to liver and kidney invasive disease respectively. Blood cultures are positive in no more than 30% of cases. Conversely, a blood culture positive for *Candida* should never be interpreted as either catheter-related, transient candidemia, or a contaminant in any transplant recipient. Clinical investigation of several circulating antigenic markers for deep-seated investigation are promising but still without proven sensitivity.

Amphotericin therapy (0.6 mg/kg/day) should be initiated early on an empiric basis when the diagnosis is suspected rather than proven. Addition of 5-flucytosine (150 mg/kg/day) has shown clinical benefit in some studies (44) though in vitro susceptibility testing should be requested. Fluconazole and itraconazole have shown promising efficacy in superficial *Candida*-related infection (mucositis, cystitis, and esophagitis), however, there are no large clinical trials at the current time to justify it as a primary agent.

Aspergillus

Aspergillus are ubiquitous molds capable of causing devastating infection in the transplant recipient. The most common sites of clinically evident disease are the lungs and the central nervous system though unsuspected systemic dissemination is not uncommon. Pneumonic involvement may manifest as either a focal consolidating process or diffuse patchy infiltration with or without true cavitation. Occasionally, wedge-shaped infiltrates representing actual pulmonary infarction due to proximal vessel invasion occur and should suggest invasive aspergillosis. Other suggestive features include clinical and radiographic deterioration despite broad spectrum antibacterial therapy, hemoptysis and recent clustering of documented cases of aspergillosis in the same ICU or institutional environment (63). *Aspergillus* is inconsistently isolated from either sputum or bronchoscopic specimens since this organism spreads hematogenously rather than being shed into the alveolus (37). Isolation of *Aspergillus* either by stain or culture in the organ transplant recipient with a pneumonic illness correlates significantly with invasive disease (129). Demonstration of tissue invasion by septate hyphae with dichotomous branching provides convincing evidence of invasive aspergillosis however this requires transbronchial or open lung biopsy. Skin lesions due to invasive aspergillosis often appear as eschar-like ulcers and are easily accessible for a histologic diagnosis.

Another major clinical manifestation of *Aspergillus* following organ transplantation are brain abscesses. These may occur with or without clinically evident pulmonary disease via hematogenous dissemination. Clinical presentation is usually acute with focal neurologic signs and secondary seizures in some. Computerized tomography of the brain may have single or multiple contrast enhancing lesions, nonhemorrhagic or hemorrhagic infarction. CSF findings are usually abnormal with a mild pleocytosis and elevated protein however the organism is rarely stained or cultured. Definitive diagnosis must be accomplished with stereotactic or open biopsy. Overall, the prognosis is grim with mortality rates in excess of 90% though renal transplant recipients have fared better.

In most instances, a clinical diagnosis of invasive aspergillosis is adequate justification for initiating antifungal therapy. High dose amphotericin B (1.0 mg/kg/day) with either 5-flucytosine or rifampin is still the principal therapeutic regimen. Recent experience with itraconazole for amphotericin intolerant individuals or clinical failures on amphotericin appears favorable, however, the drug is not available in parenteral form and a direct comparative trial versus amphotericin has still not been published (23, 31). In select cases, chances for definitive cure may be increased by surgical excision of isolated lung or brain lesions (46).

Cryptococcus

This budding yeast is one of the major etiologies of CNS infection in solid-organ transplant recipients. It is ubiquitous in nature and commonly gains access to the body via inhalation with silent dissemination to the meninges and other parts of the nervous system. A clinical pulmonary syndrome can occur with transient infiltrates, however, more usually, the patient is asymptomatic. CNS clinical presentation tends to be subacute with fever, headache, and mild alterations in mental status (18). Frank meningeal signs are not commonly present. Brain CT findings are usually normal though communicating hydrocephalus and even cerebral edema may be present in those with late presentations. Analysis of CSF is initially diagnostic in the majority of cases. A mild to moderate lymphocytic pleocytosis, depressed glucose, and elevated protein levels are usually found (74). Diagnosis from CSF is made of India ink stain in 50% of cases, latex agglutination for cryptococcal antigen, or fungal culture (42, 68). Serum cryptococcal antigen is also positive in approximately 50% of cases. Poor prognostic indicators include hypoglycorrhachia, positive India ink, a poor cellular response, and elevated opening CSF pressure (25).

Amphotericin B combined with 5-flucytosine has been the mainstay of therapy with excellent clinical response rates (8). Recent trials utilizing fluconazole have demonstrated comparable initial response rates in transplant recipients though patients with more severe disease had higher early mortality rates than those treated with amphotericin (62). Response to therapy should be monitored with serial analysis of CSF cell counts, chemistries, and the cryptococcal antigen titer. Intraventricular amphotericin (0.1–0.5 mg/day) has been utilized for severe or refractory cases though its independent value in altering clinical outcome is still debatable (83). Finally, patients with significant hydrocephalus may benefit from therapeutic drainage of CSF via an intraventricular or lumbar drain.

Protozoan Infection

Pneumocystis carinii

P. carinii is a ubiquitous protozoa with inherently low pathogenicity except in the setting of impaired lymphocyte-mediated immunity where it is capable of causing severe pneumonitis and respiratory failure. The frequency of pneumonia due to this organism had remained at a remarkably constant rate of 5–10% in all solid-organ recipients with the highest attack rate seen in the heart-lung recipient group. Over the past several years, the widespread use of chemoprophylaxis with TMP/SMX or aerosolized pentamidine has greatly reduced the incidence of this infection in all solid-organ recipients (50). Nevertheless, *P. carinii* pneumonia must be in the differential diagnosis of any immunosuppressed solid-organ recipient who presents with a diffuse or atypical pneumonitis since sporadic cases still occur due either to chemoprophylaxis failure from patient noncompliance, physician oversight in initiating appropriate chemoprophylaxis, or rarely, ineffectiveness of the chemoprophylaxis regimen itself.

Clinical manifestations of pneumonia most commonly include fever, dyspnea, and cough. Acute presentations are more common in solid-organ recipients in contrast to the more indolent course of onset affecting AIDS patients. The degree of respiratory insufficiency may be unimpressive initially with tachypnea and hypocapnia, however, rapid progression to refractory arterial hypoxemia may occur early. The most common radiographic findings when the clinical syndrome is already well established are bilateral diffuse interstitial and/or alveolar infiltrates (114). Early in the clinical course the chest film may appear atypical with predominantly unilateral or perihilar infiltrates and even lobar consolidation (115). Patients receiving aerosolized pentamidine prophylaxis who ultimately develop *P. carinii* pneumonia may even present with only bilateral apical involvement apparently due to the poor distribution of aerosolized pentamidine to the apical lung zones.

The diagnosis of *Pneumocystis* pneumonia is established by the microscopic demonstration of either the cyst or trophozoite forms from respiratory specimens or rarely lung tissue. The sensitivity of bronchoalveolar lavage in the transplant recipient does not equal the near 100% sensitivity in the AIDS population due to the smaller number of alveolar organisms present (124). Thus, the early institution of empiric anti-*Pneumocystis* therapy clouds the meaning of a negative bronchoalveolar lavage result obtained after several days of treatment. If clinical suspicion remains high, an open lung biopsy may be necessary to distinguish *Pneumocystis* pneumonia from other common similar entities including ARDS and CMV pneumonitis in the transplant recipient.

Early initiation of therapy drastically lowers *Pneumocystis* related mortality to less than 10%. Delaying empiric therapy in the hope of boosting the diagnostic yield of bronchoalveolar lavage is often poorly tolerated in the critically ill transplant recipient and unwarranted due to the excellent diagnostic sensitivity of the bronchoalveolar lavage method. Trimethoprim/sulfamethoxasole (20 mg/kg/day of trimethoprim i.v.) or pentamidine (4 mg/kg/day i.v.) are the two first line regimens for serious cases of *P. carinii* pneumonia. Response rates to both drugs are equivalent though pentamidine toxicity may be more serious, i.e., pancreatitis, hypoglycemia, and renal failure. An adequate clinical trial for either drug requires 3–5 days since both defervescence and improvement in the alveolararterial oxygen gradient may be delayed (20). Adjunctive therapy with high dose corticosteroids has recently been shown to reduce supplemental oxygen requirements and overall mortality in AIDS patients with severe *Pneumocystis* pneumonia, however, its efficacy in the solid-organ transplant recipient is as yet unproven (38).

Immunosuppressive Strategy with Concomitant Infection

The utilization of combination immunosuppressive therapy permits immunologic acceptance of the allograft tissue and has been instrumental in prolonging both patient and graft survival. Since there are no existing immunosuppressive agents which abort the immune response to donor-specific antigens all immunosuppressive therapy is by definition, nonspecific, with deleterious effects on host defense mechanisms against bacterial, viral, fungal, and protozoal infectious pathogens. Indeed, the risk of many infectious complications are either related to specific immunosuppressive agents, i.e., CMV disease and OKT3, or the total dose of others, i.e., corticosteroids and opportunistic bacterial or fungal infection. Reciprocally, well-intentioned tapering or withdrawal of baseline immunosuppression in order to promote immunologic recovery against the infectious process may precipitate florid allograft rejection and organ failure. Since rejection directly or indirectly comprises the second most common cause of mortality in organ recipients, an individualized and judicious approach is definitely warranted. Infections which are self limited or easily treated usually should not necessitate major reductions in immunosuppressive therapy.

For serious and or life-threatening infections, immunosuppression should be decreased to the minimally tolerable level while closely monitoring for clinical or laboratory signs of allograft rejection. Reduction of corticosteroids to the equivalent of 5 mg of prednisone may provide sufficient background immunosuppression though clinical vigilance for the symptoms and signs of adrenal insufficiency in stressed patients must be maintained. Reduction of cyclosporine dosage may be guided by daily trough blood levels into the low or even subtherapeutic range. Significant leukopenia or neutropenia due to azathioprine may potentiate bacterial or fungal infection and should be discontinued. OKT3 antilymphocyte therapy is a strong potentiator of many opportunistic pathogens including CMV, *Legionella*, *Listeria*, *Cryptococcus*, and *Pneumocystis* and should be avoided unless severe concurrent allograft rejection refractory to less potent immunosuppressive therapy ensues.

Infections which are self limited or easily treatable such as cystitis, superficial wound infection, *C. difficile* colitis probably require no adjustment in immunosuppression. Kidney recipients may tolerate low-

ering of their immunosuppression since renal dysfunction may be supplanted by hemodialysis while heart, heart-lung, and liver recipients lack such a practical artificial backup device for rejection related allograft failure. High risk subsets for acute rejection include a history of frequent or refractory acute rejection episodes, cadaveric kidney recipients, positive cytotoxic tissue crossmatch, and all organ recipients within three months of transplantation.

Overwhelming infection and superimposed allograft rejection are a relatively common scenario often precipitated by reduction in immunosuppression. Empiric misdiagnosis and treatment of allograft rejection based on nonhistologic findings will further predispose the patient to infection-related complications. Common reasons for biochemical evidence of allograft dysfunction unrelated to rejection include renal or hepatic drug toxicity, sepsis related dysfunction, and actual tissue invasion of the allograft, i.e., CMV hepatitis in allograft livers. Efficient targeting of immunosuppressive therapy in the critically ill organ recipient with serious infection must be guided by the liberal use of allograft biopsy which can provide unequivocal evidence of superimposed rejection.

References

1. Aisner J, Schimpff SC, Sutherland JC, et al. Torulopsis glabrata infections in patients with cancer: increasing incidence and relationship to colonization. Am J Med 1976;61:23–28.
2. Aisner J, Murillo J, Schimpff SC, et al. Invasive aspergillosis in acute leukemia: correlation with nose culture and antibiotic use. Ann Intern Med 1979;90:4–9.
3. Armstrong D. Listeria monocytogenes. In: Mandell GL, Douglas RG, Bennett JE, eds. Principles and practice of infectious diseases. 2nd ed. New York: Wiley, 1985:585–592.
4. Armstrong JA, Evans AS, Rao N, et al. Viral infections in renal transplant recipients. Infect Immun 1976;14:970–975.
5. Balfour HH, Chace BA, Stapleton JT. A randomized, placebo-controlled trial of oral acyclovir for the prevention of cytomegalovirus disease in recipients of renal allografts. N Engl J Med 1989;320:381.
6. Balikian JP, Herman PG, Kopit S. Pulmonary nocardiosis. Radiology 1978;126:569.
7. Bartlett JG. Diagnosis of bacterial infections of the lung. Clin Chest Med 1987;8:119–134.
8. Bennett JE, Dismukes WE, Duma RJ, et al. A comparison of amphotericin B alone and com-

bined with flucytosine in the treatment of cryptococcal meningitis. N Engl J Med 1979;301:126–131.

9. Bille J, Stockman L, Roberts GD, et al. Evaluation of a lysis-centrifugation system for recovery of yeast and filamentous fungi from blood. J Clin Microbiol 1983;18:469–473.

10. Binder HJ, Filburn B, Floch M. Bile acid elimination of intestinal anaerobic organisms. Am J Clin Nutr 1974;28:119–125.

11. Blank I, Oawaes RK. The water content of stratum corneum: the importance of water in promoting bacterial multiplication on cornified epithelium. J Invest Dermatol 1958;31:141–145.

12. Blazar BR, Hurd DD, Snover DC, et al. Invasive fusarium infections in bone marrow transplant recipients. Am J Med 1984;77:645–651.

13. Bodey GP, Alvarez ME, Jones PG, et al. Imipenem-cilastatin as initial therapy for febrile cancer patients. Antimicrob Agents Chemother 1986;30:211.

14. Centers for Disease Control. Aseptic meningitis among kidney transplant recipients receiving a newly marketed murine monoclonal antibody preparation. MMWR 1986;35:551–552.

15. Chatterje SN, Fiola M, Weiner J, et al. Primary cytomegalovirus and opportunistic infections: incidence in renal transplant recipients. JAMA 1978;240:2446–2449.

16. Chou S, Gallagher JC, Merigan TC. Controlled clinical trial of intravenous acyclovir to treat mucocutaneous herpes simplex virus infection after marrow transplantation. Lancet 1981;1:1392–1394.

17. Cluff LE, Reynolds RC, Page DL, et al. Staphylococcal bacteremia and altered host resistance. Ann Intern Med 1968;69:859.

18. Conti DJ, Rubin RH. Infection of the central nervous system in organ transplant recipients. Neurol Clin 1988; vol 6.

19. Crawford J, Ozer H, Stoller R et al. Reduction by granulocyte colony stimulating factor of fever and neutropenia induced by chemotherapy in patients with small cell lung cancer. N Engl J Med 1991;325:164–170.

20. Davey RT Jr, Masur H. Recent advances in the diagnosis, treatment and prevention of Pneumocystis carinii pneumonia. Antimicrob Agents Chemother 1990;34:499–504.

21. DeGregorio MW, Lee WMF, Linder CA, et al. Fungal infections in patients with acute leukemia. Am J Med 1982;73:543–548.

22. Dekker AW, Rozenberg-Arska M, Sixma JJ, et al. Prevention of infection by trimethoprim-sulfamethoxasole plus amphotericin B in patients with acute nonlymphocytic leukemia. Ann Intern Med 1981;95:555–559.

23. Denning DW, Tucker RM, Hanson LH. Treatment of invasive aspergillosis with itraconazole. Am J Med 1989;86:791–800.

24. Derbes SJ. Trimethoprim-induced aseptic meningitis. JAMA 1984;252:2865–2866.

25. Diamond RD, Bennett JE. Prognostic factors in cryptococcal meningitis: a study in 111 cases. Ann Intern Med 1974;80:176–181.

26. Du Moulin GJC, Paterson DG, Hedley-White J, et al. Aspirations of gastric bacteria in antacid-treated patients: A frequent cause of post-operative colonization of the airway. Lancet 1982;1:242.

27. Dummer JS, Armstrong J, Ho M, et al. Transmission of infection with herpes simplex virus by renal transplantation. J Infect Dis 1987;155:202–206.

28. Dunn DL, Simmons RL. Opportunistic infections after renal transplant. Part I. Viral and bacterial infections. Infect Surg 1989;8:164.

29. EORTC Antimicrobial therapy project group: Combination of amikacin and carbenicillin with or without cefazolin as empirical treatment of febrile neutropenic patients. J Clin Oncol 1983;1:597–603.

30. Erice A, Jordan MC, Chase BA, et al. Ganciclovir treatment of cytomegalovirus disease in transplant recipients and other immunocompromised hosts. JAMA 1987;257:3082–3087.

31. Faggian G, Livi U, Bortolotti U, et al. Itraconazole therapy for acute invasive pulmonary aspergillosis in heart transplantation. Transplant Proc 1989;21:2506–2507.

32. Fainstein V, Bodey GP, Elting L, et al. Amphotericin B or ketoconazole therapy of fungal infections in neutropenic cancer patients. Antimicrob Agents Chemother 1987;31:11.

33. Fairbank JT, Mamourian AC, Dietrich PA, et al. The chest radiograph in Legionnaires' disease. Radiology 1983;147:33–34.

34. Fanta CH, Pennington JE. Fever and new lung infiltrates in the immunocompromised host. Clin Chest Med 1981;2:19–39.

35. Felices FJ. Use of the central venous catheter to obtain blood cultures. Crit Care Med 1979;7:78.

36. Finland M. Changing ecology of bacterial infections as related to antibacterial therapy. J Infect Dis 1970;122:419–431.

37. Fischer BS, Armstrong D, Yu B, et al. Invasive aspergillosis. Progress in early diagnosis and treatment. Am J Med 1981;71:571–577.

38. Gagnon S, Boota AM, Fischl MA, et al. Corticosteroids as adjunctive therapy for severe pneumocystis carinii pneumonia in the acquired immunodeficiency syndrome. N Engl J Med 1990;323:1444.

39. Gerson SL, Talbot GH, Hurwitz S, et al. Prolonged granulocytopenia: the major risk factor for invasive pulmonary aspergillosis in patients with acute leukemia. Ann Intern Med 1984;100:345–351.

40. Gill FA, Robinson R, MacIowry JD, et al. The relationship of fever, granulocytopenia and antimicrobial therapy to bacteremia in cancer patients. Cancer 1977;39:1704.

41. Gombert ME, Josephson A, Goldstein EJC, et al. Cavitary Legionnaires' pneumonia: nosocomial infection in renal transplant recipients. Am J Surg 1984;147:402–405.

42. Goodman JS, Kaufman L, Keonig MG. Diagnosis of cryptococcal meningitis: value of immunologic detection of cryptococcal antigen. N Engl J Med 1971;285:434–436.

43. Hart PO, Russel E, Remington JS. The compromised host and infection. Deep fungal infection. J Infect Dis 1969;120:169–191.

44. Hawkins C, Armstrong D. Fungal infections in

the immunocompromised host. Clin Haematol. 1984;13:599–630.

45. Henry NK, McLimans CA, Wright AJ, et al. Microbiological and clinical evaluation of an isolator-lysis centrifugation blood culture tube. J Clin Microbiol 1983;17:864–869.

46. Henze G, Aldenhoff P, Stephani U, et al. Successful treatment of pulmonary and cerebral aspergillosis in an immunosuppressed child. Eur J Pediatr 1982;138:263.

47. Hinman F Jr, Cox, CE. The voiding vesical defense mechanism: the mathematical effect of residual urine, voiding interval and volume on bacteriuria. J Urol 1966;96:491–498.

48. Holleran WM, Wilbur JR, DeGregorio MW. Empiric amphotericin B therapy with acute leukemia. Rev Infect Dis 1985;7:619–624.

49. Horn R, Wong B, Kiehn TE, et al. Fungemia in a cancer hospital: changing frequency, earlier onset and results of therapy. Rev Infect Dis 1985;7:646–655.

50. Hughes WT, Kuhn S, Chaudhary S, et al. Successful chemoprophylaxis of Pneumocystis carinii pneumonia in adults. N Engl J Med 1977;297:1419–1426.

51. Hughes WT, Bodey GP, Meyers JD, et al. Guidelines for the use of antimicrobial agents in neutropenic patients with fever. J Infect Dis 1990;161:381.

52. Jensen S, Torben KG, Bacher T, et al. Ibuprofen-induced meningitis in a male with systemic lupus erythematosus. Acta Med Scand 1987;221:509–511.

53. Johanson WG, Pierce AK, Sanford JP. Changing pharyngeal bacterial flora of hospitalized patients. N Engl J Med 1969;281:1137–1140.

54. Johanson WG, Pierce AK, Sandord JP, et al. Nosocomial respiratory infections with gram negative bacilli. Ann Intern Med 1972;77:701.

55. Johanson WG Jr., Seidenfeld JJ, Gomez P, et al. Bacteriologic diagnosis of nosocomial pneumonia following prolonged mechanical ventilation. Am Rev Respir Dis 1988;137:259–264.

56. Kaye D. Host defense mechanisms of the urinary tract. Urol Clin North Am 1975;2:407.

57. Klastersky J, Zinner SH, Calandra T, et al. Empiric antimicrobial therapy for febrile granulocytopenic cancer patients: lessons from four EORTC trials. Eur J Cancer Clin Oncol 1988;24:S35–S45.

58. Klintmalm G, Lonnquist B, Oberg B, et al. Intravenous foscarnet for the treatment of severe cytomegalovirus infection in allograft recipients. Scand J Infect Dis 1985;17:157–163.

59. Kramer BS, Pizzo PA, Robichaud KJ, et al. Role of serial microbiological surveillance and clinical evaluation in the management of patients with fever and granulocytopenia. Am J Med 1982;72:561–567.

60. Krick J, Remington, J. Opportunistic fungal infection in patients with leukemia and lymphoma. Clin Haematol 1976;5:249–310.

61. Kusne S, Dummer JS, Ho M, et al. Infections after liver transplantation: an analysis of 101 consecutive cases. Medicine 1988;67:132–143.

62. Larsen RA, Leal MA, Chan LS. Fluconazole compared with amphotericin B and flucytosine for cryptococcal meningitis in the acquired immunodeficiency syndrome. Ann Intern Med 1990;113:183–187.

63. Lentino JR, Rosenkranz MA, Michaels JA, et al. Nosocomial aspergillosis: a retrospective review of airborne disease secondary to road construction and contaminated air conditioners. Am J Epidemiol 1982;116:430–437.

64. Lockshin MD, Kagen LJ. Meningitic reactions after azathioprine. N Engl J Med 1972;286:1321–1322.

65. Love LJ, Schimpff SC, Schiffer CA, et al. Improved prognosis for granulocytopenic patients with gram-negative bacteremia. Am J Med 1980;68:643.

66. Masur H, Shelhamer J, Parrillo JE. The management of pneumonia in immunocompromised patients. JAMA 1985;253:1769–1773.

67. Meduri GU. Ventilator associated pneumonia in patients with respiratory failure: a diagnostic approach. Chest 1990;97:1208–1209.

68. Meunier-Carpentier F. Cryptococcal meningitis: a case report and review of diagnostic procedures and therapy. Acta Clin Belg 1981;36:300–302.

69. Meunier-Carpentier F, Kiehn TE, Armstrong D. Fungemia in the immunocompromised host. Changing patterns, antigenemia, high mortality. Am J Med 1981;1:363–370.

70. Moellering RC Jr, Medoff G, Leech I, et al. Antibiotic synergism against Listeria monocytogenes. Antimicrob Agents Chemother 1972;1:30.

71. Parker MM, Parrillo JE. Septic shock. Hemodynamics and pathogenesis. JAMA. 1983;250:3324–3327.

72. Parrillo JE. The cardiovascular response to human septic shock. In: Fuhrman BP, Shoemaker WC, eds. Critical care: state of the art. Vol 10. Fullerton, California: Critical Care Medicine; 1989:285–314.

73. Parrillo JE. Septic shock in humans: clinical evaluation, pathophysiology, and therapeutic approach. In: Shoemaker WC, Thompson WL, Holbrook P, et al, eds. Textbook of critical care. 2nd ed. Philadelphia: WB Saunders, 1989:1006–1023.

74. Perfect JR. Cryptococcosis. In: Moellering RC Jr, Drutz DJ, eds. Fungal infections: diagnosis and treatment II. Infect Dis Clin North Am 1989;3(1):77–102.

75. Peterson EA, Nash ML, Mammana RB, et al. Minocycline treatment of pulmonary nocardiosis. JAMA 1983;250:930.

76. Peterson PK, Balfour HH Jr, Marker SC, et al. Cytomegalovirus disease in renal allograft recipients: a prospective study of the clinical features, risk factors and impact on renal transplantation. Medicine 1980;59:283–300.

77. Pizzo PA, Ladisch S, Simon R, et al. Increasing incidence of gram positive sepsis in cancer patients. Med Pediatr Oncol 1978;5:241.

78. Pizzo PA, Robichaud KJ, Gill FA, et al. Duration of empiric antibiotic in granulocytopenic cancer patient. Am J Med 1979;67:194.

79. Pizzo PA, Commers J, Cotton D, et al. Approaching the controversies in the antibacterial management of cancer patients. Am J Med 1981;76:436–439.

80. Pizzo PA, Robichaud KJ, Gill A, et al. Empiric antibiotic and antifungal therapy for cancer patients with prolonged fever and granulocytopenia. Am J Med 1982;72:101.
81. Pizzo PA, Robichaud KJ, Wesley R, et al. Fever in the pediatric and young adult patient with cancer: a prospective study of 1001 episodes. Medicine 1982;61:153.
82. Pizzo PA, Hathorn J, Hiemenz J, et al. A randomized trial comparing ceftazidime alone with combination antibiotic therapy in cancer patients with fever and neutropenia. N Engl J Med 1986;315:552–558.
83. Polsky B, Depman MR, Gold JWM, et al. Intraventricular therapy of cryptococcal meningitis via a subcutaneous reservoir. Am J Med 1986;81:24–28.
84. Press OW, Ramsey PG, Larson EB, et al. Hickman catheter infections in patients with malignancies. Medicine 63;1989:189.
85. Proctor DF, Andersen I, Lundgvist G. Clearance of inhaled particles from the human nose. Arch Intern Med 1973;131:132.
86. Rhodin JAG. Ultrastructure and function of the human tracheal mucosa. Am Rev Respir Dis 1966;(Suppl):1.
87. Robertson MJ, Larson RA. Recurrent fungal pneumonias in patients with acute nonlymphocytic leukemia undergoing multiple courses of intensive chemotherapy. Am J Med 1988;84:233–239.
88. Rubin RH, Levin M, Cohen C, et al. Summary of workshop on cytomegalovirus infections during organ transplantation. J Infect Dis 1979;139:728–734.
89. Rubin M, Hathorn JW, Marshall D, et al. Gram positive infections and the use of vancomycin in 550 episodes of fever and neutropenia. Ann Intern Med 1988;108:30.
90. Saravolatz LD, Burch KH, Fisher E, et al. The compromised host and Legionnaires' disease. Ann Intern Med 1979;90:533.
91. Schimpff SC. Diagnosis of infection in patients with cancer. Eur J Cancer 1975;11:S29–S38.
92. Schimpff SC, Moody MM, Young VM. Relationship of colonization with Pseudomonas aeruginosa to development of Pseudomonas bacteremia in cancer patients. Antimicrob Agents Chemother 1970;10:240–244.
93. Schimpff SC, Satterlee W, Young VM, et al. Empiric therapy with carbenicillin and gentamicin for febrile patients with cancer and granulocytopenia. N Engl J Med 1971;284:1061–1065.
94. Schimpff SC, Young VM, Greene WH, et al. Origin of infection in acute nonlymphocytic leukemia: significance of hospital acquisition of potential pathogens. Ann Intern Med 1972;77:707.
95. Schooley RT, Hirsch MS, Colvin RB, et al. Association of herpes virus infections with T-lymphocyte subset alterations, glomerulopathy, and opportunistic infection following renal transplantation. N Engl J Med 1983;308:307–313.
96. Simpson GL, Stinson EB, Egger MJ, et al. Nocardial infections in the immunocompromised host: A detailed study in a defined population. Rev Infect Dis 1981;3:492–507.
97. Singer C, Kaplan MH, Armstrong D. Bacteremia and fungemia complicating neoplastic disease. A study of 364 cases. Am J Med 1977;62:731–742.
98. Singh N, Dummer JS, Ho M, et al. Infections with cytomegalovirus and other herpes viruses in 121 liver transplant recipients: transmission by donated organs and the effect of OKT3 antibodies. J Infect Dis 1988;158:124–131.
99. Smith RF. Lactic acid utilization by the cutaneous Micrococcaceae. Microbiology 1971;21:777–779.
100. Stamm AM, Dismukes WE, Simmons BP, et al. Listeriosis in renal transplant recipients: report of an outbreak and review of 102 cases. Rev Infect Dis 1982;4:665.
101. Stein RS, Kayser J, Flexner JM. Clinical value of empirical amphotericin B in patients with acute myelogenous leukemia. Cancer 1982;50:2247–2251.
102. Stout J, Yu VL, Vickers RM, et al. Ubiquitousness of Legionella pneumophila in the water supply of a hospital with endemic Legionnaires' disease. N Engl J Med 1982;306:466–468.
103. Suwansirikul S, Rao N, Dowling JN, et al. Primary and secondary cytomegalovirus infection: clinical manifestations after renal transplantation. Arch Intern Med 1977;137:1026–1029.
104. Thorpe JE, Baughman RP, Frame PT, et al. Bronchoalveolar lavage for diagnosing acute bacterial pneumonia. J Infect Dis 1987;155:855–861.
105. Todd JK, Roe MH. Rapid detection of bacteremia by an early subculture technic. Am J Clin Pathol 1975;64:694–699.
106. Tomasi TB, Plaut AG. Humoral aspects of mucosal immunity. In: Gallin JI, Fauci AS eds. Advances in host defense mechanisms. Vol 4. New York: Raven, 1985:31–61.
107. Tonnesen A, Peuler M, Lackwood WR. Cultures of blood drawn by catheters vs venipuncture. JAMA 1976;235:1877.
108. van der Waay D, Berghuis-de Vries JM, Lekkerkerk-van der Wees JEC. Colonization resistance of the digestive tract and the spread of bacteria to the lymphatic organs in mice. J Hyg 1972;70:335–342.
109. Wade JC, Schimpff SC, Hargadon MT, et al. A comparison of trimethoprim-sulfamethoxazole plus nystatin with gentamicin in the prevention of infection in acute leukemia. N Engl J Med 1981;304:1067–1071.
110. Wade JC, Schimpff SC, Newman PA. Staphylococcus epidermidis: an increasing cause of infection in patients with granulocytopenia. Ann Intern Med 1982;97:503–508.
111. Wade JC, de Jongh CA, Newman KA, et al. Selective antimicrobial modulation as prophylaxis against infection during granulocytopenia: trimethoprim-sulfamethoxazole vs nalidixic acid. J Infect Dis 1983;147:624–634.
112. Wallace RJ Jr, Septimus EJ, Williams TW Jr, et al. Use of trimethoprim-sulfamethoxasole for treatment of infections due to Nocardia. Rev Infect Dis 1982;4:315.
113. Walling DM, McGraw DJ, Merz WG, et al. Dis-

seminated infection with Trichosporon beigelii. Rev Infect Dis 1987;9:1013–1019.

114. Walzer PD, Perl DP, Krogstad DJ, et al. Pneumocystis carinii pneumonia in the United States: epidemiologic, diagnostic and clinical features. Ann Intern Med 1974;80:83–93.

115. Walzer PD, Kim CK, Cushion MT. Pneumocystis carinii. In: Walzer PD, Genta RM, eds. Parasitic infections in the compromised host. New York: Marcel Dekker, 1989:83–178.

116. Washington JA II. Blood cultures–principles and techniques. Mayo Clin Proc 1975;59:91–98.

117. Washington JA II. Blood cultures: issues and controversies. Rev Infect Dis 1986;8:792–802.

118. Wiesner RH, Hermans PE, Rakela J, et al. Selective bowel decontamination to decrease gram negative aerobic colonization and prevent infection after orthotopic liver transplantation. Transplantation 1988;45:570.

119. Wing EJ, Norden CW, Shadduck RK, et al. Use of quantitative bacteriologic techniques to diagnose catheter related sepsis. Arch Intern Med 1979;139:482–488.

120. Wingard JR, Merz WG, Saral R. Candida tropicalis: a major pathogen in immunocompromised patients. Ann Intern Med 1979;91:539–543.

121. Winston DJ, Barnes RC, Ho WG, et al. Moxalactam plus piperacillin versus moxalactam plus amikacin in febrile granulocytopenic patients. Am J Med 1984;77:442–450.

122. Winston DJ, Gale RP, Meyer DV, et al. Infectious complications of human bone marrow transplantation. Medicine 1989;58:1–59.

123. Yoo D, Lee HS, Kwong-Chung KJ. Brain abscess due to Pseudallescheria boydii associated with primary non-Hodgkin's lymphoma of the central nervous system: a case report and literature review. Rev Infect Dis 1985;7:272–277.

124. Young JA, Hopkin JM, Cuthbertson WP. Pulmonary infiltrates in immunocompromised patients: diagnosis by cytological examination of bronchoalveolar lavage fluid. J Clin Pathol 1984;37:390–397.

125. Young LS. Amikacin: experience in a comparative clinical trial with gentamicin in leukopenic subjects. In: Luthy R, Siegenthaler W, eds. Current chemotherapy. Washington, DC: American Society for Microbiology, 1978:246–248.

126. Young LS: Combination or single drug therapy for gram negative sepsis. In: Mandell G, Douglas JG, Bennett JV, et al, eds. Hospital infections. Boston: Little, Brown, 1979:489–506.

127. Young LS. Treatment of infections due to gram negative bacilli: a perspective of past, present and future. Rev Infect Dis. 1985;7(suppl 4):572–578.

128. Yu VL, Gjoetz A, Wagener M, et al. Staphylococcus aureus nasal carriage and infections in patients on hemodialysis. Efficacy of antibiotic prophylaxis. N Engl J Med 1986;2:91–96.

129. Yu VL, Muder RR, Poorsattar A. Significance of isolation of Aspergillus from the respiratory tract in diagnosis of invasive pulmonary aspergillosis. Am J Med 1986;81:249–254.

130. Zervos MJ, Dembinki S, Mikesell TS, et al. High-level gentamicin resistance in Streptococcus faecalis: risk factors and evidence for exogenous acquisition of infection. J Infect Dis 1986;153:1075–1083.

131. Ziegler EJ, Fisher CJ, Sprung CL, et al. Treatment of gram negative bacteremia and septic shock with HA-1A human monoclonal antibody against endotoxin. A randomized double blind placebo controlled trial. N Engl J Med 1991;324:429–436.

132. Zuravleff JJ, Yu VL, Shonnard JW, et al. Diagnosis of Legionnaires' disease. An update of laboratory methods with new emphasis on isolation by culture. JAMA 1983;1981–1985.

51

HIV Infection and Acquired Immunodeficiency Syndrome

Mary B. Ramundo
Bruce F. Farber

The Centers for Disease Control estimates that there are one million people infected with the human immunodeficiency virus (HIV) in the United States. Physicians in all specialties will be called upon to care for HIV-infected patients. Our knowledge of this infection and its effects is increasing every day. In keeping with the theme of this text, this chapter focuses on the pathophysiology of HIV infection and some of the critical care problems that are common to patients infected with this virus.

Human immunodeficiency virus I (HIV-I) has been clearly identified as the cause of the acquired immunodeficiency syndrome (AIDS). This virus is a member of a subfamily of retroviruses, the lentiviruses, which includes simian immunodeficiency virus, the visna virus of sheep, feline immunodeficiency virus, and equine infectious anemia virus. All of these viruses have a long incubation period, a tropism for hematopoietic and nervous system tissues, and an association with immune suppression. HIV is endemic throughout the world. Two HIVs have been identified. HIV-II is found mostly in western Africa, and it is more closely related to the simian immunodeficiency virus. There is less than 50% homology between the genomes of HIV-I and HIV-II (21). The following discussion is based on information on HIV-I.

PATHOGENESIS

Like other retroviruses, the HIV-I RNA genome is divided into *gag, pol,* and *env* coding regions. The genome also codes for at least six regulatory proteins. The *gag* and *env* genes code for the major structural proteins of the virus, and the *pol* region codes for the enzyme reverse transcriptase. The virus has an icosahedral structure with 72 external spikes. Each spike is formed by two major viral proteins: gp120 and gp41. The virus core is composed of four nucleocapsid proteins of which p24 is the chief component (21). The core also contains two copies of single-stranded RNA, with the viral enzymes closely associated with the genetic material. The CD4 membrane antigen serves as a high-affinity receptor for HIV, and cells that express the CD4 molecule are the targets of HIV infection. CD4-positive lymphocytes (T4 or T helper cells) and monocytes are the major cellular targets for HIV, but it may also infect Langerhans cells, microglial cells, gastrointestinal epithelial cells, and bone marrow progenitor cells. This may help to explain the hematological abnormalities, the neurological disease, and the diarrheal-wasting syndrome that can be seen in HIV-infected patients. A gp120 molecule binds to the CD4 membrane receptor and gp41-mediated membrane fusion occurs (36). The HIV RNA genome enters the cell where reverse transcriptase acts to produce a double-stranded DNA product from the RNA template. The double-stranded DNA is integrated into the cellular genome and the viral DNA is then referred to as a provirus. In this manner, HIV establishes a latent or persistent infection. This may account for the long latency period between seroconversion to HIV and the development of AIDS.

The basis of viral latency is unclear, but

it may be related to the state of cellular activation as many viruses do not replicate in resting T cells. Activation of T cells promotes HIV replication; therefore chronic infection with microbes may activate HIV expression (20). Transcription of the host cell genome results in transcription of the provirus. The viral RNA drives production of viral proteins and the formation of virions that may bud from the cell membrane. HIV infection may procede differently in different cell populations. In macrophages, the virus replicates continuously, but slowly, resulting in alteration of cell function without cell lysis. In T helper cells, the virus can lay dormant for an indefinite period of time, but when the T cells are stimulated the virus destroys the cell with a burst of viral replication (24). New virus, which buds from macrophage membrane or is released with lysis of T cells, can in turn infect other CD4-bearing cells. Viral replication alone cannot account for destruction of T4 cells. HIV replication can be demonstrated only in a small percentage of T4 cells isolated from HIV-infected patients. Infected cells can express gp120 on their surface. This gp120 may bind with the CD4 of one or more uninfected cells resulting in syncytial formation and death of the uninfected cells. Free gp120 may bind to the CD4 receptor of uninfected cells targeting these cells for attack by the immune system (36). It is the killing of the CD4-positive subset of T cells that leads to the immunodeficiency syndrome characteristic of HIV infection.

CD4-positive T lymphocytes serve as regulators and effectors of the normal immune response. These cells recognize foreign antigen on infected cells and help activate B lymphocytes to multiply and produce antibodies. The presence of HIV effects an overstimulation of B cells, resulting in elevated antibody production and enlargement of the lymph nodes. Therefore, there is a decrease in the number of resting B cells that can differentiate to produce antibody in response to new pathogens. T4 lymphocytes are also important in cell-mediated immunity: the killing of infected cells by cytotoxic T cells and NK cells. Macrophages are influenced by T4 lymphocytes to secrete cytokines,

Table 51.1
Functional Abnormalities of T4 Lymphocytes in HIV Infection

Defective induction of B cells to secrete Ig
Defective response to alloantigens and soluble Ag
Decreased expression of interleukin-2 receptors
Decreased Ag or mitogen-induced IL-2 production
Decreased ability to form T cell colonies in vitro

which modulate the activity of many other cell populations. T4 lymphocytes also secret cytokines that stimulate proliferation of T cells, so a decrease in the number of T4 cells may serve to alter the amount and function of cytokines. In addition to the fall in the total number of T4 cells, there are functional abnormalities of T4 lymphocytes in HIV infection (Table 51.1) (38). Therefore, both qualitative and quantitative changes in the T4 lymphocyte population results in impairment of multiple aspects of the immune systems.

CLINICAL MANIFESTATIONS

HIV-infected patients are most susceptible to infections that require functional cell-mediated immunity for eradication of the organisms. The reduction in the quantity of T4 lymphocytes especially impairs the body's defense against viruses, fungi, parasites, and certain bacteria, including mycobacteria. Although HIV can damage organs directly, most of the illness and death associated with AIDS results from progressive damage of the immune system and the development of opportunistic infections. Opportunistic infections are defined as infections with organisms that rarely cause disease in people with normal immune systems. These infections often represent reactivation of quiescent infection that was previously held in check by the patient's immune system. Stimulation of the immune system by infection can increase HIV expression. Therefore, the main goal of therapy in these patients is the treatment and prevention of opportunistic infections. At the present time, antiretroviral therapy can slow the HIV-related damage to the immune system, but it does not eradicate the virus. Therapies such as soluble CD4 may interfere with the binding of the viral gp120 with CD4 on cells. Most of the other available agents such as 3'-azido-2',3'-dideoxythymidine (AZT), 2',3'-dideoxycytidine (ddC), and 2',3'-dideoxyinosine (ddI) act by interfering with reverse transcriptase. These drugs are phosphorylated intracellularly to the triphosphate form, which competes with the normal deoxynucleoside 5'-triphosphate (21). Incorporation of the drug triphosphate results in chain termination. A discussion of antiretroviral therapy is beyond the scope of this chapter.

People are exposed to HIV via three main routes: sexual, perinatal, or parenteral (through sharing needles for drug use, transfusion of HIV-positive blood products, or accidental needle stick). Usually within 6 months of exposure, antibodies to HIV can be detected in the patient's blood. There is an asymptomatic phase, with the median incubation period being 10 years before the patient shows clinical signs of immunodeficiency. A healthy individual has an average of 1000 T4 lymphocytes/mm^3 of blood. In an HIV-infected patient, when the T4 count is between 200 and 400 cells/mm^3, the patient may begin to experience infections such as thrush, shingles, and severe dermatophyte infection. Patients may develop fever, weight loss, and diarrhea, and this symptom complex is referred to as ARC (AIDS-related complex). When the T4 count is below 200 cells/mm^3, patients are at increased risk for developing infections with *Pneumocystis carinii*, *Toxoplasma gondii*, and *Cryptococcus neoformans*. It is often infections with these organisms that place HIV-infected patients in the realm of the critical care physician.

PULMONARY DISEASE

Pneumocystis carinii

The most common indication for admission of AIDS patients to the ICU is for respiratory failure secondary to *Pneumocystis carinii* pneumonia (PCP). It is not clear if *Pneumocystis carinii* is a parasite or a fungus. It is probably transmitted by droplet infection, and most adults are thought to harbor this organism in the lung although person-to-person transmission has never been documented (32). The pathophysiology of this infection is unclear.

Pneumocystis carinii pneumonia is developed in an animal model by exposing the animal to the organism and treating the animal with high doses of corticosteroids. Pathological studies show evidence for an active inflammatory response in the lung. Biopsy specimens reveal alveoli filled with white blood cells, protein, and trophozoites and cysts of *Pneumocystis carinii*. There is hyperplasia of type II pneumocytes. The spectrum of lung injury with PCP is similar to that seen in adult respiratory distress syndrome (ARDS). Hyaline membranes and pulmonary hemorrhage are less likely to be demonstrated in biopsies from patients with PCP (13, 31). Fibrosis is seen in biopsies from patients who died from PCP.

Pneumocystis carinii pneumonia occurs in up to 80% of patients with AIDS at some time during their illness. Approximately 25% of these patients develop respiratory failure (19). The most common presenting symptoms are fever, cough, shortness of breath, and pleuritic chest pain. The most common chest x-ray finding is bilateral interstitial infiltrates. A wide variety of x-ray patterns have been reported with PCP including: a localized infiltrate, cystic or honeycomb lesions, hilar adenopathy, and a spontaneous pneumothorax (11). Bronchoscopic alveolar lavage (BAL) reveals the organisms in approximately 90% of patients. The addition of transbronchial biopsy increases the yield to greater than 95% (27). Even with treatment, the organism is not completely eradicated and patients are at risk of developing recurrent PCP. Patients with T4 counts of less than 200 cells/mm^3 or a history of PCP are put on prophylactic therapy for PCP. In patients receiving aerosolized pentamidine therapy for PCP prophylaxis, breakthrough PCP does occur, but the symptoms are milder and it is more difficult to diagnose. The yield on bronchoscopic alveolar lavage is decreased to approximately 62%, but approaches 100% in patients with their third or fourth episode of PCP. The yield on transbronchial biopsy in patients on aerosol pentamidine is equal to the yield in untreated patients (27).

In intubated patients, nonbronchoscopic or endotracheal lung lavage can be performed for diagnosis. This procedure has an overall sensitivity of 86%, and there is no significant oxygen desaturation as is often seen with bronchoscopic lavage (29). In nonintubated patients, a sputum sample may be obtained after inhalation of 3% saline via a nebulizer. These specimens have a 56% sensitivity, although the sensitivity varies from institution to institution (5).

The two main drugs used to treat PCP are pentamidine and trimethoprim/sulfamethoxazole (TMP/SMX). These two drugs are equally effective; however, they both have side effects that frequently require change in therapy. Approximately 50% of patients on TMP/SMX and 20% of patients on pentamidine have their therapy discontinued because of adverse effects (43). Trimethoprim/sulfamethoxazole is given in a total daily dose of 15–20 mg/kg, which is divided into three or four doses. The duration of therapy is 2–3 weeks. Side effects include: anorexia, nausea, vomiting, neutropenia, thrombocytopenia, fever, rash, hepatitis, nephritis, toxic epidermal necrolysis, and Stevens-Johnson syndrome. Pentamidine is used in patients who are sulfa-allergic or who fail to respond to intravenous TMP/SMX within 5–7 days. Pentamidine is given in a single daily intravenous dose of 4 mg/kg infused over 1–2 hr. The duration of therapy is 2–3 weeks. Sterile abscesses form at the injection in patients who receive the drug intramuscularly. The major side effects include: hypotension, renal failure, hypoglycemia, hyperglycemia, leukopenia, thrombocytopenia, pancreatitis, and ventricular arrhythmias. In patients who fail pentamidine or TMP/SMX, other compounds have been tried such as trimetrexate and clindamycin.

Recently there has been a great amount of discussion regarding the use of steroids in the treatment of PCP. There have been several recent studies to evaluate the possible benefit of adjunctive steroids in the treatment of PCP. The general concensus is that steroids are beneficial in moderately severe PCP. Two studies (7, 18) demonstrated that steroids used as early adjuvant therapy for PCP resulted in a decreased risk of respiratory failure and a decreased risk of death. Neither study demonstrated a significant increase in infections or neoplasms in the steroid-treated group. One study did report a 25% relapse rate on withdrawal of the steroids (18). In patients with PCP and a Pao_2 less than 70 mm Hg on room air, the equivalent of prednisone, 40 mg every 12 hr or 60 mg every 24 hr, should be given for 5–7 days with the dose tapered to zero by day 21. It is unclear why steroids are beneficial in PCP. It may be that TMP/SMX or pentamidine kill the organisms, resulting in an increased inflammatory response. This is consistent with the fact that many patients show increased oxygen desaturation during the first 4 days of anti-*Pneumocystis* therapy. Steroids may help suppress this inflammatory response.

Another consideration in patients with moderate to severe PCP is the use of continuous positive airway pressure (CPAP) by face mask instead of by endotracheal intubation and mechanical ventilation. Gregg and his coworkers used CPAP in 18 patients with PCP who were in hypoxic respiratory failure. The mean change in Pao_2 ranged from 62 to 158 mm Hg and the respiratory rate decreased from 51 to 32 breaths/min. There was no significant change in the $Paco_2$ in these patients. The patients were on CPAP for a mean of 4.5 days. In general, CPAP was effective and well tolerated with no aspiration complications in any of the patients. One patient developed a pneumothorax and five patients had progressive deterioration in their respiratory status, requiring endotracheal intubation. The overall hospital mortality was 55% (22). CPAP may be an alternative to intubation in patients with PCP who are not hypercarbic and who are conscious and able to protect their airway.

Survival rates in patients with PCP and respiratory failure vary in different studies. Friedman and associates studied patients with PCP who had a $Paco_2 < 60$ mm Hg with a Fio_2 of at least 40%. They reported a survival rate to discharge of 36% (17). The survival rate was not different in patients receiving pentamidine versus TMP/SMX. Another study reported an overall survival rate of 54.5% in patients requiring mechanical ventilation for their first episode of PCP, and a 25% survival rate for patients with a second episode of PCP and respiratory failure (12). Although it was not statistically significant, survivors had a shorter duration of symptoms prior to admission. In a retrospective study by El-Sadr and Simberkoff, there was no difference between survivors and nonsurvivors in terms of age, risk factor, drug therapy, or use of steroids. Survivors had a shorter duration of symptoms prior to admission, better Pao_2 levels on admission, and a history of deterioration occurring shortly after bronchoscopy (13).

Other Pathogens

There are a multitude of other pathogens that can cause serious pulmonary disease in patients with HIV infection: cytomegalovirus (CMV), *Cryptococcus*, *Aspergillus*, *Mycobacterium tuberculosis*, and a wide variety of bacteria. These, however, are much less likely to result in disease causing respiratory failure. Patients with AIDS can also have extensive pulmonary involvement with Kaposi's sarcoma, which can result in respiratory compromise.

Pneumothorax

Another pulmonary problem that is occurring with increased frequency in patients with AIDS is spontaneous pneumothorax. There have been an increasing number of reports of pneumothoraces in patients with PCP or in patients on prophylactic aerosol pentamidine. In 1988 Martinez and his coinvestigators reported on 6 cases of spontaneous pneumothoraces in AIDS patients without active PCP. All of the patients had at least one previous episode of PCP and all were on aerosol pentamidine for PCP prophylaxis (30). More recently Sepkowitz and associates looked at pneumothoraces in AIDS. They noted an increased risk of developing a pneumothorax with an increase in the number of past episodes of PCP; however, the num-

bers did not reach statistical significance. They concluded that aerosol pentamidine alone was a significant risk factor for the development of pneumothorax. Ninety-five percent of the patients with pneumothorax had evidence for concurrent PCP. The overall mortality in this group was 10%, but there was significant morbidity. Most patients responded to chest tube placement of sclerotherapy, but 25% of the patients required thoracotomy. Pneumothorax recurred in 65%, most commonly occurring in the contralateral lung (41).

Pathological studies have helped to elucidate the etiology of these pneumothoraces. In patients who die from PCP, the lungs show an interstitial inflammatory process with tissue destruction, which is most pronounced in the periphery of the lungs (4). Radiotracer aerosol studies confirm poor apical delivery of aerosol in the lungs (39). Therefore a persistent focal infection with *Pneumocystis carinii* may exist in the apices or periphery of the lungs. The tissue destruction and fibrosis results in the formation of blebs or pneumatoceles, which may rupture, resulting in a spontaneous pneumothorax.

One study compared spontaneous pneumothoraces in non-AIDS patients and AIDs patients. Ninety-seven percent of non-AIDS patients with spontaneous pneumothoraces survived to hospital discharge, whereas 40% of AIDS patients with spontaneous pneumothoraces (unrelated to mechanical ventilation) died. All of the AIDS patients with spontaneous pneumothoraces had a documented pulmonary infection, most commonly PCP. Non-AIDS patients required tube thoracostomy for an average of 5.7 days, whereas AIDS patients required 8–12 days for their air leak to resolve (8). No patient who had a tension pneumothorax, or an air leak for >12 days, was successfully treated. Therefore, it is important to rule out active PCP in any AIDS patient who presents with a pneumothorax. Closed tube thoracostomy is the treatment of choice, but if an air leak is present for more than 7 days pleurectomy should be considered in patients who can tolerate thoracotomy (16). Some surgeons recommend a midline incision with oversewing of apical blebs on both sides.

This is recommended because of the significant incidence of recurrent pneumothorax on the contralateral side.

NEUROLOGICAL DYSFUNCTION

Toxoplasma

Neurological disease is probably the second most common reason for AIDS patients to be admitted to the ICU. The most common presentation of neurological disease requiring intensive care management is seizures. There is a multitude of central nervous system (CNS) disease in AIDS that can present as seizures. *Toxoplasma gondii* is the most common cause of CNS disease in people with AIDS. *T. gondii* is a parasite that is transmitted by contact with feces from an infected cat, or ingestion of undercooked meat from an infected animal. In the United States, approximately 20% of adults harbor *T. gondii* in their brain or muscle tissue. *Toxoplasma* encephalitis occurs in 30–40% of AIDS patients with positive antibodies to *T. gondii* (32). These patients can present with nonlocalizing symptoms such as myoclonus, asterixis, coma, confusion, or lethargy, but focal hemiparesis and seizures may also occur. Although negative *Toxoplasma* serology does not rule out *Toxoplasma* disease, it makes it unlikely. There have been reports of biopsy-proven *Toxoplasma* encephalitis in patients with negative *Toxoplasma* serology. A CT scan or MRI usually shows single or multiple nodular or ring-enhancing lesions with edema or mass effect. This CT scan pattern is not diagnostic for *Toxoplasma* infection. The use of steroids can cause a false-negative scan. Cohn and coworkers evaluated empiric therapy of suspected *Toxoplasma* encephalitis in patients with AIDS. They reported a sensitivity of 100% for positive *Toxoplasma* serology. There was no difference in response rates in biopsy-proven cases versus empirically treated cases. No relapses were seen in patients who were continued on antitoxoplasma therapy. Fifty-three percent of the treated patients developed toxicities that required a change in the therapeutic regimen (10). Lumbar puncture is usually not helpful in making the diagnosis.

Toxoplasma encephalitis is treated with combination therapy of pyrimethamine and sulfadiazine. Pyrimethamine is usually given in a single daily dose of 25–50 mg. Some people recommend an initial loading dose of up to 200 mg. The daily dose may need to be increased depending on patient response. Sulfadiazine is used in doses of 2–4 g/day given in divided doses every 6 hr. Both of these drugs affect folic acid metabolism. They are effective against only the trophozoite stage of *Toxoplasma*, so cysts remain viable (45). This may account for the high rate of relapse. Levcovorin (folinic acid), 10 mg/day, should be given in combination with this treatment regimen to alleviate bone marrow suppression. Toxicities of pyrimethamine and sulfadiazine include: neutropenia, fever, hepatitis, renal insufficiency, rash, anemia, and thrombocytopenia. Clindamycin (300–600 mg p.o. or i.v. every 6 hr) can be substituted for sulfadiazine in patients that are sulfa-allergic. Steroids may be used transiently in patients with evidence of mass effect, but no difference in survival has been demonstrated in patients who did or did not receive steroids (10). Most patients will show a clinical and roentgenographic response after 1–3 weeks of therapy. Because of the high rate of relapse, lifelong therapy is required. Patients with positive *Toxoplasma* serology and a consistent picture on CT scan should be treated empirically with pyrimethamine and sulfadiazine. Brain biopsy should be considered if there is no clinical response in 10–14 days, new lesions develop on therapy, or the CT scan pattern is atypical for *Toxoplasma* encephalitis.

Cryptococcus

Another central nervous system infection that can present with seizures is cryptococcal meningitis. This infection occurs in approximately 10% of patients with AIDS, and it has a high mortality (32). The yeast *Cryptococcus neoformans* usually enters the body via the lungs, and disseminates via the bloodstream to the meninges. Patients usually present with fever, headache, and stiff neck. A serum cryptococcal antigen is usually positive. Cerebrospinal fluid (CSF) reveals pleocytosis with 5–50 mononuclear cells/mm³, slightly elevated protein, and a normal glucose. India ink examination of the CSF reveals organisms in 50–90% of cases and cryptococcal antigen is positive in more than 95% of patients. Cultures of the CSF are usually positive. Cryptococcal meningitis is treated with intravenous amphotericin B with or without flucytosine. Amphotericin B binds to the cholesterol-like substance that is unique to the cell membrane of fungi, resulting in a leaky membrane and death of the organism. Patients receiving amphotericin B may experience fever and chills. Intravenous hydrocortisone (25–50 mg), used as a premedication, may decrease the intensity of these reactions. Pretreatment with ibuprofen, or acetaminophen, and benadryl, may also help to minimize the adverse effects. Dose-dependent azotemia is observed in most patients, but this is usually transient, and minimal permanent renal damage occurs. Improved hydration, dose reduction, and discontinuation of other nephrotoxic agents will help improve renal function. Flucytosine may cause bone marrow suppression and gastrointestinal distress. As with other infections in AIDS, there is a significant relapse rate, so patients need lifelong treatment for cryptococcal meningitis. A newer antifungal agent, fluconazole, given at doses of 200–400 mg daily, can be effective for maintenance therapy. This drug has been well tolerated with minimal side effects.

Other Entities

Progressive multifocal leukoencephalopathy is a reactivation of infection with the JC papovavirus. Patients with AIDS have a higher incidence of central nervous system lymphoma. Both of these entities can cause focal lesions on CT scan, and they are more likely to present as focal neurological deficits and not seizures. There is limited therapy available for these lesions. Bacterial meningitis can cause seizures, but these infections are in no way unique to patients with AIDS.

Holtzman and coworkers evaluated new onset seizures in HIV infection. They found that mass lesions were the major cause of

seizures. In approximately 25% of the patients, HIV-induced dementia was the only neurological abnormality. Atrophy with subcortical white matter abnormalities is seen on CT scan, and cerebrospinal fluid reveals a mild lymphocytic pleocytosis. In patients with a normal interictal neurological examination, there was a low probability of identifying a cause for seizures. The seizures were often recurrent, even in patients in which no cause could be identified. The researchers concluded that HIV encephalopathy was the most common cause of seizures in patients infected with HIV (25). Mass lesions should be suspected in patients with status epilepticus or with seizures that are difficult to control. All patients should be treated with anticonvulsants and evaluated with a CT scan with intravenous contrast material or MRI and to rule out structural lesion. In addition, lumbar puncture should be performed to look for infectious pathogens. These patients may require intubation to protect their airway until the seizures are adequately controlled.

Patients with HIV disease are at increased risk of cerebral infarction or transient neurological deficits (14). It should be noted that these entities are often associated with a treatable, underlying infection. Therefore, these patients should be evaluated with a CT scan and lumbar puncture to look for a potentially treatable lesion.

CARDIAC MANIFESTATIONS

There have been an increasing number of articles published on the cardiac manifestations of HIV infection. These manifestations should be mentioned briefly, as they fall into the realm of ICU care of HIV-positive patients. Postmortem studies have revealed more cardiac disease in HIV-positive patients than was suspected clinically antemortem. The percent of HIV-positive patients with cardiac abnormalities varies in different studies. Several studies have shown that there is a greater prevalence of cardiac disease in patients with low T4 counts or AIDS versus patients that have asymptomatic HIV infection (28, 34).

There is a wide range of myocardial

pathology reported. Myocardial involvement has been demonstrated with *T. gondii*, *Mycobacterium avium intracellulare*, *Histoplasma capsulatum*, *Cryptococcus neoformans*, *Pneumocystis carinii*, cytomegalovirus, HIV, Kaposi's sarcoma, and lymphoma. Chest x-ray reveals cardiomegaly and echocardiogram demonstrates mono- or biventricular dilatation. Right ventricular hypertrophy can be seen in patients with repeated pulmonary infections. On pathological examination, the myocardium exhibits lymphocytic myocarditis with or without necrosis. There are many theories as to the pathogenesis of the myocarditis: anemia, malnutrition, catecholamine excess, or direct effect of HIV. Pericardial disease in patients with HIV is also common, and pericardial effusion is the most common cardiac abnormality seen. The list of infectious and neoplastic etiologies is similar to the above list for myocarditis. Endocarditis is also seen in this population. Obviously, patients with a history of intravenous drug use are at high risk for infectious endocarditis with bacteria or fungi; however, thrombotic endocarditis may be more common. Vascular lesions described as fibrocalcific arteriopathy with or without aneurysms have also been reported (1).

There are also drug-related, cardiovascular problems seen in AIDS. Amphotericin B may cause hypotension and it may predispose patients to arrhythmias because of its effect on potassium and magnesium levels. Pentamidine can cause recurrent, ventricular tachycardia that has a torsades pattern (33). Pentamidine is similar in structure to procainamide, and it may cause bradycardia and prolongation of the Q-T interval. Torsades in this situation is treated with isoproterenol, CaCl, MgSO$_4$, and a temporary pacemaker if necessary. The arrhythmia usually resolves with discontinuation of pentamidine therapy.

RENAL DYSFUNCTION

Nephrotoxicity secondary to pentamidine and other drugs used in the management of AIDS patients is just one of the many renal complications seen in HIV disease. Knowledge of the renal complications of HIV infection is important in the critical care management of these patients. The renal manifestations of HIV infection include proteinuria, focal segmental glomerulosclerosis, acute renal insufficiency, and fluid and electrolyte disturbances. HIV nephropathy may be an early manifestation of disease. This entity is defined by heavy proteinuria (more than 2 g/24 hr) or nephrotic syndrome with focal segmental glomerulosclerosis (FSGS) on pathological examination. Focal segmental glomerulosclerosis is the most common pathological lesion, with mesangial hyperplasia the second most common (6). Other lesions that are observed include: acute tubular necrosis, interstitial nephritis, and nephrocalcinosis. Invasion of the kidneys by opportunistic pathogens or neoplasms has also been reported. HIV nephropathy most commonly presents as decreased renal function or proteinuria. Renal ultrasound demonstrates increased echogenicity of the kidneys. More than 50% of patients with HIV infection and nephrotic syndrome or FSGS are otherwise asymptomatic HIV carriers (6). The prevalence of HIV nephropathy is lower in white homosexuals than in other risk groups. It is much more common in blacks.

There has been a great deal of debate whether intravenous drug use is an independent risk factor for renal disease. A large study by Pardo found that patients with FSGS were more likely to have clinical manifestations of renal disease than were patients with mesangial hyperplasia. Fifty percent of the addicts in their study had renal disease. The high incidence of renal disease in the pediatric patients suggests that HIV nephropathy exists independent of intravenous drug use. The incidence of renal pathology in intravenous drug users with AIDS was much greater than the incidence of renal disease in intravenous drug users without AIDS (35). Humphreys and Schoenfeld observed no difference in the time to progression to uremia in AIDS patients with a history of intravenous drug use versus AIDS patients without a history of intravenous drug use (26). This supports the theory that AIDS nephropathy and the nephropathy associated with intravenous drug use are discrete entities. Carbone and his coworkers studied HIV-positive patients with FSGS on renal biopsy (group I) and compared them to AIDS patients with no evidence of glomerular disease on biopsy (group II). The average time to the development of renal failure in group I was 10.9 weeks. There was no correlation between the rate of progression to renal insufficiency and the stage of HIV infection. The median survival time from the diagnosis of renal disease to death was 4.5 months in patients with HIV-associated nephropathy. The survival time differed depending on the stage of HIV infection: asymptomatic, 9.7 months; ARC, 3.6 months; and AIDS, 1.9 months (9). Feinfeld and his coinvestigators analyzed the survival of HIV-infected patients on maintenance dialysis. They found that the life expectancy of AIDS patients on dialysis is shorter than that of other dialysis patients, but similar to the survival of AIDS patients in New York City in general (15).

The role of other viral infections or the role of drugs in the development of renal failure in this patient population is not clear. Many of the drugs used in HIV-infected patients are nephrotoxic (Table 51.2). In patients treated with intramuscular or intravenous pentamidine at 4 mg/kg/day for more than 7 days, the creatinine increased by 0.5 mg/dl in 64% of cases. The creatinine increased by more than 2 mg/dl in 23% of these patients (6). The mechanism of the nephrotoxicity is unknown, but the renal failure is usually transient. Trimethoprim/sulfamethoxazole can cause interstitial nephritis, but it can also cause a false elevation of the creatinine because it competes with creatinine for tubular secretion. AZT is not nephrotoxic but it can cause rhabdomyolysis. In general, unless acute renal failure is associated with overwhelming infection; respiratory or other organ failure; or massive

proteinuria, severe hypoalbuminemia, and prerenal azotemia, the renal function can be expected to recover (6). The role of renal biopsy in HIV-infected patients with abnormal renal function has been debated. Since the most common lesion is FSGS, which responds poorly to steroid therapy, and physicians are reluctant to use steroids in this patient population, biopsy is usually not recommended.

There are a multitude of electrolyte abnormalities that occur in HIV-infected patients, but hyponatremia is the most common electrolyte abnormality. Hyponatremia and volume depletion are seen in patients with tubular defects in sodium reabsorption or adrenal insufficiency. Adrenal disease rarely results in insufficiency because less than 70% of the gland is involved (6). Euvolemic patients with a low sodium are seen with the syndrome of inappropriate antidiuretic hormone (SIADH) secretion. This is common in AIDS patients as a consequence of the frequent pulmonary or central nervous system pathology. These patients need to have normal renal, adrenal, and thyroid function to fulfill the definition of SIADH. Agarwal and associates studied 36 patients with AIDS and an admission serum sodium level of less than 130 mEq/liter. Twelve cases were associated with volume depletion and were corrected with saline replacement. Twenty-three cases were attributed to SIADH, and only one case was secondary to adrenal insufficiency. Hyponatremia was observed in 35% of the hospitalized AIDS patients (2). Other electrolyte abnormalities such as hyperuricemia, hypocalcemia, and hypokalemia are also seen in HIV-infected patients.

OTHER MANIFESTATIONS

Gastrointestinal Manifestations

There is no real gastrointestinal pathology specific to HIV-infected patients that would require critical care management. These patients can develop severe volume depletion and hyponatremia from chronic diarrhea. The list of etiologic agents for the diarrhea is extensive including: CMV, Gram-negative enteric pathogens, parasites, mycobacteria, and HIV itself. Kap-

Table 51.2
Nephrotoxic Drugs Used in HIV Infection

Pentamidine	Acyclovir
TMP/SMX	Dapsone
Amphotericin B	Foscarnet

osi's sarcoma can involve the bowel, resulting in gastrointestinal bleeding, which may be difficult to control.

Endocrine Manifestations

Endocrine dysfunction in AIDS results from: involvement of the glands by infectious agents, drugs, or the generalized debilitated state of the patients. Although endocrine complications are not prominent, they should be recognized. The adrenal gland is the most commonly affected endocrine organ. Pathologic studies demonstrate involvement of the glands with Kaposi's sarcoma or opportunistic pathogens such as CMV, *Crytococcus*, and *M. avium intracellulare*. Ninety-two percent of these patients have a normal cortisol response to corticotropin injection (3). Adrenal insufficiency secondary to ketoconazole is dose-related and reversible. Rifampin decreases the bioavailability of cortisol.

Abnormalities of glucose metabolism are also seen in AIDS. These are most often related to specific medications. Approximately 8% of patients receiving intravenous pentamidine therapy develop hypoglycemia (42). It is more common in patients that develop renal dysfunction. This is thought to be secondary to direct toxicity of pentamidine on the pancreatic islet cells, resulting in cytolytic release of insulin. Unrecognized hypoglycemia can be complicated by seizures. The hypoglycemic period may be followed by hyperglycemia resulting from insulin deficiency. The diabetogenic effect of pentamidine may be permanent, and it may occur as late as 11 months following pentamidine therapy. Other endocrine abnormalities have been reported in HIV-infected patients, but these are much less common.

Hematological Manifestations

Hematological abnormalities in HIV infection may be complex in etiology. Infiltration of the bone marrow with infection or neoplasm, production of cytokines that inhibit hematopoesis, ineffective hematopoesis, and direct infection of stem cells with HIV may each play a role in the cytopenias seen in HIV-infected patients

(23). Drugs such as AZT, ganciclovir, pentamidine, Bactrim, and pyrimethamine can cause cytopenias. There can also be peripheral destruction of blood components. Approximately 21% of HIV-infected patients demonstrate a positive direct antiglobulin test (47). Clinically significant anemia, thrombocytopenia, and neutropenia may be seen. Non-Hodgkin's lymphomas and Kaposi's sarcoma are the two main neoplasms that are seen in HIV-infected patients. Treatment of aggressive lymphoma can result in tumor lysis syndrome, sepsis, hemorrhage, and other complications that are not unique to HIV-infected individuals.

Sepsis

HIV-infected patients can develop sepsis secondary to a wide variety of pathogens that may cause disease in immunocompetent hosts. Septicemia with organisms such as *Salmonella* and *Listeria* may be more common in HIV-infected patients. Because of the need for prolonged intravenous therapy for conditions such as CMV retinitis, *M. avium intracellulare* infection, and cryptococcal meningitis, many AIDS patients have permanent intravenous access devices. These catheters provide another possible source for sepsis.

ICU SURVIVAL

Physicians must possess accurate information on prognosis, risks and benefits of treatment, and availability of alternate modes of therapy in order to make decisions in the critical care management of AIDS patients. Older studies reported dismal ICU survival statistics for patients with HIV disease. Schein and his associates quoted an overall ICU mortality of 77% for patients with AIDS. Seventy-four percent of their patients were admitted to the ICU for respiratory failure and the mortality was 91% in that group (40). Smith and coworkers used the APACHE II scoring system to try to predict outcome of AIDS patients requiring ICU care. The mean APACHE II score of AIDS patients who survived their ICU course did not differ from those that did not survive (44). The

AIDS patients had a higher observed mortality than that predicted by the APACHE II score.

More recent studies demonstrate improvement in the ICU survival of AIDS patients. This may be a function of improvement in therapies, but it may reflect a selection bias in the patients admitted to the ICU. Perhaps more "end-stage" HIV patients are electing to forego ICU care. Wachter and coworkers reported a survival rate to discharge of 20–43% for AIDS patients admitted to the ICU for reasons other than respiratory failure. Two recent studies of *Pneumocystis carinii* pneumonia and respiratory failure report survival rates to discharge of 50–58% (46). These studies did not look at functional status or quality of life in the survivors. When survival was defined as the patient's status 3 months postdischarge, the survival rate in one study fell to 15% for patients requiring mechanical ventilation and 26% for all AIDS patients requiring ICU care (37).

CONCLUSION

This chapter has tried to focus on the pathophysiology of HIV infection and the critical care problems that are common in HIV-infected patients. It is difficult for many physicians to deal with death in such a young patient population, and discussions on life-sustaining therapy are often postponed. The data suggests that survival in certain critical care situations such as in acute respiratory failure secondary to PCP or in seizures secondary to *Toxoplasma* or *Cryptococcus* is improving. At the present time, however, there is no cure for AIDS. Therefore, it is up to us as physicians to counsel our patients using the information we have available.

In this day of diminishing health care resources, it is important to gather statistics on new therapies and survival so that we can use our ICUs efficiently and appropriately.

References

1. Acierno LJ. Cardiac complications in acquired immunodeficiency syndrome (AIDS). J Am Coll Cardio 1989;13(5):1144–1154.
2. Agarwal A, Soni A, Ciechanowsky M, Chander P, Tester G. Hyponatremia in patients with the acquired immunodeficiency syndrome. Nephron 1989;53:317–321.
3. Aron DC. Endocrine complications of the acquired immunodeficiency syndrome. Arch Intern Med 1989;149:330–333.
4. Beers MF, Sohn M, Swartz M. Recurrent pneumothorax in AIDS patients with pneumocystis pneumonia. Chest 1990;98(2):267–270.
5. Bigby TD, Margolskee D, Curtis JL, et al. The usefulness of induced sputum in diagnosis of *Pneumocystis carinii* pneumonia in patients with acquired immunodeficiency syndrome. Am Rev Respir Dis 1986;133:515–518.
6. Bourgoignie JJ. Renal complications of human immunodeficiency virus type 1. Kidney Int 1990;37:1571–1584.
7. Bozzette SA, Sattler FR, Chiu J, et al. A controlled trial of early adjunctive treatment with corticosteroids for *Pneumocystis carinii* pneumonia in the acquired immunodeficiency syndrome. N Engl J Med 1990;323(21):1451–1457.
8. Byrnes TA, Brevig JK, Yeoh CB. Pneumothorax in patients with acquired immunodeficiency syndrome. J Thorac Cardiovasc Surg 1989;98:546–550.
9. Carbone L, D'Agati V, Cheng JT, Appel GB. Course and prognosis of human immunodeficiency virus-associated nephropathy. Am J Med 1989;87:389–395.
10. Cohn JA, McMeeking A, Cohen W, Jacobs J, Holzman R. Evaluation of the policy of empiric treatment of suspected toxoplasma encephalitis in patients with acquired immunodeficiency syndrome. Am J Med 1989;86:521–527.
11. DeLorenzo LJ, Huang CT, Stone DJ. Roentgenographic patterns of *Pneumocystis carinii* pneumonia in 104 patients with AIDS. Chest 1987;91(3):323–327.
12. Efferen LS, Nadarajah D, Palat DS. Survival following mechanical ventilation for *Pneumocystis carinii* pneumonia in patients with the acquired immunodeficiency syndrome. Am J Med 1989;87:401–404.
13. El-Sadr W, Simberkoff MS. Survival and prognostic factors in severe *Pneumocystis carinii* pneumonia requiring mechanical ventilation. Am Rev Respir Dis 1988;137:1264–1267.
14. Engstrom JW, Lowenstein DH, Bredesen DE. Cerebral infarctions and transient neurologic deficits associated with acquired immunodeficiency syndrome. Am J Med 1989;86:528–531.
15. Feinfeld DA, Kaplan R, Dressler R, Lynn RI. Survival of human immunodeficiency virus-infected patients on maintenance dialysis. Clin Nephrol 1989;32(5):221–224.
16. Fleisher AG, McElvaney G, Lawson L, Gerein AN, Grant D, Tyers GFO. Surgical management of spontaneous pneumothorax in patients with acquired immunodeficiency syndrome. Ann Thorac Surg 1988;45:21–23.
17. Friedman Y, Franklin C, Rackow EC, Weil MH. Improved survival in patients with AIDS, *Pneumocystis carinii* pneumonia, and severe respiratory failure. Chest 1989;96(4):862–866.
18. Gagnon S, Boota AM, Fischl MA, Baier H, Kirk-

sey OW, LaVoie L. Corticosteroids as adjunctive therapy for severe *Pneumocystis carinii* pneumonia in the acquired immunodeficiency syndrome. N Engl J Med 1990;323(21):1444–1450.

19. Gallacher BP, Gallacher WN, MacFadden DK. Treatment of acute *Pneumocystis carinii* pneumonia with corticosteroids in a patient with acquired immunodeficiency syndrome. Crit Care Med 1989;17(1):104–105.

20. Gallo RC. Mechanism of disease induction by HIV. AIDS 1990;3(4):380–389.

21. Greene WC. The molecular biology of human immunodeficiency virus type I infection. N Engl J Med 1991;324(5):308–316.

22. Gregg RW, Friedman BC, Williams JF, McGrath B, Zimmerman JE. Continuous positive airway pressure by face mask in *Pneumocystis carinii* pneumonia. Crit Care Med 1990;18(1):21–24.

23. Groopman JE. Management of the hematologic complications of the human immunodeficiency virus infection. Rev Infect Dis 1990;12(5):932–937.

24. Haseltine WA, Wong-Staal F. The molecular biology of the AIDS virus. Sci Am 1988:52–62.

25. Holtzman DM, Kaku DA, So YT. New-onset seizures associated with human immunodeficiency virus infection. Am J Med 1989;87:173–177.

26. Humphreys MH, Schoenfeld PY. Renal complications in patients with the acquired immune deficiency syndrome (AIDS). Am J Nephrol 1987;7:1–7.

27. Jules-Elysee KM, Stover DE, Zaman MB, Bernard EM, White DA. Aerosolized pentamidine: effect on diagnosis and presentation of *Pneumocystis carinii* pneumonia. Ann Intern Med 1990;112(10):750–757.

28. Levy WS, Simon GL, Rios JC, Ross AM. Prevalence of cardiac abnormalities in human immunodeficiency virus infection. Am J Cardiol 1989;63:86–89.

29. Mann JM, Altos CS, Webber CA, Smith PR, Muto R, Heurich AE. Nonbronchoscopic lung lavage for diagnosis of opportunistic infection in AIDS. Chest 1987;91(3):319–322.

30. Martinez CM, Romanelli A, Mullen MP, Lee M. Spontaneous pneumothoraces in AIDS patients receiving aerosolized pentamidine. Chest 1988;94(6):1317–1318.

31. Maxfield RA, Sorkin IB, Fazzini EP, et al. Respiratory failure in patients with acquired immu-

nodeficiency syndrome and *Pneumocystis carinii* pneumonia. Crit Care Med 1986;14(5):443–449.

32. Mills J, Masur H. AIDS-related infections. Sci Am 1990;50–57.

33. Mitchell P, Dodek P, Lawson L, Kiess M, Russel J. Torsades de pointes during intravenous pentamidine isethionate therapy. Can Med Assoc J 1989;140:173–174.

34. Monsuez JJ, Kinney EL, Vittecoq D, et al. Comparison among acquired immune deficiency syndrome with and without clinical evidence of cardiac disease. Am J Cardiol 1988;62:1311–1313.

35. Pardo V, Meneses R, Ossa L, et al. AIDS-related glomerulopathy. Kidney Int 1987;31:1167–1173.

36. Redfield RR, Burke DS. HIV infection: the clinical picture. Sci Am 1988:90–98.

37. Rogers PL, Lane C, Henderson DK, Parrillo, J, Masur H. Admission of AIDS patients to a medical intensive care unit. Crit Care Med 1989;17(2):113–117.

38. Rosenberg ZF, Fauci AS. Immunopathology and pathogenesis of human immunodeficiency virus infection. Pediatr Infect Dis J 1991;10:230–238.

39. Scannell KA. Pneumothoraces and *Pneumocystis carinii* pneumonia in two AIDS patients receiving aerosolized pentamidine. Chest 1990;97(2):479.

40. Schein RMH, Fischl MA, Pitchenik AE, Sprung CL. ICU survival of patients with the acquired immunodeficiency syndrome. Crit Care Med 1986;14(12):1026–1027.

41. Sepkowitz KA, Telzak EE, Gold JWM, et al. Pneumothorax in AIDS. Ann Intern Med 1991;114:455–459.

42. Shen M, Orwoll E, Conte J, Prince MJ. Pentamidine-induced pancreatic beta-cell dysfunction. Am J Med 1989;86:726–728.

43. Singer P, Askanazi J, Akiva L, Bursztein S, Kvetan V. Reassessing intensive care for patients with acquired immunodeficiency syndrome. Heart Lung 1990;19:387–394.

44. Smith RL, Levine SM, Lewis ML. Prognosis of patients with AIDS requiring intensive care. Chest 1989;96(4):857–861.

45. Tuazon CU. Toxoplasmosis in AIDS patients. J Antimicrob Chemother 1989;23(suppl A):77–82.

46. Wachter RM, Luce JM, Lo B, Raffin TA. Life-sustaining treatment for patients with AIDS. Chest 1989;95(3):647–652.

47. Zon LI, Arkin C, Groopman JE. Hematologic manifestations of the human immune deficiency virus (HIV). Br J Haematol 1987;66:251–256.

52

Diabetes

Gérard Slama
Jean-Louis Selam

The diabetic patient is menaced by acute complications that can be life-threatening. These complications include hypoglycemia, ketoacidosis, nonketosis hyperosmolar coma, lactic acidosis, and tissue necrosis of the lower extremities (infectious or ischemic). These complications are neither rare nor specific to patients with diabetes. All these complications can be observed in nondiabetic subjects. The above complications can lead to grave diagnostic errors whenever diabetes is over- or underdiagnosed. We will develop these basic concepts first and then discuss their management.

DIABETES MELLITUS AND ITS ACUTE COMPLICATIONS: A DISEASE MORE FREQUENT THAN USUALLY THOUGHT

Diabetes is a common disease, afflicting 2–5% of Caucasians; 0.3–1% are type I diabetics (insulin-dependent diabetes mellitus, IDDM), the remainder are mostly type II (non-IDDM, NIDDM) subjects with or without insulin treatment. The proportion of type II diabetes treated with insulin varies from one country to another depending on habits, oral drug availability, and legal considerations and ranges from 5% in Southern Europe to 50–75% in Northern Europe and North America. Although some complications are associated with type I diabetes (hypoglycemia and

diabetic ketoacidosis (DKA) and others are associated with type II diabetes (nonketotic hyperosmolar coma, lactic acidosis, critical ischemia of the lower limbs), in fact any of the above complications can occur with either type of diabetes, depending on the precipitating circumstances.

Some interesting facts are developing in the epidemiology of this disease. The incidence of diabetes mellitus is becoming more and more frequent, roughly doubling every decade.

Diabetes mellitus is becoming more prevalent (10–30%) in some non-Caucasian populations: Native Americans, inhabitants of the Pacific islands, Hispanic Americans, and other populations living in or migrating to western countries.

Many epidemiological studies have shown that for every two people diagnosed with NIDDM, there are one to two others ignoring their disease. (The patient being treated in an emergency room does not always come with a medical alert tag.)

Perhaps 30% of the Caucasian population carries the genetic trait of diabetes, which will never express itself in most people but can emerge in certain acute situations (enormous physical or psychological stress, massive corticotherapy, β_2 stimulant administration, severe trauma, or surgical intervention). Thus, anyone admitted to an intensive care unit can become severely diabetic, even after having been diagnosed as "normal" the day before.

Acute complications observed in diabetes are not specific to this disease.

Hypoglycemia can occur in nondiabetic subjects either spontaneously (with B-cell tumors, cancer, and pituitary or corticosurrenal insufficiency) or after absorption or injection of exogenous compounds or drugs (with alcohol and certain drugs, whether antidiabetic or not). Treatment of such hypoglycemia may differ from that used for insulin-treated diabetic patients (see below for more details).

Ketoacidosis can result from alcohol abuse.

Nonketotic hyperosmolar coma can be observed in nondiabetic patients and can result from molecules other than glucose (sodium) or from glucose in essentially nondiabetic subjects (as in massive perfusion of dextrose-extended burns). Moreover, varying combinations of the above situations can occur.

Hyperglycemia, even severe, is not diagnostic of diabetes.

Lactic acidosis occurs as frequently in nondiabetic as in diabetic patients. Hyperglycemia can erroneously be taken as indicative of diabetes when it actually results from a technical mistake, for example, when blood sampling is done in a patient perfused with concentrated dextrose solution (downstream sampling). Significant hyperglycemia can be observed in severely ill patients during and a few days after a myocardial infarction. This hyperglycemia results from an enormous secretion of catecholamines and insulin secretion inhibition. Further, severe hyperglycemia nearly always occurs after surgery under hypothermia.

Over- or under diagnosis of diabetes may lead to fatal errors.

Undetected hypoglycemia in a patient assumed to be nondiabetic may be fatal.

Administering parenteral glucagon to a patient with an insulinoma or who is being treated with sulfonylurea may be dangerous.

Administering insulin to an alcoholic patient with ketoacidosis would be disastrous.

Administering insulin to a patient affected with an acute myocardial infarction may be useless or potentially dangerous.

It should be emphasized that all of the above-cited acute complications (metabolic, infectious, or ischemic) are either totally preventable, with the patient education playing an important role, or can at least be limited to the early warning signs. In many cases, the development of acute complications may indicate malpractice at some stage of the process.

HYPOGLYCEMIA

Acute hypoglycemia is the most frequent complication observed in diabetes mellitus (2) and can be considered a nearly unavoidable consequence of insulin therapy; it may also be observed after the administration of sulfonylurea, but this life-threatening occurrence can be prevented. Diabetes mellitus is, by far, the most common form of hypoglycemia, and this etiology should be the first to come to mind when this condition occurs. Many other causes of hypoglycemia are also known (7, 24) or suspected. Some differences in the treatment of hypoglycemia may depend on the etiology. In most cases, determining the exact cause of the hypoglycemia does not affect its emergency treatment; however, correct early diagnosis(ses) with adequate diagnostic techniques is of utmost importance for future therapy. It may be the best or only way to ensure that exact etiological diagnosis and appropriate long-term treatment are rendered.

Two items are critical for correct diagnosis of hypoglycemia: (a) accurate measurement of blood glucose levels using proper laboratory equipment, not determination based solely on a blood glucose strip; and (b) freeze-storage of 5 ml of the patient's plasma if the blood glucose level is ≤2.5 mmol, assuming that the patient is not insulin treated and no obvious etiology is found. This stored plasma sample may be analyzed later for insulin levels if necessary.

Pathophysiology

Most of the signs and symptoms of hypoglycemia reflect altered neuronal function. The oxidative metabolism in the brain is one of the highest in the human body (7, 42). A constant supply of fuel is mandatory to maintain continuous production of ATP necessary for neuronal biosynthesis, secretion of neurotransmitter, and membrane potential. Acute fuel deprivation leads to the suspension of neuronal function followed by cell edema and, eventually, irreversible cell destruction. *Total* fuel deprivation is only observed in vascular obliteration, or acute anoxia, leading to cell death within a few minutes; in hypoglycemia, fuel deprivation is only *partial*, explaining the potential for recovery after hours of coma.

The energy requirement of an adult brain is approximately 2500 kJ/day, drawn mainly from circulating glucose, because glucose storage as glycogen is modest (<10 min of functional autonomy) (42). Other substrates derive from oxidation of amino acids (7) (modest contribution) and metabolism of ketone bodies (modest contribution under normal conditions, but a very good substrate after a few days of adaptation to a prolonged carbohydrate fast) and lactate (small contribution).

To regulate the substrate pathways in the neuron, one must take into consideration the blood concentration of the substrate, the rate of blood flow, and the transport and consumption rate of the given substrate. The consumption rate depends on the enzyme concentration (41). The overall rate of consumption of glucose by the brain is approximately 70 mg/min with local fluctuations related to functional variations. The transmembrane transport of glucose is dependent on a glucose transport mechanism with a very high K_m, whereas that of hexokinase is very low (11 mM versus 0.04). As a result, under conditions of normal blood glucose levels, glucose utilization by the brain depends on its needs and is not limited by its transport system. At 50 mg/dl, transport equals utilization and the intracellular concentration of glucose approaches zero; below this approximate concentration, transport does not meet utilization, and the cell suffers. A long-term adaptation to chronically low blood glucose levels is possible with a comparative increase in brain glucose transport activity. This explains, in part, the progressive neuronal adaptation to low blood glucose levels and the enzymatic adjustments to optimize ketone body utilization.

The symptoms observed during hypoglycemia result partly from neuroglucopenia and partly from the adrenergic response to hypoglycemia (Table 52.1) (6, 7, 28). The order in which symptoms appear seems to be related to the degree of dependence of the given neurons to glucose. The first areas to suffer are the cortex,

Table 52.1
Signs and Symptoms of Hypoglycemia

Signs due to the adrenergic reaction
  Sensation of imperative hunger
  Palor
  Tremor (objective or subjective)
  Palpitations, tachycardia
  Moist palms
  Abundant sweating
Signs due to neuroglucopenia
  Blurred vision
  Peribuccal tingling
  Sluggish speech
  Difficulty with concentration
  Dullness
  Bizarre behavior
  Aggressiveness, violence, agitation
  Abnormal facial movements (grimacing, sucking)
  Uncoordinated movements
  Neurological symptoms (facial palsy, hemiplegia)
  Seizures, coma

cerebellum, and mesencephalon followed by the myelencephalon.

The adrenergic response to hypoglycemia is part of the complex contraregulatory hormone response (ACTH, cortisol, glucagon, growth hormone), which is implicated in correcting hypoglycemia.

Clinical Manifestations

The symptoms of a hypoglycemic coma can be either highly evocative or totally misleading. The most characteristic presentations are: acute psychiatric disorders (which might be falsely attributed to alcohol abuse) or focal neurological defects (monoplegia, hemiplegia, and the like). Another recognizable symptom is coma with agitation, seizures, abundant diaphoresis, bilateral extension of the big toes (Babinski sign), and deep reflex hyperreactivity. The EEG may be profoundly altered (8).

Profound hypoglycemia can be associated with stage IV coma with complete absence of encephalic or pyramidal excitation. Such symptoms may lead to a diagnosis of toxic ingestion of, for example, tranquilizers. Only the systematic search for hypoglycemia, including measurement of blood glucose, will lead to a correct diagnosis.

Depending on the stage and duration of hypoglycemia, mydriasis or miosis, tachycardia or bradycardia, or even hypothermia may be observed (28).

Complications and Sequelae

Complications and sequelae include:

Contusions, severe musculoskeletal injuries, and fractures (in particular those of the spine) due to falls or to seizures
Cardiac arrhythmia
Post-hypoglycemic coma due to cerebral edema
Persistent neurological or psychological defects (dementia, Parkinson's syndrome) (46)
Death (The role of hypoglycemia in this complication is difficult to appreciate and there is a lack of reliable epidemiological studies (56).)

These symptoms can be transient or intractable for weeks or even months. Particular care should be taken not to consider patients in a prolonged coma as being definitively and irreversibly comatose; appropriate corrective treatment should be provided for a sufficient period (up to 1 year).

Causes of Hypoglycemic Coma

Hypoglycemia can result from a number of different causes. Hypoglycemia occurring within 3–5 hr after a meal (functional hypoglycemia) never leads to severe hypoglycemia; therefore, this type of patient (32) is rarely seen in an emergency unit. Hypoglycemic comas are either drug-induced or spontaneous (Table 52.2). Analysis of patient records shows that most are drug-induced hypoglycemias; and, in this group, diabetic patients represent the largest portion (mainly insulin-treated patients, particularly children (30, 46), and less frequently, those treated with sulfonylureas). In most cases, the cause of the neurological syndrome and its mechanism are known soon after the patient is examined in the emergency unit. Information can be revealed by a relative, inspection of the patient or the contents of the patient's purse or pockets, or the circumstances in which the patient was found (prescription bottles containing insulin or sulfonylureas

Table 52.2
Main Causes of Hypoglycemic Coma[a]

Drug-induced hypoglycemia (very frequent)
 Insulin injection (in diabetic subject (A) or facticious (C))
 Sulfonylurea (in diabetic subject (A) or facticious (C))
 Alcohol (A)
 Acetyl salicylic acid and derivatives (A)
 Other drugs (see specific table) (A to C)
Spontaneous hypoglycemia (relatively rare)
 Islet cell tumors (benign or malignant) (B)
 Nonpancreatic tumors (benign or malignant) (A)
 Contraregulatory hormone(s) deficiency
  Adrenal insufficiency (peripheral or hypopituitary) (A, B, or C)
  (Severe) hypothyroidism (myxedematous coma) (A)
 Severe hepatocellular failure (A) and some alimentary intoxications (amanite phalloide, Lakee fruit, some Mediterranean plants (*Bighia sapida*) (C) (Ref. 7)
 Massive cell proliferation (neoplasia or circulating cells) (A)
 Autoimmune
  Spontaneous antiinsulin antibodies (C) (Ref. 23)
  Antiinsulin receptor antibodies (C)
 Excessive circulating substrate consumption (anecdotal in terms of frequency)
  Exhausting physical exercise (A to C)
  Terminal denutrition (A)
  Severe sepsis (38) (C)
  Terminal end-stage renal failure (B)
  Terminal heart failure (B)
 Acute paludism; trypanosomiasis (B)
 Abnormal cerebral glucose transporters (glut 4 deficiency) (21) (C) (2 cases reported in 1991)

[a] The letters in parentheses indicate the increasing difficulty of diagnosis: A, very easy; B, relatively difficult, needing specialized investigations; C, very difficult.

surrounding the patient). Sometimes such clues are lacking but, after treatment and recovery, the patient will be aware that certain medications or drugs are known to potentially induce hypoglycemia (see list on Table 52.3). Certain rare conditions known to induce hypoglycemia are easy to diagnose at first glance. These include Addison's disease, severe icteric hepatitis, obvious metastatic cancer, and profound denutrition. Sometimes no obvious cause

Table 52.3
Main Toxics and Compounds That May Lead to Hypoglycemia in Adults (Nonexhaustive List)[a]

Alcohol (large intake or lesser intake, but associated with other drugs)
Aspirin and derivatives (at very high dosage)
Acetaminophen
Ketoconazol
Pentamidine (Ref. 55)
β-Blockers (massive intake or in association with other drugs; antidiabetic or others)
Quinine (i.v. or acute paludism) (Ref. 59)
Disopyramid (Rythmodan)
Propoxyphen (Antalvic, Di-Antalvic, Propophan)
Some monoaminoxidase inhibitors
Perhexiline maleate (Pexid)
Oxytetracyclin
Haloperidol
Penicillamine
Cibenzolin (Cipralan)
Metformin (massive dose only, self-poisoning)
Tranylcipromine
Drugs containing a thiol moiety (such as pyrithinol) can induce spontaneous antiinsulin antibodies with hypoglycemic comas (Ref. 23)
Error in prescription delivery, i.e., sulfonylurea instead of antihypertensive tablets (examine any ingested drug, whatever its supposed nature)

[a] In nondiabetic as well as in diabetic subjects; not including insulin and sulfonylureas.

of the hypoglycemia may be found. It is nevertheless essential to determine the correct physiopathological diagnosis, which may require sophisticated investigations in a specialized center. The principal causes for such hypoglycemias are:

Drug induction (Table 52.3)
Nonpancreatic tumors
Factitious insulin or sulfonylurea administration
β-Cell tumors
Incomplete forms of adrenal insufficiency (primary or secondary)
Autoimmune diseases

Treatment of Hypoglycemic Coma

The primary treatment for a hypoglycemic coma is the administration of dextrose (15–30 g i.v. as a prime dose). This treatment, however, is not always easy to perform in a convulsive or agitated patient and requires the intervention of a doctor or a nurse. Parenteral glucagon (1 mg s.c. or i.m.) is the preferred drug for treating hypoglycemia in patients taking insulin (except when alcohol has been taken concomitantly). The intranasal route may become the preferred route in the future (52). Glucagon, which stimulates endogenous insulin secretion, is contraindicated in sulfonylurea-induced hypoglycemia or in patients with β-cell tumors; hypoglycemia can be aggravated by such an injection. This treatment should also be avoided in hypoglycemia due to alcohol abuse because glucagon is unable to stimulate neoglycogenesis and glycogenolysis in such a functionally or organically altered liver. However, when no other therapy is available, parenteral glucagon can always be used and will correct the situation long enough to permit oral carbohydrate administration. Intrarectal glucose is ineffective.

After recuperation of mental functions, clinical attitude thereafter depends on the suspected cause for the hypoglycemia (Table 52.4).

If hypoglycemia is due, in an insulin-treated patient, to insulin overdosage or any other "error" such as unplanned exercise or insufficient carbohydrate intake, the patient should then eat 20–30 g of any food high in carbohydrates such as bread (53). After 1–3 hr of observation, the patient can be discharged and referred to his or her doctor or diabetologist. Admittance to the ICU is unwarranted in these patients.

If hypoglycemia is due to sulfonylurea intake, particular care should be taken. A continuous infusion of dextrose should be given at a rate of 200–600 mg/min i.v. according to frequent monitoring of blood glucose levels (extreme care should be taken in the manipulation of the glucose strips to avoid contamination by dextrose on the fingers of the patient or staff). Hypoglycemia caused by sulfonylurea is often severe when it occurs in elderly patients who have "delicate" vascular systems and are often affected by some degree of renal insufficiency. In these patients, recurring hypoglycemic attacks must be anticipated, and adequate monitoring and corrective measures ensured. Hypoglycemia can recur from 1 to 4 days after entry. Continuous i.v. ad-

Table 52.4
Attitude When a Hypoglycemic Attack Is Suspected (Psychiatric or Neurological Disorders)

Systematic Suspicion for Hypoglycemia
1. Determine blood glucose level using a glucose-oxidase strip
2. Withdraw 5–10 ml of blood for laboratory blood glucose determination and eventual freezing of the remaining plasma (if blood glucose ≤ 2.5 mmol/liter).
3. Treat without waiting for the result of step 2 only if blood glucose strip ≤ 2.5 mmol/liter, or systematically if no strip determination is available
    If the patient is known to be an insulin-treated diabetic (and alcohol has not been overconsumed) give 1 mg of glucagon s.c. or i.m.
In all other situations give dextrose, 15–20 g i.v. (i.e., 50–70 ml of 30% solution)

| | Mental Recovery | |
Patient Is Insulin-Treated	Patient Is Diabetic and Takes Sulfonylureas	Other Cases
Give about 20–30 g of carbohydrate as a food	Recurrent hypoglycemia highly suspected	Admit to hospital
Advise to contact the MD in charge	Admit to hospital	Treatment depends on the suspected etiology
Quick discharge (immediate to 2 hr)	Give continuous i.v. dextrose infusion on the basis of 200–600 mg/min (may need 1–4 days)	Plasma creatinine may be a good indicator of risk

ministration of diazoxide may be an alternate treatment to i.v. dextrose; however, this is a pathophysiological approach and nothing more.

When hypoglycemia is induced by any drug known to produce such a reaction, monitoring, as with sulfonylurea overdosage, is recommended.

When hypoglycemia is corrected and no cause is found, the patient should be rapidly transferred to a specialized unit to determine the exact cause of the event.

Prolonged Coma

A sufficient amount of dextrose injected i.v. should partially or totally correct the neurological (glucopenic) symptoms within minutes, sometimes even before the injection has been completed. However, the patient may remain abated for 15 min or so. If drastic clinical improvement does not occur, one must determine whether treatment is effective (by checking blood glucose level with a glucose strip) or cerebral edema exists (by observing a normal or high blood glucose level). Parenteral glucocorticoids or hypertonic i.v. solutions can be used. It should again be stressed that a spectacular recovery can be ob-

served months after prolonged coma and subsequent cerebral edema resulting from severe hypoglycemia. In such patients, sustained conservative treatment must be ensured.

HYPEROSMOLAR COMA

Hyperosmolar hyperglycemic nonketotic coma has only recently been identified (19, 47) and prospectively studied (5). It occurs at about one tenth as often as diabetic ketoacidosis; however, it results in a much higher mortality rate (20–50%). It usually occurs in elderly patients with NIDDM. The syndrome is defined as: hyperglycemia >33 mmol/liter, plasma osmolarity >350 mosm/liter, pH >7.20, serum bicarbonates >15 mmol/liter, and no ketonemia (5).

Causes

The precipitating factors for hyperosmolar hyperglycemic nonketotic coma are multiple and are summarized in Table 52.5 (60). Hyperosmolar hyperglycemic nonketotic coma usually results from a combination of factors, such as a respiratory

Table 52.5
Main Etiologic Factors for Hyperosmolar
Hyperglycemic Nonketotic Coma in Diabetic
Patients[a]

Variable	% of Patients
Age >80	29
Female	71
Unknown NIDDM	32
NIDDM	58
Acute infections	39
Diuretics	38
Retirement home resident	28
Senile dementia	18

[a]Watchel TJ, Silliman RA, Lamberton P. Predisposing factors for the diabetic hyperosmolar state. Arch Intern Med 1987;147:499–501.

infection, in an elderly patient with senile dementia and unknown NIDDM complicated by dehydration caused by inability to drink.

Pathophysiology

The precise mechanisms of hyperosmolar hyperglycemia nonketotic coma have only recently been clarified (6). The sequence of events may be as follows: a factor such as infection, gastrointestinal hemorrhage, or cerebral ischemia occurs; counterregulatory hormones are secreted; and hyperglycemia and hyperosmolarity are generated. Hyperosmolarity may often be aggravated by the consumption of hyperglycemic drugs such as diuretics and corticoids or of a large volume of soft drinks with a high sugar content in response to thirst. In most cases, though, thirst mechanisms that would ordinarily compensate for plasma hyperosmolarity are defective, or such drinks are inaccessible (elderly, comatose, or psychiatric patients), and hyperosmolarity increases.

Sodium movements are more complex: osmotic diuresis represents a hypotonic loss of water and salts, particularly sodium. Nonreabsorbed glucose reduces the fraction of water after sodium reabsorption. The hypotonicity of urine remaining in the renal tubules reduces sodium reabsorption. However, in plasma the net result is either a dilution hyponatremia with hypovolemia or, at a more advanced stage, a hypernatremia with hypovolemia and hyperglycemia.

The consequences of hyperosmolarity are numerous: at the renal level, hypovolemia induces functional renal failure, which in turn aggravates glucose retention. At the cerebral level, in an effort to maintain brain volume despite extracellular hyperosmolarity, cerebral cells produce "idiogenetic" osmoles, which then transfer water from intracellular to extracellular compartments (6). These idiogenetic osmoles include glucose, ions, amino acids (e.g., taurin, alanin, aspartate, and glutamate), and aminobutyric acid. Other consequences of hyperosmolarity include reduced cardiac output, increased blood viscosity, increased hepatic synthesis of triglycerides, increased risk of rhabdomyolysis (48), and impaired insulin secretion. The last explains the transient hyperglycemia seen in most nondiabetic hyperosmolar comas. In diabetic patients, because of some persistent insulin secretion, DKA is absent (27). However, ketone bodies generally are moderately increased, suggesting a continuum rather than two separate conditions (DKA and hyperosmolar hyperglycemic nonketotic coma).

Cerebral edema is the most frequent iatrogenic complication. The mechanism of cerebral edema involves the rapid extracellular correction of hyperosmolarity (e.g., with hypotonic fluids) and the slow, spontaneous disappearance of intracerebral idiogenetic osmoles. Another iatrogenic complication is cardiovascular collapse caused by hypovolemia aggravated by a too rapid transfer of glucose-associated water into the cells during intensive insulin administration. Finally, the risk of insulin-induced hypoglycemia is increased during treatment because of dilution of extracellular glucose with i.v. fluids, restoration of normal renal function including glucose filtration, and improvement of better insulin secretion when hyperosmolarity is reduced.

Signs and Symptoms

Prodromal Phase

This phase is longer in hyperosmolar hyperglycemia nonketotic coma (from a few

Table 52.6
Mechanism of Cerebral Edema during Hyperosmolar Hyperglycemic Nonketotic Coma
Treatment: Comparison with Events in Nondiabetic Hyperosmolar Comas

Condition	Serum Osmolality (mmol/kg)	Deficit	Cerebral Osmolality (mmol/kg)	Effect
Nondiabetic rapid hyperosmolarity, e.g., NaCl intoxication	350	Water ⟵	300	Cerebral collapse
Gradual hyperosmolarity, i.e., hyperosmolar hyperglycemic nonketotic coma	350	Water ⟷	350	Brain volume maintained via production of idiogenetic osmoles
Rapid treatment of hyperosmolar hyperglycemic nonketotic coma	300	Water ⟶	350	Brain osmolarity cannot follow plasma osmolarity decrease: cerebral edema

days to a few weeks) than in DKA. The duration of the prodromal phase explains the magnitude of dehydration. The patient becomes gradually lethargic. Other symptoms such as polyuria and fatigue are similar to DKA, but hyperventilation is not present and the breath does not smell of acetone.

Hyperosmolar Hyperglycemic Nonketotic Coma Phase

The major symptoms include varying levels of consciousness with focal neurological signs and intense dehydration with paradoxic polyuria. Consciousness constantly varies from stupor to deep coma. Focal signs such as myoclonus and local epilepsy are frequent. Dehydration is massive and predominantly intracellular. Intracellular symptoms of dehydration include massive weight loss (often >10 kg), dry skin, and hyperthermia (note that, in contrast, DKA is associated with hypothermia). Extracellular dehydration causes hypotension, with or without shock. At this phase, paradoxic polyuria is replaced by oliguria (Table 52.6).

Laboratory Investigations

Blood glucose levels often are higher in hyperosmolar hyperglycemic nonketotic coma than in DKA, often greater than 1000 mg/dl (up to 3000 mg/dl). Plasma sodium levels may be low in the initial phase, then usually increase to the upper range of nor-

mal or higher. The hypernatremia requires correction according to the degree of hyperglycemia (see "Diabetic Ketoacidosis"). Hypernatremia does not reflect sodium loss, which may reach 500 mmol, but water loss, which may exceed 10 liters. Osmolarity is often greater than 400 mosm/liter. Water loss as well as osmolarity may be calculated using blood chemistry results and formulas (see "Diabetic Ketoacidosis"). Arterial pH is at the lower end of the normal range (usually >7.2) as a result of moderate hyperlactacidemia and ketonemia. The latter is made essentially of 3β-hydroxybutyrate and is undetected by the usual test strips (see "Diabetic Ketoacidosis"). Increased lactates and 3β-hydroxybutyrate account for the slightly increased anion gap. The serum potassium level is usually normal, but total potassium depletion is constant. Hematocrit and serum creatinine levels are usually increased.

Evolution

Monitoring of evolution of hyperosmolar hyperglycemic nonketotic coma is critical and similar to that for DKA (see "Diabetic Ketoacidosis"). With adequate monitoring and treatment, hyperosmolar hyperglycemic nonketotic coma regresses with a parallel return of consciousness and osmolarity. However, the mortality rate is high (20–40%) usually within the first 2–3 days, and there is a risk of cerebral sequellae such as the extrapyramidal syndrome, cognitive impairment, and, in some cases, subdural hematoma (5).

Complications may occur during therapy. Hypotension may be aggravated during insulin therapy as the result of intracellular shift of glucose and glucose-associated water. Cerebral edema may occur if hyperglycemia is corrected too rapidly because of a slower intracellular correction of hyperosmolarity. As in DKA, potassium levels must be monitored carefully because of the constant potassium depletion and intracellular shift with insulin therapy. Other complications include iatrogenic infections, arterial and venous thrombosis (justifying preventive low-dose heparin therapy), rhabdomyolysis due to dehydration (48), pulmonary collapse due to bronchial obstruction by dehydrated secretions, and hemoglobinuria due to hypotonic fluids (11).

Treatment

The general principles of treatment are similar to those outlined for DKA (3).

Preventive Treatment

Most hyperosmolar hyperglycemic nonketotic coma can be prevented if blood glucose is measured in any patient older than 50 years who is undergoing surgery or being given diuretics or corticosteroids. Elderly diabetic patients should be adequately rehydrated, even if they are not thirsty, especially when fever or infection is present.

Curative Treatment

As in DKA, fluids, insulin, and electrolytes are the major elements of hyperosmolar hyperglycemic nonketotic coma treatment.

Fluids and Electrolytes

The priority in treatment is the correction of hypovolemia to prevent shock. Volume replacement can be obtained with plasma expanders or isotonic saline, 1–2 liters in 1–2 hr or until the blood pressure is acceptable. Then, rehydration is prudently commenced. If the patient is hypernatremic, half-strength saline may be preferred to normal saline; 6–8 liters should

be given in the first 12 hr. Because potassium loss is not as critical as in DKA, potassium replacement may be given in the saline vials (1–2 g of potassium chloride/liter, i.e., 13–26 mmol/liter). However, potassium levels should be as carefully monitored as in DKA. Once blood glucose levels reach 250 mg/dl, half-strength saline should be replaced by 5 or 10% dextrose to keep blood glucose levels in the 200–250 mg/dl range (not below 200 mg/dl) (see DKA).

Insulin

Patients with hyperosmolar hyperglycemic nonketotic coma are sensitive to low doses of insulin. Nevertheless, the rules are similar to DKA: ideally 0.1 unit/kg/hr of insulin by constant i.v. infusion, eventually decreased by one third to one half when blood glucose levels reach 250 mg/dl.

It must be remembered that most hyperosmolar hyperglycemic nonketotic coma patients do not require insulin after the acute episode, and a trial period without insulin should be attempted before the patient is discharged from the hospital.

Other Measures

Antibiotics and preventive low-dose heparin are highly recommended, regardless of the corresponding complication. In elderly patients or those with cardiopulmonary deficiency, a central catheter should be inserted to monitor central venous pressure.

DIABETIC KETOACIDOSIS

Precise definitions are more important for surveys and research than for clinical use. Nevertheless, some relevant definitions are outlined in the Diabetes Control and Complication Trial (a very large clinical study currently being performed in the United States) (18): Diabetic ketoacidosis is considered present if (a) clinical symptoms, (b) positive serum ketones or large or moderate urine ketones, (c) pH less than 7.25 or bicarbonates less than 15 mEq/liter, and (d) nonambulatory therapy occur at the same time. This definition was intended to exclude minor prodromal states, called "ketosis" or "diabetic precoma," which are usually restored promptly by a simple adjustment in insulin treatment.

No recent data exist on the incidence of DKA. In the 1980s the number usually quoted was about 4% events per patient per year, with no trend to decrease (33). On the contrary, because the prevalence of type I diabetes is steadily increasing, the number of new cases is approximately doubling every decade; and because newly diagnosed diabetes is responsible for almost one third of all DKA, the total cases of DKA may increase in the future. Whether the widespread use of home blood glucose monitoring and the discovery of new types of insulin and improved treatment regimens such as multiple injections will reduce the impact of DKS remains uncertain.

Causes

DKA may be the consequence of an absolute or relative deficiency in insulin. An imbalance is created when insulin is insufficient to mitigate the effects of a predominance of counterregulatory hormones (glucagon, adrenaline, cortisol, and growth hormone).

Absolute Insulin Deficiency

Thirty percent of new patients with type I diabetes have DKA as their initial presentation. In established type I diabetes, insulin interruption is frequent in negligent or manipulative patients. Manipulation may represent the major cause of so-called "brittle" diabetes, a form of diabetes predominantly seen in young women whose lives are severely disrupted by frequent episodes of hypoglycemia or ketoacidosis. Involuntary interruption of insulin delivery is the major cause of DKA in patients treated with insulin pumps (50). The risk of DKA is increased three- to fivefold in such patients. Obstruction or leakage of the subcutaneous catheter, failure of the pumps, and local inflammation are the most common mechanisms of insulin flow interruption. The increased risk of DKA, long-term discomfort, and minimal if any glycemic superiority over insulin injections have been the major reasons for the

current decline in the utilization of portable insulin pumps (50). According to a recent survey among pump users in the United States, the current incidence of DKA has decreased to 7% per patient per year as a result of increased knowledge of potential problems, use of buffered insulins that are less likely to precipitate in the catheter, better prevention of skin infections by the use of local antiseptics and more compatible catheters, and, probably, selection of more compliant patients (17). Notably, the increased risk of DKA has not been seen with implantable insulin pumps, probably for the same reasons mentioned above in addition to the reliability of the devices and the safety of full implantability (51).

Other causes of absolute insulin deficiency include islet paralysis by pharmacologic agents such as betamimetic drugs, diazoxide, hydantoins, and pentamidine.

Relative Insulin Deficiency

This situation may theoretically occur in both type I and II diabetes. However, type II diabetic patients are usually DKA-resistant. Infection, either minor or severe, is the leading cause of DKA. Diabetic ketoacidosis may be precipitated by inappropriate manipulation by the patient such as reducing or omitting an insulin dose to "compensate" for inappetence due to illness, or by failure to test for urine ketones in patients habituated to blood glucose testing only. Other precipitating factors include pregnancy, myocardial infarction, trauma, hyperthyroidism, hyperadrenocorticism and steroid administration, and pheochromocytoma. In most cases, however, the increased hyperglycemic hormones are balanced by appropriate insulin dosage. A specific cause remains unidentified in 25% of patients with DKA.

Pathophysiology

Carbohydrate and fat metabolism are perturbed by the abnormal balance of insulin and counterregulatory hormones during DKA as a catabolic state evolves (Fig. 52.1)(3).

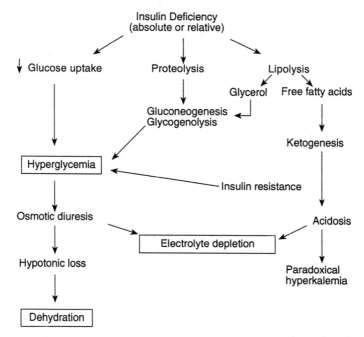

Figure 52.1. Pathophysiology of diabetic ketoacidosis.

Carbohydrate Metabolism

Hepatic, and less importantly, renal, glucose production is increased three- to five-fold (up to 20 μmol/kg/min, i.e., approximately 15 g/hr), as a result of increased glycogenolysis, decreased glycolysis, and increased neoglucogenesis. The major impact of glucagon and epinephrine is the inhibition of fructose 2,6-biphosphate, which, when uninhibited, stimulates phosphofructokinase and inhibits fructose 1,6-diphosphatase, thereby increasing flux along the glycolytic pathway. Another major mechanism is the increase in the flux of neoglucogenic substrates such as amino acids, lactate, and glycerol to the liver.

In addition to increased glucose production by the liver, DKA is associated with decreased peripheral glucose through several mechanisms: excess ketone bodies are utilized by brain tissue instead of glucose, and insulin-dependent tissues such as muscles have a lower uptake and oxidation of glucose in the presence of circulating free fatty acids and excess ketones. The only protective mechanism is the massive renal elimination of glucose,

which usually partially compensates for the effects of the other hyperglycemic mechanisms and thus limits the increase in blood glucose levels.

Fat Metabolism

Lipolysis is increased during DKA. Circulating fatty acids are taken up by the liver, where they are turned into triglycerides and ketones. Circulating amino acids produced by peripheral proteolysis also participate in up to 20% of ketogenesis. Ketone bodies (acetoacetic acid, β-hydroxybutyric acid, and acetone) may accumulate in the circulation at levels of up to 30 mmol/liter because their peripheral oxidation in the Krebs cycle is blocked as a result of lack of oxaloacetate, which is being fully utilized for gluconeogenesis (Fig. 52.2). Circulating ketones have major consequences: as weak acids, they are completely dissociated. Excess hydrogen ions (H^+) are partly eliminated by the kidneys after being buffered by phosphates, whereas elimination of ketones in the urine is responsible for the loss of sodium and po-

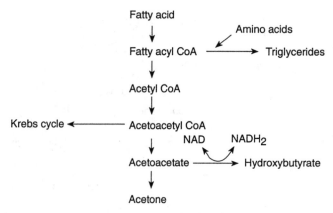

Figure 52.2. Ketone bodies formation.

tassium and the prevention of uric acid elimination.

Excess H^+ accelerates the respiratory rate, permitting elimination of some H^+ and volatile acetone. Excess H^+ is also responsible for peripheral vasodilation, and thus hypothermia, negative cardiac inotropic effects, displacement of potassium from intracellular to extracellular fluid, peripheral insulin resistance, and poor dissociation of oxyhemoglobin at the tissue level resulting from a decreased formation of 2,3-diphosphoglycerate due to phosphate deficiency. This may aggravate ischemic situations such as infarction or cerebral attack.

Excess H^+ has a complex central effect during DKA, depending on the level and rate of change. For example, massive acidosis depresses the respiratory centers, and rapid correction of circulating acidosis may provoke a paradoxical cerebral acidosis because of the premature arrest of polypnea causing slower diffusion of bicarbonates than of carbon dioxide throughout the cerebrovascular barrier.

Finally, both carbohydrate and fat metabolism disorders result in extreme hydroelectrolytic abnormalities: 50–150 ml/kg of water or about 10% of body weight may be lost, mostly by osmotic diuresis following excess glucose elimination and by vomiting. Sodium losses may reach 7–10 mEq/kg and cause hypovolemia, which in turn may cause renal impairment and accompanying lactic acidosis. Lactate acidosis may be responsible for as much as 25% of total acidosis during DKA. A paradoxical circulating hyponatremia is a common consequence of the osmotic presence of excess plasma glucose. As a rule, true natremia may be calculated by knowing that for every 50 mg/dl increase in plasma glucose, plasma sodium is decreased by 1 mmol/liter. Potassium losses may reach 3–12 mmol/kg and are not reflected initially by kaliuresis, because of the intra- to extracellular potassium shift. Vomiting aggravates potassium deficiency, which in turn aggravates gastric stasis. Other major losses include phosphates (0.5–1.5 mmol/kg), magnesium, and calcium (0.25–0.75 mmol/kg each).

Signs and Symptoms

Ketosis Phase

The ketosis (pre-DKA) phase may last a few hours to a few days. Initial symptoms include fatigue, thirst, anorexia, nausea, and polyuria. These symptoms should warn the patient to check the level of urine ketones and supplement with regular insulin (see "Preventive Treatment," p. 876).

Diabetic Ketoacidosis Phase

The classic presentation of DKA includes a series of symptoms. Kussmaul respiration, or deep-sighing hyperventilation, is a major sign. Respiration frequency parallels the degree of acidosis, except when acidosis is extreme and depresses the respiratory centers. Consciousness is altered but is usually limited to confusion and stupor. Only 10% of DKA is associated with unconsciousness. Symptoms of intracellular and extracellular dehydration are present and parallel the severity of DKA, especially hypotension. Others symptoms include hypothermia, peripheral vasodilation (facial rubor contrasts with the palor seen in hypoglycemic coma). Occasionally, abdominal symptoms may predominate including pain, gastric paresis, and absence of bowel sounds.

Laboratory Investigations

Ketosis resulting from DKA should be diagnosed at bedside (Table 52.7). The use of plasma is preferable to urine to detect ketones, because the degree of ketonuria correlates poorly with the degree of ketonemia. Both tablets (Acetest) and test strips (Ketodiastix, Ketostix, Ketodiabur) made to detect ketones in urine can also detect them in plasma. A measurement of 1+ on a test strip is considered positive. The level of normal total ketone bodies is usually lower than 0.15 mmol/liter and may reach 30 mmol/liter during DKA. It should be noted that, with severe anoxia and acidemia, β-hydroxybutyrate levels may predominate to such an extent that a false-negative test may result.

Hyperglycemia should be diagnosed at bedside, using blood glucose test strips rather than urine test strips. However, Ketodiastix strips may give false-negative urine glucose readings because of ketones in the urine, whereas Ketodiabur test strips are not influenced.

Blood glucose levels are usually in the 300–500 mg/dl range. Values higher than 500 mg/dl are more common in hyperosmolar coma, and values lower than 300 mg/dl are more common in lactic acidosis. The distinction is sometimes difficult, because ketones can be present in either state. However, blood glucose levels outside this range may be seen in DKA, as in so-called "euglycemic" DKA (actually about 200 mg/dl), a situation not infrequent in patients treated with insulin pumps.

While other immediate measures such as ECG (see below) are taken, the most urgent laboratory test is arterial blood pH, because the extent of acidemia will influence treatment. Analysis of blood chemistry is also essential: blood glucose will confirm test strip results and creatinine levels will determine the degree of prerenal failure. Plasma sodium levels are generally low despite a total body deficit of hypotonic saline. As mentioned before, true natremia must be corrected according to the degree of hyperglycemia. Serum chloride levels may be normal or excessive. Plasma potassium levels may be low, normal, or high, despite a constant major body deficit. As mentioned before, plasma potassium levels increase by 1 mmol/liter independent of potassium loss for every 0.1-pH decrement; therefore, initial hyperkalemia may be seen in 30% of DKA cases. Normokalemia indicates significant deficit. Initial hypokalemia, although rare, indicates massive deficit and may be seen in DKA with insidious onset or with concomitant treatment with diuretics. Electrolyte levels allow calculation of the anion gap by using the following formula:

$$(Na^+ + K^+) - (Cl^- + HCO_3^-) - 17$$

The normal anion gap (<3 mEq/liter) increases during DKA. If the level of plasma ketones is insufficient to explain the increased anion gap, lactic acidosis or renal insufficiency should be suspected. Electrolyte levels also permit calculation of osmolarity:

$$2(Na^+ + K^+) + glycemia \ (mmol/liter) + urea \ (mmol/liter)$$

Table 52.7
Initial Tests for the Diagnostic and Management of DKA

Bedside
  Blood glucose
  Plasma ketones
  ECG
  Chest x-ray
  Urine volume and ketonuria
Laboratory
  Arterial pH
  Blood chemistry (glucose, urea, creatinine, electrolytes)
  Urinalysis and culture
  Blood and throat swab culture ($\pm$)
  CBC ($\pm$)

The converting factors from mg/dl to mmol/liter are 1/18 for glucose and 1/2.8 for urea.

Bacterial cultures of urine, throat swab, and blood are optional, but should be ordered if there is the least suspicion of infection. Pyrexia is usually absent even with infection, and leukocytosis is present even without infection. A chest radiograph should also be ordered routinely because pulmonary infections are frequent, and the risk of subsequent iatrogenic pulmonary disorders is high.

Evolution

With adequate treatment, DKA regresses usually within 12–48 hr. Positive urinary ketones may be found several hours after ketogenesis is normalized. Ketosis may also be aggravated after 6–10 hr of therapy because of a shift in the acetoacetate/β-hydroxybutyrate ratio while the total ketone bodies continue to decrease. The decision to discontinue DKA treatment should therefore depend only on the regression of blood acidosis.

Monitoring of evolution is critical. Vital signs and bedside tests (blood glucose, urine volume, urine ketones) should be repeated at least every hour for the first 6 hr, then every 2 hr. Potassium should be monitored ideally by both continuous ECG and urgent laboratory determination of electrolytes repeated at least at 2 hr, 6 hr, and then every 12 hr. Arterial pH should be rechecked within the first hours if no clinical improvement is seen. After more than 6 hr of treatment and when clear clinical regression of DKA is indicated by correction of clinical symptoms, hyperglycemia, and dehydration and diminution of urine ketones, arterial pH can be used to determine when to stop first-phase DKA treatment. In clinical practice, the determination of urine ketones may be omitted, and the decision to discontinue DKA therapy decided if electrolytes, including bicarbonates, are normalized.

Treatment

Preventive Treatment

Most DKA could be prevented if adequate instructions were given to insulin-treated diabetic patients regarding such issues as management of hyperglycemia and sick-day rules.

Management of Hyperglycemia

If blood glucose is above 250/dl, check urine ketones.
If urine ketones + or greater, supplement the usual insulin regimen with regular insulin, 10 units s.c. every 4 hr.
Check blood glucose every 2 hr. Reinject if necessary. Stop supplementing when blood glucose is lower than 250 mg/dl. Call doctor or go to emergency room if problem persists more than 12 hr.

Sick-day Rules

Never omit usual insulin injections. DO NOT decrease doses.
Absorb fractionated carbohydrates (six meals or more). Take sugar containing a glucide equivalent (milk, soft drink) if gastric intolerance exists. Take a second meal if vomiting occurs.
Check blood glucose four times a day and urine ketones two times a day.
Supplement with s.c. rapid insulin if necessary every 4 hr, as follows:
Blood glucose > 150 and urine ketones 2 +: 4 units + 20 g carbohydrates
Blood glucose > 250 regardless urine ketones: 8 units
Blood glucose > 400 regardless urine ketones: 12 units
Call doctor or go to emergency room if problem persists more than 24 hr, or sooner if clinical symptoms such as vomiting occur.

Curative Treatment

Fluid insulin and electrolytes are the major elements of DKA treatment. Because of the need for precise adjustments and the risk of dramatic iatrogenic complications such as hypoglycemia or hypokalemia, treatment in a hospital unit accustomed to metabolic intensive care is highly recommended.

Fluids

Fluid replacement is the first priority, even to correct hyperglycemia, because the patient will be more sensitive to insulin if rehydrated, and hemodilution by fluid replacement may account for as much as

23% of the decrease in blood glucose. An infusion of isotonic saline (154 mmol/liter; 0.9%) is initially given as 1 liter in 30 min, then 1 liter in the next hour, and then 1 liter every 2–4 hr, so that one half of the fluid deficit is replaced in 8–12 hr, and the second half in 16–24 hr.

Only if pH is less than 7.0 is i.v. bicarbonate administration justified. Isotonic 1.4% bicarbonate, 500–750 ml (80–120 mmol), is administered in the first hour, rather than normal saline. It must be remembered that bicarbonate administration carries a high risk of aggravated hypokalemia, paradoxical cerebral acidosis, and tissue hypoxia. Plasma expanders are indicated at the start of fluid replacement if blood pressure is below 90 mm Hg. Half-normal saline (0.45%) should be administered only when hypernatremia is definite (>155 mmol), and administration should be at a slower rate than with normal saline. Saline administration should be replaced by 5% dextrose (with sodium chloride to keep solution at 0.9%) when the blood glucose level reaches 250 mg/dl. The 5% dextrose solution should be replaced by 10% dextrose if the blood glucose level falls below 200 mg/dl. Blood glucose levels should be maintained in the 200–250 mg/dl range.

Insulin

Regular insulin should be administered as a continuous i.v. infusion using a bedside infusion pump. Insulin may be diluted in normal saline or water at a concentration of 1 unit/ml. Insulin absorption on syringe and catheter walls is minimal. However, the first 5 ml of solution should be flushed from the syringe-catheter apparatus. After a loading dose of 0.1 unit/kg, a constant infusion of 0.1 unit/kg/hr is begun. When the blood glucose level falls below 250 mg/dl, the insulin infusion is maintained at 0.05 unit/kg/hr, and dextrose infusion is started. The blood glucose level is subsequently maintained in the 200–250 mg/dl range by adjusting i.v. dextrose concentrations. Others prefer to maintain the dextrose concentration (e.g., 5%) and adjust (usually down to 2–3 units/hr) the insulin rate. The former procedure is preferable because it allows more insulin and dextrose administration per unit of time, which provides more calories and may accelerate the clearance of ketosis and acidemia. However, one should not hesitate to double the initial insulin rates if blood glucose remains unchanged after the first 2 hr.

Other Electrolytes

Potassium is the most critical electrolyte to replace during DKA. Ten percent potassium chloride (one 10-ml ampule contains 1 g of potassium chloride, i.e., 13 mmol of K^+) should be added to fluids, starting with 20 mmol/hr until laboratory results are known (if ECG is normal), then frequently readjusted according to laboratory potassium values as follows:

If K^+ > 6 mmol/liter: no potassium administration
If K^+ 5–6 mmol/liter: 10 mmol/hr
If K^+ 4–5 mmol/liter: 20 mmol/hr
If K^+ 3–4 mmol/liter: 30 mmol/hr
If K^+ < 3 mmol/liter: 40 mmol/hr

A central catheter is mandatory for high-rate potassium administration, to avoid irritation to the vein, pain, and tissue reactions. Therefore, an i.v. central catheter should be placed at the start of treatment if the potassium level is below 4 mmol/liter.

Other Measures

Existing or restored diuresis is a critical condition for safe fluid and potassium administration.

If no urine is obtained after 2 hr of rehydration and therapy, a urinary catheter should be inserted. If no urine is found, potassium administration should be stopped, and fluid administration decreased. Furosemide (40 mg) may help to restore impaired diuresis. If no urine appears after 4 hr of rehydration, a central venous catheter must be placed and used to adjust fluid administration. Other measures include nasogastric suction if the patient is comatose, prudent heparinization if osmolarity is greater than 360 mosm/liter, and oxygen if Po_2 is lower than 80 mm Hg. Intravenous phosphate replacement (e.g., potassium phosphate) is unnecessary and is therefore not recommended. Antibiotics should always be considered and used more liberally than usual, starting with broad-spectrum antibiotics after the culture samples have been taken.

Post-DKA Phase

Intravenous therapy (insulin, fluids, and electrolytes) should be discontinued only if all the following criteria are met: the patient is conscious and eating if the usual time for a meal is reached, dehydration is corrected by 75% or more, the level of plasma electrolytes is normal, and the level of blood glucose is in the 150–250 mg/dl range. Remember that it is less harmful to the patient to prolong i.v. treatment unnecessarily rather than to stop it prematurely and thus to induce a DKA recurrence. Oral caloric and carbohydrate intake may be reinstated, preferably in a semiliquid or soft form. Potassium replacement should be continued with oral potassium supplements for 1 week. Initially, s.c. insulin should be reinstated as rapid insulin, although NPH insulin may be used at night. The usual insulin regimen is restored after 2–3 days of convalescence.

Complications of Therapy

Hypoglycemia, hyper- and hypokalemia, and fluid overload constitute the major iatrogenic complications (see above).

Cerebral edema is a severe iatrogenic complication and is indicated by the recurrence of coma during an apparently successful therapy (34). The prognosis is poor. The mechanism is unclear, but may involve an imbalance between intra- and extracerebral osmolarity caused by a too-rapid fall in plasma osmolarity. This is usually seen with hypotonic rehydration in both adults and children. Prevention includes preferential use of isotonic saline, even if hypernatremia is present, and stabilization of blood glucose values in the 200–250 mg/dl range.

Adult respiratory distress syndrome is another severe complication, possibly resulting from overadministration of hypotonic fluids. Post-DKA metabolic alkylosis can result from overuse of i.v. bicarbonate

during the first-phase treatment. Infections are frequent in diabetic patients. Iatrogenic infections include inhalation pneumonia, urinary infection, and opportunistic infections such as mucormycosis. Thromboembolic risk is increased in DKA because of hypovolemia and hyperviscosity. This complication warrants routine administration of anticoagulants in more severely affected patients.

Conclusion

DKA remains a significant complication of type I diabetes and has a persistently high mortality rate. Major efforts should be directed toward prevention by education of patients and health-care providers. Treatment is urgent and complex, but is currently well standardized, a factor that should improve the prognosis of this complication.

ALCOHOLIC KETOACIDOSIS

Alcoholic ketoacidosis is a state of metabolic acidosis associated with excessive ketone-body formation that can be mistaken for DKA. Such a misjudgment can lead to improper therapeutic measures that could be potentially fatal. Typically, however, alcoholic ketoacidosis and DKA present with striking differences that, in principle, make them easy to distinguish (Table 52.8). In particular, the blood glucose level is low, normal, or moderately high in alcoholic ketacidosis, but is mostly high in DKA. However, many reasons explain why alcoholic ketoacidosis and DKS may be confused.

Alcoholism and diabetes are frequently associated. It may be difficult to distinguish between the moderately increased blood glucose values observed in alcoholic ketoacidosis and some cases of true DKA with so-called "normal blood glucose values" or with only "slight hyperglycemia" such as that seen after abrupt interruption of a continuous subcutaneous insulin infusion by pump (50).

Bedside measurements of blood glucose with test strips, particularly when performed by inexperienced hands, are not accurate enough to distinguish between "slightly" increased (alcoholic ketoaci-

Table 52.8
Differential Diagnosis of Acidosis and Coma in a Diabetic Subject[a]

Type of Disturbance	Blood Glucose (mmol/liter)	Plasma Ketone Bodies	Arterial pH	Plasma Osmolarity (mosm/liter)	Serum HCO₃ (mmol/liter)	Anion Gap (mosm/liter)
Hypoglycemic coma	<2.5	0/+	Normal	Normal	Normal	0
DKA[b]	15–50+	++/++++	<7.25	<350	<15	>12
AKA	≈5.5 (3–9)	+/++	Variable ↑ N ↓	Normal	7–14	<20
Hyperosmolar nonketotic coma	30–150	0/+	>7.2	>350	>15	<12
Lactic acidosis	≈5.5 (2.5–10)	0/+	<7.1	Normal	<10	>20

[a]Modified from Kreisberg RA. Acidosis and coma in the diabetic. In: Brodoff BN, Bleicher SJ, eds. Diabetes mellitus and obesity. Baltimore: Williams & Wilkins, 1982:526–535.
[b]DKA, diabetic ketoacidosis; AKA, alcoholic ketoacidosis.

dosis) and "moderately" increased (DKA) blood glucose values.

A modest glycosuria may be observed in alcoholic ketoacidosis.

Alcoholic ketoacidosis is mainly due to β-OH-butyrate accumulation undetected by conventional methods of urine analysis. However, DKA with predominant β-OH-butyrate formation has also been described (40).

Diabetic ketoacidosis is more familiar to young doctors (because they are better taught) than is alcoholic ketoacidosis, facilitating misdiagnosis of alcoholic ketoacidosis by young physicians.

Clinical Manifestation

Alcoholic ketoacidosis was first described by Dillon in 1940 (22). Since then, fewer than 100 observations have been published. However, the real prevalence of alcoholic ketoacidosis may be underestimated, as nonspecific supportive or corrective therapeutic measures often reverse the situation.

Alcoholic ketoacidosis is observed in subjects suffering from chronic alcoholism who have a history of a recent heavy alcohol intake followed by abrupt cessation (14, 22, 25, 43). In two thirds of the cases, the patients are women; pregnancy may be a factor. Throughout the time of heavy drinking, patients undereat and weight loss is a common feature. When admitted, the patient is dehydrated (intra- and extracellular dehydration); abdominal pain, nausea, vomiting are usually observed; hyperventilation resulting from a metabolic acidotic state may be noted; and clinical signs of chronic alcoholism are often present.

Biological Features

Blood glucose ranges from hypoglycemic (40–60 mg/dl) to slight hyperglycemic levels (140–190 mg/dl) (14). Alcoholic ketoacidosis may be associated with acidemia, alkalemia, or a normal pH (25, 35, 43). Complex acid-base disorders are very common and may be responsible for confusing laboratory values. Usually, pH is acidotic; however, normal or near-normal pH values can be observed when metabolic alkalosis caused by vomiting and chloride depletion is present, or when hyperventilation caused by stress or fever leads to respiratory alkalosis. Hypokalemia and hypochloremia are frequently seen in alcoholic ketoacidosis (but are uncommon in DKA). When vomiting leads to hypochloremic metabolic alkalosis, the increase in anion gap is greater than the decrease in the bicarbonate concentration (35). (The anion gap (AG) can be estimated by using the following formula: $AG = [Na - (HCO_3^{2+}$

+Cl⁻)−12]. In the published case reports, pH values were found between 7.03 (25) and 7.25 (14); Paco₂ was between 19 and 21 mm Hg; plasma HCO_3^{2-} was between 7 and 14 mmol/liter, and β-OH-butyrate was in the range of 8–9 mmol/liter.

Because alcohol produces a more reduced cellular redox state than is generally encountered in DKA, quantitative tests for ketone bodies tend to indicate a lesser degree of ketonuria and ketonemia than actually exists (35). Indeed, nitroprusside reagent reacts with acetoacetate and, to a lesser degree, with acetone, but not with β-OH-butyrate. Plasma β-OH-butyrate assay is thus necessary to clearly identify the situation.

Pathophysiology

Alcohol ketoacidosis is associated with a large production of ketone bodies resulting from starvation, carbohydrate deprivation, and stress, consequently leading to the hypersecretion of glucagon, growth hormone, ACTH, cortisol, and catecholamines (Fig. 52.3). Insulin secretion is depressed, and lipolysis is stimulated. Ethanol and its oxidative derivatives cause an increase in the NADH/NAD⁺ ratio and the preferential formation of β-OH-butyrate.

Associated with the increased formation of ketone bodies is a decrease in their peripheral uptake and in urinary excretion (caused by vomiting-induced hypovolemia). The increased NADH/NAD⁺ ratio is associated in the liver with decreased neoglucogenesis, explaining the absence of severe hyperglycemia in this state of hypercatabolism.

Treatment

Management relies on rehydration and infusion of 5 or 10% dextrose solution. The rate of infusion and amount of liquid depend on the severity of dehydration; 3–5 liters/day are usually necessary. Intravenous bicarbonate is usually not necessary to correct the acidotic state. Insulin infusion is not indicated and may be dangerous, increasing the risks of hypokalemia and severe hypoglycemia. If diagnosis is difficult, however, small amounts of insulin (≤5 units/hr i.v.) can be used if blood glucose is carefully monitored (one strip every 15–30 min). Complete recovery occurs in less than 12 hr.

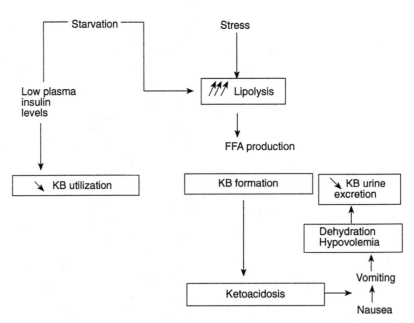

Figure 52.3. Alcoholic ketoacidosis pathophysiology. *FFA*, free fatty acids; *KB*, ketone bodies.

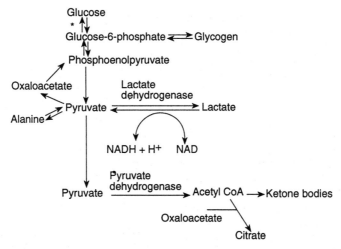

Figure 52.4. Lactate metabolism. *, in liver and kidney.

LACTIC ACIDOSIS

Lactic acidosis is the most frequent cause of metabolic acidosis, but is often undiagnosed or diagnosed too late. There has been considerable argument over the definition. According to Alberti and Nattrass (4), lactic acidosis is present when blood lactate levels are greater than 5 mmol/liter and arterial blood pH is less than 7.25. Interest has recently been renewed because drug-induced lactic acidosis has been identified in diabetic patients treated with biguanides, especially phenformin. The prognosis remains poor.

Pathophysiology

Biochemistry

Normal lactate levels at rest are 0.75 mmol/liter. Normal pyruvate levels are 0.07 mmol/liter. Therefore, the lactate/pyruvate (L/P) ratio is normally 10. Blood lactate levels may reach 22 mmol/liter during intense exercise. Otherwise, lactate levels remain stable over the day. Lactate levels remain balanced as a result of production and elimination.

Lactate Production

Pyruvate from glycolysis and amino acids, particularly alanine, are transformed into lactate. This conversion is controlled by a specific enzyme, lactate dehydrogenase (Fig. 52.4). This reaction occurs in the cytoplasm of most human cells, especially in the skin, red blood cells, brain, muscles, and, with anoxia, in the liver as well. This lactate diffuses rapidly into the blood in an ionized form.

Lactate Elimination

Lactate metabolism occurs in the liver predominantly (70%) and in the kidney (30%). Lactate is converted back into pyruvate when NAD^+ is present. Pyruvate is then directed into the tricarboxylic cycle, a reaction that occurs in the mitochrondria and is controlled by a key enzyme: pyruvate dehydrogenase. The activity of this enzyme is, in turn, regulated by a number of factors, including insulin and thiamine (vitamin B_1).

Other elimination pathways include neoglucogenesis; oxidation in muscles, myocardium, liver, and kidney; and excretion in urine. Urine excretion is responsible for only 0.5 mmol/24 hr in the basal state. Ketone bodies and uric acid are competitors of lactic acid in tubular excretion.

The overall turnover of lactate is 1500 mmol/24 hr. Lactate elimination is highly dependent on the redox equilibrium, the $NADH/NAD^+$ ratio. Therefore, the L/P ratio increases as $NADH/NAD^+$ increases (e.g., if dehydrogenases are increased). This occurs with anoxia (glyceraldehyde dehydrogenase) or alcohol intoxication (alcohol

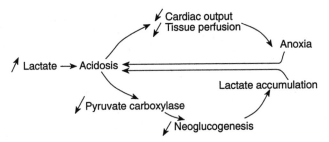

Figure 52.5. The vicious circle of lactic acidosis.

dehydrogenase). The NADH/NAD$^+$ ratio is also increased when NADH is not utilized because neoglucogenesis is blocked, as occurs with alcohol or biguanides or when the electron cascades are blocked, as with anoxia. As a result of a vicious circle (Fig. 52.5), the above mechanisms tend to accelerate once lactic acidosis has begun. Renal neoglucogenesis, however, is not blocked by acidosis. Therefore, when acute tubulopathy is associated with lactate excess, this protective mechanism is lost.

Classification

Overproduction and decreased elimination of lactate often coexist in clinical situations. However, according to Cohen and Woods (12), type A lactic acidosis is present when anoxia or shock occur before lactic acidosis. In type B lactic acidosis, anoxia or shock occur after lactic acidosis. Table 52.9 shows the classifications and causes of lactic acidosis. The most frequent form of lactic acidosis is Type A although it is frequently ignored. Diabetes is the most frequent cause of type B lactic acidosis, either directly (type B1) or indirectly (type B2). Diabetes predisposes to type 1 lactic acidosis because of factors such as poor tissue perfusion and epinephrine and cortisol abnormalities. Indeed, some lactic acidosis (>5 mmol/liter) is present in 10–15% of diabetic ketoacidotic states. Alcohol and biguanides intoxication cause type B2 lactic acidosis in diabetics. The high incidence of lactic acidosis in patients treated with phenformin and buformin has resulted in a general ban on all biguanides in the United States for the last 20 years (9). In European countries, metformin is

Table 52.9
Classification of Lactic Acidosis[a]

Type	Description
Type A	Hypoxic, poor tissue perfusion, shock
Type B1	Associated with common disorders: diabetes mellitus, renal failure, liver failure, infection, leukemia
Type B2	Due to drugs or toxins: phenformin, metformin, buformin, ethanol, salicylates, fructose, methanol
Type B3	Hereditary forms: glucose 6-phosphatase deficiency, infantile lactic acidosis
Type B4	Miscellaneous

[a]From Cohen RD, Woods HF. Clinical and biochemical aspects of lactic acidosis. Oxford: Blackwell, 1976: 42.

used because of the much lower incidence of lactic acidosis than with phenformin (10, 36). In an extensive report published in 1978, 285 cases of lactic acidosis were associated with phenformin uses versus 12 with metformin associated in every case to nonobservance of contraindications like renal insufficiency (36). Biguanides block transfer of reduced equivalents from the mitochondria to the cytosol, therefore preventing neoglucogenesis and promoting lactate accumulation. This effect is potentiated by alcohol intake or fructose or sorbitol administration. Biguanides in excess are necessary to induce lactic acidosis. This may be the consequence of overdosage or reduced elimination. Phenformin is excreted by the liver and kidneys, whereas metformin is excreted by the kidneys only, without being metabolized. Therefore, phenformin may accumulate with either hepatic or renal insufficiency, whereas metformin accumulates only with renal impairment.

Consequences of Excess Lactate

As long as pH is greater than 7.10 (i.e., bicarbonates > 10 mmol/liter), the stimulatory effects of acidosis occur predominantly via catecholamines causing tachycardia. When pH is less than 7.10, cardiac output decreases, venoconstriction and arterial vasodilation occur, and blood pressure drops. Respiratory depression and nodal bradycardia are signs of profound acidosis.

Signs and Symptoms

Prodromal Phase

A prelactic acidosis phase is irregular and of variable duration (a few hours to a few days). Symptoms include abdominal and thoracic cramps, asthenia, and anorexia.

Lactic Acidotic Phase

Consciousness is altered, but this is usually limited to anxiety and agitation. Major symptoms include hyperventilation, minor dehydration, oligoanuria, and hypotension. Hypothermia is common. Cardiac arrhythmia, bradycardia, and cardiovascular collapse are symptoms of advanced lactic acidosis.

Laboratory Investigations

Metabolic acidosis is usually massive. A pH less than 7.0 is common. Ketone bodies are usually slightly positive or negative. However, β-hydroxybutyrate levels are increased. Blood glucose is likely to be low or normal. Blood electrolytes exhibit a major anion gap, usually of 15–40 mmol/liter, resulting from the accumulation of blood lactate, β-hydroxybutyrate, phosphates, and sulfates. Plasma potassium may be normal or slightly increased. Creatinine and urea levels are frequently increased, but not enough to explain the above abnormalities. Blood lactate may be measured immediately, preferably in arterial blood. Values vary between 5 and 40 mmol/liter (normal values: <1 mmol/liter). Blood pyruvate is increased, and the L/P ratio is usually greater than 20 (normal L/P ratio: 10).

In clinical practice, lactic acidosis should be suspected when there is metabolic acidosis with a large anion gap and no major diabetes decompensation. Measurement of blood lactate and, if present, plasma biguanide levels will confirm the diagnosis.

Treatment

Treatment of lactic acidosis is unsatisfactory, with a mortality rate of about 50% in biguanide-associated cases and 60–80% in others. Lower mortality rates have been reported with metformin-associated cases (10).

Symptomatic Treatment

Symptomatic treatment includes correction of acidosis and hyperlactacidemia, restoration of hemodynamic stability, and treatment or prevention of anuria. Consciousness, vital signs, levels of bicarbonates, lactate, creatinine, and electrolytes, and the anion gap should be closely monitored.

Vascular support and reversal of hypotension must be provided immediately for treatment to be successful. Vasodilatory drugs (e.g., nitroprussiate) and drugs with positive inotropic effects (e.g., dopamine or dobutamine) should be used.

Correction of acidosis is equally important. However, the risk of paradoxical intracellular acidosis may increase because carbon dioxide diffuses more readily than bicarbonates within the cells. On the other hand, as long as pH remains below 7.0, the liver will produce, rather than clear, lactate, resulting in a vicious circle. Alkalinizing substances other than bicarbonates (e.g., THAM) have been proposed, but prospective comparative studies remain to be done. Therefore, i.v. bicarbonate should be given to increase pH to no higher than 7.20 and blood bicarbonates to no higher than 10 to avoid overloading of bicarbonates and the risk of paradoxical aggravation.

Correction of hyperlactacidemia has been successful with dichloroacetate, which activates pyruvate dehydrogenase. However, dicloroacetate is not freely available, and studies on humans are still rare (54).

Treatment or prevention of anuria is critical to avoid the inevitable sodium load that occurs with bicarbonate administration. Diuretics may help, but hemodialysis is the preferred treatment. In addition, hemodialysis treats acidosis and lactacidemia and clears biguanides. Symptomatic treatment can also include insulin therapy. However, insulin therapy should be carefully considered. The beneficial effect resulting from activation of pyruvate dehydrogenase is offset by the activation of glycolysis and the inhibition of glucogenesis, which tend to increase lactate production.

Preventive Treatment

Although lactic acidosis is a potential complication of biguanide therapy, the least toxic of biguanides (i.e., metformin) can be used because it has been proved to effectively treat type II diabetes. However, the contraindications must be carefully reviewed when using metformin. These include existing or potential hepatopathy (e.g., alcoholism), existing or potential nephropathy (e.g., in patients age >65), acute tubulopathy, surgery, x-ray procedures (implying dye opacification), and dextran administration. Biguanides should not be given with drugs such as diuretics, aminosides, or antiinflammatory compounds. Clinical conditions such as circulatory problems, septicemia, and pregnancy are also contraindications because of the potential hemodynamic changes.

THE DIABETIC PATIENT IN AN INTENSIVE CARE UNIT

Diabetes mellitus is a common disease affecting 5–10% of the general population and 20–30% of patients older than 60 years admitted to the hospital. Often, patients admitted with diabetic complications are unaware of their disease. It is not surprising, therefore, that the medical treatment for such acute situations frequently is unrelated to the disease. The patient may then be faced with severe, and sometimes life-threatening metabolic complications.

Conditions leading to admittance to an emergency room are usually severe, both physically and psychologically. This enormous challenge to the normal islet cells of the pancreas causes metabolic control to deteriorate profoundly and rapidly. Severe hyperglycemia or DKA can appear in a few hours, even in patients with no history of diabetes or whose blood glucose values were "normal" in the recent past.

The following situations offer some answers to pragmatic clinical questions.

The patient is a known diabetic and has been on treatment. How should the patient's treatment be handled during hospitalization?

If the patient is insulin treated, insulin therapy must be maintained; however, regardless of previous insulin regimen, the patient should be given either multiple s.c. insulin injections or a continuous i.v. insulin infusion. The choice between the two depends on the severity of the underlying situation.

If the clinical situation is relatively stable and there is no immediate threat such as a planned, extensive surgical procedure or a life-threatening and rapidly evolving infection, the s.c. route is preferred. One injection of intermediate insulin (isophane, NPH), repeated every 12 hr, is given at the patient's normal daily dosage. This method is used, not to obtain near-normoglycemia (as it is usually), but to contain blood glucose levels between 180 and 200 mg/dl. Concomitantly, and if the patient is unable to take meals and snacks, a continuous dextrose i.v. infusion must be initiated at the rate of 200–250 g of dextrose/24 hr. Blood glucose monitoring every 1–3 hr, depending on the severity of the situation, will indicate the need for supplementary bolus injections of regular insulin. These boluses can be delivered s.c. every 3 hr or i.v. every hour, when blood glucose values are above 250–300 mg/dl (at a rate of 5 units of regular insulin when the blood glucose level is above 250 mg/liter and 10 units above 300 mg/liter). Up to half of the total amount of regular insulin injected as boluses should be used to determine the amount of intermediate insulin planned for the following day. For example, if 40 IU regular insulin have been injected as supplements in addition to the s.c. dosage of intermediate insulin, the following day's dosage should be increased by 16–20 units of isophane given in two equal amounts (8–10 units in the morning and again in the evening).

Urine should also be carefully monitored for ketone bodies. The appearance of significant numbers of ketone bodies (++ or +++) should be treated with extra boluses of s.c. or i.v. insulin, regardless of blood glucose values. However, if blood glucose values are below 200 mg, the dextrose infusion rate should be increased to accommodate the insulin boluses without risk of hypoglycemic reactions. Boluses should be repeated every hour i.v. or every 2–3 hr s.c. until ketone bodies equal 0 or trace amounts.

If the clinical situation is excessively unstable or if major events can be foreseen, then continuous i.v. infusions are preferable to the s.c. route. The only risk with i.v. insulin infusion is that its discontinuation can be detrimental, even after a short interruption of a few hours. Electric syringes, or even small pumps used for s.c. insulin infusion, are preferable to insulin added to the i.v. drip bottle, which is subject to wide and unpredictable rate variations. This method should not be used unless insulin and dextrose are mixed (with some potassium) in the same bottle. Nevertheless, this procedure requires careful monitoring so that the total amount of insulin and dextrose planned for the following 24-hr period is effectively administered. For this reason, insulin administered by means of a syringe-pump may be preferable. Of course, only regular insulin can be used for i.v. infusion. The rate of infusion, in units/hour, is calculated according to the previous total daily insulin need. The main advantage of this method is that the pump rate can be quickly adapted according to the hourly blood glucose measurements as determined by test strips. If blood glucose values are above 200, 250, or 350 mg/100 ml, the hourly basal rate can be increased by 50, 60, or 80%, respectively; if blood glucose values are below 150 or 100 mg/liter, the initial rate should be decreased by 20–50%, respectively. This simple rule is often sufficient to maintain blood glucose values between 180 and 200 mg/liter. More sophisticated rules can be described that not only take into account the actual blood glucose values, but also earlier values. Such rules are described in Table 52.10.

If the patient is treated by oral drugs, biguanides must be stopped whether the situation is severe or not. Sulfonylureas may be continued at the same dosage only if the medical situation is not severe, the patient is able to eat, and blood glucose

Table 52.10
Changes (in %) in the Current Intravenous Insulin Infusion Rate Taking into Account the Actual Blood Glucose Value and the Increment/Decrement in Blood Glucose (in mg/100 ml) Observed Over One Hour[a]

Actual Blood Glucose Value (mg/100 ml)	ΔG (mg/100 ml)			0 or Unknown	+30	+60	+90
	−90	−60	−30				
0.50–1	−80%	−80%	−80%	−50%	NC[b]	NC	
100/150	−60%	−40%	−30%	−20%	NC	+10%	+50%
150–200	−50%	−30%	−20%	NC	+10%	+20%	+30%
200–250	−40%	−20%	NC	+20%	+20%	+40%	+60%
250–350	−30%	NC	+10%	+50%	+60%	+70%	+80%
350–450	NC	NC	+60%	+80%	+80%	+80%	+80%

[a] This scheme implies hourly blood glucose measurements and target blood glucose values in the range of 150–200 mg/100 ml. When starting, the insulin infusion rate is calculated as follows: IIR (units/hour) = total daily SC dosage (in units)/24 hr. After setting this initial value, changes are cumulative. For example: at 10:00 AM the insulin infusion rate was 1.8 unit/hr and had to be increased by 20% (i.e., became 2.2); if at 11:00 AM the blood glucose is now 270 mg/100 ml and the ΔG is +30 mg, the rate should be increased by 60%, making the new rate 3.5 units/hr. A cumulative increase of up to 1000% over 24 hr is conceivable in very severe stress or infectious situations.
[b] NC, no change.

values are 200 mg/dl or lower. In all other situations, a transient insulin therapy is preferable. The method of s.c. or i.v. therapy is similar to that previously described. The initial total insulin dosage can be rated at 0.5–0.7 units/kg/day.

If the diabetic patient undergoes surgery, surgical stress causes additional suppression of insulin secretion and an aggravated-state of insulin resistance (hormone-induced) that can further deteriorate the metabolic control. As can be expected, the degree of foreseen deterioration is proportional to the degree of surgical trauma. The previously described rules for diabetic management when a patient is hospitalized in an ICU should remain the same when a patient undergoes surgery.

If the diabetic patient has not been given insulin, is moderately hyperglycemic (≤250 mg/dl), and is undergoing a minor surgical procedure, simple observation can suffice, and taking care to avoid dextrose perfusion.

If the patient is already insulin-treated with twice daily s.c. intermediate insulin and the surgical procedure is minor, i.v. dextrose infusion (200–250 g/24 hr) with the same s.c. insulin regime will suffice.

If the surgical procedure is a major one, i.v. insulin and i.v. dextrose are recommended (as already described); blood glucose monitoring is mandatory.

When emergency, not elective, surgery is needed, correction of preexisting significant ketonuria/ketonemia or, more importantly, DKA is mandatory. No patient should be operated upon before absolute correction of DKA, unless it is necessary to stop a bleeding artery. Abdomens appearing to require surgery are often "cured" by the correction of DKA!

Heart surgery with cardiopulmonary bypass, particularly with hypothermia, in a nondiabetic patient is frequently associated with some degree of pre- and postoperative hyperglycemia resulting from insulin secretion shutoff, and decreased peripheral utilization due to hypothermia. Even in nondiabetic patients, this hyperglycemia is highly insulin-resistant, but does not significantly influence outcome and quickly corrects itself. The best treatment to prevent this hyperglycemic state in non-

diabetic patients is to avoid dextrose infusion.

If the patient is not identified as a diabetic but presents with hyperglycemia, how can diabetes be confirmed? This question is more theoretical than pragmatic. Any major stress can transform an individual with normal blood glucose values into a diabetic, with even insulin dependency or ketoacidosis, all within only a few hours. The decision to treat with insulin depends on the level of hyperglycemia or associated metabolic disturbances such as ketonuria. However, caution should be taken not to misinterpret the presence of ketone bodies in the urine or plasma, which may be a result of fasting or stress-induced lipolysis. Acidosis may be due to many different causes, including severe shock.

Mild hyperglycemia (up to 200 mg/100 ml) is frequently observed in the early phase of myocardial infarction. Knowing whether the patient was previously diabetic or not is of some importance. Diabetic patients with myocardial infarction should be maintained in the ICU for a longer period than nondiabetics because a higher incidence of sudden death has been observed in these patients between 2 and 3 weeks postinfarct. To retrospectively diagnose diabetes, the immediate measurement of glycated hemoglobin ($HbA1_c$) levels is recommended; this variable reflects the mean blood glucose levels over the preceding 2–3 months, and its use should be encouraged.

What diabetogenic treatments can induce or aggravate moderate hyperglycemia? Exacerbation of hyperglycemia in patients with diabetes or slightly impaired glucose tolerance may be induced by many drugs or compounds. Three are particularly "effective": parenteral β-adrenergic stimulants, corticosteroids, and dextrose infusion.

β-Adrenergic stimulants such as salbutamol and ritodrin are used to treat asthma and premature labor. In their parenteral form, they can induce a ketoacidosis within a few hours (see below). The oral and respiratory forms are less detrimental, but caution is advised. These drugs increase glycogenolysis in the liver and in skeletal muscles, but they also stimulate insulin secretion. The net result is hyperglycemia, particularly when insulin secretion is impaired.

Corticosteroids are the most commonly used drugs and are capable of severely impairing glucose metabolism. They stimulate gluconeogenesis and decrease hepatic and peripheral tissue sensitivity to insulin. Corticosteroids can induce hyperglycemia regardless of the route of administration; however, the parenteral and oral routes are the most detrimental and can induce severe hyperglycemia.

Dextrose infusion in massive (hypertonic) or prolonged i.v. doses can induce hyperglycemia in glucose-intolerant patients and can aggravate metabolic control in diabetic patients. These facts are well known and need no further expansion. However, nonketotic hyperosmolar coma is frequently observed after massive or prolonged dextrose infusion, particularly in patients with impaired consciousness, diminished glomerular filtration, or who are elderly.

Two treatments that lead to false diagnosis of hyperglycemia should be avoided:

Performing a venopuncture for blood glucose measurement on the same side as, or through a three-way stopcock valve into which dextrose has been infused.
Using blood glucose test strips when fingers have been contaminated with dextrose infusion solutions (very careful hand washing is necessary to remove all trace of dextrose).

The list of other hyperglycemic drugs or compounds able to deteriorate blood glucose metabolism is long. However, few have the potential to cause acute problems in ICU.

The most common hyperglycemic drugs are epinephrine, asparaginase, phenytoin, pentamidine (which can induce hypoglycemia and, secondarily, true diabetes), and diazoxide. Less significant for ICU use are thiazidic diuretics, indomethacin, azathioprine, and phenothiazine derivatives.

The patient is a pregnant woman (known to be diabetic or not) in premature labor. The obstetrician has decided to infuse i.v. a β-adrenergic stimulant with or without a corticosteroid (to accelerate fetal pulmonary maturation). Severe metabolic deterioration is rapid. Severe ketosis, or even ketoacidosis, can be induced within a few hours. Such patients must receive continuous i.v. insulin infusion at a high flow rate and infusion rates must be rapidly adapted to blood glucose monitoring (every 15 min if necessary). Flow rates as high as 6–10 UI/hr and even higher are often necessary.

The pregnant diabetic woman is to deliver. What should be done with her insulin therapy? The difficulty of the situation lies in the dramatic decrease in insulin needs in the few minutes after delivery. A sharp decrease ($\approx$50%) in insulin dosage is mandatory to prevent severe hypoglycemia.

If the delivery is scheduled in advance, one approach to insulin therapy is to (*a*) omit the morning s.c. injection of intermediate insulin; (*b*) begin a continuous i.v. insulin infusion, the rate of which is based on the total insulin need of the previous day before rate of infusion (in units/hour) to equal the total s.c. insulin needs for the next 24 hr; (*c*) begin a 10% dextrose i.v. infusion at the rate of 150–180 mg/min (about 250 g/day); and (*d*) adapt the insulin infusion rate (usually between 1 and 3 units/hr) to hourly blood glucose determinations using test strips.

If the delivery is spontaneous and unscheduled and the patient has received her s.c. insulin injection, there is a risk of severe hypoglycemia just after delivery. This situation can be prevented by starting a 10% dextrose infusion at the lowest rate possible and monitoring blood glucose levels to determine when to increase it after delivery.

Intravascular infusion of radiographic contrast medium is one of the major causes of induced renal failure in the hospital. The most commonly accepted risk factor seems to be that of preexisting renal insufficiency. Some studies have also implicated diabetes mellitus as an independent risk factor, as well as the volume of the ioded material injected, and the nature (ionic or nonionic), and presence or absence of a contracted extracellular volume.

Acute renal failure after a radiologic examination does not prove that the contrast agent used was the cause of renal function derangement. A recent, controlled study (44) in diabetic patients has shown that clinically important renal failure (+50% increase of basal plasma creatinin levels) did not occur in nondiabetic patients with preexisting renal insufficiency or in diabetic patients with normal renal function. The incidence in diabetic patients with impaired renal function was about 9% (and about 2% in the corresponding control group). If an increase of +25% plasma creatinin was taken as a criterion, the percentage became 12%, with 5.5% of the cases where contrast material was the only unusual factor found. In the same study, the authors found no difference according to the osmolarity (high or low) of the material used.

The risk of developing renal insufficiency after an i.v. injection of contrast medium is present not only in patients with diabetes, but when associated with dehydration and hypovolemia (as observed in the nephrotic syndrome, cirrhosis, or congestive heart failure).

In any case, such a risk demands careful monitoring of diuresis throughout the 24–48-hr period after the radiologic exploration (even after a CT scan or cholangiography). Plasma creatinin levels should be monitored before and 72 hr after the i.v injection. True or falsely positive proteinuria may be noted for a few days, with no deleterious prognostic significance.

Prevention of acute renal failure relies on the following measures (20):

Stop, if possible, any nephrotoxic drug, and perhaps nonsteroidal antiinflammatory drugs as well.
Correct dehydration, hypovolemia, abnormal low blood pressure.
Avoid repetitive injection (within 5 days after the first one), if possible.
Stop biguanides to avoid lactic acidosis.

According to these authors, furosemide or osmotic diuresis has no preventive or protective value, but may be of help when natriuresis and diuresis tend to decrease after the radiological examination, or in a patient with heart failure or liver cirrhosis.

Hemodialysis soon after the injection of contrast material may prevent acute renal insufficiency in subjects at high risk for this problem; however, this procedure has not been validated.

Once hemodialysis begins, the renal failure usually improves within 1 week or so. Transient or definitive hemodialysis is however possible.

References

1. Anonyme. Uraemic hypoglycaemia. Lancet 1986;i:660–661.
2. Anonymous. Hypoglycaemia and diabetes control. Lancet 1991;338:853–855.
3. Alberti KGMM. Diabetic acidosis, hyperosmolar coma and lactic acidosis. In: Becker KL, ed. Principles and practice of endocrinology and metabolism. Philadelphia: JB Lippincott, 1990:1175–1184.
4. Alberti KGMM, Natrass M. Lactic acidosis. Lancet 1977;ii:25–29.
5. Arieff AI, Carroll HJ. Nonketotic hyperosmolar coma with hyperglycemia: clinical features, pathophysiology, renal function, acid-base balance, plasma-cerebrospinal fluid equilibria and the effects of therapy in 37 cases. Medicine 1972;51:73–94.
6. Arieff AI, Kleeman CR. Studies on mechanism of cerebral edema in diabetic comas. Effects of hyperglycemia and rapid lowering of plasma glucose in normal rabbits. J Clin Invest 1973;52:571–83.
7. Assan R, Girard J, Guillausseau PJ, Lesobre B. Hypoglycémies de l'adulte. In: G Tchobroutsky, G Slama, R Assan, P Freychet, eds. Traité de Diabétologie. Paris: Pradel 1990:867–883.
8. Bendtson I, Gade J, Rosenfalck AM, Thomsen CE, Wildschiodtz, Binder C. Nocturnal electroencephalogram registrations in Type 1 (insulin-dependent) diabetic patients with hypoglycaemia. Diabetologia 1991;34:750–756.
9. Berger W. Present status of biguanides. Pharma-Kritik, 1972;1:9–12.
10. Bergman U, Boman G, Wiholm BE. Epidemiology of adverse drug reactions to phenformin and metformin. Br Med J 1978;2:464–466.
11. Blackwell SW, Burns-Cox CJ. Intravascular haemolysis complicating treated non-ketotic hyperglycaemic diabetic coma. Postgrad Med J 1973;49:656–657.
12. Cohen RD, Woods HF. Clinical and biochemical aspects of lactic acidosis. Oxford: Blackwell, 1976:267.
13. Connell F, Vadhein C, Emanuel I. Diabetes in pregnancy: a population based study of incidence, referral for care and perinatal mortality. Am J Obstet Gynecol 1985;151:598–603.
14. Cooperman MT, Davidoff F, Spark R, Paccota J. Clinical studies of alcoholic ketoacidosis. Diabetes 1974;23:433–439.
15. Crock PA, Ley CJ, Martin IK, Alford FP, Best JD. Hormonal and metabolic changes during hypothermic coronary artery bypass surgery in diabetic and non-diabetic subjects. Diabetic Med 1988;5:47–52.
16. Cronin RE. Radiocontrast media-induced acute renal failure. In: Schrier, RW, ed. Diseases of the

kidney. 4th ed. Boston: Little Brown, 1988:1301–1317.

17. Davidson PC, Steed DR, Bode BW. A 1990 nationwide survey of CSII pump use in USA. Diabetes 1991;40(suppl 1):453A.

18. The DCCT Research Group. Diabetes control and complications trial (DCCT): results of feasibility study. Diabetes Care 1987;10:1–19.

19. DeGraeff J, Lips JB. Hypernatremia in diabetes mellitus. Acta Med Scand 1957;157:71–75.

20. Deray G, Dubois M, Baumelou A, Jacobs C. Risques rénaux lors de l'administration de produits de contraste iodès chez les patients diabétiques. Diabete Metab 1991;17:379–382.

21. De Vivo DC, Trifiletti RR, Jacobson RI, Ronen GM, Behmand RA, Harik SI. Defective glucose transport across the blood-brain barrier as a cause of persistent hypoglycorrhachia, seizures, and developmental delay. N Engl J Med 1991;325:703–709.

22. Dillon ES, Dyer WW, Smelo LS. Ketone acidosis in non diabetic adults. Med Clin North Am 1940;24:1813–1822.

23. Faguer de Moustier B, Burgard M, Boitard C, Desplanque N, Fanjoux J, Tchobroutsky G. Syndrome hypoglycémique auto-immun induit par le pyritinol. Diabete Metab 1988;14:423–430.

24. Fischer KF, Lees JA, Newman JH. Hypoglycemia in hospitalized patients. Causes and outcomes. N Engl J Med 1986;315:1245–1250.

25. Fulop M, Hoberman HD. Alcoholic ketosis. Diabetes 1975;24:785–790.

26. Gerich JE. Glucose counterregulation and its impact on diabetes mellitus. Diabetes 1988;37:1608–1617.

27. Gerich JE, Martin MM, Recant L. Clinical and metabolic characteristics of hyperosmolar nonketotic coma. Diabetes 1971;20:228–238.

28. Goldgewicht C, Slama G, Papoz L, Tchobroutsky G. Hypoglycaemic reactions in 172 type 1 (insulin-dependent) diabetic patients. Diabetologia 1983;24:95–99.

29. Grimm JJ, Haardt MJ, Thibult N, Goicolea I, Tchobroutsky G, Slama G. Lifestyle, metabolic control and social implications of pump therapy in 54 routine type 1 diabetic patients. Diabete Metab 1987;13:3–11.

30. Hepburn DA, Deary IJ, Frier BM, Patrick AW, Quinn JD, Fisher BM. Symptoms of acute insulin-induced hypoglycemia in humans with and without IDDM. Diabetes Care 1991;14:949–957.

31. Husband DJ, Thai AC, Alberti KGMM. Management of diabetes during surgery with glucose-insulin-potassium infusion. Diabetic Med 1986;3:69–74.

32. Johnson DD, Dorr KE, Swenson WM, Service FJ. Reactive hypoglycemia. JAMA 1980;243:1151–1155.

33. Keller U. Diabetic keto acidosis: current views on pathogenesis and treatment. Diabetologia 1986;29:71–77.

34. Krane E.J. Diabetic keto acidosis: biochemistry, physiology, treatment and prevention. Pediatr Clin North Am 1987;34:935–59.

35. Kreisberg RA. Acidosis and coma in the diabetic. In: Brodoff BN, Bleicher SJ, eds. Diabetes mellitus

and obesity. Baltimore: Williams & Wilkins, 1982:526–535.

36. Luft D, Schmulling RM, Eggstein M. Lactic acidosis in biguanide-treated diabetics. Diabetologia 1978;14:75–87.

37. Manske CL, Sprafica JM, Strony JT, Wang Y. Contrast nephropathy in azotemic patients undergoing coronary angiography. Am J Med 1990;89:615–620.

38. Miller SI, Wallace RJ, Musher DM, Septimus EJ, Kohl S, Baughn RE. Hypoglycemia as a manifestation of sepsis. Am J Med 1980;68:649–654.

39. Miodovnik M, Peros N, Holroyde JC, Siddiqi TA. Treatment of premature labor in insulin-dependent diabetic women. Obstet Gynecol 1985;65:521–528.

40. Mosnier-Pudar H. Acidocétose alcoolique. In: Tchobroutsky G, Slama G, Assan R, Freychet P, eds. Traité de diabétologie. Paris: Pradel, 1990:435–437.

41. Namba H, Lucignani G, Nehlig A, et al. Effects of insulin on hexose transport across blood-brain barrier in normoglycemia. Am J Physiol 1987;252:E299–303.

42. Owen OE, Morgan AP, Kemp HG, Sullivan JM, Herrera MG, Cahill GR Jr. Brain metabolism during fasting. J Clin Invest 1967;46:1589–1595.

43. Palmer JP. Alcoholic ketoacidosis: Clinical and laboratory presentation, pathophysiology and treatment. Ballieres Clin Endocrinol Metab 1983;12:381–389.

44. Parfrey PS, Griffiths SM, Barrett BJ, Paul MD, Genge M, Withers J, Farid N, McManamon PJ. Contrast material induced renal failure in patients with diabetes mellitus, renal insufficiency or both: a prospective controlled study. N Engl J Med 1989;320:143–149.

45. Pedersen J. The pregnant diabetic and her newborn. Copenhagen: Munksgaard, 1967:219.

46. Ryan CM. Neurobehavioral complications of type 1 diabetes: examination of possible risk factors. Diabetes Care 1988;11:86–93.

47. Sament S, Schwartz MB. Severe diabetic stupor without ketosis. S Afr Med J 1957;31:893–894.

48. Schlepphorst E, Levin ME. Rhabdomyolysis associated with hyperosmolar nonketotic coma (letter). Diabetes Care 1985;8:198–200.

49. Schwab SJ, Hlatky MA, Pieper KS, Davidson CJ, Morris KG, Skelton TN, Bashorf TM. Contrast nephrotoxicity: a randomized controlled trial of a non-ionic and an ionic radiographic contrast agent. N Engl J Med 1989;320:149–153.

50. Selam JL, Charles MA. Devices for insulin administration. Diabetes Care 1990;13:955–979.

51. Selam JL, Micossi P, Dunn FL, Nathan DM. Clinical trial of a programmable implantable insulin pump for type I diabetes. Diabetes Care 1992;15:877–885.

52. Slama G, Alamowitch C, Desplanque N, Letanoux M, Zirinis PH. A new non-invasive method for treating insulin-reaction: intranasal lyophylised glucagon. Diabetologia 1990;33:671–674.

53. Slama G, Traynard PY, Desplanque N, et al. The search for an optimized treatment of hypoglycemia: carbohydrates in tablets, solution or gel

for the correction of insulin reactions. Arch Intern Med 1990;150:589–593.

54. Stacpoole PW, Lorenz AC, Thomas RG, Harman EM. Dichloracetate in the treatment of lactic acidosis. Ann Intern Med 1988;108:58–63.

55. Stahl-Bayliss CM, Kalman CM, Laskin OL. Pentamidine-induced hypoglycemia in patients with the acquired immune deficiency syndrome. Clin Pharmacol Ther 1986;39:271–275.

56. Stephenson J, Fuller J. Hypoglycaemia as cause of death in human insulin era [letter]. Lancet 1990;335:661.

57. Tallroth G, Lindgren M, Stenberg G, Rosen I, Agardh C-D. Neurophysiological changes during insulin-induced hypoglycaemia and in the recovery period following glucose infusion of type 1 (insulin-dependent) diabetes mellitus and in normal man. Diabetologia 1990;33:319–323.

58. Taylor R. Drugs and diabetes mellitus. In: Pickup JC, Williams G, eds. Textbook of diabetes mellitus. Oxford: Blackwell Scientific Publication, 1991:803–809.

59. Taylor TE, Molyneux ME, Wirima JJ, Fletcher KA, Morris K. Blood glucose levels in Malawian children before and during the administration of intravenous quinine for severe falciparum malaria. N Engl J Med 1988;319:1040–1047.

60. Watchel TJ, Silliman RA, Lamberton P. Predisposing factors for the diabetic hyperosmolar state. Arch Intern Med 1987;147:499–501.

53

Thyroid Dysfunction

Pierre Thomopoulos

Two special and infrequent complications of thyroid diseases require emergency treatment in a department of critical care medicine: myxedema coma and thyroid storm. These are life-threatening complications of undiagnosed or ill-treated hypo- or hyperthyroidism. Their mortality rate has improved during the last 20 years, but it remains unacceptably high. Their incidence has also decreased. This is related to the availability of radioimmunoassays of thyroid hormones and thyroid stimulating hormone (TSH) with increasing sensitivity that has greatly facilitated the diagnosis and follow-up of thyroid diseases. Such progress has resulted in better prevention of myxedema coma and thyroid storm.

On the other hand, modern radioimmunoassays also made possible the description of disturbances in the production and metabolism of thyroid hormones induced by nonthyroidal diseases. This situation is almost constantly observed in critically ill patients and raises diagnostic problems with the identification of primary thyroid dysfunction.

THE NORMAL THYROID

The Hypothalamic-Pituitary Thyroid Axis

Thyrotropin, a 28,000-dalton glycoprotein synthetized by the anterior pituitary, holds a central position in the regulation of this axis. Its secretion is controlled mainly by the hypothalamus (and central nervous system) and by the feedback action of thyroid hormones.

Thyrotropin-releasing hormone (TRH) is a tripeptide produced in the hypothalamus that stimulates the pituitary thyrotrophs (16). Its concentration in the portal vein hypothalamo-hypophyseal system is 10 times higher than in peripheral plasma. In addition to TRH, dopamine (25) and somatostatin (3), produced in the hypothalamus, act directly on the thyrotrophs to inhibit the basal and TRH-stimulated TSH secretion.

The feedback action of thyroid hormones is the main regulator of TSH production. Both triiodothyronine (T_3) and thyroxine (T_4) (through its intrapituitary conversion to T_3) act directly on the thyrotrophs to inhibit TSH synthesis and to decrease the number of TRH receptors (21, 25). They do not modify the hypothalamic TRH content; however, they increase the secretion of somatostatin (and dopamine). The pituitary is very sensitive to small modifications of the concentration of plasma T_3 and T_4, even within the normal range. On the other hand, after a prolonged inhibition (during hyperthyroidism) or stimulation (during primary hypothyroidism) of TSH production, the adaptation of the thyrotroph is sluggish. Thus, TSH plasma levels may remain abnormal for several weeks after successful treatment and normalization of the T_4 and T_3 concentrations.

Glucocorticoids modulate TSH secretion directly at the pituitary level (25). They may also modify the production of TRH. Thus, hypercorticism, either spontaneous or iatrogenic, decreases the basal and TRH-stimulated TSH levels, while adrenal insufficiency is accompanied by increased serum TSH. In addition, these hormones act on the plasma transport and peripheral metabolism of thyroid hormones.

Due to its central position in the physiology of the pituitary-thyroid axis, the TSH concentration has became one of the most important parameters in the investigation of thyroid diseases. Modern assays, using the immunometric "sandwich" methodology (27), allow measurement of the upper and lower level of the normal range: approximately 0.25–6 μU/ml. The new "third generation" assays are 10 times more sensitive.

Thus, in primary hypothyroidism, TSH concentration is high, while in hyperthyroidism, it is low to undetectable. Stimulation by intravenous administration of TRH might be useful: the TSH response is increased in primary hypothyroidism and it remains flat in hyperthyroidism. In the rare patient with hypothyroidism secondary to an hypothalamic or pituitary lesion, the basal TSH is normal or low and the response to TRH is below normal and/or delayed.

Secretion and Peripheral Metabolism of Thyroid Hormones

TSH stimulates the release of thyroid hormones. The main secretion product is T_4. Its extrathyroidal pool contains 1000 μg, mostly extracellular. Its turnover rate is 10%/day, so that its daily production is 100 μg. On the contrary, only 20% of T_3 is directly secreted by the thyroid. The majority (80%) is produced through the extrathyroidal deiodination of T_4 that gives rise to equal amounts of T_3 and reverse triiodothyronine (rT3) (12). The latter has no biological activity. The extrathyroidal pool of T_3 contains 50 μg, mostly intracellular. Its turnover rate is 75%/day, so that its daily production is 30–40 μg.

There are several $T_4$5'-deiodinases. The type I is mainly located in the liver and the kidneys. Most of the circulating T_3 is produced by this enzyme. Its activity is decreased in starvation, various debilitating illnesses, and hypothyroidism. It is also inhibited by glucocorticoids, propranolol, amiodarone, cholecystographic agents (iopanoic acid), and propylthiouracil. On the contrary, hyperthyroidism and high caloric intake increase its activity. Another deiodinase (type II) predominates in the brain, is unaffected by starvation, and increases during thyroid deficiency. Thus, it protects the availability of T_3 to brain cells.

Circulating thyroid hormones are almost totally bound to specific plasma proteins and to albumin (1). Thyroxine-binding globulin (TBG) binds 80% of T_4 and 90% of T_3; thyroxine-binding prealbumin (TBPA) binds 15% of T_4 and 5% of T_3; and albumin binds 5% of both iodothyronines. Only a tiny fraction is free (0.05% of T_4 and 0.5% of T_3). This fraction, as well as the albumin-bound hormones, is available to tissues.

Increased levels of thyroid hormone binding protein may occur as familial hereditary disorders. The most common cause of high TBG levels is, however, related to estrogens: pregnancy and contraceptive pills. In addition, clofibrate and 5-fluorouracil can increase serum TBG. Pathological increases occur also in acute hepatitis (14) and, to a lesser degree, in chronic hepatitis, in biliary cirrhosis, and in intermittent acute porphyria.

Decreased TBG concentration may occur as a X-linked recessive trait. It is also observed in hypercorticism (spontaneous or iatrogenic) and during administration of androgens and anabolic steroids. During acute and chronic nonthyroidal illnesses, TBG, TBPA, and albumin may decrease by up to 30%. In addition, in these situations a decrease of the binding capacity and/or affinity of TBG is observed, probably related to the appearance of ill-defined circulating inhibitors. Some pharmacologic agents (salicylates, phenytoin, furosemide) can also competitively inhibit T_4 binding to TBG; in vitro, phenylbutazone, sulfonylureas, and penicillin G have a similar effect, which is not observed in vivo at the usual serum drug concentrations.

The serum T_4 and T_3 concentrations are measured by reliable and specific radioimmunoassays. Normal values are: 4.5–12.5 μg/dl (58–161 nmol/liter) for total T_4; 0.8–2.3 ng/dl (10.3–29.7 pmol/liter) for free T_4; 80–220 ng/dl (1.23–3.39 nmol/liter) for total T_3; 1.3–5.5 ng/liter (2–8.47 pmol/liter) for free T_3. The observed values depend on thyroid hormone production and on the serum concentration and affinity of thyroid hormone-binding proteins. For this reason, several assays have been developed that measure, indirectly or directly, free T_4 or T_3 (17). Indirect methods, like free T_4 index or free T_3 index, have recently been replaced by direct measurements. These are nonequilibrium, two-step radioimmunoassays. Their results are reliable in patients with thyroid disease. However, in the nonthyroidal illnesses or in primary abnormalities of thyroid hormone-binding proteins, the values obtained may be misleading and show no correlation with data from direct equilibrium measurement of free hormones (equilibrium dialysis or ultrafiltration) (13, 32).

Thyroid Hormones Action

Thyroid hormones act upon almost every tissue, with specific effects depending on the cell type. One of their most universal actions is the stimulation of oxygen consumption and thermogenesis, by mechanisms which remain controversial. The present overview will be limited to the influence of thyroid hormones on the cardiovascular system (19, 22).

One of their earliest effects is a peripheral vasodilation and a decrease in systemic vascular resistance. This is accompanied by a fall of the diastolic blood pressure that causes a reflex increase in heart rate and in cardiac output. The latter is reinforced by an increase in blood volume and in erythropoiesis. In addition, thyroid hormones directly stimulate cardiac contractility. They induce the transcription of myosin heavy chain α which has a high ATPase activity and allows an increase in the velocity of contraction. They also stimulate the synthesis of the calcium ATPase pump of the sarcoplasmic reticulum, which results in a faster sequestration of calcium (released in the cytosol during the systole) and a more rapid relaxation of cardiac muscle. Both modifications lead to an increased hydrolysis of ATP. In addition, the chemical energy of this hydrolysis is used less efficiently and is converted into heat.

Finally, thyroid hormones increase the density of β-adrenergic receptors in the heart and might sensitize this organ to the effects of catecholamines.

THYROID FUNCTION IN NONTHYROID ILLNESSES

Alterations of Serum Hormone Levels

Thyroid hormone production and metabolism are almost constantly altered in euthyroid subjects during systemic nonthyroidal illnesses or caloric deprivation. The importance of the observed changes depends on the severity of the disease (7, 9).

In mild illnesses or caloric deprivation, total and free T_4 are high normal or slightly increased, while total and free T_3 are low normal or slightly decreased. The rT3 is increased. The basal serum TSH remains normal and its response to TRH stimulation is normal or blunted.

In diseases of moderate severity, total T_4 is normal and free T_4 is slightly increased or normal (13, 32). Total and free T_3 are frankly decreased and rT3 remains high. The serum TSH is as above.

In severe illnesses or prolonged total starvation, total T_4 and indirect free T_4 index are low. However, free T_4 measured by equilibrium dialysis or ultrafiltration remains normal. Total and free T_3 are very low to unmeasurable, while rT3 is high. The basal serum TSH may be normal, low or high (almost never greater than 20 μU/ml) and the response to TRH is normal or blunted. In these hypothyroxinemic situations, the level of serum total T_4 is highly correlated with the mortality rate, while this is not the case for total or free T_3 (31).

During the evolution from a mild to a severe illness, the spectrum of the described changes may be sequentially observed, although this is not always the case. The high T_4 state is particularly transient. On the other hand, during recovery the pattern of hormonal changes is reversed. In some situations a special profile may be observed. Thus, the serum total rT3 remains normal in renal diseases and in primary hyperparathyroidism. After a head trauma with prolonged coma, a true hypothalamic hypothyroidism may develop, with low total and free T_4, low TSH and increased (and delayed) TSH response to TRH, which superimpose the previ-

Table 53.1
Drugs Interfering with the Level of Thyroid Hormones and TSH

	TSH	Total T_4	Free T_4	Total T_3	Free T_3	
Corticosteroids	↓	N^a or ↓	N	N or ↓	N or ↓	Decreased TSH secretion, TBG levels and T_4 5'-deiodinase
Dopamine Somatostatin	↓	N	N	N	N	Decreased TSH secretion
Estrogens	N	↑	N	↑	N	Increased TBG
Salicylates Furosemide	↓	↓	↑	↓	↑	Competitive inhibition of TBG binding
Diphenylhydantoin Carbamazepine Rifampin	N	↓	↓	N	N	Increased hepatic metabolism of T_4
Ipodate[b] Iopanoic acid[b] Amiodarone[b]	↑	↑	↑	↓	↓	Inhibition of T_4 5'-deiodinase
Propranolol	N	↑	↑	↓	↓	Inhibition of T_4 5'-deiodinase
Lithium[c]	↑	N	N	N	N	Inhibition of T_4 and T_3 secretion

[a] N, normal.
[b] May induce primary hypo- or hyperthyroidism.
[c] May induce goiter and hypothyroidism.

ously described "nonthyroidal illness" changes.

In addition, physiological or pharmacological factors may modify the hormone levels (7, 33). The basal and TRH stimulated TSH may be decreased in elderly people (28) in the absence of caloric deprivation or concomitant disease; total and free T_4 and T_3 remain normal. Moreover, the production, binding to serum proteins, and metabolism of thyroid hormone may be modified by several medications, listed in Table 53.1.

Pathophysiology

Three modifications appear sequentially or concurrently in nonthyroidal illnesses:

Inhibition of 5'-deiodinase (18),
Suppression of pituitary TSH secretion,
Formation of a circulating inhibitor of TBG binding affinity (8).

In mild diseases, the increase of serum T_4 and rT3 and the decrease of T_3 are probably related to the inhibition of 5'-deiodination, which impairs T_4 and rT3 clearance and T_3 extrathyroidal production. Simultaneous pituitary suppression leads to a blunted TSH response to TRH.

With increasing severity of the disease, the 5'-deiodinase is more strongly blocked, so that serum rT3 remains high and T_3 further decreases. However, there appears a circulating inhibitor of TBG binding, of unknown structure. Its action is additive to the previously described decrease of the concentration of serum thyroid hormone-binding proteins. As a consequence, T_4 clearance rate increases, total T_4 decreases to normal, then to frankly low concentrations, while free T_4 is normal. T_4 production rate remains normal or low normal, independently of the level of serum total and free T_4.

The biochemical mechanism of the observed changes are still ill-defined. The hypercortisolemia accompanying the stress of the illness, as well as the associated caloric deprivation, may contribute to their appearance.

Another important unresolved problem is the thyroid hormone status of the tissues of these patients in the face of low serum T_3 (total and free) levels. The answer is probably complex because of the probable existence of tissue heterogeneity for the metabolism and effects of thyroid hormones (34). The clinical and laboratory indexes (basal metabolic rate, Achilles tendon reflex relaxation time, systolic time interval) are normal in the euthyroid sick.

However, these evaluations lack specificity and sensitivity. It has been reported that the serum angiotensin-converting enzyme is low in severe nonthyroidal illnesses with low serum total T_4 (6). Since this enzyme may reflect the action of thyroid hormones, the above data suggest the existence of tissular "hypothyroidism" in this case. The point remains controversial and requires the description of more precise and specific methods to measure the end-organ hormone response.

In any case, attempts to normalize the serum T_3, by administrating oral T_3 to the patients, induced an increase of protein breakdown. Thus, such a treatment is probably detrimental and should be avoided (5, 23). This point stresses the importance of the diagnostic evaluation of such patients, in order to differentiate their situation from primary thyroidal disorders.

Evaluation of the Euthyroid Sick

The diagnosis of concurrent primary thyroid disease may be suspected in an acutely ill patient in the presence of specific clinical manifestations.

In a patient with mildly severe illness the symptoms and signs of hyperthyroidism or hypothyroidism are not masked. An elevated total and free T_4 may be due to hyperthyroidism or the nonthyroidal illness itself. If total or free T_3 is elevated, thyrotoxicosis is confirmed. However, T_3 may be normal or reduced. In this case a normal TSH, with normal or simply blunted response to TRH, eliminates the suspicion of hyperthyroidism. In the latter TSH is low and is not stimulated by TRH.

On the contrary, the recognition of hyperthyroidism may be difficult in patients with severe, concurrent nonthyroidal illness. The usual symptoms of thyrotoxicosis may be masked and the diagnosis is usually suspected in the presence of unexplained weight loss, tachyarrhythmia or intractable congestive heart failure. Total T_4, indirect free T_4 indexes, and total and free T_3 are normal or low. Again, the diagnosis will be confirmed by the measurement of basal and TRH-stimulated TSH. However, in elderly patients (28) or during administration of glucocorticoids or dopamine, TSH may be low in the absence of hyperthyroidism. It should be stressed that the availability of the "third generation" TSH immunoassays will probably greatly facilitate these diagnostic problems (27).

When hypothyroidism is suspected, the low values of total and free T_3 and total T_4 (in the severe illnesses) make these results uninformative. The measurement of serum rT3 should be of value since it is low in hypothyroidism and high in the nonthyroidal illnesses. However in 30% of the latter rT3 remains normal and its assay is not available except in a few research laboratories. Thus, the diagnosis will mostly rely upon the TSH measurement. If TSH is higher than 20 μU/ml, primary hypothyroidism is highly likely. For values between the upper limit of normal (approximately 6 μU/ml) and 20 μU/ml a TRH-stimulation test becomes necessary. The TSH response is normal or blunted in the euthyroid sick and increased in primary hypothyroidism. Finally, a normal basal TSH is compatible with the diagnosis of hypothalamic or pituitary hypothyroidism. These etiologies account for 5% of all cases of hypothyroidism. They are frequently associated with deficiencies of other pituitary hormones, which should be ruled out by clinical and laboratory investigations. TSH response to TRH is not informative since it is often normal or blunted in this situation. If a direct assay of free T_4 is available it might be helpful, since its value is normal in the euthyroid sick.

This diagnostic evaluation of such patients has important therapeutic consequences. It is unnecessary and probably detrimental to administrate T_4 or T_3 to the euthyroid sick. On the other hand, concurrent hypothyroidism or hyperthyroidism should receive appropriate therapy, which will improve the course of the nonthyroidal disease and prevent the occurrence of such life-threatening complications as myxedema coma or thyroid storm.

THYROTOXIC STORM

This is a relatively rare syndrome. Its incidence has decreased due to a better prevention and may be less than one percent of admissions for thyrotoxicosis (15, 26).

Pathogenesis Precipitating Events

The occurrence of thyrotoxic storm is related to the decompensation of the adaptation mechanisms to the increased production of thyroid hormones. As described in the section "Thyroid Hormone Action," one of the main consequences is increased thermogenesis. A major part of the cardiovascular changes induced by hyperthyroidism is the requirement to promote heat dissipation (19, 20, 22). Thus, hyperthermia, which is an essential feature of thyroid storm, develops if the adaptative mechanisms are overriden. It is constantly accompanied by hypothalamic and brain dysfunction leading to altered mental status.

This situation occurs in undiagnosed or ill-treated hyperthyroidism, especially in the aged. However, there is always one or more precipitating factors leading to the decompensation. These factors include:

An augmentated hormonal release, after thyroidectomy, ^{131}I therapy, thiourea withdrawal, or administration of iodinated drugs or contrast dyes.
A "surgical stress": nonthyroid surgery, trauma, parturition.
A "medical stress": infection, pulmonary thromboembolism and others.

Clinical Features

The diagnosis of thyrotoxic storm is based largely on clinical presentation. In most cases, either thyrotoxicosis is already known or its signs and symptoms are obvious, including goiter and ophthalmopathy (Graves disease). However, the masked or "apathetic" thyrotoxicosis of the aged may pose difficult diagnostic problems.

The suspicion of impending or established thyrotoxic storm is based on the occurrence of hyperthermia, altered mental status, and the presence of a precipitating factor. Since infection is very commonly such a factor, it may be difficult to determine whether hyperpyrexia is merely related to the associated illness or is announcing the storm. In the latter case, fever is elevated out of proportion to the infection and it is associated with altered mental status and excessive tachycardia or tachyarrhythmias. These patients are rest-less, agitated, confused, and even psychotic. They present with severe tremor. Thus, normal mentation makes the diagnosis highly unlikely. Sinus tachycardia is constant and unrelated to the level of fever. In some patients, atrial fibrillation and symptoms of congestive heart failure may be present, even in the absence of underlying heart disease. In most cases systolic hypertension is observed. However, in the absence of vigorous treatment, particularly after vomiting or diarrhea, volume depletion and vascular collapse may supervene. It should be stressed that pulmonary embolism may be an initiating factor or a complication of thyroid storm, which goes often unrecognized.

Gastrointestinal manifestations include diarrhea, vomiting, abdominal pain (diffuse or localized to the liver), hepatomegaly, and splenomegaly. Liver damage resulting from congestive failure or hepatic ischaemia may lead to jaundice, which is a poor prognostic finding.

Laboratory Findings

Given the poor prognosis of thyrotoxic storm, therapy should be initiated as soon as the diagnosis is suspected without waiting for confirmation by the laboratory tests. Serum total or free T_4 and T_3 are elevated and TSH is suppressed. The results in storm are not different from the values observed in severe uncomplicated thyrotoxicosis.

Other laboratory findings include mild hyperglycemia in the absence of diabetes mellitus. It probably results from catecholamine mediated glycogenolysis and inhibition of insulin release. Hypercalcemia with increase of alkaline phosphatase may exist as a result of increased bone resorption by thyroid hormones. Bilirubin, lactate dehydrogenase and glutamic oxaloacetate transaminase are often increased. A leukocytosis may be observed, but any leftward shift in the differential white count should suggest the presence of an infection.

Treatment

Early diagnosis and control of thyrotoxicosis is the best prevention of thyroid storm.

Preparation with thionamide drugs in order to obtain a euthyroid state before operation or before radioiodine administration as well as use of beta-blocking drugs have greatly contributed to the decreased prevalence of this complication.

The treatment of impending or established crisis is an emergency. Several simultaneous approaches are necessary in order to:

Control systemic decompensation,
Decrease circulating thyroid hormones and block their cellular actions,
Treat any underlying precipitating illness.

Control of hyperthermia and agitation is achieved by external cooling (hypothermia blanket, ice packs, and so forth) and administration of sedatives (chlorpromazine 25–50 mg and meperidine 25–50 mg intravenously every 4–6 hr). The latter are also important to prevent shivering in response to cooling. Their effect is followed by monitoring central body temperature and the mental status in order to avoid excessive sedation. It has been reported that dantrolene (100 mg i.v.) is useful for the control of hyperthermia in thyroid storm (2, 10) and in malignant hyperthermia of anesthesia. It may be tried if the previous measures are unsuccessful. In addition, adequate hydration must be supported by intravenous administration of fluids containing 5–10% glucose and electrolytes. Vitamin supplements may be advisable.

Decrease of circulating thyroid hormones, in particular normalization of total or free T_3 in 48 hr, is obtained by blocking their synthesis and release and by inhibiting peripheral conversion of T_4 to T_3. Intrathyroidal hormone synthesis is inhibited by thionamide drugs, propylthiouracil (PTU) 200 mg every 4 hr or methimazole 30 mg every 6 hr given by mouth or via nasogastric tube. The former is preferred because it blocks peripheral deiodination of T_4 to T_3. In addition, iodine is administrated in order to block proteolysis of thyroglobulin and release of thyroid hormones, either orally (5 drops of saturated solution of iodine 4 times a day or equivalent doses of Lugol's solution), by intravenous drip of sodium iodine (0.5 g every 12 hr), or intravenously (1 g every 8 hr).

It should be given 1 hour after initiation of PTU therapy to avoid organification of the iodide and enrichment of thyroglobulin stores within the gland. Similar effects are obtained by sodium ipodate or iopanoic acid (1 g orally 3 times a day) which also block the conversion of T_4 to T_3. In the case of allergy to iodine, lithium carbonate (300 mg every 6 hr) can be used to inhibit thyroid hormone release. Its serum levels must be monitored and maintained at 1mEq/liter to avoid cardiac toxicity.

Additional inhibition of peripheral T_4 to T_3 conversion is obtained by glucocorticoids such as dexamethasone, 2 mg every 6 hr.

In cases resistant to treatment, some have employed plasmapheresis and have obtained a rapid decrease of thyroid hormones (30).

Control of the cellular effects of thyroid hormones is partly reached by drugs blocking β-adrenergic receptors. Propranolol is the drug of choice because it also inhibits conversion of T_4 to T_3. Its beneficial effects are obvious in the cardiovascular system, but it also improves tremor, agitation, and psychotic behavior. Oral doses of 40–120 mg every 6 hr are needed to obtain a heart rate between 90–110 beats/min after fever has been controlled. When a rapid effect is needed, 1 mg of intravenous propranolol may be given and repeated every 5 min until response. Contraindications include asthma and, mainly, the existence of moderate to severe congestive heart failure. These patients require close monitoring of their hemodynamics and judicious administration of β-blockers, in addition to digitalis and diuretics.

Finally, a search for a precipitating factor (infection, thromboembolism, etc.) is needed in order to initiate specific treatment.

After complete resolution of the crisis, corticosteroids and iodine are stopped, while β-blockers are continued as long as needed and PTU is maintained for the long-term normalization of the thyroid status. Definitive therapy of hyperthyroidism will require, most of the time, surgical thyroidectomy or administration of radioiodine.

MYXEDEMA COMA

This is a rare complication of hypothyroidism. However, it is possible that cases remain unrecognized and seriously ill aged persons with various medical problems, especially infections and respiratory failure, may have undiagnosed thyroid insufficiency (15, 26).

Precipitating Events: Pathogenesis

External cold may be an aggravating factor, since cases of myxedema coma occur more frequently during the winter. Precipitating factors include any surgical or medical injury. A special mention should be made of pulmonary infections, which compromise the fragile respiratory function of these patients, and of loss of blood volume, since this parameter is already decreased in hypothyroidism. Similar problems may be initiated by the administration of tranquilizers, sedatives, antidepressants, narcotics, or diuretics, as the metabolism of many drugs is prolonged in such patients.

The above factors lead to the decompensation of the cardiovascular and metabolic adaptations, which are the reverse of those observed in hyperthyroidism. The primary problem of hypothyroid patients is decreased thermogenesis and the subsequent efforts for heat conservation. A marked peripheral vasoconstriction is observed, with diastolic hypertension, reduced total blood volume and decreased cardiac output and heart rate (19, 20). The direct action of thyroid hormones on the synthesis of myosine heavy chains is also responsible for these findings. In addition to compromised thermoregulation, there exists a depression of the respiratory center with reduction of the respiratory drive (4, 11, 24, 37).

Clinical Features

Myxedema coma not infrequently occurs in a patient with unrecognized hypothyroidism. In that case, examination may reveal a goiter or a surgical scar of the neck. The classical signs of myxedema are usually present including dry, coarse, yellowish and cold skin, puffy facies with periorbial edema, sparse or coarse hair, large tongue and hoarseness. Hypothermia and unconsciousness are the basic findings for the establishment of diagnosis. The former may remain unrecognized if a special thermometer is not used for confirmation. Unconsciousness may have been preceded by disorientation or paranoia. In some patients minor seizures or convulsions may occur (35). Examination may reveal myotonia-like contractions. Reflexes are diminished or absent and their recovery phase is prolonged. In addition, directly tapping a muscle induces a transient local swelling (myoedema) which is characteristic of hypothyroidism. The patients are often cyanotic, since hypoventilation with hypoxia and hypercarbia is one of the most prominent features of myxedema coma. The main cause is the depression of hypoxic respiratory drive that is accompanied by depressed response to hypercarbia, myopathy of the respiratory muscles, possible concomitant pleural effusion, and upper airway partial obstruction by edema and macroglossia. Bradycardia with heart sounds of decreased intensity is a constant finding. It is associated with cardiac enlargement, which is mainly due to pericardial effusions. Congestive heart failure is unusual, although extracellular fluid volume is often increased. The reduced effective intravascular volume contributes to a propensity to hypotension, which may develop into collapse and shock in the untreated patient. A frequent finding is decreased intestinal mobility and gastric atony that affects the absorption of oral medications and should not be diagnosed as mechanical obstruction, since its regression is obtained after reversal of the hypothyroid state. Easy bruising and prolonged bleeding time are also observed and may add to the difficulty in the management of these patients.

Electrocardiographic abnormalities include low voltage, prolonged QT interval, flattened or inversed T waves and varying degrees of block. Chest radiograph reveals the cardiomegaly and may show the existence of pleural effusions, or an infiltrate (pneumonia) which could be a precipitating factor of the coma.

Laboratory Findings

Routine laboratory evaluation frequently indicates anemia with normal white cell count. If a leftward shift in the differential white count is observed, the presence of infection should be considered. Hypercholesterolemia and hypertriglyceridemia are usual findings. Hypoglycemia may exist even in isolated primary hypothyroidism. Serum creatinine may be high, due to the decreased glomerular filtration rate. A frequent and important finding is hyponatremia, which may aggravate the mental disturbances of the patient. It is mainly related to diminished glomerular filtration, decreased delivery of water to the distal tubule, and, to a lesser degree, to the coexistence of inappropriate secretion of antidiuretic hormone and decreased secretion of atrial natriuretic factor (36). Transaminases (SGOT, SGPT), lactate dehydrogenase, and creatine phosphate kinase may be abnormal and raise diagnostic problems with myocardial infarction. Arterial blood gas analysis reveals the presence of respiratory acidosis with hypoxemia and hypercapnia.

Specific laboratory tests measuring the thyroid function are obtained in order to confirm the diagnosis. Treatment, however, should be instituted immediately upon clinical suspicion. Serum total and free T_4 are low. Total or free T_3 are not useful when hypothyroidism is suspected, because they may be only slightly decreased while they are constantly low in the euthyroid sick. In primary hypothyroidism TSH is invariably elevated, although previous administration of corticosteroids or dopamine might decrease its value. In secondary hypothyroidism, serum TSH is normal or low. Serum cortisol (and ACTH) measurement may be performed, if concomitant adrenal insufficiency is suspected. However, specific treatment should be initiated without delay.

Treatment

In patients with myxedema coma, respiratory and cardiovascular problems are major causes of death. Respiratory assistance should be initiated without delay, as soon as clinical findings and/or blood gas determinations show evidence for hypoxia and hypercapnia. Endotracheal intubation and mechanical respiratory assistance are needed in such cases. Tissue hypoxia may be worsened by the existence of anemia, so transfusions of red packed cells may be indicated if hematocrit is lower than 30%.

If hypotension is present, it is best treated by administration of plasma expanders or transfusions of whole blood, with monitoring of central venous pressure. Vasoconstriction already exists in such patients, so α-adrenergic agents are not indicated and may induce tachyarrhythmias.

Correction of hypoglycemia should be obtained by infusion of concentrated glucose solution in order to minimize input of free water and prevent the appearance or worsening of hyponatremia. However, if serum sodium is below 120 mEq/liter, administration of a small amount of hypertonic saline should be considered (50–100 ml of 5% NaCl).

Adrenal steroids (hydrocortisone hemisuccinate 200–300 mg/day, intravenously) are routinely given since association with hypopituitarism or primary adrenal failure is observed in some patients. Their dosage is tapered after 7–10 days, according to clinical response, in order to obtain a diagnostic evaluation.

Hypothermia should not be treated aggressively. External warming may induce excessive vasodilation and hypotension. Covering the patient with blankets is all that is required to avoid further heat loss and to allow spontaneous warming.

Thyroid hormone is the specific treatment of hypothyroidism. In myxedema coma it is given intravenously because of the gastric atonia observed in this situation. The dose and nature of the hormone is still a matter of debate. Many authors recommend the intravenous administration of 500 µg (300 µg/m²) of L-thyroxine in one single dose, followed by 75–100 µg/day for the next few days until proper dosage can be individualized by measuring serum TSH and T_4 levels. This dosage is sufficient to saturate serum binding proteins and obtain circulating values close to the low normal limit. Peripheral deiodination of thyroxine will ensure a steady production of triiodothyronine. However, generation of triiodothyronine may be compromised by an associated illness. In addition, triiodothyronine has a much quicker onset of action than thyroxine. For these reasons, some authors advocate the use of triiodothyronine, 50 μg/day as an infusion, to avoid excessive elevations of serum T_3 concentrations (29).

If intravenous preparations of thyroxine or triiodothyronine are not available, one can prepare them by dissolving T_4 or T_3 powder in 1–2 ml of 0.1 N NaOH and diluting this solution with sterile normal saline containing 2% albumin. This preparation is then sterilized by passage through a 0.22-μm filter and used when fresh.

References

1. Bartalena L. Recent achievements in studies on thyroid hormone-binding proteins. Endocr Rev 1990;11:47–64.
2. Bennett MH, Wainwright AP. Acute thyroid crisis on induction of anesthesia. Anaesthesia 1989; 44:28–30.
3. Berelowitz M, Maeda K, Harris S, Frohman LA. The effect of alterations in the pituitary thyroid axis on hypothalamic content and in vitro release of somatostatin-like immunoreactivity. Endocrinology 1980;107:24–29.
4. Bertrand Y, Roels J, Sondag JP. Respiratory, haemodynamic and haematologic characteristics in two patients with myxoedema coma and hypothermia. Acta Clin Belg 1986;41:96–101.
5. Brent GA, Hershman JM. Thyroxine therapy in patients with severe nonthyroidal illnesses and low serum thyroxine concentrations. J Clin Endocrinol Metab 1986;63:1–8.
6. Brent GA, Hershman JM, Reed AW, Sastre A, Lieberman J. Serum angiotensin-converting enzyme in severe nonthyroidal illnesses associated with low serum thyroxine concentration. Ann Intern Med 1984;100:680–683.
7. Cavalieri RR. The effects of nonthyroidal disease and drugs on thyroid function tests. Med Clin North Am 1991;75:27–39.
8. Chopra IJ, Solomon DH, Teco GNC, Eisenberg JB. An inhibitor of the binding of thyroid hormones to serum proteins is present in extrathyroidal tissues. Science 1982;215:407–409.
9. Chopra IJ, Hershman JM, Partridge WM, Nicoloff JT. Thyroid function in nonthyroidal illnesses. Ann Intern Med 1983;98:946–957.
10. Christensen PA, Nissen LR. Treatment of thyroid storm in a child with dantrolene. Br J Anaesth 1987;59:523.
11. Domm BM. Vasallo CL. Myxedema coma with respiratory failure. Am Rev Respir Dis 1973;107:842–845.
12. Engler D, Burger AG. The deiodination of io-
dothyronines and of their derivatives in man. Endocr Rev 1984;5:151–184.
13. Faber J, Kirkegaard C, Rasmussen B, Westh H, Busch-Sorensen M, Jensen IW. Pituitary thyroid axis in critical illness. J Clin Endocrinol Metab 1987;65:315–320.
14. Gardner DF, Carithers RL, Utiger RD. Thyroid function tests in patients with acute and resolved hepatitis B virus infection. Ann Intern Med 1982;96:450–452.
15. Gavin LA. Thyroid crises. Med Clin North Am 1991;75:179–193.
16. Jackson IMD. Thyrotropin-releasing hormone. N Engl J Med 1982;306:145–155.
17. Kaptein EM, MacIntyre SS, Weiner JM, Spencer CA, Nicoloff JT. Free thyroxine estimates in nonthyroidal illness: comparison of eight methods. J Clin Endocrinol Metab 1981;52:1073–1077.
18. Kaptein EM, Robinson WJ, Grieb DA, Nicoloff JT. Peripheral serum thyroxine, triiodothyronine and reverse triiodothyronine kinetics in the low thyroxine state of acute nonthyroidal illnesses. A noncompartmental analysis. J Clin Invest 1982;69:526–535.
19. Klein I. Thyroid hormone and the cardiovascular system. Am J Med 1990;88:631–637.
20. Ladenson PW. Recognition and management of cardiovascular disease related to thyroid dysfunction. Am J Med 1990;88:638–641.
21. Larsen PR. Thyroid pituitary interaction. Feedback regulation of thyrotropin secretion by thyroid hormones. N Engl J Med 1982;306:23–32.
22. Levey SG. Catecholamine thyroid hormone interactions and the cardiovascular manifestations of hyperthyroidism. Am J Med 1990;88:642–646.
23. Little JS. Effects of thyroid hormone supplementation on survival after bacterial infection. Endocrinology 1985;117:1431–1435.
24. Massumi RA, Winnacker JL. Severe depression of the respiratory center in myxoedema. Am J Med 1964;36:876–878.
25. Morley JE. Neuroendocrine control of thyrotropin secretion. Endocr Rev 1981;2:396–436.
26. Nicoloff JT. Thyroid storm and myxedema coma. Med Clin North Am 1985;69:1005–1017.
27. Nicoloff JT, Spencer CA. The use and misuse of the sensitive thyrotropin assay. J Clin Endocrinol Metab 1990;71:553–558.
28. Parle JV, Franklyn JA, Cross KW, Jones SC, Sheppard MC. Prevalence and follow up of abnormal thyrotrophin (TSH) concentrations in the elderly in the United Kingdom. Clin Endocrinol 1991;34:77–83.
29. Pereira VG, Haron ES, Linea-Neto N, Madeiros-Neto GA. Management of myxedema coma: report on three successfully treated cases with nasogastric or intravenous administration of triiodothyronine. J Endocrinol Invest 1982;5:331–334.
30. Schlienger JL, Faradji A, Sapin R, Blickle JF, Chabrier G, Simon C, Imler M. Traitement de l'hyperthyroidie grave par échange plasmatique. Presse Med 1985;14:1271–1274.
31. Slag MF, Morley JE, Elson MK, Crowson TW, Nattall FQ, Shafer RB. Hypothyroxinemia in crit-

ically ill patients as a predictor of high mortality. JAMA 1981;245:43–45.

32. Surks MI, Hupart KH, Pan C, Shapiro LE. Normal free thyroxine in critical nonthyroidal illnesses measured by ultrafiltration of undiluted serum and equilibrium dialysis. J Clin Endocrinol Metab 1988;67:1031–1039.

33. Wenzel KW. Pharmacological interference with in vitro tests of thyroid function. Metabolism 1981;30:717–732.

34. Williams GR, Franklyn JA, Neuberger JM, Sheppard MC. Thyroid hormone receptor expression in the "sick euthyroid" syndrome. Lancet 1989;2:1477–1481.

35. Woods KL, Holmes GKT. Myxoedema coma presenting in status epilepticus. Postgrad Med J 1977;53:46–48.

36. Zimmerman RS, Gharib H, Zimmerman D, Heublein D, Burnett JC. Atrial natriuretic peptide in hypothyroidism. J Clin Endocrinol Metab 1987;64:353–355.

37. Zwillich CW, Pierson DJ, Hofeldt FD, Lafkin EG, Weil JV. Ventilatory control in myxedema and hypothyroidism. N Engl J Med 1975;292:662–665.

54

Acute Adrenal Insufficiency

Marie Emilie Chauveau

Acute loss of adrenocortical function is a rare and life-threatening emergency. It includes isolated glucocorticoid deficiency, secondary to ACTH insufficiency, and combined glucocorticoid and mineralocorticoid deficiency, in the case of primary adrenocortical insufficiency. Early clinical diagnosis is of utmost importance, since treatment is specific, simple, and rapidly efficacious. In fact, careful education of patients with Addison's disease and after withdrawal of glucocorticoid therapy should prevent the appearance of acute adrenocortical insufficiency.

PHYSIOLOGICAL ASPECTS

Adrenocortical Hormones: Synthesis and Release

Adrenal cortex is composed of three zones:

The outer zone (zona glomerulosa) produces aldosterone and is primarily regulated by the renin angiotensin system,

The inner two zones (zona fasciculata and zona reticularis) produce cortisol and androgens and are regulated by ACTH (1, 2).

All adrenal steroids are derived from cholesterol (Fig. 54.1). The cleavage of cholesterol side chain leads to the formation of Δ5-pregnenolone, which is the common precursor of three different pathways. This initial step is the rate-limiting step and is the major site of action of ACTH.

Glucocorticoid Pathway

Cortisol is the major glucocorticoid. Its daily secretory rate is 20–30 mg/24 hr. About 10% of the circulating cortisol is free and biologically active. The remainder is bound to a cortisol binding globulin (transcortin) and to albumin. Hepatic synthesis of transcortin is increased by estrogen. Conversely, transcortin concentration is reduced in protein deficiency states (cirrhosis of the liver, nephrotic syndrome). Half-life of cortisol is 70–90 min. A small fraction of free cortisol is excreted into the urine (less than 100 μg/day in normal people).

Mineralocorticoid Pathway

Aldosterone is the primary mineralocorticoid. It is produced exclusively in the zona glomerulosa. The secretion of aldosterone varies from 50 to 250 μg daily on normal sodium intake. Approximately 30% of the circulating aldosterone is free. Its half-life is 15–20 min and it is metabolized mainly in the liver.

Sex Steroids

Their secretion and physiology are beyond the scope of this review, since they are not involved in the pathogenesis of acute adrenal crisis.

Regulation of Adrenal Secretion

Glucocorticoid Secretion

ACTH is the main regulator of cortisol secretion (1). It is itself under the control of the hypothalamus through corticotropin-releasing hormone (CRH). The neuroendocrine control of CRH and ACTH secretion involves three mechanisms: a circadian rhythm, stress, and negative feedback.

ACTH is secreted by the corticotrophs of the anterior pituitary. It is a 39-amino acid peptide hormone processed from a large precursor molecule, proopiomelanocortin. ACTH exerts rapid and chronic ef-

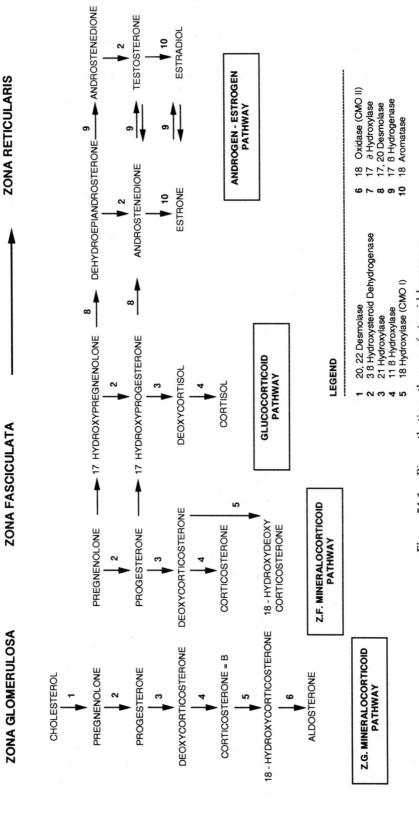

Figure 54.1. Biosynthetic pathways of steroid hormones.

fects on the adrenal cortex. It rapidly stimulates synthesis and secretion of steroids. As a consequence, plasma cortisol levels closely parallel those of ACTH. Chronic effects of ACTH include: a trophic role on zona fasciculata and reticularis and a sustained stimulation of all the enzymes involved in cortisol synthesis.

CRH is a hypothalamic peptide that stimulates the release of ACTH and its related peptides. It is secreted in a pulsatile manner and is submitted to a circadian rhythm under central nervous system control.

Thus, the release of ACTH and cortisol follows a circadian rhythm. There is a major burst of activity in the early morning hours before awakening. At this time, plasma cortisol level is high, 10–20 μg/dl. Then it gradually declines during the day and may be undetectable in the late evening and first hours of sleep.

This pattern of secretion is modulated by feedback inhibition. Circulating free cortisol and synthetic glucocorticoids exert a negative feedback at both the hypothalamic and pituitary levels.

Thus, exogenous glucocorticoid therapy prescribed for more than 5 days in suppressive doses (more than 30 mg of cortisol equivalent/day) induces a reversible inhibition of ACTH secretion. The duration of this inhibition depends on the duration and importance of steroid therapy. Following a high dose regimen administered for more than 1 month, the suppression of the hypothalamopituitary adrenal axis induces an atrophy of the adrenal cortex. CRH and ACTH secretion recover first, followed by the adrenal hormone. However, even after a progressive decrease of steroid treatment, these patients may develop acute adrenal insufficiency induced by stress during the next 12 months (15).

Stress can override both the feedback mechanism and the circadian rhythm. Acute hypoglycemia, pain, trauma, surgery, emotional stress, and fever induce a rapid stimulation of cortisol secretion mediated through the hypothalamic pituitary axis. The production of cortisol may be increased sixfold and its serum concentration more than 25 μg/dl and may reach 100 μg/dl.

Mineralocorticoid

The major regulators of aldosterone production are the renin-angiotensin system, potassium ion, and ACTH.

Renin is a proteolytic enzyme released from the juxtaglomerular cells of the kidney, which converts angiotensinogen to angiotensin I. This inactive decapeptide is rapidly transformed into the octapeptide angiotensin II by converting enzyme located in the vascular bed. Angiotensin II is a powerful vasoconstrictor and the major stimulator of aldosterone secretion.

Renin release is stimulated mainly by depletion of the intravascular volume, through decreased sodium delivery to macula densa of the kidney and decreased renal perfusion pressure. In addition, increased renal sympathetic activity mediates the renin secretory response to exercise and upright posture.

Hyperkalemia increases aldosterone production and hypokalemia reduces it.

Finally, stressful situations stimulate the renin-angiotensin-aldosterone pathway, through the sympathetic nervous system, as well as through ACTH. This hormone stimulates transiently aldosterone secretion.

Glucocorticoid Effects

Glucocorticoids exert a variety of effects in almost all body tissues. Three systems are mainly involved in the pathogenesis of acute adrenal insufficiency (1): cardiovascular, salt and water balance, and carbohydrate metabolism.

Cortisol increases total peripheral vascular resistance (4). It stimulates the production of prorenin and of angiotensinogen and it enhances vascular reactivity to vasoconstrictor substances such as catecholamines and angiotensin II. In addition, glucocorticoids increase cardiac output by a direct action on the heart, by increasing the synthesis of epinephrine in the adrenal medulla, and by a permissive role on catecholamine effects at the receptor and postreceptor level. On the other hand, cortisol inhibits the vasodilator systems by decreasing the synthesis by the vascular endothelium of prostaglandins prostacyclin (PGI_2) and nitric oxide. Thus, in the absence of cortisol, abnormal vasodilation and hypotension occur even in the absence of dehydration.

The effects of glucocorticoids on salt and water balance include enhanced glomerular filtration rate, increased water excretion, and a raised osmotic threshold for vasopressin release (12). Furthermore, cortisol is a weak mineralocorticoid. When administered at supraphysiological doses, it induces significant aldosterone-like effects. In addition, it modulates intracellular/extracellular distribution of salt and water by inducing a shift of sodium and fluids from the intra- to extracellular compartment, which increases plasma volume. Thus, acute cortisol deficiency results in a shift of about 200 mmol of sodium with a corresponding 1.3 liters of water from extracellular to intracellular spaces, even when total sodium balance is unchanged (14); the dilutional hyponatremia observed in this situation involves increased vasopressin (antidiuretic hormone (ADH)) release, as well as an ADH-independent pathway, probably related to a decreased medullary tonicity.

The action on carbohydrate metabolism contributes to the maintenance of plasma glucose, particularly during fasting, through several mechanisms: increased hepatic glycogen synthesis and storage, enhanced hepatic glucose production (gluconeogenesis), and decreased glucose uptake in muscle and adipose tissue (insulin-resistant state).

As a result of these effects, a deficiency of cortisol leads to hypoglycemia, which is precipitated by prolonged fast and is associated with poor adrenergic response and decreased recovery.

Mineralocorticoid Effects

Aldosterone's primary action is to increase sodium reabsorption in the collecting duct and maintain a very precise control over sodium balance. Thus, it plays a key role in the control of extracellular fluid and plasma volume. Aldosterone also increases potassium excretion. This action depends on the sodium delivery to the distal tube (a high sodium load increases K^+ excretion). In addition, it increases hydrogen secretion in the medulla collecting tubule independently of sodium reabsorption.

Mineralocorticoid deficiency leads to renal sodium wasting with hyponatremia, decreased extracellular fluid and blood volume, and clinical features of dehydration. This is associated with potassium retention and metabolic acidosis.

In Addison's disease, these effects are additive to those of glucocorticoid deficiency and increase the risk of cardiovascular collapse.

CLINICAL ASPECTS

Clinical presentation of acute adrenal insufficiency depends on the nature of the underlying disease (1, 2, 11). This situation may present itself:

As a complication of chronic primary adrenocortical insufficiency,
After bilateral adrenal hemorrhage, or
As the acute decompensation of ACTH deficiency.

Acute Primary Adrenocortical Insufficiency (Addison's Disease)

Precipitating Factors

Adrenal insufficiency may be undiagnosed; cortisol secretion remains sufficient in the basal state but the patient is unable to increase steroid output during a situation of increased requirements. Thus, acute adrenal crisis may reveal Addison's disease as a result of intercurrent disease.

More commonly, Addison's disease is already known and treated. In such patients, adrenal crisis occurs when replacement steroid dosage is not appropriately increased during a stressful situation.

These precipitating factors are usually:

Withdrawal of substitutive therapy because of vomiting or noncompliance of the patient;
Infection (Even an apparently minor upper respiratory viral infection may induce a rapid decompensation.);
All kind of febrile illnesses;
Trauma, surgery, labor and delivery;
Any cause of dehydration: salt deprivation, diarrhea, vomiting, excess of diuretics or laxatives, skin fluid losses during hot weather, etc.

Intercurrent therapy that modifies steroid metabolism such as hepatic enzyme inducers. Rifampicin has been reported to induce adrenal crisis in an Addisonian patient receiving replacement therapy (5, 8). Barbiturates and phenytoin may also increase patient's steroid requirement.

Clinical Features

Clinical symptoms are due to both gluco- and mineralocorticoid deficiency. They usually appear gradually over a few hours, but in acutely stressed patients collapse may occur suddenly. Fever is always present and may be high even in the absence of underlying infection. It is due to hypoadrenalism per se. Anorexia, nausea, vomiting, and diarrhea are frequent symptoms. They may worsen dehydration and are associated with massive recent weight loss. Diffuse abdominal pain may be mistaken for an acute abdominal emergency. Myalgia, joint pains, and headache are frequent complaints of impending crisis. Extreme weakness and apathy may lead to coma without local neurological defect. Sometimes patients present with psychiatric symptoms: agitation, confusion, and delirium (1, 2, 3, 11).

Physical examination shows symptoms of massive dehydration and hypovolemia with fall in blood pressure and tachycardia. Hyperpigmentation of the skin and mucous membranes is a classical sign of primary adrenocortical deficiency and may be useful in the presence of an acutely ill patient. ECG may reveal low voltage and abnormalities due to hyperkalemia (peaked T waves). If treatment is not rapidly instituted, vascular collapse and then refractory shock occur.

Biologic Features

Hyponatremia is present in about 90% of patients and is seldom lower than 120 mmol/liter (because of volume depletion). Hyperkalemia is not constant (65% of the patients) and is usually mild, between 4.5 and 5 mmol/liter. It is exceptionally severe and life-threatening. Metabolic acidosis with low serum bicarbonate (15–20 mmol/liter) is observed. Increased blood urea and creatinine are related to massive dehydration and prerenal failure. In urine specimens, sodium concentration is greater than 20 mmol/liter and potassium is low. Hypoglycemia is not constant and appears after a prolonged fast. Mild hypercalcemia occurs in few patients (11). Other symptoms may be suggestive: eosinophilia, lymphocytosis, and normocytic normochromic anemia.

Bilateral Massive Adrenal Hemorrhage (BMAH) (13)

Adrenal hemorrhage induces an acute adrenal destruction, and the classic clinical features of Addison's disease are absent.

Precipitating Factors

BMAH occurs in patients with severe concurrent disease and leads to a dramatic deteriorating course. The major risk factors are thromboembolic disease, coagulopathy (spontaneous or iatrogenic), postoperative state, and severe infection. Quite often, several risk factors are present.

Clinical Features

In the early stages, symptoms are rather progressive: pain localized to the abdomen, flank, lower chest, or back with abdominal tenderness or rebound. Hypotension is not constant, fever is the only reliable sign.

These manifestations are not specific and may be mistaken for a complication of the underlying disease. They should be viewed as highly suspicious in the context of patients at risk for developing BMAH.

If these premonitory features are ignored, the patient will develop an acute adrenal crisis with catastrophic hypotension and progression to refractory shock despite of maximal inotropic support.

Biologic Features

Biologic features are first characterized by a drop in hemoglobin and hematocrit. Signs due to adrenal failure appear later (see above).

Diagnosis

Specific diagnosis will be confirmed after the treatment of the acute adrenal crisis and stabilization of the clinical picture.

Anatomic evidence of hemorrhage is obtained then by ultrasound or computed tomography showing bilateral enlargment of adrenal glands with hyperdense areas. Magnetic resonance imaging is actually the best diagnostic procedure. It shows specific signs of hemorrhage in addition to the increased volume of the adrenals.

Long-Term Prognosis

BMAH results in complete and irreversible loss of adrenal function associated with progressive adrenal atrophy.

ACTH Deficiency

Pathophysiology and Clinical Aspects

The predominant effect of ACTH deficiency is decreased cortisol and adrenal androgen secretion (1). Aldosterone secretion may be diminished, probably through the action of cortisol on the renin-angiotensin system (9). Thus, acute presentation of ACTH deficiency is similar to that of primary hypoadrenalism. However, hyperpigmentation is absent and dehydration is much less important. Severe hypotension and shock may occur. Hypoglycemia is frequent and may be severe, especially if there is growth hormone deficiency. Hyponatremia is usually moderate and is mainly due to inappropriate ADH secretion. Urea and kalemia are normal (12).

Etiologic Aspects

Isolated ACTH deficiency most commonly occurs after long-term corticosteroid therapy. Acute adrenal crisis, although rare, is a result of abrupt cessation of therapy or severe stress. It should be avoided by systematic steroid covering therapy and by careful follow-up and education of the patients.

The other causes of ACTH deficiencies are tumors of the pituitary and/or hypothalamus, surgery and radiation of these regions, and pituitary apoplexy.

Cortisol deficiency is the most important endocrine defect but is clinically associated with features of panhypopituitarism. In growth hormone secreting adenoma or prolactinoma, hypersecretion of these hormones may coexist with partial or complete deficiency of the rest of the pituitary (1).

Sheehan's Syndrome

Sheehan's syndrome (postpartum ischemic necrosis of the pituitary) may occur abruptly, so that vascular collapse, shock, and hypoglycemia postpartum should strongly suggest the diagnosis of acute ACTH deficiency.

DIAGNOSIS OF ACUTE ADRENAL INSUFFICIENCY

As soon as the acute adrenal crisis is clinically suspected, plasma samples are obtained for the measurement of basal cortisol level. Therapy is instituted without delay and may use dexamethasone for the first 30 min in order to allow a rapid ACTH stimulation test: 0.25 mg of cosyntropin (tetracosactrin) are injected intravenously and a sample for plasma cortisol is obtained 30 min later. The increase of cortisol is subnormal in primary and in most of the cases of secondary adrenal insufficiency. Normal values are higher than 20 μg/dl after stimulation. If the ACTH assay is available, it may be performed in the basal plasma sample. Its value is higher than 250 pg/ml in primary adrenal failure (in the presence of low cortisol level), while it is inappropriately low (0–50 pg/ml) in secondary adrenal deficiency. In the absence of ACTH assays, the response of plasma aldosterone to the rapid ACTH stimulation test may be discriminating: it is subnormal in primary adrenal deficiency and normal in pituitary failure (1–3).

THERAPY OF ACUTE ADDISONIAN CRISIS

Since acute adrenal crisis may be fatal, treatment should be started as soon as the diagnosis has been suspected and blood samples drawn for hormone measurement (1, 2, 10).

The aims of treatment are:

Correction of dehydration and volume depletion with massive saline infusion;
Hormone substitution, mainly using glucocor-

ticoids in large amounts that reverse hypotension and shock;
Treatment of associated conditions.

Fluid Restoration

A large bore intravenous line must be established.
Fluids that are generally used are: 5% glucose
containing sodium chloride (6 g/liter); isotonic saline infusion may be used after initial
hypoglycemia has been corrected.
Perfusion rate is always rapid at the beginning
of therapy: 1 liter/30 min, and further saline
is given according to the patient's hemodynamic condition. Generally, 4 liters are needed
approximately during the first 24 hr of treatment.
Hypokalemia and acidosis do not generally require specific therapy.
Late administration of potassium depends on
electrolyte changes during therapy.

Hormonal Replacement Therapy

Glucocorticoids are given intravenously at
the very beginning of fluid restoration.
The drug of choice is a soluble form of
cortisol (hydrocortisone hemisuccinate).
One hundred milligrams of hydrocortisone hemisuccinate should be given intravenously and then repeated every 6 hr
during the first day.

The use of lower dosages of hydrocortisone, 100 mg/day, in a continuous intravenous perfusion preceded by an intravenous bolus of 50 mg has recently been
proposed (7).

Dexamethasone (2 mg intravenously)
may be used for the first 30 min in order
to allow the ACTH stimulation test.

Mineralocorticoid therapy is theoretically not required at this time of treatment
(1, 10). (When hydrocortisone is used in
large amounts (>100 mg/day) it has a sufficient sodium-retaining capacity). However, some authors treat aldosterone deficiency with desoxycorticosterone acetate
administered intramuscularly. Its action
begins 2 hr after injection and persists for
24 hr. The initial dose is 2–5 mg and may
be repeated 12–24 hr later if oral intake is
not possible and/or electrolytic abnormalities persist.

Follow-up

After institution of the appropriate treatment, improvement is dramatic in less than

12 hr. Glucocorticoid dosage is adapted
according to the precipitating illness. High
dose intravenous therapy (hydrocortisone
hemisuccinate, 200–400 mg/day) is maintained until clinical improvement and resolution of the aggravating factors are obtained. It is then progressively tapered to
100, 75, then 50 mg/day. Maintenance
treatment requires oral administration of
30 mg of hydrocortisone/day and 50–200
μg of the mineralocorticoid 9 α-fluorohy-
drocortisone/day in divided doses.

THERAPY OF ACUTE SECONDARY ADRENAL INSUFFICIENCY

Glucocorticoid

Glucocorticoid replacement is the major
requirement in this situation. Prevention
and treatment of hypoglycemia with intravenous glucose are especially required. On
the other hand, care should be taken to
avoid overloading the patient with fluids,
since dehydration is less severe than in
the case of addisonian crisis.

Other Endocrine Deficiencies

Thyroxine replacement should never be
instituted in hypoadrenal patients until
steroid replacement is instituted.

Finally, it should be stressed that in
some patients with suprasellar lesion or
Sheehan's syndrome, hydrocortisone therapy may unmask diabetes insipidus.

PREVENTION

Adrenal crisis in patients with known
adrenal or pituitary deficiency is easily
prevented by appropriate increases of hydrocortisone treatment.

In case of surgery (1, 6, 16), the usual
dose of hydrocortisone should be doubled
the day before operation. Before induction
of anesthesia, 100 mg of soluble hydrocortisone is administered intravenously.
During surgery and in the immediate postoperative period, 50 mg are given intramuscularly or intravenously every 4 hr
and dosage increased if hypotension occurs. If the patient's course is satisfactory,
the dosages are reduced to 50 mg every 6
hr and gradually reduced to the maintenance regimen.

Doubling the usual dose of hydrocortisone is also required for a few days in the case of febrile illnesses. If oral intake becomes impossible, intramuscular hydrocortisone hemisuccinate should be instituted in divided doses (every 6 hr).

References

1. Baxter, JD, Tyrrel JB. The adrenal cortex. In: Felig P, Baxter JD, Broadus AE, Frohman LA, eds. Endocrinology and metabolism. New York: McGraw Hill 1986:511–650.
2. Bethune JE. The diagnosis and treatment of adrenal insufficiency. In: De Groot LJ, ed. Endocrinology. Philadelphia: WB Saunders, 1989.
3. Burke CW. Adrenocortical insufficiency. Clin Endocrinol Metab 1985;14:948–976.
4. Grunfeld JP, Eloy L, Moura AM, Ganeval D, Ramos-Frando B, Worcel M. Effects of antiglucocorticoids on glucocorticoid hypertension in the rat. Hypertension 1985;7:292.
5. Kyriazopouou V, Paparousis O, Vagenakis AG. Rifampicin-induced adrenal crisis in Addisonian patients receiving corticosteroid replacement therapy. J Clin Endocrinol Metab 1984;59:1204–1206.
6. Lampe GH, Roizen MF. Anesthesia for patients with abnormal function of the adrenal cortex. Anesth Clin North Am 1987;5:245–267.
7. Lefebvre J, Vantyghem MC. Le traitement de l'insuffisance corticosurrénale aigue. Rev Prat Med Gen (Paris) 1989;47:7–11.
8. McAllister AC, Thompson PJ, Al-Habet SM, Rogers HJ. Rifampicin reduces effectiveness and bioavailability of prednisolone. Br Med J 1983;286:923–925.
9. Merriam GR, Baer L. Adrenocorticotropin deficiency: correction of hyponatremia and hypoaldosteronism with chronic glucocorticoid therapy. J Clin Endocrinol Metab 1980;50:10–14.
10. Muir A, Maclaren N. Adrenocortical insufficiency. In: Bardin CW, ed. Current therapy in endocrinology and metabolism. Philadelphia: BC Decker, 1991:124–129.
11. Nerup J. Addison's Disease—clinical studies—report of 108 cases. Acta Endocrinol (Copenh) 1974;76:127–141.
12. Oelkers W. Hyponatremia and inappropriate secretion of vasopressin (antidiuretic hormone) in patients with hypopituitarism. N Engl J Med 1989;321:492–496.
13. Rao RH, Vagnucci AH, Amico JA. Bilateral massive adrenal hemorrhage: early recognition and treatment. Ann Intern Med 1989;110:227–235.
14. Skrabal F, Arnot RN, Jopling F, Fraser TR. The effect of glucocorticoid withdrawal on body water and electrolytes in hypopituitary patients with adrenocortical insufficiency as investigated with ^{77}Br, ^{43}K, ^{24}Na and ^{3}H$_2$O. Clin Sci 1972;43:79–90.
15. Tyrell JB, Baxter JD. Glucocorticoid therapy. In: Felig P, Baxter JD, Broadus AE, Frohman LA, eds. Endocrinology and metabolism. New York: McGraw Hill, 1986;809–813.
16. Udelman R, Ramp J, Gallucci WT, Gordon A, Lipfond E, Norton JA, Loriaux DL, Chrousos GP. Adaptation during surgical stress. A reevaluation of the role of glucocorticoids. J Clin Invest 1986;77:1377–1381.

55

Pathology of Posterior Pituitary

Marie Emilie Chauveau

PHYSIOLOGICAL ASPECTS

The posterior pituitary gland secretes two nonapeptides of very similar structure: vasopressin (also called antidiuretic hormone (ADH)) and oxytocin. Only the former has important effects on water balance.

Vasopressin Synthesis and Secretion

Vasopressin and oxytocin are synthesized (5, 14, 15) in magnocellular neurons of supraoptic and paraventricular nuclei of the hypothalamus. Each hormone is produced by a different population of neurons and is associated to a specific protein carrier called neurophysin.

Thus, ADH is derived from a large precursor molecule that consists of the vasopressin nonapeptide, its specific neurophysin, and a glycoprotein moiety.

This precursor migrates along neuronal axons that end mainly in the neurohypophysis close to the capillary sinusoid. Cleavage occurs during this transport. Both cleaved and uncleaved products are then stored in neurosecretory granules. ADH itself has a molecular mass of 1084 daltons and is characterized by a ring structure with a disulfide linkage.

After synthesis, ADH is released into the systemic circulation with its specific neurophysin by a process of exocytosis following electrical activation of the neuron. Circulating neurophysin has no known biological function.

ADH circulates unbound to protein but is largely associated with platelets. It is rapidly cleaved by aminopeptidases and its half-life is short (5–10 min).

Biologic Effects

The major target organ of ADH is the kidney. Vasopressin increases water reabsorption by selectively increasing the water permeability of the collecting duct epithelium. This action is mediated by specific receptors located on the peritubular side of the cell called V2 receptors. This receptor is coupled to adenylate cyclase.

The action of ADH depends on two preexisting conditions: the corticopapillary gradient and the transepithelial osmotic pressure differences between relative "hypotonic" luminal fluid and relative "hypertonic" interstitium.

In the presence of ADH, water is reabsorbed in excess of solute and a hypertonic urine is excreted (maximal urine osm: 1200 mosm/kg). In the absence of ADH, the lumen fluid remains dilute throughout its entire course in the collecting tube, water is excreted in excess of solute, and urine osmolality is low (<100 mosm/kg).

Extra renal effects of ADH are mediated by V1 receptors, which stimulate influx of calcium into the cells and are independent of adenylate cyclase. They are mainly located in vascular smooth muscle and are associated with vasoconstriction. This pressor action requires very high levels of ADH and is probably not significant in physiological conditions but might be important in the maintenance of blood pressure during acute hypovolemia.

Control of Secretion

Under normal circumstances, vasopressin secretion as well as thirst is primarily regulated by plasma osmolality (5, 14, 15). When plasma osmolality increases, ADH is released. On the other hand, a decrease of osmolality reduces ADH release. This mechanism involves osmoreceptors located in the anterior hypothalamus in close proximity to thirst "osmoreception."

They are mainly sensitive to sodium and its anions, which contribute to more than 95% of the plasma osmotic pressure. Such solute as urea or glucose permeate cell membranes and have little effect, if any. Conversely, mannitol is as potent as sodium.

This mechanism is extraordinarily sensitive. A change in plasma osmolality as small as 1% is enough to produce a readily detectable change in plasma ADH.

When plasma osmolality falls below a threshold value of approximately 280 mosm/kg H_2O, plasma vasopressin is suppressed to low or undetectable levels. Urine is maximally diluted (osmolality <100 mosm/kg). Water diuresis increases significantly and prevents further decrease in plasma osmolality.

When plasma osmolality rises above a threshold value of approximately 295 mosm/kg, plasma vasopressin reaches sufficient levels for maximal antidiuresis. In normal conditions, this high osmolality also activates thirst and water intake preventing further dehydration.

Thus, osmoregulation of thirst and arginine vasopressin (AVP) secretion maintains plasma osmolality within a narrow range (280–295 mosm/kg).

Other nonosmotic factors may also modulate ADH release mainly in pathologic states. Blood volume and pressure modification influence vasopressin secretion through baroreceptors located in the left atrium and sinoaortic region.

A reduction of at least 5–10% of blood pressure or volume is required to induce significant change in ADH level. A significant decrease of pressure (20–30%), raises ADH to very high levels and produces arteriolar vasoconstriction.

This baroregulatory system is much less sensitive than the osmoregulatory system. It has little significance in normal conditions, but may override the osmoregulation when severe hypovolemia occurs.

Lastly many neuromediators and other factors have been implicated in the control of ADH release. Nausea and emesis are the most potent defined stimuli.

SYNDROME OF INAPPROPRIATE SECRETION OF ANTIDIURETIC HORMONE (SIADH)

The SIADH is by far the most common cause of hyponatremia encountered in clinical practice (1). It was first described by Bartter and Schwartz (4) and is characterized by an inappropriate persistent secretion of ADH in the face of hypoosmolality of body fluids.

Fixed antidiuresis initially results in free water retention and dilutional hyponatremia. Natriuresis then increases by a mechanism involving increased natriuretic atrial peptide. This effect prevents the occurrence of significant hypervolemia and edema. Sodium balance is essentially normal in this syndrome.

Etiologies

Many conditions are associated with SIADH: malignant tumors, diseases of the lung and central nervous system, and administration of certain drugs. (Etiologies are listed in Table 55.1).

The mechanism of AVP secretion is not always clearly established. Ectopic production of the hormone has been demonstrated in many tumors associated with SIADH but not all of them. On the other hand, in pulmonary diseases and central nervous system disorders, AVP is released from neurohypophysis but with abnormal osmoregulation mechanism.

Clinical Features

Hyponatremia is often asymptomatic, but if present, clinical manifestations are largely of central nervous system origin and reflect brain edema (2). Symptoms occur when plasma sodium level falls below 125 mmol/liter and/or when hyponatremia develops rapidly. Symptoms include lethargy, apathy, confusion, disorientation, seizures, and coma. These symptoms may be wrongly linked to the underlying neurological disease. Nausea and vomiting have

Table 55.1
Etiologies of SIADH

Tumors
  Bronchial carcinoma (particularly small cell type)
  Other carcinomas: duodenum, pancreas, bladder, ureter, prostate
  Leukemia lymphoma
  Thymoma, sarcoma
Central nervous system disorders
  Mass lesions: tumors, abscess, hematoma
  Infections: encephalitis, meningitis
  Cerebrovascular accident
  Senile cerebral atrophy
  Hydrocephalus
  Trauma
  Delirium tremens, acute psychosis
  Demyelinating and degenerative disease
  Inflammatory disease
Pulmonary disorders
  Infections: tuberculosis, pneumonia, abscess
  Acute respiratory failure
  Positive pressure ventilation
Drugs
  Vasopressin DDAVP
  Chlorpropamide
  Cloribrate
  Carbamazepine
  Others: vincristine, vinblastine, tricyclics, phenothiazine
Idiopathic
  Diagnosis of exclusion

Table 55.2
Criteria for the Diagnosis of SIADH

Hypoosmolality (P osm <275 mosm/kg of H_2O)
  Corrected plasma Na+ < 135 mmol/liter
Inappropriate urinary osmolality
  U osm > 100 mosm/kg of H_2O
Elevated urinary sodium concentration (>20 mEq/liter)
Absence of clinically detectable hypovolemia or hypervolemia
Absence of hypothyroidism, hypocortisolism, diuretic therapy

solutes are present in extracellular fluid (mannitol, radiographic contrast agent, etc.).
Inappropriate urinary osmolality for the plasma hypoosmolality: Uosm > 100 mosm/kg of H_2O
Urinary sodium concentration is generally greater than 20 mEq/liter. Natriuresis reflects sodium intake. This biologic feature excludes many other causes of hyponatremia, but may be absent if the patient's water and sodium intake is restricted.
Blood urea nitrogen and serum uric acid are normal (or low because of increased renal excretion of each metabolite).

Diagnostic Procedure

Dilutional hyponatremia with inappropriate natriuresis in clinically euvolemic patients strongly suggests the diagnosis of SIADH. But this diagnosis remains essentially a diagnosis of exclusion, and all other causes of hyponatremia should be investigated (20).

Clinically Euvolemic Hyponatremia

If the hyponatremic patient appears clinically euvolemic, three other diagnoses should be first excluded because they may exactly mimic SIADH: glucocorticoid deficiency, hypothyroidism and diuretic-induced hyponatremia.

Hypocortisolism can cause elevated plasma AVP levels as well as impaired water excretion through an AVP-independent pathway (12). This diagnosis is easily excluded by a rapid ACTH stimulation test.

Hypothyroidism also causes impaired water excretion (16) by at least two mech-

the same significance as other neurological symptoms.

An important clinical feature in diagnosing SIADH is the absence of hypovolemic symptoms as well as edema. There is no recent history of diuretic intake.

Biological Features

Biological features (Table 55.2) include:

Hyponatremia below 135 mmol/liter. Pseudohyponatremia due to hyperlipidemia or hyperglycemia are excluded. If hyperglycemia is concomitant, corrected natremia may be calculated as follows: Na corrected = Na measured + 1.5 (Gly − 5)/5.
Effective hypoosmolality. Plasma osm < 275 mosm/kg of H_2O). Plasma osmolality may be calculated with the formula: P osm (mosm/kg of H_2O) = $2 \times Na^+$ (mmol/liter) + glucose (mmol/liter). A direct measurement of osmolality is useful when unmeasured osmotic

anisms: a diminished distal fluid delivery and a persistent AVP release. Diagnosis is based on measurement of free thyroxine and thyroid-stimulating hormone.

Diuretic-induced hyponatremia is very frequent. Despite substantial urinary sodium loss, patients often appear clinically euvolemic. Hyponatremia results from mild volume depletion, and enhanced ADH secretion. In practice, if diuretic use is known or suspected, the patient should be first considered as being solute depleted and treated accordingly.

Hypovolemic Hyponatremia

Suggestive symptoms of hypovolemia (low blood pressure, tachycardia, raised blood urea nitrogen, and uric acid) indicate sodium depletion and hypovolemic hyponatremia. Measurement of urinary sodium concentration distinguishes renal from extrarenal losses (Table 55.3).

Mechanisms of depletional hyponatremia involve increased thirst and water intake, nonosmotic release of vasopressin, and replacement of extracelluar fluid losses by hypotonic fluid, which dilutes the remaining body sodium.

Hypervolemic Hyponatremia

Diagnosis is easy on clinical grounds in a patient in an edematous state and/or with ascites. Natriuresis is usually low (less than 10 mEq/liter) except if associated with diuretic therapy. Causes are listed in Table 55.4. This type of hyponatremia is linked

Table 55.3
Causes of hypovolemic hyponatremia

Urinary sodium concentration >20 mmol/
  liter = renal solute loss
  Diuretic therapy
  Mineralocorticoid deficiency
  Salt wasting nephropathy
  (Solute diuresis: mannitol, glucose)
Urinary sodium concentration < 10 mmol/liter
  = Nonrenal solute loss
  Gastrointestinal (diarrhea, vomiting, pancreatitis)
  Cutaneous (sweatings, burns)

Table 55.4
Hypervolemic Hyponatremia

Urinary sodium < 20 mEq/liter
  Nephrotic syndrome
  Cirrhosis
  Cardiac failure
Urinary sodium > 20 mEq/liter
  Renal failure

to an increase of total body sodium content and higher increase in total body water but a relative decreased vascular volume.

This disorder produces three consequences that contribute to hyponatremia: a nonosmotic release of ADH, a secondary hyperaldosteronism (increased sodium reabsorption), and a decrease in glomerular filtration rate. This later mechanism leads to increased reabsorption of both sodium and water in the proximal tubular fluid, a decreased delivery of tubular fluid to the distal nephron, and an inability to dilute the urine.

Therapy of SIADH

Treatment of SIADH depends on the presence or absence of neurological symptoms.

Asymptomatic Patients

These patients probably have chronic hyponatremia. Therapy should induce a slow correction of hypoosmolality and avoid the neurological risks encountered by rapid correction.

Fluid restriction is the only appropriate therapy. All fluids must be included in the restriction and should be limited to 500–800 ml/day according to the daily urine volume (500 ml less than the average urine volume).

Several days are usually needed before a significant increase in plasma osmolality occurs.

Salt should not be restricted since natriuresis balances sodium intake.

Symptomatic Patients

Severe hyponatremia (generally <115 mmol/liter) with significant central nervous system symptoms requires emergency therapy. How quickly the plasma sodium should be corrected (2, 3, 11) is controversial because of the risk of developing central pontine myelinolysis when sodium level increases rapidly. This is a rare complication but it may result in death or permanent brain damage. Alcoholism, hepatic encephalopathy, and hypoxia, as well as chronic preexisting hyponatremia, increase the risk. Conversely, untreated severe hyponatremia may also be fatal, as reported in a recent description of severe complications of untreated hyponatremia in healthy young women recovering from anesthesia for benign disease. Autopsy revealed brain edema and cerebral herniation (10).

So, the rate of correction should vary from 0.7 mmol/liter/hr in mild symptomatic patients or chronic hyponatremia to 2 mmol/liter/hr in comatose patients (3, 17).

This can be achieved by intravenous infusion of hypertonic saline solution with a slow initial rate of approximately 3 ml/kg/hr of 5% NaCl or 5 ml/kg/hr of 3% NaCl during the first 2 hr.

Then the plasma sodium level is monitored every 2 hr, and treatment is stopped when the patient becomes asymptomatic and/or when the patient's Na^+ level has reached 125 mmol/liter. The magnitude of correction should never be more than 25 mmol/liter, at a rate of 1–4 mosm/kg of water per hour.

When these therapeutic aims are reached, the patient is placed on fluid restriction alone.

The simultaneous use of intravenous furosemide (1 mg/kg) is reserved by most authors to patients at risk of fluid overload (underlying cardiac disease).

Follow-up

Long-term therapy includes, first, the treatment of the underlying disease by surgery, radiotherapy, chemotherapy in the case of carcinoma, treatment of an infection, and cessation of a drug known to be associated with SIADH.

Then, fluid restriction is maintained but it may be difficult for long periods. In this case, demeclocycline can be used as an adjuvant therapy (9). This tetracyclin an-

tibiotic inhibits ADH action (via post receptor mechanism) and induces an acquired nephrogenic diabetes insipidus with excretion of an isotonic urine of increased volume. Daily 600–1200 mg should be given in divided doses. Efficiency of action usually occurs within 5–14 days. This drug can cause nephrotoxicity particularly in patients with hepatic disease or heart failure. Renal function must be monitored closely.

Lithium produces polyuria, but is no longer used because of side effects and inconsistent results (9).

Urea administration has been proposed by Decaux et al. (8) at the dose of 30 g/day orally.

VASOPRESSIN HYPOFUNCTION

Hypotonic polyuria can be defined as an increased urine output more than 2.5 liters/day or 30 ml/kg/day with low urinary osmolality (<200 mosm/kg of H_2O) and/or low specific gravity (< 1005). It may result from three basic abnormalities: decreased or absent secretion of ADH (neurogenic diabetes insipidus), renal resistance to ADH action (nephrogenic diabetes insipidus), and primary polydipsia.

In neurogenic diabetes insipidus fixed hypotonic polyuria tends to increase plasma osmolality and sodium levels, which in turn activate thirst. The result is increased water intake, which prevents dehydration. Finally, plasma osmolality remains in the normal range. Etiologies of diabetes insipidus are listed in Table 55.5.

The physiopathology of nephrogenic diabetes insipidus is the same despite normal osmotic stimulation of ADH release. Etiologies are listed in Table 55.5.

In primary polydipsia, the initial anomaly is an inappropriate fluid intake in large amounts leading to lower plasma osmolality, which in turn suppresses ADH release. Polyuria ensues and prevents hypoosmolality. Primary polydipsia may be due to an abnormally low threshold for thirst (dipsogenic polydipsia) or be associated with psychological disturbances (psychogenic polydipsia).

In all these circumstances, clinical fea-

Table 55.5
Etiologies of Diabetes Insipidus and Primary Polydipsia

Neurogenic diabetes insipidus
  Trauma
  Neurosurgery
  Tumors and cysts of hypothalamic region
  Granulomas (sarcoidosis, histiocytosis)
  Infections (meningitis, encephalitis)
  Vascular disorders (Sheehan's syndrome,
    aneurysms)
  Idiopathic (autoimmune?)
  Familial
Nephrogenic diabetes insipidus
  Metabolic (hypercalcemia, hypokalemia)
  Drugs: lithium, demeclocycline
  Sickle cell anemia
  Chronic pyelonephritis
  Postobstructive
  Sarcoidosis
  Idiopathic: familial or sporadic
Primary polydipsia
  Psychogenic
  Dipsogenic (idiopathic, sarcoidosis,
    hypothalamic lesion)

tures are limited to polyuria and polydipsia. These patients should not be treated in the critical care unit. A major exception is the rare association of central diabetes insipidus with abnormalities of thirst mechanisms. If hypodipsia coexists or if the patient is unable to request fluids, vasopressin deficiency may lead to life-threatening hypernatremic dehydration.

Diagnostic Procedure

Context of Neurosurgery or Head Trauma

The most frequent cause of neurogenic diabetes insipidus is a consequence of severe head trauma or surgery of sellar and suprasellar lesions. On the other hand, if polyuria is common after neurosurgery, causes other than diabetes insipidus should be first excluded, e.g., delayed excretion of fluid given during the operative period, osmotic polyuria due to hyperglycemia, or use of mannitol (hyperglycemia is frequently associated with a high dose of corticosteroid).

The diagnosis of acute cranial diabetes insipidus requires rigorous criteria: polyuria > 2 ml/kg/hr, inappropriately dilute urine (specific gravity < 1.005) with concomitant plasma hyperosmolality or sodium levels above 143 mEq/liter. Diagnosis is of primary importance since these patients are often unable to respond to thirst and thus are at high risk of rapid hypernatremic dehydration.

Context of Chronic Polyuria

The first step should be to exclude glycosuria, hypercalcemia, hypokalemia, chronic renal failure, and lithium therapy. Then it is necessary to ensure that hypotonic polyuria exists by monitoring each day's intake and output and measuring plasma osmolality, sodium level, and urinary osmolality (18). If plasma osmolality is high (above 295 mosm/kg) and natremia is > 145 mmol/liter in the presence of hypotonic polyuria, primary polydipsia is excluded. Administration of desmopressin distinguishes neurogenic from nephrogenic diabetes insipidus.

In the other nonemergency conditions, diagnosis of diabetes insipidus or primary polydipsia requires a standard dehydration test and, if it is noncontributory, direct measurement of ADH during osmotic stimulation, which is the most reliable method, but it is rarely available.

Therapy of Central Diabetes Insipidus

Acute Therapy

Short-term therapy is required in postoperative or posttraumatic diabetes insipidus and in all circumstances of inability to respond to thirst.

Administration of ADH analogs should start only when the diagnosis of diabetes insipidus is certain (6, 19). 1-Desamino-8-D-arginine vasopressin (DDAVP or desmopressin) is the drug of choice because of its sustained action and its absence of pressor effects. Most often the intranasal route is not available because of nasal packing or nasotracheal intubation. So DDAVP is given intramuscularly (about 2 μg). The dose can be repeated when hypotonic polyuria recurs, generally within 12 hr as long as diabetes insipidus persists.

It should be stressed that most cases of postoperative diabetes insipidus are transitory and resolve spontaneously within a few days.

To avoid over treatment, some authors have proposed intravenous continous administration of an ultra low dose of vasopressin (1–2 IU/24 hr). The advantage is a regular urine output and a rapidly reversible effect. Polyuria recurs 3 hr after the cessation of infusion (7).

Fluid replacement of urinary losses is strictly controlled and must be kept at the same level as, or below, diuresis. Water ingestion is possible because of the patient's thirst if he or she is awake. Fluid intake should be carefully monitored, especially after transsphenoidal neurosurgery because of nasal packing and congestion that may artifactually increase thirst.

If the patient is unable to request fluid, because of decreased consciousness or damage to the hypothalamic thirst center, intravenous administration of a low sodium solution is required (19).

Frequent monitoring of intake, urine output, and natremia is necessary to avoid water overload and hyponatremia.

Chronic Therapy

In persistent diabetes insipidus, DDAVP is given intranasally. A twice daily dose of 5–20 μg usually controls diuresis.

References

1. Anderson RJ, Chung HM, Kluce RK, Schrier RW. Hyponatremia: a prospective analysis of its epidemiology and the pathogenetic role of vasopressin. Ann Intern Med 1985;102:163–168.
2. Arieff AI. Central nervous system manifestations of disordered sodium metabolism. Clin Endocrinol Metab 1984;13:269–294.
3. Ayus JC, Krothapalli RK, Arieff AI. Treatment of symptomatic hyponatremia and its relation to brain damage. N Engl J Med 1987;317:1190–1195.
4. Bartter FC, Schwartz WB. The syndrome of inappropriate secretion of antidiuretic hormone. Am J Med 1967;42:790–806.
5. Baylis PH. Vasopressin and its neurophysin. In de Groot LJ, ed. Endocrinology. Philadelphia: WB Saunders, 1989:213–229.
6. Chanson P, Jedynak CP, Dabrowski G, et al. Ultra-low doses of vasopressin in the management of diabetes insipidus. Crit Care Med 1987;15:44–46.
7. Chanson P, Jedynak CP, Czernichow P. Management of early postoperative diabetes insipidus with parenteral desmopressin. Acta Endocrinol (Copenh) 1988;117:513–516.
8. Decaux G, Brimioulle S, Genette F, Mockel J. Treatment of the syndrome of inappropriate secretion of antidiuretic hormone by urea. Am J Med 1980;69:99–106.
9. Forrest JN, Cox M, Hong C, et al. Superiority of demeclocycline over lithium in the treatment of chronic syndrome of inappropriate secretion of antidiuretic hormone. N Engl J Med 1978;298:173–177.
10. Fraser CL, Arieff AI. Fatal central diabetes mellitus and insipidus resulting from untreated hyponatremia: a new syndrome. Ann Intern Med 1990;112:113–119.
11. Laureno R. Central pontine myelinolysis following rapid correction of hyponatremia. Ann Neurol 1983;13:232.
12. Linas SL, Berl T, Robertson GL, Aisenbrey GA, Schrier RW, Anderson RJ. Role of vasopressin in the impaired water excretion of glucocorticoid deficiency. Kidney Int 1980;18:58–67.
13. Robertson GL. Diagnosis of diabetes insipidus. In: Czernichow P, Robinson AG, eds. Diabetes insipidus in man. Front Horm Res 1985;13:176–189.
14. Robertson GL. Diseases of the posterior pituitary. In: Felig P, Baxter JD, Broadus AE, Frohman LA, eds. Endocrinology and Metabolism. New York: McGraw Hill, 1987:338–385.
15. Robertson GL, Berl T. Pathophysiology of water metabolism. In: Brenner BM, Rector FC, eds. The Kidney. Philadelphia: WB Saunders, 1991:677–736.
16. Robinson AG, De Rubertis FR. Disorders of sodium and water balance associated with adrenal, thyroid and pituitary disease. In: Schrier RW, Gottschalg C, eds. Disease of the kidney. Boston: Little, Brown, 1988:2795–2822.
17. Sterns RH. Severe symptomatic hyponatremia: treatment and outcome. Ann Intern Med 1987;107:656–664.
18. Thompson CJ. Polyuric states in man. Clin Endocrinol Metab 1989;3(2):473–497.
19. Verbalis JG, Robinson AG. Moses AM. Postoperative and posttraumatic diabetes insipidus. In: Czernichow P, Robinson AG, eds. Diabetes insipidus in man. Front Horm Res 1985;13:247–265.
20. Verbalis JG. Inappropriate antidiuresis and other hypo-osmolar states. In: Becker KL, ed. Principles and practices of endocrinology and metabolism. Philadelphia: JB Lippincott, 1990:237–247.

56

The Pathophysiological Basis of Current Pheochromocytoma Management

Pierre-François Plouin
Michel Azizi
Martin Day
Jean-Marc Duclos
Pierre Corvol

Pheochromocytoma (PH) is a neoplasm of chromaffin tissue, which secretes catecholamines. It is a dramatic, potentially fatal, rare cause of hypertension (3). Tumor growth is malignant in over 10% of cases and catecholamine secretion is unpredictable and often massive, resulting in sustained or paroxysmal hypertension, arrhythmias, and/or diabetes. Despite the availability of specific α- and β-adrenergic antagonists, the only effective treatment is tumoral resection because the large variation in catecholamine output does not allow a stable pharmacologic control of blood pressure (BP). Treatments which prepare for, or complement, surgery, e.g., adrenergic antagonists, antihypertensive or antiarrhythmic agents, and, in malignant cases, therapeutic embolization, antineoplastic therapy, or local radiotherapy using radioiodinated meta-Iodo-benzyl-guanidine (^{131}I-MIBG), are therefore necessary but never sufficient.

Recent advances in the understanding of inherited diseases and in imaging techniques now allow the diagnosis of PH in asymptomatic patients, either as a result of active screening in families with multiple endocrine neoplasia type 2 (MEN 2)(10) or phakomatoses (18), or following the biochemical investigation of an incidentally discovered adrenal mass (32). Asymptomatic cases of PH still require surgical extirpation of the tumor because abstention would expose the patient to acute cardiovascular crisis, either spontaneously or provoked by incidental parturition, endoscopy, or surgery. Unfortunately, undiagnosed PH may be found at autopsy in these subjects who die suddenly with collapse, pulmonary edema, or acute cardiac arrythmia (1).

PH is a rare disease with an estimated prevalence in hypertensive patients of 0.1% or less (39). Therefore, clinicians, anesthetists, and surgeons working in a general hospital might never see a case in a lifetime of clinical practice. Since preoperative management, anesthesia, and surgery may be complex and involve large and acute variations in BP and heart rate, patients with PH should be entrusted to referral centers with regular experience with the disease.

THE MECHANISM OF HYPERTENSION IN PHEOCHROMOCYTOMA

Increased total peripheral resistance is primarily responsible for the hypertension in PH (19). The mechanism of this increase seems straightforward because noradrenaline, a catecholamine secreted by the vast majority of PH, is a potent vasoconstrictor. As early as 1922, the hypertension in PH was attributed to the release of chromaffin cell amines, based on the contemporary knowledge of noradrenaline's and adrenaline's physiological effects (17). This assumption was later confirmed by the demonstration of high concentrations of tumoral (13) and urinary (8) noradrenaline. However, when plasma catecholamines were measured in subjects with PH, a poor correlation was found between BP and circulating adrenaline or noradrenaline levels (4, 22, 26). Several explanations for this poor correlation have been proposed, such as the simultaneous release of noradrenaline and of the vasodilator dopamine (20), variations in the inactivation of adrenaline and noradrenaline by conjugation (16), the down-regulation of α-adrenergic receptors (37), and, in some patients with PH, the concomitant tumoral release of neuropeptide Y and catecholamines (7).

In addition to the vascular effects of tumoral amines or neuropeptides, the increase in vascular resistance may also be linked to neurogenic or endocrine mechanisms not directly related to tumoral secretions. Bravo et al. (5) compared the effects of a single oral dose of 0.3 mg of clonidine, a centrally acting antihypertensive agent that inhibits neurally mediated catecholamine release, in 15 patients with essential hypertension and 15 with PH. Although clonidine produced significant and similar decreases in PB in both groups, plasma noradrenaline was sharply reduced in patients with essential hypertension but unchanged in patients with PH. The authors concluded that the "reduction in BP by clonidine must mean that biologically effective release of noradrenaline from the axon terminal is maintained in PH and could contribute to the hypertension. In addition, the demonstration that BP in PH was lowered despite persistently high levels of circulating catecholamines suggests that the noradrenaline released from axon terminals of sympathetic postganglionic neurons is biologically more significant than circulating catecholamines." This hypothesis was confirmed in an experimental model by Prokocimer et al. (30). They found that clonidine and chlorisondamine, a ganglionic blocker, markedly decreased BP without altering the plasma concentration of noradrenaline in rats harboring a transplanted PH, whereas both drugs had no effect on the BP of control rats made acutely hypertensive by an infusion of noradrenaline.

In addition to the tumoral production of catecholamines and the role of the central nervous system, the renin-angiotensin system may be involved in the hypertension of PH (27). We measured plasma renin activity and plasma catecholamines in 26 untreated patients with PH, 18 untreated patients with primary hypertension, and 10 normal volunteers. We found that, in PH, hypertension is accompanied by high renin levels and that renin release is stimulated in response to noradrenaline overflow: plasma renin activity was higher in the subjects with PH than in those with primary hypertension or in the volunteers and was closely correlated with noradrenaline levels in the subjects with PH but not in the subjects with primary hypertension or in the volunteers. In addition, the hypotension observed in response to β-blockade and captopril provided indirect support for the possibility that renin-dependent mechanisms are involved in the hypertension of PH (27). The cardioselective β-blocker acebutolol reduced heart rate, mean BP, and renin activity by averages of 20, 12, and 89%, respectively, in the 7 pheochromocytoma patients given this drug. The angiotensin converting enzyme inhibitor captopril decreased mean BP by 19% and raised renin activity by 293% in the 9 pheochromocytoma patients tested. The therapeutic relevance of these findings is discussed below.

PREOPERATIVE DIAGNOSIS AND EVALUATION

The techniques of biochemical diagnosis and tumor location in PH have been described in detail elsewhere (3, 4, 26, 28) and will be briefly summarized. Biochemical investigation for PH is usually confined to hypertensive patients reporting bouts of headaches, palpitations, and sweating (25), to those with severe hypertension resistant to treatment, and to those with MEN 2, phakomatosis, or familial PH. Positive diagnosis of PH is chiefly based on urinary metanephrine quantification, as this test is more sensitive than urinary catecholamine or vanillylmandelic acid quantification (23) or plasma catecholamines (26) or neuropeptide Y (29) determination. If the patient is hypertensive at the time of urinary collection for metanephrine quantification, pathological or normal excretion will confirm or refute, respectively, the diagnosis of PH. If the hypertension is paroxysmal and the metanephrines are measured during a period of normotension, pathological excretion will confirm the diagnosis, but normal excretion will not enable it to be refuted. In such cases, urinary catecholamines should be quantified during the hours following paroxysmal manifestations. It is not logical to quantify urinary metanephrines in these cases because catecholamine degradation to metanephrines is not significant in the shortened urine-collection period. With accurate urinary assays readily available, there is little need to subject patients to the hazards of provocative pharmacologic tests.

A clear biochemical diagnosis of PH is necessary before surgery. Paroxysmal vasomotor symptoms are reported by 5–10% of hypertensive patients (25). The frequency of incidentally discovered adrenal masses, mostly nonfunctional cortical adenomas, is 2–12% (32, 35) in hypertensive patients. These figures are tenfold higher than the actual prevalence of PH, and so surgery should not be considered solely on the basis of "suggestive" signs and symptoms associated wtih an adrenal mass.

The purpose of preoperative topographical exploration is to locate the PH, ascertain whether it is unique or multiple, adrenal or ectopic, benign or malignant, and isolated or present with other neoplasms in the context of MEN 2 or phakomatosis. A significant minority of cases have either multiple, ectopic, or malignant tumors or are associated with other diseases. Among the 120 consecutive cases of PH we have treated between 1976 and 1990, 20 harbored ectopic tumors, 18 were malignant, 11 were associated with phakomatosis and 9 with MEN 2, some patients combining several of these features. Computerized tomography and ^{131}I-MIBG scintigraphy have allowed dramatic diagnostic advances in the last 10 years (3, 28). We found that the combination of the two techniques yielded a sensitivity of 100% when the tumors were intraabdominal (28). When these imaging methods give negative or discordant results, the investigation should be completed by magnetic resonance imaging of the posterior mediastinum and retroperitoneal area and, if necessary, by cystoscopy and digitalized arteriography.

PREOPERATIVE MANAGEMENT

The specific objectives of preoperative treatment are hypertensive control, correction of hypovolemia, and prevention of arrhythmias (Fig. 56.1).

The control of the hypertension in PH requires α- and β-adrenergic antagonists. Since the vast majority of PH secrete predominantly the α-agonist noradrenaline (4, 22, 26), α-adrenergic antagonists are the cornerstone of hypertensive control. Noncompetitive α-blockers such as phenoxybenzamine or dibenamide bind covalently to α-receptors producing an irreversible blockade that lasts for several days. They are therefore useful for the prolonged antihypertensive treatment of malignant PH, where surgery is not feasible, but should be avoided preoperatively because they increase the risk of acute hypotension during tumor removal and the immediate postoperative period. Competitive pure α-blockers such as prazosine are more suitable. Since the first dose of prazosine may induce a sharp drop in BP, this agent should be increased progressively from 0.5 to 5 mg t.i.d. α-Adrenergic blockade generally gives rise to a tachycardia, secondary to catecholamine β-receptor stimulation. This requires the subsequent addition of a β-blocker (propranolol, 20–60 mg t.i.d.), or, alternatively, the use of a combined α- and β-receptor antagonist, such as labetalol (100–200 mg b.i.d.). Labetalol has been proposed as a firstline treatment in PH (31). However, the conventional combination of α-blockade with subsequent sep-

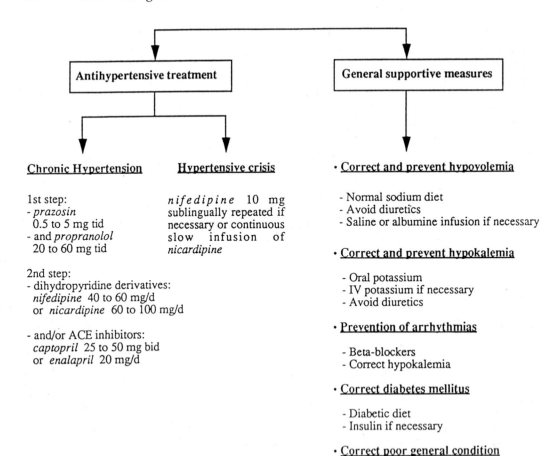

Figure 56.1. Preoperative management of pheochromocytoma. *ACE,* angiotensin-converting eyzyme.

arate β-blockade seems preferable because labetalol has predominantly β-blocking activity and may induce paradoxical rises in BP (9), at least if the tumor is predominantly adrenaline-secreting (24). When adrenergic blockade is insufficient, the antihypertensive therapy may be completed by a dihydropyridine (34) (extended release nifedipine, 20 mg b.i.d.) and/or, after correction of hypovolemia, a converting enzyme inhibitor (27) (captopril, 20 mg b.i.d.). Considering the variability of BP in PH, it may be useful to document the response to antihypertensive treatment with a 24-hr noninvasive ambulatory BP monitor. It must be noted that antihypertensive treatment aims at suppressing sustained hypertension but cannot prevent paroxysmal rises in BP. If these paroxysmal surges in BP are symptomatic, they should be treated (sublingual nifedipine, 10 mg,

or intravenous nicardipine). Antihypertensive therapy must be considered a short-term preparation for, and not an alternative to, surgery.

The hypovolemia associated with PH is a nonspecific consequence of the hypertension, a result of the pressure-diuresis regulation (3, 19). Correction of hypovolemia, therefore, relies on BP control per se, a normal sodium diet, and the avoidance of any diuretic agent. While Bravo and Gifford (3) recommend one or two whole-blood transfusions within 12–18 hr before surgery, we routinely measure total blood volume the day before surgery and infuse saline and albumin when necessary.

Prevention of arrhythmias is based on β-blockade (see above) and careful correction of hypokalemia. PH causes a state of marked secondary hyperaldosteronism, resulting in increased urinary potassium excretion (27). This involvement of the renin-aldosterone system can be partly suppressed by β-blockade and/or angiotensin converting enzyme inhibition (27). When necessary, this pharmacologic approach is completed by oral or intravenous potassium supplementation. Plasma potassium should be carefully monitored, including the day prior to surgery and at the beginning of the operation.

Similar to thyrotoxic patients, patients with PH are frequently in poor condition after months or years of a hypermetabolic state. They are therefore vulnerable to various nonspecific complications, such as infections. In addition to the specific treatments listed above, preoperative management should disclose any associated disease that might be acutely complicated by surgery, e.g., brainstem hemangioblastoma associated with Von Hippel-Lindau disease, which would expose to the risk of hemorrhagic stroke.

ANESTHESIA

Large variations in BP and cardiac rhythm may be expected during the anesthetic management of patients with PH, particularly during induction, intubation, peritoneal incision, and tumor handling and devascularization. The most critical phase is tumor devascularization, which, due to removal of circulating catecholamines, induces a simultaneous drop in BP and in cardiac contractility. Hemodynamic variations may be provoked by the anesthetic agents: whereas nitrous oxide, fentanyl, etomidate, enflurane, vecuronium, and their derivatives may be used safely, droperidol, atropine, suxamethonium, tubocurarine, pancuronium, and halothane may induce pressor or arrhythmic responses and should be avoided (14).

We currently use a combination of flunitrazepam, fentanyl and thiopental, and curarize with vecuronium. Radial artery pressure, pulmonary artery pressure through a Swan-Ganz catheter, and ECG are monitored continuously. Infusions of short-acting vasodilator (nitroprusside or nicardipine) or antiarrhythmic agents (lignocaine, amiodarone, esmolol) are pre-

pared in advance and begun as soon as necessary. Controlled ventilation is estabished, enabling a positive end-expiratory pressure to be performed if pulmonary wedge pressure rises. Volume replacement is determined by pulmonary wedge pressure levels.

SURGICAL MANAGEMENT

Although the vast majority of PH are found in the abdomen, the tumor(s) may be extraadrenal or multiple. Even if a tumor location is obvious preoperatively, a complete exploration of the abdomen is required, including the contralateral adrenal, the organ of Zuckerkandl, the urinary bladder, and the periaortic and pericaval lymphatic chains. The tumor approach, handling, devascularization, and excision must be performed step by step to limit BP and heart rate variations and to allow adequate hemostasis. Our currently preferred technique is as follows (in the usual case of an adrenal PH):

Abdominal incision. A xiphopubic incision is performed, followed by division of the round and falciform hepatic ligaments.

Peritumoral dissection. A thorough dissection enables the tumor to be kept separate from the aorta, the vena cava, and the kidney vessels. Great care is taken to avoid moving the tumor at this stage.

Tumor cleavage. Because the posterior aspect of the tumor is generally devoid of vessels, a gentle posterior digital cleavage is used to mobilize the tumor, draw its upper pole downward, and gain access to the upper pedicle, which is clamped immediately. Clamping is followed by a pause to monitor the hemodynamics. If a precipitous drop in BP ensues, temporary unclamping is necessary.

Tumor extirpation is then followed by careful hemostasis, exploration of the opposite adrenal and the other possible tumor sites, and a careful search for lymph node or visceral metastases.

POSTOPERATIVE PERIOD

Volume replacement may be gradually discontinued if hypovolemia has been adequately corrected preoperatively and blood loss has been adequately compensated. The use of competitive, short-acting antagonists permits a rapid waning of α- and β-blockade, and stable BP and heart rate are achieved within a few hours. Blood glucose must be monitored closely because hypoglycemia may occur as a consequence of rebound hypersecretion of insulin and reduction of glycogenolysis (14).

Biochemical evidence of the cure of the PH cannot be obtained immediately: a high-but-decreasing output of catecholamines and catecholamine metabolites remains during the first week following tumor resection (4). This output represents the emptying of extratumoral pools of catecholamines and should not be interpreted as reflecting incomplete cure. We routinely check the normalization of urinary metanephrine excretion 10 days after surgery. If metanephrine excretion is normalized, the patient is discharged and BP, glucose tolerance, and urinary hormones are controlled 6 months later. If the metanephrines remain high 10 days postoperatively, ^{131}I-MIBG scintigraphy is performed. This may show a persistence of fixation at the primary tumor site or disclose metastases whose ^{131}I-MIBG uptake was masked preoperatively by the primary tumor's higher metabolic activity.

LONG-TERM FOLLOW-UP

Any patient operated on for PH should have a detailed follow-up for 15 years (21) or more, the minimum annual workup in asymptomatic subjects comprising BP measurement, glycemia, and urinary metanephrines. The reason for this is that PH is a borderline tumor whose benign character cannot be definitely proven by any clinical, biochemical, or histopathological criteria (12, 21). Nevertheless, malignant PH tends to be more frequently ectopic (36) and to exhibit higher levels of plasma neuropeptide Y and neuron-specific enolase (11) than does benign PH. However, the only rigorous definition of malignancy is the occurrence of tumor cells at a site where chromaffin tissue is not otherwise present (12, 21, 33, 36). This criterion may be met either at the primary operation, or several months or years later at the time of recurrent signs and symp-toms of PH and/or the occurrence of symptomatic metastases.

Malignant PH is compatible with prolonged survival with symptom-free or tumor-free intervals varying from months to decades. Factors associated with a longer survival (12, 21) seem to be (a) early diagnosis and excision of the primary tumor; (b) adjunctive lymphadenectomy at the initial operation when one or more lymph nodes contain tumor; (c) close follow-up; and (d) whenever possible, aggressive excision of any recurrence or soft-tissue metastases. We have operated on some of our patients 5 times in 15 years with excellent remissions. When recurrences are small with an accessible vascular pedicle, surgical excision may be preceded, or replaced, by therapeutic embolization (38). In cases where soft-tissue or skeletal metastases are too widespread to make surgery or embolization feasible, several palliative therapies may be considered. Pharmacologic treatment aimed at the long-term blockade of catecholamine synthesis with α-methyl-p-tyrosine (6), or irreversible α-receptor blockade with phenoxybenzamine, may permit a good quality of life but does not affect tumor progression. Conventional radiotherapy may provide good palliation in cases of painful metastases (33). In situ radiotherapy with ^{131}I-MIBG and chemotherapy may provide clinical, hormonal, and sometimes tumoral improvement: a reduction of the number and/or the volume of metastases has been reported in 5/15 patients given ^{131}I-MIBG (15) and in 8/14 patients treated with a combination of cyclophosphamide, vincristine, and dacarbazine (2). Such therapies have been evaluated only in limited uncontrolled trials and their effect on survival is not known. They should, therefore, be considered only after the surgical excision of primary or recurrent tumors.

References

1. Anonymous. Phaeochromocytoma still surprises. Lancet 1990;335:1189–1190.
2. Averbuch SD, Steakley CS, Young RC, et al. Malignant pheochromocytoma: effective treatment with a combination of cyclophosphamide, vincristine and dacarbazine. Ann Intern Med 1988;109:267–273.

3. Bravo EL, Gifford RW. Pheochromocytoma: diagnosis, localization and management. N Engl J Med 1984;311:1298–1303.

4. Bravo EL, Tarazi RC, Gifford RW, Stewart BH. Circulating and urinary catecholamines in pheochromocytoma. Diagnostic and pathophysiologic implications. N Engl J Med 1979;301:682–686.

5. Bravo EL, Tarazi RC, Fouad F, Textor SC, Gifford R, Vidt DG. Blood pressure regulation in pheochromocytoma. Hypertension 1982;4(suppl II): 193–199.

6. Brogden RN, Heel RC, Speight TM, Avery GS. Alpha-methyl-p-tyrosine: a review of its pharmacology and clinical use. Drugs 1981;21:81–89.

7. Corder R, Shapiro B, Lowry PJ, et al. Relationship between tumour and plasma concentrations of neuropeptide Y in patients with adrenal medullary phaeochromocytoma. J Hypertens 1986; 4(suppl 6):S193–S195.

8. Engel A, Von Euler US. Diagnostic value of increased urinary output of noradrenaline and adrenaline in phaeochromocytoma. Lancet 1950;2:387.

9. Feek CM, Earnshaw PM. Hypertensive response to labetalol in phaeochromocytoma. Br Med J 1980;2:387.

10. Gagel RF, Tashjian AH, Cummings T, et al. The clinical outcome of prospective screening for multiple endocrine neoplasia type 2a. N Engl J Med 1988;318:478–484.

11. Grouzmann E, Gicquel C, Plouin PF, Schlumberger M, Comoy E, Bohuon C. Neuropeptide Y and neuron specific enolase levels in benign and malignant pheochromocytomas. Cancer 1990; 66:1833–1835.

12. Guo JZ, Gong LS, Chan SX, Luo BY, Xu MY. Malignant pheochromocytoma: diagnosis and treatment in fifteen cases. J Hypertens 1989;7:261–266.

13. Holton P. Noradrenaline in tumour of the adrenal medulla. J Physiol (Lond) 1949;108:525–529.

14. Hull CJ. Phaeochromocytoma: diagnosis, preoperative preparation and anaesthetic management. Br J Anaesth 1986;58:1453–1468.

15. Krempf M, Lumbroso J, Mornex R, et al. Use of ^{131}Im-Iodobenzyl-guanidine (^{131}I MIBG) in the treatment of malignant pheochromocytoma. J Clin Endocrinol Metab 1991;72:455–461.

16. Kuchel O, Buu NT, Fontaine A, et al. Free and conjugated plasma catecholamines in hypertensive patients with or without pheochromocytoma. Hypertension 1980;2:177–186.

17. Labbé M, Tinel J, Doumer A. Crises solaires et hypertension paroxystique en rapport avec une tumeur surrénale. Bull Soc Med Hop Paris 1922;46:982–990.

18. Lamiell JM, Salazar FG, Hsia YE. Von Hippel-Lindau disease affecting 43 members of a single kindred. Medicine 1989;68:1–29.

19. Levenson JA, Safar ME, London GM, Simon AC. Haemodynamics in patients with phaeochromocytoma. Clin Sci 1980;58:349–356.

20. Louis WJ, Doyle AE, Heath WC, Robinson MJ. Secretion of dopa in phaeochromocytoma. Br Med J 1972;4:325–327.

21. Mahoney EM, Harrison JH. Malignant pheochromocytoma: clinical course and treatment. J Urol 1877;118:225–229.

22. Manger WM. Plasma and tumor catecholamines and blood pressure in 38 patients with pheochromocytoma. In: Usdin E, Kopin IJ, Barchas J, (eds.) Catecholamines, basic and clinical frontiers. New York: Pergamon Press 1979:1476–1478.

23. Manu P, Runge LA. Biochemical screening for pheochromocytoma: superiority of urinary metanephrine measurements. Am J Epidemiol 1984;120:788–790.

24. Plouin PF, Ménard J, Corvol P. Norepinephrine producing phaeochromocytomas with absent pressor response to beta-blockade. Br Heart J 1979;3:359–361.

25. Plouin PF, Degoulet P, Tugayé A, Ducrocq MB, Ménard J. Dépistage du phéochromocytome: chez quels hypertendus? Etude sémiologique chez 2585 hypertendus dont 11 ayant un phéochromocytome. Nouv Presse Med 1981;10:869–872.

26. Plouin PF, Duclos JM, Ménard J, Comoy E, Bohuon C, Alexandre JM. Biochemical tests for diagnosis of phaeochromocytoma: urinary versus plasma determinations. Br Med J 1981;282:853–854.

27. Plouin PF, Chatellier G, Rougeot MA, Comoy E, Ménard J, Corvol P. Plasma renin activity in phaeochromocytoma: effects of beta-blockade and converting enzyme inhibition. J Hypertens 1988;6:579–785.

28. Plouin PF, Chatellier G, Rougeot, MA, et al. Recent developments in pheochromocytoma diagnosis and imaging. Adv Nephrol 1988;17:275–286.

29. Plouin PF, Chatellier G, Billaud E, Grouzmann E, Comoy E, Corvol P. Biochemical tests for phaeochromocytoma: diagnostic yield of the determination of urinary metanephrines, plasma catecholamines, and neuropeptide Y. In: Calmettes C, Giuliana JM, eds. Medullary cancer of thyroid. Paris, INSERM/ John Libbey Eurotext 1991;211:115–119.

30. Prokocimer PG, Maze M, Hoffman BB. Role of sympathetic nervous system in the maintenance of hypertension in rats harbouring pheochromocytoma. J Pharmacol Exp Ther 1987;241:870–874.

31. Réach G, Thibonnier M, Chevillard C, Corvol P, Milliez P. Effects of labetalol on blood pressure and plasma catecholamine concentrations in patients with phaeochromocytoma. Br Med J 1980;1:1300–1301.

32. Ross NS, Aron DC. Hormonal evaluation of the patient with an incidentally discovered adrenal mass. N Engl J Med 1990;323:1401–1405.

33. Scott HW, Reynolds V, Green N, et al. Clinical experience with malignant pheochromocytomas. Surg Gynecol Obstet 1982;154:801–818.

34. Serfas D, Shoback DM, Lorell BH. Phaeochromocytoma and hypertrophic cardiomyopathy: apparent suppression of symptoms and noradrenaline secretion by calcium-channel blockade. Lancet 1983;2:711–713.

35. Shamma AH, Goddard JW, Sommers SC. A study

of adrenal status in hypertension. J. Chronic Dis 1958;8:587–595.

36. Shapiro B, Sisson JC, Lloyd R, Nakajo M, Satterlee W, Beierwaltes WH. Malignant phaeochromocytoma: clinical, biochemical and scintigraphic characterization. Clin Endocrinol 1984;20:189–203.

37. Snavely MD, Mahan LC, O'Connor DT, Insel PA. Selective down-regulation of adrenergic receptor subtypes in tissues from rats with pheo-

chromocytoma. Endocrinology 1983;113:354–361.

38. Timmis JB, Brown MJ, Allison DJ. Therapeutic embolization of phaeochromocytoma. Br J Radiol 1981;54:420–422.

39. Tucker RM, Labarth DR. Frequency of surgical treatment for hypertension in adults at the Mayo Clinic from 1973–1975. Mayo Clin Proc 1977;52:549–555.

57

Abnormalities in Calcium Metabolism

Michel Paillard
Jean Paul Gardin
Pascale Borensztein
Pascal Houillier

HYPERCALCEMIA

Mechanisms of Hypercalcemia

Steady-state extracellular fluid (ECF) calcium concentration is normally controlled by movements of calcium that occur between plasma and bone, and plasma and kidney (see Refs. 47 and 52 for review) (Fig. 57.1). Usually calcium absorption from the gut affects ECF calcium only transiently. In a normal adult subject, the physiological circulating values of parathyroid hormone (PTH) and 1,25-dihydroxy-vitamin D_3 ($1,25-(OH)_2D_3$) (calcitriol) maintain plasma calcium to about 2.4 mmol/liter. These hormones are responsible for osteoclastic bone resorption of active bone surfaces, but because of the normal coupling of osteoblastic bone formation, net bone resorption is minimal, and bone mass and calcium balance remain essentially unchanged. Most important is the fact that these two hormones regulate the exchange system of calcium through bone lining cell membrane between quiescent bone surfaces and ECF, so that the set point for

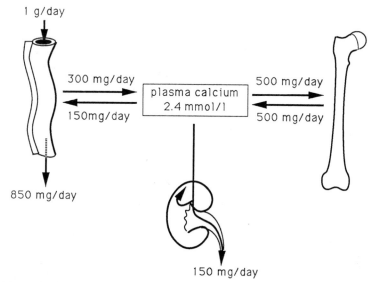

Figure 57.1. Normal adult in zero calcium balance. The *numbers* are estimates of the daily amount of calcium exchanged between the extracellular fluid and gut, kidney, and bone. The exchange system between bone fluid and the extracellular fluid is not taken into account.

calcium equilibrium between ECF and bone (i.e., no net flux of calcium) is about 2.4 mmol/liter. Note that in an aparathyroid patient the set point value for calcium equilibrium is about 1.2 mmol/liter. Finally, PTH and calcitriol regulate the calcium reabsorption in the distal nephron of the kidney, and the set point for calcium equilibrium between ECF and the kidney is also 2.4 mmol/liter.

Schematically, two situations may be responsible for persistent hypercalcemia (52). The first is a shift of the calcium set points for bone-ECF and kidney-ECF equilibrium to the same abnormally elevated value. In this event, minimal net flux of calcium from bone occurs in the new steady state as in a normal situation, and bone mass and calcium balance remain unaltered. The resultant stable hypercalcemia is called "equilibrium" hypercalcemia (52). An example is represented by primary hyperparathyroidism in its usual presentation (Fig. 57.2). The second situation is a disturbance of the bone remodeling system resulting in dramatically increased net bone resorption, decrease in bone mass, and negative calcium balance. This occurs when an increase in osteoclastic bone resorption is associated with an uncoupling of osteoblastic bone formation (i.e., bone formation not increased). In this situation, the permanent dramatic net influx of calcium into plasma from bone may exceed the capacity for the kidney to clear calcium, which results in a progressive hypercalcemia ("disequilibrium" hypercal-

cemia) (52). Indeed, in this situation, an ECF volume depletion frequently occurs, due to vomiting and renal loss of sodium by diminution of reabsorption of NaCl in the proximal tubule of the kidney. This ECF volume depletion progressively decreases the glomerular filtration rate and stimulates calcium reabsorption in the renal proximal tubule, which worsens hypercalcemia (52). An example of this disequilibrium hypercalcemia is malignancy (Fig. 57.3). Hypercalcemic states may be divided into three groups: primary hyperparathyroidism and related diseases (45%), malignancies (45%), and other causes (10%). Manifestations of hypercalcemia are listed in Table 57.1.

Primary Hyperparathyroidism and Related Diseases

Hypercalcemia in primary hyperparathyroidism (HPT) is usually moderate (serum

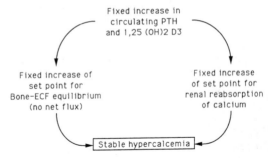

Figure 57.2. Example of equilibrium hypercalcemia in the usual presentation of primary hyperparathyroidism. *ECF*, extracellular fluid.

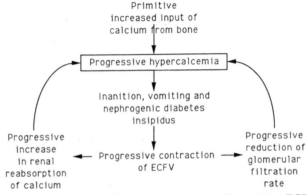

Figure 57.3. Example of disequilibrium hypercalcemia in malignancies. *ECFV*, extracellular fluid volume.

Table 57.1
Manifestations of Hypercalcemia

Gastrointestinal
  Anorexia
  Nausea
  Vomiting
  Pancreatitis
Neuromuscular
  Asthenia
  Depression
  Confusion
Cardiovascular
  Shortening of QT interval
  Increased toxicity of cardiac glycosides
  Arrhythmias
Renal
  Renal failure
  Salt wasting
  Nephrogenic diabetes insipidus
  K wasting
  Metabolic alkalosis
  Renal calculi and nephrocalcinosis
  Metabolic acidosis associated with nephro-
    calcinosis
Metastatic calcifications

calcium ~ 2.8–3 mmol/liter) and remains stable for many years (equilibrium hypercalcemia) (see Refs. 8, 32, 33, 51, and 64 for review). Circulating PTH(1–84) is usually abnormally increased, as well as nephrogenous cAMP. Renal reabsorption of phosphate is frequently decreased with hypophosphatemia due to PTH hypersecretion, while 24-hr calciuria is usually moderately increased due to elevated serum calcitriol, which enhances calcium absorption from the gut. Plasma acid-base status is usually normal, and metabolic acidosis occurs occasionally, when nephrocalcinosis (renal tubular acidosis), renal failure, or severe bone disease is present. Hypercalcemia in primary HPT results essentially from the combined effects of PTH and calcitriol on calcium fluxes from bone and kidney into the ECF volume. The increase in bone resorption is due to the activation of osteoclasts by PTH and calcitriol, but the secondary increase in bone formation attenuates the effect on net bone resorption. Finally, PTH hypersecretion increases the calcium reabsorption in the distal nephron. The relative contribution of calcium fluxes from bone, kidney, and gut is difficult to evaluate in primary HPT. The role of enhanced calcium gut absorption in hypercalcemia is probably small, since no correlation has been found between the circulating values of calcitriol and the degree of hypercalcemia (22). The role of net bone resorption is also probably limited (22) and hypercalcemia is not significantly improved by drugs inhibiting the osteoclastic activity, such as bisphosphonate (1). The main mechanisms responsible for hypercalcemia in primary HPT are probably the reset of the ECF-bone equilibrium to an abnormally high value (without continuing net loss of calcium from bone) together with an increase in renal reabsorption of calcium (equilibrium hypercalcemia). Indeed, it has been clearly shown that the degree of hypercalcemia is positively correlated with the magnitude of the renal tubular reabsorption of calcium in primary HPT (22). The increased secretion of PTH in primary HPT is explained by both a decreased sensitivity of parathyroid cells to calcium (referred to as an increase in set point for PTH secretion, i.e., an abnormal high value of plasma calcium is necessary to inhibit PTH secretion) and an increase in parathyroid cellular mass (hyperplasia) (23, 50). Moreover, primary hyperparathyroidism is present in the syndromes of multiple endocrine neoplasia (see Ref. 64 for review).

Two particular and rare presentations of primary HPT are hyperparathyroid bone disease (osteitis fibrosa cystica) and parathyroid crisis. The subacute severe bone disease presentation is associated with a very high degree of PTH hypersecretion probably related to a relative or absolute vitamin D deficiency (54, 55), important net bone resorption, and often progressive hypercalcemia mimicking that observed in malignancies (disequilibrium hypercalcemia). Parathyroid crisis is an urgent presentation of the disorder, with extreme hypercalcemia (150 mg/liter).

The syndrome of familial benign hypercalcemia also called familial hypocalciuria-hypercalcemia (FHH) is characterized by a stable asymptomatic moderate hypercalcemia (~ 2.8–3 mmol/liter) present from early childhood (see Ref. 34 for review). The pathophysiology of this syndrome is unknown. Plasma immunoreactive PTH, nephrogenous cAMP, maximum reabsorption rate of phosphate by unit of glomerular filtration rate (TmPi/GFR) are usually not different from those of normals. These parameters are, however, abnormal considering the degree of hypercalcemia, which should cause suppression of PTH secretion by normal parathyroid glands. The set point for PTH secretion in the syndrome is therefore abnormally high. Hypercalcemia is probably explained by an increase in set points for bone-ECF, and kidney-ECF equilibrium (equilibrium hypercalcemia). Daily urinary calcium excretion is usually normal in agreement with a normal value of serum calcitriol, which contrasts with primary HPT, where hypercalciuria is usually present. Fractional excretion of calcium $FE_{Ca^{2+}}$) is more discriminating, remaining usually less than 0.01 in FHH, in contrast with primary HPT, where fractional excretions of calcium is higher (34). A characteristic feature of FHH is an autosomal dominant inheritance pattern with complete penetrance, and hypercalcemia is present in half of the first degree relatives. Thus, FHH can be definitively diagnosed by measuring plasma calcium in family members.

Malignancies

Solid Tumors

The main determinant of hypercalcemia in patients with malignancies is a dramatic osteolysis (see Refs. 39 and 40 for review). This osteolysis may be due to circulating factors in the humoral hypercalcemia of malignancies or may be associated with widespread osteolytic bone metastases. Note that about half of patients with humoral hypercalcemia of malignancies (HHM) have localized bone metastases.

Humoral Hypercalcemia of Malignancies. The malignancies most frequently associated with HHM are the squamous cell carcinomas of the lung, head, and neck. Hypercalcemia is usually rapidly progressive in HHM (disequilibrum hypercalcemia). This syndrome is associated with a dramatically increased net bone resorption, appropriately decreased level of plasma PTH(1–84), increases in nephro-

genous cAMP and renal tubular reabsorption of calcium, decrease in renal tubular reabsorption of phosphate, low to normal serum calcitriol and calcium absorption from gut, and frequently multifactorial metabolic alkalosis (mostly due to vomiting and ECF contraction) (see Refs. 41 and 64 for review).

Progressive hypercalcemia results from a dramatic increase in net bone resorption responsible for a permanent net influx of calcium usually exceeding the capacity for the kidney to clear this increased input. Net bone resorption is accounted for by an abnormal uncoupling of bone resorption (which is stimulated) from bone formation (which is inhibited). The role of this abnormally elevated net bone resorption is demonstrated by the improvement of hypercalcemia by drugs inhibiting osteoclastic activity, such as bisphosphonate and plicamycin (26). In addition, the decreased capacity of the kidney to excrete calcium contributes to hypercalcemia. First, circulating PTH related peptide (PTHrp) stimulates renal reabsorption of calcium (40). Second, the frequently ECF volume depletion observed in these patients (due to vomiting and renal loss of sodium), decreases GFR and stimulates reabsorption of calcium in the renal proximal tubule, and worsens hypercalcemia (disequilibrium hypercalcemia) (26).

The circulating factors responsible for hypercalcemia are produced by the tumor itself or by host cells in response to the tumor (39–41). The identified factors are PTHrp, transforming growth factor-α(TGF-α), tumor necrosis factors (TNFs), colony stimulating factors (CSFs), and interleukin-1. Most patients have elevated circulating PTHrp. This factor has many of the biological effects of PTH. It stimulates cAMP production by the kidney, decreases renal reabsorption of phosphate, and increases net bone resorption, renal tubular calcium reabsorption, and renal 1α-hydroxylase activity. However, the presence of elevated circulating values of PTHrp does not account for all the manifestations of HHM. The very high degree of hypercalcemia may be due to the other circulating factors, which also increase bone resorption and possibly decrease bone formation. In addition, these factors could oppose the stimulating effect of PTHrp on calcitriol production, and explain the low to normal circulating values of calcitriol and calcium absorption from gut.

Osteolytic Metastases. Solid tumors that are widely metastatic to bone may be associated with hypercalcemia (see Refs. 39–41 and 64 for review). In this group, breast cancer is the most common cause. Hypercalcemia is essentially a consequence of primitively increased bone resorption, with a suppressed PTH(1–84) secretion. However, despite low circulating PTH activity, the capacity of the kidney to excrete calcium is often progressively reduced, probably because of ECF volume depletion, which lowers GFR and enhances renal calcium reabsorption (disequilibrium hypercalcemia) (26).

Two mechanisms have been identified. First, tumor cells may directly resorb bone, presumably by production of acid proteases, which would be responsible for removing mineral from bone and then causing resorption of bone matrix (17). Second, there is increasing evidence suggesting that osteoclast activity may be the major mechanism of bone resorption (6), which explains that drugs decreasing osteoclast activity, such as plicamycin or the combination of calcitonin and corticosteroids, improve hypercalcemia. This suggests a production of local osteoclast stimulating factors by tumor cells. Breast cancer cells have also been found to release TGF-α and prostaglandins, which all stimulate osteoclast activity. Breast cancer cells have been found recently to produce procathepsin D, which stimulates mature osteoclasts.

Hematologic Malignancies

Myelomas. Myeloma is one of the malignancies most frequently associated with hypercalcemia and suppressed PTH secretion (20–40% of patients develop hypercalcemia at some time during the course of their disease) (see Refs. 39, 40, and 42 for review). Hypercalcemia needs two conditions to occur: an increased net bone resorption and a reduction in glomerular filtration rate (GFR) (Bence Jones nephropathy, uric acid nephropathy, or amyloid).

A false hypercalcemia must be ruled out by measurement of plasma ionized calcium, since the abnormal plasma protein may bind calcium.

Bone resorption in myeloma is accounted for by an increase in osteoclast activity occurring adjacent to the collections of myeloma cells, while osteoblast activity is reduced. A bone resorbing activity has been found in culture media of lymphoid cell line derived from marrow myeloma cells. This osteoclast activating factor has been further identified as lymphotoxin (24). Other factors, such as interleukins, may be involved in the stimulation of osteoclast activity.

Lymphomas. Patients with T-cell, B-cell or histiocytic lymphomas may occasionally develop hypercalcemia with suppressed PTH secretion (39, 40, 42). In some cases, increased circulating levels of calcitriol have been found, and lymphoma cells have recently shown to convert 25-(OH)D_3 to calcitriol (38). In other cases, lymphomas have been shown to produce interleukins and PTHrp. Hypercalcemia has been occasionally reported in patients having Hodgkin's disease or acute or chronic leukemias.

Other Causes of Hypercalcemia

Thyrotoxicosis

About 10–20% of patients with thyrotoxicosis develop mild hypercalcemia (110 mg or 2.75 mmol/liter) at some time during the course of their disease (see Refs. 2, 45, and 64 for review). Frequencies of hypercalcemia as high as 50% have been reported using ionized plasma calcium determinations. Elevated thyroid hormones cause a marked increase in bone turnover with a predominant stimulation of osteoclast activity, which accounts for hypercalciuria. Moderate hyperphosphatemia is common, secondary to the stimulation of renal phosphate reabsorption by thyroid hormones. PTH secretion is suppressed, and the PTH-dependent renal reabsorption of calcium is thus decreased, explaining the frequently mild hypercalcemia. PTH-dependent production of calcitriol is also decreased, which lowers calcium absorption from gut. Hypercalcemia may be corrected by propranolol or the combination of calcitonin and glucocorticoids, before the antithyroid drugs become effective (up to 8 weeks).

Adrenal Insufficiency

Hypercalcemia has occasionally been described in patients with acute adrenal failure, and its mechanism is unknown (73). One possibility is an increase in sodium-dependent reabsorption of calcium in the renal proximal tubule, secondary to the dramatic ECF-volume contraction present in acute adrenal failure.

Pheochromocytomas

Hypercalcemia is an unusual but well-documented complication of pheochromocytomas (66). Most often, hypercalcemia is due to a coexistent primary hyperparathyroidism in a patient with multiple endocrine neoplasia type IIa. Occasionally, hypercalcemia appears to occur as a direct result of the pheochromocytoma, as evidenced by the prompt reversal of hypercalcemia following surgical excision of the adrenal tumor. The mechanism is unclear, and the possibility of the secretion by the tumor of bone-resorbing factors similar to those of HHM has been suggested.

Neoplasms of Vasoactive Intestinal Polypeptide-Secreting Cells ("VIP-OMA Syndromes")

Hypercalcemia has been reported in some patients having VIP-oma syndromes, with reversal of hypercalcemia after resection of the islet cell tumor suggesting the secretion of bone-resorbing factors by the tumor other than VIP (72).

Sarcoidosis and Other Granulomatous Diseases

More than 50% of patients with sarcoidosis have hypercalciuria, and about 10–15% develop hypercalcemia (see Refs. 37 and 61 for review). Circulating values of calcitriol are increased, while serum 25-(OH)D$_3$ remains normal, and serum PTH is suppressed (if elevated, concomitant primary HPT should be suspected). Calcitriol is produced extrarenally by granuloma tissue

and alveolar macrophages. Hypercalcemia is due, in part, to the increase in calcitriol-dependent calcium absorption from gut, and reduction of calcium intake may improve hypercalcemia. The lack of regulation of extrarenal production of calcitriol explains the increased sensitivity to vitamin D and exposure to sunlight. Calcitriol-dependent net bone resorption also contributes to hypercalcemia. When osteolytic bone lesions are present, the sarcoid granulomas may release directly or not bone-resorbing cytokines. Finally, hypercalcemia occurs mainly when an impaired renal function is present, such as sarcoidosis interstitial nephropathy. Hypercalcemia occurs occasionally in patients with other granulomatous diseases and tuberculosis.

Hypercalcemia may be reduced by limiting the calcium intake and exposure to sunlight. Hypercalcemia responds dramatically within a week to daily administration of 40 mg of prednisone, which limits calcium absorption from gut, probably interferes with production of calcitriol by granuloma tissue (serum calcitriol falls rapidly), and improves renal interstitial nephropathy.

Vitamin D Intoxication

Vitamin D intoxication occurs generally in patients treated with vitamin D derivatives for chronic renal failure, hypoparathyroidism, rickets, or osteomalacia (see Refs. 14 and 35 for review). These patients often take more than 50,000 units of vitamin D/day, although they vary considerably in their tolerance to the drug. Hypercalcemia may be severe. Circulating 25-(OH)D$_3$ may be increased by a factor by 20 for several weeks once vitamin D is discontinued, while calcitriol remains normal or moderately increased. With the new vitamin D derivatives of shorter half-lives, such as 1α-hydroxyvitamin D or Rocaltrol, toxicity is of shorter duration, and serum calcitriol is proportionally increased.

Hypercalcemia is associated with suppressed PTH secretion, hyperphosphatemia, and nephrocalcinosis or metastatic calcifications in the kidneys responsible for impairment in GFR. Hypercalcemia is due to the combined effects of enhanced calcium absorption from gut and net bone resorption. The renal impairment, which reduces the ability for kidney to excrete calcium, contributes to the severity of hypercalcemia.

After withdrawal of vitamin D derivatives, the duration of hypercalcemia depends on the half life of the compound. When hypercalcemia is severe, glucocorticoids are rapidly effective. In addition to their effects limiting calcium absorption from gut and bone resorption, glucocorticoids may impair the conversion of vitamin D to its active metabolites.

Vitamin A Intoxication

Vitamin A intoxication is a rare cause of hypercalcemia (48). Patients who ingest vitamin A excessively are usually food faddists who take megavitamin preparations, or who are treated inadvertently with vitamin A in excessive amounts. Vitamin A stimulates osteoclastic bone resorption. The receptors for retinoids belong to the family that includes the receptors of the steroid hormones, thyroid hormones, and calcitriol. Vitamin A withdrawal and glucocorticoids are rapidly effective.

Milk Alkali Syndrome

Hypercalcemia, which may be severe, sometimes occurs in patients taking absorbable antacids such as calcium carbonate in excessive amounts (more than 4 g of elemental calcium/day) (see Ref. 49 for review). The resulting increase in calcium absorbed from the gut may cause hypercalcemia when there is an impairment of renal handling of calcium: first, these patients have a metabolic alkalosis, which stimulates per se renal tubular calcium reabsorption; second, a nephrocalcinosis may occur, which decreases GFR. Discontinuing the ingestion of calcium and alkali is generally effective.

Thiazide Diuretics

Thiazide diuretics are well known to aggravate hypercalcemia in patients with primary HPT, and they have been suggested as a provocative diagnosis test. In fact, thiazides may induce hypercalcemia in patients with high bone turnover, such as patients with hypoparathyroidism treated with high doses of vitamin D derivatives. This suggests that effects of PTH and vitamin D metabolites on bone and kidney are enhanced by thiazides. In a normal subjects, thiazide diuretics occasionally induce a borderline ionized plasma calcium concentration (a discrete hypercalcemia may also be due to hyperproteinemia by hemoconcentration) (69). Thiazide diuretics may increase serum calcium by stimulating renal tubular reabsorption. They enhance the sodium-dependent calcium reabsorption in proximal tubules, secondary to ECF volume contraction, and more directly the calcium reabsorption in the distal tubule.

Lithium Therapy

Lithium therapy has been reported to cause hypercalcemia (20). The responsibility of lithium is not clearly established since primary hyperparathyroidism has been found in some of these patients.

Immobilization

Most patients who are completely immobilized have hypercalciuria, and 10% develop usually mild hypercalcemia (see Ref. 65 for review). Hypercalcemia, which is principally due to net bone resorption, occurs most commonly in patients with underlying high rates of bone turnover, i.e., adolescent boys, particularly those suffering spinal cord injuries, or adult patients with Paget's disease, thyrotoxicosis, primary HPT, and cancers.

Hypercalcemia associated with immobilization is due to increased bone resorption relative to bone formation, with resulting osteopenia. The uncoupling between bone formation and resorption could be due to the lack of mechanical loading. Circulating PTH(1–84) is suppressed (as nephrogenous cAMP), which reduces renal reabsorption of calcium, and limits the importance of hypercalcemia. Hypercalcemia together with urinary tract infections are responsible for recurrent renal calculi. In some patients, a reduction in GFR may explain severe hypercalcemia.

Hypercalcemia should be treated with agents that inhibit osteoclastic bone resorption (calcitonin and glucocorticoids, bisphosphonates). Vigorous fluid treatment is required to limit urinary tract infections and renal calculi. Hypercalcemia responds rapidly to effective mobilization of the patient.

Renal Failure

Hypercalcemia occasionally occurs in acute renal failure, during the polyuric phase and probably only in association with acute rhabdomyolysis. The mechanism is not known. It has been suggested that, as serum phosphorus falls during the polyuric phase of acute renal failure, calcium and phosphate salts that have been deposited in soft tissue may be liberated, causing a transient hypercalcemia. Moreover, an inappropriate calcitriol synthesis has been suggested but not confirmed.

The majority of patients with chronic renal failure have a decrease in plasma calcium. However, 10–20% of patients develop hypercalcemia (see Ref. 12 for review). Several mechanisms may explain the occurrence of hypercalcemia in patients before renal transplantation. In some patients, hypercalcemia is due to excessive administration of vitamin D derivatives and calcium supplements. In other patients, hypercalcemia has been attributed to the "tertiary hyperparathyroidism." In fact, hypercalcemia may occur during secondary hyperparathyroidism of renal failure (instead of the common hypocalcemia) when the target tissues of PTH become more sensitive to PTH, such as therapeutic reduction of plasma phosphate or administration of vitamin D metabolites, for example. A third cause of hypercalcemia is aluminum intoxication. Some patients with chronic renal failure have a state of low bone turnover (called "aplastic osteomalacia") and increased content of aluminum in the skeleton. The mechanism of hypercalcemia in patients taking normal supplements of calcium or vitamin D derivatives may be related to an impaired uptake of calcium into the skeleton.

Following renal transplantation, a period of hypercalcemia frequently occurs, which is usually mild and does not last for more than 1 year. This period of hyper-calcemia is caused by hyperparathyroidism occurring as a consequence of the slow involution of hyperplastic parathyroid glands.

Total Parenteral Nutrition

Some patients receiving total parenteral nutrition (TPN) may develop hypercalcemia and hypercalciuria, which resolve 1–2 months after discontinuing TPN (60). Bone contains considerable quantity of aluminum, which presumably enters the body via the protein source casein, which is present in the infusate. This syndrome is similar to that seen in uremic patients with low turnover osteomalacia due to aluminum.

Idiopathic Hypercalcemia of Infancy

This term has been given to hypercalcemia occurring during the first year of life. It includes hypercalcemia occurring in Williams syndrome. In this syndrome, hypercalcemia may be due to an abnormality in vitamin D metabolism. Indeed an increased sensitivity to vitamin D when administered orally, together with accumulation of calcitriol in the plasma, have been reported (21). Renal insufficiency is frequent. Hypercalcemia responds to glucocorticoids and to suppression of vitamin D supplements.

Serum Protein Abnormalities

False hypercalcemia may result from hyperalbuminemia, as in patients with a severe dehydration, with an attendant increase in albumin-bound calcium and thus total serum calcium concentration. The ionized serum calcium is either normal or slightly increased, and in the latter case an underlying disorder of calcium must be invoked. False hypercalcemia must reverse with rehydration. An increase in total serum calcium concentration, with normal ionized serum calcium, has been reported in occasional patients with multiple myeloma due to calcium binding by the myeloma protein (36).

The disorders associated with hypercalcemia are summarized in Table 57.2.

Table 57.2
Disorders Associated with Hypercalcemia

Primary hyperparathyroidism and related
   diseases
   Sporadic
   Familial endocrine neoplasia and familial
     hypocalciuric hypercalcemia
Tertiary hyperparathyroidism
   Chronic renal failure
Malignancy-associated hypercalcemia
   Humoral hypercalcemia of malignancy
   Local osteolytic hypercalcemia
   Myeloma-associated hypercalcemia
   Lymphoma-associated hypercalcemia
Endocrinopathies
   Thyrotoxicosis
   Adrenal insufficiency
   Pheochromocytoma
   VIP-oma syndrome
Medications
   Vitamins A and D
   Milk-alkali syndrome
   Thiazide diuretics
   Lithium
Sarcoidosis and other granulomatous diseases
Miscellaneous conditions
   Immobilization
   Acute and chronic renal failure
   Total parenteral nutrition
   Idiopathic hypercalcemia of infancy
   Serum protein abnormalities

Treatment of Hypercalcemia

The serum calcium can be adequately lowered in the great majority of patients with hypercalcemia due to malignancy or to any other cause. Indication for active treatment of hypercalcemia depends upon several factors. All patients who are symptomatic or have a plasma calcium greater than 130 mg/liter (or 3.25 mmol/liter) require immediate and active therapy. Patients who are asymptomatic or have a plasma calcium less than 3.25 mmol/liter, and stable, should not require immediate antihypercalcemic therapy. However patients with malignancies should be treated even if calcemia is less than 3.25 mmol/liter since hypercalcemia is rapidly progressive (disequilibrium hypercalcemia). The therapy for hypercalcemia should be individualized after careful considerations of a number of issues. These issues include the

cause of hypercalcemia, the specific contraindications to particular form of therapy (renal failure), the underlying objective of therapy, and the pathogenetic mechanism responsible for hypercalcemia, i.e., increased bone resorption, increased calcium absorption from gut, and increased renal tubular calcium reabsorption. The specific treatment of the disease responsible for hypercalcemia is not considered here.

Calciuretic Measures

Patients with symptomatic hypercalcemia are usually dehydrated and should be vigorously rehydrated (26, 27). Indeed, these patients are dehydrated because of vomiting, inanition, and hypercalcemia-induced defect in urinary concentrating ability. Dehydration decreases GFR and enhances the sodium-dependent calcium reabsorption in the renal proximal tubule, which aggravates hypercalcemia. The amount of NaCl required to normalize ECF volume varies from 200–300 mmol/day per os to more than 6 liters of isotonic NaCl solution/day intravenously. Rehydration alone may reduce plasma calcium by 20 mg/liter or 0.5 mmol/liter.

The combination of i.v. infusion of isotonic NaCl solutions and intravenous doses of a calciuretic loop diuretic (furosemide) has been frequently used in the past when hypercalcemia is symptomatic or higher than 3.25 mmol/liter (70). The initial rate of saline infusion is determined by the degree of dehydration and the cardiovascular status of the patient, but is usually in the range of 200–300 ml/hr. The initial doses of furosemide are 80 mg every 2 hr, with a reduction in dosage and spacing of doses to every 4 hr as plasma calcium begins to decrease. The use of large doses of furosemide is not a convenient form of therapy and requires the facilities of an intensive case unit and careful monitoring of fluid and electrolytes losses. The major place of loop diuretics in the treatment of hypercalcemia is in patients who require fluid therapy but have been overhydrated or have cardiac failure, with a careful monitoring of the central venous pressure.

Medications that Inhibit Bone Resorption

Bisphosphonates

The bisphosphonates are a family of synthetic compounds that are stable analogs of pyrophosphate (see Refs. 43 and 64 for review). These drugs, which have been initially shown to inhibit mineralization, are potent inhibitors of osteoclastic bone resorption, but the mechanism of the latter effect is not known. They may prevent mature osteoclasts to resorb bone, or inhibit the proliferation of osteoclast precursors. Three compounds are available: etidronate, clodronate, and pamidronate. These compounds are poorly absorbed by the gut (less than 10%) and are more effective intravenously. Plasma calcium is returned toward normal range between 3 and 7 days. Etidronate may be used in doses of 5–10 mg/kg body weight/day orally, but is more often given intravenously in doses of 7.5 mg/kg body weight/day for 3–7 days, followed by oral therapy (46). Clodronate may be used orally in doses of 0.8–3.2 g/day, but is also more often used intravenously in doses of either single infusion of 600 mg or 100–300 mg/day for periods of between 3 and 10 days (10, 28, 62). Pamidronate is usually given intravenously, 15–90 mg/day, either in single dose or daily for 2–3 days, rather than orally, because the orally administered drug is often associated with mouth ulceration (5, 46, 71). This latter compound is very effective, normalizing plasma calcium in 90% of patients with osteolysis within 3 weeks. Treatment with bisphosphonate should be monitored by following plasma calcium and fasting urinary calcium/creatinine ratios, which reflects net bone resorption. Bisphosphonates are relatively safe therapy for hypercalcemia. The short durations for treatment and the doses used do not appreciably impair mineralization. Pamidronate administration may be associated with transient fever and lymphopenia.

Plicamycin (or Mithramycin)

Plicamycin is a cytotoxic agent which inhibits DNA-dependent RNA synthesis. It probably inhibits the formation of new osteoclasts by impairment of replication and thus depletes the pool of cells available to respond to osteoclast-stimulating agents (see Refs. 43, 46, and 64 for review). A unique dose of 20 μg/kg body weight is recommended, administered intravenously over 4 hr. The maximum effect occurs between 24 and 36 hr after administration of the drug, which is effective in 80% of patients with hypercalcemia in malignancies. A possible rebound effect is possible. Plicamycin has considerable toxicity, which requires a careful monitoring: liver cytolysis, renal failure, and bleeding with or without thromobocytopenia. This major drug in hypercalcemia in malignancies should not be used in patients with impaired renal function.

Calcitonin

Calcitonin inhibits rapidly (in a few hours) osteoclastic bone resorption, but this effect does not persist for more than 24–48 hr (escape phenomenon). The effects are more prolonged when calcitonin is used with corticosteroids (4). Salmon calcitonin is most often used, in doses of 50–200 MRC (Medical Research Council) units intramuscularly or subcutaneously every 12 hr. With these high doses, an inhibition of renal tubular calcium reabsorption is initially observed, which contributes to the hypocalcemic effect of the drug. (Human calcitonin is also now available.) About half of hypercalcemias are responsive to calcitonin. The drug has little toxicity and occasionally causes skin rashes and allergic reactions or nausea and vomiting. Intranasal or intrarectal preparations will be available soon for ambulant patients.

Glucocorticoids

Glucocortacoids are particularly effective in inhibiting bone resorbing activity in hematologic malignancies (myeloma) at least in part by their antitumor effects (4, 43). They are also effective in diseases with abnormal vitamin D metabolism (lymphoma, granulomatous diseases, and vitamin D and A intoxications) (43). The short-term toxicity of glucocorticoids is low, but they are effective in only 30% of resorptive hypercalcemic states.

Anticancer Drugs

Cytotoxic agents other than plicamycin, have been recently proposed, such as gallium nitrate and cisplatin, but the use of these drugs is limited by their nephrotoxicity (31, 74). WR2721 is an organic trisphosphate compound, originally used as an anticancer agent. It inhibits PTH secretion, renal tubular calcium reabsorption, and osteoclastic bone resorption (25). It has been used to lower serum calcium in parathyroid carcinoma and malignant hypercalcemia and has little toxicity (nausea, vomiting, somnolence, and sneezing). The role of these drugs is not yet established.

Medications used for the treatment of hypercalcemia are summarized in Table 57.3.

Urgent Therapy

Urgent therapy for hypercalcemia is required when patients are symptomatic or have a serum calcium of >3.25 mmol/liter (see Ref. 43 and 64 for review). A vigorous rehydration is always urgently required (at least 6 liters of isotonic NaCl solution/day intravenously), together with calcitonin alone or in combination with glucocorticoids (100 mg of cortisol hemisuccinate every 6 hr). This initial therapy often lowers serum calcium by 0.75 mmol/liter within 24 hr, and the rehydration corrects the reversible impairment in glomerular filtration. Therapy using bisphosphonates may be started when patients are well hydrated and serum creatinine is <200 μmol/liter. In patients who respond to bisphosphonates, urinary calcium/creatinine ratios decrease while hypercalcemia improves. In patients whose hypercalcemia does not improve clearly and fasting calcium/creatinine ratios remain increased, indicating uncontrolled osteolysis, higher doses of bisphosphonates or plicamycin should be given. Finally, in patients whose hypercalcemia does not improve sufficiently while fasting calcium/creatinine ratios decrease, the pathogenetic mechanism for persistent hypercalcemia is the increased renal reabsorption of calcium. In this case, furosemide may be used only after having carefully checked that patients are well hydrated.

Maintenance Therapy

Nonurgent therapy is discussed for patients who are asymptomatic and have a serum calcium lower than 3.25 mmol/liter

Table 57.3
Medications Used in the Treatment of Hypercalcemia with Net Bone Resorption

Compound	Parenteral Therapy	Oral Therapy
Isotonic saline	6 liters/day (i.v.)	300 mmol NaCl/day
Etidronate	7.5 mg/kg BW/day in 500 ml over 2 hr for 3–7 days (i.v.)[a]	5–10 mg/kg BW/ day
Clodronate	300 mg/day in 500 ml for 3–10 days or single dose of 600 mg in 500 ml over 2–8 hr (i.v.)	0.8–3.2 g/day
Pamidronate	30 mg/day in 500 ml over 4 hr for 2–3 days or single dose of 30 mg in 300 ml over 4 hr (i.v.)	
Calcitonin	50–200 MRC every 12 hr (i.m. or s.c.)	
Glucocorticoids	100 mg of cortisol hemisuccinate every 6 hr (i.v.)	40–80 mg/day
Mithramycin	20 μg/kg BW over 4 hr (i.v.)	
Furosemide[b]	80 mg every 2 hr (i.v.)	

[a]BW, body weight.
[b]May be indicated only in patients overhydrated or with cardiac failure.

(see Refs. 43 and 64 for review). This therapy is always required for patients with malignancies, since hypercalcemia is progressive (disequilibrium hypercalcemia).

A daily intake of 200–300 mmol of NaCl and 3 liters of fluid is necessary to avoid progressive dehydration. Bisphosphonates or a combination of glucocorticoids and calcitonin should be used when net bone resorption is the main mechanism for hypercalcemia. Glucocorticoids are particularly indicated for hematologic malignancies, granulomatous diseases and vitamin D and vitamin A intoxications.

Restriction of oral intake of calcium to 400 mg of elemental calcium (suppression of dairy products) is indicated for the milk alkali syndrome, sarcoidosis, and vitamin D intoxication since increased absorption of calcium from gut is thought to contribute to hypercalcemia. Propranolol may be used initially for hypercalcemia of thyrotoxicosis. In primary HPT, patients who are asymptomatic (more than 50%) and have a serum calcium less then 3.25 mM do not need anticalcemic therapy before cervical surgery. In addition, a large prospective study from the Mayo Clinic has indicated that more than 50% of patients with mild primary HPT (plasma calcium lower than 2.87 mmol/liter) remained asymptomatic with a stable hypercalcemia (59). Thus, the decision not to treat these patients by surgery may be particularly justified in elderly patients or after an unsuccessful previous surgical treatment. Chronic medical therapy including oral phosphate, bisphosphonates, and sex steroids (estrogens) has been proposed. However, the effectiveness and harmlessness of these drugs is not well documented, and a periodic evaluation without medical treatment may be justified.

HYPOCALCEMIA

Mechanisms of Hypocalcemia

As outlined previously in this chapter, steady-state ECF calcium concentration is essentially controlled by movements of calcium occurring between plasma and bone, and plasma and the kidney. When dietary calcium is restricted in a normal subject, the increased PTH secretion leads

Table 57.4
Clinical Manifestations of Hypocalcemia

Neuromuscular
  Paresthesias
  Tetany
  Seizures
  Dementia
  Movement disorders
  Papilledema
  Anxiety, depression, psychosis
  Myopathy in vitamin D deficiency
Cardiovascular
  Hypotension
  Arrhythmias
  Heart failure
Miscellaneous
  Dry skin
  Hair loss
  Brittle nails, moniliasis
  Cataracts
  Steatorrhea

to net fluxes of calcium from bone to ECF and increased renal tubular reabsorption of calcium, so that plasma calcium is maintained in the normal range.

Persistent hypercalcemia can occur only as a result of either primitive decrease in PTH secretion (primitive hypoparathyroidism) or resistance of target tissues to PTH effects, i.e., pseudohypoparathyroidism or vitamin D metabolites deficiency. Indeed, the presence of calcitriol is necessary for PTH to have full effects on bone and kidney (30).

Manifestations of hypocalcemia are listed in Table 57.4.

Hypoparathyroidism and Pseudohypoparathyroidism

Hypoparathyroidism

Hypoparathyroidism, which is uncommon, results from an impaired synthesis and secretion of PTH (see Refs. 7, 53, and 64 for review). Serum calcium is usually less than 2 mmol/liter and may decrease to a value as low as 1.2 mmol/liter in aparathyroid patients. Circulating PTH(1–84) (as well as nephrogenous cAMP) varies from undetectable to slightly decreased, i.e., always inappropriate to hypocalcemia. Renal reabsorption of phosphate is increased with hyperphosphatemia (usual plasma phosphate about 2 mmol/liter). Serum calcitriol is decreased despite hypocalcemia, since the reduced PTH secretion and hyperphosphatemia inhibit the renal 1α-hydroxylase. Consequently, the calcium absorption from gut is decreased and 24-hr calciuria is reduced, although moderately (about 1–2 mmol). Hypocalcemia is accounted for by a reset to low values of bone-ECF equilibrium and a decrease in renal reabsorption of calcium. PTH-dependent bone turnover is decreased, but the coupling between osteoclastic bone resorption and osteoblastic bone formation remains unaltered, so that the fasting calciuria is low-normal, and bone mass usually unchanged. When acutely challenged by an exogenous PTH administration, PTH-dependent adenylate cyclase in kidney is stimulated, as shown by a marked increase in nephrogenous cAMP and phosphaturic response. Hypoparathyroidism may be postoperative, idiopathic, or acquired.

Pseudohypoparathyroidism

Pseudohypoparathyroidism is characterized by the resistance of the target tissues (bone and kidney) to the action of PTH (see Refs. 16 and 64 for review). Hypocalcemia is thus associated with an appropriately increased circulating PTH(1–84). The other biological abnormalities are similar to those observed in hypoparathyroidism. Many patients have a number of somatic abnormalities, which are referred to as the phenotype of Albright's hereditary osteodystrophy.

Most patients, when acutely challenged by exogenous PTH administration, have a subnormal increment in nephrogenous cAMP and subnormal phosphaturic response. In some patients (pseudohypoparathyroidism type 2), a normal cAMP response is observed, while the phosphaturic response remains subnormal. Note that patients with absolute vitamin D deficiency may exhibit the same biological abnormalities, probably explained by a complete resistance of target tissues to PTH, which reversed after correction of vitamin D deficiency (68).

Severe Magnesium Deficiency

Severe chronic hypomagnesemia (<0.5 mmol/liter) may be responsible for hypocalcemia, which can be corrected only when magnesium supplements are given (see Ref. 58 for review). Two mechanisms may explain hypocalcemia. Indeed, severe hypomagnesemia has been shown to decrease PTH secretion and impair the PTH and vitamin D responsiveness of bone and kidney.

Neonatal Hypocalcemia

A moderate hypocalcemia may occur in the first week of postnatal life in premature children (64). The mechanisms are not clear and may be related to low serum PTH and high serum calcitonin, secondary to high plasma calcium during fetal life (due to an active placental transfer of calcium from the mother to the fetus). A more severe hypocalcemia may occur after the first week of life in infants born to mothers with primary HPT, probably related to transient suppression of PTH secretion in the infant (64).

The diseases associated with hypoparathyroidism or pseudohypoparathyroidism are listed in Table 57.5.

Table 57.5
Hypoparathyroidism and Pseudohypoparathyroidism

Postoperative hypocalcemia and hypoparathyroidism
Idiopathic hypoparathyroidism
  Isolated
  Associated with atrophic polyendocrine failure
Other acquired forms of functional hypoparathyroidism
  Nonsurgical parathyroid damage
  Parathyroid infiltration
  Hypomagnesemia
Pseudohypoparathyroidism
Neonatal hypocalcemic syndromes
  Early and late neonatal hypocalcemia
  Secondary hypoparathyroidism
  DiGeorge's syndrome and idiopathic hypoparathyroidism

Nonparathyroid Hypocalcemia

Vitamin D Deficiency

In moderate vitamin D deficiency 24-hr hypocalciuria is present, but the secondary hypersecretion of PTH allows plasma calcium to be maintained near normal values. In more severe vitamin D deficiency, hypocalcemia appears, since in addition to the decreased calcitriol-dependent absorption of calcium from gut, there is a bone resistance to PTH and an incomplete increase in renal reabsorption of calcium (see Ref. 19 for review). Indeed, severe deficiency in calcitriol has been shown to impair the action of PTH on bone and kidney. The 24-hr calciuria is dramatically reduced, because of both decrease in calcium absorption from gut and bone resistance to PTH. Hypophosphatemia is usually present, due to both impaired absorption of phosphate from gut due to calcitriol deficiency and decreased renal reabsorption of phosphate due to secondary HPT. Circulating $25\text{-}(OH)D_3$ is dramatically decreased in vitamin D deficiency and near normal in the rare syndrome of vitamin D-dependent rickets or osteomalacia. In a few patients with severe vitamin D deficiency, features similar to pseudohypoparathyroidism type 2 may be observed, which disappear after correction of vitamin D deficiency.

Chronic Renal Failure (CRF)

A moderate hypocalcemia (serum calcium about 1.8 mmol/liter) may be observed in 50% of patients with CRF (see Refs. 13 and 63 for review). In severe CRF, hyperphosphatemia may contribute to hypocalcemia by precipitation of calcium salts. In moderate CRF, other mechanisms must be invoked to explain hypocalcemia. The decrease in renal production of calcitriol (due to reduced renal mass and phosphate retention) reduces calcium absorption from the gut, which explains, at least in part, 24-hr hypocalciuria. This decrement in calcium entry into ECF may be a factor of hypocalcemia, which is, however, offset by low GRF value, which reduces the capacity of the kidney to excrete calcium. In fact, as outlined above, a resistance of tar-

get tissues to PTH must be present for hypocalcemia to occur. The resistance to PTH effect on bone may be due, at least in part, to phosphate retention and calcitriol deficiency, since phosphate restriction and calcitriol administration limit this resistance. The mechanism of the resistance to PTH effect on renal reabsorption of calcium is also not clear, and metabolic acidosis, which is known to reduce per se renal calcium reabsorption and to impair PTH-dependent cAMP production by renal cells may play a role.

Other Hypocalcemic Conditions

Rapid or excessive skeletal mineralization may lead to transient hypocalcemia, with secondary hyperparathyroidism (64). Severe hypocalcemia may be observed in the hungry bone syndrome, which occurs during healing of osteitis fibrosa following surgical treatment of primary HPT, of hyperthyroid bone disease, and of vitamin D deficiency with rickets or osteomalacia. Moderate hypocalcemia may also be observed in osteoblastic skeletal metastasis of prostate or breast cancer (57).

A rapid hyperphosphatemia due to parenteral, oral, or rectal (enema) phosphorus administration, particularly in patients with renal failure, leads to hypocalcemia by precipitation of calcium salts in tissues and bone. Similarly, the release of endogenous intracellular phosphorus may lead to severe hyperphosphatemia and hypocalcemia in patients with extensive "crush injuries" and patients with leukemia and lymphoma following successful chemotherapy (9).

Hypocalcemia may be observed in patients with acute pancreatitis (67). Hypocalcemia correlates with severe pancreatitis and is a poor prognostic sign. Proposed mechanisms of hypocalcemia include incorporation of calcium into intra- and retroperitoneal free fatty acid complexes, associated hypomagnesemia, and hypoparathyroidism due to the destruction of PTH by circulating proteases.

Hypocalcemia may be observed in the toxic-shock syndrome, described in young women who use tampons during menstruation (11). Hypocalcemia may be related to acute renal failure. Alternatively, toxin produced by bacteria could induce mediators leading to hypocalcemia.

The rapid infusion of citrated whole blood chelates calcium and lowers serum ionized calcium concentration. Since citrate is metabolized by the liver, patients with hepatic dysfunction are particularly prone to accumulate citrate and experience reduction in ionized plasma calcium (64).

Acute fluoride intoxication is associated with marked hypocalcemia due to the formation of an insoluble precipitate with calcium (64).

Hypocalcemia may be observed following administration of mithramycin and also large doses of bisphosphonates or calcitonin in patients with increased bone turn over (Paget's disease).

Treatment of Hypocalcemia

Acute Hypocalcemia

The goal is to prevent or suppress the complications of hypocalcemia. Acute symptomatic hypocalcemia (frank tetany, seizures, or congestive heart failure) requires immediate correction by intravenous calcium therapy (see Refs. 44 and 64 for review). Initial treatment consists of intravenous administration of approximately 200–300 mg of elemental calcium (available solutions include calcium chloride, calcium gluconate, and calcium gluceptate). Concentrated calcium solutions are irritating to veins and may cause extensive inflammation if they extravasate into soft tissues, and so it is preferable to dilute the calcium solutions into 50 or 100 ml of dextrose and administer the dose over 15 min by a secure intravenous route. Calcium should be administered very cautiously in patients receiving digitalis, since hypercalcemia predisposes to digitalis intoxication and arrhythmias. Persistent recurrent severe symptomatic hypocalcemia may be treated with repeated doses at 6–8-hr intervals or by continuous infusion of a dilute calcium solution, the exact dosage being determined by serial measurements of serum calcium.

Acute hypocalcemia in the range of 2 mmol/liter (or 80 mg/liter) with or without mild neuromuscular symptoms can usually be managed with oral calcium supplements alone (1–2 g of elemental calcium daily in four divided doses).

Chronic Hypocalcemia

The principles of the chronic treatment of hypocalcemia are to give oral calcium supplements and vitamin D derivatives to increase serum calcium toward normal range and render the patient asymptomatic (see Refs. 44 and 64 for review). Oral calcium supplements are available as gluconate and carbonate salts. They should be taken as 3–4 divided doses daily. Milk products have an approximately equivalent calcium and phosphorus contents and should be avoided as calcium supplements. Several vitamin D derivatives are available. Their efficacy is based on their capacity to enhance calcium absorption from gut, set point for calcium between ECF and bone, and to some extent renal calcium reabsorption. Ergocalciferol (vitamin D_2) or calciferol can exert its effects only through conversion to $25\text{-}(OH)D_3$ in patients with aparathyroidism or severe chronic renal failure, who cannot convert $25\text{-}(OH)D_3$ into calcitriol (in these cases, high circulating concentrations of $25\text{-}(OH)D_3$ may probably activate the calcitriol receptors). In contrast, in patients with mild hypoparathyroidism or with vitamin D deficiency an entire profile of vitamin D metabolites is produced. More recent vitamin D derivatives are available, such as calcifediol ($25\text{-}(OH)D_3$) (calderol), which is the hepatic metabolite of vitamin D, calcitriol (Rocaltrol), which is the renal metabolite of vitamin D_3, and α-calcidiol ($1\alpha\text{-}(OH)_2D_3$) (one alpha), which undergoes 25-hydroxylation in the liver.

The efficacy of vitamin D and derivative preparations varies from one patient to another, and from time to time in an individual patient. Changes in vitamin D requirements may occur as a consequence of concomitant administration of drugs such as anticonvulsants, thiazide diuretics, and antacids, or the development of electolyte disturbances such as hypomagnesemia or hyperphosphatemia. Episodes of vitamin D and derivatives intoxication may occur in a totally unpredictable manner, often in a patient who has been on a stable regime for a prolonged period. Unfortunately, there is a small window between the therapeutic levels and toxic levels with all the vitamin D and derivative preparations. Moreover, toxicity may persist for several weeks with vitamin D_2, 2 weeks with calcifediol, and a few days with calcitriol (this is explained by the different half-lives). The major side effects associated with vitamin D and derivatives are hypercalcemia, hypercalciuria, soft tissue calcifications, and nephrocalcinosis.

Calcium preparations and vitamin D derivatives used for the treatment of hypercalcemia are listed in Tables 57.7 and 57.8.

Table 57.6
Causes of Nonparathyroid Hypocalcemia

Vitamin D disorders
  Vitamin D deficiency
  Intestinal malabsorption
  Hepatic and biliary disorders
  Anticonvulsant therapy
  Vitamin D-dependent rickets
Renal insufficiency
  Reduced $1,25\text{-}(OH)_2D_3$
  Hyperphosphatemia
  Metabolic acidosis
Hypomagnesemia
Hypoalbuminemia
Rapid or excessive skeletal mineralization
  Hungry bone syndrome
  Osteoblastic metastases
Acute hyperphosphatemia
  Excessive phosphate administration
  Crush injuries
  Rapid tumor lysis
Toxic shock syndrome
Medications
  Mithramycin
  Calcitonin
  Biphosphonates
  Citrated whole blood
  Acute fluoride intoxication

Hypoparathyroidism and Pseudohypoparathyroidism

The combination of vitamin D therapy and oral calcium supplements increases serum calcium only by enhancing gut absorption, bone resorption, the renal reabsorption of calcium remaining low in the absence of circulating PTH (see Refs. 3 and 7 for review). The increment in serum calcium is thus associated with hypercalciuria, with the risk of renal stones and nephrocalcinosis. Thus, the goal of the therapy is to maintain serum calcium between 80 and 90 mg/liter (2 and 2.25 mmol/liter), which suppresses symptoms of hypocalcemia and limits hypercalciuria and the risk of vitamin D intoxication. Effective daily doses of vitamin D or derivatives are progressively obtained and maintained, the patient being then followed at regular intervals (every 1 or 2 months). Pharmacological doses of vitamin D_2 (1250–2500 μg or 50,000–100,000 IU daily) or $25\text{-}(OH)D_3$ (50–200 μg daily) are necessary to correct hy-

Table 57.7
Calcium Preparations for the Treatment of Hypocalcemia

Compound	Content	Dose
Intravenous therapy		
Calcium chloride	10% solution: 272 mg of elemental calcium/10-ml ampule	10 ml[a]
Calcium gluconate	10% solution: 90 mg of elemental calcium/10-ml ampule	30 ml[a]
Calcium gluceptate	23% solution: 90 mg of elemental calcium/5-ml ampule	15 ml[a]
Oral preparations		
Calcium carbonate	500 mg of elemental calcium in 1250-mg tablet	2–4 tablets/day
Calcium gluconate	45 mg of elemental calcium in 500-mg tablet, or 90 mg in 1000-mg tablet	22 tablets/day 11 tablets/day

[a]Single injection i.v. over 10 min or continuous i.v. infusion of solution diluted in 500 ml of 5% glucose over 4 hr.

Table 57.8
Vitamin D Derivatives Used for the Treatment of Chronic Hypocalcemia

Compound	Abbreviations	Relative Potencies	Effective Daily Doses		Time for Reversal of Effects
			Vitamin D Deficiency	Hypo- and Pseudo-Hypoparathyroidism	
			μg	μg	days
Ergocalciferol (calciferol)	Vitamin D_2	1	12.5–250	1250–2500	17–60
Calcifediol (calderol)	25-(OH)D_3	10–15	2–5	50–200	7–30
Dihydrotachysterol	DHT	3	20–100	500–1000	3–14
α-Calcidiol (one alpha)	1α-(OH)D_3	1000–1500	0.5–2[a]	0.5–2	5–10
Calcitriol (Rocaltrol)	1,25-(OH)$_2D_3$	1000–5000	0.5–2[a]	0.5–2	2–10

[a]Only in Vitamin D dependency and chronic renal failure. Ergocalciferol contains 40,000 USP units or IU/1000 μg.

pocalcemia, which indicates a resistance to vitamin D due to impaired renal 1α-hydroxylase (29). In contrast, physiological doses of calcitriol or α-calcidiol (0.5–2 μg daily) are sufficient to control serum calcium. A supplement of elemental calcium per day is recommended, about 1–2 g. In some selected patients (aparathyroidism), thiazide diuretics (25–50 mg daily), which enhance renal reabsorption of calcium, may be used to reduce the doses of vitamin D derivatives necessary to obtain serum calcium between 80 and 90 mg/liter, without worsening hypercalciuria (56). Finally phosphate binding gels are not necessary since the correction of hypocalcemia by vitamin D derivatives normalizes serum phosphate.

Vitamin D Deficiency

Daily administration of physiological doses of vitamin D_2 (12.5–25 μg or 500–1000 IU) or of 25-(OH)D_3 (2–5 μg) are sufficient to correct hypocalcemia and rickets or osteomalacia (see Ref. 19 for review). However, higher doses are often recommended to restore vitamin D stores (125–250 μg or 5,000–10,000 IU daily of vitamin D_2) although there is no evidence for this view. Higher pharmacologic doses render the patient at risk for intoxication and should be avoided. Daily oral supplement of elemental calcium is necessary, usually 1 g,

and sometimes more, 2–3 g in the event of hungry bone syndrome. Directly active vitamin D derivatives, calcitriol or α-calcidiol are not recommended (except in vitamin D dependency), since they do not replete vitamin D stores, and increase the risk of toxicity since there is no feedback regulatory system (19).

Chronic Renal Failure

The goal is to correct hypocalcemia and principally to limit the degree of secondary hyperparathyroidism (see Ref. 15 for review). Physiological doses of calcitriol (0.5–2 μg daily) or its analog α-calcidiol are usually used to prevent or correct secondary HPT directly by raising circulating calcitriol and indirectly by normalizing serum calcium.

Hyperphosphatemia (serum phosphorus >1.5 mmol/liter), when present, should be corrected first by administration of oral preparations binding phosphate in the intestine. Aluminum hydroxide is useful, but doses higher than 6 g/day should be avoided to limit the risk of osteomalacia and encephalopathy secondary to aluminum accumulation. High doses of calcium carbonate (4–6 g/day) bind intestinal phosphate and correct hypocalcemia and metabolic acidosis. However, high doses of calcium carbonate together with vitamin D derivatives render the patient at a high risk for hypercalcemia. A new analog of calcitriol, 22-oxa-1,25-(OH)$_2$D$_3$, which inhibits PTH secretion with little calcemic effect, is of potential interest.

Magnesium Therapy

Symptomatic or severe hypomagnesemia (plasma Mg <0.5 mmol/liter) should be treated wtih intravenous magnesium administration (see Ref. 18 for review). Magnesium sulfate and magnesium chloride are the most widely used preparations and are available in aqueous solutions. Recommended initial doses are approximately 600 mg (24 mmol) of elemental magnesium during the first 6 hr in dextrose solutions, followed by the same dose administered throughout the remainder of the first day. The quantity of magnesium administered on the second day approximates one-half of the total dose during the initial 24 hr, and subsequent doses are determined empirically. Serum magnesium should be kept between 1 and 1.25 mmol/liter. Magnesium should be administered cautiously in patients with renal impairment. In urgent situations (seizures), a loading dose of approximately 200–500 mg of elemental magnesium may be administered intravenously over 15 min. Chronic oral magnesium may be useful in certain patients, and supplements of 20–30 mmol/day may be necessary, especially in the presence of intestinal malabsorption. When renal loss of magnesium is present, it should be noted that oral supplements cannot normalize serum magnesium.

Acknowledgments. We thank Chantal Nicolas for her assistance in the preparation of the manuscript. This work was supported by grants from the Institut National de la Santé et de la Recherche Médicale, the Université Paris 6, the Fondation pour la Recherche Médicale Française, and the Fondation de France.

References

1. Adami S, Mian M, Bertoldo F, et al. Regulation of calcium-parathyroid hormone feedback in primary hyperparathyroidism: effects of biphosphonate treatment. Clin Endocrinol 1990;33:391–397.
2. Auwerx J, Bouillon R. Mineral and bone metabolism in thyroid disease: a review. Q J Med 1986;232:737–752.
3. Avioli LV. The therapeutic approach to hypoparathyroidism. Am J Med 1974;57:34–42.
4. Binstock ML, Mundy GR. Effect of calcitonin and glucocorticoids in combination on the hypercalcemia of malignancy. Ann Intern Med 1980;93:269–272.
5. Body JJ, Borkowski A, Cleeren A, et al. Treatment of malignancy-associated hypercalcaemia with intravenous aminohydroxypropylidene diphosphonate. J Clin Oncol 1986;8:1177–1183.
6. Boyde A, Macconachie E, Reid SA, et al. Scanning electron microscopy in bone pathology: review of methods. Potential and applications. Scanning Electron Microsc 1986;4:1537–1554.
7. Breslau NA, Pak CYC. Hypoparathyroidism. Metabolism 1979;28:1261–1276.
8. Broadus AE. Primary hyperparathyroidism viewed as a bihormonal disease process. Miner Electrolyte Metab 1982;8:199–214.
9. Cadman EL, Lundberg WB, Bertino JR. Hyperphosphatemia and hypocalcemia accompanying rapid cell lysis in a patient with Burkitt's lymphoma and Burkitt cell leukemia. Am J Med 1977;62:283.
10. Chapuy MC, Meunier PJ, Alexandre CM, et al. Effects of disodium dichloromethylene diphosphonate on the hypercalcemia produced by bone metastases. J Clin Invest 1980;65:1243–1247.
11. Chesney RW, McCarron DM, Haddad JG, et al. Pathogenic mechanisms of the hypocalcemia of the staphylococcal toxic shock syndrome. J Lab Clin Med 1983;101:576.
12. Coburn JW, Slatopolsky E. Vitamin D, parathyroid hormone and the renal osteodystrophies. In: Brenner BM, Rector FC, ed. The kidney. 4th ed. Philadelphia: WB Saunders, 1991;2:2036–2120.
13. Cochran M, Nordin BEC. The causes of hypocalcaemia in chronic renal failure. Clin Sci 1971;40:305–315.
14. Davies M, Mawer EB, Freemont AJ. The osteodystrophy of hypervitaminosis D: a metabolic study. Q J Med 1986;61:911–919.
15. Delmez JA, Slatopolsky E. Recent advances in the pathogenesis and therapy of uremia secondary hyperparathyroidism. J Clin Endocrinol Metab 1991;72:735–739.
16. Drezner MK, Neelon FA. Pseudohypoparathyroidism. In: Stanbury JB, Wyngaarden JB, Fredrickson DS, Goldstein JL, Brown MS, eds. 5th ed. The metabolic basis of inherited disease. New York: McGraw-Hill, 1983;1508–1528.
17. Eilon G, Mundy GR. Direct resorption of bone by human breast cancer cells in vitro. Nature 1978;276:726–728.
18. Fenik EF. Therapy of magnesium deficiency. Ann NY Acad Sci 1969;162:901.
19. Frame B, Parfitt M. Osteomalacia: current concepts. Ann Intern Med 1978;89:966–982.
20. Fu-Hsiung S, Sherrard DJ. Lithium-induced hyperparathyroidism: an alteration of the "set point." Ann Intern Med 1982;96:63–65.
21. Garabedian M, Jacoz E, Guillozo H, et al. Elevated plasma 1,25-dihydroxyvitamin D concentrations in infants with hypercalcemia and elfin facies. N Engl J Med 1985;312:948–952.
22. Gardin JP, Paillard M. Normocalcemic primary hyperparathyroidism: resistance to PTH effect on

tubular reabsorption of calcium. Miner Electrolyte Metab 1984;10:301–308.

23. Gardin JP, Patron P, Fouqueray B, et al. Maximal PTH secretory rate and set point for calcium in normal subjects and patients with primary hyperparathyroidism. In vivo studies. Miner Electrolyte Metab 1988;14:221–228.

24. Garrett IR, Durie BGM, Nedwin GE, et al., Production of the bone resorbing cytokine lymphotoxin by cultured human myeloma cells. N Engl J Med 1987;317:526–532.

25. Glover D, Riley L, Carmichael K, et al. Hypocalcemia and inhibition of parathyroid hormone secretion after administration of WR-2721 (a radioprotective and chemoprotective agent). N Engl J Med 1983;309:1137–1141.

26. Harinck HIJ, Bijvoet OLM, Plantingh AST. Role of bone and kidney in tumor-induced hypercalcemia and its treatment with bisphosponate and sodium chloride. Am J Med 1987;82:1133–1142.

27. Hosking DJ, Cowley A, Bucknall CA. Rehydration in the treatment of severe hypercalcemia. Q J Med 1981;ser L:473–481.

28. Jacobs TP, Siris ES, Bilezikian JP, et al. Hypercalcemia of malignancy. Treatment with intravenous dichloromethylene diphosphonate. Ann Intern Med 1981;94:312–316.

29. Kooh SW, Fraser D, DeLuca HF, et al. Treatment of hypoparathyroidism and pseudohypoparathyroidism with metabolites of vitamin D: evidence for impaired conversion of 25-OH-D to 1-25 (OH)$_2$D. N Engl J Med 1979;293:840–844.

30. Kurokawa K. Calcium-regulating hormones and the kidney. Kidney Int 1987;32:700–771.

31. Lad TE, Mishoulam HM, Shevrin DH, et al. Treatment of cancer-associated hypercalcemia with cisplatin. Arch Intern Med 1987;147:329–332.

32. Mallette LE. Primary hyperparathyroidism, an update: incidence, etiology, diagnosis and treatment. Am J Med Sci 1987;293:239–249.

33. Mallette LE, Bilezikian JP, Heath DA, et al. Primary hyperparathyroidism: clinical and biochemical features. Medicine 1974;53:127–146.

34. Marx SJ, Spiegel AM, Levine MA, et al. Familial hypocalciuric hypercalcemia. N Engl J Med 1982;307:416–426.

35. Mawer EB, Hann JT, Berry JL, et al. Vitamin D metabolism in patients intoxicated with ergocalciferol. Clin Sci 1985;68:141–145.

36. Merlini G, Fitzpatrick LA, Siris ES, et al. A human myeloma immunoglobulin G binding four moles of calcium associated with asymptomatic hypercalcemia. J Clin Immunol 1984;4:185–196.

37. Meyrier A, Valeyre D, Bouillon R, et al. Resorptive versus absorptive hypercalciuria in sarcoidosis: correlations with 25-hydroxyvitamin D3 and 1,25-dihydroxyvitamin D3 and parameters of disease activity. Q J Med 1985;54:269–281.

38. Mudde AH, Van der Berg H, Boshuis PG, et al. Ectopic production of 1,25-dihydroxyvitamin D by B-cell lymphoma as a cause of hypercalcemia. Cancer 1987;59:1543–1546.

39. Mundy GR. Hypercalcemia of malignancy. Kidney Int 1987;31:142–155.

40. Mundy GR. Hypercalcemia of malignancy revisited. J Clin Invest 1988;82:1–6.

41. Mundy GR. Malignancy and hypercalcemia: humoral hypercalcemia of malignancy, hypercalcemia associated with osteolytic metastases. In: Mundy GR, ed. Calcium homeostasis: hypercalcemia and hypocalcemia. 2nd ed. London: Martin Dunitz, 1990:69–99.

42. Mundy GR, Hypercalcemia associated with hematologic malignancies. In: Mundy GR, ed. Calcium homeostasis: hypercalcemia and hypocalcemia. 2nd ed. London: Martin Dunitz, 1990:100–116.

43. Mundy GR. Treatment of hypercalcemia due to malignancy. In: Mundy GR, ed. Calcium homeostasis: hypercalcemia and hypocalcemia. 2nd ed. London: Martin Dunitz, 1990:116–136.

44. Mundy GR. Treatment of hypocalcemia. In: Mundy GR, ed. Calcium homeostasis: hypercalcemia and hypocalcemia. 2nd ed. London: Martin Dunitz, 1990:215–219.

45. Mundy GR, Raisz LG. Thyrotoxicosis and calcium metabolism. Miner Electrolyte Metab 1979; 2:285–292.

46. Mundy GR, Wilkinson R, Heath DA. Comparative study of available medical therapy for hypercalcemia of malignancy. Am J Med 1983;74:421–432.

47. Nordin BEC. Plasma calcium and plasma magnesium homeostasis. In: Nordin BEC, ed. Phosphate and magnesium metabolism. Edinburgh: Churchill Livingstone, 1976:186–216.

48. Oreffo ROC, Teti A, Triffitt JT, et al. Effect of vitamin A on bone resorption: evidence for direct stimulation of isolated chicken osteoclasts by retinol and retinoic acid. J Bone Miner Res 1988; 3:203–210.

49. Orwoll ES. The milk-alkali syndrome: current concepts. Ann Intern Med 1982;97:242–248.

50. Paillard M, Gardin JP, Borensztein P, et al. Determinants of parathormone secretion in primary hyperparathyroidism. Hormone Res 1989;32:89–92.

51. Paillard M, Patron P, Gardin JP, et al. Physiological and clinical aspects of primary hyperparathyroidism. In: Valker VR, Sutton RAL, Cameron ECB, Pak CYC, Robertson WG, eds. Urolithiasis. New York, Plenum Press, 1989:619–625.

52. Parfitt AM. Equilibrium and disequilibrium hypercalcemia: new light on an old concept. Metab Bone Dis Relat Res 1989;1:279–293.

53. Parfitt MA. Surgical, idiopathic, and other varieties of parathyroid hormone-deficient hypoparathyroidism. In: DeGroot LJ, et al, eds. Endocrinology. Vol 2. New York: Grune and Stratton, 1989:755–768.

54. Patron P, Gardin JP, Paillard M. Renal mass and reserve of vitamin D: determinants in primary hyperparathyroidism. Kidney Int 1987;31:1174–1180.

55. Patron P, Gardin JP, Borensztein P, et al. Marked direct suppression of primary hyperparathyroidism with osteitis fibrosa cystica by intravenous administration of 1,25 dihydroxycholecalciferol. Miner Electrolyte Metab 1989;15:321–325.

56. Porter RH, Cox BG, Heaney D, et al. Treatment of hypoparathyroid patients with chlorthalidone. N Engl J Med 1978; 298:577–581.

57. Raskin P, McClain CJ, Medsger TA. Hypocal-

cemia associated with metastatic bone disease. Arch Intern Med 1973;132:539–543.

58. Rude RK, Oldham SB, Singer FR. Functional hypoparathyroidism and parathyroid hormone end-organ resistance in human magnesium deficiency. Clin Endocrinol 1976;5:209–224.

59. Scholz DA, Purnell DC. Asymptomatic primary hyperparathyroidism. 10 year prospective study. Mayo Clin Proc 1981;56:473–478.

60. Shike M, Harrison JE, Strutridge WC, et al. Metabolic bone disease in patients receiving long-term parenteral nutrition. Ann Intern Med 1980;92:343–350.

61. Singer FR, Adams JS. Abnormal calcium homeostasis in sarcoidosis. N Engl J Med 1986;315:755–757.

62. Siris ES, Sherman WH, Baquiran DC, et al. Effects of dichloromethylene diphosphonate on skeletal mobilization of multiple myeloma. N Engl J Med 1980;302:310–315.

63. Slatopolsky E, Lopez-Hilker S, Delmez J, et al. The parathyroid-calcitriol axis in health and chronic renal failure. Kidney Int 1990;38:S41–S47.

64. Stewart AF, Broadus AE. Mineral metabolism. In: Felig P, Baxter JD, Broadus AE, Frohman LA, eds. Endocrinology and Metabolism. 2nd ed. New York: MacGraw-Hill, 1987:1317–1453.

65. Stewart AF, Alder M, Byers CM, et al. Calcium homeostasis in immobilization: an example of resorptive hypercalciuria. N Engl J Med 1982; 306:1136–1140.

66. Stewart AF, Hocker Jr., Mallette LE, et al. Hy-

percalcemia in pheochromocytoma. Ann Intern Med 1985;102:776.

67. Stewart AF, Longo W, Kreutter D, et al. Hypocalcemia associated with calcium soap formation in a patient with a pancreatic fistula. N Engl J Med 1986;315:496–498.

68. Stögmann W, Fischer JA. Pseudohypoparathyroidism. Disappearance of the resistance to parathyroid extract during treatment with vitamin D. Am J Med 1975;59:140–144.

69. Stote RM, Smith H, Wilson DM et al. Hydrochlorothiazide effects on serum calcium and immunoreactive parathyroid hormone concentrations. Ann Intern Med 1972;77:587–591.

70. Suki WN, Yium JJ, von Minden M, et al. Acute treatment of hypercalcemia with furosemide. N Engl J Med 1970;283:836–840.

71. Thiebaud D, Jaeger P, Jacquet AF, et al. A single-day treatment of tumor-induced hypercalcemia by intravenous amino-hydroxypropylidene bisphosphonate. J Bone Miner Res 1986;6:555–562.

72. Verner JV, Morrison AB. Endocrine pancreatic islet disease with diarrhea. Arch Intern Med 1974;133:492.

73. Walser M, Robinson BHB, Duckett JW. The hypercalcemia of adrenal insufficiency. J Clin Invest 1963;42:456–465.

74. Warrell RP Jr, Bockman RS, Coonley CJ, et al. Gallium nitrate inhibits calcium resorption from bone and is effective treatment for cancer-related hypercalcemia. J Clin Invest 1984;73:1487–1490.

Index

Page numbers followed by "*f*" denote figures; those followed by "*t*" denote tables.

ABCs of trauma assessment, 792
Abdomen
    acute processes of
        cholangitis, 720–721
        cholecystitis, 718–720
        intraabdominal abscesses, 724
        large bowel obstruction, 717
        mechanical intestinal obstruction, 716–717
        pancreatitis, 724–727*t*
        peritonitis, 721–724
    complications of, in end-stage renal failure,
        685–687
    trauma of, 800–801*t*
Abdominal binding, cardiopulmonary resuscitation
    and, 513
Abdominal compressions, interposed, 513–515
Abnormal carrier state, 82
Abscesses
    brain, posttransplant, 844
    intraabdominal, 724
    perivascular, in endocarditis, 379
Absolute neutrophil count (ANC), 836
Absorption, intestinal, 729
Acalculous cholecystitis, 718–720
Acetate
    dialysis, 623–626
    intolerance, in kidney dialysis, 690
    metabolism of, 623–624
Acetylsalicylic acid, for bacterial pneumonia, 407
Acid-base balance
    acetate dialysis and, 624
    acid-base load and, 611–612*t*
    bicarbonate dialysis and, 626
    buffers, 610–611*t*
        closed system of, 612–614
        intracellular, 614
        of bicarbonate load, 614
        of fixed base load, 613*f*
        of volatile acid load, 613–614
        open system of, 614–618*f*
        respiratory, 614–618*f*
    disorders of (*see also* Acidosis; Alkalosis)
        compensatory responses in, 619–620*t*
        continuous arteriovenous hemofiltration
            therapy for, 664–665
        correction by renal replacement therapy, 636

    in acute renal failure, 620–621
        treatment of, 621–627
    in acute renal failure, 633
Acid load
    definition of, 611–612*t*
    fixed
        buffering of, 612–613
        respiratory buffering of, 615
    volatile, buffering of, 613–614
Acid maltase deficiency, 786
Acidosis
    intracerebral, in brain injury, 770–771
    lactic. (*see* Lactic acidosis)
    left ventricular performance and, 223
    metabolic. (*see* Metabolic acidosis)
    respiratory
        compensatory responses, 619, 620*t*
        treatment of, 438
        with acute renal failure, 621
    systemic, in brain injury, 770–771
Acids, net excretion of, 618
Acquired immunodeficiency syndrome (AIDS)
    cardiac manifestations of, 857–858
    clinical manifestations of, 852–853
    endocarditis risk and, 374
    endocrine manifestations of, 860
    etiology of, 851. (*see also* Human
        immunodeficiency virus I (HIV-I))
    gastrointestinal manifestations of, 859–860
    hematological manifestations of, 860
    ICU survival and, 860–861
    neurological dysfunction in, 856–857
    pathogenesis of, 851–852*t*
    pneumocystis carinii pneumonia in, 853–855
    pneumothorax in, 855–856
    pulmonary disease in, 853–856
    renal dysfunction in, 858–859*t*
    sepsis and, 860
    therapies for, 853
Acquired infection, SDD and, 89
ACTH (adrenocorticotrophic hormone), 902, 904,
    907
Actin, inotropic agents and, 252*f*, 352
Acute interstitial nephritis, 581
Acute renal failure (ARF)
    acid-base balance in, 633

Acute renal failure (ARF)—(*continued*)
  acid-base derangements in, 610
    treatment of, 621–627
    types of, 620–621
  biochemical disturbances in, 586–588
  calcium abnormalities of, 588–589
  cardiovascular complications of, 590–591
  cellular pathophysiology of, 581
  clinical features of, 630
  complicated, acid-base derangements of, 621
  definition of, 571
  diabetes and, 887–888
  diagnosis of, 575–577*f*
  diagnostic imaging in, 576–577
  electrolyte balance in, 633
  energy metabolism management, 632–633
  etiology of, 572–577*f*
  fluid balance, management of, 631–632
  gastrointestinal complications of, 593–594
  hematologic abnormalities of, 596–597
  hemodialysis for, 623–627
  hepatorenal syndrome and, 582
  history of, 575
  hypercalcemia in, 607–608, 932
  hyperkalemia in
    clinical manifestations of, 606–607
    treatment of, 607*t*
  hypermagnesemia in, 607–608
  hyperphosphatemia in, 607
  hypocalcemia in, 607–608
  hyponatremia in
    clinical manifestations of, 603–604
    treatment of, 604–605*t*
  in multiple organ failure, 582–583*f*
  in renal transplant, 581–582
  infectious complications of, 597–598
  interstitial causes of, 572–573*f*
  magnesium abnormalities of, 590
  management, conservative, 631–633*t*
  nervous system complications of, 594–596
  nutritional support for, 64–66
  outcome of, 668–669*t*
  parenchymal disease, 572–574*f*
  pathophysiology of, 577–581
  phosphorus abnormalities of, 589–590
  physical examination of, 575–576
  prevention of, 630–631
  pulmonary complications of, 591–593
  renal replacement therapy
    choice of, 634
    continuous, 646–648*f*
    initiation of, 633–634
    intermittent hemodialysis. (*see* Intermittent
      hemodialysis)
    peritoneal dialysis. (*see* Peritoneal dialysis)
    requirements for, 634–636*t*
    solute and water transport mechanisms,
      636–638*f*
  risk of, 571–572
  toxic causes of, 572–573*f*
  uncomplicated, acid-base derangements of,
    620–621
Acute renal failure syndrome, 571
Acute tubular necrosis, 572, 579–581, 631
Acyclovir, 840
Addisonian crisis, acute, therapy for, 907–908
Addison's disease
  clinical aspects of, 905–907
  precipitating factors, 905–906

ADH (antidiuretic hormone). (*see* Vasopressin)
Adrenal cortex, anatomy of, 902
Adrenal insufficiency, acute
  Addisonian crisis, therapy for, 907–908
  diagnosis of, 907
  hypercalcemia of, 930
  prevention of, 908–909
  primary, clinical aspects of, 905–907
  secondary, therapy for, 908
α-Adrenergic agonists, 117, 919
ß-Adrenergic agonists, 353–355*t*, 497
α-Adrenergic blockers, 359
ß-Adrenergic blockers
  for hypertension control in pheochromocytoma,
    919
  for hypertension in brain injury, 767
  for myocardial ischemia, 252
  with calcium antagonists, for unstable angina, 249
  with thrombolysis, 254
ß-Adrenergic receptors, 116–117, 117, 152
ß-Adrenergic stimulants, 441, 886–887
Adrenocortical hormones
  release of, 902
  secretion, regulation of, 902, 904
  synthesis of, 902, 903*f*
Adrenocorticotrophic hormone (ACTH), 902, 904, 907
Adult respiratory distress syndrome (ARDS)
  associated conditions, 414–415*t*
  auto-PEEP in, 457
  clinical characteristics of, 416–418
  complications and, 423
  diagnosis of, 416–418
  difficult-to-wean patients, 422–423
  etiology of, 414–415
  gas exchange and, 395–399*f*
  in diabetic ketoacidosis, 878
  in multiple organ failure, 72, 73
  incidence of, 414
  liver and, 99
  management of, 292–293
    mechanical ventilation for, 419–420
    new approaches for, 423–425
    overview for, 418–419*f*
    oxygenation for, 419*f*
    supportive care for, 420–422
  mechanisms of, 416
  mimicking infection, 83
  100% oxygen for, 402–403
  pathophysiology of, 415–417*f*
  pneumonia and, 555
  positive end-expiratory pressure for, 399–402*f*,
    420
  prevention of, 62
  prognosis for, 423
  right ventricular dysfunction in, 285
  structure-function correlations in, 395–399*f*
  therapeutic implications of right ventricular
    failure, 291–293
  vasoactive agents for, 403–406*f*
  ventilation-perfusion mismatch in, 390
  vitamin E deficiency and, 53
Afterload
  cardiac function and, 141
  in left ventricular failure, 234–236*f*
  left ventricular performance and, 281
  myocardial performance and, 365
  right ventricular performance and, 281, 286–287
AIDS. (*see* Acquired immunodeficiency syndrome
  (AIDS))

AIDS-related complex (ARC), 853
Air embolism, from continuous arteriovenous
    hemofiltration therapy, 666
Air space pneumonia, 534–535f
Air-trapping, 474–475
Airflow obstruction, pathophysiology of, 453–454f
Airway(s)
  chronic obstruction of. (*see* Chronic airway
    obstruction)
  dynamics of, in asthma, 435–436
  management of
    in trauma, 794–798t
    muscle relaxants and, 798
    narcotic sedation, 798
  narrowing of, in asthma, 491–492
  obstruction of
    partial ventilatory support for, 463–468f
    practical management of, 461–463f
    weaning from ventilatory support and,
      468–470f
Airway pressure, 486
Albumin, serum, in anorexia nervosa, 37
Alcoholic ketoacidosis
  biologic features of, 879–880
  clinical manifestations of, 879
  pathophysiology of, 880f
  treatment of, 880
Alcoholism, diabetes and, 878
Aldosterone, 905. (*see* Renin-angiotensin-
    aldosterone system)
Alkali ingestion, esophagitis of, 697
Alkalosis, metabolic
  compensatory responses, 619, 620t
  with acute renal failure, 621
Almitrine
  for adult respiratory distress syndrome, 405f
  for chronic obstructive pulmonary disease, 409
Amino acid formulas
  adverse consequences of, 33
  for acute renal failure, 66
Amino acids
  catabolism of, 29f, 34
  for postoperative period, 72
  metabolism of
    during stress, 33
    normal, 30–31
  oxidative deamination of, 28, 29f
  ventilatory drive and, 64
Aminoglycosides, for nosocomial pneumonia, 563
Aminophylline
  diaphragmatic contractility and, 440
  for asthma, 497
  for septic syndrome, 182
Ammonia formation, 587
Amphotericin B, 580, 843, 844
Ampicillin, for *Listeria monocytogenes* infections, 841
Amrinone
  for heart failure, 242–243
  for right heart failure, 332
  pharmacology of, 355
  side effects of, 355
AMV (assisted mechanical ventilation), 463
Amylase, in pancreatitis, 725
Amyotrophic lateral sclerosis, 785–786
Anabolic proteins, 50
Anaerobic microorganisms, in community-acquire
    pneumonia, 529–530
Analgesics, for end-stage renal failure, 693
Anaphylactic shock, epinephrine for, 157

ANC (absolute neutrophil count), 836
Anemia
  causes of, 817
  cellular oxygen delivery and, 364
Anesthesia, for pheochromocytoma surgery, 921
Angina, unstable
  classification of, 245
  definition of, 245
  diagnosis of, 245–246
  intervention strategies
    bypass surgery, 250
    emergency angioplasty, 250
    goal of, 248
    pharmacologic, 248–250
  pathogenesis of, 246–248f
Angiography, of coronary artery disease, 247–248f
Angioplasty, emergency, for unstable angina, 250
Angiotensin. (*see* Renin-angiotensin-aldosterone
    system)
Animal exposure, infective endocarditis of, 374
Anion gap, 875
Anisoylated plasminogen streptokinase activator
    complex (APSAC), 253
Anorexia nervosa, serum albumin and, 37
Antacids
  adverse effects of, 705
  for nosocomial pneumonia prophylaxis, 554f
  for stress ulcer prophylaxis, 699, 702–705t
Anti-factor VIII antibody, 807
Antiarrhythmic drugs
  classification of, 348–350t
  for end-stage renal failure, 694
  pharmacokinetic characteristics of, 351t
  pharmacology of, 348–350t
  postoperative use of, 365
Antibiotics
  broad-spectrum, for nosocomial pneumonia, 562
  combinations therapy, for endocarditis, 383
  continuous arteriovenous hemofiltration therapy
    and, 667
  diarrhea and, 735
  for acute respiratory failure, in COPD, 438–439
  for central nervous system infections, 748–749
  for end-stage renal failure, 693–694t
  for endocarditis, 383–385t
  for granulocytopenia, 835t, 836–838t
  for hyperosmolar coma, 871
  for infection in ICU, 83
  for SDD, 87–88t
  for sepsis, 107–108
  of cholecystitis, 719
  prophylactic, 827
    for nosocomial pneumonia, 566
Anticancer drugs, for hypercalcemia, 935
Anticarriage regimen, SDD as, 86–87
Anticoagulation
  for continuous arteriovenous hemofiltration
    therapy, 659–661
  for hemodialysis, 642
Antidiarrheal drugs, 736–737
Antidiuretic hormone. (*see* Vasopressin)
Antiendotoxin antibodies, 108–109
Antifibrinolytic agents, 808
Antihypertensive therapy, with brain injury, 767
Antihypertonics, for end-stage renal failure, 694
Antimicrobial agents. (*see* Antibiotics)
Antisepsis, topical, 83
Antithrombin III concentrate, 822
Antithrombin III deficiency, 812

Anxiety, in asthma, 497–498
Aortic dissection, acute, 275
Aortic input impedance, in left ventricular failure, 234–236f
Aortic insufficiency, acute
  diagnosis of, 262–263
  noninfective causes, timing of surgery, 276
  timing of surgical repair, 275–276
Aortic pressure, in pulmonary hypertension, 332
Aortic valve disorders
  leaks, 266–267f
  regurgitation
    clinical examination of, 262–263
    left-sided heart catheterization findings, 272
    postoperative care, 368–369
    quantitation of regurgitant volume, 268–270
  stenosis, postoperative care for, 368
  transthoracic echocardiography of, 264–265
Aortogram, in blunt trauma, 794
APACHE scores, midrange, SDD and, 89–90
Apneustic breathing, 768–769
APSAC (anisoylated plasminogen streptokinase activator complex), 253
Arachidonic acid, free, 59, 60f
Arachidonic acid metabolites, 319, 416
ARC (AIDS-related complex), 853
ARDS. (*see* Adult respiratory distress syndrome (ARDS))
Arginine, 61–62
Arginine-vasopressin (AVP), 222, 911
Arrhythmias. (*see also specific arrhythmias*)
  after cardiac transplantation, 367
  in acute renal failure, 591
  in brain injury, 766
  in end-stage renal failure, 683–684
  in intermittent hemodialysis, 645
  in pheochromocytoma, 920–921
  pharmacologic treatment of, 350–352
  reperfusion injury and, 254
Arterial blood sampling, of acute valve regurgitation, 263
Arterial circulation, coupling with heart, 236–239f
Arterial oxygenation, 482–484
Arterial pressure-flow relationship, in septic shock, 174f
Arterial resistance, 140, 157
Artifacts, in pressure monitoring, 5–8f, 7t
Ascitic fluid, in cirrhotic patients with primary peritonitis, 721
Aspergillus infections
  granulocytopenia of, 835
  posttransplant, 843–844
Aspirin
  for unstable angina, 249
  platelet dysfunction and, 810
  with streptokinase, 253
Assisted mechanical ventilation (AMV), 463
Asthma
  acute respiratory failure in, pathophysiology of, 435–436
  airway dynamics of, 435–436
  clinical presentation of, 495–497f
  epidemiology of, 491
  gas exchange in, 436
  hemodynamic consequences of, 493–495f
  lung volumes in, 435–436
  paradoxical pulse in, 495
  pathophysiology of, 491–492
  pulmonary hypertension in, 493–494

  respiratory consequences of, 492–493
  respiratory mechanics of, 492
  right ventricular failure in, 494–495f
  structure-function correlations, 428–429
  treatment of, 497–500f
    therapeutic goals for, 497
    with right ventricular failure, 295–297
  ventilation-perfusion mismatch, 492–493
  ventilation-perfusion relationship, 409–410f
  work of breathing in, 436
Ataxic breathing, 769
Atenolol, for arrhythmias after head injury, 766
ATP, 58, 112, 132
Atrial contraction, left ventricular performance and, 215
Atrial fibrillation, pharmacologic treatment of, 351
Atrial flutter, pharmacologic treatment of, 351
Atrial natriuretic factor, release of, 290
Atrial vasodilation, hemodynamics of, 358f
Atriopeptin, 223
Atrioventricular nodal reentrant tachycardia, pharmacologic treatment of, 351
Atrioventricular synchronism, 286
Atypical pneumonia syndrome, 532–533
Auto-PEEP
  breathing patterns and, 456f
  definition of, 454
  determinants of, 454–456f
  tidal volume and, 461f
  types of, 456–457
  with proportionate hyperinflation, 457
  without proportionate hyperinflation, 456–457f
Autocannibalism, 42
Autocrine functions, of heart, 223
Autoimmune thrombocytopenia, 809–810
Autonomic nervous system, neurohormone release, 221–222f
Autonomic neuropathy, 682
Autoregulatory escape, 115
Autotransfusion, 144, 817
AVP (arginine-vasopressin), 911
Azathioprine, 691
Azotemia
  amino acid/protein administration and, 33
  definition of, 586, 677
  in uremia, 677, 681t
  postrenal, 571, 574–575f
  prerenal, 571, 572

Backward failure, 231
Bacteremia, definition of, 96, 97t
Bacteria, pathogenic, in granulocytopenia, 834–835
Bacterial monitoring policy, 565
Bacterial peritonitis, 722–723
Balance, metabolic, 23–24
Barbiturates, cerebral metabolism and, 759
Barium enema, toxic megacolon and, 732
Baroreceptor reflex, 140
Base load, fixed
  buffering of, 613f
  respiratory buffering of, 615–616
Basophils, 815
BCAAs. (*see* Branched-chain amino acids (BCAAs))
Beneficence, 196–197
Benzodiazepine, 759
Bezold-Jarisch reflex, 223–224
Bicarbonate
  dialysis of, 626–627
  for cardiopulmonary resuscitation, 520

loss of, in CAVH, 664–665
reabsorption of, 618, 622
Bicarbonate buffers, 611t, 614
Bicarbonate load, respiratory buffering, 617f
Bidirectional effects, of cytokines, 175
Biguanides, 882
Bilateral massive adrenal hemorrhage (BMAH),
  906–907
Biliary tree, infection of, 720–721
Biocompatibility, in renal replacement therapy, 636
Biologic value, of nutritional support, 23
Biphasic $\dot{V}O_2$-$\dot{D}O_2$ model, 120–131f
Bisphosphonates, for hypercalcemia, 934
Bleeding
  clotting factor analysis, 806–808
  from continuous arteriovenous hemofiltration
    therapy, 665–666t
  from stress ulcers, 699–702t
    risk factors for, 702
  gastrointestinal. (*see* Gastrointestinal bleeding)
  general approach to, 806
  in acute renal failure, 596–597
  in end-stage renal failure, 687
  in intermittent hemodialysis, 645–646
  postoperative control of, 366–367t
ß-Blockers. (*see* ß-Adrenergic blockers)
Blood access, in end-stage renal failure, 692
Blood cultures
  for immunocompromised patients, 830–831
  for pneumonia diagnosis, 537
  of infective endocarditis, 376–377
Blood doping, 817
Blood flow
  cerebral. (*see* Cerebral blood flow)
  data interpretation, 14–16t
  distribution of
    in bacterial pneumonia, 406–407f
    venous return and, 146–147
    ventilation and, 478–479
  effects on ventilation, 484
  from venous return, 144
  generation, by cardiopulmonary resuscitation,
    503–507f
  in beating heart, 504
  in CPR, theoretical considerations, 504–506f
  in shock, 161
  in tissue, control of, 114–117
  intrapulmonary gas exchange and, 482–484t
  systemic, physiologic regulation of, 112–118
  vasoactive drugs and, 117–118
Blood gases, arterial
  abnormal, principle mechanisms of, 389t
  for monitoring, of cardiopulmonary resuscitation,
    519–520
  in adult respiratory distress syndrome, 395–399f
  regulatory factors of, 389–395f
Blood lactate, 133–135
Blood oxygen content, 120
Blood pressure
  arterial
    determinants of, 7–8t
    regulation of, 114
  blood volume and, 143f
  cardiac output and, 113
  data interpretation, 7–12f
  determinants of, 7–8t
  in brain injury, 767
  measurement, by restoration of flow, 8
  monitoring

pitfalls of, 5–7f
technology for, 4–5
restoration of, 156–157
systolic, determinants of, 7–8t
tissue perfusion and, 140
Blood products, for transfusion, 820–822
Blood urea nitrogen (BUN)
  in acute renal failure, 64–65, 586–588
  nitrogen balance and, 38
Blood volume
  cardiopulmonary resuscitation and, 512
  of pulmonary circulation, in pulmonary
    hypertension, 325
  static blood pressure and, 113
Blunt trauma
  definitive care for, 793–794t
  primary survey of, 792–793
  resuscitation of, 792–793t
  secondary survey of, 793
BMAH (bilateral massive adrenal hemorrhage),
  906–907
Body size, energy requirements and, 503
Body weight, maintenance, in renal replacement
  therapy, 635
Boerhaave's syndrome, 697–698
Bone marrow transplantation, SDD for, 91
Bone remodeling, hypercalcemia and, 926
Bone resorption, inhibition of, pharmacologic,
  934–935
Bradyarrhythmias
  after cardiac transplantation, 367
  control of, in brain dead patient, 190
Brain abscesses, posttransplant, 844
Brain death
  criteria for, 189t, 749–750t
  definition of, 188–189
  electrolyte balance and, 190
  fluid balance and, 190
  hemodynamic monitoring of, 190
  hormonal changes of, 190
  in adults, 188–189t
  of organ donors, care for, 189–190
  ventilatory support and, 190
Brain edema, types of, 746
Brain herniation syndrome, 745
Brain injury
  cardiac abnormalities in, 765–767
  central nervous system infections and, 748–749
  cerebral blood flow disorders and, 743–744
  diagnostic considerations for, 763–764
  gastrointestinal bleeding and, 772
  general considerations for, 760–772f
  hypertension and, 767
  hypotension and, 767–768
  intracranial pressure and, 744–746
  maintenance of cerebral blood flow and, 740–744f
  mechanisms of, 738–740t
  primary, 738, 750, 772
  prognostic factors of, 763–764
  resuscitation for. (*see* Cerebral resuscitation)
  secondary, 738, 750, 772–773
  somatic resuscitation and, 760–772f
Brain metabolism, in normal and injured brain,
  746–748
Branched-chain amino acids (BCAAs)
  as fuel in critical illness, 136
  enriched formulas of, 33, 51, 68
  in hepatic failure, 66–67, 68
  protein catabolism and, 27–28

Branched-chain amino acids (BCAAs)—*(continued)*
  ventilatory drive and, 64
Branhamella catarrhalis, in community-acquired
      pneumonia, 529
Breathing
  mouth-to-mouth, 502
  patterns of
    auto-PEEP and, 456*f*
    in chronic obstructive pulmonary disease,
        429–430*f*, 433
    work-cost of, 478*t*, 486–487
  work of
    hyperinflation and, 454*f*
    in asthma, 436, 493
    in dynamic hyperinflation, 457–458*f*
Breathing circuit, in airway obstruction, 463
Brescia-Cimino fistula, 692
Brittle diabetes, 872
Bronchiolitis, airflow limitation and, 428
Bronchoalveolar lavage
  in diagnosis of pneumonia, 539–540*f*
  of nosocomial pneumonia, 558–560*f*
Bronchodilators
  for asthma, 497
  for chronic obstructive pulmonary disease,
      293–294, 439–441
Bronchomotor tone, 491–492
Bronchopneumonia, 534*f*
Bronchopulmonary infection, diagnosis of, in ICU,
      83–84
Bronchoscopy specimens, in diagnosis of
      nosocomial pneumonia, 556–560
Bronchospasm, triggering of, 492
Budd-Chiari syndrome, 813
Buffers, physiologic, 610–611*t*, 623
Buformin, 882
BUN. (*see* Blood urea nitrogen (BUN))
Burn patients, SDD for, 91
Bypass surgery
  for cardiogenic shock, 255
  for unstable angina, 250

Caffeine, for acute respiratory failure, in COPD, 440
Calcitonin, for hypercalcemia, 934
Calcitrol, 925
Calcium
  abnormalities of, in acute renal failure, 588–589,
      595
  balance of, 925–926*f*
  decreased levels of. (*see* Hypocalcemia)
  increased levels of. (*see* Hypercalcemia)
  myocardial relaxation and, 210
  myocyte contractility and, 217
  oral intake, hypercalcemia and, 935–936
  reuptake of, 212
Calcium antagonists
  for myocardial ischemia, 252
  for unstable angina, 248–249
  pharmacology of, 360
Calcium channel blockers
  for unstable angina, 248–249
  hypotension of, 157
  in brain resuscitation, 760
Calcium preparations, for hypocalcemia, 939–940*t*
Calciuretic measures, for hypercalcemia, 933
Calculous cholecystitis, 718–720
Candida infections
  esophagitis, 696
  granulocytopenia of, 835

posttransplant, 843
Carbohydrate metabolism
  diabetic ketoacidosis and, 873
  in hepatic failure, 67–68
  in stress, 31–32
  normal, 28, 29*f*
Carbon dioxide
  end-tidal, monitoring of, in CPR, 519–520
  excretion of, 484
Carbon dioxide tension, arterial, cerebral blood flow
      and, 741*f*
Carbon monoxide poisoning, 817
Carbonic acid buffer, 611*t*, 613–614
Carbonic acid load, respiratory buffering of,
      616–617
Cardiac arrest, intracranial pressure increase and,
      745
Cardiac catheterization. (*see* Heart catheterization)
Cardiac chamber compliance, in pericardial
      restraint, 338
Cardiac chamber volume, in pericardial restraint,
      338
Cardiac function curve, interaction with venous
      return curve, 147–149*f*
Cardiac index, 15, 48*f*
Cardiac ischemia, in acute renal failure, 591
Cardiac-lung interaction, left ventricular
      performance and, 216
Cardiac output
  adequacy of, 19–20
  blood flow and, 14–15
  end-diastolic volume of right ventricle and, in
      adult respiratory distress syndrome, 291–292*f*
  in cardiogenic shock, 153
  in septic shock, 154–155
  increasing, 157
  low, 20
    mechanism in pulmonary hypertension,
        321–325*f*
  mixed venous oxygen saturation and, 17
  regulation of, 113–114, 140
  thermodilution measurement, 3, 12–13*f*, 330
    pitfalls of, 13–14
  variables of, 140
Cardiac performance, in sepsis syndrome, 170–173*t*
Cardiac pump theory, 504
Cardiac surgery, postoperative right ventricular
      failure, 300–301
Cardiac tamponade
  classic
    deviations from pathophysiology of, 340–341
    hemodynamics of, 338–340*f*
    pathophysiology of, 338–340*f*
  clinical presentation of, 341–342
  diagnosis of, 342–344
  echocardiography of, 343
  etiology of, 341*t*
  low-pressure, 340–341
  medical therapy for, 345
  noninvasive testing for, 343
  regional, 340
  treatment of, 344–345
Cardiac transplantation. (*see* Heart transplantation)
Cardiac valves, prosthetic, 810
Cardiogenic shock
  definition of, 162
  pathophysiology of, 152–154
  ventricular filling pressure and, 20
Cardioplegia, right ventricle and, 301

Cardiopulmonary bypass, cellular oxygen demand and, 363
Cardiopulmonary resuscitation
  blood flow generation and, 503–507*f*
  case illustration of, 502
  catecholamines for, 517–519
  closed chest technique vs. open chest, 515–517
  defibrillation and, 503*f*
  for sepsis syndrome, 180–183
  history of, 502–503
  in sepsis, 104–105
  in trauma system, 789
  monitoring during, 519–520
  open chest vs. closed chest technique, 515–517
  peripheral vs. thoracic limitations of, 508–515*f*
  sodium bicarbonate for, 520
  theoretical modeling of, implications for, 506–507
  thoracic pump vs. direct compression models, 507–507*f*
Cardiopulmonary system
  interactions
    assessment of, 472–473
    clinical correlates, 474–475
    mechanical, 474
  support, after cardiac transplantation, 367–368
Cardiothoracic surgery, SDD for, 91–92
Cardiovascular medications
  antiarrhythmic. (*see* Antiarrhythmic drugs)
  considerations for, 348
  inotropic agents. (*see* Inotropic agents)
  vasodilators. (*see* Vasodilators)
Cardiovascular system
  acetate dialysis and, 625–626
  bicarbonate dialysis and, 626–627
  complications of
    in acute renal failure, 590–591
    in end-stage renal failure, 683–684
  during cerebral resuscitation, 765–768
  function of, in sepsis, 100–101
  functions of, 119
  homeostasis, right ventricular performance and, 281–282
  reflex changes, 473
  regulation, categories of, 162
  status
    ventilation and, 481–482*t*
    ventilatory strategies for, 485*t*
  support of
    general principles for, 363–365*t*
    in airway obstruction, 462
    in sepsis, 104–105
  variables, altered by ventilation, 479–481*t*
Carriage state, 83
Catabolism, 24
Catecholaminergic blockade, in cerebral resuscitation, 769
Catecholamines
  for sepsis management, 181
  in cerebral injury, 766
  mechanisms, in cardiopulmonary resuscitation, 517–519
Catheters, arterial
  design of, 5
  flush devices, 5, 6–7
  thrombotic/embolic complications, 5
Caustic esophagitis, 696–697
CAVH. (*see* Continuous arteriovenous hemofiltration therapy)

CAVH (continuous arteriovenous hemofiltration), 106
CAVHD (continuous arteriovenous hemofiltration therapy with dialysis), 648. (*see also* Continuous arteriovenous hemofiltration therapy)
CCK (cholecystokinin), 593, 731
Cell-mediated immunity, 825–826
Cell mediators, 43
Cell membrane depolarization, in hypovolemic shock, 165
Cellular redox state, 132
Central blood pressure, regulation of, 140
Central nervous system
  complications of, in endocarditis, 380–381
  in sepsis, 101
  infections of
    brain injury and, 748–749
    in immunocompromised patients, 833–834*t*
  injuries of, heart abnormalities in, 765–767
  neurohormone release, 221–222*f*
  toxicity, medium-chain triglycerides and, 32
Central respiratory drive, in chronic obstructive pulmonary disease, 430
Central venous pressure (CVP), 9, 150–151
Cerebral blood flow
  autoregulation of, 741–742*f*
  disorders of, 743–744*t*
  increasing, 757–758
  maintenance of, 740–744*f*
  measurement of, 743
  oxygen consumption and, 747–748
  reduction of, 740*f*
  regulation of, 741–743*f*
Cerebral edema
  hyperosmolar coma and, 869, 870*t*
  in diabetic ketoacidosis, 878
Cerebral hemorrhage, in end-stage renal failure, 682
Cerebral ischemia, reperfusion, 739–740
Cerebral metabolism
  decreasing demand of, 758–760
  monitoring of, 746
  regulation of, 747–748
Cerebral perfusion pressure (CPP), 741–742
Cerebral resuscitation
  cardiovascular considerations, 765–768
  endocrinologic concerns, 770–772
  evaluation of neurologic injury, 761–764*f*
  goals of, 754*t*, 773
  metabolic concerns, 770–772
  pharmacologic considerations of, 764–765*t*
  pulmonary aspects of, 768–770
  secondary injury minimization and, 753, 754*t*
  therapeutic strategies, 755*t*
    to decrease cerebral metabolic demand, 758–760
    to decrease intracranial pressure, 753, 755–757*t*
    to increase cerebral blood flow and cerebral oxygen delivery, 757–758
    to protect and preserve the neuronal environment, 759–760
Cerebral salt wasting, 772
Cerebrospinal fluid (CSF)
  analysis of
    in central nervous system infection, 833
    in *Cryptococcus neoformans* infection, 856–857
    in endocarditis, 380–381
  production of, 756–757
Cerebrovascular accidents, in endocarditis, 381
Cervical spine evaluation, in blunt trauma, 794*t*

Cervical spine injury, nasotracheal intubation and, 795–796, 797f
Chamber stiffness, 213, 216
Characteristic impedance, 315–316f
Chemical ingestion, caustic, esophagitis of, 696–697
Chemoreceptors, 223
Chest compression, 503, 504
Chest radiograph
    of acute valve regurgitation, 263–264
    of adult respiratory distress syndrome, 418
    of asthma, 496f
    of pulmonary hypertension, 328
Cheyne-Stokes respiration, 768
CHFD (continuous high-flux dialysis), 656f
Chlamydia pneumoniae, in community-acquired pneumonia, 530
Cholangitis, 720–721
Cholecystectomy, 719–720
Cholecystitis
    acalculous, 718–720
    calculous, 718–720
Cholecystokinin (CCK), 593, 731
Cholestasis, 102
Christmas disease, 807
Chronic airway obstruction
    consequences of, 429–435f
    in asthma, structure-function correlations, 428–429
    structure-function correlations, 427–428. (see also Chronic obstructive pulmonary disease)
    ventilation-perfusion mismatching and, 432–435f
Chronic lymphocytic leukemia, 818
Chronic obstructive pulmonary disease (COPD)
    acute respiratory failure of
        antibiotics for, 438–439
        heparin for, 439
        treatment of, 436–442
    breathing pattern, 429–430f
    central respiratory drive, 430
    gas exchange abnormalities, 432–433
    oxygen therapy, with oxygen-enriched air, 433–434t
    pathologic studies of, 427–428
    pathophysiology, of acute respiratory failure, 429–435f
    pulmonary hypertension of, 319
    respiratory muscle fatigue, 430–432
    structure-function correlations, 427–428
    therapeutic implications, of right ventricular failure, 293–295f
    ventilation-perfusion mismatching, 432–435f
    ventilation-perfusion relationship, 407–409f
    weaning and, gas exchange improvement and, 449
Chronic renal failure. (see End-stage renal failure)
Cimetidine
    adverse effects of, 705
    for stress ulcer prophylaxis, 703–704t
    for upper gastrointestinal bleeding, 593–594
Circulation
    effects on ventilation, 482–485t
    failure, 230
        nutritional support for, 68–69
    ventilation and, 473–482f
Cirrhosis, primary peritonitis and, 721
Cisplatin nephrotoxicity, 588–589
Clinical care
    trauma elements of, 193–195f

trauma team response, 194f, 195, 204
Clinical decision making, beneficence and, 196–198f
Clinical outcomes research, 198–200f
Closed-chest cardiac massage
    technique, 504, 507–508
    vs. open chest, 515–517
Clostridium perfringens, 819
Coagulation
    cascade, 805–806f, 811f
    disorders
        in acute renal failure, 596–597
        in sepsis, 102
        of platelets, 808–811
    in acute coronary syndromes, 247
    postoperative support, 366–367t
Coagulation factors analysis, in bleeding, 806–808
Cold agglutinin disease, 818–819
Cold calorics, 762
Cold cardioplegia, 132
Colloid resuscitation
    for adult respiratory distress syndrome, 420–421
    for immunocompromised patient, 104
    for sepsis, 181
    vs. crystalloid, 168
Colonization
    in intensive care unit, 83
    in stomach, gastric pH and, 86
    mechanisms of, in nosocomial pneumonia, 552–554t
Colonization defense
    definition of, 85
    in intensive care unit, 85–86
Community-acquired pneumonia
    clinical evaluation of, 531–533
    definition of, 525
    diagnostic techniques
        bacteriologic noninvasive, 535–537
        invasive, 537–540f
    etiologic agents of, 526–531t
    laboratory evaluation of, 532t
    mortality of, 532t
    pathogenesis of, 525–526
    physical signs of, 532t
    prognostic factors of, 532t
    radiologic examination of, 533–535f
    treatment, 540–542t
    underlying conditions of, 532t
Compartment syndromes, 803
Compensated shock, 164, 165f
Complement activation, adult respiratory distress syndrome and, 416
Compliance, vascular
    cardiac output and, 113
    cardiopulmonary resuscitation and, 509
    total, 113, 143
    venous return and, 142–144f
Compressions
    chest, 503, 504
    interposed abdominal, 513–515
    rate of, in cardiopulmonary resuscitation, 509
Computerized axial tomography
    in endocarditis, 380
    vs. peritoneal lavage, in blunt trauma, 793
Congenital heart disease, endocarditis and, 372
Congestive heart failure, 230
Consciousness, assessment of, 761
Continuous arteriovenous hemofiltration therapy
    accidental disconnection, 666
    anticoagulation for, 659–661

clearances, 650–653f
clinical indications, 661–665t
description of, 646–648f
efficiency and quality of treatment, 654–657f
extracorporeal circuit for, 649–650f
for sepsis, 666–667
hemofilters, 653–654t
in sepsis, 106
maximal urea clearance, 655f
membranes, 650–653f
reinfusion of substitution fluid, 661
risks and complications of, 665–666t
treatment monitoring and automation, 657–659f
ultrafiltration, 650–653f
vascular access for, 648–649f
vs. intermittent hemodialysis, 661t
Continuous high-flux dialysis (CHFD), 656f
Continuous positive airway pressure (CPAP), 419,
449
Continuous venovenous hemofiltration (CVVH),
106, 648. (*see also* Continuous arteriovenous
hemofiltration therapy)
Continuous venovenous hemofiltration with
dialysis (CVVHD), 648. (*see also* Continuous
arteriovenous hemofiltration therapy)
Contractility, ventricular, 16, 141, 289–290
Contrast angiography, of right ventricle
performance, 301–302
Contrast media, for end-stage renal failure, 695
Contrast ventriculography, 330
Convection, 637–638f
Coomb's test, 819
COPD. (*see* Chronic obstructive pulmonary disease)
Copper sulfate ingestion, 819
Cor pulmonale, 294
Cori cycle, 47, 134
Coronary artery disease, morphology of, 247–248f
Coronary circulation, left ventricular performance
and, 220
Coronary heart disease, in end-stage renal failure,
683
Coronary syndromes, acute, 246–247f
Corticosteroids
for acute respiratory failure, in COPD, 441
hyperglycemia and, 887
intracranial pressure reduction and, 757
Corticotropin-releasing hormone (CRH), 902, 904
Cortisol, 27, 904–905
Coumadin, 806–808, 812
Counterimmunoelectrophoresis, 537
CPAP (continuous positive airway pressure), 419,
449
CPP (cerebral perfusion pressure), 741–742
CPR. (*see* Cardiopulmonary resuscitation)
Creatinine, serum, in acute renal failure, 588
Cricothyrotomy, 797–798
Critical illness. (*see also specific aspects of*)
metabolic support for, 73
use of term, 42
withholding or withdrawal of life-sustaining
therapy, 190–192
Cryoprecipitate, 820–821
Cryptococcal infection
in acquired immunodeficiency syndrome, 856–857
post-organ transplant, 844
Crystalloid resuscitation
for adult respiratory distress syndrome, 420–421
for hemorrhagic shock, 163
for sepsis, 181

vs. colloid, 168
CSF. (*see* Cerebrospinal fluid (CSF))
Cushing's response, 767
Cushing's triad, 767
CVP (central venous pressure), 9, 150–151
CVVH (continuous venovenous hemofiltration),
106, 648. (*see also* Continuous arteriovenous
hemofiltration therapy)
CVVHD (continuous venovenous hemofiltration
with dialysis), 648. (*see also* Continuous
arteriovenous hemofiltration therapy)
Cyanide toxicity, 819
Cyclooxygenase inhibitors, 62, 319
Cyclosporin
and graft and patient survival, 839
potassium metabolism and, 606
side effects of, 691
toxicity of, 582
Cystic fibrosis, 531
Cytokine-eicosanoid network, 175–176f
Cytokines
in sepsis syndrome, 178–180
interaction with noncytokine-dependent
pathways, 175
muscle proteolysis and, 27–28
overlapping actions of, 175
Cytomegalovirus infections, posttransplant, 842–843
Cytoprotective agents, 759–760
Cytotoxic brain edema, 746

DDAVP (Desmopressin), 597, 915–916
Dead space to tidal volume ratio, 36
Dead space ventilation, 453
Decerebrate posturing, 763
Decorticate posturing, 763
Defibrillation, 503f, 505f
Definitive care
for blunt trauma, 793–794t
in trauma system, 789–790
Delayed hypersensitivity, 44
Demeclocycline, 772
Dental procedures, endocarditis and, 372–373
Desmopressin (DDAVP), 597, 915–916
Dexamethasone, 748–749, 908
Dextrose
for hypoglycemic coma, 867
for myocardial infarction, 136
hyperglycemia and, 887
isocaloric, 31–32
protein catabolism and, 28, 31
Diabetes insipidus
diagnosis of, 914–915t
therapy for, 915–916
Diabetes mellitus
acute complications of, 863–864
acute renal failure and, 887–888
alcoholic ketoacidosis and, 878–880f
diagnostic errors of, 864
epidemiology of, 863–864
hyperosmolar coma of, 868–871t
hypoglycemia in
clinical manifestations of, 865–866t
complications and sequelae of, 866
pathophysiology of, 864–865
hypoglycemic coma
causes of, 866–867t
prolonged, 868
treatment of, 867–868t
in intensive care unit, 884–888t

Diabetes mellitus—(*continued*)
  insulin-dependent type I, 863
  lactic acidosis and, 881–884*f*
  non-insulin-dependent type II, 863
  surgical considerations for, 886
Diabetic ketoacidosis (DKA)
  causes of, 872
  definition of, 871–872
  epidemiology of, 872
  euglycemic, 875
  evolution of, 876
  hyperosmolar coma and, 869, 870
  laboratory investigations for, 875–876*t*
  pathophysiology, 872–874*f*
  post-DKA phase, 878
  sick day rules, 876
  signs and symptoms of, 874–875
  treatment of, 876–878
    complications of, 878
Dialysis
  acetate, 623–626
  bicarbonate, 626–627
  diffusion and, 636–637*f*
  for end-stage renal failure, complications of,
      689–690
  peritoneal. (*see* Peritoneal dialysis)
  primary peritonitis and, 721–722
  use of term, 636
Dialysis dementia, in end-stage renal failure, 682
Diaphragm fatigue, 430–432
Diaphragm mechanics, in asthma, 492
Diarrhea
  acute disease of, 731–732
  in critically ill patients, 55, 57, 734–737
  management of, in critically ill patient, 736–737
  osmotic, 730
  pathogenic mechanisms for, 730–731
  pathophysiology of, 729–731
  products of, 731
  secondary, 730–731
  toxic megacolon and, 732–734
Diastolic blood pressure, determinants, 8*t*
Diastolic compliance curve, 232
Diastolic ventricular interaction, left ventricular
      performance and, 215–216
DIC (disseminated intravascular coagulation), 808,
      809, 814
Diffusion, in dialysis, 636–637*f*
Diffusion barriers, 136
Digitalis glycosides, 352–353
Digoxin, 294, 352–353
1,25-Dihydroxyvitamin D$_3$, in acute renal failure,
      588, 589
Diltiazem, for unstable angina, 249
2,3-Diphosphoglycerate (2,3-DPG), 364
Direct closed compression, vs. thoracic pump
      model, 507–508*f*
Direct immunofluorescence, of sputum samples, 536
Disseminated candidiasis, 843
Disseminated intravascular coagulation (DIC), 808,
      809, 814
Diuresis
  for diabetic ketoacidosis, 877–878
  for end-stage renal failure, 695
  for left ventricular dysfunction, 294
  for postoperative management, 366
Divalent ions (*see also specific divalent ions*),
      metabolism, pathophysiology of, 607–608
Diverticulitis, in end-stage renal failure, 686

DKA. (*see* Diabetic ketoacidosis (DKA))
Dobutamine
  for ARDS-induced right ventricular failure, 293
  for cardiogenic shock, 153–154
  for low cardiac output, 364–365
  for sepsis syndrome, 181
  mechanism of action, 354
  tissue oxygen extraction and, 117
Doll's eye reflex, 762
Doll's head maneuver, 762
Dopamine
  for cardiogenic shock, 153
  for sepsis control, 105
  in heart failure treatment, 241
  pharmacology of, 354
Dopexamine, pharmacology of, 355
Doppler echocardiography
  of infective endocarditis, 378
  of regurgitant volume, 268–270
  of valve leaks, 266–268*f*
  of valve regurgitation, 264–265*f*
Drug abusers, parenteral, endocarditis in, 374–375
Drugs. (*see also specific drugs*)
  lupus anticoagulant and, 813
  nephrotoxic, for HIV infection, 858–859*t*
  neutropenia and, 816
Duty cycle, 505, 509, 510*f*
Dynamic hyperinflation, 474–475. (*see also* Auto-
      PEEP)
  definition of, 454
  physiologic consequences of, 457–461
Dysoxia, 120, 133, 136
Dysoxic threshold, 136–137
Dysoxyic injury, 136

ECF. (*see* Extracellular fluid (ECF))
ECG. (*see* Electrocardiography (ECG))
Echocardiography
  of cardiac tamponade, 343
  of infective endocarditis, 377–378*f*
  of left ventricular function, 270–271
  of right ventricle performance, 302–303
Edema, peripheral, in endothelial injury, 175
EDRF (endothelium-derived relaxing factor), 357
Edrophonium test (Tensilon test), 782–783
EEG (electroencephalography), 595
Eicosanoids, 180, 730–731
Elastic recoil, 211
Electrocardiography (ECG)
  abnormalities of
    in myxedema coma, 898–899
    in pulmonary embolism, 328–329*t*
    in unstable angina, 245–246
  for V-wave confirmation, 10, 12*f*
  in brain injury, 766
  in myocardial infarction, 250
  in pulmonary hypertension, 328–329*f*
  of acute valve regurgitation, 263
Electroencephalography (EEG), 595
Electrolyte balance
  brain death and, 190
  cellular, 32
  disorders of
    continuous arteriovenous hemofiltration
        therapy for, 664–665
    in acquired immunodeficiency syndrome, 859
    in acute renal failure, 595, 601–608
    in acute respiratory failure, treatment of, 438*f*
    in end-stage renal failure, 686

in lactic acidosis, 883
in sepsis, 105–106
in uremia, 681–682
renal replacement therapy for, 635–636
enteral/parenteral nutrition and, 53–54t
in acute renal failure, 633
Electrolyte replacement therapy
for diabetic ketoacidosis, 877
for hyperosmolar coma, 871
Electromechanical pressure transducer, 4–5, 6–7f
Electromyography (EMG), 431–432
Electrophysiology, of class I antiarrhythmics, 350t
Emax (maximum elastance), 234
Embden-Meyerhof pathway, 25, 29f
Embolectomy, surgical, 332
Emergency room trilogy, of acute valve
regurgitation, 263–264
EMG (electromyography), 431–432
Emotional support and sleep, difficult-to-wean
ARDS patients and, 423
Emphysema, 293, 319
Encephalopathy
hypertensive, hypertension control and, 767
uremic
in end-stage renal failure, 682
in renal failure, 594
End-organ dysfunction, 100t
End-stage renal failure
abdominal complications of, 685–687
clinical picture of, 677, 678t–680t
dialysis treatment, induced complications of,
689–690
drugs for, 693–695t
emergencies following renal transplantation,
690–691
hemostatic complications of, 687
hypercalcemia and, 932
hypocalcemia of, 938, 941–942
infections in, 687, 689
intensive care treatment for, 692–695t
neurologic complications of, 682
parenteral nutrition for, 692–693t
pulmonary complications of, 684–685t
shunt-induced complications of, 690
single organ failure in, 682–689t
End-systolic volume, 144
Endocarditis, infective
acute aortic insufficiency, 275
acute mitral regurgitation and, timing of surgical
repair, 273–275
antimicrobial therapy for, 383–385t
blood cultures of, 376–377
cardiac complications of, 379–380
cardiac surgery, indications for, 381–383t
clinical features of, 376–377
definition of, 376
diagnosis of, 376–379f
end-stage renal failure and, 687, 689
etiology of, 372–376t
extracardiac complications of, 380–381
hospital-acquired, 373
in acquired immunodeficiency syndrome, 858
in parenteral drug abusers, 374–375
management of, 379–381
native valve, in nonaddicts, 372–373
predisposing factors of, 372
prosthetic valve, 375–376t
risk factors for, 372–376t
Staphylococcus aureus, 372

vegetations, antibiotic activity and diffusion into,
383–384
Endocrine dysfunction
in acquired immunodeficiency syndrome, 860
in brain injury, 772
secondary adrenal insufficiency therapy and, 908
Endocrine functions, of heart, 223
Endocrine organ, heart as, 290
Endogenous infection, 82, 84, 87
Endogenous mediators, 178–180
Endogenous nephrotoxins, 572
Endothelial-dependent vasodilation, 357
Endothelin, 223
Endothelium-derived relaxing factor (EDRF), 357
Endotoxemia, in septic shock, 178
Endotoxin, Gram-negative, 171–172
Endotracheal tube extubation, timing for, 451
Energy expenditure, 45, 46t
Energy supply, substrate preference for, 47–50f
Energy transfer, between ventricle and aorta, 235
Enoximone
for heart failure, 242–243
pharmacology of, 355–356
Enteral nutrition
contraindications for, 57
diarrhea from, 735
electrolytes and, 53–54t
energy supply adjustments, 58–59
formulas, classification of, 57f
hormonal manipulations, 61–62
immediate postoperative, 54, 56f
immunological manipulations, 61–62
intolerance to, 57
nitrogen substrate preference and, 51–53f
protein and, 33
vs. intravenous administration, 24
vs. parenteral nutrition, 54–58f
Enterocolitis in end-stage renal failure, 686
Enterotoxin, diarrhea and, 730
Enzymes, cardiac, in unstable angina, 246
Eosinophilia, 816–817
Eosinophils, 815
Epidermal growth factor, 62
Epinephrine
catabolic rate and, 27
for anaphylactic shock, 157
for cardiopulmonary resuscitation, 518–519
for sepsis syndrome, 181
in heart failure treatment, 241
lipolysis and, 25
pharmacology of, 354
Esophageal surgery, SDD for, 91
Esophagus
infections of, 696–697
perforation of, 697–698
Ethics, withdrawal or withholding of life-support,
190–193
Euthyroid sick, evaluation of, 895
Evoked potentials, sensory, of brain injury, 764
Exercise, difficult-to-wean ARDS patients and,
422–423
Exogenous infection, 82, 84, 87
Exploratory laparotomy, 803
Extracellular fluid (ECF)
calcium balance and, 925–926f
sodium balance and, 601
Extracorporeal membrane oxygenation, for adult
respiratory distress syndrome, 424
Extrinsic coagulation pathway, 805–806

Eye movements, in unconscious patients, 762*f*

Facial fractures, 798
Factor concentrate, 821–822
Factor IX concentrate, 813
Factor VII deficiency, 806–807
Factor VIII deficiency, 807
False hypercalcemia, 932
Familial hypocalciuria-hypercalcemia, 927–928
Fanconi's syndrome, 590
Fat emulsions, intravenous, free fatty acids and, 69
Fat metabolism, diabetic ketoacidosis and, 873–874*f*
Fever
  in granulocytopenia, 836
  in immunocompromised patients, 831–833
  in kidney dialysis, 689
FFP (fresh frozen plasma), 820–821
Fiberoptic bronchoscopy, for diagnosis of
      community-acquired pneumonia, 538–540*f*
Fiberoptic intubation, 796
Fibrinolysis, primary, 808
Fick equation, 16, 17
Fick principle, 392
Fitz-Hugh and Curtis syndrome, 722
5-2 rule, 150–151
Flail chest, 504
Fluid balance
  continuous arteriovenous hemofiltration therapy
      and, 668
  in hypovolemic shock, 165–166*f*
  management of, in acute renal failure, 631–632
Fluid lung, in end-stage renal failure, 684–685
Fluid overload, 661, 662*f*, 666
Fluid retention
  in weaning, 450–451
  nutritional assessment and, 43–44
Fluid therapy
  difficult-to-wean ARDS patients and, 423
  for Addisonian crisis, 908
  for adult respiratory distress syndrome, 420–421
  for brain dead patient, 190
  for brain injury, 767–768
  for diabetic ketoacidosis, 876–877
  for hyperosmolar coma, 871
  for hypovolemic shock, 167–168
  in hemorrhagic shock, 150–151
  in pulmonary embolism in RV failure, 298
Focal segmental glomerulosclerosis (FSGS), 858–859
Force, applied in cardiopulmonary resuscitation,
      510–512*f*
Forward failure, 231
Frank-Starling law, 210
FRC (functional residual capacity), 320, 474, 487
Free fatty acids, 48, 69
Free radical scavengers, 760
Fresh frozen plasma (FFP), 820–821
Functional residual capacity (FRC), 320, 474, 487
Fungal infections
  antibiotic therapy for, 107–108
  community-acquired pneumonia, 530
  drug addiction and, 375
  granulocytopenia of, 835
  posttransplant, 843–844
Furosemide, 132

Gallbladder inflammation, 718–719
Gallium scans, in infective endocarditis, 378–379
Gallstones, with pancreatitis, 727
Ganciclovir, 843

Gas exchange
  blood flow and, 482–484*t*
  failure of, 389
  in acute renal failure, 592
  in adult respiratory distress syndrome, 395–399*f*
  in asthma, 436
  in cerebral resuscitation, 768–769
  in chronic obstructive pulmonary disease,
      432–433
  in pulmonary hypertension, 327
  in weaning, improvement of, 448–450
Gastric pH
  colonization in stomach and, 86
  nosocomial pneumonia and, 553–554*t*, 706
  pulmonary infections and, 706
  stress ulcer prophylaxis and, 706–710*f*
Gastritis, uremic, in end-stage renal failure, 685–686
Gastrointestinal bleeding. (*see also* Stress ulcer(s))
  in acute renal failure, 593–594
  in brain injury, 772
  in end-stage renal failure, 685–686
  incidence, in stress ulceration, 711
  risk factors for, 702
Gastrointestinal inhibitory polypeptide, 593
Gastrointestinal system
  in acquired immunodeficiency syndrome, 859–860
  in acute renal failure, 593–594
  in sepsis, 102
  lesions, endocarditis and, 373
  manifestations, in thyrotoxic storm, 896
  procedures, endocarditis and, 373
  support of, in sepsis, 106
Glasgow Coma Scale, 763*t*, 771, 791*t*, 802–803*t*
Glomerular filtration rate, reduction in acute renal
      failure, 577–579
Glucagon, 27
Glucocorticoids
  effects of, 904–905
  for Addisonian crisis, 908
  for hypercalcemia, 934
  for secondary adrenal insufficiency, 908
  pathway, 902, 903*f*
  secretion, regulation of, 902, 904
  TSH secretion and, 891
Glucocorticosteroids, side effects of, 691
Glucogenic amino acids, 25
Glucose
  blood levels
    in alcoholic ketoacidosis, 878–879
    in diabetic ketoacidosis, 875
  hepatocytic conversion to lipid, 35
  metabolic abnormalities, in acquired
      immunodeficiency syndrome, 860
  oxidation, 48
  oxidative phosphorylation and, 25
  preferential oxidation of, 28
Glutamine
  in postaggression conditions, 59–60
  intestinal infusion and, 136
  muscle proteolysis and, 28, 58
Goblet cell metaplasia, 428
Gram-negative bacteria, 82, 89, 667
Gram-negative rod pneumonia, in community-
      acquire pneumonia, 529
Gram-positive cocci endocarditis, antibiotic therapy
      for, 383–385*t*
Gram-stained smears, of sputum, 536–537
Granulocyte abnormalities, in acute renal failure,
      597–598

Granulocyte colony stimulating factor, 838
Granulocyte transfusion, 821
Granulocytopenia, management of, 834–838*t*
Granulomatous diseases, hypercalcemia of, 930
Graves disease, 896
Growth factors, 62
Growth hormone, 62, 164
Guillain-Barré syndrome, 781, 784–785
Gut failure, enteral nutrition and, 57
Gut hypothesis, 99
Gut motility, abnormal, colonization and, 86
Guyton's venous return curve, 232–233*f*

HA-1A, for adult respiratory distress syndrome, 424–425
Hard water syndrome, 689
Harris-Benedict formula, 34–35
Head and neck cancer, SDD for, 91
Head position, intracranial pressure and, 753, 756
Head trauma, 802–803*t*
Health care costs, 193
Health care quality, reevaluation of, 193
Health Evaluation through Logical Processing (HELP)
  input information overload and, 200–203*f*
  protocol development methods, 198–200*f*
Heart. (*see also cardiac entries*)
  abnormalities of
    in acquired immunodeficiency syndrome, 857–858
    in central nervous system injury, 765–767
  as endocrine organ, 290
  autocrine functions of, 223
  blood flow in, 504
  coupling with arterial circulation, 236–239*f*
  endocrine functions of, 223
  enlargement, 342. (*see also* Cardiac tamponade)
  function of, variables in, 141
  paracrine functions of, 223
Heart block, endocarditis and, 379–380
Heart catheterization
  left-sided, 271–272
  of acute valve regurgitation, 271–272
  right-sided, 271, 303–304*f*, 344
Heart disease
  nutritional support for, 68–69
  structural, alteration of classic cardiac tamponade and, 340
Heart failure
  backward, 231
  definition of, 230
  etiologies, pathophysiologic classification of, 230*t*, 231*t*
  forward, 231
  nitroprusside for, 242
  signs, acute vs. chronic, 231
  treatment
    pathophysiologic rationale for, 231–239*f*
    vasodilators for, 242–243
    ventricular performance and, 231–236*f*
    ventriculoarterial coupling and, 236–239*t*
Heart-lung interactions. (*see* Cardiopulmonary system, interactions)
Heart-lung transplantation patients, infections of, 838–846*t*
  in early posttransplant period, 840
Heart murmur, in mitral regurgitation, 262
Heart rate
  cardiac function and, 141

  changes in, 157
  left ventricular performance and, 220
Heart transplantation
  postoperative infections of, 838–846*t*
  postoperative period, 367–368
HELP (Health Evaluation through Logical Processing)
  input information overload and, 200–203*f*
  protocol development methods, 198–200*f*
Hematocrit, elevated, causes of, 817
Hematology disorders
  hypercalcemia and, 929
  in acquired immunodeficiency syndrome, 860
  in acute renal failure, 596–597
  in sepsis, 102
Hemodiafiltration, 642*f*, 643–644
Hemodialysis. (*see also* Intermittent hemodialysis)
  hemolysis and, 819
  immunologic function and, 598
  technique, 642–643*f*
Hemodilution, 757–758
Hemodynamics
  continuous arteriovenous hemofiltration therapy and, 668
  determinants of, in sepsis syndrome, 170–175
  in pulmonary hypertension, 327*f*
  management of, in sepsis, 108
  monitoring
    goals of, 3–4*t*
    history of, 3
    of blood flow, 12–16
    of blood pressure. (*see* Blood pressure, monitoring)
    of brain death, 190
    of oxygen transport, 16–21*f*, 17*t*
  of acute renal failure, 578
  of aortic insufficiency, 272
  of classic cardiac tamponade, 338–340*f*
  of intrathoracic pressure changes, 475–477*f*
  of lung volume changes, 473–475*f*
  of ventilation, 479–482*t*
  right ventricle role in, 284–286
  supportive care, in asthma, 500
  variables of, 15*t*
  vasodilation effects, 358–359*f*
Hemofilters, 653–654*t*
Hemofiltration, 627, 642*f*, 643
Hemoglobin, 17, 612–613
Hemolysis
  diagnosis of, 819–820
  drug-induced, 819
Hemolytic uremic syndrome, 809–810
Hemophilia A, 807, 813
Hemophilia B, 807, 813
Hemophilus influenzae, in community-acquired pneumonia, 526–527, 529
Hemorrhage
  gastrointestinal. (*see* Gastrointestinal bleeding)
  in trauma, 798–799
Hemorrhagic shock
  categories of, 163
  clinical manifestations of, 163
  pathophysiology of, 149–152, 161
  treatment goals for, 163
  uptake phase of, 166–167
Hemostatic abnormalities, transtracheal aspiration and, 538
Hemostatic complications, in end-stage renal failure, 687

Hemothorax, 799
Henderson-Hasselbalch equation, 610
Heparin
    after thrombolysis, 253–254
    for acute respiratory failure, in chronic
        obstructive pulmonary disease, 439
    for pulmonary embolus, 331–332
    for unstable angina, 249
    prolonged PTT and, 807–808
    thrombocytopenia of, 809
Hepatic encephalopathy, 33, 66
Hepatic failure, nutritional support for, 66–68
Hepatic gluconeogenesis, 28
Hepatobiliary disease, in acute renal failure, 594
Hepatocellular dysfunction, 99
Hepatorenal syndrome, 582
Hering-Breuer reflex, 223
Herpes simplex virus infections
    posttransplant, 840
    ulcerative esophagitis, 696
Herpetic esophagitis, 696
High risk surgical groups, SDD for, 91–92
Histamine-2-receptor antagonists
    adverse effects of, 705
    for stress ulcer prophylaxis, efficacy of, 702–705t
Histidine deficiency syndrome, 66
Homeostatic mechanisms, 163
Homocystinuria, thrombosis and, 813
Hormonal replacement therapy, for Addisonian
        crisis, 908
Hormones. (see also specific hormones)
    brain death and, 190
    responses to acute hypovolemia, 164–165f
Host defense mechanisms
    age extremes and, 85
    cellular, 825–826
    description of, 823–826t
    humoral-mediated, 825–826
    immunocompromised. (see Immunocompromised
        patients)
    in lung, 525–526
    invasive instrumentation and, 85
    nature of disease, colonization defense and, 85
Human immunodeficiency virus I (HIV-I)
    acquired immunodeficiency syndrome and, 851.
        (see also Acquired immunodeficiency
        syndrome (AIDS))
    renal dysfunction and, 858–859
    RNA genome, 851–852
Human immunodeficiency virus II (HIV-II), 851
Human monoclonal antiendotoxin antibody
        (HA-1A), 838
Humoral hypercalcemia of malignancies, 928–929
Humoral immunity, 825–826
Hydralazine, 294, 330–331
ß-Hydroxybutyrate, 58, 879
ß-Hydroxybutyrate/acetoacetate ratio, 135
Hyperamylasemia, in acute renal failure, 594
Hyperbilirubinemia, in acute renal failure, 594
Hypercalcemia
    disorders of, 933t
    false, 932
    familial benign, 927–928
    idiopathic, of infancy, 932
    in acute renal failure, 589, 607–608
    in renal failure, 932
    in thyrotoxicosis, 929–930
    malignancies and, 928–929
    mechanisms of, 925–926f

    of vitamin A intoxication, 931
    of vitamin D intoxication, 930–931
    primary hyperparathyroidism and, 926–928f
    total parenteral nutrition and, 932
    treatment of, 933–936t
        by calciuretic measures, 933
        by pharmacologic inhibition of bone resorption,
            934–935
        drugs for, 935t
        maintenance therapy, 935–936
        urgent therapy, 935
Hypercapnia
    in asthma, 496
    in heart failure, 231
    treatment of, 366
Hypercapnic respiratory failure, predisposing
        factors, 427
Hypercarbia, in brain injury, 770
Hypercatabolism, in acute renal failure, 587
Hyperdynamic shock, 20
Hyperemia, 744t
Hypergastrinemia, in acute renal failure, 593
Hyperglycemia
    diabetes mellitus and, 864
    diagnosis of, 875
    false diagnosis of, 887
    in aggression, 47
    in brain injury, 771
    in diabetes mellitus, 886–887
    in hypovolemia, 164
    in renal failure, 66
    management of, in diabetic ketoacidosis, 876
    postinsult, 48
Hyperglycemic drugs, 887
Hyperglycemic glucose clamp technique, 47f
Hyperhydration, in end-stage renal failure, 684–685
Hyperinflation
    auto-PEEP with, 457
    dynamic
        detrimental effects on respiratory muscles,
            458–459f
        hemodynamic importance of, 459–460
        monitoring cardiac and ventilatory function in,
            461f
        panic cycle and, 460–461f
    prevention of, 485–486
Hyperinsulinemia, postinsult, 48
Hyperkalemia
    aldosterone and, 904
    causes of, 606
    clinical manifestations of, 606–607
    in uremia, 681–682
Hypermagnesemia, in acute renal failure, 590,
        607–608
Hypermetabolic syndrome, nutritional and
        metabolic recommendations, 54t
Hypermetabolism, in brain injury, 771–772
Hypernatremia
    in hyperosmolar coma, 870
    in uremia, 681
    treatment of, 605
Hyperosmolar coma
    causes of, 868–869t
    evolution of, 870–871
    hyperglycemic nonketotic coma phase of, 870
    laboratory investigations of, 870
    pathophysiology of, 869, 870t
    prodromal phase of, 869–870
    signs and symptoms of, 869–870

treatment of, 871
Hyperparathyroidism
  primary
    hypercalcemia and, 926–928f
    manifestations of, 927t
  secondary, hypocalcemia of, 938
Hyperphosphatemia
  hypocalcemia of, 938
  in acute renal failure, 589, 607
  in chronic renal failure, treatment of, 941–942
Hypertension
  after cerebral injury, 767
  iatrogenic, 757–758
  in end-stage renal failure, 684
  in pheochromocytoma, 917–918
    preoperative control of, 919–921f
  postoperative, 365
  spontaneous, after brain injury, 769
  systolic, 8
Hyperthyroidism
  diagnosis of, 895
  thyrotoxic storm, 895–897
Hyperventilation, iatrogenic, intracranial pressure
    reduction and, 756
Hypervolemia, in uremia, 677, 681
Hypervolemic hyponatremia, 913t
Hypoalbuminemia, 104
Hypocalcemia
  clinical manifestations of, 936t
  in acute renal failure, 588–589, 607–608
  in hypoparathyroidism, 936–937
  in pseudohypoparathyroidism, 937t
  mechanisms of, 936
  neonatal, 937
  nonparathyroid types of, 938–939, 940t
  treatment of, 939–942t
Hypocarbia, spontaneous, after brain injury,
    769
Hypodynamic shock
  hemodynamic manifestations of, 20
  low cardiac output of, 20
Hypoglycemia
  diagnosis of, 864
  in diabetes mellitus, 864
    clinical manifestations of, 865–866t
    pathophysiology of, 864–865
  in myxedema coma, 899
  pancreas and, 25
Hypoglycemic coma
  causes of, 866–867t
  prolonged, 868
  treatment of, 867–868t
Hypokalemia, in uremia, 682
Hypomagnesemia, 366, 590
Hyponatremia
  causes of, 601–602t
  clinical euvolemic, diagnosis of, 912–913
  clinical manifestations of, 603–604
  hypervolemic, diagnosis of, 913t
  hypovolemic, diagnosis of, 913t
  in acute primary adrenal insufficiency, 906
  in acute renal failure
    clinical manifestations of, 603–604
    treatment of, 604–605t
  in brain injury, 772
  in uremia, 681
Hyponatremic hypoosmolar syndromes, 772
Hypoparathyroidism, hypocalcemia of, 936–937t
  treatment of, 940–941t

Hypoperfusion, systemic inflammatory response
    and, 161
Hypophosphatemia, 364, 589–590
  from continuous arteriovenous hemofiltration
    therapy, 666
Hypotension
  hypovolemia and, 603
  in blunt trauma, 792
  in brain injury, 767–768
  in end-stage renal failure, 684
  in myxedema coma, 899
  in septic shock, 100
  management of, 157
  of intermittent hemodialysis, 644–645f
Hypothalamic-pituitary thyroid axis, normal
    function of, 891–892
Hypothermia
  cerebral oxygen consumption and, 747
  from continuous arteriovenous hemofiltration
    therapy, 666
  in myxedema coma, 898, 899
Hypothyroidism
  diagnosis of, 895
  primary, 892
Hypovolemia
  acute, hormonal responses to, 164–165f
  in pheochromocytoma, 920
  normal response to, 163–164
Hypovolemic hyponatremia, 913t
Hypovolemic shock
  activators of, 161–162f
  cellular changes of, 165–166f
  definition of, 162
  fluid shifts in, 165–166f
  hemorrhagic. (*see* Hemorrhagic shock)
  irreversible stage of, 166–167
  pharmacologic interventions for, 152
  treatment of, 167–168
Hypoxanthine, 739
Hypoxemia, in asthma, 436, 496
Hypoxemic respiratory failure, acute
  associated conditions, 414–415t
  causes of, 414
  etiology of, 414–415t
  of adult respiratory distress syndrome. (*see* Adult
    respiratory distress syndrome)
  pathophysiology of, 415–416
Hypoxia
  calcium reuptake and, 212
  cellular responses, 112
  left ventricular performance and, 223
  pulmonary vasoconstriction and, 317t
  vasoconstriction and, 140
Hypoxic pulmonary parenchymal failure, weaning
    from respiratory support, pathophysiology
    of, 447–448

Iatrogenic hypotension, in brain injury, 767
ICP. (*see* Intracranial pressure (ICP))
Idiogenic osmoles, 603
Idiopathic hypercalcemia of infancy, 932
Idiopathic thrombocytopenic purpura, 809
Ileus, in end-stage renal failure, 686
Imidazoles, 108
Immobilization, hypercalcemia and, 931–932
Immune response, suppression, 182
Immune thrombocytopenia, 821
Immunocompromised patients
  categories of, 825–826t

Immunocompromised patients—(*continued*)
  diagnostic approach, 826–834*t*
  evaluation
    of fever, 831–833
    of pulmonary infiltrates, 831–833*t*
    of suspected central nervous system infection, 833–834*t*
  granulocytopenic, management of, 834–836*t*
  infections of organ transplant recipients, 838–846
  initial evaluation, database for, 827*t*
  laboratory tests for ICU admission, 830*t*
  opportunistic pulmonary infections of, diagnosis of, 539
  symptoms of common infectious etiologies, 829*t*
  with granulocytopenia, antibiotic therapy for, 836–838*t*
Immunosuppressant drugs, side effects of, 691
Immunosuppression
  endocarditis risk and, 374
  for renal transplantation, complications of, 691
  postoperative, 368
  with concomitant infection, 845–846
IMV (intermittent mandatory ventilation), 449–450
Inactivation system, 210
Indicator dilution technology, 12–13*f*
Indium scans, in infective endocarditis, 378–379
Indocyanine green dye dilution method, 12
Infections
  adaptation, 63*f*
  after renal transplantation, 691
  anatomic barriers to, 823–825*t*
  causality of, 178
  concomitant, immunosuppressive therapy for, 845–846
  from continuous arteriovenous hemofiltration therapy, 666
  Gram-negative, 178
  in end-stage renal failure, 687, 689
  neutropenia and, 816
  of central nervous system, in immunocompromised patients, 833–834*t*
  posttransplant, 840–842
  rate of, in traditionally managed ICUs, 84–86
  vs. sepsis, 170
Infectious agents
  common, 825
  hemolysis and, 819
Infectious complications, in acute renal failure, 597–598
Inferior vena cava, plethora, in cardiac tamponade, 343
Inflammation
  products of, 731
  signs of, 836
Inflammatory proteins, 50
Inflammatory response
  blocking, for sepsis management, 181
  in sepsis, 183
Injury(ies)
  energy expenditure and, 45–46*f*
  initial period of, 42
  protein catabolism and, 45–46*f*
  response phases of, 161
  with hepatic failure, nutritional support for, 67
Inotropic agents
  ß-adrenergic agonists, 353–355
  digitalis glycosides, 352–353
  for adult respiratory distress syndrome, 421
  for cardiac tamponade, 345
  for right heart failure, 332

  phosphodiesterase inhibitors, 355–356
Inotropic agents, mechanisms of action, cellular, 352, 353*f*
Insect bites, hematologic disorders of, 819
Inspiratory pressure support, in weaning, 450
Insulin, blood
  in normal starvation, 25–26
  in stressed starvation, 27
  lipoprotein lipase and, 29
Insulin clamp technique, 31
Insulin deficiency
  absolute, diabetic ketoacidosis and, 872
  relative, diabetic ketoacidosis and, 872
Insulin resistance, 47, 66
Insulin therapy
  for diabetes mellitus, in intensive care unit, 884–886*t*
  for diabetic ketoacidosis, 877
  for hyperosmolar coma, 871
  for myocardial infarction, 136
Intensive care units (ICUs)
  clinical decision making process of, 196–198*f*
  colonization defense in, 85–86
  colonization in, 83
  design of, for prevention of nosocomial pneumonia, 565
  diabetic patients in, 884–888*t*
  diarrhea in critically ill patients, 734–737
  end-stage renal failure treatment in, 692–695*t*
  infection control measures, 82
  infection in, 83–84
  infection rate in, 82
  nosocomial pneumonia incidence in, 545–547*t*
  rationale for SDD usage, 86–87
  SDD trials, 88–90
  sepsis in, 84
  survival, of AIDS patients, 860–861
  traditionally managed, colonization and infection rates in, 84–86
Interleukin-1
  acute phase response and, 771
  in diarrheal disorders, 731
  in sepsis syndrome, 179
  muscle proteolysis and, 27–28
  properties and interactions of, 176*t*
Interleukin-6, 176*t*, 179
Interleukin-8, 176*t*, 179
Interleukin-9, 176*t*
Intermittent hemodialysis
  anticoagulation for, 642
  biocompatibility, 644
  complications, 644–646*t*
  dialysate composition, 644
  efficiency and prescription, 643*f*, 644
  for acid-base disorders in acute renal failure, 623–627
  techniques for, 642–644*f*
  vascular access for, 641–642
  vs. continuous arteriovenous hemofiltration therapy, 661*t*
Intermittent mandatory ventilation (IMV), 449–450
Interposed abdominal compressions, 513–515
Interstitial brain edema, 746
Interstitial pneumonia, 534, 535*f*
Intestines
  absorption process of, 729
  mechanical obstruction of, 716–717
  secretion of, 729–730
Intraabdominal abscesses, 724

Intraaortic balloon pump, for cardiogenic shock, 153
Intraaortic counterpulsation, aortic regurgitation and, 273
Intracerebral steal syndrome, 742
Intracranial hematomas, 761
Intracranial hemorrhage, hypertension control and, 767
Intracranial hypertension, 745
Intracranial pressure (ICP)
  compliance, 744–745
  decreasing, therapeutic measures for, 753, 755–757t
  increased, 741–742f
  monitoring of, 745–746
  regulation of, 744–745
Intrathoracic pressure (ITP), 473, 475–477f, 486–488
Intravenous lipid emulsions, 32–33
Intravenous nutrition, hepatic parenchymal abnormalities and, 24
Intrinsic coagulation pathway, 805
Intubation
  fiberoptic, 796
  in cerebral resuscitation, 769–770
  nasotracheal, 795–796, 797f
  of trauma patients, 794–795t
  stabilized oral endotracheal, 795, 796f
  standard oral, 796
Inverse ratio ventilation (IRV), 200–203F
Iodine contrast medias, for end-stage renal failure, 695
Ionic channels, vasoregulation and, 357
Iron deficiency anemia, 818
Irreversible shock, 164–165f, 166–167
Ischemia, calcium reuptake and, 212
Ischemic brain edema, 746
Ischemic heart disease, acute mitral regurgitation and, timing of surgical repair, 275
Ischemic penumbra, 747
Isoproterenol, 241–242, 355
Isosorbide dinitrate, 248
ITP (intrathoracic pressure), 473, 486–488

Jaundice, in acute renal failure, 594
Jejunostomy "a minima" technique, 54, 56f
Jugular venous oxygen saturation, monitoring of, 747

Ketanserin, 403
Ketoacidosis, 25, 864. (*see also* Alcoholic ketoacidosis; Diabetic ketoacidosis (DKA))
α-Ketoisocaproate, 51
Ketone bodies, 26, 873–874f, 883
Ketonuria, 25
Kidney(s). (*see also renal entries*)
  buffering response of, 618
  diseases of
    coagulation disorders and, 808
    platelet dysfunction and, 811
  dysfunction of, in acquired immunodeficiency syndrome, 858–859t
  failure. (*see* Renal failure, acute; End-stage renal failure)
  functions of, 586, 610
    in sepsis, 101
  hypoperfusion, in acute renal failure, 577–579
  nonmuscular variable oxygen demand and, 129–131f
  postoperative support, 366t
  rejection of, after renal transplantation, 691
  rupture, after renal transplantation, 691
  support, for sepsis, 105–106
Kidney transplantation
  acute renal failure in, 581–582
  postoperative infections of, 838–846t
Klebsiella outbreak, SDD and, 90–91
Kupffer cells, 99, 108
Kupfferian hepatic steatosis, 48
Kussmaul's sign, 328f, 344
Kwashiorkor, 25

Labetalol, 919–920
ß-Lactam antibiotics
  for endocarditis, 383–385
  for granulocytopenia, 836–837
Lactate
  elimination of, 881–882f
  excess, consequences of, 883
  production of, 881f
Lactic acid, 19, 20, 739
Lactic acidosis
  classification of, 882t
  focal ischemia and, 134
  in asthma, 436
  in diabetes mellitus, 864
  in diabetic ketoacidosis, 874
  laboratory investigations of, 883
  oxygen consumption and, 19–21
  pathophysiology of, 881–882f
  signs and symptoms of, 883
  treatment of, 883–884
Lactose ingestion, in lactase-deficient subjects, 730
Landry-Guillain-Barré syndrome, 784–785
Laparotomy, 181, 717
Large bowel obstruction, 717
Latex agglutination techniques, 537
LCT (long-chain triglycerides), 48, 59
Le Fort fractures, 798
Lead poisoning, 818
Lean body mass, 24
Left-sided heart catheterization
  in acute aortic regurgitation, 272
  in acute mitral regurgitation, 272
  indications for, 271–272
Left ventricle
  after, intrathoracic pressure changes and, 477
  afterload, left ventricular performance and, 218–220
  contraction of, 217
  ejected blood volume of, 15
  failure. (*see* Left ventricular failure)
  function
    echocardiographic assessment, 270–271
    increased pulmonary artery pressure and, 321
    geometry, during pulmonary hypertension, 327f
    hypertrophy, 221
    mechanical efficiency of, 219–220f
    passive properties of, 213–215f
    performance. (*see* Left ventricular performance)
  preload
    in asthma, 495
    intrathoracic pressure changes and, 476–477
  relaxation load of, 210–211
  viscoelastic properties of, 215
Left ventricle end-systolic volume, 142
Left ventricular ejection, intrathoracic pressure changes and, 476
Left ventricular ejection fraction, 100–101
Left ventricular end-diastolic pressure, 9

Left ventricular failure
 digitalis glycosides for, 352–353
 treatment
  by volume loading, 240–242
  general considerations of, 239–240
  vasodilators for, 242–243
  ventriculoarterial coupling and, 236–239t
Left ventricular filling
 factors, 216t
 left ventricular performance and, 209–210
Left ventricular performance
 afterload and, 281
 definition of, 209
 determinants
  afterload, 218–220
  atrial contraction and, 215
  cardiac-lung interaction and, 216
  coronary circulation, 220
  diastolic ventricular interaction and, 215–216
  heart rate, 220
  left ventricular contraction, 217
  left ventricular filling and preload, 209–217f
  left ventricular hypertrophy, 221
  myocardial contractility, 217
  myocardial perfusion, 220
  neurohormonal and hormonal interactions,
   221–224
  pericardium and, 215–216
  preload, 209–210
  rapid filling and, 210–213f
  relaxation and, 210–213f, 214f
  systolic ventricular interaction, 220–221
  ventriculoarterial coupling, 218–220f
  vs. right ventricular performance determinants,
   280–281
 myocardial contractility and, 280
 preload and, 280–281
 representation of, 224f
Legionella infections, posttransplant, 841–842
Legionella pneumonia, 532t
Legionella sp., in community-acquired pneumonia,
 529
Legionnaires' disease, 535, 536
Leucine, 51
Leukocyte intercellular adhesion molecule
 (ICAM-1), 175
Leukocyte-reduced red blood cells, for transfusion,
 820
Leukoencephalopathy, in acquired
 immunodeficiency syndrome, 857
Leukotrienes, 180
Lidocaine, toxicity of, 365
Life-sustaining therapy, withholding or withdrawal
 of, 190–192
Lipid emulsions, 48
Lipid infusion, PMN chemotaxis and, 49f
Lipids
 hepatocytic conversion from glucose, 35
 metabolism of
  during stress, 32–33
  in hepatic failure, 67–68
  normal, 28–30f
  postinsult, 48
 supply adjustments, for enteral and parenteral
  nutrition, 59, 60f
Lipolysis, 25, 42
Lipooxygenase products, 180
Lipoprotein lipase, 29
Lipoprotein X, 67

Listeria monocytogenes infections, posttransplant, 841
Lithium therapy, hypercalcemia and, 931
Liver
 end-stage disease, 99
 failure, nutritional support for, 66–68
 function of, in sepsis, 102
 hemostasis and, 808
Liver function tests
 in sepsis, 106
 septic state and, 99
Liver transplantation
 postoperative infections of, 838–846t
 SDD for, 91
Lobar pneumonia, 534f
Long-chain triglycerides (LCT), 48, 59
Loop diuretics, 631
Lumbar puncture, for central nervous system
 infection, 833
Lung
 defenses against infection, 525–526
 fluid accumulation, in end-stage renal failure,
  684–685
 function of, in sepsis, 101
 vascular injuries of, pulmonary hypertension
  and, 319
Lung compliance, in adult respiratory distress
 syndrome, 417
Lung volumes
 changes, hemodynamics, 473–475f
 end-expiratory, 487
 in asthma, 435–436
 pulmonary vascular resistance and, in adult
  respiratory distress syndrome, 291–292
Lupus anticoagulant, 807, 813
Lusitropy, 213, 214f
Luxury perfusion, 744t
Lymphocytes, 815, 825
Lymphokines, 825
Lymphomas, hypercalcemia and, 929

M-mode echocardiography, of valve regurgitation,
 264–265f
Macrophage inhibitory protein (MIP), 176t
Magnesium, abnormalities of, in renal failure, 590
Magnesium therapy, for hypocalcemia, 942
Magnetic resonance imaging, of brain injury, 764
Magnetic resonance spectroscopy, for cerebral
 metabolism monitoring, 747
Malignancies, cardiac tamponade and, 341
Mallory-Weiss syndrome, 697
Malnutrition
 in respiratory failure, 62–64
 preoperative support for, 70
Mannitol, intracranial pressure reduction and, 756
Marasmus, 25
Marfan's syndrome, 372
MAST (military antishock trousers), 168
MCT (medium-chain triglyceride), 32–33, 48, 59
Mean circulatory filling pressure, 113–114
Mean pulmonary arterial pressure (MPAP), 64
Mean right atrial pressure (MRAP), 329
Mean systemic pressure, 143–144
Mechanical trauma, hemolysis and, 819
Mechanical ventilation
 continuous arteriovenous hemofiltration therapy
  and, 667–668
 for adult respiratory distress syndrome, 419–420
  right ventricular failure and, 291–292
 for asthma, 498–500f

for brain dead patient, 190
for COPD-induced right ventricular failure, 294–295
in airway obstruction, 462
in cerebral resuscitation, 769–770
partial, for airway obstruction, 463–468f
patient-ventilator interface, 485–488t
positive end-expiratory pressure. (*see* Positive end-expiratory pressure)
weaning. (*see* Weaning)
withdrawal or withholding of, 190–193
Mechanoreceptors, 223
Medial longitudinal fasciculus (MLF), 762f
Mediators
antagonism of, 182–183
endogenous, 178–180
exogenous, 178
of hypoxic pulmonary vasoconstriction, 317t
pulmonary circulation regulation and, 316
Medical care costs, reevaluation of, 193
Medical practice
content of, 195–196
process of, 196–198f
standardization, impact of, 203–205f
Medium-chain triglyceride (MCT), 32–33, 48, 59
Metabolic acidosis
alcoholic ketoacidosis, 878–880f
compensatory responses, 619, 620t
in asthma, 496–497
in uremia, 681
treatment of, 437
with acute renal failure, 621
Metabolic alkalosis
compensatory responses, 619, 620t
treatment of, in acute renal failure, 622–623
with acute renal failure, 621
Metabolic disorders. (*see also specific disorders*)
in chronic obstructive pulmonary disease, treatment of, 437–438f
Metabolic theory of microvascular control, 114–115
Metabolism, postoperative support and, 366t
Methemoglobinemia, 819
Methoxamine
for cardiopulmonary resuscitation, 518
tissue oxygen extraction and, 117
Methylxanthines
diaphragmatic contractility and, 440
for acute respiratory failure, in COPD, 440
Microbial resistance, SDD and, 90
Microorganisms
in nosocomial pneumonia, 548–550t
in septic shock, 176
Microvascular consequences, of septic shock, 174–175
Mid-arm muscle circumference, 37
MIGET (multiple inert gas elimination technique), 394–395, 398
Migratory thrombophlebitis, 813
Military antishock trousers (MAST), 168
Milk alkali syndrome, hypercalcemia of, 931
Milrinone, pharmacology of, 355
Mineralocorticoids
effects of, 905
for Addisonian crisis, 908
pathway, 902, 903f
secretion of, 904
Minute ventilation, 36f, 429
MIP (macrophage inhibitory protein), 176t
Mithramycin, for hypercalcemia, 934

Mitral valve disorders
leaks, 266–267f
postoperative care for, 369
prolapse, 275
endocarditis and, 372
regurgitation
clinical examination of, 262–263
diagnosis of, 262
left-sided heart catheterization findings, 272
quantitation of regurgitant volume, 268–270
timing of surgical repair, 273–275
transthoracic approach, 265–267f
transthoracic echocardiography of, 264
MLF (medial longitudinal fasciculus), 762f
MOF. (*see* Multiple organ failure (MOF))
Monroe-Kellie doctrine, 744
Moraxella catarrhalis, in community-acquired pneumonia, 529
Mortality rates, SDD and, 89–90
Motor neuron disease, 785–786
Motor posturing, 771
Motor system, anatomy of, 779f
MPAP (mean pulmonary arterial pressure), 64
MRAP (mean right atrial pressure), 329
MSOF. (*see* Multiple organ failure (MOF))
Multiple endocrine neoplasia type 2 (MEN 2), 917, 919
Multiple inert gas elimination technique (MIGET), 394–395, 398
Multiple organ failure (MOF)
acute renal failure and, 582–583f
continuous arteriovenous hemofiltration therapy for, 666–667
diarrhea and, 735–736
in hypovolemic shock, 161
liver and, 99
metabolic and nutritional support for, 72–73
mortality of, 177
nosocomial infection and, 82
nutritional support delay and, 42
oxygen deprivation and, 119
prevention, 62
SDD and, 92
sepsis-induced, 170, 177
Muscle cramps, in kidney dialysis, 690
Muscle hypercatabolism, 42
Muscle phosphocreatine-to-phosphorus ratio, 132
Muscle power grading scale, 781t
Muscle relaxants, airway management and, 798
Myasthenia gravis
causes of, 784t
clinical features, 781–782
diagnosis of, 782–783
lid changes in, 783f
management of, 783
physical examination maneuvers in, 782–783t
Myasthenic crisis, 781, 783–784t
Mycoplasma pneumoniae, in community-acquired pneumonia, 530
Myelomas, hypercalcemia and, 929
Myeloproliferative disorders, 813
Myocardial contractility
alteration, assessment in heart failure, 239–240
left ventricular performance and, 280
right ventricular performance and, 280
Myocardial infarction
in acute renal failure, 591
in end-stage renal failure, 683
non-Q wave, 250

Myocardial infarction—(*continued*)
  Q wave, 250
  with right ventricular failure, treatment of, 299–300*f*
Myocardial ischemia
  demand type, 251
  functional impairment of, 250–251
  intervention strategies
    myocardial-specific pharmacologic, 251–253
    primary coronary angioplasty, emergency, 254–255
    surgical revascularization, 254–255
  intervention strategies to minimize myocardial injury, 251–254
  myocardial infarction, 250
  reperfusion injury and, 254
  supply type, 251
  thrombolysis for, 251–255
  unstable angina, 245–250*f*
  ventricular compliance and, 16
Myocardial perfusion, left ventricular performance and, 220
Myocardial stiffness, 213, 216
Myocarditis, in acquired immunodeficiency syndrome, 858
Myocardium
  function
    depression of, in septic shock, 171–173
    echocardiographic assessment, 270–271
    in percutaneous transluminal coronary angioplasty, 251
  in acquired immunodeficiency syndrome, 857–858
  injury of, in cerebral injury, 766–767
  oxygen transport, decline of, 363
  relaxation, left ventricular performance and, 210–213*f*, 214*f*
  viscoelastic properties of, 211
Myocyte contractility, basic determinants of, 217
Myopathy, 778
Myosin, inotropic agents and, 252*f*, 352
Myxedema coma
  clinical features of, 898–899
  laboratory findings, 899
  pathogenesis of, 898
  treatment of, 899–900

NADH, 112, 132, 133*f*
Naloxone
  for opiate overdose, 761
  for septic syndrome, 182–183
Narcotic sedation, in airway management, 798
Nasogastric feeding, diarrhea and, 735
Nasotracheal intubation, 795–796, 797*f*
Near-infrared spectroscopy, of cerebral blood flow, 743
Neck cancer. (*see* Head and neck cancer)
Necrotizing pancreatitis, 724, 726
Needle aspiration, of pulmonary infiltrate, 560
Neoglucogenesis, 881–882*f*
Neonatal hypocalcemia, 937
Nephritis, acute interstitial, 581
Nephrotic syndrome, thrombosis and, 813
Nephrotoxicity, acute renal failure and, 579–581
Nephrotoxins, exogenous, 572
Nerve conduction velocities, 782*f*
Nervous system
  complications of, in acute renal failure, 594–596
  response to injury, 164
Neuroendocrine system, response to injury, 164
Neurogenic diabetes insipidus, 914–916*t*

Neurogenic shock, definition of, 162
Neurogenic vasoregulation, 356–357
Neurohormonal influences, on pulmonary circulation, 316
Neurologic complications
  in acquired immunodeficiency syndrome, 856–857
  of end-stage renal failure, 682
  of endocarditis, 380–381
Neurologic injuries
  diagnostic considerations for, 763–764
  evaluation of, 761–764*f*
  prognostic factors of, 763–764
Neurological disease, with weakness, 780*t*
Neurological examination, 761–764*f*
Neuromuscular disease
  acid maltase deficiency, 786
  Guillain-Barré syndrome, 784–785
  motor neuron disease, 785–786
  myasthenia gravis, 781–784*f*
  polyneuropathy of critical illness, 786–787
  respiratory failure and, 781, 783*t*
Neuromuscular dysfunction
  clinical symptoms of, 778
  ventilatory failure and, 778–781*t*
Neuronal damage, excitotoxic hypothesis of, 760
Neuropathy, uremic, in end-stage renal failure, 682
Neutropenia, causes of, 816
Neutrophil aggregation, in acute lung injury, 416
Neutrophil count, absolute, 836
Neutrophilia, causes of, 815–816
Newborns, continuous arteriovenous hemofiltration therapy for, 665
Nicardipine, 760
Nicotine adenine dinucleotide (NAD), 132, 133*f*
Nifedipine, 249, 294
Niroscopy, of cerebral blood flow, 743
Nitrates
  for myocardial ischemia, 251–252
  for unstable angina, 248
  pharmacology of, 360
Nitric oxide, for adult respiratory distress syndrome, 405
Nitrogen, 23
Nitrogen balance measurements, 38
Nitrogen excretion, during postinjury wasting, 42
Nitrogen substrate, selection of, 51–53*f*
Nitrogen supply, high, rationale for, 50–51*t*
Nitroglycerin
  for pulmonary hypertension, 331*t*
  for unstable angina, 248
  pharmacology of, 360
Nitroprusside
  for heart failure, 242
  for pulmonary hypertension, 331
  pharmacology of, 360
  thiocyanate toxicity and, 242
  tissue oxygen extraction and, 117
  venous return and, 232–233*f*
No-reflow phenomenon, 254, 743
Nocardia, in community-acquired pneumonia, 531
Nocardia infections, posttransplant, 840–841
Noninvasive ventilatory support (NIV), for airway obstruction, 467–468*f*
Nonketotic hyperosmolar coma, in diabetes mellitus, 864
Nonosmotic diuresis, intracranial pressure reduction and, 756–757
Nonresponder, 799
Nonsteroidal antiinflammatory drug (NSAID), 810

Nonvolatile acids, 611
Noradrenaline, in pheochromocytoma, 918
Norepinephrine
    for cardiogenic shock, 153
    for cardiopulmonary resuscitation, 518
    for shock refractory to volume loading, 180
    in heart failure treatment, 241
    in hemorrhagic shock, 152
    pharmacology of, 354
    tissue oxygen extraction and, 117
Nosocomial infections
    alteration of colonizing microflora, 824–825
    endocarditis, 373
    exogenous vs. endogenous, 84
    in intensive care unit, 83–84
    incidence of, 82
    pneumonia. (*see* Nosocomial pneumonia)
Nosocomial pneumonia
    acquisition, sources and modes of, 552–554*t*
    diagnosis of, 554–562*f*
        bronchoscopy specimens for, 556–560
        by nonbronchoscopic procedures, 560–562
    epidemiology of, 545–551*t*
    etiologic agents of, 548–550*t*
    gastric pH and, 706
    incidence of, 545–547*f*
    monotherapy vs. combination therapy, 562–564*t*
    morbidity of, 547–548
    mortality of, 547–548*t*
    pathogenesis of, 551–554*f*
        intubation and oropharyngeal colonization and,
            555*t*
    predisposing factors, 550–551*t*
    prevention of, 565–566
    prophylaxis
        gastric pH and, 553–554*t*, 706–710*f*
        sucralfate or antacids and, 554*f*
    stress ulcer prophylaxis and, 706–710
    susceptibility of, 551*t*
    treatment of, 562–565*t*
        duration for, 563
NSAIDs (nonsteroidal antiinflammatory drugs), 810
Nucleotides, 62
Nutrition
    continuous arteriovenous hemofiltration therapy
        and, 668
    difficult-to-wean ARDS patients and, 423
Nutritional assessment, parameters of, 37–38,
        43–45*t*
Nutritional depletion
    energy expenditure and, 45–46*f*
    protein catabolism and, 45–46*f*
Nutritional pharmacology, 73
Nutritional support
    decision tree for, 55*f*
    during respiratory failure, 62–64
    enteral. (*see* Enteral nutrition)
    for acute renal failure, 64–66
    for acute respiratory failure, in COPD, 441–442
    for circulatory failure, 68–69
    for hepatic failure, 66–68
    for perioperative period, 69–72*f*
    high nitrogen supply, rationale for, 50–51*t*
    improvements, future, 54
    in brain injury, 771–772
    in postoperative period, 70, 72
    in preoperative period, 70, 71*f*
    parenteral. (*see* Parenteral nutrition)
    rationale for, 42–43

response to, 37–38
    therapeutic approaches, 45–54*f*
Obstruction
    of intestines, 716–717
    of large bowel, 717
Obstructive shock, 20, 162–163
Occult bleeding, from stress ulcers, 699–702*t*
Oculocephalic reflexes, 762*f*
Oculomotor abnormalities, asymmetric, 762
Oculovestibular reflexes, 762*f*
Ohm's law, 312
OKG (ornithine α-ketoglutarate), 61*f*
OKT3, side effects of, 691
Oleic acid, 48
Oliguric renal failure, nutritional support for, 64–65
Open chest direct cardiac massage
    complications of, 517
    technique, 507
    vs. closed chest technique, 515–517
Open lung biopsy, in pneumonia diagnosis, 540
Opiate overdose, naloxone for, 761
Opportunistic infections. (*see also specific infections*)
    in acquired immunodeficiency syndrome, 852
    in immunocompromised patients, 827
    posttransplant, 840–845
Optimal energy supply, 45–47
Oral contraceptives, thrombosis and, 814
Organ donors, care of, with brain death, 189–190
Ornithine α-ketoglutarate (OKG), 61*f*
Orthopaedic trauma, 803
Osmolality, plasma, vasopressin and, 911
Osmosis, 637*f*, 638
Osmotic diarrhea, 730
Osmotic disequilibrium syndrome, 689
Osmotic diuresis, intracranial pressure reduction
    and, 756–757
Osteitis fibrosa cystica, 927
Osteolytic metastases, hypercalcemia of, 929
Overdamping, 5–7*f*
Overlapping actions, of cytokines, 175
Oxidative phosphorylation, 25, 34*f*
Oxygen
    adequacy, limits of, 136
    content in blood, 120
    during shock, 135–136
    extraction, 115, 181
    extrinsic conformity, 131
    pathologic supply dependency, 129
    regulation, 121
    supply dependency, 122
    supply independency, 121
    utilization, microvascular parameters of, 120
Oxygen conformity, 131
Oxygen consumption
    assessment of, 18–19*f*
    in pathologic states, 20
    in sepsis, 101
    in shock, 20–21
    metabolic stress/treatment modifications, 46*t*
    oxygen uptake and, 16–17
Oxygen delivery
    biphasic $\dot{V}O_2$-$\dot{D}O_2$ model and, 120–131*f*
    calculation of, 120
    cerebral, 738–740*t*
    critical, of whole body vs. individual organs,
        125–127*f*
    improvement in hemorrhagic shock, 150
    in sepsis syndrome, 181

Oxygen delivery—(*continued*)
 in septic shock, 175
 increasing, therapy for, 363–364
 pulmonary support and, 365–366
Oxygen demand
 dependency, 124
 of muscles, tissue blood flow and, 115
 of tissues, dysoxic injury and, 131–132
 oxygen use and, 17
 variable muscular, 122–125f
 variable nonmuscular, 129–131f
Oxygen deprivation
 brain injury from, 738–740t
 multiple organ failure and, 119
Oxygen extraction ratio, 17–19, 120
Oxygen free radicals, brain injury and, 739
Oxygen saturation, mixed venous, 17–18
Oxygen supply/demand ratio, 132
Oxygen tension, arterial, cerebral blood flow and, 741f
Oxygen therapy
 for acute respiratory failure, in COPD, 438
 for adult respiratory distress syndrome, 417
 for asthma, 497
 for pulmonary hypoxic vasoconstriction, 330
 in cerebral resuscitation, 769
 with 100% oxygen
  for adult respiratory distress syndrome, 402–403
  for bacterial pneumonia, 407
  for chronic obstructive pulmonary disease, 434–435t
  ventilation-perfusion relationship and, 391
 with oxygen-enriched air, for chronic obstructive pulmonary disease, 433–434t
Oxygen transport
 balance, determinants of, 18–19
 data interpretation, 18–19
 enhancement, by estimation of tissue redox state, 131–135
 hemodynamic monitoring of, 16–21f, 17t
 oxygen demand and, 112
 terminology, 16–17t
 treatment priorities, 19–21
Oxygen uptake
 blood lactate and, 133–135
 changes, effects of, 392–393
 definition of, 119
 diffusion vs. convection limitation, 127–129f
 macrovascular parameters of, 119–120
 oxygen consumption and, 16–17
Oxygen utilization coefficient, 17–19
Oxyhemoglobin dissociation curve, 20, 419f
Oxyhemoglobin saturation, 17–18
Oxytocin, 910

Packed red blood cells, for transfusion, 820
PAF (platelet-activating factor), 178, 180
Pancreatitis, acute
 biological features of, 725
 clinical features of, 725
 hypocalcemia of, 938
 in acute renal failure, 594
 in end-stage renal failure, 686
 pathology of, 724–725
 prognostic factors, 725–726t
 radiological findings, 725
 treatment of, 726–727
Paracrine functions, of heart, 223
Paradigms

 therapy content, 195–196
 therapy process, 196–198f
Paradoxical pulse
 in asthma, 495
 in cardiac tamponade, 340
Paralysis, in airway obstruction, 462–463
Paralytic ileus, 716
Parasympathetic stimulation, 221, 222f
Parathyroid crisis, 927
Parathyroid hormone
 abnormalities of, in acute renal failure, 595
 in hypercalcemia, 925–930
 in hypoparathyroidism, 936–937
 in primary hyperparathyroidism, 926–928f
 in pseudohypoparathyroidism, 937
Parathyroid hormone related peptide, 928–929
Parenchymal disease, acute renal failure and, 572–574f
Parenteral nutrition
 electrolytes and, 53–54t
 energy supply adjustments, 58–59
 hormonal manipulations, 61–62
 immunological manipulations, 61–62
 in end-stage renal failure, 692–693t
 lipid supply adjustments, 59, 60f
 nitrogen substrate preference and, 51–53f
 vs. enteral nutrition, 54–58
Paroxysmal nocturnal hemoglobinuria, 813, 819
Partial thromboplastin time (PTT), 805–806
Patient-disease complex, 194–195f
Patient outcome
 signal-to-noise ratio, 194–195
 value of medical care and, 194f
PAV (proportional assist ventilation), 466–467f
PCR (protein catabolic rate), 633
PCV (pressure-controlled ventilation), 463–465f
Peak systolic gradient (PSG), 329–330
PEEP. (*see* Positive end-expiratory pressure (PEEP))
Pelvic fractures, 801
Penetrating trauma, 803–804
Pentamidine, 858
Pentobarbital coma, 759
Pentoxifylline, 182, 757
Percutaneous transluminal coronary angioplasty, myocardial function, 251
Perforation, toxic megacolon and, 733
Pericardial effusion
 drainage of, 344–345
 in cardiac tamponade, 342, 343
Pericardial tamponade
 in acute renal failure, 591
 in end-stage renal failure, 683
 obstructive shock and, 20
Pericardiectomy, 337–338f, 345
Pericarditis
 cardiac tamponade and, 341
 in acute renal failure, 591
 in end-stage renal failure, 683
Pericardium
 anatomy of, 337–338f
 left ventricular performance and, 215–216
 physiology of, normal, 338
 pressure-volume relationship, in classic cardiac tamponade, 339f
 restraint, pathologic consequences of, 338
 ventricular interaction and, 323–325f
Perioperative period, nutritional support for, 69–72f
Peripheral nervous system, in sepsis, 101–102
Peripheral reflex vasoconstriction, 20

Peripheral resistance
  cardiopulmonary resuscitation and, 512
  in septic shock, 154
Peripheral vasodilation, in prerenal azotemia, 572
Peripheral vasomotor tone, in septic shock,
    173–174*f*
Peritoneal dialysis, 627
  advantages and disadvantages, 640*t*
  clinical results of, 639–640
  complications of, 640*t*, 646*t*
  description of, 638, 639*f*
  efficiency of, 638–639
  for acute renal failure, 627
  indications, 640–641
  peritonitis of, in end-stage renal failure,
    686–687
Peritoneal lavage
  for pancreatitis, 726
  in abdominal trauma, 800–801*t*
  vs. computerized axial tomography, in blunt
    trauma, 793
Peritonitis
  in end-stage renal failure, 686
  in peritoneal dialysis, in end-stage renal failure,
    686–687
  primary, 721–722
  secondary, 722–723
  tertiary, 723–724
Perivascular abscess, in endocarditis, 379
PET (positron-emission tomography), 743, 747
Phenformin, 882
Pheochromocytoma
  anesthesia and, 921
  description of, 917
  epidemiology of, 917
  evaluation of, 918–919
  hypercalcemia of, 930
  hypertension in, mechanism of, 917–918
  long-term follow-up for, 922
  postoperative period, 921–922
  preoperative diagnosis of, 918–919
  preoperative management of, 919–921*f*
  surgical management of, 921
Phlebotomy, 294, 758
Phosphodiesterase inhibitors, 242–243, 355–356. (*see
    also* Amrinone; Enoximone)
Phospholipase A₂, in sepsis syndrome, 179
Phosphorus
  hemolysis and, 819
  in acute renal failure, 589–590
  requirements, 53
Physician-patient relationship, basis of, 188
Physiologic dead space, blood gases and, 391–395*f*
PINI (Prognostic Inflammatory and Nutritional
    Index), 50–51
PLA1 antigen, 810
Plasma expanders, for end-stage renal failure, 695
Plasmapheresis
  for autoimmune thrombocytopenia, 809–810
  for sepsis management, 181–182
  in myasthenia gravis, 784
Platelet-activating factor (PAF), 178, 180, 416
Platelet count, critical, 821
Platelet dosing, 821
Platelets
  dysfunction of, 808–811
    causes of, 810–811
    in acute renal failure, 596–597
  in coagulation, 806

transfusions of, 821
Pleiotropic actions, of cytokines, 175
Pleural pressure, 9–10, 296
Plicamycin, for hypercalcemia, 934
PMN chemotaxis, lipid infusion and, 49*f*
Pneumatoceles, 534
Pneumococcal capsular antigen, 537
Pneumocystis carinii pneumonia
  diagnosis of
    in TMP/SMX prophylaxis, 827–828
    sputum samples and, 832
  in acquired immunodeficiency syndrome, 531,
    853–855
    ICU survival and, 861
  in post-organ transplant patients, 845
Pneumonia
  acute infectious, definition of, 525
  community-acquired. (*see* Community-acquired
    pneumonia)
  diagnosis of, in immunocompromised patient,
    832–833
  hospital-acquired. (*see* Nosocomial pneumonia)
  in end-stage renal failure, 685*t*
  mortality of, 525
  of *Legionella pneumophila*, posttransplant, 841–842
  of *Pneumocystis carinii*. (*see Pneumocystis carinii*
    pneumonia)
  weaning and, 451
Pneumothorax, 799, 855–856
Poiseuille's law, 140, 317
Polycythemia vera, 817
Polydipsia, with diabetes insipidus, 914–916*t*
Polymyxin E, 88
Polyneuropathy of critical illness, 786–787
Polyunsaturated fatty acids (PUFAs), 57, 59
Pontine infarction, 768–769
Portosystemic collateral blood, 99
Positive end-expiratory pressure (PEEP)
  assisted control, for airway obstruction, 463
  cardiac tamponade and, 345
  for shock, 155–156
  in adult respiratory distress syndrome, 395–396,
    398–399, 402*f*, 420
  in cerebral resuscitation, 769–770
  in chronic obstructive pulmonary disease, 432
  intrinsic. (*see* Auto-PEEP)
  postoperative, 365–366
  pulmonary artery occlusion pressure and,
    421–422
  weaning and, 447
Positive pressure ventilation, for shock, 155–156
Positron-emission tomography (PET), 743, 747
Posterior pituitary gland, physiological aspects of,
    910–911
Postinjury wasting, nitrogen excretion and, 42
Postinsult hypermetabolism, 73
Postoperative period
  bleeding control and, 366–367*t*
  cardiovascular support and, 363–365*t*
  coagulation support, 366–367*t*
  for cardiac transplant recipients, 367–368
  for valvular heart disease patients, 368–369
  nosocomial pneumonia and, 550
  pulmonary support, 365–366*t*
  renal and metabolic considerations, 366*t*
Posttransfusion purpura, 810
Potassium
  imbalance of, in uremia, 681–682
  metabolism, pathophysiology of, 605–606

Potassium—(continued)
  total-body, 45
Prazosin, 359
Pregnancy
  diabetes mellitus and, 887
  thrombocytopenia of, 810
  thrombosis and, 814
Preload
  as positive inotropic factor, 217
  cardiac function and, 141
  definition of, 15
  left ventricular performance and, 209–210, 280–281
  right ventricular performance and, 280–281, 286–287
  ventricular compliance and, 16
  ventricular function in heart failure and, 232
Preload-afterload mismatch, 152
Preoperative period, nutritional support for, 70, 71f
Pressure-controlled ventilation (PCV), 463–465f
Pressure overload, right ventricular, 288–289
Pressure support ventilation (PSV), 465–467f
Pressure-volume loop, ventricular, 209, 210f, 234f, 236–238
Primary coronary angioplasty, emergency, in myocardial ischemia, 254–255
Primary endogenous infection, SDD and, 87
Primary fibrinolysis, 808
Primary graft anuria, 582
Prognostic Inflammatory and Nutritional Index (PINI), 50–51
Progressive shock, 164, 165f
Proportional assist ventilation (PAV), 466–467f
Prostacyclins, 179–180, 294, 757
Prostaglandin E_1, 368, 403, 424
Prostaglandin E_2, 575
Prostaglandin I_2, 403
Prostaglandins, 64
Prosthetic valve endocarditis
  cardiac complications of, 379–380
  incidence of, 375
  risk factors for, 375
  source and microbiology, 375–376t
  surgical outcome, 381–383t
  valve ring abscess and, 379
Protamine, 367
Protected specimen brush bacterial culture, of nosocomial pneumonia, 556–558t, 559, 561f
Protected specimen brush technique, 538–539t
  in pneumonia diagnosis, 560–561
Protein C deficiency, 812
Protein C system, vitamin K-dependent, 811f
Protein-calorie malnutrition, 25
Protein catabolic rate (PCR), 633
Protein catabolism
  exogenous dextrose and, 28
  in acute renal failure, 587–588
  in brain injury, 771
  in starvation, 26, 27
Protein S, 811, 812
Proteins
  adverse consequences of administration, 33
  metabolism of
    during stress, 33
    normal, 30–31
  serum abnormalities, hypercalcemia and, 932
  supply adjustments, for enteral and parenteral nutrition, 59–61
  synthesis, branched-chain amino acids formulas and, 51

turnover, 23, 24f
Prothrombin time (PT), 805–806
Protozoan infection, post-organ transplant, 845
Prourokinase, for myocardial ischemia, 253
PSAP (pulmonary artery systolic pressure), 330
Pseudohypoparathyroidism, hypocalcemia of, 937t
Pseudohypoparathyroidism hypocalcemia of, treatment of, 940–941t
Pseudoperitonitis, uremic, in end-stage renal failure, 686
PSG (peak systolic gradient), 329–330
PSV (pressure support ventilation), 465–467f
PT (prothrombin time), 805–806
PTA regimen, 88t
PTT (partial thromboplastin time), 805–806
PUFAs (polyunsaturated fatty acids), 57, 59
Pulmonary artery
  constriction, 315, 322–323f
  pressure flow relationships, 314–315f
Pulmonary artery catheter
  flow-directed, 3
  placement, V-waves and, 10
  tip positioning
    mixed venous oxygen saturation monitoring and, 18
    proper, 10
    transverse segment, confirmation of placement, 10
Pulmonary artery catheterization, for adult respiratory distress syndrome, 421–422
Pulmonary artery input resistance, stroke volume and, 323–324f
Pulmonary artery occlusion pressure
  in fluid challenge, 151–152
  monitoring of, 9–12f, 15
Pulmonary artery pressure
  ancillary tests for, 328–329f
  determinants of, 317–318
  increased
    clinical identification of, 327–330f
    left ventricle function and, 321
    right ventricle function and, 321
Pulmonary artery systolic pressure (PSAP), 330
Pulmonary blood distribution, West zones of, 313–314f
Pulmonary blood volume, in pulmonary hypertension, 325
Pulmonary capillary endothelial damage, mechanisms of, 416
Pulmonary circulation
  active regulation of, 316–317
  dynamic view of, 315–316f
  hypoxic vasoconstriction of, 317t
  in pulmonary hypertension, 320–327f
  nature of, 312–317f
  neurohormonal influences, 316
  passive regulation of, 312–316f
  postoperative support for, 365–366t
Pulmonary complications, of end-stage renal failure, 684–685t
Pulmonary disease
  acute renal failure and, 592–593
  in acquired immunodeficiency syndrome, 853–856
  of immunocompromised patient, 832–833
Pulmonary edema
  in acute renal failure, 592
  in adult respiratory distress syndrome, 397–398
  neurogenic, 769
Pulmonary embolism

electrocardiographic abnormalities of, 328–329t
hemodynamic management, in right ventricular failure, 297–298
in cardiogenic shock, 153–154
Pulmonary function, in sepsis, 101
Pulmonary hypertension
    ancillary tests for, 328–329f
    causes of, 317–320t
    circulatory consequences, 320–327f
    classification of, 317–320t
    definition of, 312
    electrocardiogram of, 328–329f
    gas exchange and, 327
    hemodynamic changes of, 327f
    history of, 327–328
    in stable chronic obstructive pulmonary disease, 293–294
    incidence of, 312
    management of, 330–332t
    mechanism of low cardiac output in, 321–325f
    noninvasive studies of, 329–330
    of cardiac transplant recipients, 368
    physical examination of, 327–328f
    pressure flow relationships in, 314–315f
    pulmonary blood volume in, 325
    right heart failure, management of, 332
    right ventricle myocardial supply:demand ratio, 325, 326f
    right ventricular dysfunction in, 285–286
    right ventricular failure in, 325, 326f
    right ventricular filling and, 153
    transseptal pressure gradient and, 325
    two-dimensional echocardiogram of, 325f
    ventricular diastolic function and, 323–325f
    ventricular geometry of, 327f
Pulmonary infarction, 10, 11f
Pulmonary infections
    delayed, in brain injury, 770
    gastric pH and, 706
Pulmonary infiltrates, in immunocompromised patients, 831–833t
Pulmonary system
    cerebral resuscitation and, 768–770
    complications of, in acute renal failure, 591–593
Pulmonary vascular disease, in cardiogenic shock, 153–154
Pulmonary vascular pressure, 404
Pulmonary vascular resistance
    calculation of, 312–314f
    limitations of, 312–314f
    lung volume changes and, 473–474f
    reduction of, 330–332t
Pulmonary vascular tone, in adult respiratory distress syndrome, 404–405
Pulmonary vasodilators, in COPD-induced right ventricular failure, 294
Pulsus paradoxus, 340–342, 344
Pupils, size and responsiveness of, 761–762
Pyrogenic reactions, in kidney dialysis, 689

Quinolones, for end-stage renal failure, 693

Radionuclide angiography
    equilibrium-gated technique, 302
    of right ventricle performance, 302
Randle's cycle, 47
Rapid eye movement (REM), 459
Rapid-response thermistor, 330
Red blood cells

abnormalities, clinical approach for, 817–820
decreased production of, 817–818
destruction of, causes for, 818
function of, 817
leukocyte-reduced or washed, for transfusion, 820
packed, for transfusion, 820
Red cell aplasia, 818
Reflexes, left ventricular performance and, 223–224
Refractory shock, definition of, 97t
Rehabilitation, in trauma system, 790–791
Rejection, organ, after renal transplantation, 691
Relaxation, left ventricular performance and, 210–213f, 214f
Renal failure index, in acute renal failure, 576
Renal failure (*see* Renal failure, acute; End-stage renal failure)
Renal failure/uremia, cardiac tamponade and, 341
Renal hypoperfusion syndrome, 571
Renal replacement therapy.(*see also* Dialysis; Hemodialysis)
    continuous, 646–648f
    for acute renal failure
        choice of, 634
        initiation of, 633–634
        requirements for, 634–636t
    solute and water transport mechanisms, 636–638f
Renal system, postoperative support, 366t
Renal transplantation, emergencies after, 690–691
Renin, 904, 918
Renin-angiotensin-aldosterone system
    in acute renal failure, 578
    in cardiac tamponade, 339
    in hypovolemia, 164
    left ventricular performance and, 222–223
    suppression of, 606
Resistance
    systemic vascular, 16
    ventricular, 233
Respiratory acidosis
    compensatory responses, 619, 620t
    treatment of, 438
    with acute renal failure, 621
Respiratory alkalosis, compensatory responses, 619–620t
Respiratory cycle, in chronic obstructive pulmonary disease, 429–430f, 433–434f
Respiratory failure, acute
    electrolyte disorders, treatment of, 438f
    in asthma, pathophysiology of, 435–436
    in chronic obstructive pulmonary disease
        bronchodilators for, 439–441
        treatment of, 436–442
    in COPD, corticosteroids for, 441
    metabolic disorders, treatment of, 437–438f
    neuromuscular causes of, 781, 783t
    nutritional support for, 62–64, 441–442
    oxygen therapy for, 438
    pathophysiology of, in chronic obstructive pulmonary disease, 429–435f
Respiratory muscles
    fatigue of, 430–432, 493
    function of, in dynamic hyperinflation, 458–459f
Respiratory quotient (RQ), 35–37f, 48, 63–64
Respiratory sinus arrhythmia, 473
Respiratory system
    buffering of, 614–618f
    compromise of, in acute renal failure, 592
    mechanics of, in asthma, 492
    support of, in sepsis, 104

Responder, 798–799
Resting energy expenditure, 34–35f, 45
Reticuloendothelial system, 825
Retinol-binding protein, 44
Retroperitoneal injuries, 800
Reye's syndrome, 32, 745, 746
Rhabdomyolysis, in acute renal failure, 588
Right atrial pressure
   in pulmonary hypertension, 328f
   venous return and, 141–142
Right heart failure, management of, 332
Right-sided heart catheterization
   findings, 271
   for cardiac tamponade, 344
   indications for, 271
   of right ventricle performance, 303–304f
Right ventricle
   afterload, in pulmonary hypertension, 320–321f
   anatomy of, 284–285
   contractility impairment, 289–290
     in septic shock, 298–299
   conus region, 285
   failure. (see Right ventricular failure)
   filling, in cardiac tamponade, 340
   function
     evaluation and monitoring, 301–304f
     in shock, 484–485
     increased pulmonary artery pressure and, 321
     invasive studies of, 330
     noninvasive studies of, 329–330
     vascular lesion site of pulmonary hypertension
      and, 320
   function of, 284
   geometry, during pulmonary hypertension, 327f
   hemodynamic role of, 284–286
   in systole, 285
   ischemia, in pulmonary hypertension, 322
   myocardial supply:demand ratio, in pulmonary
     hypertension, 325, 326f
   performance. (see Right ventricular performance)
   preload
     septic shock and, 171
   preload, in pulmonary hypertension, 320–321f
   response
     to decreased contractile state, 289–290
     to decreased contractility, 286–290
     to wall stress, 286–290
   sinus region, 285
   structural and functional changes
     in pressure overload, 288–289
     in volume overload, 287
Right ventricle ejection fraction, calculation,
   303–304f
Right ventricle infarct, with right ventricular failure,
   treatment of, 299–300f
Right ventricle overload, right coronary circulation
   and, 289
Right ventricular ejection fraction, 364
Right ventricular end-systolic volume, 142
Right ventricular failure
   death from, 282
   in asthma, 494–495f
   in pulmonary hypertension, 325, 326f
   postoperative cardiac surgery, 300–301
   therapeutic implications, 290–291
     for septic shock, 298–299f
     in adult respiratory distress syndrome, 291–293
     in asthma, 295–297
     in pulmonary embolism, 297–298

   of chronic obstructive pulmonary disease,
     293–295F
Right ventricular invagination, for cardiac
   tamponade diagnosis, 343
Right ventricular performance
   afterload and, 281
   assessment variables, 301
   cardiovascular homeostasis and, 281–282
   contrast angiography of, 301–302
   determinants, 280–282
     vs. left ventricular performance determinants,
     280–281
   evaluation and monitoring, 301–304f
   myocardial contractility and, 280
   preload and, 280–281
   radionuclide angiography of, 302
RQ (respiratory quotient), 35–37f, 48, 63–64

Sarcoidosis, hypercalcemia of, 930
Scribner shunt, 692
SDD. (see Selective decontamination of digestive
   tract (SDD))
Secondary endogenous infection, SDD and, 87
Sedation, in airway obstruction, 462–463
Sedatives, for end-stage renal failure, 695
Seizures, cerebral metabolism and, 758–759
Seldinger guidewire, 5
Selective decontamination of digestive tract (SDD)
   acquired infection and, 89
   antimicrobial agents for, 87–88t
   as outbreak control method, 90–91
   colonization and infection rates in ICUs and,
     84–86
   definition of, 82–83
   for high risk surgical groups, 91–92
   gastrointestinal carriage of GNBs and, 89
   in sepsis, 108
   microbial resistance and, 90
   mortality rates and, 89–90
   multiple organ failure and, 92
   rationale for, 86–87
   trials in ICU practice, 88–90
Sensory evoked potentials, of brain injury, 764
Sepsis. (see also Sepsis syndrome; Septic shock)
   cardiovascular function in, 100–101
   cardiovascular support for, 104–105
   clinical features of, 99–102t
   clinical investigations, 106–107
   continuous arteriovenous hemofiltration therapy
     for, 666–667
   definition of, 96, 97t
   end-stage renal failure, 687
   endogenous inflammatory mediators of, 175–176t
   energy expenditure and, 45–46f
   epidemiology of, 97–98
   etiology of, 98–99t
   future considerations, 108–109
   gastrointestinal function in, 102
   gastrointestinal support for, 106
   hematologic function in, 102
   hepatic function in, 102
   in acquired immunodeficiency syndrome, 860
   in acute renal failure, 597–598
   in intensive care unit, 84
   initial period of, 42
   management of, 96, 102–108t
   neurological function in, 101–102
   pathophysiologic expression of, 170
   pathophysiology of, 98–99

postresuscitation support for, 107–108
protein catabolism and, 45–46*f*
pulmonary function in, 101
renal function in, 101
renal support for, 105–106
respiratory support for, 104
SDD for, 108
vs. infection, 170
Sepsis syndrome
definition of, 96, 97*t*, 176
epidemiology of, 176–177
management of, 180–183
multiple system organ failure and, 177
pathogenesis of, 177–178
pathophysiology of, 178–180
vs. infection, 170
Septic encephalopathy, 66
Septic shock. (*see also* Sepsis; Sepsis syndrome)
definition of, 96–97*t*, 162
microorganisms in, 176
microvascular consequences of, 174–175
pathophysiology of, 98–99, 154–155
peripheral vasomotor tone and, 173–174*f*
with right ventricular failure, treatment, 298–299*f*
Septicemia
definition of, 96
enteral nutrition and, 58
Serologic tests, for pneumonia diagnosis, 537
Serotonin, vasoconstriction of, 315, 316*f*
7-3 rule, 150–151
Sex steroids, 902
SGA (subjective global assessment), 44
Sheehan's syndrome, 907
Shock
cardiogenic, pathophysiology of, 152–154
classification of, 162–163
definition of, 3, 140, 161
hemorrhagic, pathophysiology of, 149–152
pathophysiology of
classification of, 141*t*
positive pressure ventilation and, 155–156
systemic vascular resistance decrease and, 156–157
positive pressure ventilation for, 155–156
resuscitation, brain injury and, 768
right ventricular function and, 484–485
septic, pathophysiology of, 154–155
Shock mediators, antagonism of, 182
Shock pants, 157
Shunt complications, in end-stage renal failure, 690
SIADH. (*see* Syndrome of inappropriate antidiuretic hormone secretion (SIADH))
Sickle cell anemia, thrombosis and, 813
Sideroblastic anemia, 818
SIMV (synchronized intermittent mandatory ventilation), 458, 466
Single photon emission computed tomography (SPECT), 743
Sinus tachycardia, pharmacologic treatment of, 350–351
Skin
as infection barrier, 823–824*t*
colonizing microflora of, 824
in infective endocarditis, 377
Skin fold measurements, 37
Small intestines, obstruction of, 716–717
Smoking, carbon monoxide blood level and, 817
Sodium
decreased levels of. (*see* Hyponatremia)

fractional excretion, in acute renal failure, 576
imbalances of
in acute renal failure, 601–602*t*
in uremia, 681
increased levels of. (*see* Hypernatremia)
metabolism, pathophysiology of, 601–603*t*
Sodium bicarbonate. (*see* Bicarbonate)
Sodium nitroprusside, 403, 404
Solid tumors, hypercalcemia of, 928–929
Solute removal, continuous arteriovenous hemofiltration therapy for, 662–664
Solute transport, in renal replacement therapy, 636–638*f*
Source control, continuous arteriovenous hemofiltration therapy for, 667
SPECT (single photon emission computed tomography), 743
Spinal cord injury, 801–802*t*
Spinal shock, 156
Splenic septic emboli, in endocarditis, 381
Sputum analysis
in community-acquired pneumonia, 535–537
in immunocompromised patient, 832
Stabilized oral endotracheal intubation, 795, 796*f*
Standardization of therapy, 203–205*f*
Staphylococcus, coagulase-negative, 83
Staphylococcus aureus endocarditis, 372, 374–375, 383
Staphylococcus aureus pneumonia, 529, 534*f*
Starling curve, 232, 287
Starling resistors, 312–314*f*, 320
Starling's Law, 16
Starvation
body protein and, 30–31
during stressed states, 26–28
metabolic alterations of, 43*t*
normal, 25–27*f*
Status asthmaticus, ventilation-perfusion relationship, 409*f*
Steroids
for ARDS treatment, 423–424
for asthma, 497
Stewart-Hamilton equation, 12
β₂-Stimulants, for acute respiratory failure, in COPD, 440
Stomach, colonization, gastric pH and, 86
Streptococcus, endocarditis and, 372–373
Streptococcus pneumoniae, 107
in community-acquired pneumonia, 526
Streptokinase, for myocardial ischemia, 252
Stress
adaptation, 63*f*
amino acid metabolism and, 33
carbohydrate metabolism and, 31–32
definition of, 24
exogenous substrate utilization and, 31–33
initial phase of, 73
metabolic alterations of, 43*t*
protein metabolism and, 33
starvation during, 26–28
Stress ulcer(s)
bleeding from
definition of, 699–702*t*
risk factors for, 702
incidence of gastrointestinal bleeding, 711
pathophysiology of, 699
prophylaxis, 699
disadvantages of, 705–706, 710–711
efficacy of, 702–705*t*
future research and, 712

Stress ulcer(s)—(continued)
    gastric pH and, 706–710f
    nosocomial pneumonia and, 706–710
    patient selection for, 711–712
    policy recommendations, 710–712
    selection of agent for, 710–711
Stressed volume, 143f, 145, 157
Stroke volume, 15, 101, 323–324f
Stroke work index, 16
Subarachnoid space inflammation, 748
Subjective global assessment, 44
Substrate utilization, exogenous. (see also specific
    exogenous substrates)
    during stress, 31–33
    normal, 28–31f
Sucralfate, 554f, 705
Superinfection, 451, 550
Surrogate decision-maker, 191
Swan-Ganz catheter, 240, 330
Sympathetic response, to injury, 164
Sympathetic stimulation, 221–222f
Sympathetic vasoconstrictor mechanisms, in
    hypovolemia, 164
Sympathomimetics, 16
Synchronized intermittent mandatory ventilation
    (SIMV), 458, 466
Syndrome of inappropriate antidiuretic hormone
    secretion (SIADH)
    biologic features of, 912t
    clinical features of, 911–912
    diagnosis of, 912–913t
    etiology of, 911, 912t
    in AIDS, 859
    in brain injury, 772
    in Guillain-Barré syndrome, 785
    therapy for, 913–914
Systemic inflammatory response, activators of,
    161–162f
Systemic vascular resistance, 16, 156–157
Systole, right ventricle in, 285
Systolic blood pressure, 7–8t
Systolic hypertension, treatment of, 8
Systolic ventricular elastance, in heart failure,
    233–234f
Systolic ventricular interaction, as left ventricular
    performance determinant, 220–221

T_3, 892–894t
T_4, 892–894t
T4 lymphocytes, in HIV infection, 852t
Tachypnea, in pulmonary hypertension, 328
TBG (thyroxine-binding globulin), 892
TBPA (thyroxine-binding prealbumin), 892
Temperature alterations, cerebral metabolism and, 758
Tensilon test, 784
Tension pneumothorax, 20
Theophylline, 440–441, 497
Thermodilution measurement, of cardiac output,
    12–13f, 330
Thiazide diuretics, 931
Thiocyanate toxicity, 242
Thoracic pump model, 504, 507–508f
Thoracic trauma, 799–800t
Thrombocytopenia
    causes of, 809
    drug-induced, 809
    heparin-induced, 813
    in acute renal failure, 596–597
    in sepsis, 102

Thromboemboli, from continuous arteriovenous
    hemofiltration therapy, 666
Thrombolysis
    for myocardial ischemia, 252–253, 255
        adjunctive pharmacotherapy and, 253–254
    for pulmonary embolus, 332
    in unstable angina, 249–250
Thrombolytic agents. (see also specific thrombolytic
    agents)
    categories of, 252
Thrombolytic therapy, for myocardial ischemia, 251
Thrombosis
    congenital disorders of, 812
    from continuous arteriovenous hemofiltration
        therapy, 666
    general approach, 811–812f
    in end-stage renal failure, 687
Thrombotic disorders
    primary, 812
    secondary, 812–814
Thrombotic thrombocytopenic purpura, 809
Thromboxane B_2, in pulmonary hypertension, 319
Thyroid gland
    disorders of, myxedema coma, 898–900
    function of, in nonthyroid illness, 893–895t
    normal function of, 891–893
    pathophysiology of, in nonthyroid illness,
        894–895
Thyroid hormone binding protein, 892
Thyroid hormones
    action of, 893
    control of, in thyrotoxic storm, 897
    for myxedema coma, 899–900
    in thyrotoxic storm, 896
    peripheral metabolism of, 892–893
    secretion of, 892–893
    serum levels, alterations of, in nonthyroid illness,
        893–894t
Thyroid stimulating hormone (TSH), 891, 893–894t
Thyrotoxic storm, 895–897
Thyrotoxicosis
    diarrhea and, 730
    hypercalcemia and, 929–930
Thyrotropin-releasing hormone (TRH), 891
Thyroxin-binding prealbumin, 37
Thyroxine-binding globulin (TBG), 892
Thyroxine-binding prealbumin (TBPA), 892
Tidal ventilation, 453
Tidal volume, in weaning, 448
Time constant, 146–147f
Time-varying elastance, 504
Tissue blood flow, control of, 114–117
Tissue oxygen extraction, vasoactive drugs and,
    117–118
Tissue perfusion, blood pressure and, 140
Tissue plasminogen activator, 253
Tissue redox state, 120
Torsade de pointe, 352
Total body water, 635
Total parenteral nutrition (TPN)
    for postoperative period, 72
    hypercalcemia and, 932
    preoperative, 70
Toxic megacolon
    causes of, 732
    clinical features of, 732–733
    diagnosis of, 732–733
    treatment of, 733–734
Toxic-shock syndrome, 938–939

Toxoplasma gondii infection, 856
TPN. (*see* Total parenteral nutrition (TPN))
Trace elements, enteral/parenteral nutrition and, 53–54*t*
Tracheobronchitis, weaning and, 451
Transcranial Doppler ultrasound, of cerebral blood flow, 743
Transdiaphragmatic pressure, 431
Transducers, pressure, 4–5
Transesophageal echocardiography
    of infective endocarditis, 377–378*f*
    of left-sided valvular regurgitation, diagnostic improvement of, 269*t*
    of valvular disorders, 364–365*f*
Transferrin, serum, 37
Transfusion therapy
    dilutional effect of, 809
    in trauma, 798–799
    principles of, 820–822
Transient responder, 799
Transmembrane pressure calculation, 651
Transplantation, organ. (*see also specific organ transplantations*)
    postoperative infections of, 838–846
        in early posttransplant period, 839–840
        timetable for, 839*t*
    SDD for, 91
Transseptal pressure gradient, in pulmonary hypertension, 325
Transthoracic echocardiography
    of aortic valve disorders, 264–265
    of mitral valve disorders, 264
Transthoracic needle aspiration, in pneumonia diagnosis, 540
Transthyretin (prealbumin), 44
Transtracheal aspiration
    indications for, 538
    of community-acquired pneumonia, 537–538*t*
Trauma patients
    airway management for, 794–798*t*
    cricothyrotomy for, 797–798
    fiberoptic intubation and, 796
    hemorrhage and, 798–799
    initial period of, 42
    intubation, stabilized oral endotracheal, 795, 796*f*
    morbidity and mortality of, 789
    nasotracheal intubation, 795–796, 797*f*
    standard oral intubation, 796
Trauma score, 790*t*, 791*t*
Trauma system, 789–791*t*
    scoring of injuries, 790*t*, 791*t*
    triage guidelines, 791*t*
Trauma team, 791–792
Traumatic shock, 163
Treatment priorities, 19–21
Trendelenburg position, 157, 168
TRH (thyrotropin-releasing hormone), 891
Tricuspid regurgitation
    rapid-response thermistor measurement and, 330
    right ventricle performance in, 304*f*
    treatment, stroke index and, 300*f*
Tricuspid valve annulus, in systole, 285
Triglycerides, blood, 25, 29
Trimethoprim/sulfamethoxazole (TMP/SMX), 827–828, 854
Tropomyosin, inotropic agents and, 252*f*, 352
Troponin C, 210
Trousseau's syndrome, 813
TSH (thyroid stimulating hormone), 891, 893–894*t*

Tuberculosis, community-acquired pneumonia and, 530–531
Tubular necrosis, acute, 579–581, 631
Tumor necrosis factor-α, 172, 176*t*, 179, 180
Two-dimensional echocardiography
    of infective endocarditis, 379
    of pulmonary hypertension, 325*f*
    of valve regurgitation, 264–265*f*

Ulcerative colitis, toxic megacolon and, 733
Ultrafiltration, 637*f*, 638
Underdamping, 5–8*f*
Unstable angina, 245–250*f*
Unstressed volume, 143*f*, 145
Upper gastrointestinal bleeding, in acute renal failure, 593–594
Urapidil, 294
Urea, production of, 587
Urea appearance rate, calculation of, 66
Urea nitrogen, 38
Uremia
    definition of, 677
    electrolyte imbalance in, 681–682
    problems in, 677, 681–682*t*
    therapeutic measures for, 678*t*, 680*t*
    treatment of, central nervous system dysfunction and, 595–596
Uremic encephalopathy
    in end-stage renal failure, 682
    in renal failure, 594
Uremic neuropathy, in end-stage renal failure, 682
Uremic pericarditis, in end-stage renal failure, 683
Urinalysis, in diagnosis, of acute renal failure, 576
Urinary nitrogen, 38
Urinary nitrogen efflux, 26
Urinary volume, of acute renal failure, 576
Urine
    chemical indices, in acute renal failure, 576, 577*f*
    chemistry of, in acute renal failure, 576
Urine osmolality, in acute renal failure, 576
Urine/plasma creatinine ratio, in acute renal failure, 576
Urogenital tract lesions, endocarditis and, 373
Urogenital tract procedures, endocarditis and, 373
Urokinase, for myocardial ischemia, 253

V-wave
    delayed, 10, 12, 13*f*
    identification of, 10, 12*f*
    in mitral valve regurgitation, 271
    pulmonary artery catheter placement and, 10
Valsalva maneuver, 481
Valve regurgitation, acute. (*see also specific valves*)
    causes of, 263*t*
    clinical examination of, 262–263
    echocardiography of, 264–265*f*
    immediate urgency, laboratory investigations of, 263–264
    invasive assessment, 271–272
    medical therapy
        good tolerance state, 273
        poor tolerance state, 273
    noninvasive assessment, 264–271*f*
    prognostic factors, 272–273
    severity of symptoms, 263
    surgical repair, timing of, 273–276*f*
Valve ring abscess, prosthetic valve endocarditis and, 379

Valvular regurgitation, acute left-sided, 262–276f
Vascular access
  for continuous arteriovenous hemofiltration
      therapy, 648–649f
  for intermittent hemodialysis, 641–642
Vascular compliance. (*see* Compliance, vascular)
Vascular steal phenomenon, 115.
Vasoactive drugs
  for adult respiratory distress syndrome, 403–406f
  physiologic effects of, 117–118
Vasoactive factors, in vasoregulation, 357
Vasoconstriction
  in acute renal failure, 577–579
  pulmonary hypoxic, 317t
Vasoconstrictive factors, 357
Vasoconstrictors, in septic shock, 155
Vasodilation
  endothelial-dependent, 357
  hemodynamic effects of, 358–359f
  in septic shock, 298
  systemic, coronary hemodynamics and, 358–359
  venous, 358f
    hemodynamics of, 358f
Vasodilators
  combination therapy of, 360–361t
  for heart failure treatment, 242–243
  for hypertension in brain injury, 767
  for reduction of pulmonary vascular resistance,
      330–332t
  hemodynamic effects of, 359t
  in pulmonary embolism in right ventricular
      failure, 298
  major classes, pharmacology of, 359–361t
  pulmonary, 330–332t
  systemic modulation and, 356–361f
Vasogenic brain edema, 746
Vasomotor paralysis, 104, 742
Vasopressin
  biologic effects of, 910
  dilutional hyponatremia and, 905
  duration of action, 597
  hypofunction of, 914–916t
  release of, 164
  secretion, control of, 910–911
  secretion of, 910
  synthesis of, 910
Vasoregulation
  ionic channels and, 357
  mechanisms of, 356–357f
  neurogenic, 356–357
  vasoactive factors of, 357
Vasospasm, 743–744
Venous blood admixture, blood gases and, 391–395f
Venous return
  alterations of, 147
  calculation of, 114
  curve, interaction with cardiac function curve,
      147–149f
  determinants of, 141–147f, 156–157
  distribution of flow and, 146–147
  Guyton's equation of, 144, 147
  increasing, 149–150
  intrathoracic pressure changes and, 475–476f
  maximal, 146
  regulation of, 140
  resistance to, 144–146f
  variables of, 140
  vascular compliance and, 142–144f
Ventilation. (*see also* Mechanical ventilation)

acetate dialysis and, 624–625
bicarbonate dialysis and, 626
blood flow and, 484
blood flow distribution and, 478–479
circulation and, 473–482f, 482–485t
hemodynamic effects, 479–482t
  beneficial, maximizing of, 487–488
  detrimental, minimizing of, 485–487
problems of, in cerebral resuscitation, 768–769
steady-state, 480–481
Ventilation-perfusion ratio distributions, in adult
    respiratory distress syndrome, 396–397f
positive end-expiratory pressure and, 399–401f
vasoactive agents and, 405f
Ventilation-perfusion relationship
  in bacterial pneumonia, 406–407
  in status asthmaticus, 409–410f
  in weaning, 448
  mismatch
    blood gas regulation and, 390–395f
    in asthma, 492–493
    in chronic airway obstruction, 432–435f
  physiologic perspective, 389–395f
Ventilatory failure, neuromuscular dysfunction and,
    778–781t
Ventricular afterload, definition of, 16
Ventricular compliance, preload and, 16
Ventricular diastolic function
  in heart failure, 232–233
  pulmonary hypertension and, 323–325f
Ventricular efficiency
  definition of, 209
  pressure-volume loop and, 209, 210f
Ventricular elastance
  definition of, 233
  end-systolic, 233f
Ventricular hypertrophy, 215
Ventricular interaction
  direct, 215–216
  pericardial restraint and, 338
  series, 216
Ventricular performance, in heart failure, treatment
    of, 231–236f
Ventricular relaxation, 232
  left ventricular performance and, 210–213f, 214f
Ventricular tachycardia, pharmacologic treatment
    of, 351–352
Ventricular wave, large. (*see* V-wave)
Ventriculoarterial coupling, left ventricular
    performance and, 218–220f
Ventriculoarterial coupling, 236–239f
VIP-oma syndromes, hypercalcemia of, 930
Viral infections, posttransplant, 842–843
Viral pneumonia, 530
Viscoelastic properties, of left ventricle, 215
Vital capacity, in weaning, 448
Vitamin A intoxication, hypercalcemia of, 931
Vitamin B$_1$, 53
Vitamin C, 53
Vitamin D
  deficiency
    hypocalcemia of, 938
    treatment of, 941t
  intoxication, hypercalcemia of, 930–931
  preparations, for hypocalcemia, 940–941t
Vitamin K
  deficiency of, 808
  factor VII and, 806
Vitamins, enteral/parenteral nutrition and, 53–54t

VO$_2$, mixed venous oxygen saturation and, 17
V̇O$_2$-ḊO$_2$ covariation, 131
V̇O$_2$-ḊO$_2$ model, 134*f*
Volatile acids, 611, 613–614
Volume expansion
   for cardiac tamponade, 345
   for cardiovascular support, 364
Volume loading, for left ventricular failure, 240–242
Volume overload
   in acute renal failure, 590–591
   right ventricle structural and functional changes
     in, 287
Volume repletion, in sepsis, 104–105
Von Willebrand's disease, 807, 810, 821

Washed red blood cells, for transfusion, 820
Water transport, in renal replacement therapy,
   636–638*f*
Weaning
   criteria for, 366
   during glucose-based total parenteral nutrition,
     64
   in myasthenia gravis, 784
   indications for, 447
   lipids and, 36

nonrespiratory aspects of, 450–451
pathophysiology of, 447–448
personal approach, 468–470*f*
premature, 447
protracted ventilator dependence and, 468
pulmonary gas exchange improvement in,
   448–450
respiratory support in, partial support of, 449–450
timing for extubation, 451
Wedge pressure, 9
Wernicke's encephalopathy, 53
West zones of pulmonary blood distribution,
   313–314*f*
White blood cells, abnormalities of, clinical
   approach for, 815–817
Whole blood, for transfusion, 820
Wilson's disease, 819
Windkessel concept, 495
Windkessel model, 218–219*f*

Xanthine dehydrogenase, 739
Xanthine oxidase, 739

Zinc, 53
Zollinger-Ellison syndrome, 593